Occupational Therapy for Physical Dysfunction

Fourth Edition

Occupational Therapy for Physical Dysfunction

Fourth Edition

Editor

Catherine A. Trombly
Sc.D., O.T.R., F.A.O.T.A.

Professor, Department of Occupational Therapy
Sargent College of Allied Health Professions
Boston University
Boston, Massachusetts

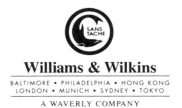

Williams & Wilkins

BALTIMORE • PHILADELPHIA • HONG KONG
LONDON • MUNICH • SYDNEY • TOKYO

A WAVERLY COMPANY

Editor: John P. Butler
Managing Editor: Linda S. Napora
Copy Editor: Candace B. Levy, Ph.D.
Designer: Wilma E. Rosenberger
Illustration Planner: Ray Lowman
Production Coordinator: Charles E. Zeller

Accurate indications, adverse reactions, and dosage schedules for drugs are provided in this book, but it is possible that they may change. The reader is urged to review the package information data of the manufacturers of the medications mentioned.

Printed in the United States of America

First Edition 1977
Second Edition 1983
Third Edition 1989

Library of Congress Cataloging-in-Publication Data
Occupational therapy of physical dysfunction / Catherine A. Trombly,
   editor. — 4th ed.
      p.   cm.
   Includes bibliographical references and index.
   ISBN 0-683-08390-2
   1. Occupational therapy.   2. Physically handicapped—
Rehabilitation.   I. Trombly, Catherine Anne.
   [DNLM: 1. Occupational Therapy.   2. Disabled.   WB 555 0143 1995]
Rm735.033   1995
615.8'515—dc20
DNLM/DLC
for Library of Congress

97 98 99
3 4 5 6 7 8 9 10

To Christopher

Preface

*T*his textbook, written for the basic professional level student and as a resource to experienced therapists, has undergone a major revision. Not only does it have a hard cover and more chapters, but it is also reorganized to better emphasize the goal of occupational therapy. That goal is to provide those services that enable patients and clients to restore or improve their occupational functioning—to be in control of their lives to the greatest extent possible—and to enjoy the concomitant sense of competence and self-efficacy. While this has always been my philosophy and was voiced in previous editions, the organization of past editions may have failed to emphasize it. In *Occupational Therapy for Physical Dysfunction—Fourth Edition*, the organization supports the emphasis on occupational performance. It receives first consideration and the performance components are examined in relation to their contributions to occupational dysfunction.

The original goals for writing this textbook are preserved in this edition. They were the transmission of current information on the evaluation and treatment of adults with occupational dysfunction secondary to physical disability and the presentation of the material within a conceptual framework rather than in a cookbook fashion. Only by having a fund of factual knowledge in combination with a framework for decision-making can the professional occupational therapist offer effective services to particular persons.

This edition is comprised of six sections with 44 chapters. The first section describes the historical and theoretical aspects and the process of the practice of occupational therapy with adults who, because of some physical problem, experience occupational dysfunction. Section II presents the areas of assessment that an occupational therapist working with adults with physical dysfunction would be responsible for, beginning with assessment of the person's occupational performance and his or her environment. Section III presents the four mechanisms used by occupational therapists to bring about therapeutic change in the individual: purposeful activity (occupation), development, learning, and rapport (therapeutic relationship). Section IV elucidates treatment principles and practices. As in earlier editions, this part does not provide treatment instructions that will apply to each patient of a particular diagnosis. It presents guidelines to assist the professional occupational therapist in choosing the best therapeutic intervention for a particular patient who has his or her own particular goals and manifestation of the diagnosis. Section V contains those adjunctive therapies that are used to facilitate the effectiveness of the therapeutic mechanisms or to enable greater levels of occupational performance. The last section includes discussions of the practice of occupational therapy for particular, major diagnostic categories written by specialists. These experts alert the therapist who is beginning practice with one or more of these populations to the various commonly encountered primary and secondary impairments and functional limitations that affect occupational performance and to the specialized evaluations and treatments that have been developed for these patients.

Another obvious, major change in this edition is the long list of contributors who are outstanding clinical and academic therapists. Forty-eight authors joined me in bringing this edition to fruition. They each did so with the desire to contribute to the profession of occupational therapy by sharing their knowledge and skills with the occupational therapists who will take this profession into the 21st century.

The format of each chapter has been changed slightly; each starts with learning objectives to help the learner focus on the major goals ("the forest") as he or she plunges into the details given in the chapter ("the trees"). Key words or terms with specialized meanings have been highlighted in the text and defined in the glossary. The study questions are again presented at the end of each chapter to help the learner validate his or her knowledge of the major points of the chapter and to provide direction for the professor and testing experts in developing examinations. Another change is the referencing style. We have adopted the American Psychological Association style used by the major journals of the profession: The *American Journal of Occupational Therapy* and *The Occupational Therapy Journal of Research*.

This text is meant to be used by learners who have prerequisite knowledge. Before studying assessment and treatment of persons who have suffered neurological trauma or disease, the reader should have knowledge of neuroanatomy, neurophysiology, and clinical neurological conditions. The prerequisite knowledge of anatomy, physiology, kinesiology and biomechanics, and clinical orthopaedic and general medical conditions is needed before studying assessment and treatment of persons who have suffered trauma or illness to their musculoskeletal, cardiopulmonary, immune, integumentary, or digestive systems. Other knowledge includes construction skills (prerequisite to making splints and adaptations) and knowledge of activities that can be used as therapeutic media. A basic physics course that includes information on mechanics and electronics and a course on computer usage are highly recommended in preparation for study of physical agent modalities, biofeedback, electronic "high-tech" adaptations, and computerized therapeutic activities.

This fourth edition utilizes *Uniform Terminology for Occupational Therapy—Third Edition* and the *International Classification of Impairments, Disabilities, and Handicaps* of the World Health Organization as amended by the National Center for Medical Rehabilitation Research of NIH.

Wherever possible, gender-neutral language has been used. When not possible, and for efficiency's sake, I have again adopted the convention of using female-gender wording to designate the therapist and male-gender wording to designate the patient or client. To those whom this offends, I apologize.

Catherine A. Trombly

Acknowledgments

Many people have contributed to the ongoing development of this textbook. The textbook and its several revisions could not have been produced without their help. To each of them, my sincere thanks and gratitude. They are:

Gail Bliss, M.O.T., O.T.R.; Anita Bundy, Sc.D., O.T.R.; Mary Ann Bush, M.S., O.T.R.; Brian Despres, O.T.R.; Mark Erickson; Anne G. Fisher, Sc.D., O.T.R.; Sam Fitzpatrick; Mauren Hayes Fleming Ed.D., O.T.R.; Alice Follows, M.S., O.T.R.; Margaret Hayes, O.T.R.; Frederic J. Kottke, M.D.; Judith La-Drew; Lucia Grochowska Littlefield; Linda S. Napora, managing editor; Lillian Hoyle Parent, M.A., O.T.R.; Deborah Yarett Slater, M.S., O.T.R.; Gayle M. Thompson, M.Ed., O.T.R.; Christopher F. Trombly.

Specific help has also been given by others to some of the contributing authors, who cite them at the end of the particular chapters.

Contributors

M. Irma Alvarado, M.A., O.T.R.
formerly, *Director of Rehabilitation Services*
Shriners Burns Institute
Galveston, Texas

Ben Atchison, M.Ed., O.T.R., F.A.O.T.A.
Associate Professor
Department of Associated Health Professions
Eastern Michigan University
Ypsilanti, Michigan

Julie Bass Haugen, Ph.D., O.T.R.
Associate Professor and Graduate Program Director
Department of Occupational Therapy
College of St. Catherine
St. Paul, Minnesota

Jane Bear-Lehman, M.S., O.T.R., F.A.O.T.A.
Assistant Professor of Clinical Occupational Therapy
Program in Occupational Therapy
Columbia University
New York, New York

Karen Bentzel, M.S., O.T.R.
Clinical Lecturer
Department of Occupational Therapy
Elizabethtown College
Elizabethtown, Pennsylvania

Bette R. Bonder, Ph.D., O.T.R./L, F.A.O.T.A
Associate Professor and Chairperson
Department of Health Sciences
Cleveland State University
Cleveland, Ohio

Felice Celikyol, M.A., O.T.R., F.A.O.T.A.
Director, Occupational Therapy Services
Kessler Institute for Rehabilitation
West Orange, New Jersey

Barbara Cooper, Ph.D. (ABD), OT(C)
Associate Dean for Health Sciences
Director of the School of Occupational Therapy and Physiotherapy
McMaster University
Hamilton, Ontario, Canada

Wendy Coster, Ph.D., O.T.R., F.A.O.T.A.
Assistant Professor
Department of Occupational Therapy
Sargent College of Allied Health Professions
Boston University
Boston, Massachusetts

Jean Deitz, Ph.D., O.T.R./L, F.A.O.T.A.
Associate Professor
Division of Occupational Therapy
Department of Rehabilitation Medicine
University of Washington
Seattle, Washington

Glenn Digman, M.S.W., M.A., O.T.R./L
Senior Occupational Therapist
National Rehabilitation Hospital
Washington, D.C.

Patricia Weber Dow, M.S., O.T.R.
Assistant Professor
Department of Occupational Therapy
LSUMC, School of Allied Health Professions
New Orleans, Louisiana

Brian Dudgeon, M.S., O.T.R./L
Lecturer
Division of Occupational Therapy
Department of Rehabilitation Medicine
University of Washington
Seattle, Washington

Maria Elena Echevarria, B.S., O.T.R./L
Occupational Therapist
Nova Care Inc.
Silver Springs, Maryland

Marilyn Ernest-Conibear, M.A., OT(C)
Retired, Vancouver, British Columbia
formerly, *Associate Professor*
Department of Occupational Therapy
Faculty of Applied Health Sciences
The University of Western Ontario
London, Ontario, Canada

Judy R. Feinberg, Ph.D., O.T.R., F.A.O.T.A.
Indianapolis Medical Center
Indianapolis, Indiana

Glenn Goodman, M.O.T., O.T.R./L
Associate Professor
Department of Health Sciences
Cleveland State University
Cleveland, Ohio

Laura Devore Hollar, M.S.O.T., O.T.R.
Occupational Therapist
Shepherd Spinal Center
Atlanta, Georgia
and
DeKalb County School System
Decatur, Georgia

Karen Jacobs, Ed.D., O.T.R./L, C.P.E., F.A.O.T.A.
Assistant Professor
Department of Occupational Therapy
Sargent College of Allied Health Professions
Boston University
Boston, Massachusetts

Lyn Jongbloed, Ph.D., OT(C)
Associate Professor
School of Rehabilitation Sciences
University of British Columbia
Vancouver, British Columbia, Canada

Katherine A. Konosky, M.S., O.T.R.
formerly, Clinical Specialist
Mary Free Bed Hospital & Rehabilitation Center
Grand Rapids, Michigan

Mary Law, Ph.D., OT(C)
Associate Professor
School of Occupational Therapy and Physiotherapy
Department of Clinical Epidemiology and Biostatistics
McMaster University
and
Research Associate
Department of Occupational Therapy
Chedoke-McMaster Hospitals
Hamilton, Ontario, Canada

Susan L. Lee, B.S., O.T.R./L
Director of Planning and Development
Advanced Rehabilitation Services, Inc.
Marietta, Georgia

Lori Letts, M.A., OT(C)
Assistant Professor
School of Occupational Therapy and Physiotherapy
McMaster University
Hamilton, Ontario, Canada

Kathryn Levit, B.S., O.T.R.
Making Progress
Physical & Occupational Therapy
Alexandria, Virginia

Cheryl A. Linden, M.S., O.T.R.
Education Coordinator
Department of Occupational Therapy
Shepherd Spinal Center
Atlanta, Georgia

Jaclyn Faglie Low, Ph.D., O.T.R.
Associate Professor and Chair, ad interim
Department of Occupational Therapy
School of Allied Health Sciences
The University of Texas Medical Branch
Galveston, Texas

Colleen T. Lowe, M.P.H., O.T.R./L, C.H.T.
Coordinator, Hand and Upper Extremity Therapy Service
Department of Occupational Therapy
Massachusetts General Hospital
Boston, Massachusetts

Virgil Mathiowetz, Ph.D., O.T.R., F.A.O.T.A.
Associate Professor and Chair
Department of Occupational Therapy
College of St. Catherine
St. Paul, Minnesota

Beverly J. Myers, M.H.P.E., O.T.R./L
Assistant Professor and Staff Therapist
Department of Occupational Therapy
Rush-Presbyterian-St. Luke's Medical Center
Chicago, Illinois

Elizabeth M. Newman, B.S., O.T.R./L
Clinical Specialist
Musculoskeletal Unit
Department of Occupational Therapy
National Rehabilitation Hospital
Washington, D.C.

Cynthia A. Philips, M.A., O.T.R./L, A.S.H.T.
Hand Therapist
New England Rehabilitation Center at Brookline
Brookline, Massachusetts

Janet L. Poole, M.A., O.T.R., F.A.O.T.A.
Lecturer III
Occupational Therapy Program
University of New Mexico
Albuquerque, New Mexico

Robert E. Post, Ph.D., PT
Assistant Professor
Department of Physical Therapy
College of Allied Health Sciences
Thomas Jefferson University
Philadelphia, Pennsylvania

Lee Ann Quintana, M.S., O.T.R.
Coordinating Therapist
Rehabilitation Medicine Unit
Catholic Medical Center
Manchester, New Hampshire

Nancy Pearson Rees, M.O.T., O.T.R.
Private Practice
Covington, Louisiana

Patricia Rigby, M.H.Sc., OT(C)
Research Occupational Therapist
Hugh MacMillan Rehabilitation Centre
Toronto, Ontario, Canada

Joyce Shapiro Sabari, Ph.D., O.T.R.
Clinical Assistant Professor
Department of Occupational Therapy
State University of New York Health Sciences Center at Brooklyn
Brooklyn, New York

Anna Deane Scott, M.Ed., O.T.R.
Associate Professor
Department of Occupational Therapy
Sargent College of Allied Health Professions
Boston University
Boston, Massachusetts

Cara Stewart, B.S., O.T.R.
Private Practice, Environmental Access Specialist
Kingsville, Maryland

Debra Stewart, B.Sc., OT(C)
Occupational Therapy Consultant in Pediatrics
Mississauga, Ontario, Canada

Susan Strong, B.Sc., OT(C)
Occupational Therapy Supervisor
Hamilton Psychiatric Hospital
Hamilton, Ontario, Canada

Dorie B. Syen, O.T.R., C.H.T.
Clinical Director
Physiotherapy Associates
Conyers, Georgia

Linda Tickle-Degnen, Ph.D., O.T.R./L
Assistant Professor
Department of Occupational Therapy
Sargent College of Allied Health Professions
Boston University
Boston, Massachusetts

Jeannette Tries, M.S., O.T.R./L
Manager, Biofeedback Center
Department of Occupational Therapy
Sacred Heart Rehabilitation Hospital
Milwaukee, Wisconsin

Catherine A. Trombly, Sc.D., O.T.R./L, F.A.O.T.A.
Professor
Department of Occupational Therapy
Sargent College of Allied Health Professions
Boston University
Boston, Massachusetts

Hilda Powers Versluys, M.Ed., O.T.R./L
Assistant Professor
Department of Occupational Therapy
Boston School of Occupational Therapy
Tufts University
Medford, Massachusetts

Anne M. Woodson, B.S., O.T.R.
Senior Clinical Specialist
Department of Occupational Therapy
The University of Texas Medical Branch at Galveston
Galveston, Texas

Ruth Zemke, Ph.D., O.T.R., F.A.O.T.A.
Associate Professor and Graduate Program Coordinator
Department of Occupational Therapy
University of Southern California
Los Angeles, California

Contents

The Practice of Occupational Therapy for Physical Dysfunction

The history of the practice of occupational therapy in the United States is presented in Chapter 1 to illustrate to the new occupational therapist that our profession does not stop at the clinic or university door. The economic trends, scientific developments, and social changes have had, are now having, and will continue to have profound influences on the practice of occupational therapy.

The practice of occupational therapy, as with any professional practice, is not carried out in disconnected bits and pieces. It is guided by theoretical systems. The theoretical foundations of practice with physical dysfunction are described in Chapter 2. The theoretical foundation that a therapist subscribes to will guide her choice of assessment (or interpretation of assessment data) and choice and method of implementation of treatment. The occupational therapy process—including an introduction to the clinical reasoning process and documentation—that is valid across all types of practices is described in Chapter 3. As professionals, occupational therapists need to be able to communicate the decision-making process they used in developing and carrying out the treatment of a particular patient and must document the outcome. Current social and economic trends mandate that outcome be documented in terms of function and consumer satisfaction.

Historical and Social Foundation for Practice

Jaclyn Faglie Low

OBJECTIVES

After studying this chapter, the reader will have had the opportunity to:
1. Appreciate the changes in hospital structure and function that facilitated the development of occupational therapy.
2. Discuss the factors that generated a concern for age-related expectations for occupational function.
3. Compare the history of occupational therapy with changes in nursing.
4. Recognize the influence of gender-based roles in the development of occupational therapy.
5. Appreciate the relationship of adaptations to social conditions at the founding of the profession to contemporary concerns in practice.

An occupational therapist with 10 years of experience ponders the offer of a new position in management. The salary increase and expanded responsibilities make the offer attractive, but she is unsure about job satisfaction with less patient contact. Two therapists debate the inclusion of physical agent modalities into their repertoire of techniques. Another considers whether she can provide better care if she leaves an inpatient setting for a job with a home health agency. Each of these therapists may believe that her concerns stem from contemporary conditions in health care and in occupational therapy. Each might be surprised, however, to find in her concerns a direct link to the early years of the profession.

Philosophers and historians advocate the study of history for the understanding of the present. Knowledge gleaned from appreciation of the past does not come from a dry recital of the chronological sequence of events. It is found in examining relationships between significant events within social, cultural, and political contexts. The evolution of occupational therapy lies within a matrix formed by these factors.

This exploration of the social and historical foundations of occupational therapy begins with a review of the history of activity in the service of health. Central to this discussion is an introduction to those credited with founding the profession. This is preparatory to the exploration of three facets of late-19th- and early-20th-century American life crucial to the development of occupational therapy.

The first is the evolution of the structure and role of the hospital. Second is a burgeoning concern for age norms for life tasks. Last, and perhaps most important, is the accommodation of traditional roles for women to careers in health care. All three factors influenced the founding of occupational therapy. This chapter concludes with speculation about their legacy to the present.

ACTIVITY AS THERAPY

Occupational therapy is based on the belief that purposeful activity (occupation) prevents or mediates dysfunction of physical or psychological origin. Although they arose in diverse cultures, the earliest beliefs in the value of occupation in the treatment of illness had common grounding in ideas about physical fitness for physical, mental, and spiritual health. Fitness was necessary for optimal functioning in one's occupational role. Occupational roles were determined by age and gender and often by socioeconomic class. Writings attributed to Hippocrates, Galen, and Aesclepias promulgated exercise, "activity treatment," and employment as important therapeutic agents.

Centuries later, physicians in European asylums for the insane instituted work therapy for inmates. They based the practice on empirical observations. They noted that lower-class patients who performed tasks while incarcerated recovered more quickly than did idle upper-class patients. The value of physical activity and productive work was central to the "moral treatment" advanced by the French physician Phillipe Pinel in the 18th century.

Ideas about the value of activity were successfully transported to colonial America. The first hospital chartered in the North American British colonies included as part of its equipment and supplies spinning wheels, wool, and flax for use by patients. Dr. Benjamin Rush, a signer of the Declaration of Independence, wrote to the managers of the Pennsylvania Hospital in 1797 and again in 1813 in support of the therapeutic value of work for patients (Dunton, 1917). In their 1941 *Syllabus for Training of Nurses in Occupational Therapy*, Eleanor Clarke Slagle and Harriet Robeson reported that Rush

> recognized occupation as a "valuable means of preventing violent outbreaks." Sewing, embroidery and flower gardens were arranged for women; and shoe repairing, carpentry and farm work provided for men. A "mono-rail" was put on the lawn for their amusement and those who did not ride in it were amused by watching the cars upset. A varied program of work and play (p. 8).

Several institutions initiated programs of work therapy. In a speech delivered at the Consolation House Conference in 1917, Dr. William Rush Dunton, a founding member of the National Society for the Promotion of Occupational Therapy, cited an earlier publication:

> In "The Story of the Bethlehem Hospital," E. G. O'Donoghue writes (page 307):
> "As early as 1822 Lord Robert Seymour had urged with great truth and force that some form of employment was one of the best medicines for certain forms of mental malady, where it is necessary to divert painful thoughts or restart the machinery of a lethargic mind. He suggested that the making of mats, paper bags, and felt slippers might be safely entrusted to the patients, but it was not till the beginning of 1844 that the workshops were completed. In them from this date for another ten or fifteen years painting, glazing, engineering, and other trades were followed by male patients under the superintendent of attendants skilled in the various handicrafts" (p. 380).

In his analysis of the Bethlehem program, Dunton (1917) noted, "for the period between 1815 and 1852 the patients admitted to this hospital were mostly of an artisan class" (p. 380).

Attitudes in the United States changed as immigrants with different values and habits swelled the population of the asylums. Mental illness was seen as a permanent condition for which little could be done

except to lock the sufferer away. Thus the use of activity as therapy in institutions for the mentally ill lay dormant for decades. Dunton (1917) surmised that the decline in work as therapy from 1860 to 1890 was related to the exigencies of post–Civil War conditions.

Hospitals for the physically ill required work of their patients. However, jobs were done in the service of the institution rather than for therapeutic benefit. As recovery progressed, women patients cared for sicker patients. In New York City's Bellevue and Charity hospitals, women's jobs required sewing and men's required maintenance skills such as carpentry, cleaning, and even rowing a boat to ferry passengers on a twice-daily schedule (Rosenberg, 1978).

The formalized idea of occupation as therapy did not emerge until the latter years of the 19th and early years of the 20th centuries. However, 19th-century Americans valued work and activity, especially outdoor activity, as vital in the acquisition of good health. Traditional medical care was, until the introduction of the germ theory of disease and asepsis, frequently more harmful than helpful. Emphasis on curing disease through bleeding, blistering, and purging to restore the balance of the body's humors was challenged by sectarian or nontraditional approaches to health care. Health reformers advocated education, regular exercise, dress reform, and dietary restrictions in addition to specific curative practices such as hydrotherapy and homeopathy.

Many practitioners and adherents to sectarian methods were women. Mary Gove Nichols (1810–1884) was a prominent health reformer and one of the first American women to practice medicine. Nichols was self-educated in hydropathy. She did not have a degree from a medical college or hold a license to practice medicine, but neither was a requirement at that time. Nichols advocated regular exercise, fresh air, and a vegetarian diet (Blake, 1984). Ellen G. White (1827–1915) founded the Seventh Day Adventists and championed reliance on "nature's remedies: fresh air, sunshine, rest, exercise, [and] proper diet" (quoted in Numbers & Schoepflin, 1984, p. 384).

THE FOUNDERS AND THE NEAR FOUNDERS

In the first decades of the 20th century, individuals in different fields of endeavor began almost simultaneously to practice and promote the use of occupation as therapy. George Barton was an architect. He endured long periods of convalescence from tuberculosis. In addition, he underwent amputation of a lower extremity because of frostbite and gangrene. Barton suffered the frostbite while in Colorado on an altruistic mission, a survey of the famine conditions among farmers along the Kansas border. Hysterical paralysis of his left side followed the amputation.

Barton received help at a hospital for convalescents in Clifton Springs, New York. There he became convinced that he could help others with problems similar to his. He opened Consolation House in Clifton Springs where he provided education, vocational assistance, and workshop activities for convalescents. On his own, Barton undertook extensive study of medicine, nursing, pharmaceutics, and related subjects to make his work more effective. He was impressed by the writings of Dunton, a psychiatrist, and initiated correspondence with him.

Barton assembled five like-minded individuals to meet with him in 1917. The purpose of the meeting was to establish the National Society for the Promotion of Occupational Therapy. The name of the organization changed to its present form—the American Occupational Therapy Association—in 1923.

Joining Barton at the 1917 meeting to establish the national society was Dunton. William Rush Dunton Jr. received his medical degree from the University of Pennsylvania in 1893. He was a descendant of Rush, an early proponent of occupation as therapy, and Dunton's middle name reflected his heritage.

Dunton took charge of the occupations program at the Sheppard and Pratt Institute in Maryland in 1912. He included instruction in printing, metalwork, and fiber arts as part of his therapy. Dunton wrote a number of books and articles on occupation as therapy and on training nurses to provide occupation. His major works included *Occupational Therapy* (1915), *Reconstruction Therapy* (1919), and *Prescribing Occupational Therapy* (1928). He coauthored, with Dr. Sidney Licht, a volume titled *Occupational Therapy: Principles and Practice* (1950, 1957).

Also present at the inaugural meeting was Eleanor Clarke Slagle. Born in 1876, she was the daughter of an architect. She married Robert Slagle who died apparently before Eleanor enrolled, at age 34, in a study program designed by Julia Lathrop and Jane Addams at the Chicago School of Civics and Philanthropy. Her studies concentrated on "invalid occupations" and curative occupations and recreation for patients in state mental hospitals. She worked with Dunton at Johns Hopkins in Baltimore, where she developed a program she called "habit training" for chronic schizophrenic patients. Patients in that program had a highly structured daily schedule. They got up at a specific time, dressed, made their beds, used good table manners, and engaged in craft activities. Slagle returned to Chicago where she directed the Henry P. Favill School of Occupations until it closed in 1920. The Favill School developed from a course offered by the Chicago School of Civics and Philanthropy for hospital attendants ("History," 1940).

Slagle was president of the Society for the Promotion of Occupational Therapy in 1919. From 1923 to 1937, she served as executive director of the American Occupational Therapy Association. Barton and Dunton preceded Slagle as president, and all presidents from 1920 until 1947 were men.

Other founding members of the National Society for the Promotion of Occupational Therapy were Susan Cox Johnson and Thomas Kidner. Johnson was born in Corsicana, Texas, in 1876. She taught school in Berkeley, California, where she wrote a textbook on textiles. She also spent 2 years as a teacher of arts and crafts in the Philippines (Licht, 1967). Upon her return to the United States, Johnson was appointed director of occupations for the New York State Department of Public Charities (Johnson, 1917).

Kidner, a London-born architect, was the vocational secretary of the Canadian Military Hospitals Commission. He was subsequently appointed as a special adviser to the U.S. government on problems of rehabilitation (Licht, 1967). Kidner served as president of the American Occupational Therapy Association from 1923 to 1928. Kidner's architectural training was reflected in his professional publications. His drawings illustrated plans for occupational therapy clinics (Peloquin, 1991b).

Isabel Newton, Barton's secretary, was also present at the 1917 meeting and was listed as a founding member. She later married Barton and worked with him as a teacher of occupations to invalids. As Barton's widow, she shared her memories of the founding of the society. She characterized Dunton as "a genial friendly person with sound ideas, although he seemed to prefer being in the quiet background" (Barton, 1968, p. 345). Kidner was "a fascinating personality, so very British. . . . Full of wit" (Barton, 1968, p. 345).

Isabel Barton (1968) described Slagle as "a person of strong personality, great charm, and a dignity that won instant admiration" (p. 345). Barton (1968) contrasted Slagle with Johnson, whom she found also to be "a strong personality although in a quiet modest manner" (p. 345).

Susan Tracy was a nurse. She believed strongly in the benefit of occupation during convalescence. Although she did not attend the organizational meeting called by Barton, she was one of the five directors of the society listed on the Certificate of Incorporation. Peloquin (1991a) more appropriately referred to Tracy and Herbert J. Hall as "near founders," because of their influence on the profession.

Tracy, born in 1864, graduated from nurse's training at the Massachusetts Homeopathic Hospital in 1889. She took courses in the manual arts department of Teachers College at Columbia University while working as a private-duty nurse. Tracy served as a training school superintendent and taught courses in invalid occupations for nursing students. She incorporated her course material into her textbook *Studies in Invalid Occupations* (1910). In 1916, she introduced an occupational therapy program for general medicine ward patients at Michael Reese Hospital in Chicago ("Occupational Therapy," 1917, p. 425).

Dunton recommended Hall, a physician, for inclusion in the founding group. However, Barton chose not to invite him (Peloquin, 1991b). Barton selected Johnson instead of Hall, because he had greater esteem for Johnson's work than for Hall's treatment of wealthy neurasthenics (Breines, 1986). Hall was the director of Devereux Mansion in Marblehead, Massachusetts, where he established an experimental workshop. In spite of his exclusion from the first meeting, Hall was an active member of the society. He served as president of the organization from 1920 to 1923 (American Occupational Therapy Association [AOTA], 1967).

The founders of occupational therapy included a nurse, teachers, a social worker, architects, a physician, and a psychiatrist. They shared a belief in the efficacy of occupation as a curative force for mental and physical problems. Their belief was empirically based, formed through observation and personal experience. Together they formed a profession, generated a body of professional literature, and introduced a new group of workers—the reconstruction aides of World War I—into military medicine.

The continuing influence of the founders and the near founders on the profession is reflected in the listing of textbooks required for the January 1920 term at the School of Diversional Occupation in Colorado Springs, Colorado:

Studies in Invalid Occupation: A Manual for Nurses and Attendants, by Susan E. Tracy
Rake Knitting, and Its Special Adaptation to Invalid Workers, by Susan E. Tracy
Occupational Therapy: A Manual for Nurses, by William R. Dunton Jr.
Occupational Nursing: How the Installation of Invalid Occupation Work in Institutions Will Affect the Nursing Profession, and a Practical Example of Its Therapeutic Value, by George Edward Barton
A View of Invalid Occupation: An Explanation of the New Idea of Providing Convalescents with Occupation, by George Edward Barton
The Work of Our Hands: A Study of Occupation for Invalids, by Herbert J. Hall and Mertice M. C. Buck ("Textbooks Required," 1920)

THE MATRIX OF PRACTICE

Changes in the late 19th and early 20th centuries fostered the development of the profession of occupational therapy. First, the organizational structure and the role of the hospital changed. Under earlier configurations, there was no role for services of the type provided by occupational therapy. Although work was required of patients, it was for the benefit of the institution rather than the patient.

Second, a concern for the timeliness of life events and codification of age-related life roles emerged. This development granted scientific authority to therapy aimed at restoring people to functional occupation in their usual life roles.

Finally, the profession of occupational therapy allowed women to enter a career that required technical competence without compromising femininity. Successful therapy required those who combined appropriate personality traits with training in the methods of occupational therapy.

The Development of Hospitals

For centuries, hospitals existed only as institutions of refuge for those without family members to care for them during illness. There was little emphasis on cure, because there was often little that could effect cure. From 1870 to 1910, two factors operated to change the role of the hospital. First, people moved to the cities in response to industrialization and thus were cut off from family support systems. Second, the introduction of aseptic techniques and anesthesia made surgery not only effective but survivable. According to Starr (1982),

> The reconstitution of the hospital involved its redefinition as an institution of medical science rather than of social welfare, its reorganization on the lines of a business rather than a charity, and its reorientation to professionals and their patients rather than to patrons and the poor (pp. 147–148).

Within the hospital, divisions of labor developed to increase efficiency. Hospitals "projected ideals of specialization and technical competence" (Starr, 1982, p. 146). Patients no longer provided their own care. The population of hospitalized patients shifted from the poor to the middle class.

Nursing as a profession emerged within the hospital setting. Nursing care was initially provided in the home by women for a family member and

> then incorporated into a market economy as women began to nurse for hire in their patients' homes; then concentrated in central plants where workers were subject to

close supervision and new forms of control (Melosh, 1982, p. 8).

During the latter decades of the 19th century, hospitals served as training programs for nursing students. Students did the ward work. Most left the institution for private duty after graduation. Middle- and upper-class patients convalesced at home under the care of the hospital-trained professional nurse. By the end of the 1930s, however, the cost of private-duty nursing was prohibitive for most middle-class families (Melosh, 1984). These patients moved to hospitals for care.

Occupational therapy has a different history. When patients were cared for in their homes, activities to pass the time during convalescence and adaptations to activities for those with permanent impairments were provided according to the resources and imagination of family and the patient himself.

Patients in hospitals of the late 19th and early 20th centuries had to work to keep the hospital functioning. There was no place and no time for occupation as therapy. Professional nurses who provided convalescent care in the home may have offered, like Susan Tracy did, invalid occupations to clients. But that was a matter of individual circumstance. It was not until hospitals became curative centers for middle-class patients that there was a place for occupational therapy.

The Timeliness of Life Events

The ancients observed that there is a predetermined and established order to changes that occur in human beings as they grow up and grow old. Observations culminated in theories dividing human life into specific periods with associated actions or behaviors. Hippocrates was credited in a Latin translation of a Greek text with describing seven seasons, or ages, in human life. During the Middle Ages, medicine adopted a four-age theory, while the astrological theory included seven stages—because astrology was considered a science, the two were not mutually exclusive. Subsequent representations of seven-age schemata were common. The most well known to the English-speaking world appeared in William Shakespeare's *As You Like It.* It begins

> All the world's a stage,
> And all the men and women merely players;
> They have their exits and their entrances;
> And one man in his time plays many parts,
> His acts being seven ages (II.7).

The 19th-century American neurologist George Miller Beard (1874) developed a six-age schema of adult life to codify his beliefs about the relationship between productivity and age.

Kern (1983) identified the introduction of standard time, which occurred at the end of the 19th century, as the event that set the stage for the development of concepts about the timeliness of life events. Chudacoff (1989) placed the origin of age grading in "the education and medical care of children" (p. 50). He traced the former to the work of Pestalozzi, a Swiss educator, and the latter to the development of pediatrics as a medical specialty in the late 19th century. Chudacoff (1989) observed:

> As the nineteenth century closed, these theories [educational and medical] were refined and applied to older age groups as well as to youths. Moreover, spokespersons in popular and professional journals and the institutions that their theories influenced began to delineate the ideal sequencing of a wide variety of experiences. Such delineations not only implied norms but also often specified them. As a result, the concept of being on, ahead of, or behind schedules referred to more than the arrival of a train or the completion of a task; it meant matching the timing of one's personal experiences and achievements to cultural standards (p. 50).

Events of the late 19th and early 20th centuries set the stage for the incorporation of concepts about the age appropriateness of occupational role into a profession. Chudacoff (1989) noted that "the proliferation of intelligence testing in the 1910s and 1920s evidences a near-obsession with age norms in American social science" (p. 81).

Implicit within the belief systems of the founders of occupational therapy was the idea that there is age and stage specificity to role and activity. For example, the acceptable role of the young adult male was that of soldier and worker. The first reconstruction aides sent to France during World War I were stationed near the front lines and were charged with the task of returning men suffering from "war neurosis" to duty as quickly as possible (Low, 1992). In the postwar years, the concern was for return to productive employment. From the beginning, occupational therapists formulated goals that focused on occupational function.

Gender and Role

As 19th-century American workers became increasingly engaged in industrial tasks, the spheres of activity for men and women moved further apart. In earlier rural societies, members of the family worked together to produce needed goods. With urbanization, men went out to work while most women stayed at home as unpaid workers. Women's work focused primarily on caring for the family. According to Morantz (1984), "The ideal of the modern family—small in size, emotionally intense, and woman supervised—made its appearance as a distinctive emblem of middle-class culture" (p. 348). This set the stage for women to expand the care taking of their families through involvement in health reform activities. Educational opportunities became available and women took advantage of them. Many took advocacy of self-help in health from family to community venues.

As women moved out of the home to paying positions, careers in health care offered an expansion of the traditional female caregiving sphere of activity rather than a complete severance from it. A special challenge existed for these women in attempting to meet societal demands for scientific approaches to care without denigrating the aspects of their care that stemmed from womanly attributes.

Nursing as a profession also struggled with these dilemmas. Conflict arose between those who attempted to professionalize the work and those who adhered to traditional ideas of selfless service. Melosh (1982) reported that "while professional leaders worked to establish uniform and objective standards in nursing practice, traditionalists defended womanly empathy and intuition as nursing methods" (p. 24).

Occupational therapists dealt with this conflict in two ways: first, by adhering to traditional male-female roles in task assignment and, second, by emphasizing equally in professional literature the goal of returning patients to productive occupational roles and the personal traits of the providers. The technical aspects of training and practice stressed the scientific aspects of practice.

As Serrett (1985), an occupational therapist, pointed out,

> the division of labor between physicians and occupational therapists followed traditional patterns regarding men and women. From its inception, occupational therapists were women, who were to act under the guidance of the physicians, predominantly men (p. 19).

The lives of the founders and near founders of the National Society for the Promotion of Occupational Therapy illustrate the differentiation between the masculine and feminine spheres by many of their activities. Men were the decision makers; the women carried out the work. There were, however, exceptions in both camps. Tracy, Slagle, and Johnson achieved high administrative positions and produced influential books and articles.

The men were planners and directors. Barton founded a treatment center and an organization. Kidner planned and designed departments. Among Dunton's works was a book titled *Prescribing Occupational Therapy*, a manual not for the practitioner but for the prescribing physician. But Barton also treated patients and wrote of his caregiving experiences.

RATIONALES FOR OCCUPATION AS THERAPY

The early practitioners of occupational therapy validated the idea of occupation as therapy in different ways. Some posited a scientific basis for their beliefs while arguing for the value of occupation in regaining, obtaining, or maintaining physical and mental health. Barton emphasized the scientific aspects of occupational therapy when he used the language of medicine in a speech presented at the First Consolation House Conference (March 15–17, 1917). The written text of his speech appeared in *The Modern Hospital* under the title "Inoculation of the Bacillus of Work." The subtitle of his article used numerous medical metaphors:

> Preparation of the Patient—The Occupational Diagnosis—Occupational "Applications," "Hypodermics," and "Lumbar Punctures"—The Therapeutic Value of Drawing and Modeling—Like Water, a Tonic and Alterative (Barton, 1917, p. 399).

Barton (1917) explained his terminology by comparing occupational dysfunction with medical conditions and interventions:

> But there are many cases where superficial stimulation is not sufficient, cases in which one has to get inside into the blood, or into the muscle itself. And for these there are occupations which I call "hypodermics."
>
> But there are still other cases so very much worse that it is necessary to go right in through the backbone of the patient, in order to find out what the real trouble is, or how to relieve abnormal tension. These I call "lumbar punctures" (p. 400).

Conversely, Dunton acknowledged the absence of a scientific basis for occupation as therapy (Serrett, 1985), yet he proposed nine principles of occupational therapy to imbue the work with greater precision:

1. Work should be carried on with cure as the main objective.
2. Work must be interesting.
3. The patient should be carefully studied.
4. One form of occupation should not be carried to the point of fatigue.
5. It should have some useful end.
6. It preferably should lead to an increase in the patient's knowledge.
7. It should be carried on with others.
8. Possible encouragement should be given the worker.
9. Work resulting in a poor or useless product is better than idleness (Dunton, 1919, p. 320).

Concurring with Barton was Elizabeth Upham, director of the art department at Milwaukee-Downer College. She referred to "the modern science of therapeutic occupations for the handicapped" (Upham, 1917, p. 409). Other authors added their views to the debate. An unsigned history of occupational therapy credited Tracy's book *Studies in Invalid Occupation* as "the first attempt to place occupational therapy on a scientific basis" ("History," 1940, p. 31). Hall defined occupational therapy as "the science of organized work for invalids" ("Definitions of Occupational Therapy," 1940, p. 37).

At an organizational level, the National Society for the Promotion of Occupational Therapy emphasized the scientific aspects of practice by selecting engineer and efficiency expert Frank Gilbreth as an honorary member in 1917 (AOTA, 1967).

THE NEW LITERATURE

It was important to the founders to disseminate information about occupational therapy. The directors of the National Society for the Promotion of Occupational Therapy selected the *Maryland Psychiatric Quarterly* as the official organ.

The Modern Hospital also carried information on occupational therapy, including reports of national and state association meetings. Articles focused equally on physical rehabilitation and mental illness. Authors emphasized returning people to productive lives. In 1915, *The Modern Hospital* began publication of the monthly column "Occupational Therapy, Vocational Re-Education and Industrial Rehabilitation."

A new journal, *Archives of Occupational Therapy*, appeared in 1922. Dunton owned and edited it along with the *Maryland Psychiatric Quarterly*. The *Archives of Occupational Therapy* was subsequently renamed *Occupational Therapy in Rehabilitation* and continued publication until the early 1950s. At the time of his retirement in 1947, Dunton offered ownership of *Occupational Therapy in Rehabilitation* to the American Occupational Therapy Association. However, it was discovered that the publisher, Williams & Wilkins, owned the copyrights to the journal name and its contents, necessitating the formation of an entirely new journal (Bone, 1971). Publication of the *American Journal of Occupational Therapy* by the American Occupational Therapy Association began in 1947.

Therapeutics and Therapists

Within the professional literature, occupational function was identified as the goal of therapy. Techniques varied with diagnostic categories. For many years, sanitariums for the treatment of tuberculosis were major employers of occupational therapists. Patients moved through a graduated regimen from bed rest to light activity to vocational training, a program

easily recognizable as work hardening. The general superintendent of the Cook County Tuberculosis Hospital proclaimed the desired outcome of treatment for tuberculosis was that the patient be "cured and fitted for work" (Bailey, 1917, p. 378).

The director of occupational therapy at a curative workshop for orthopaedic conditions and industrial injuries reported on the program of physical and occupational therapy: "Our patients report for treatment at 8:00 in the morning, so that they will continue the habit of starting out early, thus making it easier for readjustment to work later on" (Taylor, 1929, p. 337).

Occupational function was a priority regardless of the patient's age. Paisley (1929), in "Occupational Therapy Treatment for a Group of Spastic Cases; Children under Twelve Years of Age," emphasized present and future occupational function: "The value of an occupation may be twofold. It may furnish the means for physical correction and at the same time lay the foundation for future usefulness, both of mind and body" (p. 91).

A highly valued component, according to occupational therapy literature, was the character of the provider; it was essential to the success of therapy. Two examples are presented. Eunice Cates, registered occupational therapist and chief aide at the Veterans Administration Hospital in Pittsburgh, began her occupational therapy career as a reconstruction aide. She trained as a teacher and did not attend a school of occupational therapy. Cates's comments echo those of the nursing "traditionalists" described by Melosh (1982). Speaking to the newest graduates in occupational therapy, Cates (1940) said,

> A diploma does not insure success. Though you possess all the degrees in the category, and have not an understanding heart, adaptability and tact, they profit you little—or nothing. We might add also, a sense of humor as a necessary attribute. How often we have seen that save the day (p. 116).

Interestingly, she attributed to Hall words antithetical to his definition of occupational therapy:

> Dr. Herbert Hall, whom we like to call "The Father of Occupational Therapy," rated personality as eighty-five per cent, and we are more and more convinced, as the years go by, that he was one hundred per cent right. "It isn't what she does, but how she does it," said a patient recently; thus paying an enviable tribute to the therapist who had been working with him for more than a year (Cates, 1940, pp. 116–117).

Cates's comments support the valuing of "female" caring attributes over "male" scientificism.

The first volume of the *American Journal of Occupational Therapy* included an article on the treatment of patients with paraplegia. The author, occupational therapist Margaret Rood, stressed the importance of gaining rapport with a difficult patient population. To facilitate this process, she emphasized that "the therapist should be attractive preferably but more specifically she should be sweet tempered and not easily depressed" (Rood, 1948, p. 24).

Many publications addressed both the goals of therapy for occupational functioning and the value of the therapist's personal traits. A number of these stressed the importance of training in occupational therapy. In *Prescribing Occupational Therapy*, Dunton (1928) noted:

> It is difficult to say positively or exactly just what qualities of personality make the greatest appeal to children. Undoubtedly a gay, lively individual will attract the attention of the young, but we often find that such a personality is unable to hold their interest, while one who is quiet and reserved will be idolized (p. 136).

He tempered the emphasis on innate qualities with a comment on the importance of training: "Undoubtedly the aide who has had a course in kindergarten methods is better equipped to administer occupational therapy to children" (Dunton, 1928, p. 136).

Upham ascribed importance to the specificity of the work to the patient's handicap and adaptations for improved functional ability. She differentiated between simple engagement in handicrafts and craftwork under the guidance of an occupational therapist:

> As basketry is taught under the old system, its chief value is time-passing. . . . Basketry in the hands of one specially trained for occupational directing is quite different. The patient's methods of work are studied in consultation with the physician, and occupation is accordingly adapted (Upham, 1917, p. 410).

Upham confirmed the importance of training for occupational directors but contended that more was needed than skill in activities. Therapeutics must be integrated with personal characteristics. Thus rapport with the patient was the key to successful therapy. She said, "Here a keen understanding and breadth of sympathy is necessary on the part of the director who gains confidences through the medium of work" (Upham, 1917, p. 411).

Colonel James A. Mattison addressed the importance of the therapist's "magnetic personality" as well as the goals of the program. He described occupational therapy at the National Home for Disabled Volunteer Soldiers for a 1929 issue of *Occupational Therapy and Rehabilitation*:

> One of the principal aims of occupational therapy is to create morale, and to provide every opportunity for the coordination of all hospital efforts toward returning the

patient to community life and economic usefulness (p. 80).

Dr. Fred P. Clark (1917) spoke to the personal traits of successful teachers of occupation and to the need for specialized training. He averred that

> the mistake is made of trying to carry on this work with nurses who have had no special training in work therapy and who are occupied with their regular daily duties. . . . The work must be under the direction of teachers who have been trained along the proper lines. . . . The teachers should be intelligent, observant and tactful in order that they may command the respect of their pupils and be able to observe when the patients begin to tire of any special line of work (p. 392).

The ideal therapist linked both skills, according to Elnora Thomson, superintendent of the Illinois Society for Mental Hygiene. She characterized Slagle as possessing a combination of professional preparation and appropriate personal traits. She described Slagle as, "a teacher who had both vision and training" (Thomson, 1917, p. 398).

Craven (1940) similarly affirmed the importance of the therapist's personal characteristics. She argued that they should be employed in the service of therapy and not in lieu of educational preparation:

> Thorough knowledge of the patient and of the craft, sympathy, and tact are required for the successful administering of work. The "personality of the therapist" is important, not as an entity in itself but in the relation to her ability to give the patient the most therapeutic value from the work he does (Craven, 1940, p. 17).

Descriptions of training programs and schools emphasized the technical aspects of practice. They focused on the application of crafts to medical and psychological conditions. A 1916 bulletin for a course in occupations for invalids at the School of Practical Arts, Teachers College, Columbia University, reported that during the course, "the relation of the age, sex, interests, physical and mental limitations of the patient to the occupation selected will be discussed" ("Occupations for Invalids," 1916).

THE IMPACT OF WORLD WAR I

The rapid growth of occupational therapy was credited in part to the World War I experience. The reconstruction aides were appointed to help in rehabilitation efforts for servicemen suffering from battle fatigue, war neurosis, or war-related injuries. The occupational therapy aides used craft activities that were carefully selected to meet each patient's physical and psychological needs. The work of one reconstruction aide, Ora Ruggles, is recounted in *The Healing Heart* (1946) written by John Carlova and Ruggles.

Women were selected for training and service as reconstruction aides on the basis of proficiency in a variety of craft activities. Although the training courses included psychology, specific handicapping conditions, the history of occupational therapy, and hospital etiquette, the use of crafts remained the focus (Emergency Course of Instruction). An Army Medical Department circular dated March 27, 1918, described the job and the qualifications for appointment:

> trained women to furnish forms of occupation to convalescents in long illness. . . to give to patients the therapeutic benefit of activity. . . . She shall have a High School Education, or its equivalent. Applicants must have a theoretical knowledge of the following crafts and practical training in at least three of them:
> Basketry,
> Weaving (Hand and bead looms including simple forms of rugs and mat making),
> Simple wood carving,
> Block-printing (paper and textiles),
> Knitting,
> Needlework.

The seriousness of purpose of occupational therapy was subject to question because the providers of occupational therapy were women and their primary tools were craft activities and their own personalities. Colonel Frank Billings (1918) of the Office of the Surgeon General characterized the work of the reconstruction aides:

> It [ward work] has consisted frequently of work not so purposeful in its character, but rather as diversional in character, in the form of knitting, in the form of basket weaving, etc. But the work which the Surgeon-General utilizes as curative in character in the general hospital for these soldiers is more purposeful than knitting, basket weaving and the like. In other words, it is of the kind and character of curative work that will look toward the training of the soldier for employment after his discharge from the Army (p. 1925).

This differentiation between women's work and men's work culminated in a distinction between bedside activities and vocational activities. Prolonged engagement in bedside activities provided by female reconstruction aides was criticized as promoting dependence and invalidism (Sexton, 1918). Vocational activities conducted by male vocational teachers prepared the men to return to economic productivity.

PROFESSIONALISM AND THE USE OF CRAFTS

In civilian practice, concerns about the adequacy of handicrafts in preparing patients for occupational function were also apparent. Even among the founders and supporters of occupational therapy, there was self-conscious debate about the value of crafts. According to an editorial in a 1918 issue of *Maryland Psychiatric Quarterly,*

> It is a fact, well recognized by those familiar with occupational therapy, that the mind of the convalescent is "let down" similar to the physical diminution of power. So that as soon as possible efforts should be made to build up the patient's morale by means which may appear trivial but which have as their ultimate object the restoration of the orderly thinking which has been characteristic of the individual previous to his sickness ("Occupational Aides," 1918, p. 27).

Although the editorial was unsigned, it was undoubtedly the work of Dunton. The language of the editorial was similar, and in some cases identical, to the language of Dunton's 1928 book, *Prescribing Occupational Therapy.*

Hall, a near founder and several times president of the National Society for the Promotion of Occupational Therapy, commented in a 1917 article,

> The occupations that are employed therapeutically range all the way from work in the service of the institution to a virtual play in the construction of rather useless articles of the so-called arts and crafts order (p. 383).

Practicing therapists also recognized the limitations of crafts. Decrying the scarcity of crafts that required finger extension, Taylor (1929) reported, "Mechanical means are often necessary because of the limitations in occupations" (p. 337). She was equally concerned about activities for lower extremity function: "The problem ahead of us in the use of occupational therapy for functional restoration is to readapt and make jig saw, looms, etc, so that all physical exercises may be obtained through occupations" (p. 337).

After describing adaptations of loom, bicycle saw, and treadle saw for lower extremity strengthening, one director of occupational therapy made an additional suggestion:

> Mechanical appliances. As ankle flexion is usually limited, I am going to mention two ways of getting it by mechanical appliances:
> 1. The patient lies on his side on a cot which has a pulley at the end. A band around the patient's foot is fastened to the cord over the pulley, and a weight attached. Flexion of the foot uses the flexor muscles to pull up the weight, which may be gradually increased.
> 2. The foot may be strapped in the ankle circumductor, and the circumductor turned entirely by pulling the foot away from the pedal. [The term *circumductor* suggests a device that moves the ankle through full circumduction.] The handle is not used except to start. This makes a heavy exercise (Hickinson, 1934, p. 34).

Adaptive equipment for the accomplishment of occupational tasks and activities of daily living was described for a patient with paralysis from a gunshot wound. While working at Michael Reese Hospital in Chicago, Tracy

> hit upon the plan of equipping the patient with a polishing pad, fastened into his right palm by a band buttoning around the hand. With this apparatus he is able to polish articles fastened on a special bed table in front of him, using his inert hand simply as a tool driven by his arm, somewhat as a carpenter uses a plane. It is hoped that he may thus be enabled at least to contribute to his own support when he is discharged. . . . This man had not been able to put anything into his own mouth for four months, but, with the aid of a second leather palm which holds a fork or spoon, he can now feed himself ("Occupational Therapy," 1917, p. 426).

The successful emergence of occupational therapy as a profession required a compromise between the demands for a scientific approach to the work and the restricted sphere of activity available to women. This was accomplished in two ways. First, roles were assigned within the profession in a way that was consistent with culturally acceptable gender roles. Second, attribution of therapeutic success was granted equally to the scientific basis for the work and the personal characteristics of the female therapist. Despite this, the profession did not achieve total acceptance. The reliance on women as practitioners and the use of crafts as therapeutic modalities permitted differentiation between occupational therapy and "real" work, although the goals of therapy were directed toward occupational function.

SUMMARY

The founders of occupational therapy relied on observation and personal experience to develop a common belief system. Their statements and publications reflected shared convictions: the unity of body and mind and the value of occupation. The development of a profession that assists people in attaining or retaining occupational functioning required three elements. First, there had to be a physical location for practice. Hospitals had to develop into institutions that provided care for people who anticipated a return to occupational role. Second, concern for age-related normative behavior gave scientific weight to concerns about appropriate occupational function. Third, occupational therapy, like other health professions, gave women an opportunity for careers in a way that expanded the realm of feminine activity from the domestic sphere to the market economy. This required accommodation achieved through delineation of roles. Women were the providers of therapy and men gave direction and determined the course of the profession.

Hospitals are no longer the place of treatment for any but the most acutely ill or injured. Much of health care has returned to the home. The difference now is that there is a role for occupational therapy. The home is often the place where problems of function are best addressed.

Occupational function is determined by the individual's age, gender, and station in life, although there are far fewer culturally determined limitations. Failure to accomplish life tasks in a timely manner interferes with achieving or maintaining functional occupational roles. Intervention may be needed to help individuals overcome impairments that interfere with life task accomplishment. This is as true today as it was in the late 19th and early 20th centuries and authenticates the role of occupational therapy now as then.

The 19th-century health reform movement was successful because traditional medicine had little to offer; its methods often caused more harm than good. Because of the acceptance of the germ theory and asepsis and the subsequent improvements in pharmaceuticals, surgical techniques, and technological innovation, traditional medicine claimed dominance. However, we are confronted with situations that illustrate the limitations of medicine. Occupational therapists have much to offer those whose lives are changed by chronic illness or injury. The patient with a spinal cord injury cannot be cured, but he can be helped to achieve optimal functional ability.

Problems relating to gender role differentiation plague not only occupational therapy but all of contemporary society. Serrett (1985), an occupational therapist, related the inability of occupational therapists to articulate a philosophical base for practice to the role assignments determined at the founding of the profession. Women's historian Melosh (1982) asserted that no occupational group that is dominated by women can achieve true professional status. In addition, current debate over the use of crafts and of physical agent modalities are linked to earlier concerns about the scientific basis for practice and the adequacy of occupations to meet patient needs.

Our current concerns cannot be easily answered by examining our beginnings. What does emerge, however, is a constancy of concern that is not an indicator of problems unsolved but rather of continued thoughtfulness and self-examination. These are traits that foster positive change.

STUDY QUESTIONS

1. Describe the changes in hospitals that permitted the development of occupational therapy.
2. In what ways does the history of occupational therapy differ from the history of nursing?

STUDY QUESTIONS, *continued*

3. What factors facilitated the development of standards for the timeliness of life task accomplishment?
4. How do the practices of the 19th-century health reformers relate to occupational therapy in the 20th century?
5. How did the female sphere of activity differ from the male sphere of activity in the late 19th century?
6. What factors made occupational therapy an acceptable career for women?
7. How did the founders and near founders of the National Society for the Promotion of Occupational Therapy fulfill the typical male and female roles of that time? How did they differ from them?
8. Discuss early concerns about crafts as occupations.

REFERENCES

American Occupational Therapy Association. (1967). *Then—and now!* Washington DC: Author

Army Medical Department. (1918, March 27). Circular of information concerning the employment of reconstruction aides (2) (Medical Department circular A-329). American Occupational Therapy Association Archives, Series 1, Box 01, Folder 06. Rockville, MD.

Bailey, H. L. (1917). The Cook County Tuberculosis Hospital, Oak Forest, Ill. *The Modern Hospital, 8,* 377–379.

Barton, G. E. (1917). Inoculation of the bacillus of work. *The Modern Hospital, 8,* 399–402.

Barton, I. G. (1968). Consolation House, fifty years ago. *American Journal of Occupational Therapy, 22,* 340–345.

Beard, G. M. (1874). *Legal responsibility in old age.* Speech presented before the Medico-Legal Society of the City of New York.

Billings, F. (1918). Chairman's address—The national program for the reconstruction and rehabilitation of disabled soldiers. *Journal of the American Medical Association, 70,* 1924–1925.

Blake, J. B. (1984). Mary Gove Nichols, prophetess of health. In J. W. Leavitt (Ed.), *Women and health in America* (pp. 359–375). Madison: University of Wisconsin Press.

Bone, C. D. (1971). Origin of the *American Journal of Occupational Therapy. American Journal of Occupational Therapy, 25,* 48–52.

Breines, E. (1986). *Origins and adaptations: A philosophy of practice.* Lebanon, NJ: Geri-Rehab, Inc.

Carlova, J., & Ruggles, O. (1946). *The healing heart.* New York: Messner.

Cates, E. M. (1940). We dare say! *Occupational Therapy and Rehabilitation, 19,* 115–119.

Chudacoff, H. P. (1989). *How old are you? Age consciousness in American culture.* Princeton, NJ: Princeton University Press.

Clark, F. P. (1917). The beneficial effects of work therapy for the insane. *The Modern Hospital, 8,* 392–393.

Craven, L. M. (1940). Some suggested principles for occupational therapy. *Occupational Therapy and Rehabilitation, 19,* 15–18.

Definitions of Occupational Therapy. (1940). *Occupational Therapy and Rehabilitation, 19,* 35–38.

Dunton, W. R. (1915). *Occupational therapy.* Philadelphia: W. B. Saunders.

Dunton, W. R. (1917). History of occupational therapy. *The Modern Hospital, 8,* 380–382.

Dunton, W. R. (1919). *Reconstruction therapy.* Philadelphia: W. B. Saunders.

Dunton, W. R. (1928). *Prescribing occupational therapy.* Baltimore: Thomas.

Dunton, W. R., & Licht, S. (1950). *Occupational therapy, principles and practices.* Springfield, IL: Charles C. Thomas.

Dunton, W. R., & Licht, S. (1957). *Occupational therapy, principles and practices* (2nd ed.). Springfield, IL: Charles C. Thomas.

Emergency Course of Instruction for Reconstruction Aides. American Occupational Therapy Association Archives, Series 1, Box 01, Folder 06. Rockville, MD.

Hall, H. J. (1917). Remunerative occupations for the handicapped. *The Modern Hospital, 8,* 383–386.

Hickinson, L. M. (1934). Anatomical considerations and technique in using occupations as exercise for orthopedic disabilities. *Occupational Therapy and Rehabilitation, 13,* 30–34.

History. (1940). *Occupational Therapy and Rehabilitation, 19,* 27–34.

Johnson, S. (1917). Occupational therapy in New York City institutions. *The Modern Hospital, 8,* 414–415.

Kern, S. (1983). *The culture of time and space.* Cambridge, MA: Harvard University Press.

Licht, S. (1967). The founding and founders of the American Occupational Therapy Association. *American Journal of Occupational Therapy, 21,* 269–277.

Low, J. F. (1992). The reconstruction aides. *American Journal of Occupational Therapy, 46,* 45–48.

Mattison, J. S. (1929). The program of occupational therapy at the National Home for Disabled Volunteer Soldiers. *Occupational Therapy and Rehabilitation, 8,* 77–81.

Melosh, B. (1982). *The physician's hand: Work, culture and conflict in American nursing.* Philadelphia: Temple University Press.

Melosh, B. (1984). More than "the physician's hand": Skill and authority in twentieth-century nursing. In J. W. Leavitt (Ed.), *Women and health in America* (pp. 482–496). Madison: University of Wisconsin Press.

Morantz, R. M. (1984). Making women modern: Middle-class women and health reform in 19th-century America. In J. W. Leavitt (Ed.), *Women and health in America* (pp. 346–358). Madison: University of Wisconsin Press.

Numbers, R. L., & Schoepflin, R. B. (1984). Ministries of healing: Mary Baker Eddy, Ellen G. White, and the religion of health. In J. W. Leavitt (Ed.), *Women and health in America* (pp. 376–389). Madison: University of Wisconsin Press.

Occupation aides. (1918). *Maryland Psychiatric Quarterly, 8,* 27.

Occupational therapy in the general hospital. (1917). *The Modern Hospital, 8,* 425–427.

Occupations for Invalids. (1916). School of Practical Arts, Teachers College, Columbia University. American Occupational Therapy Association Archives, Series 12, Box 101, File 733. Rockville, MD.

Paisley, S. A. (1929). Occupational therapy treatment for a group of spastic cases: Children under twelve years of age. *Occupational Therapy and Rehabilitation, 8,* 83–93.

Peloquin, S. M. (1991a). Occupational therapy service: Individual and collective understandings of the founders, part 1. *American Journal of Occupational Therapy, 45,* 352–360.

Peloquin, S. M. (1991b). Occupational therapy service: Individual and collective understandings of the founders, part 2. *American Journal of Occupational Therapy, 45,* 733–744.

Rood, M. (1947). A program for paraplegics. *American Journal of Occupational Therapy, 1,* 22–25.

Rosenberg, C. E. (1978). The practice of medicine in New York a century ago. In J. W. Leavitt & R. L. Numbers (Eds.), *Sickness and health in America* (pp. 55–74). Madison: University of Wisconsin Press.

Serrett, K. D. (1985). Another look at occupational therapy's history: Paradigm or pair-of-hands? *Occupational Therapy in Mental Health, 3*, 1–31.

Sexton, F. H. (1918). Vocational rehabilitation of soldiers suffering from nervous diseases. *Mental Hygiene, 2*, 265–276.

Shakespeare, W. (1975). *The complete works of William Shakespeare.* New York: Avenel.

Slagle, E. C., & Robeson, H. (1941). *Syllabus for training of nurses in occupational therapy.* Utica, NY: State Hospitals Press.

Starr, P. (1982). *The social transformation of American medicine.* New York: Basic Books.

Taylor, M. (1929). Occupational therapy in industrial inquiries. *Occupational Therapy and Rehabilitation, 8*, 335–338.

Textbooks required for the January, 1920, term at the School of Diversional Occupation in Colorado Springs, Colorado. (1920). American Occupational Therapy Association Archives, Series 12, Box 101, File 731. Rockville, MD.

Thomson, E. E. (1917). Occupation and its relation to mental hygiene. *The Modern Hospital, 8*, 397–398.

Tracy, S. (1910). *Studies in invalid occupations: A manual for nurses and attendants.* Boston: Whitcomb & Barrows.

Upham, E. G. (1917). Some principles of occupational therapy. *The Modern Hospital, 8*, 409–413.

Theoretical Foundations for Practice

Catherine A. Trombly

How do occupational therapists know what to do when a person with a physical **impairment, functional limitation, disability,** or **handicap** is referred to them? First, they have specific knowledge gained from textbooks, journals, lectures, and workshops. They know what the diagnosis means in terms of **impairment** or **disability.** They know the **theoretical rationale** for treatments and the outcome of research on the effectiveness of those treatments. Second, they have specific skills for evaluating and treating persons with physical dysfunction obtained through instruction and practice. Third, and most important, they know how therapy is organized. That organization is found in **conceptual models of practice** and metamodels that organize more circumscribed models of practice.

ORGANIZATION OF PRACTICE OF OCCUPATIONAL THERAPY FOR PHYSICAL DYSFUNCTION

Practice with persons who have physical dysfunction has been organized hierarchically since the inception of application of occupational therapy to this population. The ability to carry out one's roles, duties, and activities of life depends on a person's basic capacities (i.e., strength, perception, motor control, ability to sequence information, etc.). This hierarchical organization assumes strong linear relationships between lower-level capacities and abilities and higher-level functioning such as activities, tasks, and roles (Fig. 2.1). These relationships are not simple. Many different capacities contribute to development of one ability; many abilities are needed to engage successfully in an activity. No single variable accounts for ability to function within a role.

This generally accepted organization further assumes that the lower-level abilities are *prerequisite to* higher-level functioning. When the basic cognitive-perceptual, socioemotional, and sensorimotor capacities and abilities are normal, the person is capable of doing those activities that he values and occupational therapy would not be needed. If the basic capacities and abilities are lacking, the occupational therapist is called on to help the person regain them or to learn new methods of achieving activities and tasks of daily life needed for competent role performance. Treatment to enable the person to accomplish the tasks of his life is preceded by treatment to increase strength and other

GLOSSARY

Conceptual model of practice—A model presents complex phenomena simply. A conceptual model organizes a number of theoretical concepts. In occupational therapy no consensus has been reached for one particular model. Each model explains a specific area of human functioning and specifies the interventions and assessments pertaining to particular kinds of problems. "Conceptual model of practice" is equivalent to Mosey's (1981) "frame of reference."

Disability—Any restriction or lack (resulting from an impairment) of ability to perform an activity in a manner or within the range considered normal for a human being (WHO, 1980, p. 143). Disability represents a person-environment–level disablement.

Functional limitation—Defined by the National Center for Medical Rehabilitation Research (NCMRR) as restriction or lack of ability to perform an action in the manner or within the range consistent with the purpose of an organ or organ system, e.g., poor hand coordination, ineffective grasping, and perceptual problems. This level of disablement probably equates to "abilities" in the theory of occupational functioning (see Table 3.1).

Handicap—A disadvantage for a given individual, resulting from an impairment or disability, that limits or prevents the fulfillment of a role that is normal (depending on age, sex, and social and cultural factors) for that individual (WHO, 1980, p. 183). Handicap represents a person-society–level disablement.

Impairment—Any loss or abnormality of psychological, physiological, or anatomical structure or function (WHO, 1980, p. 47). Impairment represents a person-level disablement.

Philosophy—A belief that guides behavior. The philosophy of occupational therapy was stated by Reilly (1962): "Man, through the use of his hands, as they are energized by mind and will, can influence the state of his own health" (p. 8). One recognizes an occupational therapist by her use of occupation (purposeful activity) as therapy and by her interest in the patient's ability to engage in occupation (meaningful interaction with his various environments).

Theory—A theory is an abstract idea or collection of ideas used to explain physical or social phenomena. A theory organizes knowledge by describing concepts or constructs pertaining to that phenomenon and the relationships between the concepts or constructs based on research evidence. It allows prediction, because the relationships are specified. Theory is dynamic and changes as hypotheses are tested. It guides thinking, observations, and action (Shepard, 1991; Van Deusen, 1993).

Theoretical rationale—The reason, based on theory or empirical evidence, for using a particular treatment for a particular patient.

capacities and abilities that contribute. The assumption is that if the lower-level **impairment** or **functional limitation** is remediated, then occupational performance will improve generally and the patient will not have to learn adapted methods for each activity separately. Whereas it was once considered that treatment of lower-level capacities and abilities would automatically result in improved occupational performance, it is now known that practice of the actual tasks and activities in the context in which they naturally occur is required. This validates the occupational therapist's practice of incorporating recovering component skills (here referred to as capacities and abilities) into occupation.

Treatment follows this "bottom-up" approach, but evaluation follows a "top-down" approach. That is, the therapist determines what roles and tasks the person was responsible for in life before the accident or disease and what he is expected to be or wants to be responsible for in postrehabilitation life. Then, based on observation of the person as he attempts to do functional activities and tasks and the probabilities established by the diagnosis and age of the person, the therapist hypothesizes which of the myriad variables assumed to be related to accomplishment of these tasks and roles might be impaired. Those variables would be assessed and, if found deficient, treated with the expectation that treatment would facilitate occupational performance.

> Occupational therapy is an open system process whereby humans interact with occupational tasks. The effects of occupational therapy are not limited to simple linear changes, such as strengthening muscles or increasing confidence. Rather, therapeutic change involves complex reorganization within the total human being and his or her environment as multiple factors are realigned, altered, coordinated into a new order (Kielhofner, 1992, p. 65).

The constructs of the occupational functioning **theory** shown in Figure 2.1 are described below.

Goal of Occupational Therapy: Sense of Efficacy and Self-Esteem

The goal of occupational therapy is the promotion of a sense of efficacy and self-esteem by developing competency, i.e., effective interaction with the environment. Competency develops by enabling the person to engage in graduated goal-directed activity that is accomplishable by that person, that produces a feeling

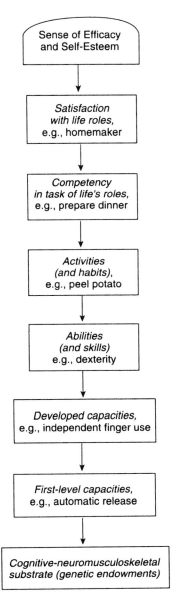

Figure 2.1. Paradigm of occupational functioning theory.

A sense of competence is a vital aspect of self-esteem. When people feel competent, they are most likely to esteem themselves. Self-esteem is that aspect of self-concept that attributes a negative or positive value to the self. Self-esteem is created by individuals' analysis of their competency in socially relevant areas (Gage & Polatajko, 1994). People's level of self-esteem depends on their confidence, based on experience, that they can make desired things happen and that others will appreciatively recognize this competence (White, 1971).

Efficacy refers both to Bandura's (1977) concept of perceived self-efficacy and to Rogers's (1983) concept of response efficacy. Bandura (1986) defined perceived self-efficacy as

> people's judgements of their capabilities to organize and execute courses of action required to attain designated types of performances. It is concerned not with the skills one has but with the judgements of what one can do with whatever skills one possesses (p. 391).

Response efficacy refers to people's judgments of the effectiveness of their responses they used to cope with a given problem. Efficacy, therefore, encompasses both the individuals' perceptions of their ability to carry out the activity and their beliefs that the recommended response will bring the desired results (Gage, 1992; Lewthwaite, 1990). The most powerful source of efficacy expectations is past performance accomplishments in similar situations. Perceived self-efficacy is influenced through an ongoing evaluation of success and failure with each task people participate in over the course of their lives (Gage & Polatajko, 1994). Therefore, therapeutic programs that build on a base of successively more difficult performance accomplishments and that promote a sense of personal responsibility for those accomplishments should be most successful in producing desired behaviors (Lewthwaite, 1990). Csikszentmihalyi (1990) might describe this sense of efficacy as one by-product of "flow," defined as a state in which the challenge of the environmental demand (task demands) matches the person's abilities. Flow is one ingredient of the "optimal experience," which is characterized as a state in which there is no threat for the self to defend against.

A sense of efficacy is derived from being in control of one's life. This means being able satisfactorily to engage in one's life roles (or voluntarily reassign a role to another). To engage satisfactorily in a life role, a person must be able to do the tasks that make up that role in his opinion. Tasks are composed of activities, which are smaller units of behavior. To be able to do a given activity, one has to have certain sensorimotor, cognitive, perceptual, emotional, and social abilities. These are referred to as "performance components"

of satisfaction (White, 1959), and that leads to the ability to live independently and to direct one's own life. To be competent means to be sufficient or adequate to meet the demands of a situation or task. It does not equate to excellence, normality, or ability to do everything, and it recognizes that there are degrees of sufficiency and adequacy in people (Mocellin, 1992; White, 1971). By competence therapists mean the experience of efficacy, of control, and of self-determination achieved through occupation (purposeful activity), development, learning, and interaction with the therapist. The sense of efficacy allows the person to believe in his own control rather than being controlled by the environment (social or physical) (Trombly, 1993a).

in the *Uniform Terminology* (American Occupational Therapy Association [AOTA], 1989). Abilities are developed from capacities that the person has gained through learning or maturation. These developed capacities depend on first-level capacities that derive from a person's genetic endowment or spared organic substrate (Trombly, 1993a).

LIFE ROLES

People occupy their lives with many different activities and tasks. They devote time to those that they value. These activities and tasks are organized into roles. Patients are motivated by their participation in their family and societal roles and will, therefore, value and engage in treatment aimed at restoring those roles.

Various thinkers have proposed different taxonomies of roles. For example, Reilly (1962) categorized occupational roles according to gender and age, identifying four: preschooler, student, housewife/paid worker, and retiree. She saw play and work roles on a continuum. Kielhofner (1992) elaborated on Reilly's work and defined three roles: play, activities of daily living (ADL), and work. Play is the developmentally earliest form of occupational behavior and includes exploration, fantasy, imagination, games, sport, and creative activities. Daily living tasks maintain one's self and lifestyle and include self-care, ordering one's life space and getting to resources (transportation, shopping) (Kielhofner, 1992). Work is productive activity that contributes some service or commodity to others. Related to work are those activities aimed at improving one's ability to produce (student, apprentice, hobbyist, volunteer, and paid worker roles) (Kielhofner, 1992). The three domains of roles (work, play, self-care), called occupational performance areas, are identified as germane to practice (AOTA, 1989).

Bränholm and Fugl-Meyer (1992) developed another taxonomy using factor analysis. They examined the value attached to roles in relation to level of life satisfaction by 210 randomly selected 25- to 55-year-old nondisabled northern Swedish people. They used the *Role Checklist* (Oakley et al., 1986) but eliminated volunteer and religious participant roles as not applicable to this population. Nine roles were grouped into four factors ("metaroles") through factor analysis: student and worker ("vocational metarole"); caregiver, partner, and family member ("family metarole"), friend and indoor and outdoor hobbyist ("leisure metarole"), and participator in organizations ("organizational participator metarole"). The 10th role, home maintainer, did not load on any of the factors. These metaroles were able correctly and significantly to classify subjects in six out of eight areas of life satisfaction. Classification accuracy varied from 62% (leisure) to 78% (family

life). Satisfaction with financial situation and sexual life were not significantly classified by role performance.

I classify roles into three domains related to aspects of self-definition (Trombly, 1993a).

Self-Maintenance Roles

Self-maintenance roles are associated with development and maintenance of the self, including family and home. This domain exceeds AOTA's (1989) occupational performance area of self-care to include care of home and family. Examples of roles in this domain are independent person, grandparent, parent, son, daughter, homemaker, home maintainer, exerciser, and caregiver. The family member, home maintainer, and caregiver roles were found to be "very valuable" to one sample of noninstitutionalized elderly (Elliott & Barris, 1987).

Self-Enhancement Roles

Self-enhancement roles add to the person's sense of accomplishment and enjoyment. This domain loosely corresponds to AOTA's (1989) occupational performance area of play/leisure in that these roles are engaged in because the person wants to do them, not because they are required, because they are chosen by the person himself, and because he is in control in doing something that absorbs his time and attention (Bundy, 1993). Examples of roles in this domain include hobbyist, friend, member/parishioner, vacationer, golfer, movie-goer, and violinist. Roles in this category that a sample of elderly persons found especially valuable were friend, religious participant, hobbyist, and participant in organizations (Elliott & Barris, 1987).

Self-Advancement Roles

The roles in the self-advancement domain are those that involve the person in productive activity of the community and add to the person's skills, possessions, or other betterment. This domain corresponds to the AOTA occupational performance area of work but extends that to include the instrumental roles that enable work. Roles that I would categorize in this domain include worker, student, commuter, shopper, investor, manager, and voter. Student, worker, and volunteer roles were found to be valued by the sample of elderly persons studied by Elliott and Barris (1987).

Using this taxonomy, some roles may be classified in the self-advancement domain for one person but in the self-enhancement domain for another, depending on the motivation, e.g., volunteer. This fact underscores the importance of assessing each person from his own point of view, letting him define his roles and their meaning to him.

It has been logically assumed that involvement in meaningful roles is critical to life satisfaction, and this was supported by results of a survey of 112 noninstitutionalized elderly persons. A low to moderate ($r = 0.29$), but significant ($P < .01$), relationship was found between meaningful role involvement and satisfaction with life (Elliott & Barris, 1987). The low correlation attests to the idea that many variables contribute to the sense of competency, mastery, life satisfaction. Performance in particular roles is only one of those variables.

TASKS OF LIFE ROLES

The tasks identified for the same role by different people may be different (Nelson & Payton, 1991; Trombly, 1993a; Yerxa & Locker, 1990), and the value ascribed to tasks varies among patients of similar situation and varies from what therapists consider important for patients of a particular diagnosis (e.g., stroke) (Chiou & Burnett, 1985). Therefore, each person needs to define his role operationally by identifying those tasks that he associates as crucial to engaging satisfactorily in that particular role. The therapist cannot assume that particular tasks are or are not important to a person's definition of his role. The therapist can determine which tasks and roles are important by engaging the person in a narrative of his life (Clark, 1993).

ACTIVITIES (AND HABITS)

Activities, in this context, are smaller units of behavior that comprise tasks. For example, one task of a gardener role is pest control. Activities included in this task are, e.g., hanging lures, spreading granular insect killer, mixing and spraying liquids, picking insects off plants, and keeping the garden area clean. Some activities, such as dressing an infant, require full attention. Others do not. Habits are chains of subroutines that are so well learned that the person does not have to pay attention to do them under ordinary circumstances. For example, brushing your teeth is a habit. You can put the paste onto the brush while talking to someone and can brush while watching TV or reading.

ABILITIES (AND SKILLS)

I, and others, assume that activities depend on more basic abilities (Clark, Czaja, & Weber, 1990; Fleishman, 1972; Fleishman & Quaintance, 1984; Kielhofner, 1992). A person with a great number of highly developed basic abilities can become proficient at a greater variety of specific tasks and activities. The term *ability* refers to a general trait that an individual brings with him when he begins to learn a new task (Fleishman, 1972). In this taxonomy, abilities are seen as a combination of endowed talents and acquired skill. A skill is an individual's ability to achieve goals under a wide variety of conditions with a degree of consistency and economy (Higgins, 1991). To accomplish the activity of hanging lures in the garden, mentioned above, the person needs certain abilities, such as gross coordination, dexterity, and ability to follow directions. There is, however, very little research characterizing the relationships between abilities and capacities and higher occupational levels of functioning.

That the relationship exists has been verified by several studies. For example, Lynch and Bridle (1989) found a moderately strong ($r = -0.65$, $P < .01$) relationship between the scores of the *Jebsen-Taylor Hand Function Test* (Jebsen et al., 1969) and the scores of the *Klein-Bell ADL Scale* (Klein & Bell, 1982). The relationship with the dressing subtest of the *Klein-Bell* was particularly good ($r = -0.69$, $P < .01$), whereas the relationship with the eating subtest was less strong ($r = -0.45$, $P < .05$). (The negative correlation occurs because the higher the score—time—on the *Jebsen-Taylor*, the worse the performance; while the higher the score on the *Klein-Bell*, the better the performance.) Filiatrault et al. (1991) found a similar relationship ($\rho = 0.60$) between the *Fugl-Meyer Motor Function Test* (upper extremity subtest) (Fugl-Meyer et al., 1975) and the *Barthel Index* (ADL) (Mahoney & Barthel, 1965).

These relationships indicate that sensorimotor control of the upper extremities is related to self-care. But because the r^2 value is only approximately 40%, some other, unidentified, variables account for the remaining 60% variance associated with ADL. This makes sense, because it is known that in addition to upper extremity coordination and dexterity ADL independence seems to require sitting and standing balance, perception of positions of objects in space, ability to sequence steps of a procedure, etc. Research needs to clarify the multivariate relationships among lower-level abilities and capacities and higher-level activities, tasks, and roles (Trombly, 1993a).

Research also needs to verify whether successful treatment of lower levels of functioning results in greater occupational role performance and development of a sense of efficacy and self-esteem than does teaching methods to accomplish activities and tasks in adapted ways. This is a key question for the practice of occupational therapy with persons having physical dysfunction. If research should indicate that satisfactory occupational performance can be obtained via encouraging functional activity alone, the treatment for patients with physical dysfunction will change from a bottom-up approach to a top-down approach. Another question for research is whether system functioning (occupation) can encourage component recovery (Anderson & Lough, 1986; Christiansen, 1991).

DEVELOPED CAPACITIES

Developed capacities reflect the organization of reflex-based responses into voluntary responses acquired through maturation. For example, to support dexterity (ability), the person needs independent use of fingers, graded release, pinch, etc., which derive from reflexive grasp and automatic release.

FIRST-LEVEL CAPACITIES

First-level capacities are the reflex-based responses. They reflect the organization of visual, sensory, and motor systems that develop prenatally and perinatally. Examples include reflexive grasp, reflexive release, primitive reaching, kicking, and stepping. They are the "subroutines" that Bruner (1973) described as underlying development of all voluntary movement. Related to cognition and perception, the ability to recognize a connection between an instrumental response (nonreflexive) given consistently within a particular perceptual situation could be a first-level capacity. In relation to the socioemotional performance component, the fascination of baby with human faces may be equivalent.

ORGANIC SUBSTRATE

The structural foundation for movement (in the neonate) cannot be learned; an innate structure that at least partly matches the structure of the adult model must be assumed (Trevarthen, 1984), including the primordial central nervous system (CNS) organization, skeleton, muscles, and nerves.

Given such an organization for practice, the therapist is still left with these questions: What assessments shall I use? and What treatments shall I choose? These choices are guided by **conceptual models of practice.**

CONCEPTUAL MODELS OF PRACTICE

Conceptual models of practice specify a domain of interest and the assessments and treatments that are applicable when using that particular model. "A good conceptual framework enables the therapist to cope with the many details of a human population by synthesizing them into a perspective of the whole" (Parham, 1987, p. 558). A therapist's theoretical perspective greatly influences what she measures, which variables she chooses to manipulate (or treat), and the conclusions she forms. It is important for clinicians to recognize the assumptions underlying their work and how their work is influenced by such assumptions

(Scholz, 1990). The **conceptual model of practice** helps the therapist name (specify) and frame (recognize the extent, explain the causes) the problem. Once the problem is identified and characterized, the clinical reasoning involved in problem solving and treatment planning begins (Kielhofner, 1992; Parham, 1987; Schön, 1983; see Chapter 3). A model of practice is not only prescriptive, i.e., guides treatment, but is also a scaffolding for creative problem solving within the therapeutic situation (Kielhofner, 1992).

The choice of which model to use comes from both the therapist's knowledge about the problem as well as her **philosophy** of health and occupational functioning. All **conceptual models of practice** used by occupational therapists must be compatible with the single official philosophic base of occupational therapy (AOTA, 1993; see Table 2.1).

The ultimate goal of a model of practice is to prescribe ways to convert states of occupational dysfunction into states of occupational function. Kielhofner (1992) noted that to do so the models typically contain several elements. First, they explain order, i.e., the normal organization and function of the phenomenon that they address. Second, they explain disorder, i.e., the process of disorganization that can occur in the phenomenon and how that causes occupational dysfunctioning. Third, the models explain the therapeutic process, i.e., how intervention positively influences disorganization to bring about organization. Some models address both remediational (change) and compensatory (adaptation) intervention, but often several models are combined to provide both aspects of therapy (Kielhofner, 1992). For example, the biomechanical approach addresses change but not compensation; the rehabilitative approach addresses compensation but not remediation. Some models are considered holistic in that they consider more than one aspect of human behavior. Even these are sometimes combined with

Table 2.1.   Philosophical Base of Occupational Therapy

1. Humans are active beings whose development is influenced by use of purposeful activity.
2. Human beings are able to influence their health and environment through purposeful activity.
3. Human life is a process of continuous adaptation.
4. Adaptation is a change in function that promotes survival and self-actualization.
5. Biological, psychological, and environmental factors may interrupt the adaptation process at any time throughout the life cycle, causing dysfunction.
6. Purposeful activity facilitates the adaptive process.
7. Purposeful activity (occupation) may be used to prevent and mediate dysfunction and to elicit maximal adaptation.
8. Activity as used by the therapist includes both an intrinsic and therapeutic purpose.

more specific models. For example, the model of human occupation, considered a holistic model, may be combined with the biomechanical approach (Kielhofner, 1992).

Furthermore, a model provides the context in which data are gathered and interpreted. If the model deals with the biomechanics of human movement, assessment must include those instruments that will provide the information about the particular biomechanical aspect of movement that the therapist needs to know, e.g., strength or endurance. The model also specifies the types of intervention procedures and materials that will be used to restore order (Kielhofner, 1992).

There are several models from which the therapist may choose in attempting to assist the person with physical injury, disease, or trauma to reach as high a level of independent functioning and life satisfaction as is possible for that person. These approaches are listed below. Three of the models were specified by the largest number of respondents (27/28) to a survey about the adult physical dysfunction content in professional curricula (Nelson, Cash, & Bauer, 1990). The model of human occupation (Kielhofner, 1985) and the occupational performance model, based on the AOTA *Uniform Terminology* (Pedretti & Pasquinelli, 1990), were the other two models cited by respondents as being taught in "phys dys" courses.

As mentioned before, models used in the practice of occupational therapy at this time are not comprehensive enough to encompass treatment of all levels of occupational functioning. Models reflect a separation between lower levels (abilities and capacities) and higher levels (activities and tasks) and between physical, cognitive, and emotional aspects of behavior. Therefore, more than one model will be chosen for use with a particular patient. However, before multiple models are used, the reflective therapist considers the compatibility of the individual models. They should not be mixed indiscriminately (Parham, 1987).

Biomechanical Approach

The biomechanical approach (or model) is applicable to the ability and capacity levels of physical function. This approach deals with increasing strength, endurance, and range of joint motion in patients who have dysfunction in the peripheral nervous system or the musculoskeletal, integumentary, or cardiopulmonary systems. It was once thought that this approach was not appropriate for the person with CNS dysfunction because resistance and stretch (two of the treatment techniques of this model) have adverse effects on movement of patients with CNS dysfunction. However, research has indicated that for persons suffering strokes, a major deficit of voluntary movement is weakness

(Bourbonnais & Noven, 1989), and researchers are considering use of strengthening activities for stroke patients who have some voluntary movement. This, of course, requires careful study.

The biomechanical approach has been used in some manner since occupational therapists began treating persons with physical dysfunction (Spackman, 1968). The basic assumption is that human movement and physical activity enable occupational function. The theoretical arguments, according to Kielhofner's (1992) scheme, are discussed below.

FUNCTION (ORDER)

Occupation requires the ability to move the limbs (range of motion and muscle strength) and the endurance to persist in movement until the goal is accomplished (central and peripheral endurance). Human movement depends on the laws of gravity (mass and acceleration), Newtonian physics (inertia, friction, and forces) (Roberts & Falkenburg, 1992), and exercise physiology. Human movement is characterized in terms of kinematics and kinetics. Kinematics refers to the description of movement in terms of displacement, d (or movement path); velocity, d/t (or speed); acceleration, d/t^2 (or the rate of change of speed); and jerk, d/t^3 (or the rate of the rate of change of speed). Kinetics refers to the forces (torques and gravity) that cause movement. Endurance depends on muscles' capacity to use oxygen, the heart's capacity to use oxygen for its own use and to pump oxygen to the muscles of the body, and the lungs' ability to provide oxygen to the system and remove waste. (Chapters 6 and 22 describe exercise physiology and the biomechanics of human movement.)

DYSFUNCTION (DISORDER)

According to the biomechanical model, dysfunction exists when there is an **impairment** of bone, joint, muscle or tendon, peripheral nerve, heart muscle, lungs, or skin that restricts range of motion, strength, and endurance that prevents the person from engaging in occupational activities or tasks. Problems such as edema, contractures, joint destruction (arthritis), cardiopulmonary disease, peripheral nerve injury, spinal cord injury, and cumulative trauma disorders are specifically treated using the biomechanical model.

MECHANISM(S) OF THERAPEUTIC CHANGE (THERAPEUTIC INTERVENTIONS)

The primary mechanisms that bring about therapeutic change within the biomechanical approach include purposeful activity and exercise that provide stretch of soft tissues, active and passive movement to preserve and restore full range of motion, resistance and other stress to strengthen weak muscles, and graduated, increasing levels of aerobic exercise to improve endurance.

Treatment is aimed at preventing and correcting loss of occupational function by preventing loss of range of motion, strength, or endurance and remediating any losses that do occur. This model does not address compensation; the rehabilitative approach is combined with this approach to compensate for permanent losses of a biomechanical nature. (The assessment and intervention techniques are described in Chapters 6, 11, and 22; adjunctive therapies that support this model are discussed in Chapters 28, 29, 32, and 33; and the application of the model, in combination with complementary models, is illustrated in Chapters 37, 38, 40, 41, 42, and 43.)

As with all models used in occupational therapy, therapeutic research is limited, although basic research by human movement scientists and exercise physiologists is sound (for examples of basic research, see Chapters 6 and 22). Therapeutically, there is some evidence that stretch to soft tissue will correct soft tissue contractures (Hallum & Medeiros, 1987), that stress to a muscle will increase its size and strength (Dons et al., 1979), and that continued physical exercise will result in lower cardiopulmonary requirements (i.e., a training effect) (Fletcher & Cantwell, 1979). However, there is little research that clarifies the relationships among function, dysfunction, and occupational function; that determines the inherent biomechanical characteristics of therapeutic activities; or that establishes the effects on occupational function of therapy applied according to the model.

Neurodevelopmental-Motor Learning Approach

The neurodevelopmental-motor learning approach (or model) is also applicable to the ability and capacity levels of function. This approach is used for persons who have been born with a dysfunctional central nervous system or who have suffered trauma or disease to their central nervous system. A therapist following this approach uses sensory input and developmental sequences to facilitate change in the sensorimotor organization of the central nervous system and motor learning principles to bring about change in voluntary movement behavior. The goal of treatment is to effect an essential change in the physiological or behavioral organization of the central nervous system and thereby improve the overall functioning of the disabled person. Treatments developed as part of the neurodevelopmental-motor learning approach are also appropriate for patients with an intact central nervous system, because this approach capitalizes on and enhances the functioning of the central nervous system.

The name of this model has been modified since the last edition of this textbook to include the newest approach to remediation of motor control, i.e., motor learning. The neurodevelopmental-motor learning approach is actually composed of several "mini-theories" relating to neurophysiologic, developmental, and motor learning aspects of acquiring motor control and voluntary human movement.

NEURODEVELOPMENTAL ASPECTS OF MOTOR CONTROL

There are four mini-theories that were developed to remediate **impairments** of motor control in persons who had suffered central nervous system disease or trauma. All are based on a hierarchical representation of the CNS and regard the lesion to result in release of reflex activity from higher control. All four use, to some extent, neurophysiologically based techniques, such as controlled sensory input to affect motor output and ontogenetic or recovery-based developmental sequences for both assessment and treatment. The approaches share the idea of the importance of the need for repetition. All emphasize the development of basic movement and postures and assume that when movement is "normalized" skilled movement occurs automatically. (The theories of Rood, Bobath, Kabat, Knott and Voss (proprioceptive neuromuscular facilitation; PNF), and Brunnstrom are described in Chapter 24.)

MOTOR LEARNING

There are two models for application of motor learning **theory** and methods to treatment of persons with CNS **impairment.** These are the Carr and Shepherd *Motor Relearning Programme for Stroke* (Chapter 25A) and the task-oriented approach described by Horak (1991) and Bass-Haugen and Mathiowetz (see Chapter 25B). Newer research on the characteristics of normal human movement, motor skill acquisition in children and adults, robotics, and the mechanisms of motor control led therapists to rethink their approach to the remediation of motor control and performance. The importance of biomechanical and environmental constraints on the patient's ability to move are being reconsidered and included in these newer approaches. For example, research on the effect of context on the organization of movement appears to support the view that practicing a skill under simplified, non–context-specific conditions is different from practicing in a context-specific situation and does not generalize (Anderson & Lough, 1986; Trombly, 1994; Wu, Trombly, & Lin, in press).

Both approaches emphasize motor performance using functional tasks, include remediation of performance components and modification of the environment to improve task performance, stress practice that fits the nature of the task, and reject assumptions of the reflex-hierarchical model of motor control and of the traditional developmental theories.

Function (Order)

Occupation requires voluntarily controlled, coordinated movements. Coordinated movement is the result of flexible stability of the head, trunk, and proximal limbs; controlled mobility of the limbs; eye-limb coordination; kinesthetic awareness; and intact motor plans. The relationships of agonist, antagonist, and synergistic muscles must be organized to allow postural stability, limb mobility, eye-hand convergence, and proper timing of limb movements. The interpretation of tactile, proprioceptive, and vestibular sensory input must be consistent and associated with response output. The CNS connections and centers need to operate to allow selection and organization of responses suitable to the environmental demand.

Dysfunction (Disorder)

According to the neurodevelopmental-motor learning model, dysfunction exists when **impairment** of the central nervous system results in an inability to move voluntarily and to effect a desired change in the physical environment. Problems such as stroke, Parkinson's disease, traumatic brain injury, and brain tumors are examples of the disorders that may be treated using this approach.

Therapeutic Mechanisms of Change (Therapeutic Interventions)

The primary mechanisms of therapeutic change associated with the neurodevelopmental-motor learning models include development, learning, and purposeful activity. The goals vary among the particular models.

Kielhofner (1992) questioned whether occupational therapy should be initiated in the early stages of development or recovery of voluntary motor control because the treatments used often cannot involve occupation. Occupation refers to "chunks of activity within the ongoing stream of behavior that are named in the lexicon of the culture and that are self-initiated, goal-directed, organized, composed of adaptive skills, and personally satisfying" (Yerxa & Locker, 1990, p. 318). Obviously, individuals who cannot move in a predictable way cannot engage in such high-level per-

formance. However, purposeful (i.e., goal-directed) activity and exercise can be used to elicit recovery of lower-level abilities (Trombly, 1992; 1993b). Once these lower-level abilities begin to return, the occupational therapist involves the patient in higher forms of purposeful activity to practice the newly gained skill.

Rehabilitative Approach

The rehabilitative approach is applicable to the **disability** and **handicap** levels of disablement (World Health Organization [WHO], 1980) or the activity, task, and role levels of occupational functioning. The rehabilitative approach aims at making the person as independent as possible in spite of residual **disability** that has resulted for any reason. If a person must live with a **disability** that decreases his independent functioning, then the occupational therapist will concentrate on helping him find ways to compensate for his losses by adapted techniques and/or equipment. The rehabilitative approach is used when remediation is complete or is not a possibility. Briefly, the theoretical arguments are as follows.

Function (Order)

The ability to maintain one's self, i.e., care for self, dependents, and home; to advance one's self through work, learning, and financial management; and to enhance the self by engaging in self-actualizing activities that add enjoyment to life represent occupational functioning. For occupational functioning to be in order, many aspects of human performance, motivation, environment, and culture must interact compatibly.

Dysfunction (Disorder)

Losses in any of the aspects of human functioning, loss of motivation, drastic changes in environment, or cultural inaccessibility result in **disability** or **handicap** (occupational dysfunction).

Therapeutic Mechanisms of Change (Therapeutic Interventions)

Interventions under the rehabilitative approach are aimed at preventing occupational dysfunction as well as restoring it, once lost. Treatments are compensatory and focus on teaching physical and emotional adaptation. The therapist teaches the patient to recognize and use his remaining abilities in adapted ways and also teaches him the principles and concepts of those methods so that he may become an independent problem solver (Trombly, 1989). Therapeutic mechanisms of change include learning, development of therapeutic rapport, and purposeful activity. The assessment and treatment procedures are described later in this text (see Chapters 4, 5, 10, 11, 13–21, 30, and 31). Societal attitudes must also be changed, but the occupational therapy technology for implementing this has not been developed.

Model of Human Occupation

Kielhofner (1992) viewed the model of human occupation (MOHO) as most applicable to the **disability** and **handicap** levels of the WHO (1980) classification of disablement for any person experiencing occupational dysfunction. The model of human occupation views the person as an open system that interacts with the social and physical environments and is changed because of that interaction. The output of the system, occupation, is achieved by interdependent functioning of three subsystems: volition, habituation, and performance (Elliott & Barris, 1987; Kielhofner, 1985). The model provides an explanation of how human behavior is motivated (volitional subsystem), organized (habitual subsystem), and carried out (performance subsystem). Therapists value its holistic approach. They combine it with other models of practice, especially when treating physical **impairments** (Kielhofner, 1992; Muñoz, Lawlor, & Kielhofner, 1993). The theoretical arguments are discussed below.

Order

There are three major elements to the concept of order in the MOHO. First, the person is conceptualized as an open system, i.e., one that interacts with the environment to cause change to the environment and that is changed by the interaction with the environment. Second, the three subsystems within the person regulate choice, lifestyle, and performance. The interaction with the environment is influenced by the state of the three subsystems, and their status reflects the internal order of the person. The third element is the environment and its effects on the individual. The environment is composed of objects, tasks, social groups, and culture. The nature of the interaction with the environment shapes the order or disorder of the system.

Disorder

A disruption in the person's ability to choose, organize, or perform occupational behavior secondary to various etiologies (developmental, psychiatric, and physical) characterizes disorder. Disorder may involve any one of the subsystems or may involve the open-systems cycle, which maintains and changes the individual (Kielhofner, 1992). Physical disabilities are, by definition, disturbances to the neurologic and/or musculoskeletal constituents of skills. Physical disabilities affect the performance subsystem, and the disorder

resonates throughout the system, constraining the higher habituation and volition subsystems (Kielhofner et al., 1985). Because habits build on skills in the performance subsystem, disruption to those skills means that habits will become disorganized. In the same way that performance limitations interfere with habits, they may also disrupt or terminate role performance. Physical disabilities confront the individual with experiences that challenge and contradict the view of self as competent and can impose a discontinuity between what persons can do and what they value or believe they should do (volitional subsystem). Physical disabilities often make it impossible or contraindicated for individuals to handle objects of everyday life, and they must learn to use new objects (object environment). Tasks are more rigidly organized (task environment). The person must alter the manner of performing tasks and learn new tasks. The temporal nature of tasks may be changed because more time is required to accomplish each step or because certain tasks can only be done when others are present to assist.

By interfering with the output of the system, physical disabilities also negatively impact the open cycle system and may lead to a maladaptive cycle of occupational dysfunction (Kielhofner et al., 1985).

Therapeutic Interventions

The occupational therapist aids the reorganization of all subsystems by engaging the disabled person in occupations and by modifying the environment to facilitate function (Kielhofner et al., 1985). Treatment focuses primarily on the performance subsystem, while relating the performance-oriented procedures to the total system. Therapy uses occupations that are volitionally relevant (meaningful) and related to the person's roles, habits, and environment. The reader is referred to Kielhofner (1985, 1992) for a more complete explanation of the model of human occupation.

Research has been done on development of assessment instruments, utility of the model to guide practice, and validation of some of the theoretical postulates. More work is needed in all these areas (Kielhofner, 1992).

Cognitive-Perceptual Model

The cognitive-perceptual model is applicable to the **functional limitation** level of the WHO (1980) classification of disablement or loss of cognitive-perceptual abilities. It focuses on treatment of cognitive and perceptual processes required for successful occupational function. The approach includes use of cognitive information processing strategies to promote learning or relearning of movement control or perceptual or cognitive functional abilities.

This is a very loosely constructed model that is undergoing development day by day. Its logical arguments, according to Kielhofner (1992), are as follows.

Order

Performance in occupations requires the ability to perceive and evaluate sensory information from the environment and the ability to conceive of, plan, and execute a purposeful action on the environment. The cognitive-perceptual model incorporates all those abilities and capacities that enable information processing required of interaction with a physical and social environment.

Disorder

Secondary to disease or injury to the central nervous system, perceptual and/or cognitive abilities (such as the ability to perceive the figure from a background, to organize and sequence information, and to perceive an object despite its spatial orientation) may be lost or disturbed.

Therapeutic Interventions

The nervous system has the characteristic of plasticity, which implies that organic or behavioral change can occur secondary to sensorimotor interventions or to relearning interventions. Interventions are, therefore, organized to try to affect the organic organization through controlled sensory input and/or to affect the behavioral organization through a teaching-learning format. Environmental adaptation is a third type of treatment and is subsumed under the rehabilitative approach. The evaluation and treatment techniques for the cognitive-perceptual model are described in Chapters 8, 9, 13, 23, 26, and 27, and application is discussed in Chapters 34, 35, and 36.

Other models for occupational therapy practice have been published, and the reader is referred to the literature for consideration of these models (Gage, 1992; Kielhofner, 1992; Llorens, 1976; Mosey, 1974; Schkade, & Schultz, 1992; Schultz & Schkade, 1992; Warren, 1993a, 1993b).

STUDY QUESTIONS

1. Compare and contrast abilities and capacities.
2. List all your roles. What percentage of them deal with self-maintenance, self-advancement, and self-enhancement?
3. What are the tasks that operationally define your role as student occupational therapist?
4. What activities are involved in the task of writing a term paper?
5. What abilities are necessary to use a computer for word processing?
6. For what type of dysfunction is the rehabilitation approach appropriate?
7. What are the therapeutic mechanisms of change used in applying the biomechanical model?
8. How might the biomechanical model and the model of human occupation be used together?

REFERENCES

American Occupational Therapy Association. (1989). Uniform terminology for occupational therapy—2nd edition. *American Journal of Occupational Therapy, 43*(12), 817–831.

American Occupational Therapy Association. (1993). The philosophical base of occupational therapy. *American Journal of Occupational Therapy, 47*(12), 1119.

Anderson, M., & Lough, S. (1986). A psychological framework for neurorehabilitation. *Physiotherapy Practice, 2*, 74–82.

Bandura, A. (1977). Self-efficacy: Toward a unifying theory of behavior change. *Psychological Review, 84*, 191–215.

Bandura, A. (1986). *Social foundations of thought and action: A social-cognitive theory.* Englewood Cliffs, NJ: Prentice Hall.

Bourbonnais, D., & Noven, S. V. (1989). Weakness in patients with hemiparesis. *American Journal of Occupational Therapy, 43*(5), 313–319.

Bränholm, I.-B., & Fugl-Meyer, A. R. (1992). Occupational role preferences and life satisfaction. *Occupational Therapy Journal of Research, 12*(3), 159–171.

Bruner, J. (1973). Organization of early skilled action. *Child Development, 44*, 1–11.

Bundy, A. C. (1993). Assessment of play and leisure: Delineation of the problem. *American Journal of Occupational Therapy, 47*(3), 217–222.

Chiou, I.-I. L., & Burnett, C. N. (1985). Values of activities of daily living: A survey of stroke patients and their home therapists. *Physical Therapy, 65*(6), 901–906.

Christiansen, C. (1991). Occupational therapy: Intervention for life performance. In C. Christiansen & C. Baum (Eds.), *Occupational therapy: Overcoming human performance deficits* (pp. 3–43). Thorofare, NJ: Slack.

Clark, F. (1993). Occupation embedded in real life: Interweaving occupational science and occupational therapy. *American Journal of Occupational Therapy, 47*(12), 1067–1078.

Clark, M. C., Czaja, S. J., & Weber, R. A. (1990). Older adults and daily living task profiles. *Human Factors, 32*(5), 537–549.

Csikszentmihalyi, M. (1990). *Flow: The psychology of optimal experience.* New York: Harper Perennial.

Dons, B., Bollerup, K., Bonde-Petersen, F., & Hancke, S. (1979). The effect of weight-lifting exercise related to muscle fiber composition and muscle cross-sectional area in humans. *European Journal of Applied Physiology, 40*, 95–106.

Elliott, M. S., & Barris, R. (1987). Occupational role performance and life satisfaction in elderly persons. *Occupational Therapy Journal of Research, 7*(4), 215–224.

Filiatrault, J., Arsenault, A. B., Dutil, E. M., & Bourbonnais, D. (1991). Motor function and activities of daily living assessments. A study of three tests for persons with hemiplegia. *American Journal of Occupational Therapy, 45*, 806–810.

Fleishman, E. A. (1972). On the relation between ability, learning, and human performance. *American Psychologist, 27*, 1017–1032.

Fleishman, E. A., & Quaintance, M. K. (1984). *Taxonomies of human performance.* New York: Academic Press.

Fletcher, G. F., & Cantwell, J. D. (1979). *Exercise and coronary heart disease: Role in prevention, diagnosis and treatment* (2nd ed.). Springfield, IL: Charles C. Thomas.

Fugl-Meyer, A. R., Jääskö, L., Leyman, I., Olsson, S., & Steglind, S. (1975). The post stroke hemiplegic patient. I. A method for evaluation of physical performance. *Scandinavian Journal of Rehabilitation Medicine, 7*, 13–31.

Gage, M. (1992). The appraisal model of coping: An assessment and intervention model for occupational therapy. *American Journal of Occupational Therapy, 46*(4), 353–362.

Gage, M., & Polatajko, H. (1994). Enhancing occupational performance through an understanding of perceived self-efficacy. *American Journal of Occupational Therapy, 48*(5), 452–461.

Hallum, A. & Medeiros, J. M. (1987). Effect of duration of passive stretch on hip abduction range of motion. *Journal of Orthopedic and Sports Physical Therapy, 18*, 408–415.

Higgins, S. (1991). Motor skill acquisition. *Physical Therapy, 71*(2), 123–139.

Horak, F. B. (1991). Assumptions underlying motor control for neurologic rehabilitation. In M. Lister (Ed.), *Contemporary management of motor control problems. Proceedings of the II STEP Conference* (pp. 11–27). Alexandria, VA: The Foundation for Physical Therapy.

Jebsen, R. H., Taylor, N., Trieschmann, R., Trotter, M., Howard, L. (1969). An objective and standardized test of hand function. *Archives of Physical Medicine & Rehabilitation, 50*, 311–319.

Kielhofner, G. (Ed.). (1985). *A Model of Human Occupation: Theory and application.* Baltimore: Williams & Wilkins.

Kielhofner, G. (1992). *Conceptual foundations of occupational therapy.* Philadelphia: F. A. Davis.

Kielhofner, G., Shepherd, J., Stabenow, C. A., Bledsoe, N., Furst, G., Green, J., Harlan, B. H., McLellan, C. L., & Owens, J. (1985). Physical disabilities. In G. Kielhofner (Ed.), *A Model of Human Occupation: Theory and application* (pp. 170–247). Baltimore: Williams & Wilkins.

Klein, R. M., & Bell, B. (1982). Self-care skills: behavioral measurement with Klein-Bell ADL Scale. *Archives of Physical Medicine & Rehabilitation, 63*(7), 335–338.

Lewthwaite, R. (1990). Motivational considerations in physical activity involvement. *Physical Therapy, 70*(12), 808–819.

Llorens, L. A. (1976). *Application of a developmental theory for health and rehabilitation.* Rockville, MD: American Occupational Therapy Association.

Lynch, K. B., & Bridle, M. J. (1989). Validity of the Jebsen-Taylor Hand Function Test in predicting activities of daily living. *Occupational Therapy Journal of Research, 9*(5), 316–318.

Mahoney, F. I., & Barthel, D. W. (1965). Functional evaluation: The Barthel Index. *Maryland State Medical Journal, 14*(2), 61–65.

Mocellin, G. (1992). An overview of occupational therapy in the context of the American influence on the profession: Part 2. *British Journal of Occupational Therapy, 55*(2), 55–60.

Mosey, A. C. (1974). An alternative: The biopsychosocial model. *American Journal of Occupational Therapy, 28*(3), 137–140.

Mosey, A. C. (1981). *Occupational therapy: Configuration of a profession.* New York: Raven Press.

Muñoz, J. P., Lawlor, M., & Kielhofner, G. (1993). Use of the Model of Human Occupation: A survey of therapists in psychiatric practice. *Occupational Therapy Journal of Research, 13*(2), 117–139.

Nelson, C. E., Cash, S. H., & Bauer, D. F. (1990). Adult physical dysfunction content in professional curricula. *American Journal of Occupational Therapy, 44*(12), 1079–1087.

Nelson, C. E., & Payton, O. D. (1991). The issue is—A system for involving patients in program planning. *American Journal of Occupational Therapy, 45*, 753–755.

Oakley, F., Kielhofner, G., Barris, R., & Reichler, R. K. (1986). The Role Checklist: Development and empirical assessment of reliability. *Occupational Therapy Journal of Research, 6*(3), 157–170.

Parham, D. (1987). Toward professionalism: The reflective therapist. *American Journal of Occupational Therapy, 41*(9), 555–561.

Pedretti, L. W., & Pasquinelli, S. (1990). A frame of reference for occupational therapy in physical dysfunction. In L. W. Pedretti & B. Zoltan (Eds.), *Occupational therapy practice skills for physical dysfunction* (3rd ed., pp. 1–17). St Louis: C. V. Mosby.

Reilly, M. (1962). Occupational therapy can be one of the great ideas of 20th century medicine. *American Journal of Occupational Therapy, 16*(1), 1–9.

Roberts, S. L., & Falkenburg, S. A. (1992). *Biomechanics: Problem solving for functional activity.* St. Louis: C. V. Mosby.

Rogers, R. W. (1983). Cognitive and psychological processes in fear appeals and attitude change: A revised theory of protection motivation. In J. T. Cacioppo, R. E. Petty, & D. Shapiro (Eds.), *Social psychophysiology* (pp. 153–176). New York: Guilford Press.

Schkade, J. K., & Schultz, S. (1992). Occupational adaptation: Toward a holistic approach for contemporary practice, Part 1. *American Journal of Occupational Therapy, 46*(9), 829–837.

Scholz, J. (1990). Dynamic pattern theory—Some implications for therapeutics. *Physical Therapy, 70*(12), 827–843.

Schön, D. (1983). *The reflective practitioner.* New York: Basic Books.

Schultz, S., & Schkade, J. K. (1992). Occupational adaptation: Toward a holistic approach for contemporary practice, Part 2. *American Journal of Occupational Therapy, 46*(10), 917–925.

Shepard, K. (1991). Theory: Criteria, importance, and impact. In M. Lister (Ed.), *Contemporary management of motor control problems. Proceedings of the II STEP Conference* (pp. 5–10). Alexandria, VA: Foundation for Physical Therapy.

Spackman, C. S. (1968). A history of the practice of occupational therapy for the restoration of physical function: 1917–1967. *American Journal of Occupational Therapy, 22*, 67–71.

Trevarthen, C. (1984). How control of movement develops. In H. T. A. Whiting (Ed.), *Human motor actions—Bernstein reassessed.* Amsterdam: Elsevier.

Trombly, C. A. (Ed.). (1989). *Occupational therapy for physical dysfunction* (3rd ed.). Baltimore: Williams & Wilkins.

Trombly, C. A. (1992). Deficits of reaching in subjects with left hemiparesis: A pilot study. *American Journal of Occupational Therapy, 46*(10), 887–897.

Trombly, C. (1993a). Anticipating the future: Assessment of occupational function. *American Journal of Occupational Therapy, 47*(3), 253–257.

Trombly, C. (1993b). Observations of improvement of reaching in five subjects with left hemiparesis. *Journal of Neurology, Neurosurgery, and Psychiatry, 56*, 40–45.

Trombly, C. A. (1994, July). *Occupation: The effects of goal—directedness.* Paper presented at the American Occupational Therapy Foundation's Research Colloquium, Boston.

Van Deusen, J. (1993). An analytic approach to teaching theory at the postprofessional level. *American Journal of Occupational Therapy, 47*(10), 949–952.

Warren, M. (1993a). A hierarchical model for evaluation and treatment of visual perceptual dysfunction in adult acquired brain injury, Part 1. *American Journal of Occupational Therapy, 47*(1), 42–54.

Warren, M. (1993b). A hierarchical model for evaluation and treatment of visual perceptual dysfunction in adult acquired brain injury, Part 2. *American Journal of Occupational Therapy, 47*(1), 55–66.

White, R. W. (1959). Motivation reconsidered: The concept of competence. *Psychological Reviews, 66,* 297–333.

White, R. W. (1971). The urge towards competence. *American Journal of Occupational Therapy, 25*(6), 271–274.

World Health Organization. (1980). *International classification of impairments, disabilities, and handicaps.* Geneva: author.

Wu, C.-Y., Trombly, C., & Lin, K.-C. (in press). The relationship between occupational form and occupational performance. *American Journal of Occupational Therapy, 48*(8).

Yerxa, E. J., & Locker, S. B. (1990). Quality of time use by adults with spinal cord injuries. *American Journal of Occupational Therapy, 44*(4), 318–326.

3

Planning, Guiding, and Documenting Therapy

Catherine A. Trombly

LEARNING OBJECTIVES

After studying this chapter, the student will be able to:
1. Understand the process of planning treatment, including gathering data, identifying problems, setting and prioritizing goals, developing the plan, and evaluating the outcome.
2. Use a client-centered approach to identify goals and design treatment.
3. Appreciate the need to use valid and reliable assessment instruments.
4. Recognize the dynamic relationship among planning, treatment, and evaluation.
5. Use current terminology and accepted procedures for documentation of treatment effects.
6. Value the role of reflective practitioner.

Occupational therapists are experts in enabling people to engage in those roles, tasks, and activities that have meaning to them on a day-to-day basis and that define their lives. People who have occupational dysfunction or for whom loss of an important function is anticipated secondary to impairment, disability, or handicap are referred to an occupational therapist (Trombly, 1993). The World Health Organization ([WHO], 1980) has defined impairment as "any loss or abnormality of psychological, physiological, or anatomical structure or function" (p. 47). This person-level dysfunction would equate to deficit of one or more **performance components** of the American Occupational Therapy Association's (AOTA) *Uniform Terminology* (1994). Disability has been defined as "any restriction or lack (resulting from an impairment) of ability to perform an activity in the manner or within the range considered normal for a human being" (WHO, 1980, p. 143). This is a problem of the person-

environment interface (Tickle-Degnen et al., 1989). Handicap has been defined as "a disadvantage for a given individual, resulting from an impairment or a disability, that limits or prevents the fulfillment of a role that is normal for that individual" (WHO, 1980, p. 183). Role has been defined as a set of behaviors that are normally or culturally defined and expected of a person in a certain social position (Jongbloed, Stanton, & Fousek, 1993). One classification of roles is personal-sexual role (male or female), familial social roles (mother, father, son, etc.), and occupational role (productive roles such as homemaker, student, and worker) (Kielhofner & Burke, 1985). Another classification includes self-maintenance (independent person, parent, homemaker, etc.), self-advancement (student, worker, traveler, commuter, etc.), and self-enhancement roles (hobbyist, friend, parishioner, movie goer, etc.) (Trombly, 1993). Handicap is a person-societal interface problem (Tickle-Degnen et al., 1989). Both disability and handicap equate to deficits in **performance areas,** to use the language of occupational therapy (Table 3.1).

This textbook describes evaluation and treatment practices for patients in general according to diagnoses. The diagnosis is important in guiding treatment planning (Rogers, 1983). It indicates the types of impairments, the course, the expectations, and the types of residual disability most likely to be seen. These are all pieces of information that delimit and focus treatment planning in general. However, this information is not sufficient to plan treatment for this person at this time with these expectations and needs. Application of general treatment plans (recipes) to a person is wrong. This chapter describes the process by which treatment is individualized. Only appropriately individualized treatment is worthy of the term *professional treatment* (Redelmeier & Tversky, 1990). To individualize treat-

GLOSSARY _____

Biomechanical approach—This approach applies to impairments of the musculoskeletal, cardiopulmonary, integumentary, and nervous (except brain) systems. Goals of this approach are to increase strength, endurance, and joint range of motion and to reduce edema.

Neurodevelopmental-motor learning approach—This approach applies to motor impairments secondary to brain damage. Goals of this approach are to improve voluntary control of limb and trunk movements and postures and to reestablish coordination and dexterity by affecting the organic (neurophysiological) and behavioral (development and learning) organization of the central nervous system. This approach is undergoing major rethinking, described in later chapters.

Performance areas—These are life tasks such as activities of daily living, work, and play or leisure (AOTA, 1994).

Performance components—These are sensorimotor, cognitive, psychosocial, and psychological skills and abilities that are the elements of functional performance in which occupational therapists have expertise to assess and intervene for improved performance (AOTA, 1994).

Rehabilitative approach—This approach applies to disabilities of whatever cause. The goal of this approach is to teach the person to be as independent as possible by using new methods to accomplish functional goals, by using adapted equipment, and/or by adapting the environment.

Reliability—Reliability refers to the consistency with which a test measures the phenomenon. Test-retest (intrarater) reliability refers to consistency from time to time. Interrater reliability refers to the consistency across raters. Internal consistency refers to how well all the questions measure the same phenomenon.

Self-efficacy—Estimate of being competent, of being in charge of one's own life.

Sensitivity—Sensitivity denotes how well changes will be captured to show progress. Tests with gross sensitivity can measure large changes but will miss small gains. The selected test should have the sensitivity necessary to document the size of effect expected within time periods that reevaluation will occur.

Standardized—A standardized test is one whose administration procedure has been written down so that, by following the directions exactly, the test is administered the same each time. Standards may include what is said to the testee, what objects to use exactly, and the environment that is appropriate for administration.

Validity—Validity refers to how well the test measures what it purports to measure. For example, an ADL test should include all those activities that the person will be responsible for at home, not simply "hospital ADL."

---

ment, it is necessary to know the person; his roles, goals, and values; how he learns; his emotional status; the manifestation of the disease in this particular person; and this person's social and physical environment.

PLANNING TREATMENT

The therapist's first task is to develop a treatment plan (Rogers, 1983). Treatment planning involves clarification of the nature of the occupational dysfunction according to the patient (and family), gathering information about the patient's strengths and weaknesses, analyzing and interpreting the meaning of that information, establishing specific goals and subgoals, prioritizing the goals, planning what to do to achieve the goals, implementing the plan, and reviewing the outcome.

Every member of the treatment team uses a similar process and collaborates to plan an overall, nonconflicting program for the patient that enhances all of the patient's capabilities but does not overstress him. The composition of the team varies, depending on the particular problem and needs of the patient. In a rehabilitation center a core team of physician, rehabilitation nurse, occupational therapist, physical therapist, speech therapist, social worker, psychologist, and reha-

bilitation counselor are occasionally joined by the orthotist, prosthetist, teacher, and medical or surgical specialists (such as rheumatologists and cardiologists). Each member is responsible for developing a treatment plan related to his or her own unique area of expertise. The occupational therapy treatment plan focuses on the discrepancy between the past and present levels of the patient's functioning in his occupational performance tasks.

The Philosophy: Client-Centered

There has been a tendency to evaluate and treat individuals in component parts and isolated functions (Smith, 1992). This may be because experienced therapists are able to foresee from the diagnosis and/or observation of the person's performance that deficits of particular **performance components** will probably hamper occupational performance. However, this approach leaves the patient, who cannot foresee how the components relate to overall function, bewildered and feeling disjointed. Sometimes, unfortunately, it also focuses the therapist's attention on the **performance components** rather than occupational performance itself. The client-centered approach, on the other hand,

Table 3.1. Examples of Assessments by Category

Levels of Performance	AOTA *Uniform Terminology*	WHO International Classification	Examples of Assessments
Role	Performance areas	Handicap	Role Checklist (Oakley et al., 1986) Craig Handicap Assessment and Reporting Technique (CHART) (Whiteneck et al., 1992) Canadian Occupational Performance Measure (COPM) (Law et al., 1991)
Tasks	Performance areas	Disability	The Revised Satisfaction with Performance Scaled Questionnaire (Yerxa et al., 1988) COPM (Law et al., 1991)
Activities	Performance areas	Disability	Functional Independence Measure (FIM) (Granger, Hamilton, & Sherwin, 1988) Klein-Bell ADL Scale (Klein & Bell, 1982) Rabideau Kitchen Evaluation—Revised (Neistadt, 1992)
Abilities	Performance components	(Functional limitations[a]	Box and Block Test (Mathiowetz et al., 1985) Jebsen-Taylor Hand Function Test (Jebsen et al., 1969; Lynch & Bridle, 1989)
Developed capacities	Performance components	Impairments	Grip and pinch dynamometry (Mathiowetz, 1991; Mathiowetz et al., 1984)
First-level capacities	Performance components	Impairments	Proprioception Balance testing
Substrate	Performance components	Impairments	Range of motion Muscle testing Sensory testing

[a]The National Center for Rehabilitation Research (NCRR) modified the WHO classification to include functional limitations, defined as restriction or lack of ability to perform an action in the manner or within the range consistent with the purpose of an organ or organ system.

takes the person's point of view and invites the patient to take responsibility for his own health and quality of life (Pollock, 1993). Goals identified by the patient are the focus of therapy. Client-centered therapy is individualized therapy. Intervention is directed at those activities that are meaningful to the client (Law, 1993).

In a client-centered approach, assessment of the patient's occupational dysfunction should take a top-down approach. That is, it should begin with the patient identifying those roles that are meaningful to him and important for him to maintain and the therapist estimat-ing which of those roles seem in jeopardy of change due the trauma or illness that brought the patient to therapy (Trombly, 1993). Furthermore, a client-centered approach asks the patient to describe each role in terms of the tasks that comprise that particular role for him. Think for yourself. Are the tasks you associate with your role as housekeeper the same as those identified by your classmates? I assure you that the tasks I associate with my role as housekeeper are far different from those that a friend of mine identifies as crucial to that role!

The Process

DATA GATHERING AND PROBLEM IDENTIFICATION

To deduce what the occupational performance deficits are and their probable underlying causes, the therapist gathers information from many sources and defines (sets or frames) the problem(s).

Chart Review

The medical record should yield background information, including the person's diagnosis(es), date of onset, medical and surgical histories, precautions, medications, age, and discharge plan as well as reports of the nursing staff about the person's daily physical and psychological functioning.

Interview

The interview should yield knowledge of the person's former roles, expected roles, and the tasks that comprise them; feelings; readiness to participate in or to take responsibility for treatment; expectations for therapy; cognitive abilities such as memory; ability to sequence and organize information; orientation to time, place, and person; comprehension of directions; perception of what he can do for himself; interests; and pertinent social, educational, and vocational history. The interview may be structured using instruments such as the *Canadian Occupational Performance Measure* (Table 3.1).

Interview of family members should produce knowledge of their goals for the disabled family member and their views about how the disability has affected the person as well as how it has affected the family unit. The family is also the source of information about the patient's premorbid personality in the event there has been a change.

The goal of the interviews is to identify realistic, practical, functional goals that can be achieved by occupational therapy intervention (Wilson, 1992).

Observation

Observation of the disabled person as he attempts to perform functional activities will allow the therapist to determine the person's present functional level as well as his sense of safety and judgment. These observations are structured using instruments such as the *Klein-Bell ADL Scale* (Table 3.1).

Observation of functional performance should identify the underlying factors that limit achievement and guide the formal assessment aspect of evaluation (Wilson, 1992). For example, the disabled person may be unable to feed himself. By watching the person try to do this, the therapist observes that the patient can lift a heavy mug but cannot approach his mouth. The therapist concludes that the patient seems to have adequate strength but range of motion seems to be the limiting factor. The therapist will check out this observation by doing a cursory strength evaluation and, confirming that weakness is not the limitation, a more detailed range-of-motion evaluation.

Assessment

Assessment is limited to occupational **performance areas** and the components of occupational performance (AOTA, 1992; Rogers & Holm, 1991). Decisions regarding which **performance area** or **performance component** should be formally assessed are based on the interview concerning what is important, the observation of what aspect of occupational performance is inadequate (Wilson, 1992), known implications of the diagnosis (Rogers, 1983), and the conceptual framework the therapist employs.

Before beginning the assessment, the therapist makes an assessment plan that includes which capabilities to evaluate and which measurement procedures to use to elicit the necessary information regarding the strengths and limitations of the person. The assessment instruments chosen must be appropriate to the conceptual model the therapist has chosen to use and the person's age, gender, and education as well as his socioeconomic, cultural, and ethnic background (AOTA, 1992). Specifics of measurement are described in succeeding chapters of this book. The results are analyzed and summarized to indicate the person's current functional status and documented in the person's medical record (AOTA, 1992).

Characteristics of Assessment Instruments

There is NO good excuse for occupational therapists about to enter the 21st century to be using instruments that are not **standardized** or do not have at least the beginnings of identification of their psychometric properties. **Standardized** tests are administered according to a protocol (AOTA, 1992). **Validity, reliability,** and **sensitivity** are psychometric properties. The instrument should have norms, if appropriate, or be criterion referenced. For example, norms of grasp and pinch strength are compared with the patient's ability to determine whether he can be expected to do activities performed by other people his age and/or body size. However, there are no "norms" for ADL activities; either the person does the activity adequately (meets criterion) or he does not.

Interpreting the Data and Identifying the Problems

A profile of strengths and limitations pertaining to the person's occupational functioning will emerge from the assessment. To identify the problem(s) toward which the treatment plan will be directed, the therapist pays attention to significant data, that which reflects actual or potential limitations or indicates potential for deformity. Once the problems are identified, they are listed along with the treatment goal related to each.

DEVELOPING THE GOALS AND SETTING PRIORITIES

Medicare requires that goals be functional, measurable, and objective (Mahoney & Kannenberg, 1992). Functional means that the goal includes some **performance area,** e.g., self-care, home care, or socialization. The functional level that the patient is expected to achieve needs to be stated as part of the goal. For example, "The patient will complete transfer from wheelchair to tub with moderate assist." If one goal of therapy is to improve an occupational **performance component,** the documentation has to relate the improvement to a functional goal. For example, "The patient will demonstrate sitting balance and trunk flexion and extension required for putting on and removing shoes and stockings." Because all therapy on underlying factors (components) is thus directed toward a specific function, no treatment time is spent on those factors that do not have functional impact (Mahoney & Kannenberg, 1992).

The goal is also stated so that the person's achievement can be measured. For example, "The patient will demonstrate *independent* sitting balance and trunk flexion and extension required for *independently* putting on and removing shoes and stockings." Clearly defined levels of assistance (Tables 3.2 and 3.3) are useful in goal writing and required for Medicare documentation. Goals written in terms of "evaluate pinch strength" or "teach the family car transfers" are not patient goals; they are therapist goals and are not part of the documentation (Mahoney & Kannenberg, 1992).

Priorities

Because it is impossible to accomplish all goals at once, the goals are prioritized. There are two bases for establishing the particular order of priority. One is the client's (and his family's) view of what is most important. The other is the therapist's knowledge that some abilities must precede accomplishment of others. To help in setting priorities, therapists identify both long- and short-term goals.

Long- and Short-Term Goals

Long-term goals specify the end product of therapy. These are the types of goals cited by patient and family. They describe the expected level of functioning the patient will achieve by the termination of the therapy program. An example of this is, "The patient will be independent in self-care." Long-term goals are educated guesses that may need modification as the patient's progress is observed. The ability of eight therapists to predict sensory, cognitive-perceptual, and functional outcome for 85 stroke patients was studied (Korner-Bitensky, Mayo, & Poznanski, 1990). Accuracy of predictions for all patients ranged from 52 to 76%, with errors more likely to be overestimations of patient's discharge status. However, the therapists were accurate in predicting total independence or total dependence (91 to 100%).

To achieve long-term goals, the therapist plans a series of short-term goals that are the building blocks leading to one or more long-term goals. Short-term goals imply sequencing and priority. They state which abilities must be developed before others. The sequencing is started from the point at which the patient is functioning successfully and stopped at the point at which the long-term goal is achieved.

Several sequences of short-term goals may be ongoing concurrently. For example, to reach the long-term goal mentioned above, the patient must learn to

Table 3.2. Levels of Independence

Independent	Patient is able to complete the task, including setup, with or without adaptive equipment; note should be made of adaptive equipment used
Independent with setup	Patient is able to complete the task once someone sets it up for him (e.g., able to dress but unable to get clothes out of the closet; able to feed self once someone applies his adaptive equipment)
Supervision	Patient is able to perform the task without physical contact but needs cuing or coaxing to do so and/or cannot be left alone because of cognitive deficits, poor balance, etc.
Minimal assistance	Patient requires minimal physical assistance or verbal cues to complete the task; assistance with 25% of the task
Moderate assistance	Patient requires moderate physical assistance or verbal cues to complete the task; assistance with 50% of the task
Maximum assistance	Patient requires maximum physical assistance or verbal cues to complete the task; assistance with 75% of the task
Total assistance	Patient is unable to do any part of the task

Table 3.3.   Medicare Definitions of Level of Assistance

Total assistance	Patient needs 100% assistance by one or more persons to perform all physical activities and/or requires cognitive stimulation to elicit a functional response to an external stimulation (e.g., swallow when food is in mouth)
Maximal assistance	Patient needs 75% assistance by one person to perform physically any part of a functional activity and/or needs cognitive stimulation to perform gross motor actions in response to direction
Moderate assistance	Patient needs 50% assistance from one person to perform physical activities or constant cognitive assistance to sustain or complete simple, repetitive activities safely
Minimum assistance	Patient needs 25% assistance by one person for physical activities and/or periodic cognitive assistance to perform functional activities safely
Standby assistance	Patient needs supervision of one person to perform new activity procedures that were adapted by the therapist for safe and effective performance
Independent status	Patient requires no physical or cognitive assistance to perform functional activities

do self-care activities. If the person's disability is weakness, then one sequence of short-term goals will be to progress the person from one plateau of strength to the next. Concurrently, short-term goals related to self-care will be sequenced so that the person is taught to do those activities for which he has sufficient strength at any given time to ensure successful experiences at each stage. In terms of priority, it is seen that activity to increase strength must precede each self-care task that requires greater strength and that certain aspects of self-care must be mastered before others that depend on a prior skill. It is very important that the patient understand the relationship of each short-term goal to the long-term goals and how the treatment activity implements the short-term goal.

Labeling a goal "long-term" or "short-term" simply informs others that the goal is being aimed for eventually or is being worked on immediately. The labeling is not what is important in treatment planning; the establishment of a laddering of goals that the patient can successfully accomplish and by which he can succeedingly approach his final level of functioning is the essence of treatment planning. Once all identified goals are achieved, the person is ready for discharge.

DEVELOPING THE PLAN FOR TREATMENT

To formulate the plan for treatment, the therapist must identify the treatment approach or approaches that are appropriate. Patients may require more than one treatment approach. Selection of the appropriate treatment approach at any given time depends on the nature of the presenting problem, its causes, the state of recovery, and established priorities. For example, if the patient has a weak upper extremity secondary to a cerebral vascular accident, the therapist must choose from among three major therapeutic approaches used in occupational therapy for physical dysfunction: neuro-developmental-motor learning, biomechanical, or rehabilitative. A **rehabilitative approach** would be chosen if the weakness is long-standing and apparently unlikely to improve. The therapist's reason for choosing this approach would be to compensate for the loss of the use of this extremity to help the patient be as independent as possible.

If recovery is hoped for, a **biomechanical approach,** with its direct strengthening techniques involving maximal resistance, might appeal to the therapist and be correctly chosen if the person had voluntary control of his movements. If he is able to move only in synergistic patterns of motion, however, this approach would be rejected in favor of the **neurodevelopmental-motor learning approach.**

After identifying the treatment approach, the therapist must identify the principle of treatment to use for each of the problems. The principle is the rationale for the treatment. It, along with the theoretical and empirical research that supports it, is the explanation or justification for the choice of a particular treatment. If, for example, the therapist is asked to explain her reason for having the patient throw increasingly heavier bean bags or balls to targets, she will cite the principle of increasing stress on weak muscles to strengthen them.

Once the principle is decided on, the method of implementing the principle must then be determined. The method is the means of translating the principle into a treatment form. The treatment principles of each approach and their methods for implementation are described in the remainder of this book.

GUIDING TREATMENT

Preplanning

The beginning therapist must carefully preplan the entire treatment session. This may include a list of what will be done in the session with approximate time estimations noted. The treatment space should be prepared with the necessary supplies, equipment, and forms to carry out the planned treatment. The therapist should have a plan of what options will be offered if the planned activity proves too easy or too hard for the person or if the person has other more pressing emotional concerns that need to be addressed.

Juggling

The inexperienced therapist will probably not be able to juggle options and changes in ongoing treatment very smoothly. As experience and reflection on practice develop, the therapist will be able to respond instantly to changes in the patient's responses and will be able to offer the "just right" challenge, i.e., grade the activities to move the patient smoothly along continua of improvement and build **self-efficacy.** Assessment and treatment are intertwined. Each time the patient is challenged, he is tested. His response informs the therapist about his improving or deteriorating abilities. Deterioration in response can occur because of fatigue, excessive demands, or changing neurophysiological or emotional status; the therapist must provide the appropriate relief that will restore performance.

Reflecting

Reflection on practice refers to paying attention to what you do and what the patient does in response and thinking about it later to try to determine if there is a generalizable principle that can be derived from this encounter or if something could have been improved. It means having an hypothesis about what is limiting the person's performance, treating that limitation, and observing the outcome. It means being able to generate alternate hypotheses when the outcome is not as expected. At those points in the therapeutic process when you encounter a "stuck point" or "choice point," you are presented with the opportunity to examine your hypothesis and treatment and to explore alternative strategies (Cohn, n.d.).

The reflective therapist, as defined by Parham (1987), is one who is able clearly and critically to analyze the reasons for the actions taken and articulate the theories behind what is done. The reflective therapist can deal "with the uncertainties of practice by not only relying on technical proficiency, but also by reflecting on the nature of clinical problems as well as the potential results of treatment" (p. 556). The reflective therapist establishes the problem before using techniques to try to solve the problem—no matter how great the technical expertise, if the wrong problem is being worked on, treatment will not have an effective outcome. The reflective therapist values theory. "Theory is a key element in problem setting and problem solving" (p. 557).

Developing Expertise

Students learn the knowledge base relatively easily. The framework for decision making, or clinical reasoning skill, is less easily acquired. Mattingly (1991a) stated that the beginner therapist does not know much more than what she can state. The performance of the new therapist is characterized by starts and stops, because she must stop to think at every stuck point. The expert therapist on the other hand demonstrates fluidity of performance, because she knows much more than can be articulated ("highly tacit and embodied knowledge," p. 979) and can access that knowledge while "in action." "The expert therapist continually modifies goals and procedures to meet the individual needs of the particular patient" (p. 985) through use of explicit or intuitive clinical reasoning strategies.

Clinical reasoning is defined here as the ability to analyze patient behavior, to deduce the problem(s) manifested in that behavior, to synthesize these into problem and goal statements based on a theoretical rationale, to translate the goal statements into therapeutic principles and procedures, and to adjust ongoing therapy to keep the challenge "just right." This skill is not acquired automatically as a logical extension of the knowledge base, nor is it acquired by rote memorization of formulas. It results from reflective practice in the application of a conceptual framework to clinical problems. Skilled clinical reasoning is a major objective of the internship phase of professional education, but the rudimentary bases for it must be developed in the university.

"Clinical reasoning in practice means reasoning not only about what is wrong and how to fix it but also about how to engage the patient in that fixing process" (Mattingly, 1991a, p. 984). This requires several different reasoning strategies, or modes of thinking (Fleming, 1991). Diagnostic reasoning is a logical process based on hypotheses testing (Rogers & Holm, 1991). The occupational therapy diagnosis describes the occupational dysfunction, offers an explanatory hypothesis (reason) for this deficit based on cues detected during the assessment process, and identifies the probable pathological agent causing the deficit. For example, a person with spinal cord injury comes to occupational therapy because, among other reasons, he cannot feed himself and he wants to do that (occupational dysfunction). The therapist observes that the person cannot move his arms smoothly or fully and hypothesizes that the reason he cannot feed himself is upper extremity weakness. The therapist confirms this with a manual muscle test. Treatment is then planned to increase muscle strength. Another name for diagnostic reasoning is procedural reasoning. It is employed when the therapist attends to the patient's impairments and what procedures are appropriate to alleviate them (Fleming, 1991).

Interactive reasoning helps the therapist interact with the person to understand the person better, engage him in the treatment session, and otherwise to develop the therapeutic relationship (Fleming, 1991). Conditional reasoning is a complex type of social reasoning used to help the patient reconstruct his life, changed forever by the injury or disease (Fleming, 1991).

> In using conditional reasoning, the therapist appears to reflect on the success or failure of the clinical encounter from both the procedural and interactive standpoints and attempts to integrate the two. . . . The therapist interprets the meaning of therapy in the context of a possible [imagined] future for the person (p. 1012).

Narrative reasoning is taking the patient's perspective and developing stories concerning how he makes sense of his situation and the meaning that the disability has in his life (Cohn, 1991; Mattingly, 1991b). This type of thinking is employed when the therapist is attending to the patient as a person. Clinical reasoning is a skill gained through reflective and supervised practice.

STRATEGIES TO DEVELOP EXPERTISE

Keep a Log

Treat patients of the same diagnoses and keep a record of similarities and differences (Cohn, n.d.). Which treatments work and which do not for these persons? How long does it take for such patients to improve? What is their level of function at discharge? Treat persons with similar symptoms, but different diagnoses. Which treatments work and which do not? Conclude when the diagnosis may be a valid treatment planning tool and when it should not be relied on. How does a particular person change over time? What facilitates this change and what impedes it? Are these factors seen across patients?

Practice

Practice your assessment and treatment skills. Practice your planning and documenting skills until you are confident of them. Never use a treatment or assessment without reasoning out why it should be used for this person given the hypothesis you have about the reason for this person's limitation. Read your professional journals; attend professional conferences. Learn new approaches or nuances of treatment or interpretation of assessment data. Know which treatments have documented effectiveness and which do not.

DOCUMENTING TREATMENT EFFECTS

Documentation is required by third-party payers so the facility or therapists can be reimbursed, and it is required to provide evidence of good standards of care to defend the facility and therapist in case of lawsuit for malpractice or to provide substantiation for insurance claim suits made on behalf of the patient. Medical records are evidence of treatment provided to a patient. Because of the legal standing of medical records, there are dos and don'ts regarding documentation (Table 3.4) (Steich, 1992).

The initial note, progress notes, and discharge summary need to be documented within the time frames established by the particular setting (AOTA, 1992). The initial note should contain the mutually agreed, achievable functional goals; problems amenable to occupational therapy intervention; and the treatment plan. The treatment plan should indicate the specific treatments planned for particular problems as well as the sequence, intensity, frequency, and expected duration of treatments (Agency for Health Care Policy and Research [AHCPR], 1994). Progress notes should contain progress toward each of the goals and what more needs to be accomplished toward that goal. Only if goals are changed or new goals added is it necessary to include the treatment plan in the progress notes (Wilson, 1992). Medicare requires that a *practical improvement* occur within a *reasonable time* and that the service be offered by a *skilled* service provider. The documentation should address all these issues. Discharge summaries should document the change that occurred from initial assessment, any remaining impairments or disabilities, any adaptive equipment issued or recommended, description of the home program given (if any), and whether continued therapy is recommended and why.

According to Foto et al. (1992), the principles of documentation are the following:

1. Terms used in reports should be accepted by the industry or other target audience to which the

Table 3.4. Dos and Don'ts for Documentation

DO
Be truthful, accurate, and complete.
Write the record as soon as possible after treatment is rendered.
Date and sign all records.
Use specific terms.
Make factual statements.
Record broken appointments with reasons.
Record attempts to reschedule.

DON'T
Change a record after the fact without clarifying when and why the change was made and what the nature of the change was.
Criticize another health care provider as part of the record.
Make judgmental statements about the patient or his family.
Assume that the record will not be open to scrutiny by patient, family, lawyers, and court.

therapist is directing her reports. Terms from the *Uniform Terminology* for occupational therapy are considered jargon to most outside of the profession. Rather than saying, "The patient has moderate to severe loss of proprioception," the therapist should say, "The patient is unable to do tasks such as buttoning unless he can watch his fingers." Guides for reporting to various third-party payers have been published and are available at the center where the therapist is practicing.

2. Concepts used in occupational therapy reports need to be translated for the audience. Examples of such concepts are sensory integration, model of human occupation, occupational performance, and **biomechanical approach.**

3. The reports must be accurate both in terms of writing style and editorial intent. Writing style is formal and professional, including correct grammar and logical syntax; complete and well-composed sentences; and logical, coherent, and concise composition. Editorial intent refers to reporting either in terms of positive attributes (abilities) or negative attributes (deficits) as expected by the audience. Either "The patient is able to bathe self, but requires assistance with bathtub transfer and shampoo" (positive) or "The patient is not 100% independent in bathing" (negative). Medicare requires that editorial intent convey functional deficits.

4. The reports should follow a **standardized** reporting format. The format is determined by each department or facility.

Methods of Recording

Problem-Oriented Medical Recording (POMR), developed by Weed (1971), consists of four interconnected elements: (1) the database—the results of the initial evaluation, including how the information was gained; (2) the problem list; (3) the initial plan, including a short-term goal for each problem to be addressed and the treatment strategy for each goal; and (4) progress notes (De Weerdt & Harrison, 1985; Weed, 1971). The first three elements appear in the initial note. The progress notes are written in SOAP format (i.e., Subjective information, Objective information, results of Assessment, and the Plan).

Ottenbacher, Johnson, and Hojem (1988) described several different types of graphs that can be used to convey clinical change clearly, both to motivate the patient and to provide clear documentation for administrative purposes. *Goal Attainment Scaling* is another method of evaluating the effectiveness of therapy to achieve identified goals (Ottenbacher & Cusick, 1990). A 5-point, behaviorally defined scale is constructed for each goal. Each point on the scale consists of observable and recordable behavior and is time limited. The expected level of performance (long-term goal) is rated 0, −2 and +2 indicate the least and most favorable outcomes, and −1 and +1 reflect less than expected outcome and greater than expected outcome, respectively. The authors described how this method can be used to evaluate overall progress of one or many patients.

COMPUTERIZED METHODS

The *Occupational Therapy Functional Assessment Compilation Tool* (OT FACT) is a computerized method of documentation that generates a profile of an individual's abilities and deficits in terms of the *Uniform Terminology* (Smith, 1990). Another computerized system is reported from the Medical University of South Carolina in which therapists have small bar code scanners that have additional limited word processor capabilities. The therapists record all aspects of evaluation and treatment by scanning the appropriate bar code that applies. The scanners are downloaded to the main computer at the end of the day and reports are generated using templated formats (Thiers, 1993).

CASE STUDY

Data Gathering and Identifying the Problems

1. The medical record yielded the following information: The patient is 24 years old, a high school graduate, a computer programmer, lives with his parents in a second-floor apartment, has four siblings all married and living away from home. Diagnosis is tetraplegia secondary to fracture dislocation of C6–7, incomplete lesion, C6 functional level, no medical complications, cervical fusion and laminectomy performed on the day of the accident, multiple lacerations of both hands, currently in traction with tongs.

2. Reports of other professionals indicated that the patient has a very supportive family. He does not know the implication of spinal cord injury and expects to walk out of the hospital. His general health is good.

3. Interview with the patient indicated that he is a friendly person and has many friends. He was active in sports and camping. It is important to him that he resume these interests and that he be able to care for himself. He wants to return to work, which requires an ability to keyboard. His immediate plan is to continue to live with his parents.

4. Interview of the family (parents) informed the therapist that the patient will live temporarily with a married brother and sister-in-law until his parents move to accessible housing. The family does not yet know the implications of spinal cord injury. It is important to the family that the patient be independent in self-care and employed.

5. Observation of the patient led the therapist to conclude that there is slight movement in the right toe, no motion in the left lower extremity, and sensory loss below T4. Using adapted equipment, the patient was able to brush his teeth and feed himself foods that were easily spooned.

6. Results of assessment are extensive. A summary of significant information is noted here: There is normal sensation of the upper extremities (UEs). Passive range of motion of the UEs is within normal limits. Muscles of the left shoulder, elbow, and forearm are adequate for function, being graded "good" (G) to "normal" (N) The proximal right UE, including the wrist, is graded

G to N. The left extensor carpi radialis longus and brevis are normal, the extensor carpi ulnaris is "fair plus" (F+), and the wrist flexors grade F. The right finger muscles are stronger than the left; they grade "poor plus" (P) to G−, whereas the left finger muscles grade 0 except for "trace" (T) for the extensor digitorum and the flexor digitorum profundus. Thumbs: the left grades 0, and right ranges from 0 in the opponens and long flexor to F in the extensor pollicis longus. There are some muscles of the lower extremities that grade T (see Chapter 6 for an explanation of these terms).

The problems are as follows:

1. Activities of daily living (ADL) dependency.
2. Lack of knowledge of meaning and/or permanency of the disability.
3. Weakness of the left wrist.
4. Weakness of the fingers and thumbs bilaterally.
5. Spotty weakness (G) of proximal musculature.

Setting Goals and Priorities

The long-term goal this patient has is to return to work as a computer programmer, to be independent in his parents' home, and to engage in (wheelchair) camping and sports. To reach these goals, shorter-term goals, each related to one or more of the problems, were devised and include the following:

A. Learn to prevent contractures at joints where muscles grade less than F (problems 3, 4, and 5).
B. Learn to protect the tenodesis function of the left wrist and hand (problem 3).
C. Increase strength of right hand muscles (problem 4).
D. Increase strength of left hand muscles (problem 4).
E. Increase strength of proximal muscles (problem 5).
F. Learn the prognosis and management requirements for spinal cord injury (problems 1 and 2).
G. Determine need for, and skill in use of, other rehabilitation equipment needed for independence (problems 1 and 2).
H. Relearn to drive (problems 1 and 2).
I. Redevelop work capacity (problems 1 and 2).
J. Learn recreational skills for the wheelchair-bound (problems 1 and 2).
K. Learn to use adapted equipment for greater independence in work and leisure activities (problems 1 and 2).
L. Learn to access the community as a wheelchair-bound person (problems 1 and 2).

Immediate short-term goals to achieve goal C are listed here in order from beginning to end. These goals guide the portion of the daily treatment session that is devoted to achieving goal C. Many goals may be worked on within one session. For each goal, the therapist has made such a list.

i. Increase strength of finger extensors from P+ to F−.
ii. Increase strength of finger extensors from F− to F.
iii. Increase strength of finger extensors increment by increment to N or as much as possible.
iv. Increase strength of finger flexors from F to F+.
v. Increase strength of finger flexors from F+ to G−.
vi. Increase strength of finger flexors increment by increment to N or as much as possible.
vii. Increase strength of thumb extensors from F to F+.
viii. Increase strength of thumb extensors from F+ to G−, etc.

Formulating the Treatment Plan for Each Short-Term Goal

Immediate short-term goal i is to increase strength of the finger extensors of the right hand from P+ to F−. The approach to be used is biomechanical, and the principle is graded resistance in a gravity-eliminated plane. One method to be used is as follows: Patient is side lying (due to cervical traction). The right arm is supported on a table with the forearm in midposition. A strap is placed around the fingers at the level of the proximal phalanges. A nylon fishing line is attached to the strap, run over a pulley attached to the edge of the table, and attached at the other end to a 7-g (0.24-oz) weight. This amount of weight had been determined to be the weight that could be lifted 10 times through range. Exercise is valued by this patient, and therefore, the therapist is satisfied that it is a purposeful activity for him.

This planning process is repeated for each short-term goal.

Treat the Patient

The patient lifts the weight through full range 10 times. The therapist observes that the quality of performance gradually degrades after trial 7, but all 10 trials are accomplished. Following a rest period, finger extension is used functionally by requiring the patient to extend his fingers to pick up larger and larger lightweight objects. This would combine treatment of the flexors and extensors, which is desirable. While the patient is working, the therapist engages him in conversation to keep him motivated, to get to know him better, and to gain clues about what types of activities would be motivating to use when the program can be upgraded.

Evaluating Response to Therapy

Reevaluation is ongoing within each treatment session. For example, once the patient is seen to maintain good quality of movement throughout the 10 trials, the therapist would increase the resistance. On the other hand, if performance deteriorated at trial 4, the therapist would immediately reduce the resistance.

Reevaluation before writing a progress note would involve formal assessment of each problem area being addressed in therapy. In the case of the goal under consideration in this example, muscle strength would be remeasured, and progress, or lack of it, would be recorded. Treatment would be modified based on these results, i.e., if the patient's finger extensors had increased to F−, then short-term goal ii would be next planned for and implemented. If the extensors had not improved, treatment would be changed, because it was not effective. The change may be in frequency (the number of treatments per day), duration (the amount of time spent doing one task within a treatment session), or intensity (the level of gradation according to the principle being used, e.g., increase resistance).

STUDY QUESTIONS

1. What is the occupational therapy treatment planning process?
2. What is the client-centered approach?
3. How does a therapist decide what should be assessed for a particular patient and which assessments to use?
4. How are problem statements generated from the results of assessments and other evaluative information?
5. How do the short-term goals relate to the identified problems?
6. How does the occupational therapist choose the appropriate treatment approach for a particular patient?

7. How does the therapist know where to start treatment for a particular patient?
8. List the four components of *Problem-Oriented Medical Recording.*
9. Why is documentation important?
10. Characterize the reflective therapist.

REFERENCES

Agency for Health Care Policy and Research. (1994). *Post-stroke rehabilitation clinical practice guideline.* Washington, DC: author.

American Occupational Therapy Association. (1992). Standards of practice for occupational therapy. *American Journal of Occupational Therapy, 46*(12), 1082–1088.

American Occupational Therapy Association. (1994). *Uniform terminology* (3rd ed.). Rockville, MD: Author.

Cohn, E. (n.d.). *Facilitating a foundation for clinical reasoning: Implications for fieldwork experiences.* Unpublished manuscript, Tufts University Boston School of Occupational Therapy, Medford, MA.

Cohn, E. (1991). Clinical reasoning: Explicating complexity. *American Journal of Occupational Therapy, 45*(11), 969–971.

De Weerdt, W. J. G., & Harrison, M. A. (1985). Problem list of stroke patients as identified in the problem orientated medical record. *Australian Journal of Physiotherapy, 31*(4), 146–150.

Fleming, M. (1991). The therapist with the three-track mind. *American Journal of Occupational Therapy, 45*(11), 1007–1014.

Foto, M., Allen, C., Bass, C., Moon-Speling, T., Wilson, D., & Robben Brown, S. (1992). Reports that work. In J. D. Acquaviva (Ed.), *Effective documentation for occupational therapy* (pp. 57–77). Rockville, MD: American Occupational Therapy Association.

Granger, C., Hamilton, B., & Sherwin, F. (1988). *Functional Independence Measure.* Buffalo: State University of New York Press.

Jebsen, R. H., Taylor, N., Trieschmann, R. B., Trotter, M. J., & Howard, L. A. (1969). An objective and standardized test of hand function. *Archives of Physical Medicine & Rehabilitation, 50,* 311–319.

Jongbloed, L., Stanton, S., & Fousek, B. (1993). Family adaptation to altered roles following stroke. *Canadian Journal of Occupational Therapy, 60*(2), 70–77.

Kielhofner, G. & Burke, J. P. (1985). Components and determinants of human occupation. In G. Kielhofner (Ed.), *A model of human occupation: Theory and application* (pp. 12–36). Baltimore: Williams & Wilkins.

Klein, R. M. & Bell, B. J. (1982). Self-care skills: Behavioral measurement with Klein-Bell ADL Scale. *Archives of Physical Medicine & Rehabilitation, 63,* 335–338.

Korner-Bitensky, N., Mayo, N. E., & Ponanski, S. G. (1990). Occupational therapists' accuracy in predicting sensory, perceptual-cognitive, and functional recovery post stroke. *Occupational Therapy Journal of Research, 10*(4), 237–249.

Law, M. (1993). Evaluating activities of daily living: Directions for the future. *American Journal of Occupational Therapy, 47*(3), 233–237.

Law, M., Baptiste, S., Carswell-Opzoomer, A., McColl, M. A., Polatajko, H., & Pollock, N. (1991). *Canadian Occupational Performance Measure.* Toronto: Canadian Association of Occupational Therapists.

Lynch, K. B., & Bridle, M. J. (1989). Validity of the Jebsen-Taylor Hand Function Test in predicting activities of daily living. *Occupational Therapy Journal of Research, 9*(5), 316–318.

Mahoney, P., & Kannenberg, K. (1992). Writing functional goals. In J. D. Acquaviva (Ed.), *Effective documentation for occupational therapy* (pp. 91–96). Rockville, MD: American Occupational Therapy Association.

Mathiowetz, V. (1991). Reliability and validity of grip and pinch strength measurements. *Critical Reviews in Physical and Rehabilitation Medicine, 2*(4), 201–212.

Mathiowetz, V. Volland, G., Kashman, N., & Weber, K. (1985). Adult norms for the Box and Block Test of manual dexterity. *American Journal of Occupational Therapy, 39*(6), 386–391.

Mathiowetz, V., Weber, K. D., Volland, G., & Kashman, N. (1984). Reliability and validity of grip and pinch strength evaluations. *Hand Surgery, 9A*(2), 222–226.

Mattingly, C. (1991a). What is clinical reasoning? *American Journal of Occupational Therapy, 45*(11), 979–986.

Mattingly, C. (1991b). The narrative nature of clinical reasoning. *American Journal of Occupational Therapy, 45*(11), 998–1005.

Neistadt, M. (1992). The Rabideau Kitchen Evaluation—Revised: An assessment of meal preparation skill. *Occupational Therapy Journal of Research, 12*(4), 242–253.

Oakley, F., Kielhofner, G., Barris, R., & Reichler, R. K. (1986). The Role Checklist: Development and empirical assessment of reliability. *Occupational Therapy Journal of Research, 6*(3), 157–170.

Ottenbacher, K. J., & Cusick, A. (1990). Goal attainment scaling as a method of clinical service evaluation. *American Journal of Occupational Therapy, 44*(6), 519–525.

Ottenbacher, K. J., Johnson, M. B., & Hojem, M. (1988). The significance of clinical change and clinical change of significance: Issues and methods. *American Journal of Occupational Therapy, 42*(3), 156–163.

Parham, D. (1987). Toward professionalism: The reflective therapist. *American Journal of Occupational Therapy, 41*(9), 555–561.

Pollock, N. (1993). Client-centered assessment. *American Journal of Occupational Therapy, 47*(4), 298–301.

Redelmeier, D. A., & Tversky, A. (1990, April 19). Discrepancy between medical decisions for individual patients and for groups. *New England Journal of Medicine, 322*(16), 1162–1164.

Rogers, J. C. (1983). Clinical reasoning: The ethics, science and art. *American Journal of Occupational Therapy, 37*(9), 601–616.

Rogers, J. C., & Holm, M.B. (1991). Occupational therapy diagnostic reasoning: A component of clinical reasoning. *American Journal of Occupational Therapy, 45*(11), 1045–1053.

Smith, R. O. (1990). *Occupational Therapy Functional Assessment Compilation Tool (OT FACT): Administration and tutorial manual.* Rockville, MD: American Occupational Therapy Association.

Smith, R. O. (1992). The science of occupational therapy assessment. *Occupational Therapy Journal of Research, 12*(1), 3–15.

Steich, T. (1992). Legal issues in documentation: Fraud, abuse, and confidentiality. In J. D. Acquaviva (Ed.), *Effective documentation for occupational therapy* (pp. 211–217). Rockville, MD: American Occupational Therapy Association.

Thiers, N. (1993, July 29). Entering the electronic age: Computerized recordkeeping improves practice. *OT WEEK, 7*(30), 14–15.

Tickle-Degnen, L., Trombly, C. A., Coster, W., Cermak, W., Henderson, A., & Murray, E. (1989). *Framework for research and scholarship for the Neurobehavioral Rehabilitation Research Center.* Unpublished manuscript, Boston University.

Trombly, C. (1993). Anticipating the future: Assessment of occupational function. *American Journal of Occupational Therapy, 47*(3), 253–257.

Weed, L. L. (1971). *Medical records, medical education and patient care: The problem-oriented record as a basic tool.* Chicago: Year Book.

Whiteneck, G. G., Charlifue, S. W., Gerhart, K. A., Overholser, J. D., & Richardson, G. N. (1992). Qualifying handicap: A new measure of long term rehabilitation outcomes. *Archives of Physical Medicine & Rehabilitation, 73*(6), 519–526.

Wilson, D. (1992). If I had known then what I know now . . . In J. D. Acquaviva (Ed.), *Effective documentation for occupational therapy* (pp. 1–3). Rockville, MD: American Occupational Therapy Association.

World Health Organization. (1980). *International classification of impairments, disabilities, and handicaps: A manual of classification relating to the consequences of disease.* Geneva: author.

Yerxa, E. J., Burnett-Beaulieu, S., Stocking, S., & Azen, S. P. (1988). Development of the Satisfaction with Performance Scaled Questionnaire (SPSQ). *American Journal of Occupational Therapy, 42*(4), 215–221.

Section II

Assessment

$\boldsymbol{B}$asic to any professional practice is the determination of the status of the client in terms of the services that the professional provides. Occupational therapists provide services relative to occupational performance and offer services to persons who have, or are at risk for developing, occupational dysfunction. Occupational dysfunction is defined as the inability to engage in one or more of the roles that are important to the client in the manner in which he or she wants to engage in them. Therefore, this part starts with the determination of the client's past roles, probable future roles, ability to accomplish the tasks and activities he or she associates with a given role (occupational performance), and his or her satisfaction with the performance. Later chapters proceed to the methods of assessment of the component abilities and capacities (components of occupational performance) that are required in order to be able to carry out the tasks and activities of a given role. The last chapter of this section focuses on understanding and assessing the client's socioemotional status regarding adjustment to the disability as well as his or her readiness to engage in the rehabilitation process.

4
Evaluation of Occupational Performance

Mary Law

OBJECTIVES

After studying this chapter the reader will be able to:
1. Understand the importance of the assessment process in occupational therapy.
2. Evaluate **occupational performance,** beginning with patient/client perception of occupational needs.
3. Understand the measurement criteria necessary for valid assessments of **occupational performance.**
4. Discuss and use current validated assessments of **occupational performance** in the areas of **activities of daily living, work,** and **leisure.**

The goal of occupational therapy is to enable individuals to achieve independence in areas of **occupational performance.** Such independence can be achieved through self-independence or through an individual directing others such as in an attendant care situation. **Occupational performance** areas include **activities of daily living, work,** and **leisure** (American Occupational Therapy Association [AOTA], 1989). Whenever a person experiences a trauma or disease that results in a physical impairment, independence in these tasks is usually jeopardized. The occupational therapist must determine the patient's abilities and limitations. Evaluation of **occupational performance** consists of interview and systematic observation to determine what activities can and cannot be performed and what factors limit performance. If the limiting factors can be improved or eliminated by direct intervention, the therapist chooses an intervention approach that is appropriate to the problem. If, however, the limiting factors are not amenable to change, the therapist teaches the individual to compensate for these limitations by adapting the task or by changing the environment in which it is performed.

In the past, therapists have assessed **occupational performance** by administering standardized evaluations or checklists of **activities of daily living** (ADL), **work,** and **leisure.** It has been recognized, however, that **occupational performance,** or the ability to carry out activities during daily life, depends on the individual's culture and gender and the roles that he wishes to undertake and the environment in which he lives (Law, 1991; Trombly, 1993). Thus **occupational performance** is an individual concept. The individuality of **occupational performance** makes it both difficult and time-consuming for one standardized evaluation to assess all aspects of **occupational performance.** As outlined by Trombly (Chapter 2), assessment should be a top-down approach beginning, with an evaluation of **occupational performance.** This evaluation of **occupational performance** will include consideration of the individual's roles and the environment in which he lives. Assessment of the environments in which people live, **work,** and engage in **leisure** is discussed in Chapter 5. The assessment process will not ignore components of **occupational performance,** such as strength, endurance, problem solving, and depth perception, but rather will begin with an assessment of the activities that the client needs, wants, or is expected to accomplish and is having difficulty in performing.

By beginning with a focus on the clients' needs and considering their roles and the environment in which they live, therapists recognize the values and the goals that clients bring to the occupational therapy process. This approach reflects a change in philosophy to a more client-centered approach, recognizing that it is the person who is engaged in therapy who should be articulating the goals of therapy and driving the therapy

GLOSSARY

Activities of daily living—Activities or tasks that a person does every day to maintain personal independence (Reed & Sanderson, 1980).

Instrumental activities of daily living—More complex activities or tasks that a person does to maintain independence in the home and community.

Leisure—Activities or tasks that are not obligatory and that are done for enjoyment.

Occupational performance—Ability of an individual to perform and be satisfied with performance in purposeful daily activities, within their environment, developmental stage, and societal roles.

Reliability—Consistency or reproducibility of an assessment under various assessment conditions (Streiner & Norman, 1989).

Validity—Ability of an instrument to assess the intended characteristic (Law, 1987).

Work—Activities or tasks in the areas of home management, care of others, education, vocation, and avocation (AOTA, 1989).

intervention process (Canadian Association of Occupational Therapists [CAOT], 1991).

The format of this chapter reflects this philosophy, beginning with a discussion of evaluation of an individual's perception of his **occupational performance,** using the *Canadian Occupational Performance Measure* (COPM) (Law et al., 1991, 1994), and then outlining assessments that can be used to evaluate the **occupational performance** areas of **activities of daily living, work,** and play.

MEASUREMENT CRITERIA

The format of the evaluation instrument can be an interview or a standardized list of activities on which the therapist indicates whether each item can be performed. The use of nonstandardized checklists is not recommended. It is suggested that intervention begin with an interview to determine the **occupational performance** activities important to the client. Following that, observational assessments of ADL, **work,** and **leisure** can be used to evaluate the client's current level of functional performance and to help the therapist determine why problems with that activity are occurring. Reassessment is done at the end of therapy intervention.

The level of measurement of most evaluations of **occupational performance** tasks is ordinal, i.e., the score can be located on a ranking from "dependent/is unable" to "independent/is able." Space is usually available on forms for periodic reevaluation. It is important, at a minimum, to record the level of performance at admission and at discharge, because these records may be used for program evaluation, to justify service to third-party payers, in legal actions, and in determining whether a patient will be discharged home or to an extended-care facility (Harris et al., 1986).

Evaluation instruments should be valid, reliable, and responsive enough to detect important changes (Law & Letts, 1989). A valid assessment is one that measures what it purports to measure. Most evaluations of functional performance have logical, or face, **valid-**

ity. The instrument may weight each item to ensure content **validity.** The items are samples of a universe of behavior, but some are more important than others (Hasselkus & Safrit, 1976), e.g., "can use the stove safely" is a more important item than "can stir batter" in the universe of "meal preparation."

A reliable assessment is one that measures the parameter under study consistently no matter who is scoring (interrater **reliability**) or when the scoring occurs (test-retest **reliability**). Some therapists still use unstandardized checklists that have not had **reliability** established. The tasks listed in departmentally composed checklists are rarely even operationally defined, the initial step in establishing **reliability.**

Responsiveness, the third characteristic of a good assessment, refers to the ability to detect the smallest increment of change that would be considered significant. As an example, for a therapist working on a day-to-day basis with a patient to increase his ability to dress, the assessment should be sensitive enough to allow progress to be noted when different areas of the body can be dressed or different articles of clothing applied. However, for program evaluation, the crucial piece of information is whether or not the patient is independent in dressing, and therefore, the tool used to measure can be less responsive. Responsiveness is directly related to the number of items on an assessment and to the number of categories on the scoring scale. An assessment with 50 items will likely be more responsive than one with 10 items.

After a patient identifies the activities that are important to him, then observation of those activities is the most direct method of assessing functional ability and is preferred for accuracy, detection of inefficient or unsafe methods, and determination of the underlying reason that a particular task cannot be performed. It can, however, be time-consuming and costly (Law & Letts, 1989). Self-report of actual performance through interview is the easiest, fastest, and most inexpensive method of assessing functional abilities. There is a concern, however, that such reports may not accurately reflect what the person can do. If a patient reports questionable data and does not permit observation, the therapist should verify the report with others who have knowledge of the patient's actual performance. False information is not a conscious intent to deceive but may reflect the fact that a patient is in a health care facility and does not have an accurate sense of his current ability. A study that compared results of self-report with observation of functional performance of 47 elderly patients with hip fractures found high agreement between the two, especially for self-care tasks performed daily (Harris et al., 1986). Conversely, Edwards (1990) and Sagar et al. (1992), in studies comparing observation of performance in ADL tasks with self-report, found that patients consistently overrated their ability.

Evaluation of all **occupational performance** tasks is not done at the same time. Ability to do self-care, personal mobility, and leisure-time activities within the current limits of a disability are usually done early and form the basis for the occupational therapy intervention plan that includes restorative therapy and/or adaptation to enable occupational function. As recovery continues and discharge planning decisions are being considered, evaluations concerned with access to home and community, transportation, care of the home and children, hobbies, sports and family recreation, and job/educational abilities are done as applicable. In addition to the physical requirements of these tasks, soundness of judgment and perceptual/cognitive skills are assessed, if necessary, to determine if these tasks can be safely and effectively accomplished. Figure 4.1 illustrates the process of assessment of **occupational performance.**

OCCUPATIONAL PERFORMANCE

In using a client-centered approach to occupational therapy, it is important that it is the person receiving occupational therapy who identifies the **occupational performance** issues that would benefit from occupational therapy intervention. Therefore, an assessment of **occupational performance** begins with the evaluation of what activities the client needs, wants, or is expected to accomplish and is having difficulty in performing. Such an assessment recognizes that **occupational performance** is an individual issue and that a person's perception of his **occupational performance** is the important force that drives the occupational therapy process.

Information about an individual's occupations, roles, developmental stage, and the environment in which he lives is best obtained through an interview. One assessment that can be used to assess a person's perception of his **occupational performance** is COPM.

COPM guides a client to identify problem areas

in **occupational performance** and assists in goal setting, and it measures changes in a person's perception of his **occupational performance** over the course of occupational therapy intervention. COPM measures an individual's perception of **occupational performance** among people with a variety of disabilities and across all developmental stages. It is client centered and incorporates roles and role expectations within the client's own environment.

COPM is administered using a semistructured, individualized interview. During the interview, the client (or caregiver) identifies areas of **activities of daily living, work,** and **leisure** that are important to him and are in need of occupational therapy intervention. COPM is administered in a four-step process, which includes problem definition, problem weighting, scoring, and reassessment. For each **occupational performance** area, the therapist gives several illustrations of the kinds of activities that fall in that area and determines from clients if they need to, want to, or are expected to perform any of these activities. If clients do not feel that they have a problem with daily activities in a performance area, then the next **occupational performance** area is explored. If clients must do an activity, then current performance is explored. If clients are unable to perform the activity or are not satisfied with the way in which they do it, then that activity is listed as a problem for intervention. After all **occupational performance** problems are identified, clients score the problems in terms of importance,

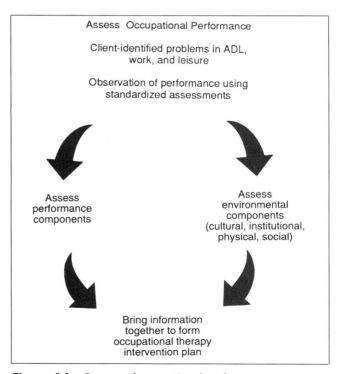

Figure 4.1. Process of occupational performance assessment.

their perception of current performance, and current satisfaction with that performance. Reassessment is completed at a time when the client and the therapist believe that it is appropriate (Fig. 4.2; see also Chapter 18).

COPM was published by the Canadian Association of Occupational Therapists and extensive testing has been completed with 268 clients in communities across Canada and in New Zealand, Greece, the UK, and the United States. Occupational therapists who have used COPM have found it helpful in setting priorities for occupational therapy intervention. The mean length of administration time for COPM was 40 min and the median length of administration time was 30 min.

Mean performance scores were 3.97 at initial assessment and 6.95 at reassessment, giving an average change score of 3.06 ($P < .0001$). Mean satisfaction score was 3.75 at initial assessment and 6.82 at reassessment, giving a change score of 3.23 ($P < .0001$). The size of these change scores is approximately 1.3 times the standard deviation of the scores, which represents a large clinical change. Studies assessing the **reliability**, criterion **validity**, and responsiveness of COPM in adults are in process.

The test-retest reliability (intraclass correlation coefficients) of COPM, in a study of 27 senior citizens attending an outpatient day care program, was 0.63 for performance and 0.84 for satisfaction (Law et al., 1994; Sanford et al., 1994). In this same population, COPM scores changed significantly after 3 months of rehabilitation. Changes on COPM correlated at a 0.55 level with overall functional change as rated by family members. Further studies of reliability and validity of COPM are ongoing.

Activities of Daily Living Skills

In the area of daily living skills, which includes self-care, mobility, and communication, observation of the activities identified on COPM as problems should be done at the time of day when these activities are normally done and in the location where the patient usually performs the tasks. Remember that people may have strong feelings of modesty regarding personal care that should be respected. If many activities are evaluated, ADL is not done at one time, because it is fatiguing. The therapist should discontinue the evaluation if fatigue occurs. Items that would be unsafe or obviously unsuccessful are postponed until the patient's physical status improves. If the patient is not independent in some required task at the time of discharge, plans must be developed to ensure that this task is done by others or that additional training is received.

Most standardized **activities of daily living** evaluations were designed for program evaluation to document the level of independence achieved by patients as the result of a particular program. The most frequently cited standardized ADL tests are the *Katz Index* (Katz et al., 1963), the *Revised Kenny Self-Care Evaluation* (Iversen et al., 1973), and the *Barthel Index* (Mahoney & Barthel, 1965). The *Barthel Index* and the *Kenny Evaluation* are more sensitive to change of a particular patient than the *Katz Index* (Gresham, Phillips, & Labi, 1980). The *Barthel Index* is more inclusive than the *Kenny Evaluation* and the *Katz Index*.

The *Katz Index* evaluates 6 functions; scoring is based on ontogenetic development of self-care skills (Gresham et al., 1980; Katz et al., 1963). The *Barthel Index* looks at 10 functions. Total score can range from 0 to 100 (total independence) in increments of 5.

Through an interview, clients identify occupational performance activities that are important to them and which they are having difficulties performing satisfactorily. These are scored on a 1-10 scale.

Activity Problems:	Importance	Performance	Satisfaction
Doing up fasteners	9	3	1
Washing face and hands	10	1	1
Preparing sandwich	5	1	4
Holding a book	7	3	5
Visiting friends	9	2	4

Figure 4.2. An example of the *Canadian Occupational Performance Measure*.

Functions are weighted according to importance to independence (Gresham et al., 1980; Mahoney & Barthel, 1965). A score of 60 seems to be the transition point from dependency to assisted independence. A modified version of the *Barthel Index* has been found to be reliable and valid when administered using a telephone interview (Shinan et al., 1987). The *Revised Kenny Self-Care Evaluation* looks at seven categories of self-care, each of which are broken down into specific tasks that define the activity. The patient achieves "independent" *(I)*, "dependent" *(D)*, "needs assistance" *(A)*, or "needs supervision" *(S)* on each task. The activity is given a number score, depending on the number of *I*'s, *D*'s, *A*'s, and *S*'s earned. The category score is an average of the activity scores. The total self-care score is a total of the category scores (Iversen et al., 1973).

The *Klein-Bell Activities of Daily Living Scale* (Klein & Bell, 1982) is even more responsive to small changes than the *Revised Kenny Self-Care Evaluation*

because of the large number of items on this assessment (Fig. 4.3). It documents basic **activities of daily living** skills, including dressing, elimination, mobility, bathing and hygiene, eating, and emergency telephone communication. Each area is broken down into tasks, and each task is broken down into step-by-step simple behavioral items. There are 170 such items on the scale, which are scored "achieved" (no physical or verbal assistance) or "failed" (assistance needed). If the person can do the item with adapted equipment, he scores "achieved." Interrater agreement of 92% has been determined from the scoring of 30 patients by three pairs of occupational therapists and three pairs of registered nurses, even without extensive training (Klein & Bell, 1982). **Validity** was established on 14 patients by comparing the total score at discharge against the hours of assistance required. A correlation of -0.86 was obtained, indicating that the amount of assistance decreases as the Klein-Bell score increases. This appears to be a useful test because it is as

Socks

8. Grasp Sock	(1)			
9. Reach sock to R foot	(2)			
10. Reach sock to L foot	(2)			
11. Pull sock over R toes	(2)			
12. Pull sock over L toes	(2)			
13. Pull sock over R foot with heel to heel	(2)			
14. Pull sock over L foot with heel to heel	(2)			
15. Pull sock up to full extension on R leg	(2)			
16. Pull sock up to full extension on L leg	(2)			

Mobility through doors

114. Operate doorknob	(1)			
115. Open door toward self	(2)			
116. Open door away from self	(2)			
117. Close door toward self	(2)			
118. Close door away from self	(1)			

Figure 4.3. An example of items on the *Klein-Bell ADL Scale.*

sensitive as a therapist needs to document daily gains and because the **validity** and **reliability** have been determined to some degree.

Two assessments developed recently have focused on evaluating functional performance and safety of ADL concurrently. The *Safety and Functional ADL Evaluation* (SAFE) (Morgan, 1992) assesses independence and degree of required supervision in bathing, dressing, feeding, bowel and bladder control, transfers, and mobility (Fig. 4.4). The *Safety Assessment of Function and the Environment for Rehabilitation* (SAFER) (Oliver et al., 1993) assesses safety in 15 areas, such as living situation, mobility, ADL tasks, and recreation. Both of these assessments are currently undergoing **reliability** testing.

The *Additive Activities Profile Test* (ADAPT) quality-of-life scale evaluates **activities of daily living** in relation to the degree of physical fitness or maximum oxygen consumption ($\dot{V}o_2$max); a correlation of 0.83 was found between maximum oxygen uptake level and the score on this test in a study of 39 patients, aged 40 to 73, who had pulmonary dysfunction (Daughton et al., 1982). ADAPT is a self-administered paper-and-pencil test that orders 105 activities according to the $\dot{V}o_2$ required for each.

The *Functional Independence Measure* (FIM) uses a 7-point scale to evaluate 18 items in the areas of self-care, sphincter control, mobility, locomotion, communication, and social cognition. FIM is intended to be a measure of disability and as such is most useful for description of disability or for program evaluation of initial rehabilitation programs. FIM is not a direct observational measure but is scored on the basis of information derived from the patient directly and from the rehabilitation team. FIM has good to excellent **reliability** and has been the subject of extensive validation (Granger & Hamilton, 1992; Granger et al., 1993).

Work

Work, including home management, child care, and employment, is another area of concern to occupational therapists (AOTA, 1989). Home management (also called **instrumental activities of daily living,** or IADL) includes meal planning, preparation, service, and cleanup; marketing for food and clothing; and routine and seasonal care of the home and one's clothing. Yard work and other maintenance tasks may have been the responsibility of the patient and may be considered homemaking tasks. While there is an overabundance of ADL evaluations, there are fewer evaluations of IADL. Reasons for this include the fact that IADL evaluations are more complex to develop and validate.

The *Assessment of Motor and Process Skills* (AMPS), developed by Fisher (1992; in press), represents an innovative assessment through which the therapist is able simultaneously to assess an individual's performance of IADL tasks along with the motor and process (organization/adaptive) performance components that contribute to completion of these tasks. AMPS was developed to provide information about the relationship between an individual's performance of IADL tasks and the underlying process and motor components that contributed to that performance in an evaluation that is less time-consuming. During the AMPS evaluation, motor and process skills are assessed concurrently with observation of functional performance. The AMPS assessment procedure involves six steps: client selection, client interview, task selection by client, preparation of the client and the test environment, administration of the assessment, and scoring. AMPS provides the most useful information for clients who need to perform IADL tasks within their living environment. Tasks that are offered to clients present a challenge to them; are not overlearned; and are appropriate to the client's environment, age, and culture (Fisher, 1993). Administration of two tasks on AMPS usually takes 10 to 20 min, with complete assessment and scoring taking approximately 1 hr.

The authors of AMPS have used many-faceted Rasch analysis (Linacre, 1989) to develop an equal-interval scale of IADL items. Rasch analysis is a scaling method designed to ensure a hierarchical, equal-interval scale. The use of Rasch analysis allows a score to be adjusted for the difficulty of the IADL item and for differences in raters observing performance. Information on functional tasks and motor and process skills can be obtained by having an individual perform a few tasks. Performance on a few tasks, once calibrated using the Rasch analysis, is used to predict performance on other tasks. Many different tasks have been included in AMPS validation studies, so that a client can choose a few tasks that are culturally and environmentally appropriate. For example, a man who does not perform complex meal preparation (perhaps because he lives with his wife) may choose tasks such as "making toast" and "brewed coffee" rather than "making a grilled cheese sandwich or an omelet." The flexibility of including client choice in the tasks that are assessed is a significant advantage of AMPS assessment.

Scoring for AMPS must be done by computer and is currently available for therapists who have received training using AMPS. The goal of the research team is to have a computer software program that therapists can use to score AMPS for individual clients. This program will be available when enough scores have

SPAULDING REHABILITATION HOSPITAL

Occupational Therapy Department

SAFE EVALUATION:

(Safety and Functional ADL Evaluation)

Adm. Date: _____

Onset Date: _____

Diagnosis: _____

FUNCTIONAL INTERPRETATION	**SAFETY INTERPRETATION**
0 to 7 = Max. Assist. to Dependent	0 to 7 = Constant Supervision
8 to 20 = Min. to Mod. Assistance	8 to 20 = Close Supervision
21 to 27 = Supervision	21 to 27 = Distant Supervision
28 = Independent	28 = Independent

ACTIVITY	TASKS	EVAL. DATE		EVAL. DATE		EVAL. DATE	
		F = __/28	S = __/28	F = __/28	S = __/28	F = __/28	S = __/28
I. **BATHING**	Washes face and hands						
	Washes upper torso						
	Washes back						
	Washes perineal area						
	Washes legs and feet						
	Brushes teeth						
	Combs hair						
	Shaving/Make-up		F S		F S		F S
	÷ 8			÷ 8		÷ 8	
II. **DRESSING**	Undershirt/bra on/off						
	Underpants on/off						
	Front opening shirt/ sweater on/off						
	Pullover on/off						
	Pants/skirt on/off						
	Stockings on/off						
	Shoes/slippers on/off						
	Belt/fasteners on/off						
	Glasses on/off						
	Equipment - splints/ sling / prosthesis		F S		F S		F S
	÷ 10			÷ 10		÷ 10	
III. **FEEDING**	Adequate reflexes/ musculature						
	Finger feed						
	Use of utensils						
	Pour from container						
	Drink (cup, glass, straw)		F S		F S		F S
	÷ 5			÷ 5		÷ 5	

Figure 4.4. *The Safety and Functional ADL Evaluation.*

Pt. Name and # _____

ACTIVITY	TASKS	EVAL. DATE		EVAL. DATE		EVAL. DATE	

IV. BOWEL & BLADDER CONTROL
- Cleansing self
- Use of equipment
- ÷ 2   F S
- ÷ 2   F S
- ÷ 2   F S

V. TUB & TOILET TRANSFERS
- Toilet Transfers
- Tub Transfers
- ÷ 2   F S
- ÷ 2   F S
- ÷ 2   F S

VI. MOBILITY
- Bed Mobility
- Transfers bed/chair
- ÷ 2   F S
- ÷ 2   F S
- ÷ 2   F S

VII. LOCOMOTION
- Wheelchair
- Ambulation
- Stairs
- ÷ 3   F S
- ÷ 3
- ÷ 3

SCORING

FUNCTIONAL:
4 = Independent
3 = Supervision
2 = Contact guard to
   minimal assist
1 = Moderate to
   maximal assist
0 = Dependent

SAFETY:
4 = Independent
3 = Distant Supervision
2 = Close Supervision
1 = Assistance
0 = Dependent

FUNCTIONAL SCORE:
I. _____
II. _____
III. _____
IV. _____
V. _____
VI. _____
VII. _____
TOTAL

SAFETY SCORE:
I. _____
II. _____
III. _____
IV. _____
V. _____
VI. _____
VII. _____
TOTAL

FUNCTIONAL SCORE:
I. _____
II. _____
III. _____
IV. _____
V. _____
VI. _____
VII. _____
TOTAL

SAFETY SCORE:
I. _____
II. _____
III. _____
IV. _____
V. _____
VI. _____
VII. _____
TOTAL

FUNCTIONAL SCORE:
I. _____
II. _____
III. _____
IV. _____
V. _____
VI. _____
VII. _____
TOTAL

SAFETY SCORE:
I. _____
II. _____
III. _____
IV. _____
V. _____
VI. _____
VII. _____
TOTAL

THERAPIST SIGNATURE: _____   _____   _____

Figure 4.4. Continued.

been obtained for each AMPS task to satisfy criteria for **reliability** and **validity.**

Interrater and test-retest **reliability** of AMPS range from 0.74 to 0.93 (Doble, 1991; Fisher, 1992). Bryze (1991) found correlations ranging from 0.62 to 0.85 between the AMPS scale and the *Scales of Independent Behavior.* In a 1991 study of 162 persons aged 16 to 87, Fisher found that the data from the AMPS assessment conformed well to the Rasch model in terms of acceptable fit. As reported, "the many-faceted equivalent of Cronbach's alpha was .83 for motor tasks, .98 for motor skill items, .96 for process tasks, and .98 for process skill items" (Fisher, 1992, p. 56). The correlation between AMPS IADL motor measures and AMPS IADL process measures was 0.58. AMPS has been shown to discriminate well between people without disabilities and those with cognitive impairments or physical disabilities. Harrison, Johansson-Charles, and Doble (1993), in a study of individuals with multiple sclerosis, found that individuals differed significantly in mean AMPS IADL motor and IADL process scores based on their overall level of independence in community living.

The *Structured Assessment of Independent Living Skills* (SAILS) is an assessment of 10 areas of daily activities: fine motor skills, gross motor skills, dressing, eating, expressive language, receptive language, time and orientation, money-related skills, instrumental activities, and social interaction. SAILS includes 50 tasks scored on a rating scale of 0 to 3 after direct observation of performance of each task. Scores are achieved for each of the 10 subdomains as well as a combined motor score, combined cognitive score, and total score. To date, research with SAILS with individuals who have Alzheimer's disease has indicated that test-retest **reliability** is excellent and that the assessment significantly discriminates between different levels of ability in daily living activities (Mahurin, DeBettignies, & Pirozzolo, 1991).

The *Kohlman Evaluation of Living Skills* (KELS) assesses daily activities in areas of self-care, safety and health, money management, transportation and telephone, and **work** and **leisure.** The assessment is administered through therapist interview and direct observation of performance. Individual items are scored as "independent," "needs assistance," or "not applicable." Interrater **reliability** of KELS has been reported to be good to excellent, and construct validation of KELS has been studied (Kohlman Thomson, 1993).

Child care and parenting includes, but is not limited to, the physical care of children and use of age-appropriate activities, communication, and behavior to facilitate child development (AOTA, 1989). Because no standard evaluations exist, the therapist must analyze the tasks, taking the age(s) and personalities of

the children into account to determine what assistance the patient may need in this area.

Employment evaluation includes determination of whether an individual has the ability to perform the necessary job skills and is otherwise prepared for employment in terms of work habits; work product quality; ability to learn or acquire new skills; and ability to work with others as a team member, supervisor, or supervisee. Velozo (1993) questioned whether current **work** evaluations reflect occupational therapists' interest in the meaning of **work** and focus on **work** environments. He described two categories of **work** evaluations: (1) standardized, commercial evaluations and (2) evaluations of physical and **work** capacity.

Standardized vocational evaluation systems use **work** samples to analyze an individual's ability to perform tasks similar to those encountered in **work** activities. Examples of such systems include the *Vocational Evaluation System; Vocational Information and Evaluation Work Samples;* and the *Vocational Interest, Temperament and Aptitude System* (Botterbusch, 1987). Other examples include the TOWER and VALPAR systems. These systems tend to be expensive and also have limited evidence of **reliability** and **validity.** However, if an occupational therapist is working in a setting in which these systems are available, she can use them as a basis for structuring observations about **work** skills and capacity.

Occupational performance evaluations of **work** have often focused on **work** and physical capacity. Evaluation of **work** capacity involves assessment of tasks such as lifting, sitting, and standing that are necessary for a specific **work** setting (see Chapter 17). Physical capacity evaluations focus on physical components necessary for **work,** such as pain, strength, and endurance. Information on assessment of the **work** environment is discussed in Chapter 5.

Occupational therapists have also been involved in specific observations of behaviors that are important for **work.** Examples of such behaviors include punctuality, communication ability, ability to work with others, and grooming. Two examples of assessments of **work** behaviors are the *Vocational Adaptive Rating Scales* (VARS), which is available from Western Psychological Services and is based on work by Malgady et al. (1980), and the *Vocational Behavior Checklist* (VBC), which is based on work by Walls, Zane, and Werner (1978).

Leisure

Leisure refers to performance and value in choosing, performing, or engaging in activities for amusement, relaxation, spontaneous enjoyment, and/ or self-expression (Hersch, 1991). Assessments evaluating **leisure** interests have been developed (Matsutsuyu, 1969; Rogers, Weinstein, & Figone, 1978), but there are fewer assessments to evaluate performance of **leisure** activities. As stated by Hersch (1991), "the concept of leisure encompasses a multitude of meanings—the leisure event itself, the amount and frequency of the activity, its meaningfulness to the participant, and the social context" (p. 55). In fact, it has been suggested by Hersch (1991) and Bundy (1993) that **leisure,** or the playfulness of an activity, depends on the characteristics of the activity rather than the classification of an activity as **leisure.** For an activity to be leisurely or playful, it must be chosen by an individual, present a challenge, and the results must be under the individual's control.

Some **leisure** assessments have focused on the amount and frequency of **leisure** activities as well as their meaningfulness to the person involved. The *Leisure Activities Inventory* by Havighurst (Mangen & Peterson, 1982) assesses the types of **leisure** activity in which an individual is engaged, the value of those activities, and the meaning of the activities to the person. In a pilot study with 10 subjects using the *Leisure Activities Inventory*, Hersch (1991) found a positive relationship between high scores on the *Leisure Activities Inventory* and a measure of life satisfaction. The revised *Activity Index* (Gregory, 1983) is a self-report assessment that determines involvement and frequency of involvement in a variety of activities, ranging from card games and theater to quiet hobbies at home. The revised *Activity Index* has been shown to have good test-retest **reliability** and is significantly correlated with life satisfaction.

Other assessments have focused on the meaning of **leisure** activities to individuals. Using the activities in the revised *Activity Index*, the *Meaningfulness of Activity Scale* measures the motivation for involvement and sense of meaning derived from involvement in **leisure** activities (Gregory, 1983). Test-retest **reliability** has been reported to be excellent, and scores on this scale are significantly related to life satisfaction (Gregory, 1983).

The *Leisure Satisfaction Questionnaire* (Beard & Ragheb, 1980) uses a self-report format with scoring on a 5-point scale to measure the agreement of individuals with 51 items that reflect points of view about **leisure.** Items are categorized into six domains: psychological, educational, social, relaxation, physiological, and aesthetic. Internal consistency of this scale is 0.96 (Beard & Ragheb, 1980). There is limited **reliability** and **validity** information for the *Leisure Satisfaction Questionnaire.*

SUMMARY

It is important that therapists investigate and use **occupational performance** assessments that are standardized and applicable to the clinical situation in which they **work.** A client-centered approach to assessment, as described in this chapter, ensures a flexible and accountable evaluation process.

STUDY QUESTIONS

1. Describe one method used to evaluate an individual's perception of his occupational performance.
2. What are the pros and cons of this method?
3. What are the necessary three characteristics of standardized evaluation instruments? Define each.
4. What are the methods used to evaluate activities of daily living, work, and leisure?
5. What is the relationship of evaluation of occupational performance to the development of the occupational therapy treatment plan?
6. Choose one of the mentioned evaluations, describe it, and state its strengths and weaknesses.
7. Define instrumental activities of daily living and basic activities of daily living.

REFERENCES

American Occupational Therapy Association. (1989). *AOTA uniform terminology system for reporting occupational therapy services.* Rockville, MD: Author.

Beard, J. G., & Ragheb, M. G. (1980). Measuring life satisfaction. *Journal of Leisure Research, 12*(1), 20–25.

Botterbusch, K. F. (1987). *Vocational assessment and evaluation systems: A comparison.* Menomonie, WI: Materials Development Center, Stout Vocational Rehabilitation Institute, School of Education and Human Services.

Bryze, K. A. (1991). *Functional assessment of adults with developmental disabilities.* Unpublished Master's thesis, University of Illinois at Chicago.

Bundy, A. C. (1993). Assessment of play and leisure: Delineation of the problem. *American Journal of Occupational Therapy, 47,* 217–222.

Canadian Association of Occupational Therapists. (1991). *Guidelines for the client-centred practice of occupational therapy.* Toronto: CAOT Publications ACE.

Daughton, D. M., Fix, A. J., Kass, I., Bell, C. W., & Patil, K. D. (1982). Maximum oxygen consumption and the ADAPT quality-of-life scale. *Archives of Physical Medicine & Rehabilitation, 63*(12), 620–622.

Doble, S. (1991). Test-retest and interrater reliability of a process skills assessment. *Occupational Therapy Journal of Research, 11,* 8–23.

Edwards, M. M. (1990). The reliability and validity of self-report activities of daily living scales. *Canadian Journal of Occupational Therapy, 57,* 273–278.

Fisher, A. G. (1992). *Assessment of motor and process skills manual* (Res. ed. 6.2). Unpublished test manual, Colorado State University, Fort Collins.

Fisher, A. G. (1993). The assessment of IADL motor skills: An application of many-faceted Rasch analysis. *American Journal of Occupational Therapy, 47,* 319–329.

Fisher, A. G. (in press). Development of a functional assessment that adjusts ability measures for task challenge and rater leniency. In M. Wilson (Ed.), *Objective measurement: Theory into practice* (Vol. 2). Norwood, NJ: Ablex.

Granger, C. V., & Hamilton, B. B. (1992). The Uniform Data System for medical rehabilitation report of first admissions for 1990. *American Journal of Physical Medicine and Rehabilitation, 71*(4), 108–113.

Granger, C. V., Hamilton, B. B., Linacre, J. M., Heinemann, A. W., & Wright, B. D. (1993). Performance profiles of the *Functional Independence Measure. American Journal of Physical Medicine & Rehabilitation, 72*(2), 84–89.

Gregory, M. D. (1983). Occupational behavior and life satisfaction among retirees. *American Journal of Occupational Therapy, 137*,(8), 548–553.

Gresham, G. E., Phillips, T. F., & Labi, M. L. C. (1980). ADL status in stroke: Relative merits of three standard indexes. *Archives of Physical Medicine & Rehabilitation, 61*(8), 355–358.

Harris, B. A., Jette, A. M., Campion, E. W., & Cleary, P. D. (1986). Validity of self-report measures of functional disability. *Topics in Geriatric Rehabilitation, 1*(3), 31–41.

Harrison, J., Johansson-Charles, E., & Doble, S. E. (1993). *Comparison of AMPS IADL motor and process ability measures of persons with multiple sclerosis and well persons.* Unpublished manuscript.

Hasselkus, B. R., & Safrit, M. J. (1976). Measurements in occupational therapy. *American Journal of Occupational Therapy, 30*(7), 429–436.

Hersch, G. (1991). Leisure and aging. *Physical and Occupational Therapy in Geriatrics, 9,* 55–78.

Iversen, I. A., Silberberg, N. E., Stever, R. C., & Schoening, H. A. (1973). *The Revised Kenny Self Care Evaluation* (Publication No. 722). Minneapolis: Abbott-Northwestern Hospital, Sister Kenny Institute.

Katz, S., Ford, A. B., Moskowitz, R. W., Jackson, B. A., & Jaffe, M. W. (1963). Studies of illness in the aged. The index of ADL: A standardized measure of biological and psychosocial function. *Journal of the American Medical Association, 185*(12), 914–919.

Klein, R. M., & Bell, B. (1982). Self-care skills: behavioral measurement with *Klein-Bell ADL Scale. Archives of Physical Medicine & Rehabilitation, 63*(7), 335–338.

Kohlman Thomson, L. (1993). *The Kohlman Evaluation of Living Skills* (3rd ed.). Rockville, MD: AOTA.

Law, M. (1987). Measurement in occupational therapy: Scientific criteria for evaluation. *Canadian Journal of Occupational Therapy, 54,* 133–138.

Law, M. (1991). The environment: A focus for occupational therapy. *Canadian Journal of Occupational Therapy, 58,* 171–179.

Law, M., Baptiste, S., Carswell, A., McColl, M., Polatajko, H., & Pollock, N. (1991). *The Canadian Occupational Performance Measure.* Toronto, Ont., Canada: CAOT Publications.

Law, M., Baptiste, S., Carswell, A., McColl, M., Polatajko, H., & Pollock, N. (1994). *Canadian Occupational Performance Measure* (2nd ed.). Toronto, Ont., Canada: CAOT Publications.

Law, M., & Letts, L. (1989). A critical review of scales of activities of daily living. *American Journal of Occupational Therapy, 43,* 522–528.

Linacre, J. M. (1989). *Many-faceted Rasch measurement.* Chicago: MESA.

Mahoney, F. I., & Barthel, D. W. (1965). Functional evaluation: The *Barthel Index. Maryland State Medical Journal, 14*(2), 61–65.

Mahurin, R. K., DeBettignies, B. H., & Pirozzolo, F. J. (1991).

Structured assessment of independent living skills: Preliminary report of a performance measure of functional abilities in dementia. *Journal of Gerontology, 46,* 58–66.

Malgady, R. G., Barcher, P. R., Towner, G., & Davis, J. (1980). Validity of the *Vocational Adaptation Rating Scale:* Prediction of mentally retarded workers' placement in sheltered workshops. *American Journal of Mental Deficiency, 84,* 633–640.

Mangen, D. J., & Peterson, W. A. (1982). *Research instruments in social gerontology: Vol. 2. Social Roles and Social Participation.* Minneapolis: University of Minnesota Press.

Matsutsuyu, J. S. (1969). Interest checklist. *American Journal of Occupational Therapy, 23*(4), 323–328.

Morgan, V. J. (1992). *The Safety and Functional ADL Evaluation.* Poster presented at the annual conference of the American Occupational Therapy Association, Houston, TX.

Oliver, R., Blathwayt, J., Brockley, C., & Tamaki, T. (1993). Development of the *Safety Assessment of Function and the Environment for Rehabilitation* (SAFER) tool. *Canadian Journal of Occupational Therapy, 60,* 78–82.

Reed, K., & Sanderson, S. R. (1980). *Concepts of occupational therapy.* Baltimore: Williams & Wilkins.

Rogers, J. C., Weinstein, J. M., & Figone, J. J. (1978). The interest checklist: An empirical assessment. *American Journal of Occupational Therapy, 32,* 628–630.

Sagar, M. A., Dunham, N. C., Schwartes, A., Mecum, L., Halverson, K., & Harlowe, D. (1992). Measurement of activities of daily living in hospitalized elderly: A comparison of self-report and performance-based methods. *Journal of American Geriatric Society, 40,* 457–462.

Sanford, J., Law, M., Swanson, L., & Guyatt, G. (1994, March). *Assessing clinically important change as an outcome of rehabilitation in older adults.* Paper presented at the Conference of the American Society on Aging, San Francisco.

Shinan, D., Gross, C., Bronstein, K. S., Licata-Gehr, E. E., Eden, D. T., Cabrera, A. R., Fishman, I. G., Roth, A. A., Barwick, J. A., & Kunitz, S. C. (1987). Reliability of the activities of daily living scale and its use in telephone interview. *Archives of Physical Medicine & Rehabilitation, 68,* 723–728.

Streiner, D. L., & Norman, G. R. (1989). *Health measurement scales: A practical guide to their development and use.* New York: Oxford University Press.

Trombly, C. (1993). Anticipating the future: Assessment of occupational function. *American Journal of Occupational Therapy, 47,* 253–257.

Velozo, C. A. (1993). Work evaluations: Critique of the states of the art of functional assessment of work. *American Journal of Occupational Therapy, 47,* 203–209.

Walls, R. T., Zane, T., & Werner, T. J. (1978). *The Vocational Behavior Checklist.* Dunbar, WV: Research and Training Center.

SUPPLEMENTARY RESOURCES

Suggested Readings

Casanova, J. S., & Ferber, J. (1976). Comprehensive evaluation of basic living skills. *American Journal of Occupational Therapy, 30*(2), 101–105.

Jacobson, N. S. (1985). Uses versus abuses of observational measures. *Behavioral Assessment, 7,* 323–330.

Kirchman, M. M. (1986). Measuring the quality of life. *Occupational Therapy Journal of Research, 6*(1), 21–32.

Klein-Parris, C., Clermont-Michel, T., & O'Neill, J. (1986). Effectiveness and efficiency of criterion testing versus interviewing for collecting functional assessment information. *American Journal of Occupational Therapy, 40*(7), 486–491.

Smith, R. O., Morrow, M. E., Heitman, J. K., Rardin, W. J.,

Powelson, J. L., & Von, T. (1986). The effects of introducing the *Klein-Bell ADL Scale* in a rehabilitation service. *American Journal of Occupational Therapy, 40*(6), 420–424.

Sources of Assessments

Assessment of Motor and Process Skills. (Available from Anne Fisher, Occupational Therapy Department, College of Applied Human Sciences, Colorado State University, 200 Occupational Therapy Building, Fort Collins, CO 80523)

Canadian Occupational Performance Measure. (Available from CAOT Publications, 110 Eglinton Avenue W, 3rd Floor, Toronto, Ont. M4R 1A3 Canada)

Klein-Bell ADL Scale. (Available from Book Store, University of Washington School of Medicine, Seattle, WA 98195)

Kohlman Evaluation of Living Skills (KELS). (Available from AOTA Products, 4720 Montgomery Lane, P.O. Box 31220, Bethesda, MD 20824-1220)

Safety and Functional ADL Evaluation (SAFE). (Available from Virginia Morgan, Director, Occupational Therapy, Spaulding Rehabilitation Hospital, 125 Nashua Street, Boston, MA 02114)

Evaluation of Access to Home, Community, and Workplace

Barbara Cooper, Patricia Rigby, and Lori Letts

OBJECTIVES

After studying this chapter, the reader will be able to:
1. Identify the role of the occupational therapist in the evaluation of access to settings within which patients and clients function.
2. Identify **environmental barriers** and **environmental supports** to occupational performance.
3. Identify assessment instruments appropriate for use in evaluating access to home, community, and workplace.
4. Evaluate the properties that make these measurement instruments useful in clinical practice.

Adaptations and modifications of both behavior and **environment** allow individuals with disabilities to function with maximum independence in the community. Traditionally, occupational therapy has played a central role in assisting disabled people to achieve this goal. This requires the occupational therapist to be able to assess the settings in which the individual functions to facilitate his ability to carry out desired activities (Mosey, 1986).

In the past, practice concerns often focused on specific issues of access, such as adapting homes for individuals (Cooper, Cohen, & Hasselkus, 1991). However, occupational therapy now considers the concept of **accessibility** more broadly, and today's assessments evaluate both **environmental barriers** and **environmental supports** to occupational performance as influenced by social, cultural, economic, institutional, and attitudinal factors as well as factors imposed by architectural elements. In addition, practice concerns in the area of access now include population needs as well as those of the individual.

Three major factors have influenced and are still shaping this broader focus in occupational therapy: the independent living movement (Cooper & Hasselkus, 1992); the increased number of frail elderly people in the population (Tiara, 1984); and legislation, such as federal and state building codes, standards issued by the American National Standards Institute (ANSI) (1980; Cooper, Cohen, & Hasselkus, 1991), and most important, the Americans with Disabilities Act of 1990 (ADA) (see Chapter 19).

The expanded role of the occupational therapist, as related to issues of access, still requires her to provide input to individuals enrolled in habilation and rehabilitation programs at various points on the continuum of care. This may include making home or workplace assessments for patients discharged from acute hospital care and/or facilitating contacts with community-based reintegration programs (see Chapter 19). Alternately, the therapist may be required to act as a consultant to an architect or to a group or community interested in implementing barrier-free design. Finally, the therapist could be called on to act as an advocate by individuals or groups with disabilities to help them gain access to necessary physical and social resources. This list is by no means exhaustive and will continue to change in response to societal needs.

ENVIRONMENTAL SUPPORTS AND BARRIERS

Supports and barriers to independence can be identified in all aspects of the **environment:** physical, social, cultural, organizational, and institutional.

Physical Factors

Physical supports and barriers of the built or natural **environment** are often the first to be addressed. There is now greater awareness of the need to

GLOSSARY

Accessibility—The ease with which an environment can be reached and utilized.

Clinical utility—Utility is based on clarity of instructions, cost of the assessment, time taken and ease in using the assessment, format used (e.g., self-report questionnaire and task performance), and examiner qualifications (e.g., skills and training necessary to use the assessment) (Law, 1991).

Environment—The physical, social, cultural, attitudinal, institutional, and organizational setting within which human function takes place.

Environmental barrier—Any component of the environment (physical, social, cultural, attitudinal, institutional, and organizational) that impedes a person's abilities to attain optimal occupational performance.

Environmental support—Any component of the environment (physical, social, cultural, attitudinal, institutional, and organizational) that encourages, facilitates, or provides assistance so that a person can achieve optimal occupational performance.

Person-environment fit—The degree to which an environment meets the functional, social, and psychological needs of an individual.

Reliability—The extent to which the results of an as-

sessment are reproducible, or give the same results, on different days (test-retest reliability) or by different observers (interrater reliability). The level of reliability is excellent when the correlation coefficient (r), or intraclass correlation, is $>.80$, is adequate when it is between .60 and .79, and is poor when it is $<.60$ (Law, 1991).

Standardization—The assessment is available in manual format and there are standard procedures for testing, scoring, and interpreting the results. Environmental assessments do not usually undergo a norming process because of the variability in environments, yet many are based on standards developed by the ANSI, government building codes, and interpretations of the ADA.

Validity—The extent to which the assessment is measuring what it is intended to measure. Content validity is most relevant to environmental assessments and is considered excellent for evaluative purposes when the assessment tool includes items that have the potential to change (e.g., physical barriers and social supports). Items selected for an assessment should be the result of a thorough review of the literature on the topic and consultation from experts in the area of study (including the input of people with physical disabilities) (Law, 1991).

provide barrier-free design features such as sufficiently wide door frames as well as ramps and curb cuts for wheelchair users. However, more subtle needs, such as the method of access available to people with disabilities, should also be considered. For example, people in wheelchairs may need to enter older public buildings through back doors, loading docks, or freight elevators. Although these allow access, the person may still require assistance and may need to plan carefully for the visit. Universal design features, such as automatic doors, should be promoted, because these facilitate access for everyone.

Social Factors

Social access considers and evaluates networks of family, neighborhood, community, and institutional groups. The social climate of an environment is critical in determining the degree of independence of someone with a disability. For example, family support, such as assistance with activities of daily living (ADL), may allow the individual to risk independent living.

Cultural Factors

The culture within which people live and work influences attitudes and role expectations. Culture relates to ethnicity, norms of behavior, traditions, and definitions of roles. All of these influence our feelings of belonging in a given **environment.** For people

with physical disabilities, cultural influences affect the expectations placed on them, the attitudes that significant others have toward them, and the roles that other people adopt in relating to them. For example, adults who become disabled may find that they are treated differently by coworkers when they return to work.

Attitudinal Factors

Attitudes in society also provide critical supports or barriers to independence. These relate to expectations and to the willingness of others to accept environmental adaptations that accommodate the needs of someone with a disability and allow him to be independent.

Organizational Factors

Finally, there are features of the environment that relate to organizations and institutions, including rules, policies, and laws. For example, the ability of a person with a disability to live independently often depends on his economic status. A person with a physical disability who has not been able to find competitive employment may receive government financial support that is barely sufficient for existence. Costs involved with disabilities, such as replacing wheelchair parts, are expensive and may be difficult to manage.

Institutions can also impose barriers or supports

to independence through their willingness to adapt their **environment** to facilitate function. However, this is not an easy issue to address: Adaptations can be costly, and seldom does a single design solution meet the needs of all disabled people. For example, a municipal transit system might be able to accommodate people with visual impairments by providing braille signage and training for transit employees but may have more difficulty creating a system that satisfies the needs of people in wheelchairs. In addition, the provision of flat ground surfaces to facilitate wheelchair travel may eliminate the crucial tactile cues required by blind people. The ADA will have a major effect on this area in the future.

ASSESSMENT OF PERSON-ENVIRONMENT FIT

The study of the relationship among personal abilities, the **environment,** and performance has interested many professional groups, including architects, social scientists, anthropologists, interior designers, biomechanical engineers, and occupational therapists and other health professionals. Common to all is the need to understand and promote **person-environment fit.** Although each discipline approaches the issue differently, many of the theoretical models developed deal with the issues broadly and in a manner relevant to occupational therapy. Assessment instruments from these disciplines and from occupational therapy are, therefore, included in this chapter.

To address the **person-environment fit,** the occupational therapist needs to assess the **environment** and the occupational functioning of the individual. In this section, we review a variety of environmental assessments and determine their usefulness to the occupational therapist. The review process addresses the following questions (Law, 1991):

1. Purpose: What is the intended use?
2. Focus: What environmental factors are addressed? In what environmental location should the assessment be used?
3. **Clinical utility:** How is this assessment carried out (e.g., questionnaire and observation)? How much time does it take to use and how easy is it to use? Are the instructions clear and comprehensive? Is the occupational therapist qualified to use it? How useful is it to occupational therapy?
4. **Standardization:** Has the assessment been published and is it available in a manual format, complete with procedures for administration, scoring, and interpretation? Did the authors consult the literature and experts to ensure that the items selected for this assessment are relevant characteristics of what is being measured? Has the assessment

undergone testing for **reliability** and **validity?** What types of tests were used and what were the results?

A total of 31 environmental assessments have been reviewed and are organized in Table 5.1 into a matrix by physical, social, cultural, and economic/institutional components, in relation to the environmental setting of home, community, and workplace. A few will be described below in more detail, organized according to the location or application in which they can be used.

Universal Assessments

Universal assessments are those that can be used to evaluate the environmental needs of any group using all sizes and types of settings. They usually do not require specific skills or knowledge of terminology to administer. Such measures are particularly useful in situations for which multidisciplinary teams are involved. The following examples may be useful.

POSTOCCUPANCY EVALUATION

Postoccupancy evaluation (POE) is a term used by architects, social scientists, and others working in the field of **environment** and behavior to describe a generic, comprehensive, and systematic approach to assessing any physical **environment** that is currently in use (Cooper, Ahrentzen, & Hasselkus, 1991; Preiser, Rabinowitz, & White, 1988).

Availability

Because this describes a process model rather than a specific assessment, no one POE is cited here. Examples of this approach are given by Preiser, Rabinowitz, and White (1988) and Cooper, Ahrentzen, and Hasselkus (1991).

Focus

The focus is to determine **person-environment fit** of a built **environment.**

Clinical Utility

A POE uses a battery of instruments to assess the congruence between the **environment** and the human functions meant to occur there. The number of instruments used, the degree of probing, and the number of people involved will vary with the objectives of the POE, but all will gather data on the **environment** and user needs using observation techniques, interviews, and site visits. Other instruments, such as cameras, questionnaires, and functional and psychometric tests may also be employed. A POE may be simple (individual home), more involved (nursing

Table 5.1.   Environmental Assessments by Attribute and Location/Application

	Physical	Social	Cultural	Economic/Institutional
Home	Accessibility Checklist (Goltsman et al., 1992) Assessment Tool (CMHC, 1989) The Enabler (Steinfeld et al., 1979) Home Modifications Workbook (Adaptive Environments Center, 1988) LIFEASE (Joe, 1992) MEAP (Moos & Lemke, 1988) SAFER Tool (Community Occupational Therapists & Associates, 1991) The Source Book (Kelly & Snell, 1989) UCP Occupational Therapy Initial Evaluation (Colvin & Korn, 1984)	Environmental Response Inventory (ERI) (McKechnie, 1974) Interpersonal Support Evaluation List (ISEL) (Cohen et al., 1985) Importance, Locus, and Range of Activities Checklist (ILRAC) (Hulicka, Morganti, & Cataldo, 1975) Life Stressors and Social Resources Inventory (LSSRI) (Moos et al., 1988) MEAP (Moos & Lemke, 1988) Multilevel Assessment Instrument (MAI) (Lawton et al., 1982) Need Satisfaction of Activity Interview (NSAI) (Tickle & Yerxa, 1981) Person-Environment Fit Scale (P-EFS) (Coulton, 1979a, 1979b)	ILRAC (Hulicka et al., 1975) LSSRI (Moos, Fenn, & Billings, 1988) MEAP (Moos & Lemke, 1988) P-EFS (Coulton, 1979a, 1979b)	MEAP (Moos & Lemke, 1988) Perceived Environmental Constraint Index (PECI) (Wolk & Telleen, 1976) P-EFS (Coulton, 1979a, 1979b)
Community	Accessibility Checklist (Goltsman et al., 1992) Disabilities Rights Guide (Goldman, 1991) The Enabler (Steinfeld et al., 1979) MEAP (Moos & Lemke, 1988) Readily Achievable Checklist (Cronburg, 1991) POE (Cooper, Ahrentzen, & Hasselkus, 1991)	Behavior Mapping (Howell, 1980) Disabilities Rights Guide (Goldman, 1991) ERI (McKechnie, 1974, 1977) MEAP (Moos & Lemke, 1988) P-EFS (Coulton, 1979a, 1979b) POE (Cooper, Ahrentzen, & Hasselkus, 1991)	P-EFS (Coulton, 1979a, 1979b)	Accessibility Checklist (Goltsman et al., 1992) MEAP (Moos & Lemke, 1988) Designing with Care (United Nations Center for Human Settlements, 1981) Planners Guide to Barrier-Free Meetings (Russell, 1980) Planning Barrier-Free Libraries (National Library Service, 1981) UFAS Accessibility Checklist (Barrier-Free Environments, 1990)
Workplace	The Enabler (Steinfeld et al., 1979) Job Analysis Schedule (U.S. Department of Labor, 1972) Job Task Analysis (Rumpel, 1991) Position Analysis Questionnaire (McPhail, Jeanneret, & Mecham, 1991) POE (Cooper, Ahrentzen, & Hasselkus, 1991) The Workplace Workbook (Mueller, 1990)	Job Analysis Schedule (U.S. Department of Labor, 1972) Work Environment Scale (Moos, 1986) Work Personality Profile (Bolton & Rossier, 1986)		POE (Cooper, Ahrentzen, & Hasselkus, 1991) Work Environment Scale (Moos, 1986) The Workplace Workbook (Mueller, 1990)

home), or highly complex (school system or several hospitals).

Standardization

The **reliability** and **validity** of the results depend on whether the total battery (e.g., Moos & Lemke, 1988) or components of the battery have been submitted to such testing. Occupational therapists often use this approach when making a home assessment. Its use in occupational therapy practice is discussed further by Cooper, Ahrentzen, and Hasselkus (1991).

PERSON-ENVIRONMENT FIT SCALE

Availability

The *Person-Environment Fit Scale* is available from C. J. Coulton, School of Applied Social Sciences, Case Western Reserve University, Cleveland, OH 44106 (see also Coulton, 1979a, 1979b).

Purpose

The purpose of the scale is to determine **person-environment fit.**

Focus

The scale focuses on social and cultural factors in the home and community environments.

Clinical Utility

This assessment involves both a self-report questionnaire and a questionnaire to be administered to someone who knows the client. The self-report questionnaire is divided into 13 subscales that address such areas as finance, family role expectations, and affiliation/acceptance. The other questionnaire addresses community functioning such as social behaviors, self-care skills, and willingness to access community resources. Both questionnaires use a 4-point Likert scale (Table 5.2). Minimal guidance for scoring and interpretation is provided. The occupational therapist may find that the opportunity to assess community and home functioning with her client provides a valuable basis for collaborative problem solving toward optimizing the client-environment fit.

Standardization

Coulton's *Person-Environment Fit Scale* was developed for research purposes and is not available in manual format from a publisher. In a study of **reliability,** the internal consistency scores for the subscales ranged from .60 to .94, with seven subscales achieving α scores of .80 and above (Coulton, 1979a). Content **validity** was established through interviews with 25 hospital patients (Coulton, 1979b). Analysis of construct **validity** reflected that the constructs of **person-environment fit** were closely correlated with the educational and economic status of the subjects in the sample (i.e., persons with high education and high income showed high capacities and aspirations in many areas) (Coulton, 1979a).

THE ENABLER

Availability

This assessment was published by Steinfeld et al. (1979) and can be obtained through HUD User P.O. Box 6091, Germantown, MD 20850.

Purpose

The Enabler provides a multidisciplinary approach to conceptualizing disability (Fig. 5.1) and

Table 5.2. Items from the *Affiliation/Acceptance Fit Subscale*

Item	Definitely True	Probably True	Probably Not True	Definitely Not True
In general, people important to me know what I can do and are satisfied with it.	1	2	3	4
My friends understand my condition.	1	2	3	4
I don't get invited out by friends as often as I would like.	1	2	3	4
There is someone I can count on to help me if I am ill.	1	2	3	4

Figure 5.1. *The Enabler.*

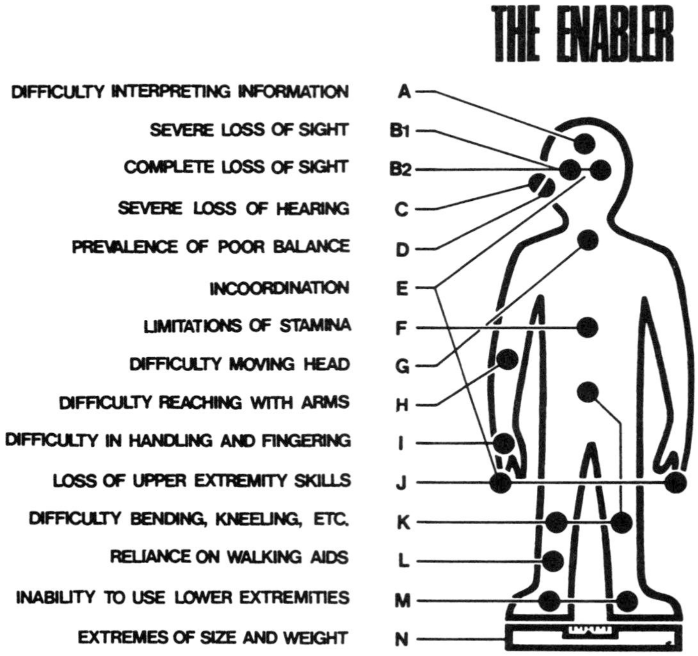

THE ENABLER

DIFFICULTY INTERPRETING INFORMATION	A
SEVERE LOSS OF SIGHT	B1
COMPLETE LOSS OF SIGHT	B2
SEVERE LOSS OF HEARING	C
PREVALENCE OF POOR BALANCE	D
INCOORDINATION	E
LIMITATIONS OF STAMINA	F
DIFFICULTY MOVING HEAD	G
DIFFICULTY REACHING WITH ARMS	H
DIFFICULTY IN HANDLING AND FINGERING	I
LOSS OF UPPER EXTREMITY SKILLS	J
DIFFICULTY BENDING, KNEELING, ETC.	K
RELIANCE ON WALKING AIDS	L
INABILITY TO USE LOWER EXTREMITIES	M
EXTREMES OF SIZE AND WEIGHT	N

Figure 5.2. An example of an *Enabler* problem matrix, using a hypothetical case. The labels for the vertical columns are defined in Figure 5.1.

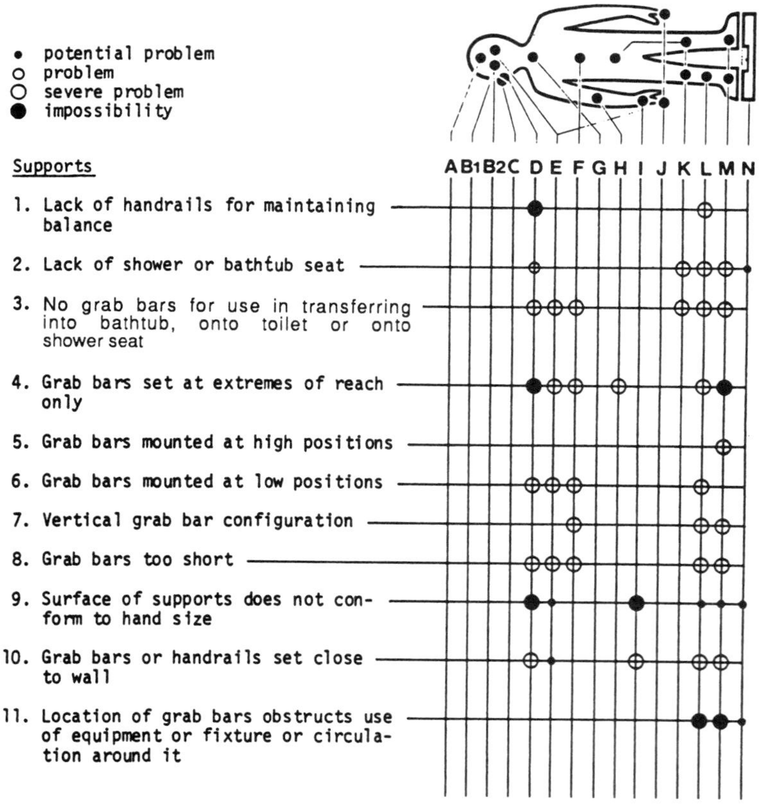

- • potential problem
- ○ problem
- ⊙ severe problem
- ● impossibility

Supports

1. Lack of handrails for maintaining balance

2. Lack of shower or bathtub seat

3. No grab bars for use in transferring into bathtub, onto toilet or onto shower seat

4. Grab bars set at extremes of reach only

5. Grab bars mounted at high positions

6. Grab bars mounted at low positions

7. Vertical grab bar configuration

8. Grab bars too short

9. Surface of supports does not conform to hand size

10. Grab bars or handrails set close to wall

11. Location of grab bars obstructs use of equipment or fixture or circulation around it

a mechanism for identifying related problems with accessing the built **environment.** The model facilitates decision making for building design.

Focus

The focus of this approach is to ensure a good fit between the built **environment** and the activity needs of people with disabilities.

Clinical Utility

This method of assessment uses language that is not specific to any one profession and is easily understood. It is, therefore, ideal for use by a multidisciplinary team or in situations involving lay or community input such as might be required by the implementation of ADA directives. Its immediate relevance to occupational therapy is discussed by Cooper, Cohen, and Hasselkus (1991).

Standardization

The Enabler was developed in 1979 by Steinfeld and colleagues who were asked by HUD to revise the ANSI standards. It is made up of 13 problem matrices (Fig. 5.2), which represent all the possible movement patterns required in the **environment** without being specific to any building type or area. To date, *The Enabler* has not undergone formal **reliability** or **validity** testing; however, content and construct **validity** were addressed at the time of development through an extensive literature review and expert consultation process (Steinfeld et al., 1979).

HOME

When evaluating a home, occupational therapists have normally used a barrier-free home assessment in the form of a checklist, which usually has been developed by members of their own occupational therapy department. Many of these checklists have great practical application and likely demonstrate acceptable interrater **reliability** and face **validity.** Yet limitations do exist, as these checklists are not available to others in a standardized format, **reliability** and **validity** have not been formally tested, and often the checklist does not address the home **environment** in relation to identified client needs.

Some standardized home assessments are now available for the occupational therapist to use with her client and his family to identify occupational performance problems in the home. The *Life Stressors and Social Resources Inventory* (Moos, Fenn, & Billings, 1988), specifically addresses the sociocultural barriers and supports that can affect client independence in the home. This tool provides a comprehensive picture of common life stressors and the social resources that influence physical and psychological functioning. It is published in manual format and has established content **validity** and **reliability** in the form of internal consistency. A few new home assessments now address social and cultural factors in the home **environment,** in addition to barrier-free factors. For example, the client and the occupational therapist can jointly determine the advantages and disadvantages of completing ADL and instrumental activities of daily living (IADL) tasks independently or with the help of community resources (Cooper & Hasselkus, 1992). The client may find that household tasks are too energy consuming to complete on his own and may decide to hire a housekeeper.

The *Assessment Tool* (Canada Mortgage and Housing Corporation [CMHC], 1989), the *Home Modification Workbook* (Adaptive Environments Center, 1988), *The Source Book* (Kelly & Snell, 1989), and *Christiansen's LIFEASE* computerized home assessment program (Joe, 1992) are four assessments that address the environmental factors in relation to clients' needs. Two of these are described below.

THE SOURCE BOOK

Availability

The Source Book is available from Barrier-Free Design Centre, 2075 Bayview Avenue, Toronto, Ont., Canada M4N 3M5 (see also Kelly & Snell, 1989).

Purpose

The purpose of this assessment is to determine the **person-environment** fit between the client with a physical disability and his physical housing requirements.

Focus

The focus is on barrier-free access of the home in relation to the client's functional abilities and needs.

Clinical Utility

The Source Book is divided into three sections: a questionnaire to determine specific problems the client experiences doing activities around the home (Table 5.3); guidelines for the measurement of physical features in the home (e.g., door widths for the passage of a wheelchair and the height of kitchen cabinets in relation to client reach from a wheelchair); and household design solutions such as ramped entrance specifications for wheelchair access. Clear examples are provided for administration, scoring, and interpretation of the assessment. It appears to be an excellent tool for the occupational therapist to use collaboratively with her client and the architects and builders.

Table 5.3. Home Assessment: Activities Checklist

Please check the box that best describes how you would normally do the activity.

This section asks questions about how you do certain activities in specific rooms in your home. Please tell us as much as you can about your abilities, and the problems or solutions you have come up with in your house.

1. The Site

I can	Does Not Apply	Can Manage Alone	Can Manage with Equipment (wheelchair, reacher, etc.)	Can Manage with Someone Helping	Cannot Manage at All
Move around outside the house	☐	☐	☐	☐	☐
Manage curbs	☐	☐	☐	☐	☐
Manage rough ground	☐	☐	☐	☐	☐
Manage slopes	☐	☐	☐	☐	☐
Manage ice/snow	☐	☐	☐	☐	☐
Carry things outdoors	☐	☐	☐	☐	☐
Get into and out of a car	☐	☐	☐	☐	☐
Load and unload things into and out of a car	☐	☐	☐	☐	☐
Use a bus, or special transportation service	☐	☐	☐	☐	☐
Drive a car	☐	☐	☐	☐	☐

Do you have any special outdoor interests or hobbies?

_____

_____

_____

Do you have any special needs when going out of doors (i.e., sensitive to sun)?

_____

_____

_____

Do you use a scooter or wheelchair when you are outside? Please describe.

_____

_____

_____

What are the biggest problems to you when you are outside or in your yard?

_____

_____

_____

Table 5.3. (Continued)

2. Front and Back Door

I can	Does Not Apply	Can Manage Alone	Can Manage with Equipment (wheelchair, reacher, etc.)	Can Manage with Someone Helping	Cannot Manage at All
Climb up stairs	☐	☐	☐	☐	☐
Go down stairs	☐	☐	☐	☐	☐
Go up a ramp	☐	☐	☐	☐	☐
Go down a ramp	☐	☐	☐	☐	☐
Use a handrail	☐	☐	☐	☐	☐
Open and go through a door	☐	☐	☐	☐	☐
Use a key	☐	☐	☐	☐	☐
Use the door lock	☐	☐	☐	☐	☐
Use the doorknob	☐	☐	☐	☐	☐
Use lever handles	☐	☐	☐	☐	☐
Reach and use the mailbox	☐	☐	☐	☐	☐
Walk, (wheel) over the lip at the door	☐	☐	☐	☐	☐

What are the biggest problems you now have when going in and/or out of your house?

_____

_____

3. Hallways and Inside Doors

I can	Does Not Apply	Can Manage Alone	Can Manage with Equipment (wheelchair, reacher, etc.)	Can Manage with Someone Helping	Cannot Manage at All
Manage carpeted areas	☐	☐	☐	☐	☐
Manage hallways	☐	☐	☐	☐	☐
Open and go through doors to rooms	☐	☐	☐	☐	☐
Manage doorknobs	☐	☐	☐	☐	☐
Manage lever handles	☐	☐	☐	☐	☐

When I move from room to room I use a:
☐ cane ☐ crutches ☐ artificial limb ☐ manual/electric wheelchair ☐ power scooter ☐ other

What are the biggest problems you now have when going from room to room in your house?

_____

_____

4. Stairs

I can	Does Not Apply	Can Manage Alone	Can Manage with Equipment (wheelchair, reacher, etc.)	Can Manage with Someone Helping	Cannot Manage at All
Climb up stairs	☐	☐	☐	☐	☐
Go down stairs	☐	☐	☐	☐	☐
Use a handrail	☐	☐	☐	☐	☐
Use elevator controls	☐	☐	☐	☐	☐
Use a lift device	☐	☐	☐	☐	☐

Table 5.3. *(Continued)*

Is going from one level up or down to another level of your house very important to you? How do you manage going up or down?

_____

_____

What are the biggest problems you now have when going from one level to another in your house?

_____

_____

5. Bathroom

I can	Does Not Apply	Can Manage Alone	Can Manage with Equipment (wheelchair, reacher, etc.)	Can Manage with Someone Helping	Cannot Manage at All
Turn the lights on and off	☐	☐	☐	☐	☐
Use the electrical outlets	☐	☐	☐	☐	☐
Use the cabinets and closets	☐	☐	☐	☐	☐
See myself in the mirror	☐	☐	☐	☐	☐
Wash hands and face and brush my teeth	☐	☐	☐	☐	☐
Use taps	☐	☐	☐	☐	☐
Use the sink	☐	☐	☐	☐	☐
Get on the toilet	☐	☐	☐	☐	☐
Get off the toilet	☐	☐	☐	☐	☐
Manage conventional toileting	☐	☐	☐	☐	☐
Reach the toilet paper	☐	☐	☐	☐	☐
Use grab bars	☐	☐	☐	☐	☐
Get into the bathtub	☐	☐	☐	☐	☐
Get out of the bathtub	☐	☐	☐	☐	☐
Take a bath	☐	☐	☐	☐	☐
Get into the shower	☐	☐	☐	☐	☐
Get out of the shower	☐	☐	☐	☐	☐
Take a shower	☐	☐	☐	☐	☐
Use taps	☐	☐	☐	☐	☐
Dry off after a bath/ shower	☐	☐	☐	☐	☐
Get dressed after a bath/shower	☐	☐	☐	☐	☐

Do you have any special needs or procedures in the bathroom?

_____

_____

_____

Table 5.3. *(Continued)*

What are the biggest problems you now have when using the bathroom in your house?

_____

_____

6. Kitchen

I can	Does Not Apply	Can Manage Alone	Can Manage with Equipment (wheelchair, reacher, etc.)	Can Manage with Someone Helping	Cannot Manage at All
Turn the lights on and off	☐	☐	☐	☐	☐
Use the electrical outlets	☐	☐	☐	☐	☐
Reach the garbage	☐	☐	☐	☐	☐
Move around in the kitchen	☐	☐	☐	☐	☐
Take food out of the refrigerator	☐	☐	☐	☐	☐
Take food out of the freezer	☐	☐	☐	☐	☐
Take things out of the cupboards	☐	☐	☐	☐	☐
Wipe the counters	☐	☐	☐	☐	☐
Wash dishes	☐	☐	☐	☐	☐
Use the dishwasher	☐	☐	☐	☐	☐
Clean the floor	☐	☐	☐	☐	☐
Open cans, bottles, boxes	☐	☐	☐	☐	☐
Mix ingredients in a bowl	☐	☐	☐	☐	☐
Fill pot with water	☐	☐	☐	☐	☐
Place pot on stove	☐	☐	☐	☐	☐
Turn stove on and off	☐	☐	☐	☐	☐
Use a microwave	☐	☐	☐	☐	☐
Open and close oven door	☐	☐	☐	☐	☐
Put pan in oven	☐	☐	☐	☐	☐
Pour hot water from a pot	☐	☐	☐	☐	☐
Cook on stovetop	☐	☐	☐	☐	☐
Use range fan	☐	☐	☐	☐	☐
Set the table	☐	☐	☐	☐	☐
Eat in the kitchen	☐	☐	☐	☐	☐
Eat in the dining room	☐	☐	☐	☐	☐
Prepare a meal	☐	☐	☐	☐	☐
Prepare a snack	☐	☐	☐	☐	☐
Feed myself	☐	☐	☐	☐	☐

Do you have any special needs in the kitchen?

_____

_____

Is using the kitchen very important to you?

_____

Table 5.3.   (Continued)

What are the biggest problems you now have when using the kitchen in your house?

_____

_____

7. Living Room or Family Room

I can	Does Not Apply	Can Manage Alone	Can Manage with Equipment (wheelchair, reacher, etc.)	Can Manage with Someone Helping	Cannot Manage at All
Get into the living room	☐	☐	☐	☐	☐
Use the television controls	☐	☐	☐	☐	☐
Use the radio/stereo controls	☐	☐	☐	☐	☐
Use the telephone	☐	☐	☐	☐	☐
Turn the lights on and off	☐	☐	☐	☐	☐
Move around in the living room	☐	☐	☐	☐	☐
Use the living room chairs	☐	☐	☐	☐	☐

What are the biggest problems you now have when using the living room or family room in your house?

_____

_____

8. Bedroom

I can	Does Not Apply	Can Manage Alone	Can Manage with Equipment (wheelchair, reacher, etc.)	Can Manage with Someone Helping	Cannot Manage at All
Turn lights on and off	☐	☐	☐	☐	☐
Use electrical outlets	☐	☐	☐	☐	☐
Open and close windows	☐	☐	☐	☐	☐
Pull drapes open and closed	☐	☐	☐	☐	☐
Get into my bedroom	☐	☐	☐	☐	☐
Reach clothes in closet	☐	☐	☐	☐	☐
Open drawers	☐	☐	☐	☐	☐
Dress myself	☐	☐	☐	☐	☐
Undress myself	☐	☐	☐	☐	☐
Get into bed	☐	☐	☐	☐	☐
Get out of bed	☐	☐	☐	☐	☐
Get into the other bedrooms in the house	☐	☐	☐	☐	☐

What are the biggest problems you now have when using your bedroom?

_____

_____

Table 5.3. *(Continued)*

9. Laundry

I can	Does Not Apply	Can Manage Alone	Can Manage with Equipment (wheelchair, reacher, etc.)	Can Manage with Someone Helping	Cannot Manage at All
Get into the laundry room	☐	☐	☐	☐	☐
Turn the lights on and off	☐	☐	☐	☐	☐
Use the electrical outlets	☐	☐	☐	☐	☐
Reach the closets and cupboards	☐	☐	☐	☐	☐
Use the washer and dryer controls	☐	☐	☐	☐	☐
Put the laundry in the machine	☐	☐	☐	☐	☐
Take the laundry out of the machine	☐	☐	☐	☐	☐
Reach the taps	☐	☐	☐	☐	☐
Do hand laundry	☐	☐	☐	☐	☐
Do the ironing	☐	☐	☐	☐	☐

What are the biggest problems you now have when doing the laundry?

_____

_____

_____

_____

Standardization

The assessment is published in manual format. Content **validity** was established through consultation with experts and the use of ANSI standards and the Ontario building code. Formal studies of **reliability** have not been undertaken.

ASSESSMENT TOOL

Availability

The *Assessment Tool* is published in CMHC (1989) and can be obtained from the CMHC National Office, 700 Montreal Road, Ottawa, Ont., Canada K1A 0P7.

Purpose

The purpose of this tool is to assess the problems the client experiences in occupational performance in relation to **environmental barriers.** It was developed for use with elderly people but is equally useful for individuals with physical disabilities.

Focus

The primary focus of the *Assessment Tool* is on the physical factors of the home **environment,** yet the occupational therapist is encouraged to think about other enabling environmental factors such as access to social supports. For example, the client who has problems buying groceries may prefer to access Meals on Wheels and/or to have his groceries delivered, rather than try to obtain them by himself (Table 5.4).

Clinical Utility

The survey questionnaire addresses functional limitations experienced by the individual, such as impairments of balance, memory, and vision, in relation to characteristics of the home **environment.** Recommendations are provided that involve adaptations and/or equipment options and the use of social supports to facilitate the performance of ADL and IADL. Throughout this excellent assessment, the occupational therapist also addresses safety features, prevention of falls, and emergency procedures, such as use of automatic

Table 5.4.   Assessing the Functional Ability to Purchase and/or Go to the Store for Groceries

Do you purchase/store groceries?
☐ No   ☐ Yes   ☐ N.A.

Functional Limitations	Home Checklist	Recommendations	
		Housing	Other
☐ Poor tolerance ☐ Muscle weakness ☐ Poor balance ☐ Reduced mobility ☐ Wheelchair dependent ☐ Poor vision	☐ Adequate/usable re-frigerator and cup-board storage space for storing items ☐ Sufficient food supply to last until next shop-ping day ☐ Bulletin board near storage for list	☐ Adequate cold storage space for 1 week (or more) of supplies ☐ Increase storage space (add pantry, shelves, baskets, etc.)	☐ Walking aids (walker with basket) ☐ Shopping cart ☐ Meals on Wheels ☐ List of local stores that deliver ☐ List of local stores that take tele-phone orders ☐ Emergency pack ☐ Escort to store ☐ Assistance

shut-off mechanisms on electric cooking appliances, strategically placed telephones, and access to an emergency call bell.

Standardization

This assessment is available in manual format. Content **validity** was established through consultation with experts (such as occupational therapists, architects, and elderly persons), using focus group methodology. In addition, home assessments were conducted to identify the modifications required to reduce difficulties in 73 activities of daily living. Interrater **reliability** was tested by two occupational therapists, assessing the same 19 individuals. The results: >80% agreement for 30 of the 72 items, and >60% agreement for 58 of the 72 items (Maltais, Trickey, & Robitaille, 1988).

Community

Accessibility to community services, programs, and social groups is as important as the implementation of barrier-free design. This category of **accessibility** assessment considers items such as the availability of adequate public transportation for frail or disabled citizens and the policies, procedures, and attitudes of workers in key community offices. Methods to assess social, cultural, and institutional **environments** are not readily available in standardized format; nevertheless, this aspect of environmental assessment should not be ignored by the occupational therapist. Checklists provided in the *Disabilities Rights Guide* (Goldman, 1991) may be helpful.

Occupational therapists provide services to sheltered care facilities in which many elderly people live. Occupational therapists should be aware of the functions of these settings and the expectations of those who work or reside there to ensure optimal **person-environment fit.** The *Multiphasic Environmental Assessment Procedure* (MEAP) (Moos & Lemke, 1988), in whole or in part, can be used to evaluate these settings.

Occupational therapists may be asked to consult on community architectural projects, e.g., housing complexes for persons with physical disabilities. The proximity of these developments to community services such as banks, grocery stores, and medical clinics is important to consider. The following assessment, which helps interpret the ADA and other relevant building codes, is an excellent comprehensive instrument to use for these purposes.

ACCESSIBILITY CHECKLIST

Availability

This assessment was published in Goltsman, Gilbert, and Wohlford (1992) and can be obtained from M.I.G. Communications, 1802 Fifth Avenue, Berkeley, CA 94710.

Purpose

The purpose of the assessment is to determine the **accessibility** and barriers to access of buildings and outdoor facilities.

Focus

This assessment primarily addresses the physical factors of the community and home **environments.** Institutional factors are also presented in community program **accessibility.**

Clinical Utility

This is a comprehensive tool that provides detailed **accessibility** checklists for many aspects of outdoor and indoor built **environments** such as stairways, play equipment, sports facilities, campsites, dining areas, retail areas, and libraries (Table 5.5). The tools recommended for conducting the site survey include tape measure, pocket ruler, graph paper, clipboard, camera (not essential), inclinometer, and stopwatch (to determine sweep time of doors with automatic door closers). The administration, scoring, and interpretation of this assessment appears clear and thorough and can be used by the occupational therapist together with professionals such as architects and designers. The occupational therapist is also encouraged to determine whether policies, procedures, and staff attitudes of the institution are discriminatory of persons with a disability.

Standardization

The assessment consists of two manuals: the survey forms and the user's guide. The survey is based on the requirements of the ADA, the Uniform Federal Accessibility Standards (UFAS), and California's Title 24 building codes. During scale construction, expert reviews were also obtained to establish content **validity**. Formal tests of **reliability** have not been undertaken by the authors.

MULTIPHASIC ENVIRONMENTAL ASSESSMENT PROCEDURE

Availability

This assessment is available from R. Moos, Center for Health Care Evaluation, Department of Psychiatry TD 114, Stanford University, Palo Alto, CA (see also Moos & Lemke, 1988).

Purpose

The purpose of this tool is to provide a comprehensive, conceptual picture of the functions of a sheltered care facility and the preferences of both the staff and the residents. It provides a well-developed procedure for evaluating sheltered care settings such as nursing homes and residential care facilities.

Focus

The tool focuses on the physical, social, and institutional factors of the home and community **environments.**

Table 5.5. Assessment of Single-User Restroom

Complies	Does Not Comply	Actual Measure	Space around Toilet
☐	☐	_____	1. Clear space from the side of the toilet to the sink is 28 inches minimum. *or* Clear space from one side of the toilet to the wall is 32 inches.
☐	☐	_____	2. Clear space from the other wall to the center of the toilet is 18 inches.
☐	☐	_____	3. Clear space in front of the toilet is 48 inches minimum.
☐	☐	_____	4. Toilet seat height is 17 to 19 inches. (Note height of lifts if provided: _____.)
☐	☐	_____	5. Flush controls are located on wide side of the toilet and 44 inches maximum above floor.
☐	☐	_____	6. Toilet paper turns freely, is 12 inches maximum in front of the toilet, and is 40 inches maximum high.
☐	☐	_____	7. Seat cover dispenser is 40 inches maximum above the floor.
			8. Grab Bars
☐	☐	_____	a. Bars are mounted 33 inches above the floor, parallel to the floor surface (36 inches rear grab bar height acceptable if tank-type toilet).
☐	☐	_____	b. Rear grab bar is 36 inches minimum long.
☐	☐	_____	c. Side grab bar is 42 inches minimum long.
☐	☐	_____	d. Side grab bars are positioned so the front end is 24 inches minimum in front of the toilet.
☐	☐	_____	e. Diameter of bars is 1¼ to 1½ inches. *or* Bars provide an equivalent gripping surface with a ⅛-inch minimum edge radius.
☐	☐	_____	f. Space between the wall and the grab bar is 1½ inches.
☐	☐		g. Grab bars do not rotate in fittings.
☐	☐		h. Grab bars have rounded and nonabrasive surfaces.
☐	☐		i. Grab bars will withstand 250-pound load.

Clinical Utility

MEAP consists of checklists and questionnaires to assess physical and architectural features, policies and programs, characteristics of the resident and staff, and the social climate. The user's guide provides item definition and instructions for organizing data collection. Clear guidelines for scoring and a scoring key are provided. The assessment can be used in part or whole to assess quality of life and quality of care in the sheltered care environment.

Standardization

MEAP is a well-constructed instrument, published in manual format. Norms from two large U.S. samples are available. The tool was developed over many years of conceptual analysis of **environmental supports** and **environmental barriers** in relation to how persons function in sheltered care settings. Excellent content **validity** for the checklists and questionnaires resulted from extensive consultation with experts and testing in sheltered care settings. Studies for **reliability** achieved the following: internal consistency scores ranged from .50 to .95; test-retest scores ranged from .61 to .99; and interrater scores using the intraclass coefficient ranged from .51 to .98 (70% of the scales achieved intraclass scores >.80) (Moos & Lemke, 1988).

Workplace

Occupational therapists commonly provide services for individuals with physical disabilities who are attempting to find work or returning to work to ensure that the workplace can successfully accommodate their disabilities. The ADA prohibits discrimination against a qualified person with a disability who can perform the "essential functions" of the job with or without reasonable accommodation.

The **environment** of the workplace is assessed to ensure a fit can be achieved between the demands of the job and the individual's mental and physical capacities (Shrey & Breslin, 1992; Velozo, 1993). For example, a complete assessment of the building is necessary to ensure barrier-free access when a client in a wheelchair will be employed in the building. The occupational therapist should use a tool such as the *Accessibility Checklist* (Goltsman et al., 1992), described earlier. In addition, the POE could be used to address further the worker's capacities in relation to the work environment. The *Work Environment Scale* (Moos, 1986), described below, can be used to assess the social factors in the work environment.

WORK ENVIRONMENT SCALE

Availability

This assessment was published in Moos (1986) and can be obtained from Consulting Psychologists Press, 3803 East Bay Shore Road, PO Box 10096, Palo Alto, CA 94303.

Purpose

The purpose of this tool is to measure the social aspects of various work settings.

Focus

This assessment focuses on the social components of the work **environment.**

Clinical Utility

This assessment is administered to the client who is currently employed or who will be employed. It has three questionnaires: one that measures perceptions of existing work **environments;** one that measures conceptions of the ideal work **environment;** and one that measures expectations about work settings. Thus the occupational therapist can choose to use the form or forms most relevant to the client's situation. The assessment is composed of three dimensions: relationships; personal growth; and system maintenance and system change.

Standardization

This assessment, available in manual format, has undergone a norming process with two samples of approximately 1500 employees each. Content **validity** has been established through consultation with experts and through observation and interviews of workers. Internal consistency, tested with a large sample ($n = 1045$), achieved Cronbach Alpha scores ranging between .69 and .86 for the 10 subscales. The 1-month test-retest reliability ($n = 75$) scores ranged from .69 to .83 (8 out of 10 subscales scored below .80).

SUMMARY

In summary, the role of the occupational therapist in evaluating access to home, community, and workplace is becoming more diverse. This expanded professional role is dynamic and will continue to be influenced by external societal factors such as demographics and legislation. Therapists should be aware of assessments designed by other professionals also interested in issues of **accessibility** and should make use of these resources when appropriate.

STUDY QUESTIONS

1. Why would an occupational therapist assess the environment?
2. List seven examples of environmental barriers that a person with a physical disability might encounter at their local grocery store.
3. List seven examples of environmental social supports that would allow a senior with arthritis to continue living at home.
4. What would you look for in an assessment tool to be sure that your results would be consistent with those of an occupational therapist colleague using the same assessment?
5. If your client has achieved functional independence yet expresses fear about his return home, what assessment(s) could you use to help him to overcome this fear?
6. What assessment tools would you use with a client who is returning to work following rehabilitation for a spinal cord injury?
7. As an occupational therapist working in a sheltered care facility, what could you offer the facility's administration regarding their plans to renovate the building?

REFERENCES

Adaptive Environments Center. (1988). *Home modification workbook*. Boston: Author.

American National Standards Institute. (1980). *American National Standards specifications for making buildings and facilities accessible to, and useable by, the physically handicapped*. New York: Author.

Barrier Free Environments & Adaptive Environments Center. (1990). *Uniform federal accessibility standards (UFAS) accessibility checklist*. Raleigh, NC: Author.

Bolton, B., & Rossier, R. (1986). *Work personality profile*. Little Rock: Arkansas Research and Training Center in Vocational Rehabilitation.

Canada Mortgage and Housing Corporation. (1989). *Maintaining seniors' independence: A guide to home adaptations*. Ottawa, Ont., Canada: Author.

Cohen, S., Mermelstein, R., Kamarck, T. & Hoberman, H. M. (1985). Measuring the functional components of social support. In I. G. Sarason & B. R. Sarason (Eds.), *Social support: Theory, research and applications* (pp. 73–94). Boston: Martinus Nijhoff.

Colvin, M. E., & Korn, T. L. (1984). Eliminating barriers to the disabled. *American Journal of Occupational Therapy, 38*, 748–753.

Community Occupational Therapists and Associates. (1991). *Safety assessment of function and the environment for rehabilitation (SAFER)*. (Available from COTA, 3101 Bathurst Street, Suite 200, Toronto, Ont. M6A 2A6 Canada)

Cooper, B. A., Ahrentzen, S., & Hasselkus, B. R. (1991). Post-occupancy evaluation: An environment-behaviour technique for assessing the built environment. *Canadian Journal of Occupational Therapy, 58*, 181–188.

Cooper, B. A., Cohen, U., & Hasselkus, B. (1991). Barrier-free design: A review and critique of the occupational therapy

perspective. *American Journal of Occupational Therapy, 45*(4), 344–350.

Cooper, B., & Hasselkus, B. R. (1992). Independent living and the physical environment: Aspects that matter to residents. *Canadian Journal of Occupational Therapy, 59*, 6–15.

Coulton, C. J. (1979a). Developing an instrument to measure person-environment fit. *Journal of Social Service Research, 3*, 159–173.

Coulton, C. J. (1979b). A study of person-environment fit among the chronically ill. *Social Work in Health Care, 5*, 5–17.

Cronburg, J. (1991). *Readily achievable checklist: A survey for accessibility*. Washington, DC: National Center for Access Unlimited.

Goldman, C. D. (1991). *Disability rights guide: Practical solutions to problems affecting people with disabilities*. Lincoln, NE: Media.

Goltsman, S. M., Gilbert, T. A., & Wohlford, S. D. (1992). *The accessibility checklist: An evaluating system for buildings and outdoor settings*. Berkeley, CA: M. I. G. Communications.

Howell, S. C. (1980). *Behavior mapping—Designing for aging: Patterns of use*. Cambridge: MIT.

Hulicka, I. M., Morganti, J. B., & Cataldo, J. F. (1975). Importance, locus and range of activities check list. *Experimental Aging Research, 1*, 27–39.

Joe, B. E. (1992, October 22). Software provides independence with EASE. *OT Week*, 14–15.

Kelly, C., & Snell, K. (1989). *The source book: Architectural guidelines for barrier-free design*. Toronto, Ont., Canada: Barrier-Free Design Centre.

Law, M. (1991). *Guidelines for reviewing clinical measures*. Hamilton, Ont., Canada: McMaster University, Neurodevelopmental Clinical Research Unit.

Lawton, M. P., Moss, M., Fulcomer, M., & Kleban, M. H. (1982). A research and service oriented multilevel assessment instrument. *Journal of Gerontology, 37*, 91–99.

Maltais, D., Trickey, F., & Robitaille, Y. (1988). *Élaboration d'une grille d'analyse du logement des personnes âgées en perte d'autonomie physique*. Ottawa, Ont.: Canada Mortgage and Housing Corp.

McKechnie, G. E. (1974). *Manual for the environmental response inventory*. Palo Alto, CA: Psychologists Press.

McKechnie, G. E. (1977). The environmental response inventory in application. *Environment and Behavior, 9*, 255–276.

McPhail, S. M., Jeanneret, P. R., & Mecham, R. C. (1991). *Position analysis questionnaire: Job analysis manual*. Palo Alto, CA: Social Ecology Laboratory.

Moos, R. H. (1986). *The work environment scale*. Palo Alto, CA: Social Ecology Laboratory.

Moos, R. H., Fenn, C. B., & Billings, A. G. (1988). Life stressors and social resources: An integrated assessment approach. *Social Science and Medicine, 27*, 999–1002.

Moos, R. H., & Lemke, S. (1988). *Multiphasic environmental assessment procedure*. Palo Alto, CA: Social Ecology Laboratory.

Mosey, A. C. (1986). *Psychosocial components of occupational therapy*. New York: Raven.

Mueller, J. (1990). *The workplace workbook: An illustrated guide to job accommodation and assistive technology*. Washington, DC: Dole Foundation.

National Library Service for the Blind and Physically Handicapped. (1981). *Planning barrier-free libraries: A guide for renovation and construction of libraries serving blind and physically handicapped readers*. Washington, DC: Library of Congress.

Preiser, W., Rabinowitz, H., & White, E. (1988). *Post-occupancy evaluation*. New York: Van Nostrand Reinhold.

Rumpel, F. (1991). Job task analysis. In F. Rumple (Ed.), *ADA management kit* (pp. 30–33). Washington, DC: Mainstream.

Russell, H. (1980). *The planner's guide to barrier free meetings.* Raleigh, NC: Barrier Free Environments.

Shrey, D. E., & Breslin, R. E. (1992). Disability management in industry: A multidisciplinary model for the accommodation of workers with disabilities. *International Journal of Industrial Ergonomics, 9,* 183–190.

Steinfeld, E., Schroeder, S., Duncan, J., Faste, R., Chollet, D., Bishop, M., Wirth, P., & Cardell, P. (1979). *Access to the built environment: A review of the literature* (HUD #660). Washington, DC: U.S. Government Printing Office.

Tickle, L. S., & Yerxa, E. J. (1981). Need satisfaction of older persons living in the community and institutions. *American Journal of Occupational Therapy, 35,* 650–655.

Tiara, E. D. (1984). An occupational therapist's perspective on environmental adaptations for the disabled elderly. *Occupational Therapy in Health Care, 1*(4), 25–33.

United Nations Centre for Human Settlements. (1981). *Designing with care: A guide to adaptation of the built environment for disabled persons* (joint project of the Swedish Development Authority, the United Nations, and the United Centre for Human Settlements). New York: United Nations.

U.S. Department of Labor. (1972). *Handbook for analyzing jobs.* Menomonie: University of Wisconsin-Stout, Stout Vocational Rehabilitation Institute, Materials Development Center.

Velozo, C. (1993). Work evaluations: Critique of the state of art of functional assessment of work. *American Journal of Occupational Therapy, 47,* 203–208.

Wolk, S., & Telleen, S. (1976). Psychological and social correlates of life satisfaction as a function of residential constraint. *Journal of Gerontology, 31,* 89–98.

6
Evaluation of Biomechanical and Physiological Aspects of Motor Performance

Catherine A. Trombly

OBJECTIVES

After studying this chapter and practicing the skills described here, the reader will be able to:
1. Evaluate range of motion of the upper extremity.
2. Determine the amount of edema of the hand.
3. Evaluate strength of the upper extremity.
4. Determine the functional strength of selected lower extremity musculature.
5. Evaluate endurance.
6. Interpret the findings of the evaluations in this chapter.

The tests that are presented in this chapter are appropriate for patients who are unable to do, or are restricted in doing, the occupational tasks and activities important to them because of impairments in range of joint motion, strength, or endurance.

RANGE OF MOTION

Each joint is potentially able to move in certain directions and to certain limits of motion as a result of its structure and the integrity of surrounding tissues. Trauma or disease that affects joint structures or the surrounding tissues can decrease the amount of motion at the joint and limit occupational performance.

Range of Motion Measurement Technique

Measurement of joint range may be done actively or passively. **Passive range of motion** (PROM) is the amount of motion at a given joint when the joint is moved by the therapist. **Active range of motion** (AROM) is the amount of motion at a given joint achieved by the patient using his own muscle strength. If AROM is less than PROM there is a problem of muscle weakness (or tendon integrity in hands). AROM measurement, used as a supplement to the measurement of the strength of muscles graded poor minus (P−) or fair minus (F−), provides documentation of small gains that would otherwise not be noted by the muscle test.

Range of motion (ROM) evaluation starts with a request to the patient to demonstrate his ability to move each joint in all motions. The therapist demonstrates the movements to the patient. If limitation is observed, the therapist attempts to move the part to its **limit of motion.** If the limit is easily achieved, the problem is one of **active range of motion,** and the therapist would go on to measure the limitation in AROM. If the limit cannot be achieved, the problem is one of **passive range of motion,** and that limitation is also measured. If the patient has no limitations in range of motion that would interfere with occupational performance, then range of motion is recorded as being within normal limits (WNL) as determined by the observation of functional movement, and no further testing is done.

Use of the universal (standard) goniometer is the most widely used method of measuring joint motion. Every goniometer has a protractor, an axis, and two arms. The stationary arm extends from the protractor on which the degrees are marked. The movable arm has a center line or pointer to indicate the degrees of the angle measured. The axis is the point at which these two arms are riveted together. A full-circle goniometer, which measures degrees from 0 to 180° in each direction, permits measurement of motion in both directions, e.g., flexion and extension, without repositioning the tool. When using a half-circle goniometer, it is neces-

GLOSSARY

Active range of motion—The amount of movement possible at a joint when the patient moves the limb himself by muscle contraction.

Anatomical position—Standing straight with feet together and flat on the floor, arms by the sides with hands facing forward. The position of "zero" for range of motion measurement.

Calibration—Determination of what the output of a measuring instrument means. The instrument's output is compared with known values.

Contracture—Inability to move a body part because of soft tissue shortening or bony ankylosis.

Limits of motion—The beginning and ending positions of movement at a joint.

Maximum voluntary contraction—The greatest amount of tension a muscle can generate and hold only for a moment, e.g., in muscle testing.

Passive range of motion—The amount of movement possible at a joint when the therapist moves the limb.

Reliability—Characteristic of a measuring instrument, indicating the stability of the instrument over time, between testers, and within its various parts when properly administered under similar circumstances (Johnston, Keith, & Hinderer, 1992). Reliability is usually defined by a correlation coefficient (r). An r of 1.0 indicates a perfect, linear relationship between one variable (e.g., Rater A's scores) and another variable (e.g., Rater B's scores). A coefficient of 0.85 is sought for measuring instruments. Reliability can be increased by controlling all the variables that affect the scores, other than the "real" variable (e.g., change in ROM). Control is gained by keeping everything the same, by deleting some variables.

Standard deviation—A measure of dispersion, indicating the variability within a set of scores. Low variability within a set of therapists' scores indicates that the therapists are following the same protocol and the phenomenon being measured is unchanging; high variability indicates that the phenomenon being measured is very unstable or that the therapists need to control better their test administration.

To interpret a score, the therapist often compares it with norms (averages and standard deviations). The SD informs you where your patient's score falls in relation to the norm score, because you can relate it to the normal curve. In the bell-shaped normal curve, ±1 SD is equal to approximately 68% of the area under the curve (34% on each side of the mean), ±2 SD is equal to approximately 95% of the area under the curve, and ±3 SD is equal to approximately 99% of the area under the curve. A score of 2 to 3 SD below the mean normative score indicates a limitation in need of treatment.

Tenodesis—The mechanical effect caused by the length of extrinsic finger flexors and extensors. When the wrist is flexed, the fingers tend to extend, because the extensors are too short to allow full finger flexion and wrist flexion at the same time. Similarly, when the wrist is extended, the fingers tend to flex.

---

sary to position the protractor opposite to the direction of motion so that the indicator remains on the face of the protractor. A finger goniometer is designed with a shorter movable arm and surfaces that are flat to fit comfortably over the finger joints. Figure 6.1 shows each of these types of goniometers.

When using the goniometer to measure joint motion, the therapist must take care to place the axis and the two arms to ensure accuracy and **reliability.** The axis of the goniometer is placed over the axis of joint motion, which is the point around which the motion occurs. The axis of motion for some joints coincides with bony landmarks, whereas for others it must be found by observing movement of the joint to determine the point around which motion occurs. In shoulder flexion, for example, the axis at the beginning of the motion is located approximately 1 inch below the acromion process, but at the end of the motion, the arm position has changed to the extent that the original axis position of the goniometer is no longer accurate.

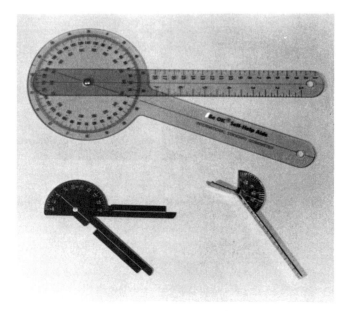

Figure 6.1.   Full-circle, half-circle, and finger goniometers.

Because it is not always possible to center the axis of the goniometer over a specific anatomical landmark, primary attention is focused on aligning the two arms of the goniometer correctly. When the two arms of the goniometer are placed correctly, they will intersect at the axis of motion (Moore, 1978). One arm is positioned parallel to the longitudinal axis of the part proximal to the joint and the other is positioned parallel to the longitudinal axis of the part distal to the joint. The tester supports both the body part and the goniometer proximally and distally to the joint, leaving the joint free to move.

In addition, accuracy and **reliability** can be influenced by patient-related and environmental factors. Patient-related factors include fear of pain, fatigue, and feelings of tension or stress. Every effort is made to make the patient physically and emotionally comfortable. Environmental variables include time of day, temperature of the room, type of goniometer used, and experience and rigor of the tester. Goniometers vary in size; large goniometers most accurately measure large joints, and small goniometers most accurately measure small joints. Goniometers should be calibrated periodically by comparing them with a standard, professional-type protractor.

Intrarater **reliability** is always higher than interrater **reliability.** In one study of shoulder motions, intrarater **reliability** ranged from 0.90 to 0.98, whereas interrater **reliability** ranged from 0.26 to 0.89 (Riddle, Rothstein, & Lamb, 1987). In a similar study of the knee, intrarater **reliability** was found to be 0.99 for flexion and 0.98 for extension, while interrater **reliability** was 0.90 and 0.86, respectively (Watkins et al., 1991). With careful adherence to technique, Horger (1990) tested interrater and intrarater **reliability** of active and passive measurement of wrist motions under clinical conditions. Intrarater **reliability** was >0.90 for the active and passive ranges; interrater **reliability** was >0.78 for the active and >0.66 for the passive range. To be reliable, original and retest measurements should be taken at the same time of day by the same person using the same kind of calibrated goniometer and technique in the same or similar setting.

RECORDING RANGE OF MOTION

Each measurement is accurately recorded on a range of motion form, which the therapist signs and dates because a medical record is a legal document. Notation is made whether scores represent AROM or PROM. A sample form is provided in Table 6.1. Any form used should allow for recording the starting and ending positions (**limits of motion**) for each movement.

The most common method of determining range of motion is the Neutral Zero Method recommended by the Committee on Joint Motion of the American Academy of Orthopaedic Surgeons (Heck, Hendryson, & Rowe, 1965). In this method, the **anatomical position** is considered to be 0, or if a given starting position is different from **anatomical position,** it is defined as 0. Measurement is taken from stated starting position to stated end position. If the patient cannot achieve the stated starting and end positions, his starting and end positions are recorded to indicate limitations in movement. An example of this, using elbow flexion, is as follows:

0 to 150°: No limitation
20 to 150°: A limitation in extension
0 to 120°: A limitation in flexion
20 to 120°: Limitations in both flexion and extension

Some therapists indicate a limitation in extension by recording the limitation negatively, for example, −20° of extension or lacks 20° of extension or −20 to 150°. On the other hand, some therapists record −20 to 150° to indicate that there are 20° of hyperextension in a joint in which hyperextension is not normally present. In the Neutral Zero Method, the term *extension* is used only for the natural motion opposite to flexion. *Hyperextension* is used only when the motion is unnatural, as is occasionally seen, for example, in the metacarpophalangeal or elbow joints. The American Academy of Orthopaedic Surgeons recommends that if 20° of hyperextension at the elbow is noted, which is an unnatural motion, it should be recorded as a separate measurement to describe fully the available range of motion without confusion and to eliminate the use of unclear negative recordings. The following notations of range would be used to describe this abnormality at the elbow:

0 to 150° of flexion
150 to 0° of extension
0 to 20° of hyperextension

In a fused joint, the starting and end positions are the same, with no range of motion. This is recorded as fused at $x°$. If a joint that normally moves in two directions is unable to be moved in one direction, the range of motion for the limited motion is recorded as *none*. For example, if wrist flexion is 15 to 80° with a 15° flexion contracture, the wrist cannot be positioned at 0 or moved into extension; therefore, wrist extension is recorded as *none*.

Because there are various systems of notations, each having its own meaning, it is important to clarify the intended meaning and to ensure consistency among therapists and physicians within the same facility.

Table 6.1. Range of Motion

Patient's Name_____
AROM_____

PROM_____

LEFT   RIGHT

		Date of Measurement			
		Tester's Name			
		SHOULDER			
		Flexion	0-180		
		Extension	0-60		
		Abduction	0-180		
		Horizontal Abduction	0-90		
		Horizontal Adduction	0-45		
		Internal Rotation	0-70		
		External Rotation	0-90		
		Internal Rotation (Alternate)	0-80		
		External Rotation (Alternate)	0-60		
		ELBOW & FOREARM			
		Flexion-Extension	0-150		
		Supination	0-80		
		Pronation	0-80		
		WRIST			
		Flexion	0-80		
		Extension	0-70		
		Ulnar Deviation	0-30		
		Radial Deviation	0-20		
		THUMB			
		CM Flexion	0-15		
		CM Extension	0-20		
		MP Flexion-Extension	0-50		
		IP Flexion-Extension	0-80		
		Abduction	cm.		
		Opposition	cm.		
		INDEX FINGER			
		MP Flexion	0-90		
		PIP Flexion-Extension	0-100		
		DIP Flexion-Extension	0-90		
		Abduction	No Norm		
		Adduction	No Norm		

Table 6.1. (continued)

LEFT   RIGHT

		Date of Measurement		
		MIDDLE FINGER		
		MP Flexion	0-90	
		PIP Flexion-Extension	0-100	
		DIP Flexion-Extension	0-90	
		Abduction (radially)	No Norm	
		Adduction (ulnarly)	No Norm	
		RING FINGER		
		MP Flexion	0-90	
		PIP Flexion-Extension	0-100	
		DIP Flexion-Extension	0-90	
		Abduction	No Norm	
		Adduction	No Norm	
		LITTLE FINGER		
		MP Flexion	0-90	
		PIP Flexion-Extension	0-100	
		DIP Flexion-Extension	0-90	
		Abduction	No Norm	
		Adduction	No Norm	

Measurement of the Upper Extremity

For the measurements given here, the patient is seated with trunk erect against the back of an armless, straight chair, although the measurements could be taken with the patient standing or supine, if necessary, unless otherwise noted.

SHOULDER FLEXION

Movement of the humerus anteriorly in the sagittal plane (0 to 180°, which represents both glenohumeral and axioscapular motion) (Figs. 6.2 and 6.3).

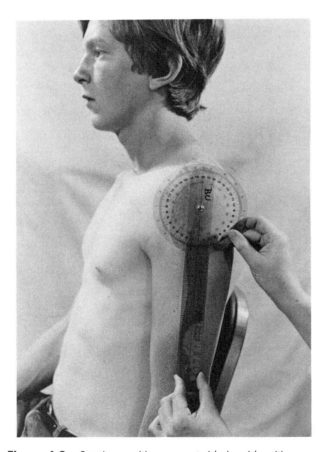

Figure 6.2. Starting position: arm at side in midposition.

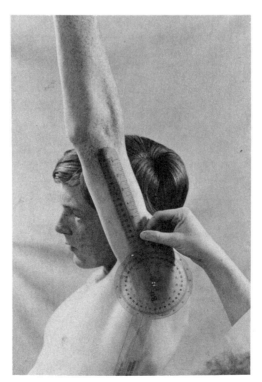

Figure 6.3. End position: arm overhead in midposition.

Goniometer Placement

Axis. A point through the lateral aspect of the glenohumeral joint around which motion occurs, located approximately 1 inch below the acromion process.

Stationary Arm. Parallel to the lateral midline of the trunk.

Movable Arm. Parallel to the longitudinal axis of the humerus on the lateral aspect.

Possible   Substitutions. Trunk   extension, shoulder abduction.

SHOULDER EXTENSION

Movement of the humerus posteriorly in a sagittal plane (0 to 60°) (Figs 6.4 and 6.5).

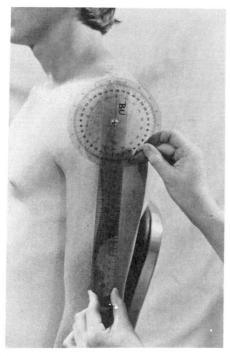

Figure 6.4. Starting position: patient seated at the edge of the chair so there is no restriction behind humerus. Arm at side in internal rotation.

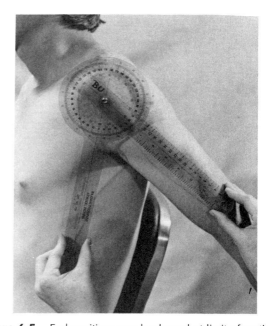

Figure 6.5. End position: arm backward at limit of motion.

Goniometer Placement

Axis. A point through the lateral aspect of the glenohumeral joint around which motion occurs, located approximately 1 inch below the acromion process.

Stationary Arm. Parallel to the lateral midline of the trunk.

Movable Arm. Parallel to the longitudinal axis of the humerus on the lateral aspect.

Possible Substitutions. Trunk flexion, scapular elevation and downward rotation, shoulder abduction.

SHOULDER ABDUCTION

Movement of the humerus laterally in a frontal plane (0 to 180°, which represents both glenohumeral and axioscapular motion) (Figs. 6.6 and 6.7).

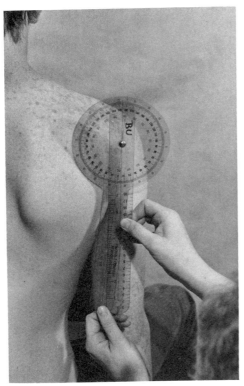

Figure 6.6. Starting position: arm at side in external rotation, which allows the humerus to clear the acromion process.

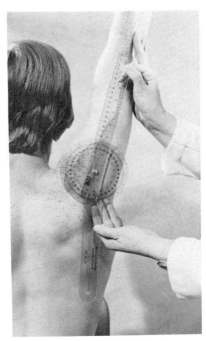

Figure 6.7. End position: arm overhead with palm facing opposite side.

Goniometer Placement

Axis. A point through the anterior or posterior aspect of the glenohumeral joint. Some people consider measurement from the anterior aspect safer, because the patient's back can be supported against the chair, but it is preferable to measure adult female patients from the posterior aspect.

Stationary Arm. Laterally along the trunk, parallel to the spine.

Movable Arm. Parallel to the longitudinal axis of the humerus.

Possible Substitutions. Lateral flexion of trunk, scapular elevation, shoulder flexion or extension.

HORIZONTAL ABDUCTION

Movement of the humerus on a horizontal plane from a position of 90° of shoulder flexion to a position of 90° of shoulder abduction and beyond to the limit of motion (0 to 90°) (Figs. 6.8 and 6.9).

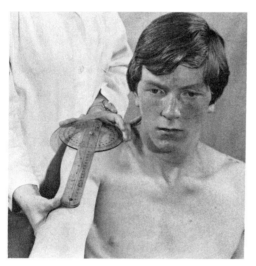

Figure 6.8.   Starting position: arm internally rotated and at 90° of shoulder flexion.

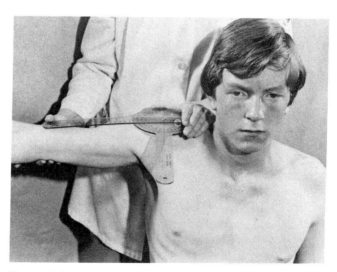

Figure 6.9.   End position: arm at 90° of shoulder abduction.

Goniometer Placement

Axis.   On top of the acromion process.

Stationary Arm.   To start, this arm is parallel to the longitudinal axis of the humerus on the superior aspect and remains in that position, perpendicular to the body, although the humerus moves away. An alternative position of the stationary arm is across the shoulder, anterior to the neck, and in line with the opposite acromion process. In this alternate position, the goniometer would read 90° at the start, and this must be considered when recording.

Movable Arm.   Parallel to the longitudinal axis of the humerus on the superior aspect.

Possible Substitution.   Trunk rotation or trunk flexion.

HORIZONTAL ADDUCTION

Movement of the humerus on a horizontal plane from a position of 90° of shoulder abduction through a position of 90° of shoulder flexion, across the trunk to the limit of motion. The 90° of return motion from horizontal abduction is not measured. The motion is measured from a position of 90° shoulder flexion across the trunk (0 to 45°) (Figs. 6.10 and 6.11).

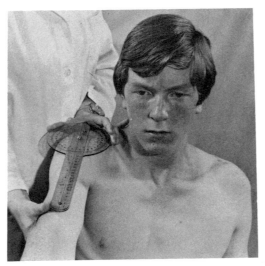

Figure 6.10. Starting position: arm internally rotated and at 90° of shoulder flexion.

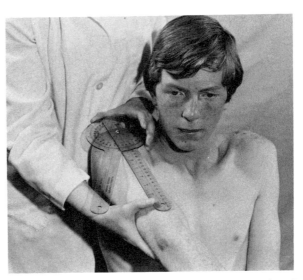

Figure 6.11. End position: arm across trunk at limit of motion.

Goniometer Placement

Axis. On top of the acromion process.

Stationary Arm. Parallel to the longitudinal axis on the superior aspect of the humerus in the starting position and remains perpendicular to the body, although the humerus moves away. The alternative placement given for horizontal abduction also applies in this case.

Movable Arm. Parallel to the longitudinal axis of the humerus on the superior aspect.

Possible Substitution. Trunk rotation.

INTERNAL ROTATION

Movement of the humerus in a medial direction around the longitudinal axis of the humerus (0 to 70°) (Figs. 6.12 and 6.13).

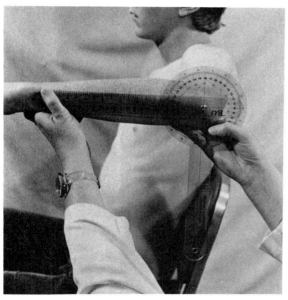

Figure 6.12. Starting position: the extremity is supported in a position of 90° of shoulder abduction and 90° of elbow flexion, with the forearm pronated and parallel to the floor.

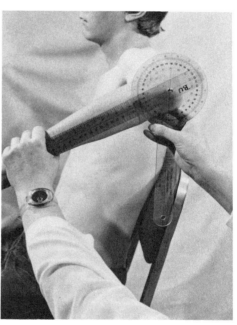

Figure 6.13. End position: the extremity is in a position of 90° of shoulder abduction and 90° of elbow flexion; forearm and hand have moved toward the floor to the limit of motion.

Goniometer Placement

Axis. Olecranon process of the ulna.

Stationary Arm. Perpendicular to the floor, which will be parallel to the lateral trunk if the patient is sitting up straight with his hips at 90°. The goniometer will read 90° at the start, and this score must be deducted from the final score when recording range of motion.

Movable Arm. Parallel to the longitudinal axis of the ulna.

Possible Substitutions. Scapular elevation and downward rotation, trunk flexion, elbow extension.

Note. In the supine position with the shoulder abducted to 90° and the elbow flexed to 90°, the stationary arm is perpendicular to the floor with the movable arm along the ulna. The goniometer will read 0° at the start (Moore, 1978).

EXTERNAL ROTATION

Movement of the humerus in a lateral direction around the longitudinal axis of the humerus (0 to 90°) (Figs. 6.14 and 6.15).

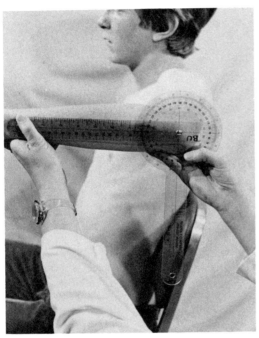

Figure 6.14. Starting position: the extremity is supported in a position of 90° of shoulder abduction and 90° of elbow flexion with the forearm pronated and parallel to the floor.

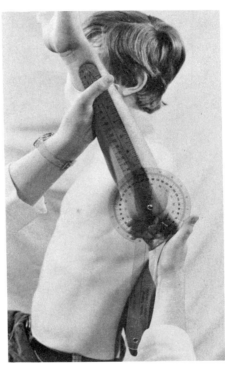

Figure 6.15. End position: the extremity is in a position of 90° of shoulder abduction and 90° of elbow flexion; forearm and hand have moved toward the ceiling to the limit of motion.

Goniometer Placement

Axis. Olecranon process of the ulna.

Stationary Arm. Perpendicular to the floor. The goniometer will read 90° at the start, and this must be considered when recording the range of motion score.

Movable Arm. Parallel to the longitudinal axis of the ulna.

Possible Substitutions. Scapular depression and upward rotation, trunk extension, elbow extension.

INTERNAL AND EXTERNAL ROTATION: ALTERNATE METHOD

If shoulder limitation prevents positioning for the previously described method, the patient may be seated with humerus adducted to the side and elbow flexed to 90° (Figs. 6.16 and 6.17). This method will be inaccurate in internal rotation if the patient has a large abdomen. (Internal rotation: 0 to 80°; external rotation: 0 to 60°).

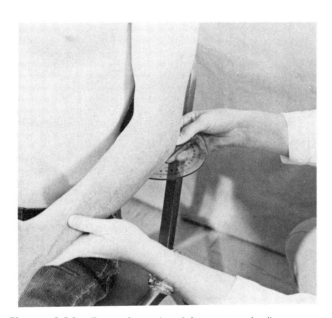

Figure 6.16. External rotation (alternate method): start position.

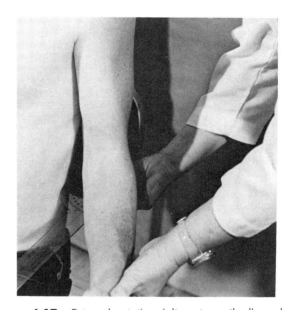

Figure 6.17. External rotation (alternate method): end position.

ELBOW FLEXION-EXTENSION

Movement of the supinated forearm anteriorly in the sagittal plane (0 to 150°) (Figs. 6.18 and 6.19).

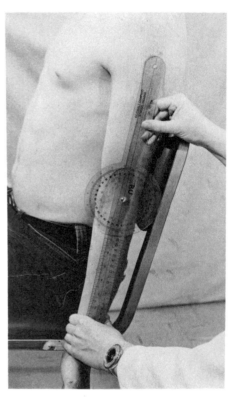

Figure 6.18. Starting position: arm in anatomical position. This measurement is recorded as the limit of extension.

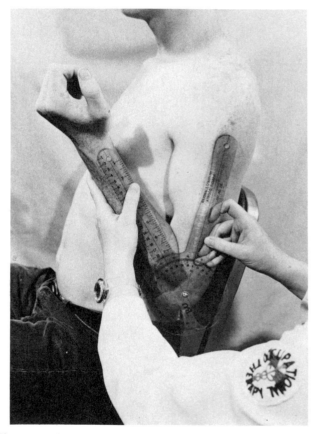

Figure 6.19. End position: forearm has moved toward the humerus so that the hand approximates the shoulder to the limit of motion of elbow flexion.

Goniometer Placement

Axis.   Lateral epicondyle of the humerus.

Stationary Arm.   Parallel to the longitudinal axis of the humerus on the lateral aspect.

Movable Arm.   Parallel to the longitudinal axis of the radius.

FOREARM SUPINATION

Rotation of the forearm laterally around its longitudinal axis from midposition so that the hand faces up (0 to 80°) (Figs. 6.20 and 6.21).

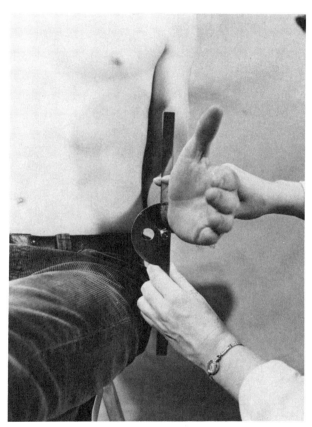

Figure 6.20. Starting position: humerus adducted to the side and elbow flexed to 90° with the forearm in midposition.

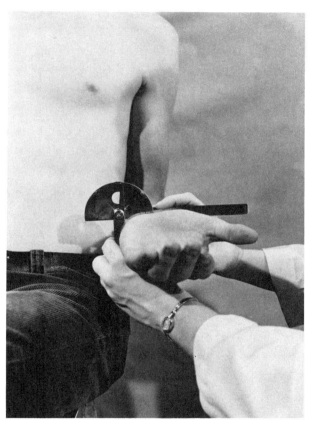

Figure 6.21. End position: forearm rotated so that the palm faces up.

Goniometer Placement

Axis. Longitudinal axis of the forearm displaced toward the ulnar side.

Stationary Arm. Perpendicular to the floor.

Movable Arm. Across the distal radius and ulna on the volar surface.

Possible Substitutions. Adduction and external rotation of the shoulder.

FOREARM PRONATION

Rotation of the forearm medially around its longitudinal axis from midposition (0 to 80°) (Figs. 6.22 and 6.23).

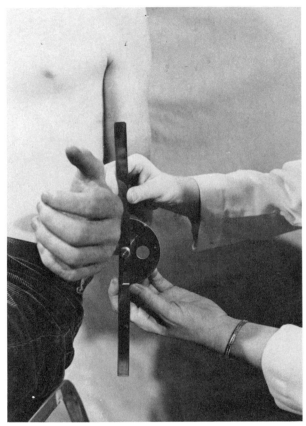

Figure 6.22. Starting position: humerus adducted to the side and elbow flexed to 90° with the forearm in midposition.

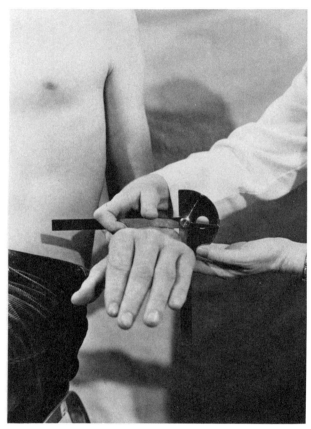

Figure 6.23. End position: forearm rotated so that the palm faces down.

Goniometer Placement

Axis. Longitudinal axis of forearm displaced toward the ulnar side.

Stationary Arm. Perpendicular to the floor.

Movable Arm. Across the distal radius and ulna on the dorsal surface.

Possible Substitutions. Abduction and internal rotation of the shoulder.

WRIST FLEXION (VOLAR FLEXION)

Movement of the hand volarly in the sagittal plane (0 to 80°) (Figs. 6.24 and 6.25).

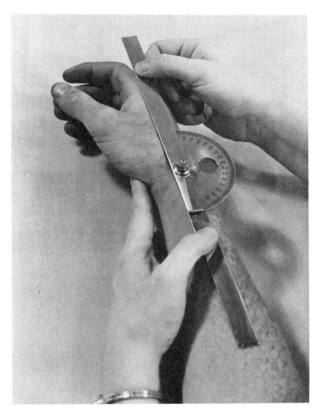

Figure 6.24. Starting position: forearm rests on the table in midposition; wrist is in neutral position. The fingers are slightly extended or relaxed to eliminate the error that could occur as a result of the tenodesis effect; the finger extensor tendons are too short to allow full wrist flexion with full finger flexion.

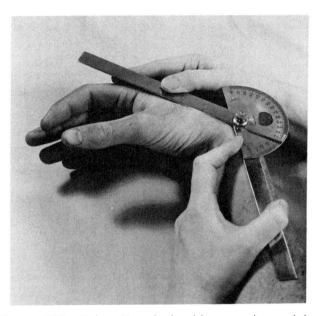

Figure 6.25. End position: the hand has moved toward the volar forearm to the limit of motion.

Goniometer Placement

Axis. Over the styloid process of the radius, which is located on the lateral aspect of the wrist at the anatomical snuff box, the indentation between the tendons of the extensor pollicis longus and the extensor pollicis brevis.

Stationary Arm. Parallel to the longitudinal axis of the radius.

Movable Arm. Parallel to the longitudinal axis of the second metacarpal.

WRIST EXTENSION (DORSIFLEXION)

Movement of the hand dorsally in the sagittal plane (0 to 70°) (Figs. 6.26 and 6.27).

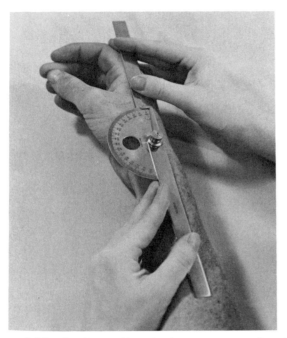

Figure 6.26. Starting position: the forearm rests on the table in midposition. The wrist is in neutral position. The fingers should be slightly flexed or relaxed to eliminate the error that could occur because the finger flexor tendons are too short to allow full wrist extension with full finger extension.

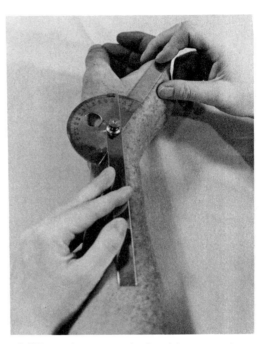

Figure 6.27. End position: the hand has moved toward the dorsal forearm to the limit of motion.

Goniometer Placement

Axis. Over the styloid process of the radius.

One Arm. Parallel to the longitudinal axis of the radius.

Other Arm. Parallel to the longitudinal axis of the second metacarpal.

WRIST ULNAR DEVIATION

Movement of the hand toward the ulnar side in a frontal plane (0 to 30°) (Figs. 6.28 and 6.29).

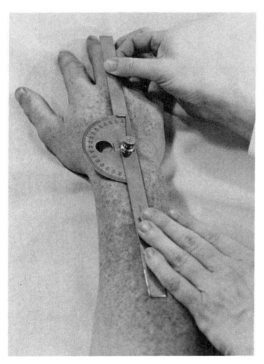

Figure 6.28. Starting position: the forearm is pronated with the volar surface of the forearm and palm resting lightly on the table. The wrist is in neutral position, with fingers relaxed.

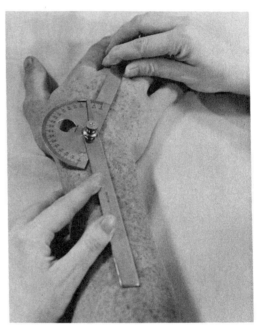

Figure 6.29. End position: the hand has moved so that the little finger approximates the ulna to the limit of motion.

Goniometer Placement

Axis. On the dorsal aspect of the wrist joint in line with the base of the third metacarpal.

One Arm. Along the midline of the forearm on the dorsal surface.

Other Arm. Along the midline of the third metacarpal.

Possible Substitutions. Wrist extension, wrist flexion.

WRIST RADIAL DEVIATION

Movement of the hand toward the radial side in a frontal plane (0 to 20°) (Figs. 6.30 and 6.31).

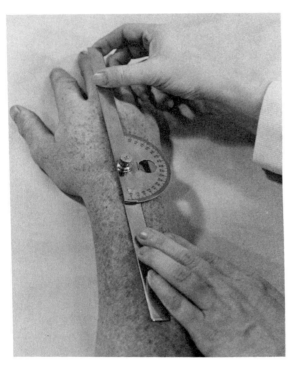

Figure 6.30. Starting position: the forearm is pronated, with the volar surface of the forearm and the palm resting lightly on the table. The wrist is in neutral position, with fingers relaxed.

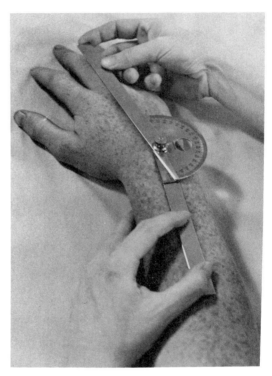

Figure 6.31. End position: the hand has moved so that the thumb approximates the radius to the limit of motion.

Goniometer Placement

Axis.   On the dorsal aspect of the wrist joint in line with the base of the third metacarpal.

Stationary Arm.   Along the midline of the forearm on the dorsal surface.

Movable Arm.   Along the midline of the third metacarpal.

Possible Substitution.   Wrist extension.

THUMB CARPOMETACARPAL FLEXION

Movement of the thumb across the palm in the frontal plane (0 to 15°) (Figs. 6.32 and 6.33).

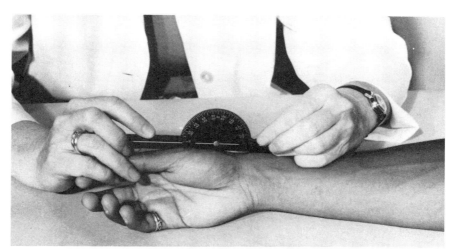

Figure 6.32. Starting position: the wrist is in neutral or slight ulnar deviation to align the second metacarpal and the radius. The carpometacarpal joint is in neutral position, with the thumb next to the volar surface of the index finger.

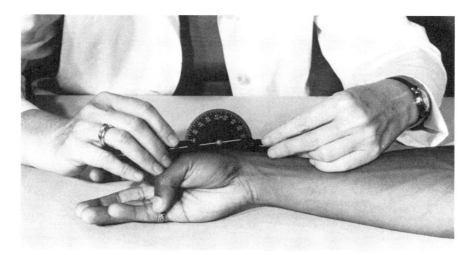

Figure 6.33. End position: the thumb has moved across the plane of the palm toward the ulnar side to the limit of motion in flexion.

Goniometer Placement

Axis. On the radial side of the wrist at the junction of the base of the first metacarpal and the trapezium.

Stationary Arm. Parallel to the longitudinal axis of the radius.

Movable Arm. Parallel to the longitudinal axis of the first metacarpal.

Note. For accuracy, the arms of the goniometer must remain in full contact with skin surface over the bones. However, excessive pressure with the edge of a half-circle goniometer must be avoided. These statements apply to all flexion-extension measurements of the thumb and fingers.

THUMB CARPOMETACARPAL
EXTENSION

Movement of the thumb away from the palm in the frontal plane (0 to 20°) (Figs. 6.34 and 6.35).

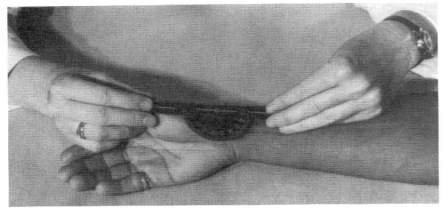

Figure 6.34. Starting position: the wrist is in neutral position or slight ulnar deviation to align the second metacarpal and the radius. The carpometacarpal joint is in neutral position with the thumb next to the volar surface of the index finger.

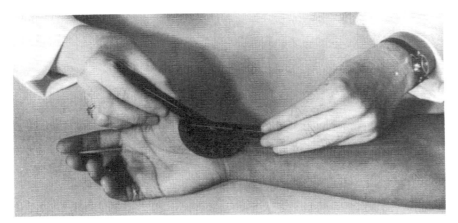

Figure 6.35. End position: the thumb has moved into full extension away from the palm toward the radial side to the limit of motion in extension.

Goniometer Placement

Axis. On the volar side of the wrist at the junction of the base of the first metacarpal and the trapezium.

One Arm. Parallel to the longitudinal axis of the radius.

Other Arm. Parallel to the longitudinal axis of the first metacarpal.

THUMB METACARPOPHALANGEAL (MP) FLEXION-EXTENSION

Movement of the thumb across the palm in the frontal plane (0 to 50°) (Figs. 6.36 and 6.37).

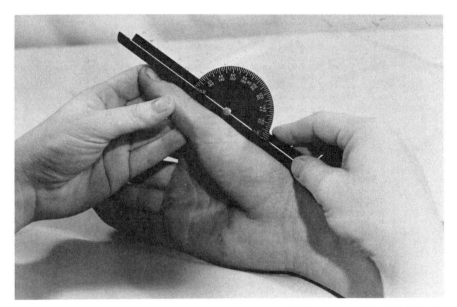

Figure 6.36. Starting position: the wrist is in neutral position or slight extension. The MP joint is in extension.

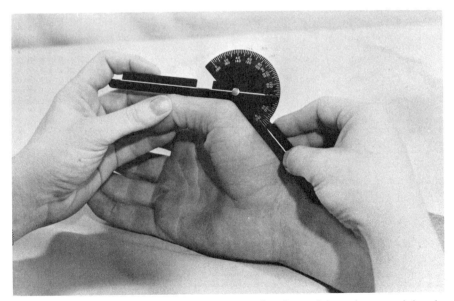

Figure 6.37. End position: the thumb has moved across the plane of the palm toward the ulnar side of the hand to the limit of motion in flexion.

Goniometer Placement

Axis. On the dorsal aspect of the MP joint.

Stationary Arm. On the dorsal surface, along the midline of the first metacarpal.

Movable Arm. On the dorsal surface, along the midline of the proximal phalanx of the thumb.

THUMB INTERPHALANGEAL (IP) FLEXION-EXTENSION

Movement of the distal phalanx of the thumb toward the volar surface of the proximal phalanx of the thumb (0 to 80°) (Figs. 6.38 and 6.39).

Figure 6.38. Starting position: the wrist is in neutral position or slight extension. The IP joint is in extension.

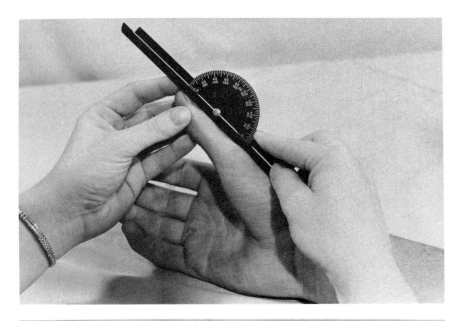

Figure 6.39. End position: the volar surface of the distal phalanx approximates the volar surface of the proximal phalanx to the limit of motion in flexion.

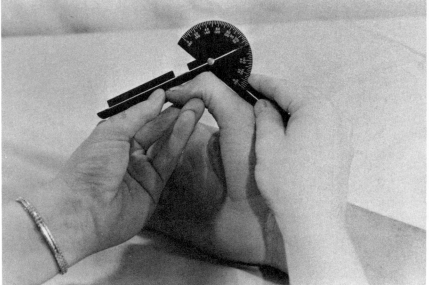

Goniometer Placement

Axis.   On the dorsal aspect of the IP joint.
Stationary Arm.   On the dorsal surface, along the proximal phalanx.

Movable Arm.   On the dorsal surface, along the distal phalanx.

Note.   If the thumbnail prevents full goniometer contact, shift the movable arm laterally to increase accuracy.

Alternate Goniometer Placement

Thumb MP and IP flexion-extension can be measured on the lateral aspect of the thumb, using lateral aspects of the same landmarks.

THUMB ABDUCTION AND OPPOSITION: RULER MEASUREMENTS

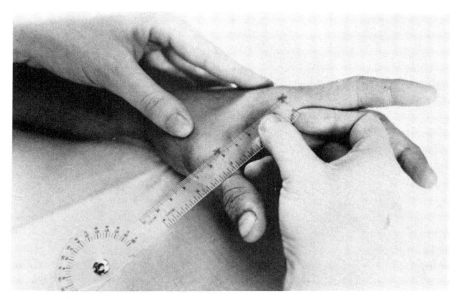

Figure 6.40.   Thumb abduction: ruler measurement of web space.

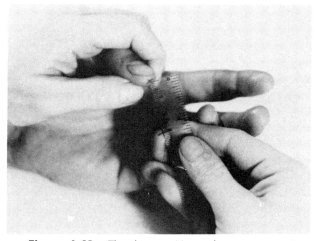

Figure 6.41.   Thumb opposition: ruler measurement.

Abduction.   Take the measurement from the midpoint of the head of the first metacarpal to the midpoint of the head of the second metacarpal while the thumb is in full abduction (Fig. 6.40).

Opposition.   Rotary movement of the thumb to approximate the pad of the thumb to pads of the fingers. Normally, a person can oppose to each of the fingers. Measure the distance from the tip of the thumb (not the thumbnail) to the tip end of the little finger to record any deficit of opposition (Fig. 6.41).

FINGER METACARPOPHALANGEAL
FLEXION-EXTENSION

Movement of the finger at the MP joint in a sagittal plane (0 to 90°) (Figs. 6.42 and 6.43).

Figure 6.42. Starting position: the wrist is in neutral position or slight hyperextension. The MP joint is in extension.

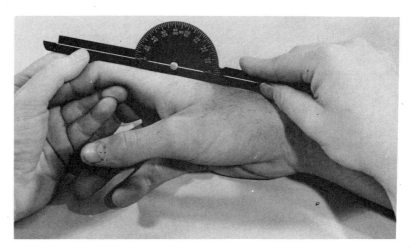

Figure 6.43. End position: the volar surface of the proximal phalanx approximates the palm to the limit of motion of flexion.

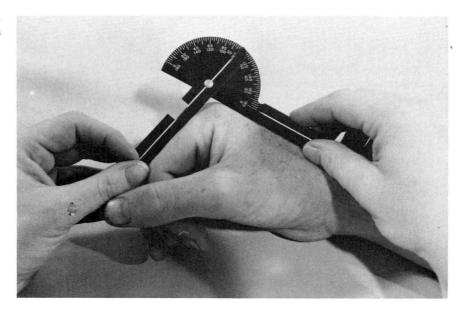

Goniometer Placement

Axis. On the dorsal aspect of the MP joint of the finger being measured.

Stationary Arm. On the dorsal surface along the midline of the metacarpal of the finger being measured.

Movable Arm. On the dorsal surface along the midline of the proximal phalanx of the finger being measured.

FINGER PROXIMAL INTERPHALANGEAL (PIP) FLEXION-EXTENSION

Movement of the middle phalanx toward the volar surface of the proximal phalanx in the sagittal plane (0 to 100°) (Figs. 6.44 and 6.45).

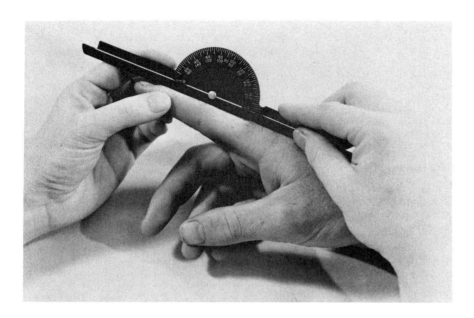

Figure 6.44. Starting position: the wrist is in neutral position or slight hyperextension. The PIP joint is in extension.

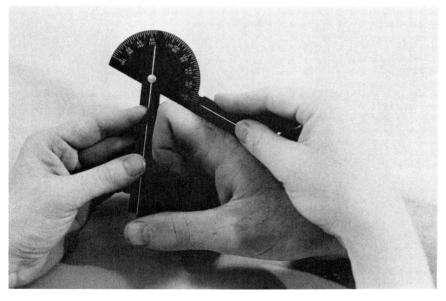

Figure 6.45. End position: the volar surface of the middle phalanx approximates the volar surface of the proximal phalanx to the limit of motion in flexion.

Goniometer Placement

Axis. On the dorsal aspect of the PIP joint of the finger being measured.

Stationary Arm. On the dorsal surface along the midline of the proximal phalanx of the finger being measured.

Movable Arm. On dorsal surface along the midline of the middle phalanx of the finger being measured.

FINGER DISTAL INTERPHALANGEAL (DIP) FLEXION-EXTENSION

Movement of the distal phalanx toward the volar surface of the middle phalanx in a sagittal plane (0 to 90°) (Figs. 6.46 and 6.47).

Figure 6.46. Starting position: the wrist is in neutral position or slight hyperextension. The DIP joint is in extension.

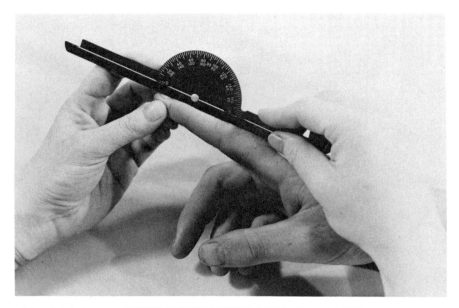

Figure 6.47. End position: the volar surface of the distal phalanx approximates the volar surface of the middle phalanx to the limit of motion in flexion. The PIP joint should flex to permit full DIP flexion.

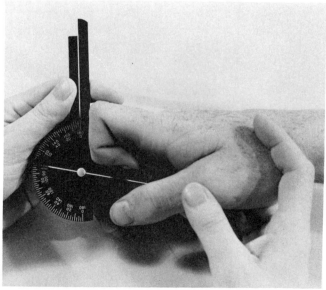

Goniometer Placement

Axis. On the dorsal aspect of the DIP joint of the finger being measured.

Stationary Arm. On the dorsal surface along the midline of the middle phalanx of the finger being measured.

Movable Arm. On the dorsal surface along the midline of the distal phalanx of the finger being measured.

Note. If the fingernail prevents full goniometer contact, shift the movable arm laterally to increase accuracy.

Alternate Goniometer Placement

Finger PIP and DIP flexion-extension can be measured from the lateral aspect of each finger, using the lateral aspect of the same landmarks. This method may be more accurate when joints are enlarged.

MEASUREMENT OF TOTAL FINGER FLEXION

PIP and DIP Flexion

Using a centimeter ruler, measure from the tip of the finger to the distal palmar crease (Fig. 6.48).

MP, PIP, and DIP Flexion

Using a centimeter ruler, measure from the tip of the finger to the base of the palm (Moore, 1978) (Fig. 6.49). An alternate, more comprehensive, method of measuring composite digital motion is to sum the values for the MP, PIP, and DIP joints, taking into consideration both flexion and extension deficits (Fess, 1990). Total active motion (TAM) or total passive motion (TPM) can then be expressed by a single number. The formula for calculating these values is as follows:

$$(MP + PIP + DIP \ \text{flexion}) - (MP + PIP + DIP \ \text{extension deficits}) = TAM \ \text{or} \ TPM$$

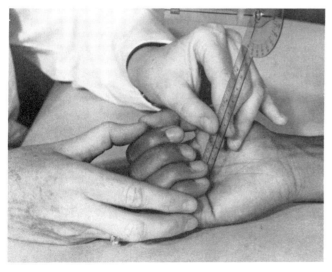

Figure 6.48. PIP and DIP flexion: ruler measurement.

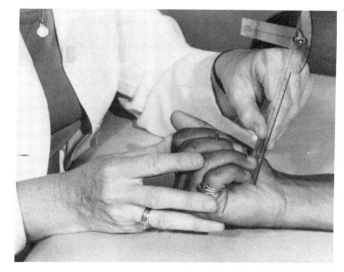

Figure 6.49. MP, PIP, and DIP flexion: ruler measurement.

FINGER ABDUCTION

Movement of the index, ring, and little fingers away from the midline of the hand in a frontal plane. The middle finger, which is the midline of the hand, abducts in both radial and ulnar directions (Figs. 6.50 and 6.51).

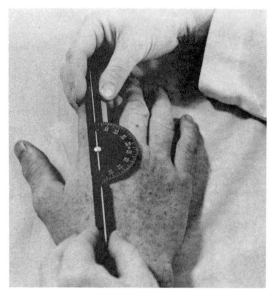

Figure 6.50. Starting position: the volar surface of the forearm and palm are resting lightly on a table. The metacarpal and the proximal phalanx of the finger being measured should be in a straight line.

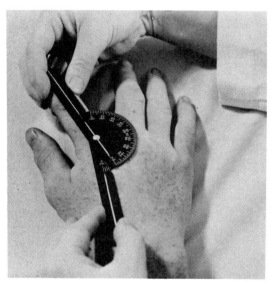

Figure 6.51. End position: the finger has moved away from the midposition to the limit of motion.

Goniometer Placement

Axis. On the dorsal aspect of the MP joint of the finger being measured.

Stationary Arm. Along the dorsal surface of the metacarpal of the finger being measured.

Movable Arm. Along the dorsal surface of the proximal phalanx of the finger being measured.

FINGER ADDUCTION

Movement of the index, ring, and little fingers toward the midline of the hand in a frontal plane (Figs. 6.52 and 6.53).

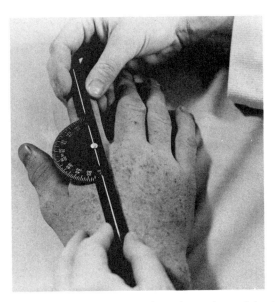

Figure 6.52. Starting position: the volar surface of the fore-arm and palm are resting lightly on a table. The metacarpal and the proximal phalanx of the finger being measured should be in a straight line.

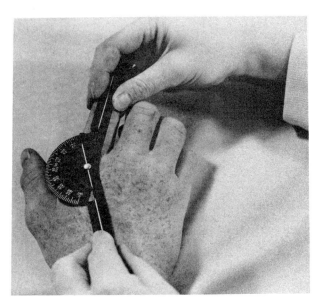

Figure 6.53. End position: the finger has moved toward the middle finger to the limit of motion. Move adjacent fingers out of the way if necessary to allow full excursion of movement.

Goniometer Placement

Axis. On the dorsal aspect of the MP joint of the finger being measured.

One Arm. Along the dorsal surface of the meta-carpal of the finger being measured. The middle finger is not measured.

Other Arm. Along the dorsal surface of the proximal phalanx of the finger being measured.

MP DEVIATION CORRECTION MEASUREMENT

When there is ulnar deviation deformity of the metacarpophalangeal joints, often seen in rheumatoid arthritis, this additional measurement is taken (Figs. 6.54 and 6.55).

Figure 6.54. Starting position: the hand and forearm rest pronated on a flat surface. The finger is in the position of ulnar deviation in which the finger normally lies.

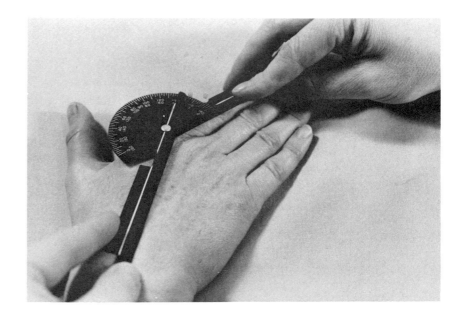

Figure 6.55. End position: radial deviation of the finger.

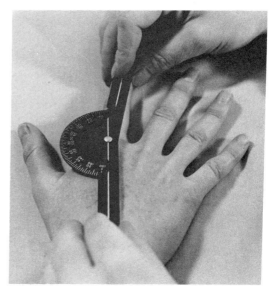

Goniometer Placement

Axis.   Over the MP joint of the finger being measured.

One Arm.   Placed along the dorsal midline of the metacarpal.

Other Arm.   Placed along the dorsal midline of the proximal phalanx.

The active range is compared with the passive range to determine if muscle weakness is present. Passive range of motion is compared with the norm of 0° deviation to determine if a fixed deformity exists.

INTERPRETING THE RESULTS

Limits of motion are compared with the noninvolved extremity or to average limits (norms) expected for each motion. The average limits that have been stated by the Committee on Joint Motion (Heck et al., 1965) are commonly used and are included here. However, patients may be functional with less range of motion than is noted in the norms for particular joints.

The initial evaluation is interpreted by reviewing the recording form to identify which joints have significant limitation. A significant limitation is one that decreases function or may lead to a deformity. Some causes of limitations are joint disease or injury, edema, pain, spasticity, skin tightness or scarring, muscle and tendon shortening caused by immobilization, muscle weakness, or excess adipose tissue. The therapist notes whether the limitation is the result of tissue changes (PROM < norms) or muscle weakness (AROM > PROM).

With the significant limitations and probable cause in mind, treatment goals that reflect the identified problem can be developed. For example, if skin, joint, and/or muscle tissues have become shortened as a result of immobilization, the goal will be to increase range through stretching these tissues. If the limitation is caused by edema, pain, spasticity, or muscle weakness, the primary goal would be to reduce or correct the underlying problem, and the secondary goal would be to prevent loss of range of motion caused by the immobility imposed by the primary condition. If the cause were bony ankylosis or long-standing **contracture,** the goal would be to teach the patient methods of compensation, since these conditions do not respond to nonsurgical treatment.

Interpretation of a reevaluation that shows improvement has occurred following treatment must be tempered with the realization of changes that could occur simply as a result of remeasurement. According to Boone et al. (1978), for a change in range of motion to be considered "true," the amount of change must exceed measurement error, which was found to be 5° for the upper extremity and 6° for the lower extremity. Horger (1990) found similar values for wrist motion. If in a reevaluation the patient has shown an increase of 10° in shoulder flexion, for example, that is a minimal improvement since only 5° of that can be considered a real change.

OTHER METHODS USED TO RECORD RANGE OF MOTION

Measuring Cone for Thumb Abduction-Extension

A yarn cone can be adapted to assess the first web space of burned hands (Schwanholt & Stern, 1984). The measurement represents the diameter around which the thumb and index finger can be positioned passively. No norms exist; it is used to compare the patient's progress from one time to another.

Torque-Angle Range of Motion

Torque-angle range of motion is used to achieve more exact conditions when measuring **passive range of motion** of one or more finger joints (Breger-Lee, 1990; Fess, 1990). A series of increasing weights (e.g., 100 g, 150 g, 200 g, etc.) are suspended at a 90° angle from the part distal to the joint being measured. The joint angle is measured after each change of weight. The results are graphed by angle versus weight, to allow visualization of the give in a stiff joint. The pretreatment graph may be compared with the posttreatment graph to document improvement.

EPM-ROM Scale

The Escola Paulista de Medicina (EPM)-ROM scale is under development to measure outcome of treatment of patients with rheumatoid arthritis (RA) (Bosi Ferraz et al., 1990). This instrument evaluates 10 movements important for function: elbow flexion and extension; wrist flexion and extension; thumb abduction and IP flexion; average MP flexion; hip flexion; knee extension; and ankle extension. The score for each motion ranges from 0 (full movement) to 3 (severe limitation). The decision regarding limitation is made based on whether the person has the minimal ROM required to do a particular activity of daily living, for example, putting on shoes and washing the face or hair. Intrarater **reliability,** based on measuring 35 RA patients 5 days apart, was fairly good ($r = 0.775$), but interrater **reliability** was less ($r = 0.69$).

Electrogoniometer

An electrogoniometer is a device that electronically measures the position of a joint or joints to which it is applied. Most electrogoniometers (elgons) use an electronic component called a potentiometer whose resistance changes with changes in position so that a voltage proportional to the angle of the joint is produced and recorded. There are two types of elgons (Fig. 6.56). One is a hinge type that is aligned with the joint to be measured similarly to the way the manual universal goniometer is aligned. In this type, the potentiometer is located at the axis of motion. The other type is a parallelogram linkage elgon used to measure the motion of the fingers and wrists in which the goniometer is placed on top of the joint. In this type, the potentiometer is located a distance from the joint and tracks the motion at the joint via the linkage.

The degrees of change can be measured from the record, based on **calibration** of the instrument. Elgons precisely measure change in exact limits of motion over the course of one treatment session, if they remain in place; however, removal and replacement decreases the accuracy of repeated measures of limits of motion, although changes in range of motion from treatment to treatment can be compared to document progress. Formerly only a research device, an elgon for the elbow or knee joints is an optional feature of at least one computerized biofeedback instrument (ORION by Self-Regulations Systems of Redmond, Washington).

Fluid Goniometer

The fluid goniometer works on the principle of a carpenter's level. The fluid is contained in a circular chamber that has a 360° scale. It is placed on the surface of the part that will move (e.g., the forearm) to measure the change in joint angle (e.g., the elbow). The scale is reset to 0 at the start position. It would

be important to place the fluid goniometer exactly for repeated measurements. In a study of active elbow range of motion, the intertester **reliability** was reported to be 0.92 for the fluid goniometer, while the value for the universal goniometer was 0.53. This indicates that the instruments cannot be used interchangeably. One drawback of the fluid goniometer is that it must be used perpendicular to gravity, which requires change of patient position, and another is that it is too big to be used for small joints (Petherick et al., 1988).

Photography

Photography was found to be more accurate than standard goniometry for measuring PROM of the elbow joint (Fish & Wingate, 1985). A single-lens reflex camera was mounted on a tripod 2.5 m (8 feet) lateral to the elbow joint at the level of the epicondyle to prevent perspective error. Landmarks (midpoint of acromion process, lateral epicondyle of the humerus, and capitate depression at the wrist) were marked with adhesive disks. To analyze the data, the film transparencies were projected directly onto a digitizer, and the angles were computed to 0.1°.

Polaroid is developing HEALTHCAM, a camera that is calibrated for certain distances to allow measurement of what has been photographed. Grid film also has been developed that would assist in estimating range of motion. The use of the camera for ROM measurements has not been standardized or validated yet, but it is a potential tool for the future.

EDEMA

Edema, one cause of limited range of motion, is quantified using circumferential or volumetric measurements. A millimeter tape measure is used to measure the circumference of a body part not easily submersed. Care must be taken to measure at exactly the same place from test to test.

Volumetric measures document changes in the mass of a body part by use of the technique of water displacement. It is most often used to measure hand edema. A water vessel that is large enough to allow submersion of the whole hand up to a given point on the wrist is used. It has a spillover spout near the top of the water level. When the hand is placed in the vessel, water is displaced and spills out into a graduated beaker. An edematous hand will displace more water than a nonedematous hand so that a lower reading is considered an improvement. A study done to determine the ability of therapists to orient the extremity consistently within the measuring device and to mea-

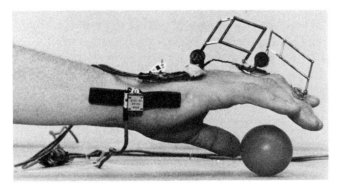

Figure 6.56. Hinge electrogoniometer placed to measure wrist flexion-extension and electrogoniometer with parallelogram linkage to measure MP and PIP flexion-extension.

sure the displaced water correctly indicated high reliability over three repeated tests on 24 hands (DeVore & Hamilton, 1968). Sitting or standing position significantly affects the score of volumetric measurement; 5.3 mL less volume was seen for the sitting position. It would be important, for that reason, to use a standardized administration procedure. Test-retest correlations of both postures were acceptable ($r = 0.91$ to 0.99) (Stern, 1991).

To interpret findings, the measurement of the affected part is compared with its contralateral counterpart to determine the extent of the edema. If edema is present, the short-term goal of treatment may be stated, for example, "to decrease edema more than 15 mL," which is slightly more than the identified within-patient variance of 10 mL (Waylett & Seibly, 1981) or "to reduce measurement by x mL."

MUSCLE STRENGTH

Muscle strength has been defined "as the capacity of a muscle to produce the tension necessary for maintaining posture, initiating movement, or controlling movement during conditions of loading on the musculoskeletal system" (Smidt & Rogers, 1982, p. 1283). Weakness is defined as a lack or reduction of this tension-producing capacity of a muscle or muscle group. When weakness limits function, it is necessary to determine the degree and distribution of the weakness. In some cases, such as Landry-Guillain-Barré syndrome, weakness will be generalized, and therefore, testing will be extensive. In other cases, such as a peripheral nerve injury, weakness will be limited to muscles innervated by the damaged nerve, and muscle testing will usually involve only these muscles. In other words, the therapist tests those muscles that are involved and toward which treatment will be directed. *If you treat it, measure it.*

The commonly measured index to assess strength is maximum tension production under voluntary effort (Darling, 1971), or **maximum voluntary contraction (MVC).** Because muscle testing is a measurement of voluntary contraction of an isolated muscle or muscle group, strength testing is inappropriate for patients who lack the ability to contract one muscle or a muscle group in isolation.

Muscle testing can be performed as a "break" test or a "make" test (Smidt & Rogers, 1982). In the *break test*, the limb is positioned so the muscle to be tested is at its greatest mechanical advantage, and the patient is asked to hold the position as the tester imparts an external force to overcome the contractile force of the muscle or muscle group using either his

hand alone or a hand-held dynamometer. In other words, the therapist tries to break the patient's isometric contraction. In the *make test*, the body segment moves through range. As it moves, it applies force against the therapist's counterresistance. Tension is estimated by the therapist or registered by the dynamometer. Changes in velocity of movement from one test to another can affect the outcome of this method.

The term *mechanical advantage* refers to the length/tension relationship of a muscle. Total tension of a muscle is the sum of the passive tension exerted by the elastic components in the lengthened muscle and surrounding tissue and the active tension generated by the contractile elements of the contracting muscle (Gowitzke & Milner, 1980). A muscle is able to generate its greatest total tension or sustain the heaviest load when positioned at a length that gives it optimal mechanical advantage. This is usually slightly (10%) longer than resting length. Developed (active) tension, which is total tension minus the elastic contribution, is greatest at resting length but decreases as the muscle is shortened or lengthened. The length/tension principle is used to elicit the best response from prime movers during muscle testing. Synergist muscles are placed at mechanical disadvantage (either lengthened or shortened) while the prime mover is asked to resist the applied force (Howell et al., 1989).

For those muscles or muscle groups too weak to resist an outside force, muscle strength is evaluated by isotonic contraction in which the muscle is required to move the mass of the body part against gravity without applied resistance or with the effect of gravity decreased (Daniels & Worthingham, 1986; Kendall, Kendall, & Wadsworth, 1971).

Reliability is essential for meaningful evaluation. Of greatest importance to the **reliability** of the scores of repeated tests is the strict adherence to the exact procedures of muscle testing. In addition, **reliability** of muscle testing scores is affected by the interest and cooperation of the patient as well as the experience and the tone of voice of the tester (Johannson, Kent, & Shepard, 1983), the ambient temperature, the temperature of the limb, distractions to the patient or tester, and other environmental conditions (Salter, 1958). Other factors known to affect outcome are ability to understand directions, posture, fatigue, and therapists' operational definitions of various grades. To increase **reliability,** these variables need to be controlled as much as possible from test to test and among therapists at the same facility. It is necessary for the therapist to develop a kinesthetic sense of what the "normal" strength for each muscle feels like. To develop a kinesthetic sense of normal, a student therapist must test many able-bodied people. Normal strength of each muscle varies according to a person's age, sex, size, body type, and occupation. When first beginning to test persons with muscle weakness, inexperienced therapists can learn the kinesthetic definitions of minimal, moderate, and maximal resistances from experienced therapists by each testing the same patient and discussing the grade to be assigned. To quantify good to normal strength of large muscle groups in a more objective way, a handheld dynamometer can be used (Bohannon, 1986). The patient pushes against the plate and piston of the dynamometer, and the therapist offers the opposing force, which must be stronger than the patient's effort. This method was found to have >.84 test-retest **reliability** when done by an experienced therapist.

MANUAL MUSCLE TESTING PROCEDURES

The method of evaluation of muscle strength presented here is the break test. Gravity as resistance is considered an important variable and is used to test all motions when practical and possible, including supination and pronation as well as motions of the fingers and toes. Standard procedures for evaluation against gravity and with gravity eliminated are described in this chapter. However, when no gravity-eliminated position was found in the literature, one was devised. Tests of the upper and lower extremities described here are, for the most part, motion tests for the purpose of evaluating strength in terms of ability to perform functionally. Tests of individual muscles in the wrist and hand are included, because of the responsibility occupational therapists have in rehabilitation of hand injuries.

The movements of head, neck, trunk, toes, leg rotation, leg abduction, and leg adduction have not been included here, because it is usually the responsibility of the physical therapist to treat this musculature in preparation for mobility and ambulation training.

The therapist moves each of the patient's joints through passive range of motion to estimate what range of motion is available at each joint. The available range is considered to be "full range of motion" for the purposes of muscle testing. However, notation is made that a limitation exists if it does.

The muscle or muscle group is assigned a grade, according to the amount of resistance it can take. Two grading systems are presented here; Table 6.2 equates the Medical Research Council (1976) (Oxford) system to the letter-grading system (Daniels & Worthingham, 1986). Each member of a particular department should learn and use the same muscle grading system. To

make this evaluation as reliable as possible, standardized procedures must be used.

1. The test procedure should be *clearly explained* and each test motion described and demonstrated to the patient. Consistency of verbal instructions is very important (Smidt & Rogers, 1982).

2. Fatigue differs for each person and each muscle; in general, however, a *rest of 2 min* between maximum effort of the same muscle is considered adequate (Caldwell et al., 1974; Milner-Brown, Mellenthin, & Miller, 1986).

3. The patient is *positioned* so that the direction of movement will be against gravity or will negate the pull of gravity (gravity eliminated) as appropriate to the strength of the muscle. As a consideration for the patient's comfort, all testing is done in one position before changing to another position. Position of head, neck and proximal parts are usually kept the same from test to test, although preliminary study results indicate that this does not affect tension development (Anderson & Bohannon, 1991; Bohannon, Warren, & Cogman, 1991).

4. For efficient movement of the part distal to the joint and to ensure isolation of the muscle or muscle group being tested, the proximal attachment must be *stabilized* (Smidt & Rogers, 1982). For weak patients, the therapist must provide this stability but must avoid placing hands over the muscles that are contracting. The supporting surface, e.g., plinth, may be used to provide stabilization for some muscles.

5. The prime movers are *palpated* to ascertain that they are functioning during the motion. Palpation is, in fact, the basis for assigning a trace grade. To palpate a muscle, the therapist places her finger pads firmly but lightly over the belly or tendon of the patient's muscle. It is sometimes necessary to have the patient try to do the motion, then relax, which causes the muscle alternately to tense and relax and allows verification that the correct muscle is being palpated.

6. *Resistance* is applied on the distal end of the moving bone i.e., the bone into which the muscle inserts. If resistance is applied at any other point, the lever arm is lengthened or shortened and, therefore, the amount of resistance is changed. For the break test, resistance is applied in a direction opposite to the motion after the patient has completed the motion (Daniels & Worthingham, 1986). The resistance should be applied as close to perpendicular as possible (Smidt & Rogers, 1982).

7. Gravity and/or synergistic muscles may substitute to cause the motion. Careful palpation and observation can identify these *substitutions* and the patient can be repositioned to eliminate them.

Table 6.2. Muscle Testing Grading Systems: Numerical Scale Equated with Letter Grading System

5	Normal	N	=	The part moves through full range of motion against maximum resistance and gravity. *Normal* differs for each muscle group and in persons of different ages, sex, and occupation.
4	Good	G	=	The part moves through full range of motion against gravity and moderate resistance.
	Good minus	G−	=	The part moves through full range of motion against gravity and less-than-moderate resistance.
	Fair plus	F+	=	The part moves through full range of motion against gravity, takes minimal resistance, and then breaks (i.e., relaxes suddenly).
3	Fair	F	=	The part moves through full range of motion against gravity with no added resistance.
	Fair minus	F−	=	The part moves less-than-full range of motion against gravity.
	Poor plus	P+	=	The part moves through full range of motion on a gravity-eliminated plane, takes minimal resistance, and then breaks.
2	Poor	P	=	The part moves through full range of motion on a gravity-eliminated plane, with no added resistance.
	Poor minus	P−	=	The part moves less-than-full range of motion on a gravity-eliminated plane.
1	Trace	T	=	Tension is palpated in the muscle or the tendon but no motion occurs at the joint.
0	Zero	0	=	No tension is palpated in the muscle or tendon.

RECORDING MUSCLE STRENGTH SCORES

The grade is accurately recorded in the appropriate place on a form that has columns to record grades for both the right and left sides of the body.

The therapist must sign and date each test; if a test continues over several days, the dates should reflect that. A sample form is presented in Table 6.3. The peripheral nerve and spinal segmental levels are listed beside each muscle to assist the therapist in interpreting the results of the muscle test.

Table 6.3. Sample Form for Recording Muscle Strength

Patient's Name:_____ Age:_____

Diagnosis:_____ Date of Onset:_____

Occupation:_____ Gender: M   F

LEFT   RIGHT

			Examiner		
			Date		
		S	ELEVATION		
			Upper Trapezius (Accessory) CR XI, C3-4		
		C	Levator Scapulae (dorsal scapular) C5, C3-4		
		A	DEPRESSION		
			Lower Trapezius (accessory) CR XI, C3-4		
		P	Latissimus Dorsi (thoraco-dorsal) C6-8		
		U	ADDUCTION		
			Middle Trapezius (accessory) CR XI, C3-4		
		L	Rhomboids (dorsal scapular) C5		
		A	ABDUCTION		
			Serratus Anterior (long thoracis) C5-7		
			FLEXION		
			Anterior Deltoid (axillary) C5-6		
			Coracobrachialis (musculocutaneous) C5-6		
			Pectoralis Major-Clavicular (pectoral) C5-T1		
		S	Biceps (musculocutaneous) C5-6		
		H	EXTENSION		
			Latissimus Dorsi (thoraco-dorsal) C6-8		
			Teres Major (lower subscapular) C5-6		
			Posterior Deltoid (axillary) C5-6		
		O	Triceps-long head (radial) C7-8		
			ABDUCTION		
		U	Supraspinatus (suprascapular) C5		
			Middle Deltoid (axillary) C5-6		
		L	ADDUCTION		
			Latissimus Dorsi (thoraco-dorsal) C6-8		
			Teres Major (lower subscapular) C5-6		
		D	Pectoralis Major (pectoral) C5-T1		
			HORIZONTAL ABDUCTION		
		E	Posterior Deltoid (Axillary) C5-6		
			HORIZONTAL ADDUCTION		
		R	Pectoralis Major (pectoral) C5-T1		
			Anterior Deltoid (axillary) C5-6		

Table 6.3. **(continued)**

LEFT   RIGHT

			Examiner	
			Date	

		S H O U L D E R	EXTERNAL ROTATION
			    Infraspinatus (suprascapular) C5-6
			    Teres Minor (axillary) C5-6
			    Posterior Deltoid (axillary) C5-6	

		C o n t . d	INTERNAL ROTATION
			    Subscapularis (upper & lower subscapular)C5-6
			    Teres Major (lowe subscapular) C5-6
			    Latissimus Dorsi (thoraco-dorsal) C6-8
			    Pectoralis Major (pectoral) C5-T1
			    Anterior Deltoid (axillary C5-6	

		E L B O W	FLEXION
			    Biceps (musculocutaneous) C5-6
			    Brachioradialis (radial) C5-6
			    Brachialis (musculocutaneous) C5-6	

			EXTENSION Triceps (radial) C7-8	

		F O R E A R M	PRONATION
			    Pronator Teres (median) C6-7
			    Pronator Quadratus (median) C8-T1	

			SUPINATION
			    Supinator (radial) C6
			    Biceps (musculocutaneous) C5-6	

			EXTENSION	
		W	Ext. Carpi Radialis Longus (radial) C6-7	
		R	Ext. Carpi Radialis Brevis (radial) C6-7	
		I	Ext. Carpi Ulnaris (radial) C7-8	
		S	FLEXION	
		T	Flexor Carpi Radialis (median) C6-7	
			Palmaris Longus (median) C8	
			Flexor Carpi Ulnaris (ulnar) C7-8	

LEFT   RIGHT

Table 6.3. (continued)

LEFT   RIGHT

				Examiner		
				Date		
				FLEXION		
			D.	Flexor Profundus 1st (median) C8-T1		
	F	I.		Flexor Profundus 2nd (median) C8-T1		
		P.		Flexor Profundus 3rd (ulnar) C8-T1		
				Flexor Profuncus 4th (ulnar) C8-T1		
	I	5th MP		Flexor Digiti Minimi (ulnar) C-T1		
		P.		Flexor Superficialis 1st (median) C7-T1		
		I.		Flexor Superficialis 1st (median) C7-T1		
	N	P.		Flexor Superficialis 3rd (median) C7-T1		
				Flexor Superficialis 4th (median) C7-T1		
				ADDUCTION		
	G			Palmar Interosseus 1st (ulnar) C8-T1		
				Palmar Interosseus 2nd (ulnar) C8-T1		
				Palmar Interosseus 3rd (ulnar) C8-T1		
	E			ABDUCTION		
				Dorsal Interosseus 1st (ulnar) C8-T1		
				Dorsal Interosseus 2nd (ulnar) C8-T1		
	R			Dorsal Interosseus 3rd (ulnar) C8-T1		
				Dorsal Interosseus 4th (ulnar) C8-T1		
				Abductor Digiti Minimi (ulnar) C8-T1		
	S			EXTENSION		
				Extensor Digitorum 1st (radial) C7-8		
		M.		Extensor Digitorum 2nd (radial) C7-8		
		P.		Extensor Digitorum 3rd (radial) C7-8		
				Extensor Digitorum 4th (radial) C7-8		
				Extensor Digiti Minimi (radial) C7-8		
				Lumbrical 1st (median) C8-T1		
		I.		Lumbrical 2nd (median) C8-T1		
		P.		Lumbrical 3rd (median) C8-T1		
				Lumbrical 4th (median) C8-T1		

Table 6.3. (continued)

LEFT   RIGHT

			Examiner		
			Date		
			EXTENSION		
		T	Extensor Pollicis Longus (radial) C7-8		
		T	Extensor Pollicis Brevis (radial) C7-8		
			ABDUCTION		
		H	Abductor Pollicis Longus (radial) C7-8		
			Abductor Pollicis Brevis (median) C8-T1		
		U	FLEXION		
		M	Flexor Pollicis Brevis (median & ulnar) C6-8 & C8-T1		
			Flexor Pollicis Longus (median) C8-T1		
		B	ADDUCTION		
			Adductor Pollicis (ulnar) C8-T1		
			OPPOSITION		
			Opponens Pollicis (median) C8-T1		
		5th	Opponens Digiti Minimi (ulnar) C8-T1		
		H	FLEXION		
		I	Iliopsoas (femoral) L2-3		
		P	EXTENSION		
			Gluteus Maximus (inf. gluteal) L5-S2		
		K	FLEXION		
		N	Hamstrings (sciatic) L5-S2		
		E	EXTENSION		
		E	Quadriceps (femoral) L2-4		
		A	DORSIFLEXION		
		N	Tibialis Anterior (deep peroneal) L4-S1		
		K	Extensor Digitorum Longus (deep peroneal) L4-S1		
		L	Extensor Hallucis Longus (deep peroneal) L4-S1		
		E	PLANTAR FLEXION		
			Gastrocnemius (tibial) S1-2		
			Soleus (tibial) S-2		

Innervations according to Lockhart, R. D., Hamilton, G. F., & Fyfe, F. W. (1959). *Anatomy of the human body.* Philadelphia: J. B. Lippincott.

Measurement of the Proximal Upper Extremity

The photograph of each against-gravity position shows the completed test motion and the application of resistance. The photograph of each gravity-eliminated position shows the support of the part during motion.

SCAPULAR ELEVATION

Prime Movers

Upper trapezius
Levator scapulae

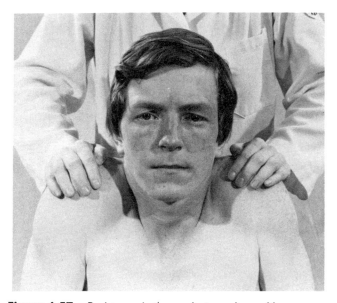

Figure 6.57. Resistance in the against-gravity position: movement starts with patient sitting erect with arms at the side. Patient raises his shoulders toward his ears.

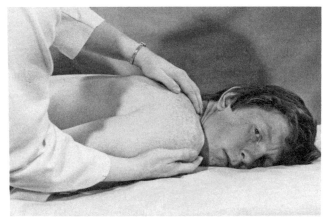

Figure 6.58. Gravity-eliminated position: with the patient prone, arms at the side, the therapist supports the shoulder as the patient attempts to move his shoulder toward his ear. The shoulder is lifted so the scapular motion will be on a gravity-eliminated plane. The therapist's left hand is palpating the upper trapezius.

Stabilize. Trunk is stabilized against the plinth or chair back.

Palpation. Upper trapezius is palpated on the shoulder at the curve of the neck. The levator scapulae is palpated posteriorly to the sternocleidomastoideus on the lateral side of the neck (Fig. 6.58).

Resistance. The therapist's hand is placed over the acromion and pushes down toward scapular depression. A normal trapezius of an adult cannot be broken (Figs. 6.57).

Substitution. Pushing on knees with hands.

SCAPULAR DEPRESSION

Prime Movers

Lower trapezius
Latissimus dorsi

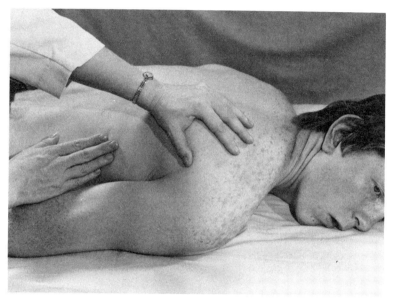

Figure 6.59.   Resistance in the gravity-eliminated position: the patient is prone with the arm internally rotated and at the side. From resting position, patient moves the scapula caudal. The therapist's right hand is palpating the latissimus dorsi.

Against-gravity position.   This is tested in the gravity-eliminated position, since the patient cannot be positioned to move against gravity.

Stabilize.   Trunk is stabilized by the plinth.

Palpation.   The lower trapezius is palpated lateral to the vertebral column as it passes diagonally from the lower thoracic vertebrae to the spine of the scapula. The latissimus dorsi is palpated along the posteriolateral rib cage (Fig. 6.59) or at its point of distal attachment in the posterior axilla.

Resistance.   The therapist's hand is cupped over the inferior angle of the scapula and pushes upward toward scapular elevation. When the inferior angle is not easily accessible because of tissue bulk, resistance can be applied at the distal humerus if the shoulder joint is stable and pain free.

Grading.   Because of the positioning, it is not possible to grade accurately shoulder depressors for against-gravity grades. Experienced therapists estimate these grades and place a question mark (?) beside the grade.

Substitutions.   In an upright position, gravity substitutes. In a prone position, the arm can be inched downward using the finger flexors.

SCAPULAR ADDUCTION

Prime Movers

Middle trapezius
Rhomboids

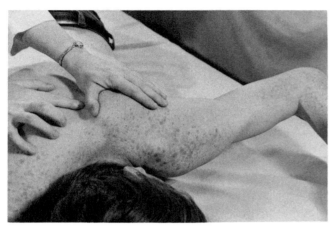

Figure 6.60. Test for middle trapezius against gravity and resistance; the shoulder is externally rotated. The patient lifts his arm up off the plinth to move the scapula toward the vertebral column. The therapist's right index finger points to the middle trapezius.

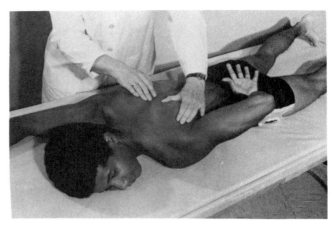

Figure 6.61. Test for rhomboids against gravity and resistance: the shoulder is internally rotated with the hand held over the lumbar region. The patient lifts his hand up off of the buttocks to move the scapula toward the vertebral column. The therapist's right hand palpates the rhomboids.

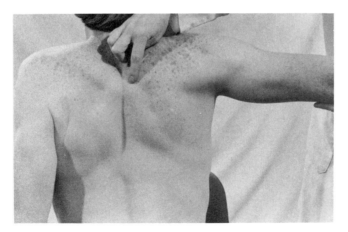

Figure 6.62. Gravity-eliminated position: the patient sits erect with the humerus abducted to 90° and supported. He attempts to move the scapula toward the vertebral column.

Stabilize. Trunk.

Palpation. Middle trapezius is palpated between the vertebral column and vertebral border of scapula at the level of the spine of the scapula (Fig. 6.62). With the arm in internal rotation and held over the back, the rhomboids are palpated along the vertebral border of the scapula, near the inferior angle.

Resistance. The whole length of the therapist's thumb is placed along the vertebral border of the scapula and the rest of the hand is placed on the dorsal surface of the scapula. The therapist pushes laterally (Figs. 6.60–6.61).

Substitutions. None.

SCAPULAR ABDUCTION

Prime Mover

Serratus anterior

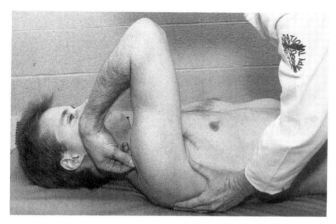

Figure 6.63. Resistance in the against-gravity position: the patient is supine with the humerus flexed to 90°; the elbow may be flexed or extended. The patient abducts the scapula so that the arm moves upward.

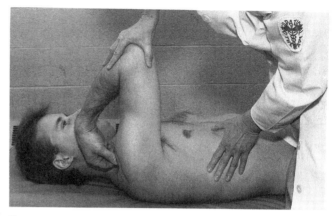

Figure 6.64. Alternative method of applying resistance in against-gravity position: the therapist's left hand palpates the digitations of the serratus anterior. See text for precautions.

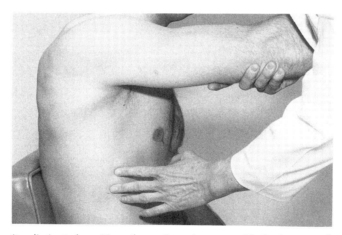

Figure 6.65. Gravity-eliminated position: the patient sits erect with the humerus flexed to 90° and supported; the elbow may be flexed or extended. He abducts the scapula so that the arm moves forward.

Stabilize. Trunk.

Palpation. Serratus anterior is palpated on the lateral ribs just lateral to the inferior angle of the scapula (Fig. 6.65).

Resistance. According to the rule, resistance should be applied along the axillary border of the scapula (Fig. 6.63). Because it is difficult to apply resistance there, therapists often resist this motion either by grasping the distal humerus or by cupping the hand over the patient's elbow and pushing down or backward toward adduction (Fig. 6.64). Of course, this is an unsafe practice if the glenohumeral joint is unstable.

Substitutions. In the gravity-eliminated position this motion can be achieved by inching the arm forward on the supportive surface using the finger flexors.

SHOULDER FLEXION

Prime Movers

Anterior deltoid
Coracobrachialis
Pectoralis major—clavicular head
Biceps—both .heads

Figure   6.66. Resistance in the against-gravity position: the patient sits erect with the arm at the side in midposition. He flexes the humerus to 90° with the elbow extended.

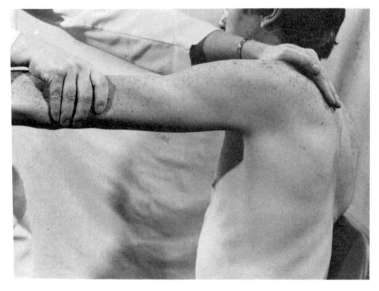

Figure   6.67. Gravity-eliminated position: the patient is side lying with the arm in midposition along the side of the body. The arm is supported by the therapist or by a smooth testing board, while the patient attempts to flex the humerus to 90° with the elbow extended. The therapist's left hand is palpating the anterior deltoid.

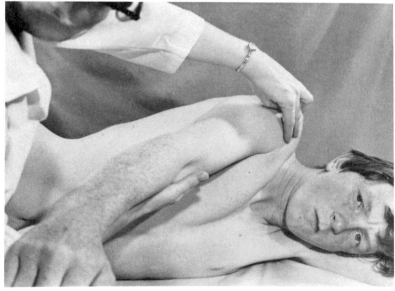

Stabilize.   Scapula.

Palpation.   Anterior deltoid is palpated immediately anterior to the glenohumeral joint. Coracobrachialis may be palpated medially to the biceps, which is palpated on the anterior aspect of the humerus (Fig. 6.67). The clavicular head of the pectoralis major may be palpated below the clavicle on its way to insert on the humerus below the anterior deltoid.

Resistance.   The therapist's hand is placed over the distal end of the humerus and pushes down toward extension. Movement above 90° involves scapular upward rotation; these motions are separated for muscle testing, although they are not separated for range of motion measurement (Figs. 6.66).

Substitutions.   Shoulder abductors, trunk extension.

SHOULDER EXTENSION

Prime Movers

Latissimus dorsi
Teres major
Posterior deltoid
Triceps—long head

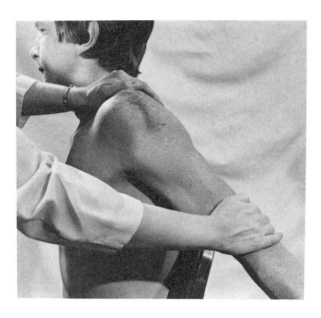

Figure 6.68. Resistance in the against-gravity position: the patient is sitting with the humerus internally rotated and the arm by the side. He extends the humerus. An alternate starting position is with the patient prone. *Note:* the therapist stands in front of the patient for safety to prevent the trunk from bending forward when resistance is applied.

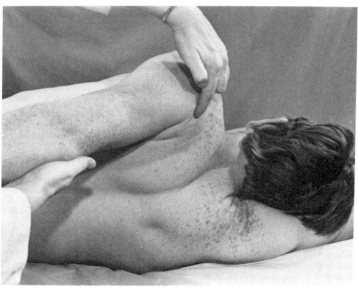

Figure 6.69. Gravity-eliminated position: the patient is lying on his side with the humerus internally rotated and the arm supported with the elbow extended. Patient attempts to extend the humerus. The therapist is pointing to the posterior deltoid.

Stabilize. Scapula.

Palpation. The latissimus dorsi and the teres major form the posterior border of the axilla. The latissimus dorsi is located inferior to the teres major. The posterior deltoid is located immediately posterior to the glenohumeral joint (Fig. 6.69). The triceps is palpated on the posterior aspect of the humerus.

Resistance. The therapist's hand is placed over the distal end of the humerus and pushes forward toward flexion (Figs. 6.68).

Substitutions. Shoulder abductors, tipping the shoulder forward.

SHOULDER ABDUCTION

Prime Movers

Supraspinatus
Middle deltoid

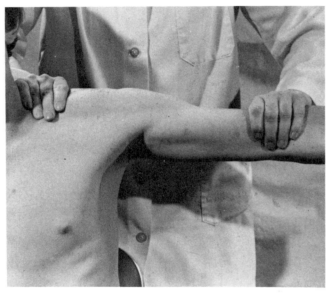

Figure 6.70. Resistance in the against-gravity position: the patient sits erect with the arm at the side in midposition. He abducts the humerus to 90° with the elbow extended.

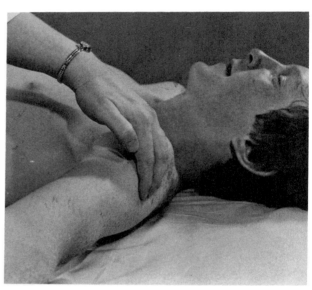

Figure 6.71. Gravity-eliminated position: the patient lies supine with the arm supported at the side in midposition. He attempts to abduct the arm to 90° with the elbow extended. The middle deltoid is palpated on top of the shoulder joint.

Stabilize.   Scapula.

Palpation.   The supraspinatus lies too deep for easy palpation. The middle deltoid is palpated below the acromion and lateral to the glenohumeral joint (Fig. 6.71).

Resistance.   The therapist's hand is placed over the distal end of the humerus and pushes the humerus down toward the body. Movement above 90° involves scapular upward rotation and is not measured (Figs. 6.70).

Substitutions.   The long head of the biceps can substitute if the humerus is allowed to be moved into external rotation; trunk lateral flexion.

SHOULDER ADDUCTION

Prime Movers

Pectoralis major
Teres major
Latissimus dorsi

Test in the gravity-eliminated position, because the patient cannot be positioned for this motion against gravity.

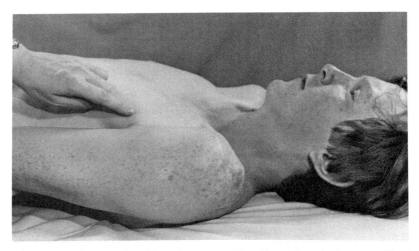

Figure 6.72. Resistance in the gravity-eliminated position: the patient is supine with the humerus abducted to 90° and in mid-position. He adducts the humerus. The therapist is pointing to the sternal portion of the pectoralis major.

Stabilize. Trunk.

Palpation. The pectoralis major forms the anterior border of the axilla where it may be easily palpated (Fig. 6.72). Palpation of the teres major and palpation of the latissimus dorsi were described earlier.

Resistance. The therapist's hand is placed on the medial side of the distal end of the humerus and pulls the humerus away from the patient's body (Fig. 6.72).

Grading. Grading for antigravity grades again can only be estimated; a question mark should be entered beside the grade on the form. With experience, the therapist develops the skill to estimate reliably.

Substitutions. In an upright position gravity substitutes. On a supporting surface, the arm can be inched down using the finger flexors.

SHOULDER HORIZONTAL ABDUCTION

Prime Mover

Posterior deltoid

Figure 6.73. Resistance in the against-gravity position: the patient is positioned prone with the arm hanging in internal rotation over the edge of the table. He horizontally abducts the humerus, allowing the elbow to flex. The therapist is pointing to the posterior deltoid.

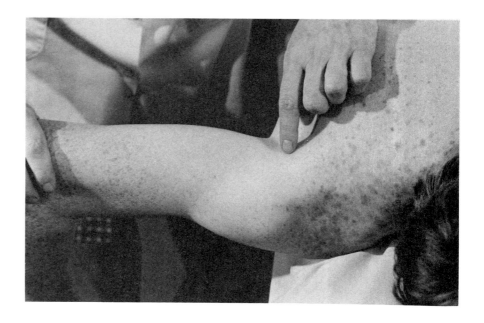

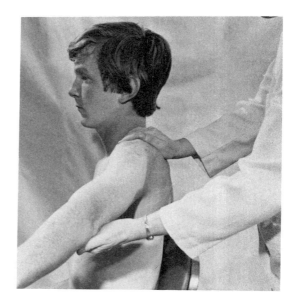

Figure 6.74. Gravity-eliminated position: the patient sits with the humerus flexed to 90° and the arm supported. He attempts horizontal abduction of the humerus.

Stabilize. Scapula. In the sitting position, stabilize the trunk against the back of the chair.

Palpation. Posterior deltoid is palpated immediately posterior to the glenohumeral joint.

Resistance. Therapist's hand is placed on the posterior surface of the distal end of the humerus and pushes the arm downward or forward toward horizontal adduction (Fig. 6.73).

Substitution. Trunk rotation in a sitting position.

SHOULDER HORIZONTAL ADDUCTION

Prime Movers

Pectoralis major
Anterior deltoid

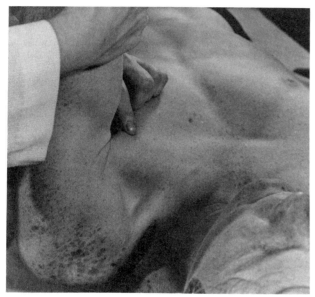

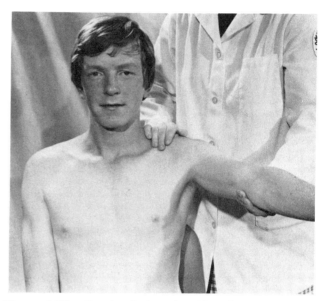

Figure 6.75. Resistance in the against-gravity position: the patient lies with the humerus abducted to 90°. The patient horizontally adducts the humerus to 90° of shoulder flexion. *Note:* in the supine position, if the triceps is weak, prevent the patient's hand from hitting his face. The therapist is pointing to the sternal portion of the pectoralis major. The clavicular portion can be seen to contract just caudal to the triangle formed by it, the clavicle, and the anterior deltoid.

Figure 6.76. Gravity-eliminated position: the patient sits with the humerus abducted to 90° and attempts horizonatal adduction of the humerus.

Stabilize.   Scapula. In the sitting position, stabilize the trunk against the back of the chair.

Palpation.   The pectoralis major can be palpated along the anterior border of the axilla. The anterior deltoid is located immediately anterior to the glenohumeral joint below the acromion process.

Resistance.   The therapist's hand is placed on the anterior surface of the distal end of the humerus and pushes the arm backward toward horizontal abduction (Fig. 6.75).

Substitutions.   In a sitting position, trunk rotation can substitute. The arm can be inched across the supporting surface using the finger flexors.

SHOULDER EXTERNAL ROTATION

Prime Movers

Infraspinatus
Teres minor
Posterior deltoid

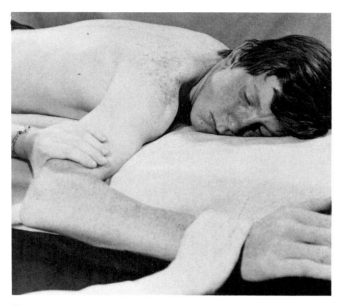

Figure 6.77. Resistance in the against-gravity position: the patient lies prone with the humerus abducted to 90° and supported on the table; the elbow is flexed to 90° with the forearm dangling over the edge of the table. The patient externally rotates the humerus, bringing the dorsal surface of the hand toward the ceiling.

Stabilize. Humerus at the elbow to allow only rotation.

Palpation. The infraspinatus is palpated inferior to the spine of the scapula. The teres minor is palpated between the posterior deltoid and the axillary border of the scapula; it is located superior to the teres major (Fig. 6.78). Palpation of the posterior deltoid was described earlier.

Resistance. Against Gravity. The therapist's hand is placed on the dorsal surface of the distal end of the forearm and pushed toward the floor, keeping the patient's elbow supported and flexed to 90° to prevent supination (Fig. 6.77).

Gravity Eliminated. The therapist's hand encircles the distal end of the humerus and turns the humerus toward internal rotation.

Alternate Gravity-Eliminated Position. The therapist's hand is placed on the dorsal surface of the distal end of the forearm and pushes forward, keeping the elbow flexed to 90° (Fig. 6.79).

Substitutions. Scapula adduction combined with downward rotation can substitute. The triceps may substitute when resistance is applied in an against-gravity position or in the alternate gravity-eliminated position. Supination may be mistaken for external rotation in a gravity-eliminated position.

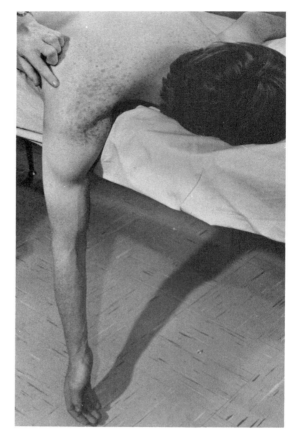

Figure 6.78. Gravity-eliminated position: the patient lies prone with the entire arm dangling over the edge of the table. He attempts to externally rotate the humerus.

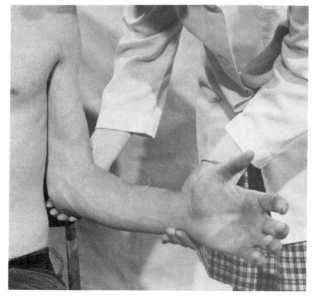

Figure 6.79. Alternate gravity-eliminated position: the patient sits with the humerus adducted and the elbow flexed to 90°. The hand moves laterally as the patient externally rotates the humerus.

SHOULDER INTERNAL ROTATION

Prime Movers

Subscapularis
Teres major
Latissimus dorsi
Pectoralis major
Anterior deltoid

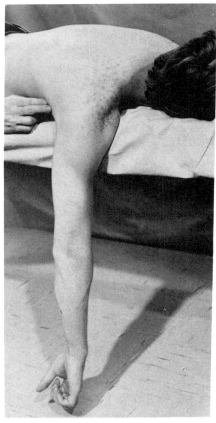

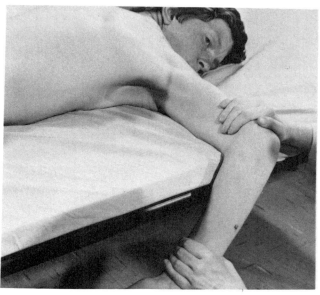

Figure 6.80. Resistance in the against-gravity position: the patient lies with the humerus abducted to 90° and supported on the table; the elbow is flexed to 90° with the forearm dangling over the edge of the table. The patient internally rotates the humerus, bringing the palmar surface of the hand toward the ceiling.

Figure 6.81. Gravity-eliminated position: the patient lies prone with the entire arm dangling over the edge of the table. He attempts to rotate the humerus internally. The therapist is palpating the teres major and latissimus dorsi.

Stabilize. Humerus at the elbow to allow only rotation.

Palpation. The subscapularis is not easily palpated but may be palpated in the posterior axilla (Fig. 6.81). The teres major, latissimus dorsi, pectoralis major, and anterior deltoid are palpated as previously described.

Resistance. Against Gravity. The therapist's hand is placed on the volar surface of the distal end of the forearm and pushes toward the floor, keeping the elbow supported and flexed to 90° (Fig. 6.80).

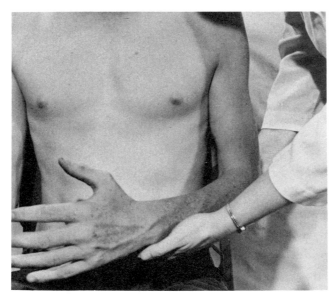

Figure 6.82. Alternate gravity-eliminated position: the patient sits with the humerus adducted and the elbow flexed to 90°. Pa-tient's hand moves toward the abdomen as he internally rotates the humerus.

Gravity Eliminated.   The therapist's hand encircles the distal end of the humerus and turns the humerus toward external rotation.

Alternate Gravity-Eliminated Position.   The therapist's hand is placed on the volar surface of the distal end of the forearm and pulls away from the abdomen, keeping the elbow flexed to 90° (Fig. 6.82).

Substitutions.   Scapula abduction combined with upward rotation can substitute. The triceps can substitute, as it did in external rotation. Pronation may be mistaken for internal rotation in a gravity-eliminated position.

ELBOW FLEXION

Prime Movers

Biceps
Brachialis
Brachioradialis

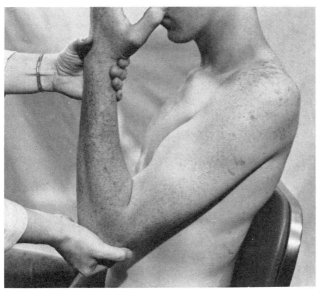

Figure 6.83. Resistance in the against-gravity position: the patient sits with his arm at the side in anatomical position. He raises his forearm so that the hand approximates the ipsilateral shoulder.

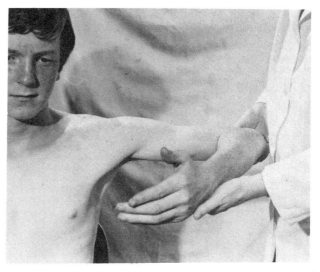

Figure 6.84. Gravity-eliminated position: the patient sits with the humerus abducted to 90° and the elbow extended, supported if necessary. The hand is relaxed. The patient attempts to flex the elbow.

Stabilize. Humerus.

Palpation. The biceps is easily palpated on the anterior surface of the humerus. With the biceps relaxed and the forearm pronated, the brachialis is palpated just medial to the distal biceps tendon. With the forearm in midposition the brachioradialis is palpated along the top of the proximal forearm.

Resistance. The therapist's hand is placed on the volar surface of the distal end of the forearm and pulls out toward extension (Fig. 6.83).

Substitution. In a gravity-eliminated plane, the wrist flexors may substitute.

ELBOW EXTENSION

Prime Mover

Triceps

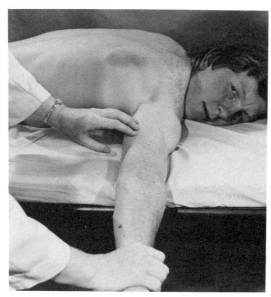

Figure 6.85. Resistance in the against-gravity position: the patient lies prone with the humerus abducted to 90° and supported on the table; the elbow is flexed and the forearm is hanging over the edge of the table. The patient extends the elbow. The therapist's left hand is palpating the long head of the triceps.

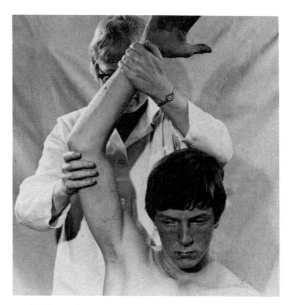

Figure 6.86. Alternate against-gravity position: the patient sits with the humerus flexed to 180° and the elbow fully flexed. He extends the elbow. *Note:* if the shoulder is flaccid, avoid shoulder abduction and external rotation when moving the arm into a position of full shoulder flexion. Without the protection of its cuff musculature, the head of the humerus may be dislocated by the stress placed on the joint capsule from abduction and rotation.

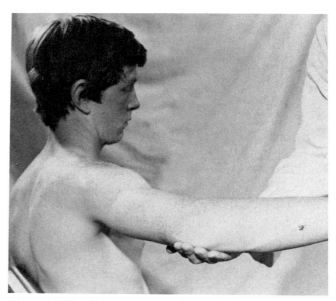

Figure 6.87. Gravity-eliminated position: the patient sits with the humerus abducted to 90° and supported if necessary; the elbow is fully flexed. The patient attempts to extend the elbow.

Stabilize. Humerus.

Palpation. The triceps is easily palpated on the posterior surface of the humerus.

Resistance. The therapist's hand is placed on the dorsal surface of the patient's forearm and pushes it toward flexion. Resistance is applied with the elbow in a position 10 to 15° less than full extension so that the elbow does not lock into position, which could unreliably indicate greater strength than really exists (Figs. 6.85).

Substitutions. Gravity may substitute in a sitting position. In the gravity-eliminated position, no external rotation of the shoulder is permitted to avoid letting extension occur as a result of the assistance of gravity. On a supporting surface, finger flexion may be used to inch the forearm across the surface.

PRONATION

Prime Movers

Pronator teres
Pronator quadratus

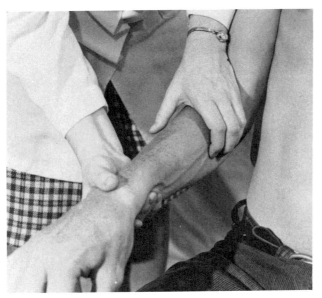

Figure 6.88. Resistance in the against-gravity position: the patient sits with the humerus adducted, the elbow flexed to 90°, the forearm supinated, and the wrist and fingers relaxed. The patient pronates to turn the palm down. *Note:* gravity assists the motion beyond midposition. The therapist is palpating the pronator teres with her left hand.

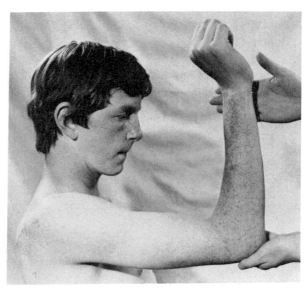

Figure 6.89. Gravity-eliminated position: the patient sits with the humerus flexed to 90° and supported, the elbow flexed to 90°, the forearm supinated, and the wrist and fingers relaxed. The patient pronates to turn the palm away from the face.

Stabilize. Humerus.

Palpation. The pronator teres is palpated medial to the distal attachment of the biceps tendon on the volar surface of the proximal forearm. Pronator quadratus is too deep to palpate.

Resistance. The therapist encircles the distal forearm by cupping the forearm between her thenar eminence and four fingers to avoid hurting the patient by applying force through the tips of the fingers and thumb. The forearm is turned in the direction of supination (Figs. 6.88).

Alternate methods of applying resistance include the following. (1) The therapist's hand encircles the patient's volar wrist with her index finger extended along the forearm. (2) The therapist interlaces the fingers of both her hands and cups the patient's distal forearm between her opposing palms.

Substitutions. The wrist and finger flexors may substitute.

SUPINATION

Prime Movers

Supinator
Biceps

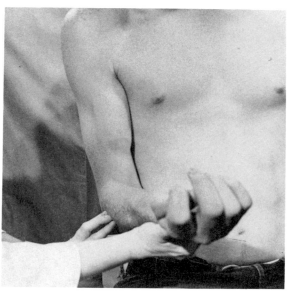

Figure 6.90. Resistance in the against-gravity position: the patient sits with the humerus adducted, the elbow flexed to 90°, the forearm pronated, and the wrist and fingers relaxed. The patient supinates to turn the palm up. *Note:* gravity assists the motion beyond midposition. The therapist's left hand is palpating the supinator.

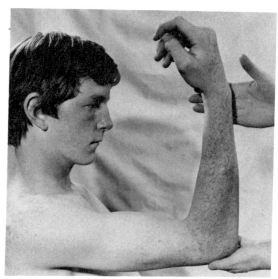

Figure 6.91. Gravity-eliminated position: the patient is positioned the same as for pronation but with the forearm pronated. He attempts to turn the palm toward his face.

Note. To differentiate the supinator from the supination function of the biceps, test the supinator with elbow extended. The biceps does not supinate the extended arm unless resisted (Basmajian & DeLuca, 1985).

Stabilize. Humerus.

Palpation. The supinator is palpated on the dorsal surface of the proximal forearm just distal to the head of the radius. Palpation of the biceps was described earlier.

Resistance. Same as for pronation except that the forearm is turned in the direction of pronation (Figs. 6.90).

Substitutions. The wrist and finger extensors may substitute.

Measurement of the Wrist and Hand

Many tendons of wrist and hand muscles cross more than one joint. For this reason, test positions for individual muscles must include ways to minimize the effect of other muscles crossing the joint. As a general rule, to minimize the effect of a muscle, place it opposite to the prime action (muscle is in its shortened range where it can develop little tension). For example, to minimize the effect of the extensor pollicis longus on extension of the proximal joint of the thumb, the distal joint is flexed.

WRIST EXTENSION

Prime Movers

Extensor carpi radialis longus (ECRL)
Extensor carpi radialis brevis (ECRB)
Extensor carpi ulnaris (ECU)

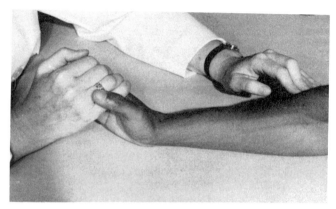

Figure 6.92. Resistance and palpation of the ECRL in the against-gravity position.

Extensor carpi radialis longus (ECRL)

Position. Against Gravity. Forearm pronated to 45°, wrist flexed and ulnarly deviated, and fingers and thumb relaxed.

Gravity Eliminated. Forearm in midposition, wrist flexed, fingers and thumb relaxed.

Stabilize. Forearm.

Test Motion. The patient extends the wrist toward the radial side.

Palpation. The tendon of the ECRL is palpated on the dorsal surface of the wrist at the base of the second metacarpal. The muscle belly is found on the dorsal proximal forearm adjacent to the brachioradialis.

Resistance. The therapist's palm is placed across the dorsum of the patient's hand on the radial side and pushes toward combined wrist flexion and ulnar deviation (Fig. 6.92).

Substitutions. Extensor pollicis longus, extensor digitorum.

Extensor carpi radialis brevis (ECRB)

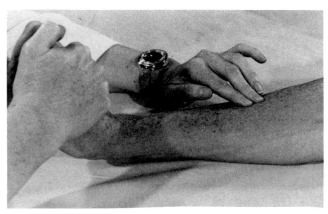

Figure 6.93. Resistance and palpation of the ECRB in the against-gravity position.

Extensor carpi ulnaris (ECU)

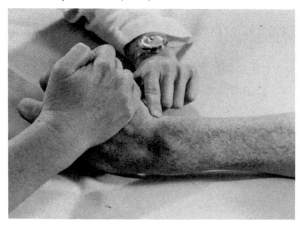

Figure 6.94. Resistance and palpation of the tendon of the ECU in the against-gravity position.

Position. *Against Gravity.* Forearm is fully pronated, wrist is flexed and undeviated, fingers and thumb are relaxed.

Gravity Eliminated. Same as for ECRL.

Stabilize. Forearm.

Test Motion. The patient extends the wrist without deviation.

Palpation. The tendon of the ECRB is palpated on the dorsal surface of the wrist at the base of the third metacarpal adjacent to the ECRL. The muscle belly of ECRB is found distal to the belly of ECRL on the dorsal surface of the proximal forearm.

Resistance. The therapist's palm is placed across the dorsum of the patient's hand and pushes directly toward flexion (Fig. 6.93).

Substitutions. Extensor pollicis longus, extensor digitorum.

Position *Against Gravity.* Shoulder internally rotated, forearm fully pronated, wrist flexed and radially deviated, and fingers relaxed.

Gravity Eliminated. Forearm pronated to 45°, wrist flexed and radially deviated, fingers relaxed.

Stabilize. Forearm.

Test Motion. Patient extends the wrist toward the ulnar side.

Palpation. The ECU tendon is palpated on the dorsal surface of the wrist between the head of the ulna and the base of the fifth metacarpal. The muscle belly is found approximately 2 inches distal to the lateral epicondyle of the humerus (Lehmkuhl & Smith, 1983).

Resistance. The therapist's palm is placed across the dorsum of the patient's hand on the ulnar side and pushes toward combined wrist flexion and radial deviation (Fig. 6.94).

Substitutions. Extensor digitorum.

WRIST FLEXION

Prime Movers

Flexor carpi radialis (FCR)
Palmaris longus
Flexor carpi ulnaris (FCU)

Flexor carpi radialis and palmaris longus

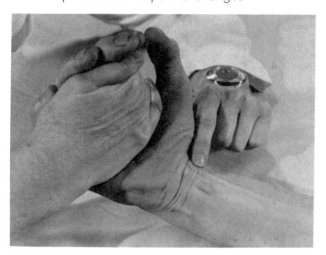

Figure 6.95. Resistance and palpation of the tendon of the FCR in the against-gravity position.

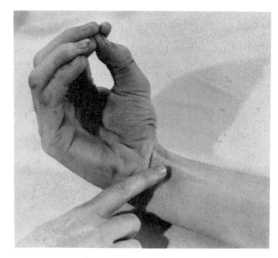

Figure 6.96. The palmaris longus.

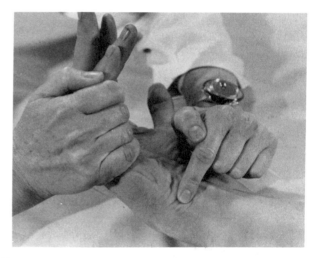

Figure 6.97. Resistance in the against-gravity position: the therapist's finger points to the tendon of the FCU.

Position. Against Gravity. Forearm supinated, wrist extended, and fingers and thumb relaxed.

Gravity Eliminated. Forearm in midposition, wrist extended, and fingers and thumb relaxed.

Stabilize. Forearm.

Test Motion. Patient flexes the wrist.

Palpation. The FCR tendon is palpated on the volar surface of the wrist in line with the second metacarpal and radial to the palmaris longus (if present). The palmaris longus is a weak wrist flexor that has a small muscle belly and long tendon. The tendon crosses the center of the volar surface of the wrist (Fig. 6.96). It is not tested for strength and may not even be present. However, if it is present, it will stand out prominently in the middle of the wrist when wrist flexion is resisted or the palm is cupped.

Resistance. The therapist's fingers are placed across the patient's palm and pull toward wrist extension (Figs. 6.95).

Substitutions. Abductor pollicis longus, flexor pollicis longus, flexor digitorum superficialis, and flexor digitorum profundus.

Flexor carpi ulnaris

Position. Against Gravity. Shoulder adducted and externally rotated, forearm fully supinated, wrist extended, and fingers relaxed.

Gravity Eliminated. Forearm supinated to 45°, wrist extended, and fingers relaxed.

Stabilize. Forearm.

Test Motion. Patient flexes the wrist toward ulnar deviation.

Palpation. The FCU tendon is palpated on the volar surface of the wrist just proximal to the pisiform bone.

Resistance. The therapist's fingers are placed across the patient's palm and pull toward wrist extension and radial deviation (Fig. 6.97).

Substitutions. Flexor digitorum superficialis, flexor digitorum profundus.

FINGER DIP FLEXION

Prime Mover

Flexor digitorum profundus (FDP)

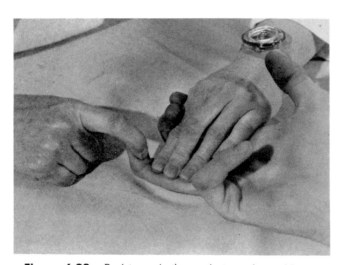

Figure 6.98. Resistance in the against-gravity position.

Position. Against Gravity. Forearm supinated and supported on a table; wrist and interphalangeal joints relaxed.

Gravity Eliminated. Forearm in midposition, resting on ulnar border on a table; wrist and interphalangeal joints relaxed in neutral position.

Stabilize. Middle phalanx of each finger as it is tested to prevent flexion of the proximal interphalangeal joint; wrist should remain in neutral position.

Test Motion. Flexion of the distal phalanx toward the middle phalanx.

Palpation. The belly of the FDP is palpated just volar to the ulna in the proximal third of the forearm. The tendons are sometimes palpable on the volar surface of the middle phalanges.

Resistance. The therapist places one finger on the pad of the patient's finger and pulls toward extension (Fig. 6.98).

Substitutions. Rebound effect of apparent flexion following contraction of extensors. Wrist extension causes **tenodesis** action.

FINGER PIP FLEXION

Prime Movers

Flexor digitorum superficialis (FDS)
Flexor digitorum profundus

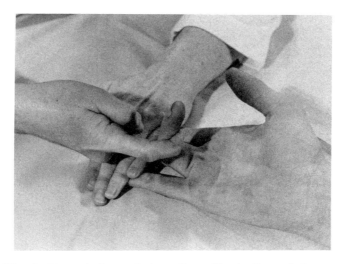

Figure 6.99. Resistance in the against-gravity position for flexor digitorum superficialis.

Position. For the flexor digitorum superficialis.

Against Gravity. Forearm supinated and supported on the table; wrist and metacarpophalangeal joints relaxed and in zero position. To rule out the influence of the profundus when testing the superficialis, hold all interphalangeal joints of the fingers not being tested into full extension. Because the profundus is essentially one muscle with four tendons, by preventing its action in three of the four fingers, it cannot work in the tested finger. In fact, the patient is unable to flex the distal joint of the tested finger at all! In some people, the profundus slip to the index finger is such that this method cannot rule out its influence on the PIP joint of the index finger. This should be noted on the test form.

Gravity Eliminated. Forearm supported in midposition, with the wrist and MP joints relaxed in neutral position. Again, rule out the influence of the FDP by holding all the joints of the nontested fingers in extension.

Stabilize. Proximal phalanx of the finger being tested.

Test Motion. Patient flexes PIP joint.

Palpation. The superficialis is palpated on the volar surface of the proximal forearm toward the ulnar side. The tendons may be palpated at the wrist between the palmaris longus and the flexor carpi ulnaris.

Resistance. Using one finger, the therapist pulls the head of the middle phalanx toward extension (Fig. 6.99).

Substitutions. Flexor digitorum profundus. Wrist extension causes **tenodesis** action.

FINGER MP FLEXION

Prime Movers

Flexor digitorum profundus
Flexor digitorum superficialis
Dorsal interossei
Volar (palmar) interossei
Flexor digiti minimi

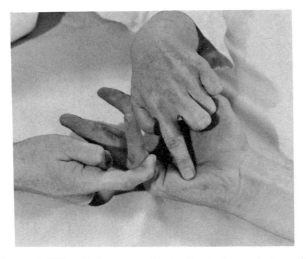

Figure 6.100. Resistance and palpation in the against-gravity position for flexor digiti minimi.

The tests for the first four muscles have been or will be discussed under their alternate actions. The flexor of the little finger has no other action and is described here.

Position.   For the flexor digiti minimi.

Against Gravity.   Forearm supported in supination.

Gravity Eliminated.   Forearm supported in midposition.

Stabilize.   Other fingers in extension.

Test Motion.   Patient flexes fifth finger at MP joint without flexing the interphalangeal joints.

Palpation.   On the volar surface of the hypothenar eminence.

Resistance.   Using one finger, the therapist pushes the head of the proximal phalanx toward extension. The therapist must be sure the interphalangeal joints remain extended (Fig. 6.100).

Substitutions.   Flexor digitorum profundus, flexor digitorum superficialis, third volar interosseus.

FINGER ADDUCTION

Prime Movers

Volar (palmar) interossei (3)

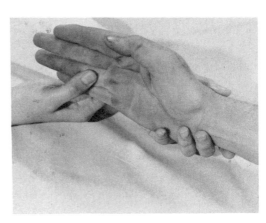

Figure 6.101. Resistance to palmar interosseus 2 in the against-gravity position.

Position.   *Against Gravity.*   For palmar interossei 2 and 3, support the forearm on the ulnar border of the wrist with the fingers extended and abducted. For palmar interosseus 1, the arm is internally rotated and the forearm is fully pronated so that the hand can be supported on the radial border, with the hand free and the fingers extended and abducted.

Gravity Eliminated.   Forearm is supinated and supported.

Stabilize.   Support the hand lightly.

Test Motion.   As each is tested, the patient moves the index, ring, or little finger toward the middle finger.

Palpation.   The palmar interossei are usually too deep to palpate with certainty. When these muscles are atrophied, the areas between the metacarpals on the volar surface appear sunken.

Resistance.   One by one, the therapist pulls the head of the proximal phalanx of each finger being tested away from the middle finger (Fig. 6.101).

Substitutions.   Extrinsic finger flexors; gravity, depending on the position of the hand, substitutes for the first palmar interosseus.

FINGER ABDUCTION

Prime Movers

Dorsal interossei (4)
Abductor digiti minimi

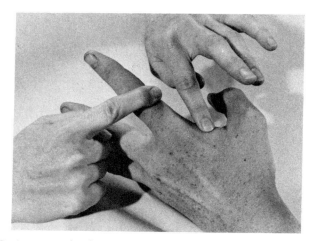

Figure 6.102.   Resistance and palpation in the against-gravity position for dorsal interosseus 1.

Position.   Against Gravity.   For dorsal interossei 1 and 2, the forearm rests on the ulnar border on a supporting surface with the hand free and MPs adducted and slightly flexed. For dorsal interossei 3 and 4 and abductor digiti minimi, the arm is internally rotated, with the forearm fully pronated so that it can be supported on the radial border. The MPs are adducted and slightly flexed. Flexion of the MPs minimizes the abduction caused by the angle of pull of the extensor digitorum.

Gravity Eliminated.   The forearm is pronated and supported with the hand free, and the MPs are adducted and slightly flexed.

Stabilize.   Support the hand lightly.

Test Motions.   One by one, the patient moves the index finger away from the middle finger, the middle finger toward the index finger, the middle finger toward the ring finger, the ring finger toward the little finger, and the little finger away from the ring finger.

Palpation.   The first dorsal interosseus fills the dorsal web space and can be easily palpated there. The abductor digiti minimi is palpated on the ulnar border of the fifth metacarpal. The other interossei lie between the metacarpals on the dorsal aspect of the hand, where they may be palpated; on some people, the tendons can be palpated as they enter the dorsal expansion near the heads of the metacarpals. When the dorsal interossei are atrophied, the spaces between the metacarpals on the dorsal surface appear sunken.

Resistance.   The therapist pushes the head of the proximal phalanx of each finger, in turn, toward the direction opposite to its test motion (Fig. 6.102).

Substitutions.   Extensor digitorum; gravity, especially for dorsal interossei 3 and 4 and the abductor digiti minimi.

FINGER MP EXTENSION

Prime Movers

Extensor digitorum (ED)
Extensor indicis proprius
Extensor digiti minimi

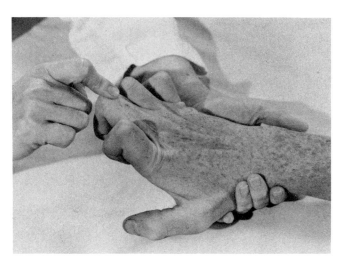

Figure 6.103. Resistance in the against-gravity position for extensor digitorum.

Position.   Against Gravity.   Forearm pronated and supported, wrist supported in neutral position, and fingers flexed at all joints.

Gravity Eliminated.   Forearm supported in midposition, wrist in neutral position, and fingers flexed.

Stabilize.   Wrist and metacarpals.

Test Motion.   Patient extends MP joints keeping the PIP and DIP joints flexed.

Palpation.   The muscle belly of the ED is palpated on the dorsal-ulnar surface of the proximal forearm. Often the separate muscle bellies can be discerned. The tendons of this muscle are readily seen and palpated on the dorsum of the hand.

The extensor indicis proprius tendon is located ulnar to the extensor digitorum tendon. The belly of this muscle is palpated on the mid- to distal dorsal forearm between the radius and ulna.

The extensor digiti minimi tendon is palpated ulnar to the ED. Actually, it is the tendon that looks as if it were the ED tendon to the little finger, because the ED to the little finger is only a slip from the ED tendon to the ring finger.

Resistance.   Using one finger, the therapist pushes the head of each proximal phalanx toward flexion, one at a time (Fig. 6.103).

Substitution.   Apparent extension of the fingers can occur due to the rebound effect of relaxation following finger flexion. Flexion of the wrist can cause finger extension through **tenodesis** action.

FINGER INTERPHALANGEAL EXTENSION

Prime Movers

Lumbricales
Interossei
Extensor digitorum
Extensor indicis proprius
Extensor digiti minimi

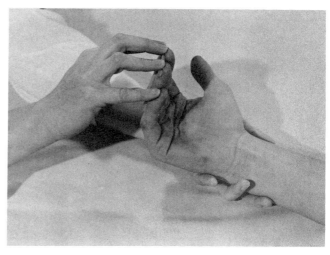

Figure 6.104. Resistance in the against-gravity position for testing lumbricales.

According to electromyographical evidence, the intrinsics, especially the lumbricales, are the primary extensors of the interphalangeal joints (Long, 1968; Long & Brown, 1962). Except for the lumbricales, the other muscles have been discussed. The lumbricales, arising as they do from the flexor profundus and inserting on the extensor digitorum, have a unique duty in regard to finger extension. Contracting against the noncontracting flexor profundus, the lumbricales pull the tendons of the profundus forward toward the fingertips. This slackens the profundus tendons distal to the insertion of the lumbricales, allowing the extensor digitorum to extend the interphalangeal joints fully, regardless of the position of the MP joints (Landsmeer & Long, 1965; Long, 1968). The interossei flex the MP joints while extending the interphalangeal joints and, in fact, operate to extend only when the MP joints are flexed or flexing (Long, 1968).

Position. For the lumbricales. There is no reliably good test for lumbrical function. Test 1 (below) is the traditional test used. Test 2 is a hypothesized test, based on electromyographical evidence.

Against Gravity. Test 1: forearm supinated and supported. Wrist in neutral position, MPs extended, IPs flexed. Test 2: (alternate) MPs flexed and IPs extended.

Gravity Eliminated. Same as above except that the forearm is supported in midposition.

Stabilize. Metacarpals.

Test Motion. *Test 1.* From the starting position, the patient simultaneously flexes his MP joints while extending his IP joints. The concept of this motion is difficult for patients to understand and will need practice.

Test 2. The patient maintains full IP extension while moving from a position of MP flexion to MP extension.

Palpation. Lumbricales lie too deep to be palpated.

Resistance. *Test 1.* The therapist holds the tip of the finger being tested and pushes it toward starting position.

Test 2. The therapist places one finger on the patient's fingernail and pushes toward flexion (Fig. 6.104).

Substitution. Nothing substitutes for DIP extension in the event of the loss of lumbrical function when the MP joint is extended. Other muscles of the dorsal expansion can substitute for DIP extension when the MP joint is flexed.

THUMB IP EXTENSION

Prime Mover

Extensor pollicis longus (EPL)

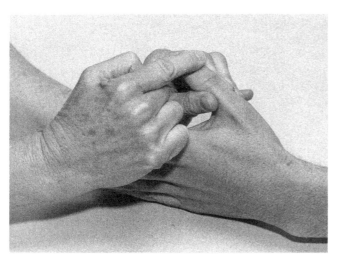

Figure 6.105. Resistance in the against-gravity position with stabilization of the proximal phalanx.

Position. Against Gravity. Forearm supported in midposition, thumb flexed.

Gravity Eliminated. Forearm pronated, thumb flexed.

Stabilize. Proximal phalanx.

Test Motion. Patient extends the IP joint of the thumb.

Palpation. The tendon of the EPL may be palpated on the ulnar border of the anatomical snuff box and also on the dorsal surface of the proximal phalanx of the thumb.

Resistance. The therapist places one finger over the dorsum of the distal phalanx (thumbnail) and pushes toward flexion (Fig. 6.105).

Substitutions. Relaxation of the flexor pollicis longus will result in apparent extensor movement as a result of rebound effect. Because the abductor pollicis brevis, adductor pollicis, and the flexor pollicis brevis insert into the lateral aspects of the dorsal expansion, they may produce thumb IP extension when the extensor pollicis longus is paralyzed. To prevent this, the position of maximal flexion of the carpometacarpal (CMC) and MP joints, wrist flexion of 10° to 20°, and full forearm supination are used to put these synergists in a shortened, disadvantaged position while testing for the EPL (Howell et al., 1989).

THUMB MP EXTENSION

Prime Movers

Extensor pollicis brevis (EPB)
Extensor pollicis longus

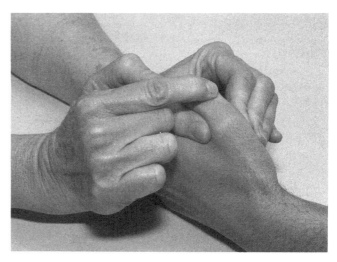

Figure 6.106. Resistance in the against-gravity position for extensor pollicis brevis with stabilization of the first metacarpal.

Position. Test for extensor pollicis brevis.

Against Gravity. Forearm supported in midposition, MP joint flexed, IP joint flexed.

Gravity Eliminated. Forearm pronated, MP joint flexed, IP joint flexed.

Stabilize. First metacarpal in abduction.

Test Motion. The patient extends the MP joint, keeping the IP joint flexed to minimize the effect of the extensor pollicis longus.

Palpation. The tendon of the EPB is palpated on the radial border of the anatomical snuff box medial to the tendon of the abductor pollicis longus. The EPB may not be present.

Resistance. The therapist's index finger is placed on the dorsal surface of the head of the proximal phalanx and pushes toward flexion (Fig. 6.106).

Substitution. Extensor pollicis longus.

THUMB ABDUCTION

Prime Movers

Abductor pollicis longus (APL)
Abductor pollicis brevis (APB)

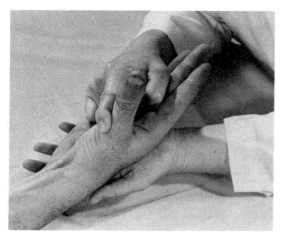

Figure 6.107. Resistance in the against-gravity position for abductor pollicis longus.

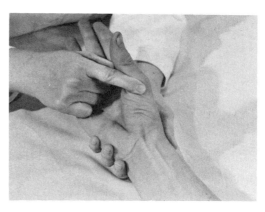

Figure 6.108. Resistance in the against-gravity position for abductor pollicis brevis.

Abductor pollicis longus (APL)

Position. Against Gravity. Forearm supinated to 45°, wrist in neutral position, thumb adducted.

Gravity Eliminated. Forearm pronated to 45°, wrist in neutral position, thumb adducted.

Stabilize. Support the wrist on the ulnar side and hold it in neutral position.

Test Motion. Patient abducts the thumb in a radial direction on a diagonal plane between extension and true abduction.

Palpation. The tendon of the APL is palpated at the wrist joint just distal to the radial styloid and lateral to the EPB.

Resistance. The therapist's finger presses the head of the first metacarpal toward adduction (Fig. 6.107).

Substitutions. Abductor pollicis brevis, extensor pollicis brevis.

Abductor pollicis brevis (APB)

Position. Against Gravity. Forearm is supported in supination, wrist in neutral position, thumb adducted.

Gravity Eliminated. Forearm is supported in midposition, wrist in neutral position, thumb adducted.

Stabilize. Support the wrist in neutral position by holding it on the dorsal and ulnar side.

Test Motion. The patient abducts the thumb, bringing it straight up from the palm.

Palpation. APB is palpated over the center of the thenar eminence.

Resistance. The therapist's finger presses the head of the first metacarpal toward adduction (Fig. 6.108).

Substitution. Abductor pollicis longus.

THUMB IP FLEXION

Prime Mover

Flexor pollicis longus (FPL)

THUMB MP FLEXION

Prime Movers

Flexor pollicis brevis (FPB)
Flexor pollicis longus (FPL)

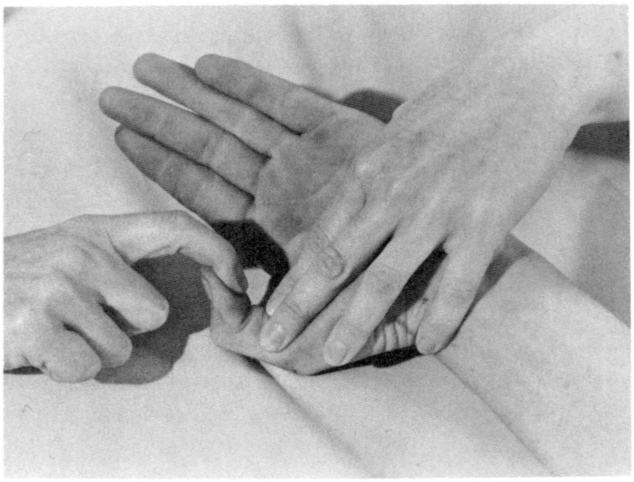

Figure 6.109. Resistance and palpation in the against-gravity position for flexor pollicis longus with stabilization of the proximal phalanx.

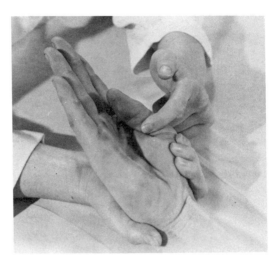

Figure 6.110. Resistance in the against-gravity position for flexor pollicis brevis with stabilization of the first metacarpal.

Position. Against Gravity. Elbow flexed and forearm supinated so that the palmar surface of the thumb faces the ceiling; thumb extended at the MP and IP joints.

Gravity Eliminated. Forearm supinated to 90° so that the thumb can flex across the palm.

Stabilize. Proximal phalanx, holding MP joint in extension.

Test Motion. Patient flexes IP joint.

Palpation. The FPL tendon is palpated on the palmar surface of the proximal phalanx.

Resistance. The therapist's finger pushes the head of the distal phalanx toward extension (Fig. 6.109).

Substitution. Relaxation of the extensor pollicis longus causes apparent, rebound movement.

Position. For flexor pollicis brevis.

Against Gravity. Elbow flexed and forearm supinated so that the palmar surface of the thumb faces the ceiling; thumb is extended at both the MP and IP joints.

Gravity Eliminated. Forearm supinated to 90° so that thumb can flex across the plane of the palm.

Stabilize. First metacarpal.

Test Motion. Patient flexes the MP joint but keeps the IP joint extended to minimize the influence of the flexor pollicis longus.

Palpation. The FPB is palpated on the thenar eminence just proximal to the MP joint, and medial to the abductor pollicis brevis.

Resistance. The therapist's finger pushes the head of the proximal phalanx toward extension (Fig. 6.110).

Substitution. Flexor pollicis longus; the abductor pollicis brevis and the adductor pollicis through insertion into the extensor hood. To rule out the effect of the flexor pollicis longus to test for the flexor pollicis brevis, a test position of maximal elbow flexion, maximal pronation, and maximal wrist flexion has been recommended (Howell et al., 1989).

THUMB ADDUCTION

Prime Mover

Adductor pollicis

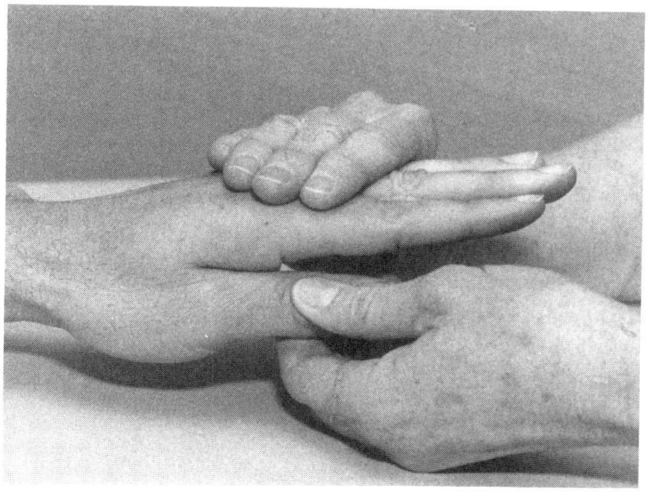

OPPOSITION

Prime Movers

Opponens pollicis
Opponens digiti minimi

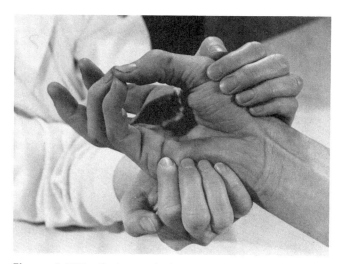

Figure 6.111. Resistance in the against-gravity position.

Figure 6.112. Resistance in the against-gravity position.

Position. Against Gravity. Forearm pronated, wrist and fingers in neutral position, thumb abducted, and MP and IP joints of the thumb in extension.

Gravity Eliminated. Same, except forearm in midposition.

Stabilize. Metacarpals of fingers, keeping the MP joints in neutral.

Test Motion. Patient brings the thumb toward the palm, without hyperextending the MP joint or flexing the MP or IP joints.

Palpation. Adductor pollicis is palpated on the palmar surface of the thumb web space.

Resistance. The therapist grasps the head of the proximal phalanx and pulls it away from the palm toward abduction (Fig. 6.111).

Substitutions. Extensor pollicis longus, flexor pollicis longus, flexor pollicis brevis.

Position. Against Gravity. Forearm supinated and supported, wrist in neutral position, thumb adducted and extended.

Gravity Eliminated. Elbow resting on the table with forearm perpendicular to the table, wrist in neutral position, thumb adducted and extended.

Stabilize. Hold the wrist in a neutral position.

Test Motion. The patient brings the thumb away from and across the palm rotating it so that the pad of the thumb approximates the pad of the little finger. The little finger rotates around to meet the thumb.

Palpation. Place fingertips along the lateral side of the shaft of the first metacarpal where the opponens pollicis may be palpated before it becomes deep to the abductor pollicis brevis. The opponens digit minimi can be palpated volar along the shaft of the fifth metacarpal.

Resistance. The therapist holds along the first metacarpal and "derotates" the thumb or holds along the fifth metacarpal and "derotates" the little finger. These can be resisted simultaneously using both hands (Fig. 6.112).

Substitutions. Abductor pollicis brevis, flexor pollicis brevis, flexor pollicis longus.

Measurement of Selected Lower Extremity Muscle Groups

Muscle testing procedures of the flexors and extensors of the three major joints of the lower extremity are described here because of their importance to functions required for completion of certain activities of daily living, such as climbing stairs or curbs, sitting down, and standing up.

HIP FLEXION

Prime Movers

Iliopsoas
Iliacus
Psoas major

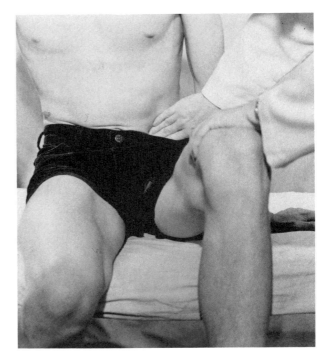

Figure 6.113. Resistance in the against-gravity position: the patient sits with his lower leg hanging over the edge of the sitting surface. He raises the thigh up from the surface; the knee remains flexed. The therapist's right hand is palpating the psoas major.

Stabilize. Pelvis.

Palpation. The iliacus is too deep to be palpated. With the patient in a sitting position, the psoas major can be palpated if the patient bends forward and relaxes the abdominal muscles. The therapist's fingers are placed at the waist between the ribs and the iliac crest and pressure is applied posteriorly to feel the contraction of the psoas major as the hip flexes (Lehmkuhl & Smith, 1983).

Resistance. The therapist's hand is placed on the distal anterior thigh and presses downward toward extension (Fig. 6.113).

Substitution. The abdominals can tilt the pelvis posteriorly to substitute for hip flexion in a gravity-eliminated position.

HIP EXTENSION

Prime Movers

Gluteus maximus
Biceps femoris

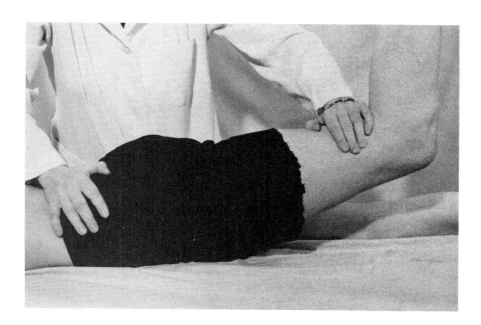

Figure 6.114. Resistance in the against-gravity position: the patient lies prone with knee flexed to 90° or more (Daniels & Worthingham, 1986; Kendall et al., 1971) to test the gluteus maximus. The biceps femoris will be tested in its alternate function of knee flexion. The patient extends the hip keeping the knee flexed.

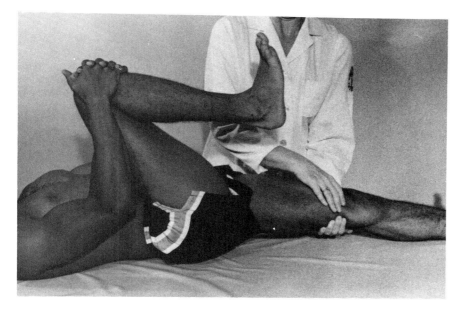

Figure 6.115. Alternate against-gravity position: gluteus maximus and biceps femoris are tested together as hip extensors with the knee extended. The patient lies supine and holds the opposite leg in flexion at the hip and knee. The therapist holds the leg to be tested just above the knee and says to the patient, "Do not let me raise your leg" (Diekmeyer, 1978). *Grading:* normal if trunk comes up from table; fair if the hip "gives" as the trunk begins to come up from the table.

Stabilize.   Pelvis and lumbar spine.

Palpation.   The gluteus maximus is the larger muscle of the buttocks and can be easily palpated. The biceps femoris (Basmajian & DeLuca, 1985) can be palpated on the posterior aspect of the thigh; its tendon bounds the popliteal fossa laterally.

Resistance.   The therapist's hand is placed over the distal posterior thigh and presses downward or forward toward flexion (Figs. 6.114 and 6.115).

Substitutions.   Extension of the lumbar spine. The semimembranosus and semitendinosus assist resisted hip extension if the hip is abducted (Basmajian & DeLuca, 1985).

KNEE FLEXION

Prime Movers

Hamstrings
  Semimembranosus
  Semitendinosus
  Biceps femoris

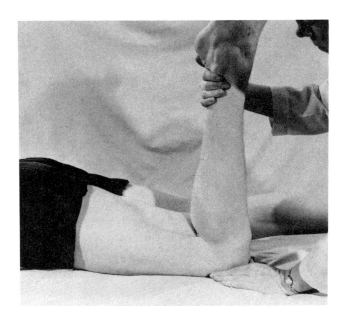

Figure 6.116. Resistance in the against-gravity position: the patient lies prone with both hips and knees extended, feet hanging free over the edge of the plinth. The patient moves the lower leg toward the back of the thigh. After the patient flexes his knee to 90°, the motion becomes gravity-assisted. In deciding between a F− or F grade, the therapist must use clinical judgment or stand the patient up to have him flex to 120° against gravity.

Stabilize.   Thigh against the plinth.

Palpation.   These three muscles can be palpated on the posterior surface of the thigh. The tendon of the biceps femoris can be palpated on the lateral side of the popliteal space, and the tendon of the semitendinosus may be palpated on the medial side of the popliteal space. Both tendons become prominent when resistance is applied (Lehmkuhl & Smith, 1983). The biceps femoris can be isolated from the other muscles by rotating the lower leg externally with respect to the femur. The semitendinosus will contract more prominently if the lower leg is rotated internally with respect to the femur. The semimembranosus lies deep to the semitendinosus, but its lower portion may be palpated on both sides of the semitendinosus tendon.

Resistance.   The therapist's hand is placed on the distal end of the posterior surface of the tibia and pushes it toward extension. If resistance is applied off to one side, medial or lateral, either the lateral or medial hamstrings will contract more strongly (Fig. 6.116).

Substitutions.   When prone, gravity assists flexion beyond 90°. When sitting, gravity can flex the knee.

KNEE EXTENSION

Prime Movers

Quadriceps
  Rectus femoris
  Vastus medialis
  Vastus intermedius
  Vastus lateralis

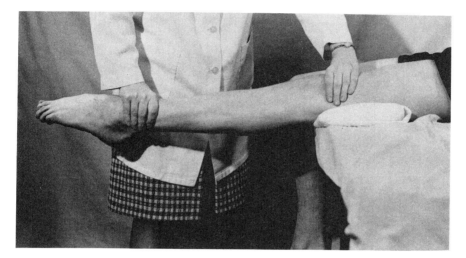

Figure 6.117. Resistance in the against-gravity position: the patient sits erect with the lower leg hanging free. A small pillow or rolled towel is placed between the edge of the plinth and the distal end of the thigh for the patient's comfort. Patient extends the knee.

Stabilize. Thigh.

Palpation. The tendon of the quadriceps may be palpated as it approaches the patella. Except for the vastus intermedius, the muscle bellies can be palpated on the anterior surface of the thigh; the rectus femoris is in the center and lies over the vastus intermedius; the other vasti are palpated medially and laterally to the rectus femoris.

Resistance. The therapist's hand is placed at the distal end of the anterior surface of the tibia. Resistance is applied slowly to build up to the patient's maximum and to avoid injury to the knee, which can result from applying sudden or excessive resistance. It is almost impossible to break a normal quadriceps (Hines, 1958) (Fig. 6.117).

Substitutions. None.

ANKLE DORSIFLEXION

Prime Movers

Tibialis anterior
Extensor hallucis longus
Extensor digitorum longus

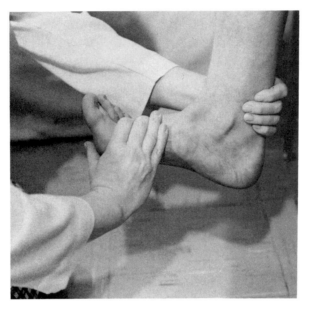

Figure 6.118. Resistance in the against-gravity position: the patient sits erect with the lower leg hanging free. The foot is in neutral position (perpendicular to lower leg). The patient moves the foot so that the dorsum of the foot approximates the anterior surface of the lower leg.

Stabilize. Lower leg.

Palpation. The belly of the tibialis anterior can be palpated immediately lateral to the shaft of the tibia. Its large tendon can be palpated on the anterior surface of the ankle, medial to the tendon of the extensor hallucis longus. The latter can be palpated in the middle of the anterior surface of the ankle. The extensor digitorum longus tendon is prominent on the lateral side of the anterior aspect of the ankle. The tendons of the extensor hallucis longus and extensor digitorum longus can be traced to their insertions on the toes.

Resistance. The therapist's hand is placed on the distal portion of the foot and pushes toward plantar flexion without allowing the foot to invert or evert (Fig. 6.118).

Substitutions. None.

ANKLE PLANTAR FLEXION

Prime Movers

Gastrocnemius
Soleus

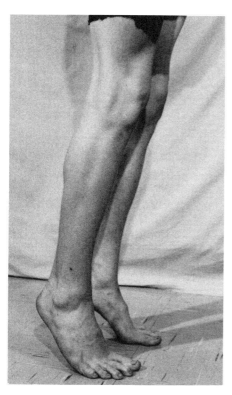

Figure 6.119. Test for plantar flexion to grade normal: standing on tiptoe.

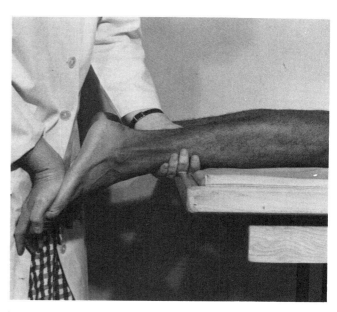

Figure 6.120. Resistance in the against-gravity position: the patient lies prone with the knee extended and the foot hanging free off the plinth. The foot is in neutral position (perpendicular to lower leg). The patient moves the foot so that the toes move away from the anterior surface of the lower leg.

Stabilize. Lower leg.

Palpation. The soleus is palpable at the distal portion of the lower leg. The gastrocnemius is the superficial muscle of the calf; the two heads can be palpated at their origin on either side of the posterior femur. The Achilles tendon is the insertion of both the soleus and gastrocnemius and is readily palpable at the back of the ankle. To minimize the influence of the gastrocnemius when testing for the soleus, the patient lies prone with his knee flexed. Slight resistance is applied to plantar flexion (Lehmkuhl & Smith, 1983).

Resistance. When the patient rises on tiptoe, the full body weight resists these muscles (Fig. 6.119). To apply manual resistance, when the patient is unable to stand, the therapist's hand is placed at the distal portion of the foot and pushes the foot toward dorsiflexion (Fig. 6.120).

Substitutions. Gravity substitutes when the person is lying supine or is sitting with feet off the supporting surface. The extrinsic toe flexors substitute weakly.

INTERPRETING THE MUSCLE TEST

After the muscle test scores have all been recorded, the therapist reviews the scores and looks for the muscles that are weak as well as the distribution and significance of the weakness. Any muscle that grades good minus (G−) or below is considered to be weak. Good plus (G+) muscles are functional and usually require no therapy. Good (G) muscles may or may not be functionally adequate for the patient, depending on his occupational task requirements. The pattern of muscle weakness is important to notice. The pattern may be one of general weakness caused by disuse secondary to immobilization. Or the pattern may reflect the level of spinal innervation in a patient after spinal cord injury or the distribution of a peripheral nerve in the case of peripheral nerve injury. A pattern of imbalance of forces in agonists and antagonists is potentially deforming; counterpositioning or splinting should be considered along with strengthening of the weak muscles.

The pattern of significant strengths is also important to notice. For example, a muscle test of a spinal cord–injured patient that indicates some strength in a muscle innervated by a segment below the diagnosed level of injury is a hopeful sign for more recovery. Or because muscles are reinnervated proximally to distally after peripheral nerve injury, muscle test results showing beginning return of strength in particular muscles help to trace the progress of nerve regeneration.

Short-term goals are set to move the patient from the level of strength determined by testing to the next higher level, e.g., if a muscle grades F, the short-term goal is to improve strength to F+; if it grades F+, the goal is to increase strength to G−, and so on.

If the muscle test is a reevaluation, the scores are compared with the previous test to note changes. The frequency of reevaluation depends on the nature of expected recovery. Expected rapid recovery requires frequent reevaluation. If the repeated muscle test shows that the patient is making gains, the therapeutic program is considered beneficial and is continued by upgrading the demands. If repeated muscle tests show no gains despite programming adaptations, the patient is considered to have reached a plateau and is no longer benefiting from remediational therapy. In that case, the patient will be taught how to compensate for his weakness to be able to do his occupational performance tasks and activities.

Patients with degenerative diseases are expected to get weaker; therefore, therapy is aimed at maintaining their strength and function as long as possible. Repeated muscle tests are done to confirm that effect of therapy. A plateau for these patients is desirable and indicates that the therapy program is effective for maintaining strength and should be continued.

MEASUREMENT OF GRASP AND PINCH

Therapists supplement manual strength testing with dynamometric evaluations of grip and pinch strength that are valid and reliable (Mathiowetz, 1991; Mathiowetz et al., 1984) and for which norms have been established (Mathiowetz et al., 1985). Abbreviated versions of the norms are listed in Tables 6.4 and 6.5.

As when using any instrument to measure, the instrument must be calibrated and set at 0 to start. Dynamometers and pinch meters can be calibrated by placing known weights on, or suspending them from, the compression part of the meter (Fess, 1987). Using this procedure, the Jamar dynamometer, designed by Bechtol (1954), was found to be accurate to within ±5% and the B & L pinch meter to within ±1% (Mathiowetz, 1990; Mathiowetz et al., 1984; Schmidt & Toews, 1970).

The standard method of measurement used in the study from which the norms were established reflects

Table 6.4. Jamar Grasp Dynamometer Norms in Pounds (Mean of Three Trials)[a]

		Norms at Age (years)											
		20	25	30	35	40	45	50	55	60	65	70	75+
Male	Right	121	121	122	120	117	110	114	101	90	91	75	66
	SD	21	23	22	24	21	23	18	27	20	21	21	21
	Left	104	110	110	113	113	101	102	83	77	77	65	55
	SD	22	16	22	22	19	23	17	23	20	20	18	17
Female	Right	70	74	79	74	70	62	66	57	55	50	50	43
	SD	14	14	19	11	13	15	12	12	10	10	12	11
	Left	61	63	68	66	62	56	57	47	46	41	41	38
	SD	13	12	18	12	14	13	11	12	10	8	10	9

[a]n = 628; age range = 20–94 years.

Table 6.5.   B & L (60) Pinchmeter Norms in Pounds (Mean of Three Trials)[a]

			20	30	40	50	60	70	75+
			— Norms at Age (years)						
Tip									
	Male	Right	18	18	18	18	16	14	14
		Left	17	18	18	18	15	13	14
	Female	Right	11	13	11	12	10	10	10
		Left	10	12	11	11	10	10	9
	(average SD: Males = 4.0; females = 2.5)								
Lateral									
	Male	Right	26	26	26	27	23	19	20
		Left	25	26	25	26	22	19	19
	Female	Right	18	19	17	17	15	14	13
		Left	16	18	16	16	14	14	11
	(average SD: males = 4.6; females = 3.0)								
Palmar									
	Male	Right	27	25	24	24	22	18	19
		Left	26	25	25	24	21	19	18
	Female	Right	17	19	17	17	15	14	12
		Left	16	18	17	16	14	14	12
	(average SD: males = 5.1; females = 3.7)								

[a] n = 628; age range = 20–94 years.

the recommendations of the American Society of Hand Therapists (ASHT) (1981). Test-retest (1 week) **reliability** of this method using the Jamar hydraulic dynamometer was found to be ≥0.88; interrater **reliability** (two raters, same time) was ≥0.99. Interrater (two raters, same time) **reliability** of averaged B & L pinch meter scores was ≥0.979; test-retest (1 week) **reliability** was ≥.81 (Mathiowetz et al., 1984).

Flood-Joy and Mathiowetz (1987) reported significant discrepancies among three different models of the Jamar hydraulic grasp meter. For this reason, it is essential that the exact same dynamometer be used when reevaluating gains as was used during the initial evaluation. Until the normative study is replicated, the data in Table 6.4 can be used with confidence for patients under 50 years of age but with slightly less confidence for patients older than 50 years (25% of the measurements were taken with a different dynamometer), if you use Model #6420—the one used in the study, which can be recognized by its off-center calibration screw. Newer versions of the dynamometer have less friction, and therefore, patients score higher and appear to be doing better than if they had been measured on the original instrument.

Grasp

The patient should be seated with his shoulder adducted and neutrally rotated, elbow flexed at 90°,

and the forearm and wrist in neutral position (Fig. 6.121). Grip strength varies with elbow position, therefore the need to adhere to a standardized position (Kuzala & Vargo, 1992). The handle of the Jamar dynamometer is set at the second position (Mathiowetz et al., 1984, 1985). The task is demonstrated to the patient. After the dynamometer is positioned in the patient's hand, the therapist says, "Ready? Squeeze as hard as you can," and then urges the patient on throughout the attempt. The patient squeezes the dynamometer with as much force as he can, three separate times with a 2- to 3-min rest between trials.

A vigorometer has been found to be an acceptable alternative hand strength–measuring device for patients whose diagnoses contraindicate stress on joints and/or skin. It requires the patient to squeeze a rubber bulb rather than a steel handle. The vigorometer is a commercially available instrument for which norms have been published (Fike & Rousseau, 1982).

Another adapted sphygmomanometer for measuring grip strength of rheumatoid arthritic patients was found to have a strong and linear relationship ($r = 0.83$ for the right hand; $r = 0.84$ for the left) to the Jamar when tested on 88 RA patients. Agnew and Maas (1991) used linear regression equations to develop conversion tables to predict scores between the Jamar and the sphygmomanometer.

The power grip attachment of the Baltimore Therapeutic Equipment Work Simulator has been evaluated for test-retest **reliability** on 30 right-dominant males and females aged 20 to 45 years (Trossman, Suleski, & Li (1990). The mean of three trials was the most reliable score. Day-to-day variability was 5% for the right hand and 3% for the left hand. Test-retest reliability was ≥0.98.

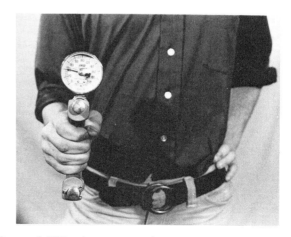

Figure 6.121. Jamar grasp dynamometer.

Pinch

TIP PINCH

The patient pinches the ends of the B & L pinch meter between the tips of his thumb and index finger (Fig. 6.122 and Table 6.5) (Mathiowetz et al., 1985) or between the thumb and the index and middle fingers (Kellor et al., 1971). The test is administered by first giving the patient instructions and a demonstration. Then the therapist says, "Ready? Pinch as hard as you can." The patient is urged on as he attempts to pinch. He does three trials with a rest between each trial. The average of three trials is recorded.

LATERAL PINCH

The patient pinches the meter between the pad of his thumb and the lateral surface of his index finger (Fig. 6.123 and Table 6.5). The instructions and procedure are the same as for tip pinch.

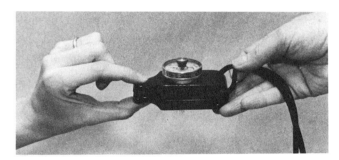

Figure 6.122. Pinch meter measuring tip pinch.

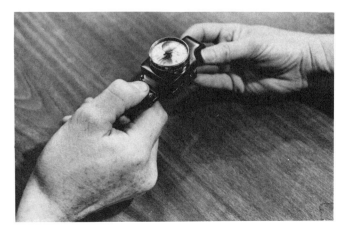

Figure 6.123. Pinch meter measuring lateral pinch.

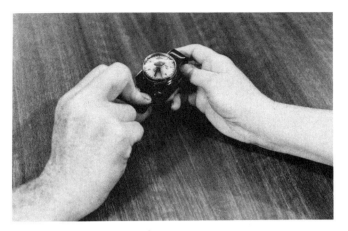

Figure 6.124. Pinch meter measuring palmar pinch.

PALMAR PINCH (THREE-JAW-CHUCK)

The patient pinches the meter between the pad of his thumb and the pads of his index and middle fingers (Fig. 6.124 and Table 6.5). The instructions and procedure are the same as for tip pinch.

Interpretation of Grasp and Pinch Scores

Scores are compared with those of the noninvolved hand or to norms to ascertain if the patient has a significant limitation. The accuracy of the Jamar dynamometer was found to be ±5% which means that if your patient scored 50 pounds, the actual strength may be somewhere between 47.5 and 52.5 pounds (Mathiowetz, 1990). Grasp and pinch scores are considered abnormal if they are associated with a functional limitation and/or if they are ±3 **standard deviations** (SD) from the mean (Mathiowetz, 1990). For example, suppose your 40-year-old male patient had a grasp score of 55 pounds when you averaged the three trials for his right, dominant hand. Looking at Table 6.4, you see that the average score for his age group is 117 pounds, thus your patient's grasp score was 62 pounds less than the mean normal score on the table. When you divide the **standard deviation** given in the table (21) into his score (62), you find that he is 2.95 SD below the mean. This is close enough to −3 SD to consider that he has a significant limitation. See Chapter 7 for another example of this method of interpretation of scores.

ENDURANCE

Endurance is the ability to sustain effort. It is related to cardiopulmonary function and to biomechanical and neuromuscular function (Asmussen, 1979; Lunsford, 1978). Persons who have cardiac or pulmonary impairments; who have suffered a major trauma or illness requiring bed rest; or who have made inefficient biomechanical adaptations secondary to pain, weakness, deformity, or use of prostheses or adapted equipment will have limited endurance.

Central (Cardiopulmonary) Aspects of Endurance

Muscular work creates a demand for oxygen (Astrand & Rodahl, 1986). As an immediate effect of exercise, the heart rate (HR) and stroke volume increase. Heart rate increases to deliver the required amount of oxygenated blood to the active muscles. Stroke volume, or amount of blood pumped per heartbeat, increases because of increased venous flow into the heart during diastole (the period of relaxation when the chambers fill) (Ellestad, 1986). As the intensity of work increases, more oxygen is required. There is, however, a maximal amount of oxygen that a person can take in and dispense to muscles during exercise. It is termed maximal oxygen uptake and is abbreviated $\dot{V}O_2$max. $\dot{V}O_2$max is a standard measure of cardiovascular fitness (Taylor, Buskirk, & Henschel, 1955). It increases with physical training and decreases with bed rest and age.

$\dot{V}O_2$max relates to the person's maximal metabolic equivalent (MET) capacity (American College of Sports Medicine, 1976); 1 MET equals basal metabolic rate (Erb et al., 1979). Basal metabolic rate is the amount of oxygen consumption necessary to maintain metabolic processes (respiration, circulation, peristalsis, temperature regulation, glandular function, etc.) of the body at rest (3.5 mL O_2/kg body weight/min). The energy cost of activities or exercise can be rated using multiples of METs.

Peripheral (Biomechanical/Neuromuscular) Aspects of Endurance

Endurance of a muscle or muscle group may be decreased because of localized trauma or reduction of innervation. In normal muscle, only a few of the available motor units are needed at any one time. The active and resting units take turns. Fatigue rarely occurs under conditions required for activities of daily life. However, if the person sustains a contraction that exceeds 15 to 20% **maximum voluntary contraction** (MVC) for the muscle group involved, blood flow to the working muscles will decrease, causing a shift to anaerobic metabolism, which limits duration (Dehn, 1980). The limitation is signaled by symptoms of muscle fatigue—cramping, burning, and tremor, which are

secondary to the accumulation of lactic acid, and slowed conduction velocity of the muscle fibers, resulting in reduced tension development and eventual inability to hold the contraction (Basmajian & DeLuca, 1985).

For neurologically disadvantaged muscle, fewer motor units or muscle fibers may be available than are required for daily activity, so each must sustain activity a greater proportion of the time. Such muscles will be contracting as much as 50 to 75% MVC to do otherwise low-intensity work (Trombly & Quintana, 1985).

THE EVALUATION

Intensity, duration, and frequency are considered when evaluating endurance. Intensity is related to both resistance and speed. The heavier the resistance or the faster the pace, the higher the intensity. Intensity of an activity is estimated in terms of light, moderate, or heavy work or number of METs. An exercise that is rated 4.0 METs requires 4 times the amount of oxygen per kilogram of body weight per minute than the basal rate. Oxygen consumption of daily living, recreational, and vocational tasks has been measured for normal subjects, and the METs required for each task have been calculated. Many charts of the metabolic cost of activities have been published (see Chapter 43). These costs do not hold for patients with chronic obstructive pulmonary disease (COPD) who, because of reduced expiration and expulsion of CO^2 waste, have greater ventilatory requirements (Whipp & Ward, 1986). These patients have limited exercise capacity (Hansen, 1986).

Endurance is reported as (1) the number of repetitions per unit of time, (2) the percent of maximal heart rate, or (3) the amount of time a contraction can be held (Milner-Brown et al., 1986). The choice of whether to measure dynamically or statically depends on the functional goal the patient is working toward and his cardiopulmonary status. If the patient's work and hobbies require only isotonic activity, endurance will be evaluated dynamically.

To measure endurance dynamically, a light, repetitive activity is used. The *Box and Block Test* (described in Chapter 7) can be adapted to measure light-work upper extremity endurance by counting the number of blocks the patient can transfer before becoming fatigued. The intensity of the test activity must be kept constant from test to test to gauge improvement.

HR is a simple means to quantify the physiological demand of a dynamic activity (McKenna & Maas, 1987). It relates linearly to $\dot{V}O_2$max, except at the upper limits (80 to 90%) of maximal capacity (Ellestad, 1986). For example, if a person's HR is 70% of maximal HR (HRmax), he is using approximately 70% of $\dot{V}O_2$max. HRmax is estimated by subtracting the person's age from 220. The pulse taken immediately after aerobic, large-muscle exercise is then related to the person's maximum HR as percent of maximum. A constant HR obtained during exercise indicates a steady state, i.e., balance of oxygen intake and consumption (Ellestad, 1986).

Heart rate is measured by placing the index and middle fingers lightly, but firmly, over the radial artery at the wrist (lateral to the flexor carpi radialis) and counting the number of beats per minute (bpm). It is most accurate to count for a full minute, but an exercise heart rate can only be counted for 10 to 15 sec, as the return to resting rate occurs quickly after stopping exercise. In that case, the obtained value is multiplied to arrive at the bpm (Lunsford, 1978).

Over time, in patients with normal lung function, a training effect will be seen, i.e., the exercise HR will be lower than previously required for the same amount of work (Fletcher & Cantwell, 1979). As the training effect occurs, the intensity of the test activity is gradually upgraded until it is equal to the demands the person expects to return to.

If the patient expects to return to a job or hobby that requires maintained grasp or holding loads and if he has a normal cardiopulmonary system, then static endurance needs to be tested. To measure statically, the amount of time a person can hold an object requiring a certain level MVC is noted. Normally, a person can hold 25% MVC for 5 to 6 min; 50% MVC for 1 to 2 min; and 100% MVC only momentarily (Dehn & Mullins, 1977).

Isometric holding increases blood pressure and stresses the cardiopulmonary system (Dehn, 1980; Ellestad, 1986). This is especially true if the person holds his breath (Valsalva maneuver) while holding the contraction. Therefore, persons being tested should talk (e.g., count or sing) while doing an isometric contraction to preclude breath holding. Isometric testing can produce arrhythmias, and therefore, electrocardiogram (ECG) and blood pressure (BP) should be monitored during isometric testing in patients with heart disease or abnormalities. The results of isometric testing cannot be extrapolated to gauge isotonic, aerobic exercise capacity (Ellestad, 1986).

Symptoms that indicate the exercise demand exceeds the person's cardiopulmonary capacity include dyspnea, weakness, changes in sensorium, angina, decreased HR for increased workload, increased ventricular arrhythmias, pallor, and cyanosis (Dehn & Mullins, 1977). Endurance testing in occupational therapy should not reach this level, but if any of these symptoms are observed or reported by the patient, the intensity of work should be immediately reduced to a comfortable level.

TOLERANCE

Amount of time that a patient can tolerate a splint, device, or posture is also a type of endurance measurement. This type of endurance is often referred to as tolerance, e.g., wearing tolerance or sitting tolerance.

STUDY QUESTIONS

1. Describe the correct placement, in general, of a goniometer.
2. What does it mean if active range of motion is less than passive range of motion?
3. ROM limitations can be caused by a number of underlying conditions. State the short-term goal for treatment of elbow flexion contracture found after removal of a cast used to immobilize a fractured humerus.
4. What is the difference between a break test and a make test?
5. Of what importance is the length/tension relationship of a muscle in manual muscle testing?
6. Name the procedures that must follow an established format in testing each muscle or motion.
7. For what muscle test grades is treatment to increase strength an appropriate goal?
8. How is dynamic endurance measured?
9. How is static endurance measured?
10. What is your maximum heart rate? What percentage of your $\dot{V}O_2$max do you use to vacuum a room? to take a shower? to wash the dishes?

REFERENCES

Agnew, P. J., & Maas, F. (1991). Jamar dynamometer and adapted sphygmomanometer for measuring grip strength in patients with rheumatoid arthritis. *Occupational Therapy Journal of Research*, *11*(5), 259–270.

American College of Sports Medicine. (1976). *Guidelines for graded exercise testing and exercise prescription.* Philadelphia: Lea & Febiger.

American Society for Hand Therapists. (1981). *Clinical assessment recommendations.* Indianapolis: American Society for Hand Therapists.

Anderson, L. R. III, & Bohannon, R. W. (1991). Head and neck position does not influence maximum static elbow extension force measured in healthy individuals tested while prone. *Occupational Therapy Journal of Research*, *11*(2), 121–126.

Asmussen, E. (1979). Muscle fatigue. *Medical Science and Sports*, *11*(4), 313–321.

Astrand, P. O., & Rodahl, K. (1986). *Textbook of work physiology: Physiological basis of exercise* (3rd ed.). New York: McGraw-Hill.

Basmajian, J. V., & DeLuca, C. J. (1985). *Muscles alive: Their functions revealed by electromyography* (5th ed.). Baltimore: Williams & Wilkins.

Bechtol, C. O. (1954). Grip test: Use of a dynamometer with adjustable handle spacing. *Journal of Bone and Joint Surgery, 36A*(7), 820–824, 832, 1954.

Bohannon, R. W. (1986). Test-retest reliability of hand-held dynamometry during a single session of strength assessment. *Physical Therapy, 66*(2), 206–209.

Bohannon, R. W., Warren, M., & Cogman, K. (1991). Influence of shoulder position on maximum voluntary elbow flexion force in stroke patients. *Occupational Therapy Journal of Research, 11*(2), 73–79.

Boone, D. C., Azen, S. P., Lin, C.-M., Spence, C., Baron, C., & Lee, L. (1978). Reliability of goniometric measurements. *Physical Therapy, 58*(11), 1355–1360.

Bosi Ferraz, M., Magalhaes Oliveira, L., Araujo, P. M. P., Atra, E., & Walter, S. D. (1990). EPM-ROM scale: An evaluative instrument to be used in rheumatoid arthritis trials. *Clinical and Experimental Rheumatology, 8*, 491–494.

Breger-Lee, D. (1990). Torque range of motion in the hand clinic. *Journal of Hand Therapy, 3*, 7–13.

Caldwell, L. S., Chaffin, D. B., Dukes-Dobos, F. N., Kroemer, K. H. E., Laubach, L. L., Snook, S. H., & Wasserman, D. E. (1974). A proposed standard procedure for static muscle strength testing. *American Industrial Hygiene Association Journal, 35*(4), 201–206.

Daniels, L., & Worthingham, C. (1986). *Muscle testing: Techniques of manual examination* (5th ed.). Philadelphia: W. B. Saunders.

Darling, R. C. (1971). Exercise. In J. A. Downey & R. C. Darling (Eds.), *Physiological basis of rehabilitation medicine* (pp. 167–183). Philadelphia: W. B. Saunders.

Dehn, M. M. (1980, March). Rehabilitation of the cardiac patient: The effects of exercise. *American Journal of Nursing, 80*, 435–440.

Dehn, M. M., & Mullins, C. B. (1977, April). Physiologic effects and importance of exercise in patients with coronary artery disease. *Cardiovascular Medicine 2*, 365–371, 377–387.

DeVore, G. L., & Hamilton, G. F. (1968). Volume measuring of the severely injured hand. *American Journal of Occupational Therapy, 22*(1), 16–18.

Diekmeyer, G., (1978). Altered test position for hip extensor muscles. *Physical Therapy, 58*(11), 1379.

Ellestad, M. H. (1986). *Stress testing: Principles and practice* (3rd ed.). Philadelphia: F. A. Davis.

Erb, B. D., Fletcher, G. F., & Sheffield, T. L. (1979). AHA Committee report: Standards for cardiovascular exercise treatment programs. *Circulation, 59*, 1084A–1090A.

Fess, E. E. (1987). A method of checking Jamar dynamometer calibration. *Journal of Hand Therapy, 1*, 28–32.

Fess, E. E. (1990). Assessment of the upper extremity: Instrumentation criteria. *Occupational Therapy Practice, 1*(4), 1–11.

Fike, M. L., & Rousseau, E. (1982). Measurement of adult hand strength: A comparison of two instruments. *Occupational Therapy Journal of Research, 2*(1), 43–49.

Fish, D. R., & Wingate, L. (1985). Sources of goniometric error at the elbow. *Physical Therapy, 65*(11), 1666–1670.

Fletcher, G. F., & Cantwell, J. D. (1979). *Exercise and coronary heart disease: Role in prevention, diagnosis and treatment* (2nd ed.). Springfield, IL: Charles C. Thomas.

Flood-Joy, M., & Mathiowetz, V. (1987). Grip-strength measurement: A comparison of three Jamar dynamometers. *Occupational Therapy Journal of Research, 7*(4), 235–243.

Gowitzke, B. A., & Milner, M. (1980). *Understanding the scientific bases of human movement* (2nd ed.). Baltimore: Williams & Wilkins.

Hansen, J.E. (1986). Respiratory abnormalities: Exercise evaluation of the dyspneic patient. In A. R. Leff (Ed.), *Cardiopulmonary exercise testing* (pp. 69–88). New York: Grune & Stratton.

Heck, C. V., Hendryson, I. E., & Rowe, C. R. (1965). Joint motion: Methods of measuring and recording. Chicago: American Academy of Orthopaedic Surgeons.

Hines, T. (1965). Manual muscle examination. In S. Licht (Ed.), *Therapeutic exercise* (2nd ed., pp. 163–256). Baltimore: Waverly Press.

Horger, M. M. (1990). The reliability of goniometric measurements of active and passive wrist motions. *American Journal of Occupational Therapy, 44*(4), 342–348.

Howell, J. W., Rothstein, J. M., Lamb, R. L., & Merritt, W. H. (1989). An experimental investigation of the validity of the manual muscle test positions for the extensor pollicis longus and flexor pollicis brevis muscles. *Journal of Hand Therapy, 3*, 20–28.

Johannson, C. A., Kent, B. E., & Shepard, K. F. (1983). Relationship between verbal command volume and magnitude of muscle contraction. *Physical Therapy, 63*, 1260–1265.

Johnston, M. V., Keith, R. A., & Hinderer, S. R. (1992). Measurement standards for interdisciplinary medical rehabilitation. *Archives of Physical Medicine and Rehabilitation, 73*(12S), S1–S22.

Kellor, M., Frost, J., Silverberg, N., Iverson, I., & Cummings, R. (1971). Hand strength and dexterity. *American Journal of Occupational Therapy, 25*(2), 77–83.

Kendall, H. O., Kendall, F. P., & Wadsworth, G. E. (1971). *Muscles: Testing and function.* Baltimore: Williams & Wilkins.

Kuzala, E. A., & Vargo, M. C. (1992). The relationship between elbow position and grip strength. *American Journal of Occupational Therapy, 46*(6), 509–512.

Landsmeer, J. M. F., & Long, C. (1965). The mechanism of finger control based on electromyograms and location analysis. *Acta Anatomica (Basel), 60*, 330–347.

Lehmkuhl, L. D., & Smith, L. K. (1983). *Brunnstrom's clinical kinesiology* (4th ed.). Philadelphia: F. A. Davis.

Long, C. (1968). Intrinsic-extrinsic muscle control of the fingers. *Journal of Bone and Joint Surgery, 50A*(5), 973–984.

Long, C., & Brown, M. E. (1962). EMG kinesiology of the hand. Part III. Lumbricales and flexor digitorum profundus to the long finger. *Archives of Physical Medicine and Rehabilitation, 43*, 450–460.

Lunsford, B. R. (1978). Clinical indicators of endurance. *Physical Therapy, 58*(6), 704–709.

Mathiowetz, V. (1990). Grip and pinch strength measurements. In L. R. Amundsen (Ed.), *Muscle strength testing: Instrumented and non-instrumented systems.* New York: Churchill Livingstone.

Mathiowetz, V. (1991). Reliability and validity of grip and pinch strength measurements. *Critical Reviews in Physical and Rehabilitation Medicine, 2*(4), 201–212.

Mathiowetz, V., Kashman, N., Volland, G., Weber, K., Dowe, M., & Rogers, S. (1985). Grip and pinch strength: Normative data for adults. *Archives of Physical Medicine and Rehabilitation, 66*(2), 69–74.

Mathiowetz, V., Weber, K., Volland, G., & Kashman, N. (1984). Reliability and validity of grip and pinch strength evaluations. *Hand Surgery, 9A*(2), 222–226.

McKenna, K. T., & Maas, F. (1987). Mean and peak heart rate prediction using estimated energy costs of jobs. *Occupational Therapy Journal of Research, 7*(6), 323–334.

Medical Research Council. (1976). *Aids to the examination of the peripheral nervous system.* London: Her Majesty's Stationary Office.

Milner-Brown, H. S., Mellenthin, M., & Miller, R. G. (1986). Quantifying human muscle strength, endurance and fatigue. *Archives of Physical Medicine and Rehabilitation, 67*(8), 530–535.

Moore, M. L. (1978). Clinical assessment of joint motion. In J. V. Basmajian (Ed.), *Therapeutic exercise* (3rd ed.). Baltimore: Williams & Wilkins

Petherick, M., Rheault, W., Kimble, S., Lechner, C., & Senear, V. (1988). Concurrent validity and intertester reliability of universal and fluid-based goniometers for active elbow range of motion. *Physical Therapy, 68*(6), 966–969.

Riddle, D. L., Rothstein, J. M., & Lamb, R. L. (1987). Goniometric reliability in a clinical setting. *Physical Therapy, 67*(5), 668–673.

Salter, N. (1958). Muscle and joint measurement. In S. Licht (Ed.), *Therapeutic exercise* (pp. 127–158). Baltimore: Waverly Press.

Schmidt, R. T., & Toews, J. V. (1970). Grip strength as measured by the Jamar dynamometer. *Archives of Physical Medicine and Rehabilitation, 51*(5), 321–327.

Schwanholt, C., & Stern, P. J. (1984). Brief or new: Measuring cone for thumb abduction/extension. *American Journal of Occupational Therapy, 38*(4), 263–264.

Smidt, G. L., & Rogers, M. W. (1982). Factors contributing to the regulation and clinical assessment of muscular strength. *Physical Therapy, 62*(9), 1283–1290.

Stern, E. (1991). Volumetric comparison of seated and standing postures. *American Journal of Occupational Therapy, 45*(9), 801–804.

Taylor, H. L., Buskirk, E., & Henschel, A. (1955). Maximal oxygen uptake as objective measure of cardiorespiratory performance. *Journal of Applied Physiology, 8*, 73–80.

Trombly, C. A., & Quintana, L. A. (1985). Differences in response to exercise by post-CVA and normal subjects. *Occupational Therapy Journal of Research, 5*(1), 39–58.

Trossman, P. B., Suleski, K. B., & Li, P.-W. (1990). Test-retest reliability and day-to-day variability of an isometric grip strength test using the work simulator. *Occupational Therapy Journal of Research, 10*(5), 266–279.

Watkins, M. A., Riddle, D. L., Lamb, R. L., & Personius, W. J. (1991). Reliability of goniometric measurements and visual estimates of knee range of motion obtained in a clinical setting. *Physical Therapy, 71*(2), 90–97.

Waylett, J., & Seibly, D. (1981). A study to determine the average deviation accuracy of a commercially available volumeter. *Journal of Hand Surgery, 6*, 300.

Whipp, B. J., & Ward, S. (1986). The normal respiratory response in exercise. In A. R. Leff (Ed.), *Cardiopulmonary exercise testing* (pp. 45–68). New York: Grune & Stratton.

SUGGESTED READINGS

Bohannon, R. W., & Andrews, A. W. (1987). Interrater reliability of hand-held dynamometry. *Physical Therapy, 67*(6), 931–933.

Boström, C., Harms-Ringdahl, K., & Nordemar, R. (1991). Clinical reliability of shoulder function assessment in patients with rheumatoid arthritis. *Scandinavian Journal of Rheumatology, 20*, 36–48.

Frese, E., Brown, M., & Norton, B. J. (1987). Clinical reliability of manual muscle testing: Middle trapezius and gluteus medius muscles. *Physical Therapy, 67*(7), 1072–1076.

Gajdosik, R. L., & Bohannon, R. W. (1987). Clinical measurement of range of motion: Review of goniometry emphasizing reliability and validity. *Physical Therapy, 67*(12), 1867–1872.

Hinson, M., & Gench, B. E. (1989). The curvilinear relationship of grip strength to age. *Occupational Therapy Journal of Research, 9*(1), 53–60.

Hinson, M., Woodard, J., & Gench, B. (1990). Reliability of the Jamar digital dynamometer Model 2A. *Occupational Therapy Journal of Research, 10*(2), 108–110.

Jarus, T., & Poremba, R. (1993). Hand function: A factor analysis study. *American Journal of Occupational Therapy, 47*(5), 439–443.

Loessin Grohmann, J. E. (1983). Comparison of two methods of goniometry. *Physical Therapy, 63*(6), 922–925.

Mayerson, N. H., & Milano, R. A. (1984). Goniometric measurement reliability in physical medicine. *Archives of Physical Medicine and Rehabilitation, 65*(2), 92–94.

Niebuhr, B. R., Marion, R., & Fike, M. L. (1984). Reliability of grip strength assessment with the computerized Jamar dynamometer. *Occupational Therapy Journal of Research, 14*(1), 3–8.

Petersen, P. Petrick, M., Connor, H., & Conklin, D. (1989). Grip strength and hand dominance: Challenging the 10% rule. *American Journal of Occupational Therapy, 43*(7), 444–447.

Reddon, J. R., Stefanyk, W. O., Gill, D. M., & Renney, C. (1985). Hand dynamometer: Effects of trials and sessions. *Perceptual and Motor Skills, 61*, 1195–1198.

Schang, S. J., & Pepine, C. J. (1977). Transient asymptomatic S-T segment depression during daily activity. *American Journal of Cardiology, 39*(3), 396–402.

Shiffman, L. M. (1992). Effects of aging on adult hand function. *American Journal of Occupational Therapy, 46*(9), 785–792.

Smith, J. R., & Walker, J. M. (1983). Knee and elbow range of motion in healthy older individuals. *Physical and Occupational Therapy in Geriatrics, 2*(4), 31–38.

Trossman, P. B., & Li, P.-W. (1989). The effect of the duration of intertrial rest periods on isometric grip strength performance in young adults. *Occupational Therapy Journal of Research, 9*(6), 362–378.

Yack, H. J. (1984). Techniques for clinical assessment of human movement. *Physical Therapy, 64*(12), 1821–1830.

Evaluation of Motor Behavior: Traditional and Contemporary Views

Virgil Mathiowetz and Julie Bass Haugen

OBJECTIVES

After studying this chapter, the reader will be able to:

1. Contrast the reflex-hierarchical and systems models of motor control.
2. Describe the traditional and contemporary theories of motor learning with an emphasis on the role of practice and feedback.
3. Compare the traditional and contemporary theories of motor development.
4. Contrast the assumptions of the traditional and contemporary views.
5. Describe how to evaluate reflex integration, muscle tone, dexterity, and hand function from a traditional perspective.
6. Describe how to evaluate a client with central nervous system dysfunction from a contemporary task-oriented perspective.

Our understanding of motor behavior—motor control, motor development, and motor learning—continues to evolve (VanSant, 1991a). Sophisticated technology has led to an explosion of information about the control, development, and acquisition of movement (Moore, 1986). Neurophysiologists, neuropsychologists, and human-movement scientists contribute to this effort. In an attempt to impose order on the many pieces of information, they deduce models and theories of motor behavior. Models represent complex phenomena in simple ways. Theories organize knowledge about a phenomenon of interest, describe relationships between concepts based on solid evidence, and allow prediction about the phenomenon (Payton, 1994). Models and theories help organize our thinking about motor behavior and thus serve as guides to our practice and research. As models and theories change, therapeutic approaches also need to change.

Abernethy and Sparrow (1992) believe that a major change—a **paradigm shift**—has occurred in motor behavior research, because most of the research on models of motor control have shifted from reflex-hierarchical models to systems models. Similar changes are seen in motor development and learning theories (Higgins, 1991; Thelen & Ulrich, 1991). As a result of these changes in the motor behavior literature, some therapists (Crutchfield & Barnes, 1993; Forssberg & Hirschfeld, 1992; Gordon, 1987; Keshner, 1981; Lister, 1991; Montgomery & Connolly, 1991; Rothstein, 1991) have questioned the assumptions underlying the traditional neurodevelopmental approaches, which include Rood's (1954) sensorimotor approach, Knott and Voss's (1968) proprioceptive neuromuscular facilitation (PNF), Brunnstrom's (1970) movement therapy, and Bobath's (1978) neurodevelopmental treatment (NDT). A contemporary task-oriented approach was proposed as an alternative to the traditional approaches (Horak, 1991). The assumptions of this new approach are derived from a systems model of motor control and from contemporary motor development and learning theories.

Figure 7.1 contrasts the traditional and the contemporary views of models and theories of motor behavior, assumptions, and evaluation strategies. We believe that the task-oriented approach will have a great influence on practice in the future. However, we also believe that some of the traditional neurodevelopmental treatment techniques are consistent with the contemporary approach. The traditional view will be discussed first.

GLOSSARY

Attractor—Preferred, but not obligatory, pattern of behavior that emerges from the interaction of a unique person with a particular task and environment.

Blocked practice—Repetition of the same task many times before moving on to the next task.

Collective variable—The fewest number of variables or dimensions that describes a unit of behavior quantitatively.

Control parameter—Variable that shifts behavior from one preferred form to another; it does not control the change but acts as an agent for reorganization of behavior; it must be a scaler quantity.

Degrees of freedom—Elements or variables that are free to vary.

Effector—The element of an open-loop control system that carries out the instructions of the executive.

Heterarchical—Control emerges from the interaction of various elements or subsystems; there is no strict order of command; subsystems in charge will vary with the tasks requirements.

Hierarchical—Control organized into several levels with each level subordinate to the one above it.

High-dimensional system—A complex system composed of many elements (subsystems, variables, dimensions, degrees of freedom).

Paradigm shift—A major change in a conceptual model and its associated theories relative to some phenomena of interest.

Phase shift—Transition, often nonlinear, from one preferred qualitative coordinated pattern to another preferred qualitative pattern.

Random practice—Repetition of various tasks in a mixed order within a practice session.

Self-organization—The system, composed of a number of subsystems, organizes spontaneously from the dynamic interaction of the subsystems; no representation, prescription, or motor program need exist.

Splinter skill—The ability to do a specific task that does not generalize to other tasks.

TRADITIONAL VIEW

Reflex-Hierarchical Models of Motor Control

The reflex-hierarchical model of motor control, which underlies the traditional neurodevelopmental approaches, was developed by integrating earlier reflex and **hierarchical** models. This combined model is able to explain a broader range of motor behaviors than the earlier models could explain individually. To provide an historical perspective, the earlier reflex and **hierarchical** models will be briefly discussed before the more detailed explanation of the integrated reflex-hierarchical model of motor control.

REFLEX MODELS OF MOTOR CONTROL

An early reflex model originated with the works of Sherrington (1906). He viewed the central nervous system (CNS) as a "black box" in which specific sensory input would elicit reflexes or stereotyped motor output (Fig. 7.2). In addition, the sensory feedback from the motor output could trigger other reflexes or stereotyped movements. This model suggested that human movement was the summation or combination of reflexes. Sherrington also originated the concept of reciprocal innervation, i.e., when an agonist muscle is activated, the antagonist is deactivated automatically. Sherrington (1906) and Magnus (1926) conducted experiments on decorticate cats that provided support for a reflex or peripheral model of motor control. A therapy example of using sensory input to elicit a motor output is the use of vibration or tapping over the triceps muscle to elicit elbow extension.

Individuals in other disciplines interested in learning have proposed some concepts similar to those of the reflex model. In psychology, Thorndike (1927) stated that rewarded responses tend to be repeated and unrewarded responses or punished responses tend not to be repeated. When therapists use behavior modification with a patient, they are using his "law of effects."

In the motor behavior field, Adams (1971), in his closed-loop model of motor learning, suggested that peripheral sensory feedback controlled movement. Schmidt (1988) defined a closed-loop system as "a control system employing feedback, a reference of correctness, a computation of error, and subsequent correction in order to maintain a desired state" (p. 184). Although the closed-loop model adds a reference of correctness, and thus recognizes a larger role for the CNS, it is similar to a reflex model of motor control because of its emphasis on peripheral sensory feedback. When therapists cue patients to focus on the "feeling" of a movement, they are encouraging patients to use peripheral sensory feedback to gain better voluntary control.

A number of studies have revealed the limitations of the reflex model. Deafferented animals have demonstrated coordinated movement without sensory input (Polit & Bizzi, 1979; Taub, 1976). Lashley (1917) reported the case of a human with severe lower extremity sensory loss who had minimal problems with coordinated movement. Thus sensory input is not necessary for all types of motor behavior. In addition, the reflex

	TRADITIONAL	CONTEMPORARY
MODELS	REFLEX-HIERARCHICAL • Movements are controlled by central programs or elicited by sensory input • Open-loop and closed-loop control are used • Feedforward and feedback influence movements • CNS is hierarchically organized with higher centers controlling lower centers • Reciprocal innervation is essential for coordinated movement	SYSTEMS • Movement emerges from interaction of many systems • Personal characteristics and environmental context interact to achieve functional goal • Systems are dynamical, self-organizing, and heterarchical • Movement patterns for a given task are stable and the preferred means for achieving a functional goal (attractor) • Control parameters or changes in one or more systems can shift behavior from one movement pattern to another
THEORIES	TRADITIONAL DEVELOPMENTAL • Changes in motor development are due to changes in CNS • Developmental sequences describe changes in motor behavior • Progression through developmental levels are invariant TRADITIONAL MOTOR LEARNING • Learning is defined as change in performance during practice • Learning is enhanced through repetition of same task, progression from part to whole task, and frequent, immediate, detailed feedback	CONTEMPORARY DEVELOPMENTAL • Changes in motor development are due to multiple factors • Normal development is the search for optimal solutions to functional problems and does not follow a rigid sequence CONTEMPORARY MOTOR LEARNING • Learning is defined as relatively permanent changes in performance due to practice or experience • Learning is enhanced through practice of whole tasks in varied contexts and summary, less frequent, feedback
ASSUMPTIONS OF THERAPEUTIC APPROACHES	TRADITIONAL NEURODEVELOPMENTAL APPROACHES (Rood, Knott & Voss, Brunnstrom, Bobath) • CNS is hierarchically organized • Behavioral changes seen after CNS damage have a neurophysiological basis • Sensory stimuli may be used to inhibit abnormal reflexes and muscle tone and facilitate specific muscles and normal movement patterns • Repetition of movement elicited by stimuli results in positive permanent changes in CNS • Recovery from CNS damage follows a predictable sequence	CONTEMPORARY TASK-ORIENTED APPROACH • Personal and environmental systems, including the CNS are heterarchically organized • Behaviors seen after CNS damage or changes in other systems reflect attempts to compensate and achieve task performance • Functional tasks help organize behavior • Occupational and role performance emerge from the interaction of multiple personal and environmental systems. • Practice and experimentation with varied strategies are needed to find the optimal motor solution and to develop skill • Recovery from CNS damage will be variable because of each client's unique personal and environmental systems
EVALUATION	• Muscle tone • Abnormal reflexes and movement patterns • Postural control • Sensation and perception • Memory and judgment • Stage of recovery or developmental level • Secondary evaluation of occupational performance	• Occupational and role performance • Client-centered identification of problematic and important tasks • Preferred movement pattern for given tasks in varied contexts (attractors) • Systems which can cause transition from one pattern to another (control parameters) • Secondary evaluation of subsystems which are interfering with performance
TREATMENT	• Remediate impaired components identified in evaluation • Inhibit spasticity and abnormal reflexes & movement patterns using sensory stimuli • Facilitate normal muscle tone & movement patterns and equilibrium responses using sensory stimuli • Progress through developmental or recovery sequence	• Help find optimal strategy for achieving functional goals • Provide opportunites to practice in varied contexts • Alter task requirements or environment to enhance performance • Remediate personal systems deficits which interfere with functional performance

Figure 7.1. Overview of the traditional and contemporary views.

model cannot account for preprogrammed instructions or anticipatory control of movement, key components of the **hierarchical** model. In conclusion, the reflex model of motor control by itself has significant limitations and is an inadequate model for explaining motor control.

HIERARCHICAL MODELS OF MOTOR CONTROL

Sir Hughlings Jackson, a neurologist, proposed one of the earliest **hierarchical** models of motor control (Jackson & Taylor, 1932). In this model, movements

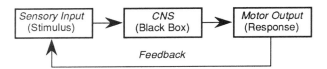

Figure 7.2. A reflex model of motor control, which emphasizes peripheral control of movement.

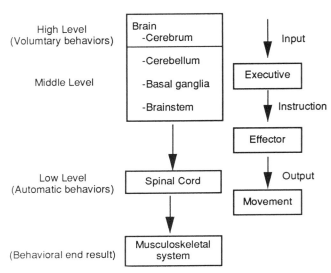

Figure 7.3. Hierarchical models of motor control, which emphasize central or top-down control of movement.

are believed to be controlled centrally in a top-down manner. The highest level of the nervous system controls the middle level, and the middle level in turn controls the lowest level (Fig. 7.3, *left*). This is similar to the **hierarchical** structure of many businesses in which the directives go from the president to vice presidents to middle managers and finally to the workers. Some **hierarchical** models of motor control (Gallistel, 1980; Keele, 1968; Schmidt, 1988) suggest that control of movement originates centrally with the executive selecting, planning, and initiating a motor program to respond to specific input (Fig. 7.3, *right*). The motor program contains the instructions for the **effector,** which carries them out without the possibility of modification if something goes wrong. The output is the observed movement (Schmidt, 1988). In patients with normal CNS function, the higher levels have control over lower levels. However, in patients with CNS dysfunction, there is loss of high-level voluntary control, resulting in the release of lower-level reflexes. In the latter case, primitive reflexes and spasticity dominate movement control.

The **hierarchical** model incorporates an open-loop system of control, rather than a closed-loop system. An open-loop system uses anticipatory or feedforward control and is defined as a system "with prepro-

grammed instructions to an effector that does not use feedback information and error-detection processes" (Schmidt, 1988, pp. 184–185). Fast movements (approximately 160 msec or less) are under open-loop control (Russell, 1976). In these cases, there is no time to use feedback information for monitoring and correcting, because the movement has ended before the feedback can be used. When a baseball player decides to swing at a pitch, it is impossible or extremely difficult to adjust the swing for an unanticipated pitch, because the movement is under open-loop control.

Feedforward, or anticipatory, control is needed for rapid movements, because there is insufficient time for sensory feedback to influence the outcome of the movement; it is defined as "the sending of information ahead in time to ready a part of the system for incoming sensory feedback or for a future motor command" (Schmidt, 1988, p. 184). Many postural adjustments that were thought to be reflexive reactions in response to sensory input have been shown to be anticipatory adjustments made before self-initiated limb movements (Belen'kii, Gurfinkel, & Pal'tsev, 1967; Cordo & Nashner, 1982; Horak et al., 1984). For example, Belen'kii et al. (1967) demonstrated that in a reaching task, electromyographic (EMG) activity occurred in the opposite leg about 60 msec before any EMG activity in the arm. Thus the subjects made postural adjustments in anticipation of changes in their centers of gravity. In the **hierarchical** model of motor control, these types of anticipatory adjustments are thought to be part of the motor program.

However, these **hierarchical** models without feedback loops cannot explain some motor behaviors documented in the motor control literature. First, how could slow, closed-loop movements that require feedback be explained by these models? Second, how could cats with transected spinal cords (Grillner, 1975; Shik & Orlovskii, 1976) locomote on a treadmill, when higher centers were unable to control lower centers responsible for the movements? Third, if voluntary and reflex levels are so distinct, why do so many voluntary movements appear similar to reflexive movements (e.g., the similarity of throwing a baseball with the asymmetrical tonic neck reflex) and why can reflex movements be modified volitionally by prior instruction (Hammond, 1956)? These limitations resulted in some models of motor control that integrated aspects of the reflex model into the **hierarchical** model.

REFLEX-HIERARCHICAL MODEL OF MOTOR CONTROL

Figure 7.4 illustrates a reflex-hierarchical model that is an adaptation of Trombly's (1989) model and synthesizes the basic science literature of the 1970s

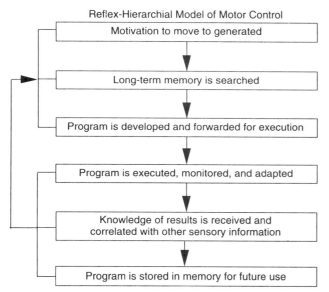

Figure 7.4. Reflex-hierarchical model of motor control, includes both open-loop and closed-loop control.

and 1980s. Each step of the model will be discussed conceptually using for an example a person reaching for a can of mineral water (refer to the references for more detail).

Motivation to Move Is Generated

Purposeful movement does not occur in the absence of a need to move (Granit, 1977). This need is generated from within the person or as a response to external stimuli (Marsden, 1982). Vision is an especially powerful sensory input to stimulate voluntary movement (Granit, 1977). The limbic system, as the seat of emotion and motivation, triggers movements from within (Cheney, 1985). Thus a person who experiences the feeling of thirst (internal stimulus) or sees a can of cold mineral water (external stimulus) becomes motivated to reach for the can of water.

Long-Term Memory Is Searched

After the will to move is generated, the executive or programming center begins to search in long-term memory (LTM) for a pattern of movement that will enable reaching for the can. All previous efforts to reach a can were stored in a generalized motor program, which contains the invariant—unchanging—features of that class of movements. More specifically, it contains an abstract representation about the order, relative timing, and relative force of the reaching movement (Schmidt, 1988). It also includes the postural adjustments that will be needed, so that the person does not lose balance as he or she reaches for the can. The most practiced movements are the ones most embedded

in memory (Schmidt, 1988) and, therefore, available as programs for future use. The generalized motor program that is closest to the reaching movement needed in this situation is selected.

A Program Is Developed and Forwarded for Execution

The reaching movement is organized and planned before its initiation, using the selected generalized motor program as a basis (Marsden, 1982). The program is adapted to take into account not only environmental factors but also the starting and ending positions of the body and its parts relative to each other and to the environment (Brooks, 1986). Specifically, the program is adapted by designating the specific muscles needed, the force of the contractions, and the overall duration of the movement. In this way, the generalized motor program is modified to meet the requirements of this specific action (i.e., reaching for a can of water on a table in front of the person).

The program can be thought of as a set of instructions of facilitation or inhibition to particular α- and γ-motoneurons and interneurons to fire at certain frequencies for certain periods of time (Brooks, 1986). If agonist and antagonist are to cocontract, the α-motoneurons of both muscles must be excited. Whereas for isotonic movements, the central program produces a triphasic muscle contraction pattern in which first the agonist contracts, then the antagonist to brake the movement, and then the agonist again to brake that countermovement (Sanes & Jennings, 1984).

To support voluntary movement, postural muscles must also contract bilaterally to provide a stable base from which movement may occur; the neurons of these muscles are activated automatically as part of the program (Keele & Summers, 1976). Also as part of the program, the γ-motoneurons are programmed so that spindle sensitivity is exactly set, and accurate information concerning the length and speed of length change can be continually monitored (Granit & Burke, 1973). Thus the α-motoneurons and the γ-motoneurons are coactivated (Granit, 1975). This coactivation, or forwarding of program for execution, is initiated by the cortex and centers in the brainstem (Evarts, 1973a). Coactivation of the α- and γ-motoneurons is not invariable; either the α- or the γ-motoneurons can be activated separately for maximal flexibility (Matthews, 1972). Very fast movement, especially of distal muscles, may in fact be the responsibility of α-motoneurons acting alone under cerebellar control via the motor cortex (Cheney, 1985). Different types of movements and environmental factors require different control strategies (Brooks, 1986). Strategies also differ among people and between trials by the same person (Abend, Bizzi, & Morasso, 1982).

Program Is Executed, Monitored, and Adapted

As the program for reaching a can of water is executed, the movements are monitored via cutaneous input; visual and auditory cues; and ongoing proprioceptive input from the muscle spindle, Golgi tendon organs, joint receptors, and the otolith organs and semicircular canals of the vestibular apparatus (Brooks, 1986). These sensory receptors provide feedback on the reaching movement to the cerebellum, basal ganglia, and cortex (Brooks, 1986; Granit, 1975). If the movement appears to be progressing successfully (i.e., the can of water is reached and picked up), the program is continued as planned. If the movement is sensed to be wrong (e.g., the hand misses the target) or an unexpected event occurs (e.g., the can is empty instead of full as expected), an adjustment is made while the movement is still in progress. In the latter case, it is the α-γ coactivation that keeps the muscle spindle sensitive to the unexpected event. The agonist lifter muscles would be preprogrammed to lift a full can. The antagonist muscles would be preprogrammed to relax enough to allow the movement and then contract to brake the movement as the can reached the mouth. Because the can was lighter than expected, the individual would lift it faster initially than what was programmed. As a result, the muscle spindles of the agonist muscles would go slack because they would shorten faster than expected while the muscle spindles of the antagonist muscles would be stretched because they would be lengthened faster than what was programmed. This information would be returned to various levels of the CNS for adjustment to this unexpected event.

The opposite circumstance would occur if the program was for lifting an empty can when in fact it was full. Then as the lift begins, nothing happens at first because too few motor units would be recruited. The muscle spindles of the agonists lifter muscles would be stretched because the muscles would not be shortening as programmed. Within 12 to 18 msec more α-motoneurons would be recruited via the monosynaptic stretch reflex (Matthews, 1972). Approximately 15 msec later, more units would be recruited via transcortical loop stretch reflexes, which are the primary basis for load compensation. Finally, at about 120 msec a cerebellar-assisted, cortically controlled adjustment in the program would occur to meet the sensed demand (Evarts, 1973b). Because this lifting movement was relatively slow, there was sufficient time for the feedback to influence the final outcome of the action. This is an example of closed-loop control (discussed earlier).

It is important to understand how the CNS adjusts for unexpected events, because it is the basis of some therapeutic procedures and illustrates why active rather than passive movement is used for therapy. When the motor program is executed, the α- and γ-motoneurons are coactivated and excite the extrafusal and intrafusal muscle fibers according to the plan. When active movement is stopped by an unexpected full can of water or a therapist's hand (i.e., external stretch), the extrafusal muscle fibers are mechanically prevented from shortening as programmed. Meanwhile, the intrafusal fibers keep contracting as programmed. Soon the discrepancy between their length and the length of the extrafusal fibers is signaled to higher centers. Because the muscle spindle is held in place by connective tissue attached to the extrafusal muscle fibers, the spindle is mechanically prevented from shortening, despite the intrafusal muscle contractions (i.e., internal stretch). As a result, external and internal stretch of the midportions of the spindle fibers are added together and the segmental and transcortical loop stretch reflexes are activated (Brooks, 1986). Therapists use this technique to enhance motor unit recruitment to increase the strength of muscle contraction.

Passive movement is used in therapy only to increase or maintain range of motion, never to improve motor control or learn new motions. There are central processing differences between active and passive movement. The cerebral readiness potential, which is an electric signal believed to reflect generalized motor cortex firing in preparation for movement, can be recorded in conjunction with voluntary movement but does not exist for passive movement (Marsden, 1982). Not only is there a lack of reflex enhancement of passive movement because no coactivation has occurred in the first place but no cortical planning takes place without the active attempt to move. There is no plan against which to match sensory feedback. Learning that requires the matching of correct sensory feedback to intent does not occur (Held, 1965). In addition, sensory feedback is reduced because the spindles are not programmed to maintain their length in relation to the length of the extrafusal muscle fibers. Therefore, when passive movement is stopped midcourse, no reflex enhancement occurs.

Knowledge of Results Is Received and Correlated with Other Sensory Information

Knowledge of results (KR) is awareness of the outcome of movement in relation to the goal. Open-loop movements are first learned as closed-loop movements in which attention is focused on the sensory feedback during the movement. Then the sensory feedback is correlated to the outcome of the movement—KR—and the plan is modified for future movements. An open-loop movement could be executed exactly as programmed and yet be inaccurate as far as accomplishing the goal (Schmidt, 1988). For example, the person reaching for the can of water could miss the target or a person throwing a bowling ball could fail to hit any of the 10 pins. These examples illustrate the importance of KR as well as sensory feedback for improving motor learning.

The Program Is Stored in Memory for Future Use

Movements are generated from past experiences if success has been recognized (Brooks, 1986). Movement memories that have been successful are stored in LTM, which seems impervious to forgetting. *Successful* indicates that the sensory feedback generated by the movement matched the sensory outflow at the time the program was generated and accomplished the goal (Gentile, 1972). If attention is directed to the movement so that information concerning it remains in short-term memory (STM) for a time, then the memory becomes stored in LTM for future use. However, if the information is lost from STM, then it does not become part of LTM and learning does not take place (Schmidt, 1988). The learned motor skill must be practiced to be retained at the same level of expertise (Brooks, 1986). Expertise is improved by practice with intention to improve. In other words, the person sets a more refined goal for himself or herself and the process of motor control restarts at step 1 of the model.

Reflex-hierarchical models of motor control have been challenged by three interrelated questions. How can the CNS control the many **degrees of freedom** of each movement (i.e., the large number of joints, planes of motion within each joint, muscles that control each joint, and single motor units within each muscle) without specifying the details of the muscle activation pattern (Bernstein, 1967)? If the CNS did specify the details, each motor program would be extremely complex. This challenge raised by Bernstein (1967) is known as the **degrees of freedom** problem. How many motor programs would be needed to perform the numerous tasks that humans perform in everyday life? It is likely an extremely large number of programs would be necessary. The size and number of motor programs needed to be stored in the CNS creates a storage problem for the brain. Finally, how many motor programs would be needed to perform a given task in varied contexts? Several studies (Marteniuk, MacKenzie, & Jeannerod, 1987; Mathiowetz, 1992) have demonstrated that small changes in environmental context can result in unique movement patterns during simple reaching tasks. Thus the environment has a larger role in motor control than the reflex-hierarchical model would suggest, and it would seem an incomprehensible number of motor programs would be necessary to re-

spond to varied contexts (i.e., the context problem). Does the brain have unlimited storage capacity to accommodate all of the motor programs, even generalized motor programs? It is believed not, and as a result, an increasing number of researchers have been exploring a systems model of motor control as an alternative explanation. This alternative will be explored after the traditional view has been presented.

MOTOR DYSFUNCTION CAUSED BY CNS DEFICITS

The traditional view is that motor deficits seen after CNS damage are understood best by knowing the site and extent of the lesions (Cheney, 1985). It is assumed that specific areas of the brain serve specific functions. Therefore, if that area of the brain is damaged, it is expected that its associated function would be impaired also. From this perspective, it is important to know the area of the CNS damage to understand fully the patient.

Cortical Lesions

Localized cortical lesions, such as occur as a result of cerebrovascular accident, gunshot, or other penetrating injuries, result in deficits in motor planning or execution of voluntary goal-directed movement. These deficits are limited to the area and function controlled by the damaged tissue. Although the patient may be unable to move a segment of a limb in isolation, he is often able to move the whole limb in a stereotyped way. The less voluntary movements are relatively spared. However, even in these patients who seem to have similar lesions, dysfunction varies as a result of the complexity of the control options available to the CNS and the way each individual uses them (Scholz & Campbell, 1980). Diffuse lesions such as may be seen after closed head injury are even more complex and can result in extensive damage to cortical areas and deeper structures of the brain. The motor dysfunction would include deficits described above plus any deficits associated with other, lower level, involved areas.

The motor deficits of cortical damage are both positive and negative. The positive or added deficits are those phenomena that are released from the inhibitory control of the cortex: exaggerated reflexes and spasticity. The negative deficits are the loss of something, in this case the loss of strength and coordination (i.e., the decreased ability to recruit sufficient motor units in the correct temporal relationship to perform normal movement). The proponents of traditional neurodevelopmental approaches believe that the positive symptoms have the most devastating effect on the motor function of cortically damaged patients. They also assume that until the positive symptoms are corrected, the negative deficits cannot be improved (Bobath, 1978). There is growing evidence to doubt these assumptions (Bourbonnais & Vanden Noven, 1989; Nwaobi, 1983), and therapists are beginning to concentrate on remediation of the positive and negative deficits simultaneously.

Another motor deficit seen in patients with cortical lesions is apraxia, which is the inability to gesture or use objects correctly without loss of motor power, sensation, or coordination. Apraxic errors are characterized as omissions, disturbed order of submovements within a sequence, clumsiness, and perseveration (Roy, 1983) (see Chapter 9).

Motor control is abnormal not only because of the motor deficits but also because of deficits in sensation, cognition, and perception. The patient with sensory loss due to a cortical lesion will not use the limb spontaneously. However, he can compensate for the loss by using intact sensory systems when directed to do so (Jeannerod, Michel, & Prablanc, 1984). The sensory loss will seriously affect the ability to sustain a constant level of force needed to hold an object or to maintain a posture. In the case of impaired sensation, movement is affected by the distortion and the patient needs to relearn the meaning of the new sensations through active movement. No relearning occurs during passive movement, even if the patient watches the movement (Gentile, 1972). Sensory problems are covered in more detail in Chapters 8 and 23.

Deficits in cognitive and perceptual processing can affect motor control as well. Perceptual processing involves accurate interpretation of sensory stimuli from the internal and external environment. A patient with a depth perception problem will have problems reaching for objects. Cognitive processing involves orientation, attention span, memory, and problem solving. A patient with impaired memory will have problems learning new tasks because he cannot remember how he was instructed to perform them or the task itself. Cognition and perception are covered in more detail in Chapters 9, 26, and 27.

CEREBELLAR LESIONS

Symptoms of cerebellar lesions reflect timing abnormalities and problems with the rate, range, and force of a movement. The basis for these deficits is a combination of delayed initiation of preprogrammed patterns and delayed termination of agonistic muscular activity, which result in delayed or missing initiation of the antagonist (Brooks, 1975). These patients are able to carry out voluntary programmed movement of a limb but lack the fine adjustments needed for end point accuracy. Common symptoms of cerebellar dysfunction that a therapist might encounter are the following.

Intention tremor occurs during voluntary movement and diminishes or is absent at rest (Bannister, 1973). Tremor is the rhythmic oscillation of joints caused by alternating contractions of opposing muscles. Tasks that require accuracy and precision of limb placement (e.g., eating and drinking) are especially difficult. The tremor usually increases as the goal is approached (Chusid, 1973). Intention tremor is common in patients with multiple sclerosis.

Dysmetria is the inability to direct or limit motions properly and is characterized by overshooting or pointing past a target toward the side of the lesion (Noback & Demarest, 1972). For example, when reaching for an object, the patient might reach past it.

Dyssynergia, or decomposition of movement, is characterized by movements that are broken up into their component parts rather than being smooth and coordinated (Chusid, 1973).

These first three symptoms may be observed by asking the patient to reach out to the therapist's finger and then touch his nose.

Dysdiadochokinesia is the impaired ability to accomplish repeated alternating movements rapidly and smoothly (Bannister, 1973). When asked to perform alternate movements such as pronation and supination or grasp and release, the patient will perform the movements slowly with an incomplete range of motion or may be unable to perform at all (adiadochokinesia).

Ataxic gait is a wide-based, unsteady, staggering gait with a tendency to veer toward the side of the lesion (Chusid, 1973). Observation of a patient walking heel to toe along a straight line or walking fast and turning quickly will elicit these symptoms (Chusid, 1973). Ataxic gait may also be caused by posterior column damage. In that case, the wide-based gait results from loss of position sense, and patients are able to compensate visually by watching the floor and the placement of their feet (Alpers & Mancall, 1971).

Hypotonia is decreased muscle tone caused by the loss of the cerebellum's facilitatory influence on the stretch reflex (Bannister, 1973).

Lesions of the Basal Ganglia

The basal ganglia control automatic, rhythmical patterned movements and the initiation of automatic (learned) movements. Lesions of the basal ganglia result in a "release phenomenon," in which the rhythmic movements are released from control and automatic movement or initiation of movement is lacking (Chusid, 1973). The major diagnosis involving basal ganglia lesions is Parkinson's disease, which is associated with the following symptoms.

Tremors at rest or nonintention tremors stop at the initiation of voluntary movement but will resume during the holding phase of a motor task when attention wanes or is diverted to another task. Tremors at rest are fatiguing to the patient, and he needs to be taught compensatory methods of stopping them.

Cogwheel rigidity is characterized by alternative contraction and relaxation of the muscles being stretched such as the elbow flexor and extensor muscles (Bannister, 1973). For example, if the therapist were to extend the patient's elbow passively, she would feel alternating periods of resistance and no resistance. Rigidity produces the typical stooped posture. Tremor and rigidity are thought to be caused by loss of inhibitory control of the basal ganglia.

Akinesia and *bradykinesia* are characterized by difficulty initiating voluntary movements and slowness in carrying out movements. These symptoms are reflected in lack of facial expression, monotone speech, reduced eye movement, diminished arm swing during walking, and decreased balance and equilibrium responses. There is evidence that these patients can develop their motor programs but have difficulty recruiting sufficient motor units to produce sufficient force of contraction to complete the task in a normal way (Marsden, 1982).

Festinating gait is characterized by small, fast, shuffling steps that propel the body forward at an increasing rate and by difficulty stopping and changing directions (Adams & Victor, 1977). These symptoms are caused by degeneration of neurons in the substantia nigra.

Other lesions of the basal ganglia may result in one or more of the following abnormal rhythmical movements.

Athetosis or athetoid movements are characterized by slow, writhing, twisting, worm-like movements, particularly involving the neck, face, and extremities. Athetosis is not present during sleep. Muscle tone may be increased or decreased. There is lack of controlled mobility in the neck, trunk, and proximal joints. Movements are involuntary and exhibit excessive mobility from one limit of motion to the other (Guess, 1978).

Dystonia is a form of athetosis in which increased muscle tone causes distorted postures of the trunk and proximal extremities. Involuntary contractions of trunk muscles result in torsion spasms, and there is increased lumbar lordosis (Bannister, 1973).

Chorea or choreiform movements are rapid, jerky, and irregular and primarily involve the face and distal extremities. The muscles are hypotonic. Chorea is related to degeneration of the putamen, as in Huntington's chorea, or may follow rheumatic fever, as in Sydenham's chorea. Chorea may occur in sleep.

Hemiballismus is unilateral chorea in which there are violent, forceful, flinging movements of the extremities on one side of the body, particularly involving the proximal musculature. It is caused by a lesion of the subthalamic nucleus (Bannister, 1973).

RECOVERY

The traditional view is that there is recovery after most types of CNS damage and that recovery is the result of changes in the CNS. Recovery from cortical lesions is believed to follow a developmental sequence from reflex to voluntary control, from mass to discrete movements, and from proximal to distal control. Recovery can stop at any level along the continua, which is not totally predictable. The speed of early spontaneous recovery offers a clue to the ultimate level of function to be gained (Twitchell, 1951).

Laurence and Stein (1978) believe that the amount of tissue damage is more disabling than specific sites of destruction because remaining healthy tissue can, with relearning, assume lost functions. However, recovery is never complete. Any cells in the brain that have been destroyed will not regenerate, and the function for which they were responsible will be diminished by the loss (Bishop, 1982). If all of the cells of the pyramidal tract are destroyed, thereby preventing the one means of control of discrete, skilled movement of the contralateral side (especially that of the fingers), then that function will not be regained. Functions served by bilateral systems may be preserved if the remaining system takes over the function (Moore, 1986).

For the most part, diseases of the cerebellum or basal ganglia are degenerative and recovery as a result of neural changes is not expected. Therefore, treatment focuses on compensation for the deficits. In contrast, some recovery is expected after traumatic injury to the cerebellum and basal ganglia.

There is insufficient evidence to determine what exactly is responsible for recovery (Craik, 1991; Moore, 1986). Some authors believe that the changes after CNS damage are caused by natural, spontaneous, neurologic recovery only (i.e., changes that occur when there are no therapeutic interventions), while others believe they are caused by therapeutic interventions. Craik (1991) suggested that recovery probably results from a combination of both. However, that does not explain the potential underlying mechanisms that can account for these changes.

Bishop (1982) suggested neuronal plasticity as an explanation for the recovery seen after CNS damage. Some examples of plasticity include use of the remaining pathways in systems with bilateral tracks, recruitment of silent synapses or latent pathways, and sprouting of axonal branches to form new synapses (Craik, 1991; Moore, 1986). Thus recovery can occur because of a takeover of function by spared tissue and/or by morphologic reorganization. There is developing evidence that neuronal plasticity may continue throughout life and can be expected to occur in the remaining living cells after trauma (Eccles, 1977). None of the recovery mechanisms seems universal for a specific type of lesion. People recover differently because no two brains are alike structurally or functionally (Moore, 1986). Therapists attempt to enhance neuronal plasticity in the rehabilitation of patients with CNS lesions.

Traditional Motor Development Theories

The neuromaturational theory of motor development (Gesell, 1954; McGraw, 1945) has influenced the traditional neurodevelopmental approaches to evaluation and treatment in various ways. The traditional theory suggests that changes in motor development are the result of maturation of the nervous system. In other words, changes in neural structures cause changes in motor function (Gesell, 1954). This implies that the environment plays a minimal role in motor development. The heavy emphasis on neural maturation to explain changes in motor development has often been overlooked by therapists; the theory implies that a child's experiences and therapist's interventions have little impact on motor development.

Developmental sequences are also an integral part of traditional developmental theory. Gesell (1954) proposed that development must progress through a particular sequence. Although he acknowledged the rate of development was variable among children, he believed the sequence was invariant and followed a particular direction: cephalo to caudal and proximal to distal. The work by Halverson (1931) added the ulnar to radial sequence in the development of prehension. Other developmental sequences have been described in terms of higher and lower centers of the CNS. In these sequences, higher centers gradually gain control over lower centers and regulate voluntary movement as the nervous system develops.

When traditional neuromaturational theory and its developmental levels are used as a guide in therapy, it is assumed treatment must start at the patient's current developmental level. Developmental and reflex testing serve as primary assessment tools (Bobath, 1978; Fiorentino, 1973; Knott & Voss, 1968; Rood, 1954). For treatment, it is assumed a patient must master the current developmental level before progressing to the next level (Rood, 1954). The normal developmental sequence becomes the organizing framework for therapy. If patients master the developmental sequence, these motor skills are assumed to generalize to task performance. There has been great concern that

working on specific functional tasks would result in **splinter skills,** which would not generalize and might in fact interfere with a child's progression through the developmental sequence. As a result, the development of movement skills was emphasized at the expense of functional performance. Some of these concepts are still used in practice, and others have been modified.

Traditional developmental theories have also been used to explain motor problems seen in adults with CNS damage. It is believed that CNS dysfunction frees lower centers from higher-level control, resulting in a release of primitive reflexes and abnormal muscle tone. Neurodevelopmental approaches focus on a progression through the developmental sequence, inhibiting primitive reflexes and spasticity and facilitating higher-level control.

Traditional Motor Learning Theories

Motor learning theories, like the developmental theories, have evolved over time. The traditional view of motor learning is that change in performance during practice reflects learning. Thus any variable that enhances performance during practice is considered important for improving motor learning. Research based on this assumption indicated that **blocked practice—** repetition of the same task—was better than **random practice,** physical and verbal guidance during practice was beneficial, and progression from part to the whole task was desirable for motor learning (Schmidt, 1988). Feedback that is more frequent, more immediate, more accurate, and more informationally rich was reported to be most effective in enhancing motor learning (Salmoni, Schmidt, & Walter, 1984). In some neurodevelopmental approaches, the repeated practice of specific movement patterns and tasks is promoted (Brunnstrom, 1970; Knott & Voss, 1968). This practice is consistent with the traditional view of motor learning.

Assumptions of the Traditional Neurodevelopmental Approaches

Figure 7.1 summarizes the assumptions of traditional approaches, which are derived from the reflex-hierarchical model of motor control and traditional motor development and motor learning theories.

Evaluations based on the Traditional Neurodevelopmental Approaches

Given the assumptions of the traditional neurodevelopmental approaches (see Fig. 7.1), the evaluations of patients from the point of view of these approaches focus primarily on components impaired by CNS damage. These include muscle tone, reflexes/abnormal movement patterns, dexterity and hand function, sensation (see Chapter 8), perception, and cognition (see Chapter 9). In addition, it is important to determine the patient's stage of recovery or developmental level. Finally, occupational performance (see Chapter 4) is evaluated secondarily with the belief that any deficits in these areas are caused by impaired components.

MUSCLE TONE EVALUATION

Muscle Tone

Muscle tone is defined as the resistance of a muscle to passive elongation or stretching (Stolov, 1966). Normal muscle tone is characterized by slight resistance in response to passive movement (Chusid, 1973). When the arm is moved, it feels relatively light and if it is dropped, it is able to maintain the position. Hypotonicity (low tone or flaccidity) is less than normal resistance to passive elongation. When the arm is moved it feels floppy, yet heavy. If the arm is dropped, it is not able to maintain the position or resist the effects of gravity. Hypertonicity (high tone) is more than normal resistance of a muscle to passive elongation. Hypertonicity has two components. The dynamic component is the resistance offered by the muscle as it is passively elongated and is caused by both neural (reflexive) and nonneural (biomechanical) factors (McPherson et al., 1985). The static component is the tendency of a muscle to return from a lengthened position to a normal resting position and is caused by nonneural factors (McPherson et al., 1985). The neural factor is the motor unit activity of a muscle that is increased in hypertonicity owing to hyperactive stretch reflexes, frequently seen after CNS damage. Spasticity (i.e., the neural factor) is characterized by hyperactive stretch reflexes, the clasp-knife phenomenon, and clonus. In a spastic muscle, there is a range of free movement, then a strong contraction of the muscle in response to stretch (i.e., stretch reflex), and free movement again when the muscle suddenly relaxes (i.e., clasp-knife phenomenon) (Chusid, 1973). Stretch may also produce spasmodic alteration of muscle contraction and relaxation occurring at a regular frequency. This is called clonus and is most commonly seen in the calf muscles. Thus spasticity is *not* synonymous with hypertonicity. The nonneural factors are the elastic properties of connective tissue and the viscoelastic properties of muscle (Wyke, 1976). There are changes in the nonneural factors if a muscle is immobilized in a shortened or lengthened position (i.e., there is increased or decreased resistance to passive elongation) (Stolov, 1966). The neural changes after CNS damage—spasticity—contribute to abnormal positioning of limbs, which causes secondary changes in the nonneural factors. Together the neural and nonneural factors account for increased resistance to passive elonga-

tion—hypertonicity—that is seen after CNS damage. A conceptual review of the physiology of muscle tone is presented here, because an understanding of it is basic to procedures of the traditional neurodevelopmental approaches (Chapter 24).

Muscle spindles are length detector mechanisms located within a muscle and are normally kept at a "zero point" by impulses from supraspinal control centers. The zero point refers to the exact match of the spindle length to the length of the muscle fibers it is monitoring. CNS dysfunction disturbs this zeroing mechanism. If too few supraspinal impulses are able to reach the spindle via γ-efferents, it goes slack (hypotonic) and is unable to detect stretch of the muscle, and movement is absent or delayed. On testing, passive movement of the joint feels "mushy" or "loose." If too many supraspinal impulses are relayed to the spindle, it becomes too taut (hypertonic) and overreacts to slight stretches. Movement is curtailed in cases of spasticity, because the spastic muscle, which is stretched by an antagonist muscle, automatically contracts and impedes the opposing movement. On passive movement, the therapist will feel a "catch" at the point in range where the spastic muscle contracts (i.e., the stretch reflex). There are two types of stretch reflexes: the static, or tonic, stretch reflex is associated with posture, whereas the dynamic, or phasic, stretch reflex is associated with movement.

The muscle spindle is mounted parallel to the muscle fibers so it can monitor their length and movement (Mitz & Winstein, 1993). It is attached to extrafusal muscle fibers or tendons by a thread of connective tissue from each of its ends. Within each spindle are the mechanisms for both static and dynamic stretch reflexes. Each spindle contains several nuclear chain fibers (static) and one to two nuclear bag fibers (dynamic) (Swash & Fox, 1972). These intrafusal muscle fibers have noncontractile midportions and contractile polar portions (Kennedy, 1970). When the contractile portions shorten in response to γ-efferent input, they pull on the midportion of the fiber, which causes that area to be stretched (internal stretch). The midportion also can be stretched by passive elongation of the muscle. Because the ends of the spindle are secured to the ends of the muscle, the spindle is stretched as well (external stretch) (Fig. 7.5). When the midportion of an intrafusal fiber is stretched, it generates a neural signal carried back to the spinal cord by afferent neurons. There are two types of afferent neurons: the primary (Ia) sensory fiber that serves the primary ending and the secondary (II) sensory fiber that serves the flower-spray ending. Tentacles of the primary ending coil or clamp around the midportions of both the bag fiber and the chain fibers (Swash & Fox, 1972). The primary ending is velocity sensitive, so its function is

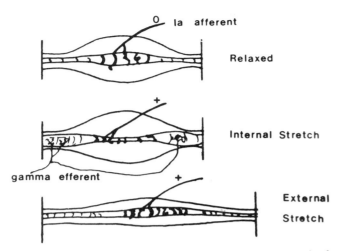

Figure 7.5. Schematic depicting two ways to cause stretch of the muscle spindle: internal and external.

to detect dynamic change of length; and it has a low threshold for stretch (i.e., it responds to a single, brief stretch and to vibration) (Matthews, 1972). The Ia afferent facilitates α-motoneurons of the muscle in which it is located and reciprocally inhibits α-motoneurons of the antagonist. Facilitation refers to a decrease of the threshold of the cell, which increases the likelihood that the cell will fire. Inhibition is the opposite; the threshold of the cell membrane is increased, making firing less likely to happen. The Ia ending around the bag fiber reacts to a single sudden stretch such as a tendon tap to produce a phasic muscle contraction (Matthews, 1972). The Ia endings around the chain fibers react to repetitive small stretches such as vibration to produce a sustained (tonic) response of the muscle (Kottke, 1975). The Ia afferent of the bag fiber has a monosynaptic connection to the α-motoneuron of the muscle stretched. The Ia's of the chain fibers connect polysynaptically to α-motoneurons. Whenever an interneuron is introduced into the chain of activation, there is increased opportunity of influence to the ongoing neural impulse from reverberating circuitry and/or other sources of neural impulses. The strength of these reflexes can be altered by other conditions within the CNS, such as an effort to overcome resistance (Clarke, 1967).

The secondary ending, or II afferent, responds exclusively and proportionately to the amount of static or maintained length of the muscle (Matthews, 1972). The classic view on which some clinical procedures have been based holds that the II afferents facilitate flexors and inhibit extensors, no matter in which muscle they are located (Scholz & Campbell, 1980). According to this view, when an extensor muscle is lengthened the II afferents of that muscle are activated, which inhibits the extensor muscle itself. This classic view is

being challenged. It is now known that the II afferent has both monosynaptic and polysynaptic connections in the spinal cord (Urbscheit, 1979). The reflex response of the II afferent varies for each type of reflex loop and between patients. The monosynaptic response, like that of the Ia, facilitates the muscle in which it lies. The predominant reflex action of the II afferent, however, is polysynaptic, mediated by interneurons whose activity is modified by supraspinal input. The variable responses seen in patients may have to do with the differences in supraspinal input due to the location of the lesion (Urbscheit, 1979).

Regulation of muscle tone requires information about muscle tension as well as muscle length (Scholz & Campbell, 1980). The Golgi tendon organs are receptors for change in muscle tension. They are located at the junction between the muscle fibers and the tendon. Impulses from Golgi tendon organs are transmitted to the spinal cord via the Ib fibers, which synapse polysynaptically with α-motoneurons (Moore, 1984). Golgi tendon organs have low thresholds for tension created by muscle contraction, but they are also activated by tension generated when a muscle is stretched beyond the maximal length it normally has in the body (Lance & Burke, 1974). When stimulated either by contraction or by excessive stretch, they inform the CNS about the amount of tension. The central control mechanisms then regulate muscle contraction or relaxation to meet environmental demands (Moore, 1984).

Evaluation of Muscle Tone

Clinically, muscle tone is measured by observing the response of a muscle to passive stretch. A problem in measuring muscle tone, especially the neural factor, is the high variability in spasticity from day to day in the same subject (Wyke, 1976). The reliability of a test is affected by the speed of the passive test movement, because the Ia response is velocity dependent (Bishop, 1977). Reliability is also affected by effort, emotional stress, temperature, changes in concurrent sensory stimulation, and head position, all of which activate brainstem reflexes (Brennan, 1959; Wyke, 1976). Rigid standardization of the test procedure must be the rule; otherwise the findings may be quite misleading. Therapeutic effectiveness may be obscured by poor evaluation techniques, which allow high test-retest variability.

A number of clinical methods of measuring spasticity or muscle tone have been proposed. Trombly and Scott (1989) described a method of measuring spasticity based on the range of resistance-free movement. It is based on data that suggest that the stretch reflex is elicited earlier in the passive range of motion (ROM) as the severity of spasticity increases (Brennan, 1959).

In this method, the amount of muscle tone is estimated for each muscle group and recorded as "normal," "absent" (flaccidity), or "increased" (spasticity). Spasticity is further described as "mild" if the muscle can be lengthened quickly through most of its range of motion before the stretch reflex occurs in the last quarter of the range, "moderate" if the stretch reflex occurs midrange, and "severe" if it occurs in the initial quarter of the range. The distribution pattern of increased, decreased, and normal tone also should be recorded. The usual distribution pattern of tone in the upper extremities of brain-injured persons is increased tone in the flexor/adductor muscle groups and decreased tone in the extensor/abductor muscle groups, and vice versa for the lower extremities.

Brennan (1959) measured the "range of normal tonus," which is defined as the range of motion that is possible before resistance to movement is felt. To take this measure, he passively moved the limb through full ROM within 1 sec and documented the point of resistance, using a goniometer. He averaged the goniometric reading of three trials as the recorded score. He also rated the degree of resistance offered to the first 10 to 15° of passive movement beyond the point of resistance. It was graded from "normal" to "intense," but the operational definitions of these terms were not published.

Ashworth (1964) proposed a scale for assessing the degree of spasticity as part of a drug study. The resistance encountered to passive movement was rated on a 5-point scale, which ranged from "no increase in muscle tone" to "limb rigid in flexion and extension." Bohannon and Smith (1987) modified the Ashworth scale (Table 7.1) by adding an additional level (1 +), by incorporating the angle at which resistance first appeared, and by controlling the speed of the passive movement with a 1-sec count. They reported a 86.7% agreement between two raters and a Kendall's τ correlation of 0.847 ($P < .001$), which support the interrater reliability of the modified scale.

Worley et al. (1991) tested the interrater reliability of three clinical measures of muscle tone in the shoulders and wrists of poststroke patients. Resting joint position, level of resistance to passive movement (on a 6-point scale), and angle within the range of movement at which the resistance appeared were measured while the patients' arms were supported in a suspension sling. Some high correlations (> 0.80) between raters were reported for particular subsets of the study. However, when all subjects were included, moderate correlations (ranging from 0.417 to 0.676) between raters were reported. These results do not support the interrater reliability of these methods.

McPherson (1986) developed a device to measure the dynamic and static components of muscle tone at

the wrist. The device measured the resistance as the wrist was moved from full flexion to full extension (dynamic reading) and the resistance of the wrist after it had been extended fully for 15 sec (static reading). McPherson believed that the 15-sec static positioning allowed the neural factors to diminish. This belief is based on the fact that EMG recordings do return to a baseline level within 15 sec after a spastic muscle has been stretched (Mathiowetz, Bolding, & Trombly, 1983; Stolov, 1966). Then McPherson computed a neural score by subtracting the static reading from the dynamic reading. Thus he was able to quantify the neural and nonneural contributions of hypertonicity. Interrater reliability (r) ranged from 0.98 to 0.99 and test-retest reliability ranged from 0.72 to 0.94, using mean weekly scores (McPherson et al., 1985). These results support the reliability of this method. Construct validity was supported by the ability of the measurements to distinguish between spastic, flaccid, and normal subjects (McPherson et al., 1985). Unfortunately, this method is limited because it measures muscle tone at the wrist only and the tool is not commercially available.

Rigidity, another form of hypertonicity, is usually noted but not measured per se. In lead pipe rigidity, muscle tone is increased in both agonist and antagonist and resistance to movement is felt throughout the range of motion. In cogwheel rigidity, as seen in Parkinson's disease, tremor is superimposed on the rigidity, causing alternate contraction and relaxation throughout the range of the muscle being stretched (Bannister, 1973). Spasticity and rigidity may both be present in a muscle group. In moving the part through the range of motion, the resistance of rigidity will be felt initially and a stretch reflex will be added later in range.

In selecting a measure for spasticity or muscle tone, these questions should be addressed (see Law

Table 7.1. Modified Ashworth Scale for Grading Spasticity

Grade	Description
0	No increase in muscle tone
1	Slight increase in muscle tone, manifested by a catch and release or by minimal resistance at the end of the ROM when the affected part(s) is moved in flexion or extension
1+	Slight increase in muscle tone, manifested by a catch, followed by minimal resistance throughout the remainder (less than half) of the ROM
2	More marked increase in muscle tone through most of the ROM, but affected part(s) easily moved
3	Considerable increase in muscle tone, passive movement difficult
4	Affected part(s) rigid in flexion or extension

and Cadman, 1988, for a more detailed selection guide): Has the measurement procedure been standardized? Is it reliable and valid for its intended uses? Is it sensitive to changes over time? and Is it clinically useful? Clearly, there is a need for better measurement tools.

Interpretation of the Results and Treatment Planning

After the severity of tone in each of the muscle groups of the involved extremity has been graded, the therapist answers these questions: What is the pattern of increased or decreased tone? Do neural and/or non-neural factors contribute to the abnormal tone? and To what degree does the abnormal tone interfere with function? Depending on the answers to these questions, the therapist devises treatment to inhibit hypertonic muscles, to facilitate hypotonic muscles, and to elongate soft tissue contracture in an effort to normalize the tone throughout the extremity.

EVALUATION OF REFLEX INTEGRATION

A reflex is an involuntary, stereotyped response to a particular stimulus. Reflex responses to stimuli begin to develop in fetal life and are apparent in motor behavior in early infancy. In adults, they reappear in motor behavior as a result of stress and/or fatigue. Reflex motor patterns continue to underlie the organized voluntary movements used in daily activities and sports (Hirt, 1967).

Reflex Evaluation

Reflex testing is done by applying the appropriate stimulus in a standardized way and observing the response. Both the intensity and quality of the response are observed. Intensity refers to the speed of the response and the degree of postural and limb changes. Quality refers to the components of the response that are present and under which conditions they are present. If the reflex is weak, the response may be a change of tone noted in the extremities rather than actual motion of the extremities (Fiorentino, 1973; Hoskins & Squires, 1973).

Reflexes can be tested with the person in any position as long as the stimulus can be applied in that position and the response can occur safely. The patient must be retested under the same conditions for reliability of scoring. If the response occurs, the reflex is positive; if the reflex does not occur, it is negative. Neither a positive nor a negative rating can be equated with "normal" without considering what is normal for the age of the person being tested. Positive spinal or brainstem (primitive) reflexes are not normal for adults.

Reflex testing procedures have been described in more detail by others (Bobath, 1971; Fiorentino, 1972, 1973; Hoskins & Squires, 1973). Table 7.2 provides a summary of the stimulus and the response of selected reflexes and the time when each reflex is present in normal development.

Interpretation of Results and Treatment Planning

Each reflex response can be recorded on a form (e.g., Fiorentino, 1973) by indicating whether the response was "positive" or "negative" or "normal" or "abnormal." The comment section on the form may be used to note any change from standard test position, the strength of the response, or other descriptions of the response. After recording the results of testing, the therapist notes the highest level of reflex control achieved. If the level is age appropriate, then reflex development is normal. However, if the level of control is lower than expected for that age, treatment is planned. Factors to consider in treatment planning include the strength of the primitive reflexes, the time since onset of damage to the CNS, and the extent of the damage. The earlier after CNS damage, the less severe the damage, and the weaker the reflex response, the greater the chances are that traditional neurodevelopmental treatment will be effective.

When brain damage occurs early in development, as in cerebral palsy, development of control of voluntary movement may be delayed. As a result, motor behavior is dominated by the spinal cord or brainstem reflexes beyond the age when these should have normally diminished. When brain damage occurs in the adult, lower-level reflexes are released from higher-level inhibitory control. In both cases, the focus of therapy is to inhibit the lower-level reflexes and to facilitate the higher-level righting and equilibrium reactions. The goal of therapy is to progress patients to their age-appropriate level of the reflex hierarchy. *A word of caution:* for some patients with severe, long-standing damage, the primitive reflexes may be the person's only means of motor function. Treatment to inhibit these reflexes as a first step toward promoting higher-level function may result in inhibition only and leave the person unable to function.

DEXTERITY AND HAND FUNCTION EVALUATION

Therapists use dexterity and hand function tests to evaluate patients with and without CNS dysfunction. Some dexterity tests such as the *Minnesota Rate of Manipulation Test* and *Purdue Pegboard* were developed to aid in the selection of employees for jobs requiring a high degree of dexterity or the ability to manipulate objects with the hands rapidly and skill-

Table 7.2.   Reflexes and Reactions Seen in Patients with CNS Dysfunction

Reflexes/Reactions	Stimulus	Response
Primitive/Spinal		
Grasp (birth to 3–4 months)	Pressure in the palm of the hand	Finger flexion with a strong grip that persists and resists object removal
Flexor withdrawal (birth to 2 months)	Noxious stimulus to sole of foot (supine or sitting)	Uncontrolled flexion of the stimulated leg
Extensor thrust (birth to 2 months)	Stimulate sole of the foot of flexed leg (supine or sitting)	Uncontrolled extension of the stimulated leg
Crossed extension (birth to 2 months)	Passively flex the extended leg while the opposite leg is flexed (supine)	Extension of the opposite leg with hip adduction and internal rotation
Brainstem Reflexes		
Asymmetrical tonic neck (ATNR) (birth to 4–6 months)	Turn head 90° to one side; repeat to the other side	Increase in extensor tone of limbs on face side and flexor tone on skull side
Symmetrical tonic neck (STNR) (birth to 4–6 months)	1. Flexion of the head 2. Extension of the head (quadruped or sitting)	1. Flexion of arms and extension of legs 2. Extension of arms and flexion of legs
Tonic labyrinthine (TLR) (birth to 4 months)	1. Prone position 2. Supine position	1. Increased flexor tone in arms and legs 2. Increased extensor tone in arms and legs
Positive supporting reaction (birth to 6 months)	Contact to the ball of the foot in upright standing	Rigid extension (cocontraction) of the legs
Associated reactions (birth to 8–9 years)	Resisted voluntary movement in any part of the body	Involuntary movement in a resting limb
Midbrain/Cortical		
Neck righting (birth to 6 months)	Head rotation to one side (supine)	Body rotates as a whole (log rolls) to align body with head
Body righting acting on the body (6–18 months)	Head rotation to one side (supine)	Segmental rotation of trunk; shoulders first and then pelvis
Labyrinthine righting (2 months throughout life)	Vision occluded; tip body in all directions	Head orients to vertical position with mouth horizontal
Optical righting (2 months throughout life)	Alter body positions by tipping in all directions	Head orients to vertical position with mouth horizontal
Protective extension (6 months throughout life)	Displace center of gravity outside the base of support	Arms and legs extend and abduct to support and to protect the body against falling
Equilibrium reactions (6–21 months throughout life)	Displace center of gravity by tilting surface of support (prone, supine, quadruped, sitting, kneel-standing, and standing)	Righting of the head and thorax; abduction and extension of the limbs on raised side; protective extension on lowered side

fully. Other dexterity tests, such as the *Box and Block Test* and *Nine-Hole Peg Test* were developed by therapists to evaluate the dexterity of patients with physical disabilities. Hand function tests such as the *Jebsen Test of Hand Function* use simulated tasks to evaluate patients' ability to use their hands for everyday, functional tasks. In all cases, the assumption is that performance on these standardized tests is representative of performance on a variety of functional tasks requiring dexterity. At this time, there is limited evidence that this assumption is true.

Fleishman and Ellison (1962) identified two types of dexterity. Manual, or gross, dexterity was defined as the ability to make skillful, controlled arm-hand manipulations of larger objects. They indicated that the *Minnesota Rate of Manipulation Test* measured this ability. Finger or fine motor dexterity was defined as the

ability to make rapid, skillful, controlled manipulative movements of small objects, using primarily the fingers. They noted that the *Purdue Pegboard* measured this ability. Tests used to evaluate various types of dexterity and hand function will be described briefly. Therapists must determine whether a specific test is valid for its intended use. All of the tests described below need additional validation studies. Therapists must use the standard procedures described in the test manuals or in the original articles to ensure reliability of their evaluations.

Box and Block Test

The *Box and Block Test* (Mathiowetz, Volland, et al., 1985) was developed to measure the manual dexterity of patients with severe coordination deficits (Fig. 7.6) (Cromwell, 1976). The test is not commercially

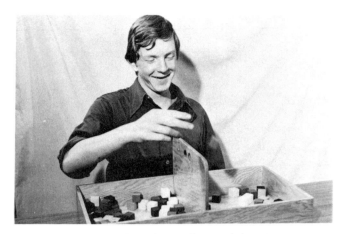

Figure 7.6. *Box and Block Test* of manual dexterity.

available. However, the construction details and standard administration protocol have been published (Mathiowetz, Volland, et al., 1985). The number of 1-inch (2.5-cm) blocks transferred from one side of the box to the other within 1 min is the score for each hand. Test-retest reliability was established at a 6-month interval and found to be high: $\rho = 0.94$ and 0.98 for left and right hands, respectively (Cromwell, 1976). Concurrent validity was established ($r = 0.91$) with the Placing subtest of the *Minnesota Rate of Manipulation Test* (Cromwell, 1976). Cromwell (1976) established norms on 124 handicapped adults using 100 blocks. In addition, norms are available based on 628 normal subjects aged 20 to 75+ years (Table 7.3) (Mathiowetz, Volland, et al., 1985) and on 471 normal subjects aged 6 to 19 years (Mathiowetz, Federman, & Wiemer, 1985) using 150 blocks. The test can be used also as an informal measure of upper extremity endurance, by counting the number of blocks the patient is able to transfer rapidly before becoming fatigued (Trombly & Scott, 1989).

Procedures for administering the *Box and Block Test* are provided in Table 7.4 to demonstrate how to use a test with standard procedures. In addition, Table 7.5 presents recommendations on how to interpret a specific patient's score relative to normative data.

Minnesota Rate of Manipulation Test

The *Minnesota Rate of Manipulation Test* (American Guidance Service, 1969) was developed to select employees for jobs requiring manual dexterity. It consists of a frame approximately 3 feet long that has four horizontal rows of openings, which are large enough to accommodate 60 round discs (approximately 1.5 inches in diameter). The complete test has five subtests: Placing, Turning, Displacing, One-hand Turning and Placing, and Two-hand Turning and Placing. Each subtest is administered in the standing position, three to five

times, the first being a practice trial. The score is the total time for the test trials for each subtest. Test-retest reliability (r) is high, ranging from 0.87 to 0.95 for two-trial administration. Norms based on older, unemployed adults ($N = 3,000$) and on young adults ($N = 11,000$) are available in percentile tables. Table 7.6 provides recommendations on how to interpret a specific patient's score relative to normative data in a percentile table. The test has also been adapted and standardized for people with visual impairments.

For most purposes, the *Box and Block Test* is recommended over the *Minnesota Rate of Manipulation Test* for measuring manual dexterity, because it is time limited, is administered in the sitting position, and has a broader range of normative data.

Purdue Pegboard

The *Purdue Pegboard* test of finger dexterity (Tiffin, 1968) was designed to aid in the selection of employees for industrial jobs requiring manual skill. The test consists of a wood board that has two centered rows of 25 small holes and reservoirs for pins, collars, and washers across the top. The four subtests are administered in the sitting position after a short practice. In the right (or preferred) hand, the left (or nonpreferred) hand, and the both hands subtests, the

Table 7.3 Average Performance of Normal Subjects on the *Box and Block Test*[a]

Age (years)	Hand	Males		Females	
		Mean	SD	Mean	SD
20–24	right	88.2	8.8	88.0	8.3
	left	86.4	8.5	83.4	7.9
25–29	right	85.0	7.5	86.0	7.4
	left	84.1	7.1	80.9	6.4
30–34	right	81.9	9.0	85.2	7.4
	left	81.3	8.1	80.2	5.6
35–39	right	81.9	9.5	84.8	6.1
	left	79.8	9.7	83.5	6.1
40–44	right	83.0	8.1	81.1	8.2
	left	80.0	8.8	79.7	8.8
45–49	right	76.9	9.2	82.1	7.5
	left	75.8	7.8	78.3	7.6
50–54	right	79.0	9.7	77.7	10.7
	left	77.0	9.2	74.3	9.9
55–59	right	75.2	11.9	74.7	8.9
	left	73.8	10.5	73.6	7.8
60–64	right	71.3	8.8	76.1	6.9
	left	70.5	8.1	73.6	6.4
65–69	right	68.4	7.1	72.0	6.2
	left	67.4	7.8	71.3	7.7
70–74	right	66.3	9.2	68.6	7.0
	left	64.3	9.8	68.3	7.0
75+	right	63.0	7.1	65.0	7.1
	left	61.3	8.4	63.6	7.4

[a]Number of cubes transferred in 1 min.

Table 7.4. Administration Procedures for the *Box and Block Test*

The test box is placed lengthwise along the edge of a standard height table (see Fig. 7.6). The 150 cubes are in the compartment of the test box to the dominant side of the patient. The therapist sits facing the patient to monitor the blocks being transported. The following instructions are given:

    I want to see how quickly you can pick up one
    block at a time with your right [left] hand [the
    therapist points to the hand]. Carry the block to the
    other side of the box and drop it. Make sure
    your fingertips cross the partition. Watch me
    while I show you how.

The therapist transports three cubes over the partition in the same direction the patient is to move them. After the demonstration the therapist says:

    If you pick up two blocks at a time, they will
    count as one. If you drop one on the floor or
    table after you have carried it across, it will
    still be counted, so do not waste time picking
    it up. If you toss the blocks without your
    fingertips crossing the partition, they will
    not be counted. Before you start you will have a
    chance to practice for 15 sec. Do you have any
    questions? Place your hands on the sides of the
    box. When it is time to start, I will say
    "Ready" and then "Go."

The stopwatch is started at the word *go*. After 15 sec, the therapist says, "Stop." If mistakes are made during the practice period, they are corrected before the actual testing begins. On completion of the practice period, the transported cubes are returned to the compartment. The therapist mixes the cubes to ensure random distribution and then says:

    This will be the actual test. The instructions
    are the same. Work as quickly as you can. Ready.
    Go! [After 1 min:] Stop!

The therapist counts the blocks transported across the partition, which is the patient's score for the dominant hand. If the patient transports two or more blocks at the same time, the number of extra blocks is subtracted from the total. After counting, the blocks are returned to the original compartment and mixed randomly. The test box is turned around, so that the blocks are on the nondominant side. The test is administered to the nondominant hand, using the same procedures given the dominant hand, including the 15-sec practice.

patient is required to put the metal pins into the holes as fast as possible. The number of pins (or pairs of pins for the both hands subtest) inserted in 30 sec is the score. In the assembly subtest, the patient is required to place a washer, a collar, and a second washer on the pin once it is in position. The score is the number of parts assembled in 1 min. Test-retest reliability (*r*) ranged from 0.60 to 0.79 for one-trial administration and from 0.82 to 0.91 for three-trial administration. The administration of three trials improves reliability but increases administration time from about 10 to 20 min for the four subtests. The

Table 7.5. Interpretation of a Score Using Normative Data from a Mean and Standard Deviation Table

After administering the test according to the standard procedures, compare the right-hand score with the right-hand normative data appropriate to the age and sex of the patient. For example, if a 23-year-old male patient transported 66 blocks within 1 min with his right hand, his score of 66 would be compared with the mean of 88.2 and the standard deviation (SD) of 8.8 (see Table 7.3). Using the formula below, it is found that he scored 2.5 SD below the mean relative to his age group and gender.

Formula to determine the SD above or below the mean for a specific patient's score:[a]

$$\frac{\text{Client's Score} - \text{Mean}}{\text{SD}} = \text{SD} \pm \text{Mean}$$

Example:

$$\frac{66 - 88.2}{8.8} = \frac{-22.2}{8.8} = -2.5 \text{ SD}^{a}$$

[a]In tests such as the *Box and Block Test,* for which a high score indicates a better performance, a negative score means "below the mean." In tests such as the *Nine-Hole Peg Test,* for which a high score indicates a poor performance, a negative score means "above the mean" (better than average performance). Thus the therapist could document objectively that the patient's right-hand performance on the *Box and Block Test* of manual dexterity was 2.5 SD below the mean. To determine the statistical meaning of the patient's score, the therapist must assume that the *Box and Block Test* scores are normally distributed (Fig. 7.7). In a standard normal distribution table, 97.7% of the sample scores are greater than 2 SD below the mean, 2.2% are between 2 and 3 SD below the mean, and 0.1% is more than 3 SD below the mean. By convention, a score that falls 2 SD below the mean or higher is usually interpreted to be "normal" or "within normal limits." A score falling between 2 and 3 SD below the mean is interpreted to be a "mild deficit." A score more than 3 SD below the mean is interpreted to be "moderate to severe deficit." Thus the example patient would be considered to have a mild deficit in manual dexterity relative to the normal distribution.

Table 7.6 Interpretation of a Score Using Normative Data from a Percentile Table

After administering the test according to the standard procedures, the therapist compares the patient's score with the most appropriate percentile table (e.g., worker category, sex, or age). A patient scoring at the 20th percentile performed better than 20% and worse than 80% of the normative sample. By convention, a score that falls at 2.3 percentiles or higher is usually interpreted to be "normal" or "within normal limits." A score falling between 2.3 and 0.1 percentiles is interpreted to be a "mild deficit." A score below 0.1 percentile is interpreted to be a "moderate to severe deficit" (see Fig. 7.7).

validity of the test in predicting work potential was much better for retarded adults (Tobias & Gorelick, 1960) than for normal subjects (Tiffin, 1968). The test manual describes the test as able to discriminate between persons with and without CNS damage. Normative data are presented in the test manual, using percentile tables for adults by various job categories and for 5- to 15-year-old children by age and sex. Normative data for preschool children (Wilson et al.,

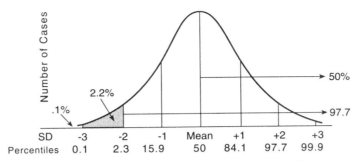

Figure 7.7. Normal probability curve with standard deviations above and below the mean and the equivalent percentiles associated with each.

1982) and for 14- to 19-year-olds (Mathiowetz et al., 1986) also are available.

Nine-Hole Peg Test

The *Nine-Hole Peg Test* (Mathiowetz, Weber, et al., 1985) was developed to measure the finger dexterity of persons with physical disabilities (Kellor et al., 1971). Construction plans and standard procedures are published (Mathiowetz, Weber, et al., 1985). The score for each hand is the time required to place nine pegs in a 5-inch (12.7-cm) square board and remove them. The test-retest reliability with normal subjects is moderate ($r = 0.43$ and 0.69 for the left and right hands, respectively), but with arthritic subjects, it is higher (interclass correlation coefficient = 0.53 and 0.85 for the left and right hands) (Backman, Mackie, & Harris, 1991). Backman et al. (1992) reported moderate correlations ($r = 0.67$ and 0.55 for the left and right hands) between the test and the aggregate applied dexterity subtests of the *Arthritis Hand Function Test*. This provides some evidence to support a relationship between the test and hand function for simulated tasks. The test is moderately correlated ($r = -0.53$ and -0.61 for the left and right hands) with the *Purdue Pegboard*, which indicates the tests are similar but not equivalent tests of finger dexterity. The *Nine-Hole Peg Test* is more sensitive in monitoring the course of multiple sclerosis than the *Kurtzke Expanded Disability Status Scale* (Goodkin, Hertsgaard, & Seminary, 1988). Normative data based on 628 males and females aged 20 to 75+ years are available (Mathiowetz, Weber, et al., 1985). Various commercial versions of the test are available. Unfortunately, there have been no studies to determine whether performance on commercial versions of this test are equivalent to the original test. Published normative data should be used only when the standard procedures to collect that data are followed.

For most purposes, the *Purdue Pegboard* is recommended over the *Nine-Hole Peg Test* for measuring finger dexterity, because it is a time-limited test, has better test-retest reliability, has bilateral as well as unilateral subtests, and has normative data for a broader age range.

Jebsen Test of Hand Function

The *Jebsen Test of Hand Function* (Jebsen et al., 1969) was developed to evaluate a patient's functional capabilities. It includes seven timed subtests: writing a sentence, turning over 3- × -5-inch cards (simulated page turning), picking up small common objects, stacking checkers, simulated eating, moving empty cans, and moving heavy cans. Test construction and standard procedures have been published (Jebsen et al., 1969). The importance of following these standard procedures is illustrated by the fact that substituting plastic checkers for wood checkers resulted in significantly slower performance (Rider & Linden, 1988). The test-retest reliability (r) of subtests based on data from 26 patients with stable hand disabilities ranged from 0.60 to 0.99. In addition, there was no significant practice effect between two sessions with these patients. This was confirmed by Stern (1992) with 20 normal subjects. However, she also reported a significant practice effect for the writing and simulated feeding subtests between the first and third sessions. The test does discriminate between subjects with and without various types of physical disabilities (Jebsen et al., 1969; Spaulding et al., 1988). The moderate correlation ($r = 0.64$) between the *Jebsen Test* and the *Klein-Bell ADL Scale* suggests it may be somewhat useful in predicting ability to do functional tasks but could not substitute for an activities of daily living (ADL) evaluation (Lynch & Bridle, 1989). Norms for adults ($N = 300$) aged 20 to 94 (Jebsen et al., 1969) and for children ($N = 378$) aged 6 to 19 have been published (Taylor, Sand, & Jebsen, 1973).

The *Jebsen Test* has a number of limitations. Mathiowetz (1993) questioned whether the subtests are representative of common, everyday tasks (e.g., stacking checkers) and whether the subtests simulated the tasks they purport to simulate. For example, he reported data that demonstrated that the movement patterns used in the simulated page-turning task are not equivalent to ones used in turning a page and movement patterns used in simulated feeding are not equivalent to ones used in eating applesauce with a spoon. Thus he suggested that subtests of a hand function test must closely simulate the functional tasks of interest. Agnew and Maas (1982) demonstrated that dividing the adult norms into only two age groups is inadequate. One could also question the importance of testing nondominant handwriting and why writing is evaluated with a timed test.

Other tests that could be considered for measuring dexterity or hand function include the *Crawford Small Parts Dexterity Test* (Crawford & Crawford, 1956), the *Bennett Hand Tool Dexterity Test* (Bennett, 1965), the *Sollerman Test of Grip Function* (Sollerman, 1984) and the *Arthritis Hand Function Test* (Backman et al., 1991).

Interpretation of Results and Treatment Planning

After determining the statistical meaning of a patient's score on a dexterity or hand function test, therapists need to compare it with their patient's observed performance on functional tasks that require dexterity (e.g., buttoning buttons, using scissors, picking up coins, or threading a needle). In most cases, patients scoring within normal limits (WNL) are expected to perform these tasks without problems, and patients scoring below normal limits are expected to have some difficulties with functional tasks. However, there may be some patients scoring WNL on a test who are not fast enough on some tasks to be successful in a specific job. Alternatively, there may be some patients who score below normal limits on a test, who are able to perform the tasks they want and need to perform. Therefore, therapists must consider both the statistical and the functional meaning of a score to interpret a patient's performance on a specific test. The functional meaning of a score should carry greater weight in determining the need for treatment. If treatment is directed at improving dexterity or hand function, one or more of the above tests can provide a relatively quick and objective measure of change in these variables. This is especially true if the requirements of the task are relatively close to the requirements of the test.

CONTEMPORARY VIEW

Systems Model of Motor Control

In the past 25 years, a new model of motor control has evolved from the ecological approach to perception and action (Bernstein, 1967; Gibson, 1966, 1979; Turvey, 1977) and from the study of complex, dynamical systems in mathematics and the sciences (Gleick, 1987). Both focus on the interaction between the person and his or her environment and suggest that motor behavior emerges from a person's multiple systems interacting with unique task and environmental contexts (Newell, 1986). Thus the systems model of motor control is more interactive or **heterarchical** and emphasizes the role of the environment more than the reflex-hierarchical model.

In the systems model, the nervous system is only one system among many that influence motor behavior (i.e., control is distributed among many systems). The nervous system itself is organized heterarchically such that higher centers interact with the lower centers but do not control them. Closed- and open-loop systems work cooperatively and both feedback and feedforward control are used to achieve task goals. The CNS interacts with multiple personal and environmental systems as a person attempts to achieve a goal.

ECOLOGICAL APPROACH TO PERCEPTION AND ACTION

The ecological approach emphasizes the study of the person-environment interaction during everyday, functional tasks and the close linkage between perception and action (i.e., purposeful movement). Gibson (1977) recognized the role of functional goals and the environment in the relationship between perception and action. He stated that direct perception involves the active search for affordances or the functional utility of objects for a person with unique personal characteristics (Warren, 1984). Thus Gibson's concept of affordances explains the close relationship between perception and action in terms of what the information available in the environment means to a specific person.

Bernstein (1967) recognized the importance of the environment and personal characteristics other than the CNS in motor behavior. He suggested that the role a particular muscle plays in a movement was dependent on the context or circumstances in which it was used (Bernstein, 1967; Turvey, Fitch, & Tuller, 1982). Bernstein (1967) identified three potential sources of variability in muscle function. There is variability due to anatomical factors. For example, from kinesiology it is known that the pectoralis major muscle will either flex or extend the shoulder, depending on the initial position of the arm. Another example relates to adducting the shoulder. If one wants to adduct it quickly, the latissimus dorsi will contract. In contrast, if one adducts the shoulder slowly, the deltoid muscles will contract eccentrically and the latissimus dorsi does not contract. In both cases, the role of the muscle depends on the context in which it is used.

A second source of variability is due to mechanical factors. There are many nonmuscular forces such as gravity and inertia that determine the degree to which a muscle needs to contract. For example, a muscle must exert much more force if contracting against gravity than if contracting in a gravity-eliminated plane. Likewise, the contraction of the elbow flexor muscles would be different if the shoulder were flexing or extending at the same time, because of the effects of inertia. Again, the impact of a muscle contraction depends on the context.

A third source of variability is the result of physiological factors. When higher centers send down a command for a muscle to contract, middle and lower centers have the opportunity to modify the command. Lower and middle centers receive peripheral sensory feedback. Thus the impact of the command on the muscle will vary depending on the context and degree of influence of the middle and lower centers. As a result, there is no one-to-one relationship between higher center or executive commands and muscle action. **Hierarchical** models cannot account for all of these sources of variability. In addition, they have not resolved Bernstein's (1967) **degrees of freedom** problem or storage problems (discussed earlier).

Coordinative structures were proposed as a solution to the **degrees of freedom** problem. Coordinative structures are groups of muscles, usually spanning several joints, that are constrained to act as a single functional unit (Turvey, 1977). Natural tenodesis grasp and release is an example of a coordinative structure. The long flexor and extensor muscles of the forearm are constrained to work together for functional grasp and release. Fitch, Tuller, and Turvey (1982) suggested that perceptual information could modulate or tune the coordinative structures without intervention from the executive or higher centers. Reed (1982) suggested that postures and movements were modulated as needed by updated perceptual information to achieve the functional goal. Thus postures and movements were not triggered by external stimulation or central commands as suggested by the reflex and **hierarchical** models but were coordinative structures capable of adapting to changing circumstances. Thus the study of motor behavior or action evolved into "the study of how organisms use available information to modulate their actions" (Reed, 1982, p. 110). Turvey and others have looked to the dynamical systems view as a means to explain the complex person-environment interactions.

DYNAMICAL SYSTEMS THEORY

The study of dynamical systems originated in the disciplines of mathematics, physics, biology, chemistry, psychology, and kinesiology; has been applied to the professions of nursing, physical therapy, adapted physical education, and some areas of medicine (Burton & Davis, 1992; Gleick, 1987; Kugler, Kelso, & Turvey, 1980; Lister, 1991; Thelen & Ulrich, 1991); and has influenced the systems model of motor control. Dynamical systems theory proposes that behavior emerges from the interaction of many systems. Because the behavior is not specified but emergent, it is considered to be self-organizing (Kamm, Thelen, & Jensen, 1990). The concept of **self-organization** is not compatible with the assumptions of the reflex-hierarchical model, which suggests that higher centers or motor programs prescribe the movements. Evidence of **self-organization** is seen in the relatively stable patterns of motor behavior observed in many tasks, in spite of the many **degrees of freedom** available to a person (Thelen & Ulrich, 1991). When we eat or write, we have many choices in how we can perform these tasks, yet we tend to use preferred patterns. The movement patterns that emerge for a given task in a given context are stable and are the preferred means of achieving the functional goal because they require the least amount of energy and are the most efficient (Kamm et al., 1990). This pattern is referred to as an **attractor** in dynamical systems theory "because the system falls into the pattern easily and returns to that pattern even when perturbed or interrupted" (Kamm et al., 1990, p. 770).

Behavior can change from being stable to being less stable as a result of aging or CNS damage. In fact, behaviors shift between periods of stability and instability throughout life. It is during unstable periods, characterized by a high variability of performance, that new types of behaviors may emerge, either gradually or abruptly. These transitions in behavior, called **phase shifts,** are changes in preferred patterns of coordinated behavior to other preferred patterns. A gradual **phase shift** occurs, e.g., when an infant decreases automatic stepping from 2 to 4 months of age. An abrupt **phase shift** occurs when a person in a hurry walks faster and faster and suddenly changes to a running pattern. How can these changes in behavior be explained?

In the dynamical systems view, a **control parameter** is a variable that shifts behavior from one form to another. It does not control the change but acts as an agent for reorganization of the behavior into a new form (Heriza, 1991). **Control parameters** are gradable in some way. In the infant example, Thelen and Fisher (1982) demonstrated that the decrease in automatic stepping was caused in part by rapid weight gain during this time. Because infants' muscles are not strong enough to move their heavier legs, automatic stepping decreases. This variable, the increase in body weight, shifted the behavior from automatic stepping to no stepping and thus is considered a **control parameter.** In the other example, increasing the speed of locomotion elicited the change from a walking to a running pattern. Consequently, speed is considered a **control parameter** as well.

Although a person is a complex, **high-dimensional system,** behaviors of interest can be described quantitatively in terms of **collective variables** (Giuliani, 1991). For example, the relationship of individual joints to each other and the timing of the movement phases have been identified as the **collective variables** for infant kicking (Thelen & Fisher, 1982), because they describe in a simple way that complex motor act.

Explanations of changes in motor behavior in the systems model of motor control are quite different from earlier models. Thelen (1989) stated that an important characteristic of a systems perspective is that the shift from one **attractor** state (preferred movement pattern) to another is marked by discrete, discontinuous transitions. These transitions in motor behavior occur as a result of changes in only one or a few personal or environmental systems (i.e., **control parameters**) (Davis & Burton, 1991). Thus important points are that systems themselves are subject to change and there is no inherent ordering of systems in terms of their influence on motor behavior. How might these ideas be applied to occupational therapy?

SYSTEM MODEL OF MOTOR CONTROL FOR OCCUPATIONAL THERAPY

A proposed systems model of motor control (Fig. 7.8) that uses occupational therapy terminology (American Occupational Therapy Association, 1989) illustrates the interaction between the personal characteristics (or systems) of the person and the performance context (or systems) of the environment. Occupational performance (i.e., activities of daily living, work, and play/leisure) emerges from the interaction between personal characteristics (cognitive, psychosocial, and sensorimotor) and performance contexts (physical, socioeconomic, and cultural). Changes in any one of these systems can affect occupational performance and, consequently, role performance. In some cases, only one primary factor might determine occupational performance. In most cases, occupational performance emerges from the interaction of many systems.

In addition, any occupational performance affects the environment in which it occurs as well as the person acting. For example, a client with hemiplegia who has just become independent in making a lunch for himself might free his spouse from coming home from work during her lunch hour. It also may mean that objects in the kitchen are positioned in accessible places and that the kitchen may not be as orderly as it could be. Thus the occupational performance of making a lunch affects people and objects in the environment. It also affects the person. The ability to be less dependent on his spouse may positively affect a client's self-esteem. The process of making lunch provides the client with the opportunity to solve problems and discover optimal strategies for performing tasks. This influences the client's cognitive and motor abilities and the ability to perform other functional tasks. This part of the model is down played here at the moment because we want to emphasize that occupational performance emerges from the interaction of the person and his environment.

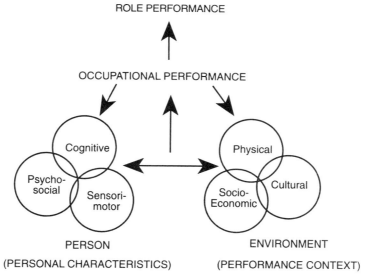

Figure 7.8. Systems model of motor control that uses occupational therapy terminology, which emphasizes that occupational and role performance emerge from an interaction of personal characteristics and performance contexts. In addition, any occupational performance affects the environment and the person in return. These interactions are ongoing.

The specific components of the systems (i.e., subsystems) that influence occupational performance may be framed in occupational therapy terminology. Strength, endurance, range of motion, coordination, sensory awareness, postural control, and perceptual skills are subsystems associated with the sensorimotor system. The psychosocial system includes a person's interests, values, self-concept, social interactions, and self-management skills that could affect occupational performance. Orientation, attention span, memory, and problem-solving skills are components of the cognitive system. The performance context includes physical, socioeconomic, and cultural characteristics of the task itself and the broader environment. The physical environment system includes objects, the natural and built environment, and the sensory environment, which could limit or enhance task performance. Societal beliefs, values, customs, and expectations are subsystems of the cultural system that also could affect occupational performance. Finally, the socioeconomic system includes family, friends, community and financial resources, and social supports, which could influence choice in activities. These examples clarify how components of each system are related to occupational performance.

Role performance is included in Figure 7.8 because it seems a natural extension of the model and is the result of successful occupational performance. However, it is deemphasized, because we believe its inclusion gives the model broader applications than are intended for a model of motor control. Because the concepts and components of the systems model may be viewed in a more general way as the model relates to occupational and role performance, the model may have applications to all areas of practice and to occupational therapy theory development.

RECOVERY

When there is CNS damage, a client attempts to compensate for the lesion to achieve functional goals. Recovery from brain damage is a process of discovering what remains to perform tasks. CNS damage will impact each system differently relative to occupational performance. Therapists need to consider all systems as potential variables to explain the behavior of each client at a specific time. For example, the flexor pattern of spasticity commonly seen after a stroke is the result of various factors in addition to spasticity (i.e., inability to recruit appropriate muscles, weakness, soft tissue tightness, and perceptual deficits) (Bourbonnais & Vanden Noven, 1989). This pattern may become obligatory because of abnormal positioning and decreased use in functional contexts. Because each client is a unique person and functions in a unique environment, thera-

pists should expect that recovery for each client will vary, even if the CNS damage is similar.

Contemporary Motor Development Theories

Contemporary theories of motor development suggest that changes over time are caused by multiple factors or systems, such as maturation of the nervous system, biomechanical constraints and resources, and the impact of the physical and social environment. Contemporary theories also suggest that normal development does not follow a rigid intertask sequence as the motor milestones would suggest (Touwen, 1976). In fact, children follow variable developmental sequences owing to their unique personal characteristics and environmental contexts. If the traditional intertask developmental sequences are no longer sufficient as a guide for working with children, then they are certainly not appropriate as a guide for working with adults with CNS dysfunction (VanSant, 1991b). In contrast, VanSant (1991b) suggested that intratask sequences—developmental sequences within a single skill such as rising without assistance—provide guides for age-appropriate movement patterns.

Contemporary Motor Learning Theories

The contemporary view of motor learning recognizes that many of the performance changes that occur during practice are only temporary and thus do not reflect learning. Schmidt's (1988) definition of motor learning reflects this thinking: "Motor learning is a set of processes associated with practice or experience leading to relatively permanent changes in the capabilities of responding" (p. 346). Contemporary research in motor learning assesses learning using transfer or retention tests, which are given after the temporary effects of the practice or acquisition phase have been allowed to dissipate. Consequently, the changes measured are thought to reflect permanent changes in motor behavior. Research using retention tests has demonstrated that **random practice** is better than **blocked practice** (Shea & Morgan, 1979). Practice on parts of a fast, discrete task or on interdependent parts of a task is less effective than practicing the whole task all at once (Schmidt, 1991a).

Research on the role of feedback suggests that physical and verbal guidance improves performance during practice but may interfere with long-term motor learning (Schmidt, 1991a). It has been demonstrated that 50% feedback—feedback after half of the trials—is better than 100% feedback (Winstein & Schmidt, 1990), faded or decreasing feedback is better than increasing feedback (Schmidt, 1991b), bandwidth knowledge of results—feedback given when a response is outside a given error range—is better than 100%

feedback (Sherwood, 1988), and summary feedback after multiple trials is better than immediate feedback after every trial (Schmidt, 1991b). Most of these results are the opposite of what one might expect and are opposite to the traditional view of motor learning.

Research on contemporary motor learning theory has some limitations and should be applied cautiously in therapeutic settings. Most of the research has been done on normal subjects in laboratory environments. Most of the tasks studied have been brief, novel tasks. Consequently, results may not generalize to subjects with disabilities in performing functional tasks in natural settings. Most of the research discussed here has been driven from a reflex-hierarchical model of motor control, in which motor learning is believed to result in a centrally represented, generalized motor program. Although most of the results could be explained with a systems model, it is premature to assume that all can be.

Higgins (1991) proposed an alternative framework for understanding motor skill acquisition based on a dynamical systems theory. She suggested that individuals are problem solvers who use their personal characteristics or resources to interact meaningfully and adaptively with their environments. If this is so, the therapist's role is to provide clients with opportunities to find optimal solutions for the functional problems that are relevant to their environmental context.

Assumptions of a Contemporary Task-oriented Approach

Figure 7.1 summarizes the assumptions of this approach, which emerge from a systems model of motor control and from contemporary motor development and motor learning/skill acquisition theories.

Evaluation Using a Contemporary Task-Oriented Approach

A framework for evaluation based on the contemporary view and relevant concepts are being explored in the literature from physical therapy (Crutchfield & Barnes, 1993; Lister, 1991; Rothstein, 1991), adapted physical education (Davis & Burton, 1991), and occupational therapy (Mathiowetz & Bass Haugen, 1994). The focus of evaluation in a contemporary task-oriented approach based on a systems model is different from traditional approaches based on a reflex-hierarchical model. Although the current literature is just beginning to discuss ideas and strategies for evaluation using a contemporary approach (Burton & Davis, 1992; Campbell, 1991; Gentile, 1992; Heriza, 1991; Thelen, 1989), functional performance of persons within their environmental contexts will certainly be an emphasis.

Currently, a standard framework for evaluation and specific measurement tools based on the contemporary perspective have not been validated for use in occupational therapy practice. We expect, however, that some existing occupational therapy instruments and some measurement tools being used in basic research have potential for use in a contemporary approach, although it is clear that we need to develop other measures. Some researchers have suggested that the evaluation process will require the use of both qualitative and quantitative measures (Davis & Burton, 1991; VanSant, 1990). In this section, we further examine the assumptions of the contemporary task-oriented approach and describe the basic principles for evaluation.

Functional tasks help organize motor behavior.

Occupational therapy is a unique profession in that the ultimate goal of intervention is to restore or enhance independence in functional tasks (self-maintenance, work and school, play and leisure) necessary to fulfill occupational roles. The roots and the future directions of the profession are consistent with this first assumption. So why is this assumption explicitly stated in the contemporary task-oriented approach? In the traditional neurodevelopmental approaches, the emphasis is on performance components and intervention techniques rather than on purposeful activities, the philosophical base of the profession. Recent research suggests that the underpinnings of motor behavior are not performance components but are in fact functional goals (Burton & Davis, 1992; Gentile, 1992; Heriza, 1991; Thelen, 1989).

In the contemporary approach, the therapist begins the evaluation process by looking at occupational performance and continues with an examination of personal and environmental systems only if she needs a further understanding of how the systems constrain or support performance. Therapists should begin (and end) by looking at occupational performance, because the primary purpose of motor behavior is to achieve functional goals. Evaluations of motor behavior should focus on function instead of general motor abilities and specific movement skills (Burton & Davis, 1992). The therapist should identify age-appropriate tasks that can and cannot be done efficiently and effectively (Heriza, 1991). This emphasis on task performance in the contemporary task-oriented approach suggests that evaluation in occupational therapy should be primarily at the disability level rather than the impairment level, using the World Health Organization (1980) taxonomy. In other words, the primary focus should be on the ability or inability to perform tasks rather than on psychological, physiological, or anatomical structures or functions. Chapter 4 provides a summary and review of occupational performance assessments.

A complete understanding of a person's tasks requires an examination of roles. The therapist should obtain a description of roles and associated tasks of each role from the perspective of the individual. Trombly (1993) stated that satisfactory fulfillment of roles is necessary for clients to achieve a sense of efficacy (i.e., competence and self-esteem). These roles may serve a variety of purposes, including development and maintenance of self (self-care), advancement of self or productivity (work), and enhancement of self (leisure). The completion of a role assessment and identification of associated tasks can serve to guide the rest of the evaluation. Until recently, there were very few evaluations of roles being used in occupational therapy practice. In the last decade, however, several instruments have been developed that have a focus on, or include an assessment of, a client's roles, including the *Occupational Therapy Functional Assessment Compilation Tool* (OT FACT) (Smith, 1990), the *Canadian Occupational Performance Measure* (COPM) (Law et al., 1990), the *Role Checklist* (Barris, Oakley, & Kielhofner, 1987), the *Role Activity Performance Scale* (RAPS) (Good-Ellis et al., 1987) and *Craig Handicap Assessment and Reporting Technique* (CHART) (Whiteneck et al., 1992).

Occupational and role performance emerge from the interaction of multiple systems that represent the unique personal characteristics of the person and the performance context.

Occupational therapists have long recognized the importance of looking at both the person and the environment in evaluation and treatment. However, the traditional approaches to evaluation of motor control emphasize the influence of sensory stimuli on the CNS. Thus CNS deficits are often used to explain occupational performance problems. The contemporary approach acknowledges the importance of the CNS but believes that it is only one of many personal and environmental systems that influence occupational performance. Thus occupational therapists examine all systems that are contributing to problems in functional performance or supporting optimal performance. An important point, however, is that the therapist examines the systems only if they are influencing occupational performance, keeping in mind the requirements of tasks that a person does now or will do in the future. Personal characteristics include sensorimotor, cognitive, and psychological status, and environmental factors considered are the physical, cultural, and socioeconomic context (Fig. 7.8). OT FACT (Smith, 1990) provides a

framework that could be consistent with these ideas. In this assessment, the therapist begins by considering a client's role integration and activities of performance. One could continue with an examination of selected integrated skills of performance—performance components—only if these components contributed to problems in role or occupational performance.

It is likely that occupational therapists will always need to use a variety of measures in their evaluation of the systems that constrain or support occupational performance. Some recently developed assessments were designed to examine one or more systems within the context of occupational performance. The *Assessment of Motor and Process Skills* (AMPS) (Fisher, 1990) allows simultaneous assessments of task performance in instrumental activities of daily living and the underlying motor and process (cognitive) systems that affect performance. The *A-One Evaluation* (Arnadattoir, 1990) facilitates evaluation of perceptual and cognitive systems within the context of ADLs. Assessment of cognitive function through a functional task is also the focus of the *Allen Cognitive Level Scale* (Allen, 1985).

Most traditional assessments have focused on personal systems (Chapters 6 and 8–10). Evaluations of environmental systems must also be completed in the contemporary approach. This requires an examination of the task itself and the broader performance context. Chapter 5 reviews assessments of the broader physical, socioeconomic, and cultural environments.

Once systems that support or constrain functional performance are identified, the therapist must assess the interactions of these systems. Consider a client who has some slight limitations in shoulder flexion. The role and tasks of client as worker may or may not be affected. If the client were a carpenter, the interaction of this personal limitation with the demands of the work environment would likely make the tasks of nailing overhead, installing cabinets, and hanging doors difficult to perform. However, if the client were a word processor, he probably could do most tasks adequately, because the interaction of personal characteristics and the performance context does not interfere with task performance. This part of the evaluation requires a qualitative assessment by the therapist and is based on the information gathered.

This assumption of interaction of multiple systems also implies that the person has an active role in the evaluation and treatment of occupational performance problems. Because the roles, tasks, and characteristics of person and environment are unique to the person, the therapist must make the client's perspective the focus of the assessment. Some describe this as a client-centered approach, because the client provides direction for the tasks that are examined and makes choices about strategies used to perform the task (Boll et al., 1992; Davis & Burton, 1991; Gentile, 1992). Client-centered assessments are being introduced in occupational therapy practice. COPM (Law et al., 1990) is an excellent example, because the client identifies his occupational performance problems and scores them in terms of performance, satisfaction with performance, and their importance to him (Chapters 4 and 18). AMPS (Fisher, 1990) is also client centered in that it assesses motor and process skills in the context of familiar tasks of the client's choice.

After CNS damage or other changes in personal or environmental systems, clients' behavioral changes reflect their attempts to compensate and to achieve functional goals.

To understand fully the movement patterns used to compensate and to achieve functional goals, the evaluation of occupational performance must include an examination of the process (i.e., the actual movement patterns), the outcome (Thelen, 1989) and the stability or instability of observed motor behaviors. Outcome measures provide information on the level of independence or performance attained. The outcome of performance on self-care tasks can be evaluated using existing activities of daily living and instrumental activities of daily living scales. Outcome measures for work and leisure tasks need to be further developed and refined.

Evaluation of the process of occupational performance will likely require use of both quantitative and qualitative measures. Some measurement tools primarily used in basic research may have application in practice. The evaluation of process involves identification of the **collective variables;** these macroscopic variables, such as time needed to complete a task, can be used to characterize the observable movement patterns (Scholz, 1990). The examination of the process used in task performance needs to be incorporated into the clinical evaluation of movement disorders. We expect that development of clinical process measures will occur in the next decade.

Personal and environmental systems are heterarchically organized.

Evaluations and interventions based on the traditional perspective have an order that usually begins at the lowest levels and ends with voluntary, isolated movements that represent the highest level of the CNS (Horak, 1991). In the contemporary task-oriented approach, there is no inherent ordering of the personal and environmental systems in terms of their influence on motor behavior. There is also no inherent ordering within these systems, even the CNS. Thus evaluation strategies consider all personal and environmental systems. Those systems, which appear to interfere with occupational performance the most, are evaluated first.

A person must practice and experiment with varied strategies to find the optimal solutions for motor problems and develop skill in performance.

This assumption emphasizes practice and experimentation, and the importance of problem solving in efforts to achieve functional goals. It would be impossible to function in our complex, ever-changing environment without being able to assess a situation and select appropriate motor behaviors to achieve the functional goal. Higgins (1991) defines motor skill as the ability to find optimal solutions for motor problems. Finding optimal solutions involves motor learning. Thus the evaluation of motor behavior is not simply a determination of whether a person can follow a predetermined routine or the occupational therapist's strategies for achieving a functional goal during the therapy session. Therapists need to know if their clients can understand the problem, select efficient and effective movements to solve the problem, and vary strategies for different situations after therapy sessions have ceased (Higgins, 1991). After all, the goal is for the clients to function successfully outside the clinical setting when the therapist is not available to structure practice or provide feedback. On the other hand, it is also important to identify clients who can perform a task only when provided with the motor solutions. In summary, the evaluation of a client's ability or inability to solve motor behavior problems is critical in planning occupational therapy interventions and selecting practice and feedback strategies. Treatment planning consists of developing and implementing learning opportunities for clients with problem-solving abilities. For the client who is unable to problem solve, however, therapists may have to provide nongeneralizable solutions or train him to perform tasks using a given routine (Higgins, 1991).

This chapter contrasted traditional and contemporary views related to models of motor control and theories of motor development and motor learning. These views provide the theoretical foundations for the evaluations used by the two approaches.

Acknowledgments—Thanks to Nancy Flinn who is exploring the use of the contemporary task-oriented approach in her clinical practice and has provided constructive feedback.

STUDY QUESTIONS

1. How is the reflex-hierarchical model of motor control different from the systems model of motor control?
2. What types of motor dysfunctions are associated with cortical, cerebellar, and basal ganglia lesions of the CNS?
3. What might account for the recovery seen after CNS damage?
4. What are at least four assumptions of the traditional neurodevelopmental approaches?
5. What is normal muscle tone, hypotonicity, hypertonicity, flaccidity, spasticity, and rigidity? How would you evaluate these?
6. What is a reflex and how are reflexes evaluated from a traditional perspective?
7. What tests would you recommend to measure finger and manual dexterity? Why?
8. If your 42-year-old female patient scored 62 on the right hand subtest of the *Box and Block Test*, how would you interpret her score relative to normative data? What else would you need to know to determine whether treatment is indicated?
9. How are contemporary motor development theories different from traditional theories?
10. From traditional and contemporary perspectives, what types of practice and feedback are most beneficial for motor learning?
11. What are at least four assumptions of the contemporary task-oriented approach?
12. How is evaluation from a contemporary task-oriented approach different from the traditional neurodevelopmental approaches?

REFERENCES

Abend, W., Bizzi, E., & Morasso, P. (1982). Human arm trajectory formation. *Brain, 105,* 331–348.

Abernethy, B., & Sparrow, W. A. (1992). The rise and fall of dominant paradigms in motor behavior research. In J. J. Summers (Ed.), *Approaches to the study of motor control and learning* (pp. 3–45). Amsterdam: Elsevier.

Adams, J. A. (1971). A closed-loop theory of motor learning. *Journal of Motor Behavior, 3,* 111–150.

Adams, R. D., & Victor, M. (1977). *Principles of neurology.* New York: McGraw-Hill.

Agnew, P. J., & Maas, F. (1982). Hand function related to age and sex. *Archives of Physical Medicine & Rehabilitation, 53,* 259–271.

Allen, C. (1985). *Occupational therapy for psychiatric diseases: Measurement and management of cognitive disabilities.* Boston: Little, Brown & Co..

Alpers, B. J., & Mancall, E. L. (1971). *Essentials of the neurological examination.* Philadelphia: F. A. Davis.

American Guidance Service. (1969). *The Minnesota Rate of Manipulation Tests: Examiner's manual.* Circle Pines, MN: Author.

American Occupational Therapy Association. (1989). Uniform terminology for occupational therapy (2nd ed.). *American Journal of Occupational Therapy, 43,* 808–815.

Arnadattoir, G. (1990). *The brain and behavior: Assessing cortical dysfunction through activities of daily living.* St. Louis: C. V. Mosby.

Ashworth, B. (1964). Preliminary trial of carisoprodol in multiple sclerosis. *Practitioner, 192,* 540–542.

Backman, C., Cork, S., Gibson, D., & Parsons, J. (1992). Assessment of hand function: The relationship between pegboard dexterity and applied dexterity. *Canadian Journal of Occupational Therapy, 59,* 208–213.

Backman, C., Mackie, H., & Harris, J. (1991). Arthritis Hand Function Test: Development of a standardized assessment tool. *Occupational Therapy Journal of Research, 11,* 245–256.

Bannister, R. (1973). *Brain's clinical neurology* (4th ed.). London: Oxford University Press.

Barris, R., Oakley, F., & Kielhofner, G. (1987). The Role Checklist. In B. J. Hemphill (Ed.), *Mental health assessment in occupational therapy* (pp. 73–92). Thorofare, NJ: Slack.

Belen'kii, V., Gurfinkel, V., & Pal'tsev, Y. (1967). Elements of control of voluntary movements. *Biophysics, 12,* 135–141.

Bennett, G. K. (1965). *Hand-Tool Dexterity Test: Manual of directions.* New York: Psychological Corp.

Bernstein, N. (1967). *The coordination and regulation of movements.* Elmsford, NY: Pergamon Press.

Bishop, B. (1977). Spasticity: Its physiology and management. Part III. Identifying and assessing the mechanisms underlying spasticity. *Physical Therapy, 57,* 385–395.

Bishop, B. (1982). Neural plasticity. Part IV. Lesion-induced reorganization of the CNS. *Physical Therapy, 62,* 1442–1451.

Bobath, B. (1971). *Abnormal postural reflex activity caused by brain lesions* (2nd ed.). London: William Heinemann Medical Books.

Bobath, B. (1978). *Adult hemiplegia: Evaluation and treatment* (2nd ed.). London: William Heinemann Medical Books.

Bohannon, R. W., & Smith, M. B. (1987). Interrater reliability of a modified Ashworth scale of muscle spasticity. *Physical Therapy, 67,* 206–207.

Boll, A., Fredriksson, M., Hellberg, G., Hirschfeld, H., Stern, M., & Weibull, J. (1992). Discussion section V. In H. Forssberg & H. Hirschfeld (Eds.), *Movement disorders in children* (pp. 284–296). Basel: S. Karger.

Bourbonnais, D., & Vanden Noven, S. (1989). Weakness in patients with hemiparesis. *American Journal of Occupational Therapy, 43,* 313–319.

Brennan, J. B. (1959). Clinical method of assessing tonus and voluntary movement in hemiplegia. *British Medical Journal, 1,* 767–768.

Brooks, V. B. (1975). Roles of cerebellum and basal ganglia in initiation and control of movements. *Canadian Journal of Neurology, 2,* 265–277.

Brooks, V. B. (1986). *The neural basis of motor control.* New York: Oxford University Press.

Brunnstrom, S. (1970). *Movement therapy in hemiplegia.* New York: Harper & Row.

Burton, A. W., & Davis, W. E. (1992). Optimizing the involvement and performance of children with physical impairments in movement activities. *Pediatric Exercise Science, 4,* 236–248.

Campbell, S. K. (1991). Framework for the measurement of neurologic impairment and disability. In M. J. Lister (Ed.), *Contemporary management of motor control problems: Proceedings of the II STEP conference* (pp. 143–154). Alexandria, VA: Foundation for Physical Therapy.

Cheney, P. D. (1985). Role of cerebral cortex in voluntary movements: A review. *Physical Therapy, 65,* 624–635.

Chusid, J. G. (1973). *Correlative neuroanatomy and functional neurology* (15th ed.). Los Altos, CA: Lange Medical Publications.

Clarke, A. M. (1967). Effect of the Jendrassik manoeuvre on a phasic stretch reflex in normal human subjects during experimental control over supraspinal influences. *Journal of Neurology, Neurosurgery, & Psychiatry, 30*, 34–42.

Cordo, P., & Nashner, L. M. (1982). Properties of postural adjustments associated with rapid arm movements. *Journal of Neurophysiology, 47*, 287–302.

Craik, R. L. (1991). Recovery processes: Maximizing function. In M. J. Lister (Ed.), *Contemporary management of motor control problems: Proceedings of the II STEP conference* (pp. 165–173). Alexandria, VA: Foundation for Physical Therapy.

Crawford, J. E., & Crawford, D. M. (1956). *Manual: Crawford Small Parts Dexterity Test.* New York: Psychological Corp.

Cromwell, F. S. (1976). *Occupational therapist's manual for basic skill assessment: Primary prevocational evaluation.* Altadena, CA: Fair Oaks Printing.

Crutchfield, C. A., & Barnes, M. R. (1993). *Motor control and motor learning in rehabilitation.* Atlanta, GA: Stokesville.

Davis, W. E., & Burton, A. W. (1991). Ecological task analysis: Translating movement behavior theory into practice. *Adapted Physical Activity Quarterly, 8*, 154–177.

Eccles, J. C. (1977). *The understanding of the brain* (2nd ed.). New York: McGraw-Hill.

Evarts, E. V. (1973a). Brain mechanisms in movement. *Scientific American, 224*, 96.

Evarts, E. V. (1973b). Motor cortex reflexes associated with learned movements. *Science, 179*, 501–503.

Fiorentino, M. R. (1972). *Normal and abnormal development.* Springfield, IL: Charles C. Thomas.

Fiorentino, M. R. (1973). *Reflex testing methods for evaluating CNS development* (2nd ed.). Springfield, IL: Charles C. Thomas.

Fisher, A. (1990). *Assessment of Motor and Process Skills* (res. ed. 6.1). Unpublished manual. (Available from 200 Occupational Therapy Building, Colorado State University, Fort Collins, CO 80523)

Fitch, H. L., Tuller, B., & Turvey, M. T. (1982). The Bernstein perspective: III. Tuning of coordinative structures with special reference to perception. In J. A. S. Kelso (Ed.), *Human motor behavior: An introduction* (pp. 271–281). Hillsdale, NJ: Erlbaum.

Fleischman, E. A., & Ellison, G.D. (1962). A factor analysis of five manipulative tests. *Journal of Applied Psychology, 46*, 96–105.

Forssberg, H., & Hirschfeld, H. (Eds.). (1992). *Movement disorders in children* (Vol. 36). Basel: S. Karger.

Gallistel, C. R. (1980). *The organization of action.* Hillsdale, NJ: Erlbaum.

Gentile, A. M. (1972). A working model of skill acquisition with application to teaching. *Quest, 17*, 3–23.

Gentile, A. M. (1992). The nature of skill acquisition: Therapeutic implications for children with movement disorders. In H. Forssberg & H. Hirschfeld (Eds.), *Movement disorders in children* (pp. 31–40). Basel: S. Karger.

Gesell, A. (1954). The ontogenesis of infant behavior. In L. Carmichael (Ed.), *Manual of child psychology* (2nd ed., pp. 335–373). New York: John Wiley & Sons.

Gibson, J. J. (1966). *The senses considered as perceptual systems.* Boston: Houghton Mifflin.

Gibson, J. J. (1977). The theory of affordances. In R. Shaw & J. Bransford (Eds.), *Perceiving, acting, and knowing* (pp. 67–82). Hillsdale, NJ: Erlbaum.

Gibson, J. J. (1979). *The ecological approach to visual perception.* Boston: Houghton Mifflin.

Giuliani, C. A. (1991). Dorsal rhizotomy for children with cerebral palsy: Support for concepts of motor control. *Physical Therapy, 71*, 248–259.

Gleick, J. (1987). *Chaos: Making a new science.* New York: Penguin.

Good-Ellis, M. A., Fine, S. B., Spencer, J. H., & Divittes, A. (1987). Developing a role activity performance scale. *American Journal of Occupational Therapy, 41*, 232–241.

Goodkin, D. E., Hertsgaard, D., & Seminary, J. (1988). Upper extremity function in multiple sclerosis: Improving assessment sensitivity with Box-and-Block and Nine-Hole Peg Tests. *Archives of Physical Medicine & Rehabilitation, 69*, 850–854.

Gordon, J. (1987). Assumptions underlying physical therapy interventions: Theoretical and historical perspectives. In J. H. Carr, R. B. Shepherd, J. Gordon, A. M. Gentile, & J. M. Held (Eds.), *Movement science: Foundations for physical therapy in rehabilitation* (pp. 1–30). Rockville, MD: Aspen.

Granit, R. (1975). The functional role of the muscle spindle— Facts and hypotheses. *Brain, 98*, 531–556.

Granit, R. (1977). *The purposive brain.* Cambridge: MIT Press.

Granit, R., & Burke, R. E. (1973). The control of movement and posture. *Brain Research, 53*, 1–28.

Grillner, S. (1975). Locomotion in vertebrates: Central mechanisms and reflex interactions. *Physiology Review, 55*, 247–307.

Guess, V. (1978). Central control insufficiency. II. Extraneous motion: A treatment approach. *Physical Therapy, 58*, 306–312.

Halverson, H. M. (1931). An experimental study of prehension in infants by means of systematic cinema records. *Genetic Psychological Monographs, 10*, 107–286.

Hammond, P. H. (1956). The influence of prior instruction to the subject on an apparently involuntary neuromuscular response. *Journal of Physiology, 132*, 17–18.

Held, R. (1965). Plasticity in sensory-motor systems. *Scientific American, 213*, 84–94.

Heriza, C. (1991). Motor development: Traditional and contemporary theories. In M. J. Lister (Ed.), *Contemporary management of motor control problems: Proceedings of the II STEP conference* (pp. 99–126). Alexandria, VA: Foundation for Physical Therapy.

Higgins, S. (1991). Motor skill acquisition. *Physical Therapy, 71*, 123–139.

Hirt, S. (1967). The tonic neck reflex mechanism in the normal human adult [NUSTEP Proceedings]. *American Journal of Physical Medicine, 46*, 362–369.

Horak, F. B. (1991). Assumptions underlying motor control for neurologic rehabilitation. In M. J. Lister (Ed.), *Contemporary management of motor control problems: Proceedings of the II STEP conference* (pp. 11–27). Alexandria, VA: Foundation for Physical Therapy.

Horak, F. B., Anderson, M., Esselman, P., & Lynch, K. (1984). The effects of movement velocity, mass displaced and task certainty on associated postural adjustments made by normal and hemiplegic individuals. *Journal of Neurology, Neurosurgery, & Psychiatry, 47*, 1020–1028.

Hoskins, T., & Squires, J. (1973). Development assessment: A test for gross motor and reflex development. *Physical Therapy, 53*, 117–126.

Jackson, J. H., & Taylor, J. (Eds.). (1932). *Selected writings of John B. Hughlings, I and II.* London: Hodder & Stoughter.

Jeannerod, M., Michel, F., & Prablanc, C. (1984). The control of hand movements in a case of hemiaesthesia following a parietal lesion. *Brain, 107*, 899–920.

Jebsen, R. H., Taylor, N., Trieschmann, R., Trotter, M., Howard, L. (1969). An objective and standardized test of hand function. *Archives of Physical Medicine & Rehabilitation, 50*, 311–319.

Kamm, K., Thelen, E., & Jensen, J. L. (1990). A dynamical systems approach to motor development. *Physical Therapy, 70*, 763–775.

Keele, S. W., & Summers, J. J. (1976). The structure of motor programs. In G. E. Stelmach (Ed.), *Motor control: Issues and trends* (pp. 109–142). New York: Academic Press.

Keele, S. W. (1968). Movement control in skilled motor performance. *Psychological Bulletin, 70,* 245–248.

Kellor, M., Frost, J., Silberberg, N., Iversen, I., & Cummings, R., (1971). Hand strength and dexterity: Norms for clinical use. *American Journal of Occupational Therapy, 25,* 77–83.

Kennedy, W. R. (1970). Innervation of normal human muscle spindles. *Neurology, 20,* 463–475.

Keshner, E. A. (1981). Reevaluating the theoretical model underlying the neurodevelopmental theory. *Physical Therapy, 61,* 1035–1040.

Knott, M., & Voss, D. E. (1968). *Proprioceptive neuromuscular facilitation* (2nd ed.). New York: Harper & Row.

Kottke, F. J. (1975). Reflex patterns initiated by the secondary sensory fiber endings of muscle spindles: A proposal. *Archives of Physical Medicine & Rehabilitation, 56,* 1–7.

Kugler, P. N. Kelso, J. A. S., & Turvey, M. T. (1980). On the concept of coordinative structures as dissipative structures: I. Theoretical lines of convergence. In G. E. Stelmach & J. Requin (Eds.), *Tutorials in motor behavior* (pp.3–47). Amsterdam: North-Holland Publishing.

Lance, J. W., & Burke, D. (1974). Mechanisms of spasticity. *Archives of Physical Medicine & Rehabilitation, 55,* 332–337.

Lashley, K. S. (1917). The accuracy of movement in the absence of excitation from the moving organ. *American Journal of Physiology, 43,* 169–194.

Laurence, S., & Stein, D. G. (1978). Recovery after brain damage and the concept of localization of function. In S. Finger (Ed.), *Recovery from brain damage: Research & theory* (pp. 369–409). New York: Plenum.

Law, M., Baptiste, S., McColl, M., Opzoomer, A., Polatajko, H., & Pollock, N. (1990). The Canadian Occupational Performance Measure: An outcome measurement protocol for occupational therapy. *Canadian Journal of Occupational Therapy, 57,* 82–87.

Law, M., & Cadman, D. (1988). Measurement of spasticity: A clinician's guide. *Physical & Occupational Therapy in Pediatrics, 8,* 77–95.

Lister, M. J. (Ed.). (1991). *Contemporary management of motor control problems: Proceedings of the II STEP conference.* Alexandria, VA: Foundation for Physical Therapy.

Lynch, K. B., & Bridle, M. J. (1989). Validity of the Jebsen-Taylor Hand Function Test in predicting activities of daily living. *Occupational Therapy Journal of Research, 9,* 316–318.

Magnus, R. (1926). Some results of studies in the physiology of posture. *Lancet, 2,* 531–585.

Marsden, C. D. (1982). The mysterious motor function of the basal ganglia [The Robert Wartenberg Lecture]. *Neurology, 32,* 514–539.

Marteniuk, R. G., MacKenzie, C. L., & Jeannerod, M. (1987). Constraints on human arm trajectories. *Canadian Journal of Psychology, 41,* 365–368.

Mathiowetz, V. G. (1992). Informational support and functional motor performance. *Dissertation Abstracts International, 52,* 11A. (University Microfilms No. #92-12071)

Mathiowetz, V. (1993). Role of physical performance component evaluations in occupational therapy functional assessment. *American Journal of Occupational Therapy, 47,* 225–230.

Mathiowetz, V., & Bass Haugen, J. (1994). Motor behavior research: Implications for therapeutic approaches to CNS dysfunction. *American Journal of Occupational Therapy, 48*(8), 733–745.

Mathiowetz, V., Bolding, D., & Trombly, C. (1983). Immediate effects of positioning devices on the normal and spastic hand measured by electromyography. *American Journal of Occupational Therapy, 37,* 247–254.

Mathiowetz, V., Federman, S., & Wiemer, D. (1985). Box and Block Test of manual dexterity: Norms for 6–19 year olds. *Canadian Journal of Occupational Therapy, 52,* 241–245.

Mathiowetz, V., Rogers, S., Dowe-Keval, M., Donahoe, L., & Rennells, C. (1986). The Purdue Pegboard: Norms for 14- to 19-year olds. *American Journal of Occupational Therapy, 40,* 174–179.

Mathiowetz, V., Volland, G., Kashman, N., & Weber, K. (1985). Adult norms for the Box and Block Test of manual dexterity. *American Journal of Occupational Therapy, 39,* 386–391.

Mathiowetz, V., Weber, K., Kashman, N., & Volland, G. (1985). Adult norms for the Nine Hole Peg Test of finger dexterity. *Occupational Therapy Journal of Research, 5,* 24–38.

Matthews, P. B. C. (1972). *Mammalian muscle receptors and their central actions.* Baltimore: Williams & Wilkins.

McGraw, M. B. (1945). *The neuromuscular maturation of the human infant.* New York: Hafner.

McPherson, J. J. (1986). *Measurement of elasticity and extensibility: A technique of assessing the static, dynamic, and reflexive components of muscle tone: A manual for occupational and physical therapists.* Menomonee Falls, WI: Smith & Nephew Rolyan.

McPherson, J. J., Mathiowetz, V., Strachota, E., Benrud, C., Ingrassia, A., & Spitz, M. L. (1985). Muscle tone: Objective evaluation of the static component at the wrist. *Archives of Physical Medicine & Rehabilitation, 66,* 670–674.

Mitz, A. R., & Winstein, C. (1993). The motor system I: Lower centers. In H. Cohen (Ed.), *Neuroscience for rehabilitation* (pp. 141–175). Philadelphia: J. B. Lippincott.

Montgomery, P. C., & Connolly, B. H. (Eds.). (1991). *Motor control and physical therapy: Theoretical framework and practical applications.* Hixson, TN: Chattanooga Group.

Moore, J. C. (1984). The Golgi tendon organ: A review and update. *American Journal of Occupational Therapy, 38,* 227–236.

Moore, J. C. (1986). Recovery potentials following CNS lesions: A brief historical perspective in relation to modern research data on neuroplasticity. *American Journal of Occupational Therapy, 40,* 459–463.

Newell, K. M. (1986). Constraints on the development of coordination. In M. G. Wade & H. T. A. Whiting (Eds.), *Motor development in children: Aspects of coordination and control* (pp. 341–360). Dordrecht: Martinus Nijhoff.

Noback, C., & Demarest, R. (1972). *The nervous system: Introduction and review.* New York: McGraw-Hill.

Nwaobi, O. M. (1983). Voluntary movement impairment in upper motor neuron lesions: Is spasticity the main cause? *Occupational Therapy Journal of Research, 3,* 131–140.

Payton, O. D. (1994). *Research: The validation of clinical practice* (3rd ed.). Philadelphia: F. A. Davis.

Polit, A., & Bizzi, E. (1979). Characteristics of motor programs underlying arm movements in monkeys. *Journal of Neurophysiology, 42,* 183–194.

Reed, E. S. (1982). An outline of a theory of action systems. *Journal of Motor Behavior, 14,* 98–134.

Rider, B., & Linden, C. (1988). Comparison of standardized and non-standardized administration of the Jebsen Hand Function Test. *Journal of Hand Therapy, 2,* 121–123.

Rood, M. S. (1954). Neurophysiological reactions as a basis for physical therapy. *Physical Therapy Review, 34,* 444–449.

Rothstein, J. M. (Ed.). (1991). *Movement science.* Alexandria, VA: American Physical Therapy Association.

Roy, E. A. (1983). Current perspectives on disruptions to limb praxis. *Physical Therapy, 63,* 1998–2003.

Russell, D. G. (1976). Spatial location cues and movement production. In G. E. Stelmach (Ed.), *Motor Control: Issues & Trends* (pp. 67–86). New York: Academic Press.

Salmoni, A. W., Schmidt, R. A., & Walter, C. B. (1984). Knowledge of results and motor learning: A review and critical reappraisal. *Psychological Bulletin, 95,* 355–386.

Sanes, J. N., & Jennings, V. A. (1984). Centrally programmed patterns of muscle activity in voluntary motor behavior of humans. *Experimental Brain Research, 54*, 23–32.

Schmidt, R. A. (1988). *Motor control and learning: A behavioral emphasis* (2nd ed.). Champaign, IL: Human Kinetics.

Schmidt, R. A. (1991a). *Motor learning and performance: From principles to practice.* Champaign, IL: Human Kinetics.

Schmidt, R. A. (1991b). Motor learning principles for physical therapy. In M. J. Lister (Ed.), *Contemporary management of motor control problems: Proceedings of the II STEP conference* (pp. 49–63). Alexandria, VA: Foundation for Physical Therapy.

Scholz, J. (1990). Dynamic pattern theory—Some implications for therapeutics. *Physical Therapy, 70*, 827–843.

Scholz, J. P., & Campbell, S. K. (1980). Muscle spindles and the regulation of movement. *Physical Therapy, 60*, 1416–1424.

Shea, J. B., & Morgan, R. (1979). Contextual interference effects on the acquisition, retention, and transfer of a motor skill. *Journal of Experimental Psychology: Human Learning and Memory, 5*, 179–187.

Sherrington, C. S. (1906). *The integrative action of the nervous system.* New Haven, CT: Yale University Press.

Sherwood, D. E. (1988). Effect of bandwidth knowledge of results on movement consistency. *Perceptual and Motor Skills, 66*, 535–542.

Shik, M. L., & Orlovskii, G. N. (1976). Neurophysiology of a locomotor automatism. *Physiological Reviews, 56*, 465–501.

Smith, R. (1990). Administration and scoring manual. *OT Fact (Occupational Therapy Functional Assessment Compilation Tool).* Rockville, MD: The American Occupational Therapy Association, Inc.

Sollerman, C. (1984). *Assessment of grip function: Evaluation of a new test method.* Sjobo, Sweden: MITAB.

Spaulding, S. J., McPherson, J. J., Strachota, E., Kuphal, M., & Ramponi, M. (1988). Jebsen Hand Function Test: Performance of the uninvolved hand in hemiplegia and of right-handed, right and left hemiplegic persons. *Archives of Physical Medicine & Rehabilitation, 69*, 419–422.

Stern, E. B. (1992). Stability of the Jebsen-Taylor Hand Function Test across three test sessions. *American Journal of Occupational Therapy, 46*, 647–649.

Stolov, W. C. (1966). The concept of normal muscle tone, hypotonia, and hypertonia. *Archives of Physical Medicine & Rehabilitation, 47*, 156–168.

Swash, M., & Fox, K. P. (1972). Muscle spindle innervation in man. *Journal of Anatomy, 112*, 61–80.

Taub, E. (1976). Motor behavior following deafferentation in the developing and motorically mature monkey. *Advances in Behavioral Biology, 18*, 675–705.

Taylor, N., Sand, P. L., & Jebsen, R. H. (1973). Evaluation of hand function in children. *Archives of Physical Medicine & Rehabilitation, 54*, 129–135.

Thelen, E. (1989). Self-organization in developmental processes: Can systems approaches work? In M. R. Gunnar, & E. Thelen (Eds.), *Systems and development* (pp. 77–117). Hillsdale, NJ: Erlbaum.

Thelen, E., & Fisher, D. M. (1982). Newborn stepping: An explanation for a "disappearing reflex." *Developmental Psychology, 18*, 760–775.

Thelen, E., & Ulrich, B. D. (1991). Hidden skills. *Monograph of the Society for Research in Child Development, 56*(Serial No. 223).

Thorndike, E. L. (1927). The law of effect. *American Journal of Psychology, 39*, 212–222.

Tiffin, J. (1968). *Purdue Pegboard: Examiner manual.* Chicago: Science Research Associates.

Tobias, J., & Gorelick, J. (1960). The effectiveness of the Purdue Pegboard in evaluating work potential of retarded adults. *Training School Bulletin, 57*, 94–104.

Touwen, B. C. (1976). *Neurological development in infancy* (Clinics in developmental medicine, No. 58). Philadelphia: J. B. Lippincott.

Trombly, C. A. (1989). Motor control therapy. In C. Trombly (Ed.), *Occupational therapy for physical dysfunction* (3rd ed., pp. 72–95). Baltimore: Williams & Wilkins.

Trombly, C. A. (1993). The issue is—Anticipating the future: Assessment of occupational function. *American Journal of Occupational Therapy, 47*, 253–257.

Trombly, C. A., & Scott, A. D. (1989). Evaluation of motor control. In C. Trombly (Ed.), *Occupational therapy for physical dysfunction* (3rd ed., pp. 55–71). Baltimore: Williams & Wilkins.

Turvey, M. T. (1977). Preliminaries to a theory of action with reference to vision. In R. Shaw & J. Bransford (Eds.), *Perceiving, acting, and knowing* (pp. 211–265). Hillsdale, NJ: Erlbaum.

Turvey, M. T., Fitch, H. L., & Tuller, B. (1982). The Bernstein perspective: I. The problems of degrees of freedom and context-conditioned variability. In J. A. S. Kelso (Ed.), *Human motor behavior: An introduction* (pp. 239–252). Hillsdale, NJ: Erlbaum.

Twitchell, T. E. (1951). The restoration of motor function following hemiplegia in man. *Brain, 74*, 443–480.

Urbscheit, N. L. (1979). Reflexes evoked by group II afferent fibers from muscle spindles. *Physical Therapy, 59*, 1083–1087.

VanSant, A. (1990). Life-span development in functional tasks. *Physical Therapy, 70*, 788–798.

VanSant, A. (1991a). Motor control, motor learning, and motor development. In P. C. Montgomery & B. H. Connolly (Eds.), *Motor control and physical therapy: Theoretical framework and practical applications* (pp. 13–28). Hixson, TN: Chattanooga Group.

VanSant, A. (1991b). Should the normal motor developmental sequence be used as a theoretical model to progress adult patients? In M. J. Lister (Ed.), *Contemporary management of motor control problems: Proceedings of the II STEP conference* (pp. 95–97). Alexandria, VA: Foundation for Physical Therapy.

Warren, W. H. (1984). Perceiving affordances: Visual guidance of stair climbing. *Journal of Experimental Psychology: Human Perception and Performance, 10*, 683–703.

Whiteneck, G., Charlifue, S., Gerhart, K., Overholser, J., & Richardson, G. (1992). Quantifying handicap: A new measure of long-term rehabilitation outcomes. *Archives of Physical Medicine & Rehabilitation, 73*, 519–526.

Wilson, B. C., Iacoviello, J., Wilson, J., & Risucci, D. (1982). Purdue Pegboard performance of normal preschool children. *Journal of Clinical Neuropsychology, 4*, 19–26.

Winstein, C. J., & Schmidt, R. A. (1990). Reduced frequency of knowledge of results enhances motor skill learning. *Journal of Experimental Psychology: Learning, Memory, and Cognition, 16*, 677–691.

World Health Organization. (1980). *International classification of impairments, disabilities, and handicaps: A manual of classification relating to the consequences of disease.* Geneva: Author.

Worley, J. S., Bennett, W., Miller, G., Miller, M., Walker, B., & Harmon, C. (1991). Reliability of three clinical measures of muscle tone in the shoulders and wrists of poststroke patients. *American Journal of Occupational Therapy, 45*, 50–58.

Wyke, B. (1976). Neurological mechanisms in spasticity: A brief review of some concepts. *Physiotherapy, 62*, 316–319.

8

Evaluation of Sensation

Karen Bentzel

OBJECTIVES

After studying this chapter, the reader should be able to:
1. Explain the importance of sensory testing.
2. Demonstrate a number of sensory testing methods.
3. Select an appropriate sensory test for a clinical application.
4. Discuss factors contributing to reliability in sensory evaluation.

Touch sensation is critical for early learning in humans. Touch sensation is probably more critical throughout life than is generally recognized (Kinnealey, 1989). Moberg (1991) stated that without sensory function, good motor function is of limited value. He credited Bunnell with describing the hand without sensation as "blind" (Dellon, 1988).

Sensation in the hand is particularly important. Any sensory loss on the volar hand surface impairs useful tactile feedback. A partial loss causes the patient to be slower and less effective at work and at play. Impaired protective sensory feedback increases the risk of injury (Bell-Krotoski, 1992). Complete loss of sensation leads to severely compromised function (Cobble et al., 1991). Without sensation, vision is needed to guide hand motion or the hand becomes virtually immobile (Dellon, 1988).

Despite the importance of tactile sensation, relatively few tests of this function exist. Sensory tests have been criticized for their subjectivity, unreliability, and lack of validity (Fess, 1990a; Kinnealey, 1989). The purposes of sensory testing (Cooke, 1991) are as follows:

1. Assess the extent of sensory loss.
2. Evaluate and document sensory recovery.
3. Assist in diagnosis.
4. Determine impairment and functional limitation.

5. Provide direction for occupational therapy intervention.
   a. Determine time to begin sensory reeducation.
   b. Determine need for education to prevent injury during occupational performance.

NEUROPHYSIOLOGICAL FOUNDATIONS OF SENSATION

Within the skin, muscles, and joints are receptors excited by somatosensory stimuli. As can be seen in Table 8.1, each receptor is connected to the central nervous system via a specific type of neuron and is primarily excited by one type of sensory input. Each sensory neuron and its distal and proximal terminations can be considered a sensory unit. Each sensory unit has a defined receptive field. A stimulus anywhere in the field may evoke a response, but stimuli applied to the central area of the receptive field will evoke responses more easily. In other words, the center of each receptive field has a lower threshold than the periphery. Adjacent receptive fields overlap; therefore, a single stimulus evokes a profile of responses from overlapping sensory units. The number of sensory units in a given area of skin varies among body parts and is referred to as innervation density. The hand and fingers have a high innervation density (Dellon, 1988).

In sensory testing, it is impossible to test separately the different types of sensory afferent fibers, because all testing involves skin deformation, which causes all types of mechanoreceptors to respond (Moberg, 1991).

Table 8.1 also shows the pathway of the second- and third-order neurons and the general area of termination of the pathway in the brain. The area of the somatosensory cortex responsible for interpreting sensation is the postcentral gyrus of the cortex. Areas of high innervation density, such as the face, lips, and hands, tend to have the largest area of representation in the brain (Dellon, 1988).

Interruption anywhere along the pathway can

GLOSSARY

Hemianesthesia—Complete loss of sensation on the left or right side of the body.

Semmes-Weinstein monofilaments—Set of nylon filaments of various diameters but constant length set at a right angle in acrylic handles and used for testing of the threshold of touch sensation. Each handle is marked with a number that is derived from the logarithm of the force of application of that particular monofilament.

Tinel's sign—Tingling or "pins and needles" sensation as a result of light tapping of the skin over a compressed or damaged peripheral nerve.

Vibrometer—Device designed to test the threshold of vibration sensation. It consists of a vibrating head that is applied to the patient's skin and a control unit that allows for gradual changes in the amplitude of vibration.

Table 8.1. Neural Pathways of Sensory Stimuli[a]

Type of Sensation	Sensory Receptor	Type of Afferent Neuron	Pathway	Termination of Pathway
Constant touch/ pressure	Merkel's cell	Type A β slowly adapting myelinated neurons	Ascend in dorsal spinal cord, cross to opposite side in medulla	Thalamus and somatosensory cortex
Moving touch/ vibration	Meissner's and Pacinian corpuscle	Type A β quickly adapting myelinated neurons		
Pain (pinprick)	Free nerve endings	Type A δ myelinated neurons	Immediately cross to opposite side and pass upward in anterolateral columns of spinal cord	Brainstem, thalamus, and somatosensory cortex
Heat	Free nerve endings specific to heat	Type C unmyelinated fibers		
Cold	Cold receptors and probably also free nerve endings	Type A δ myelinated neurons, and Type C unmyelinated fibers		

[a]Based on information in Dellon (1988) and Guyton (1992).

cause a decrease or loss of sensation. Damage to sensory receptors or sensory neurons may cause an increased threshold for touch and a decreased threshold for pain. In severe damage, these two can coincide so that only pain is elicited (Weinstein, 1993). Following compression to a nerve, the first changes to occur are increases in the threshold of touch perception; changes in innervation density follow continued nerve compression (Dellon, 1990).

In a patient with complete nerve transection, there is an absence of sensation in the area served exclusively by that nerve. Figure 8.1 depicts the typical nerve distribution for the upper extremity. Following peripheral nerve repair, there is usually an orderly progression of return of sensation as axon growth occurs. Sensation of pain generally (but not always) recovers first, followed by sensation of touch (Waylett-Rendall, 1989; Weinstein, 1993). Regrowth of pain fibers averages 1.08 mm per day; regrowth of touch fibers averages 0.78 mm per day (Waylett-Rendall, 1989). Once perception of a stimulus recovers, the perception threshold gradually diminishes, and a response is obtained with a lighter stimulus (Dellon, 1988).

Regenerating afferent fibers innervate the same class of receptors but not the same site (Rath & Green,

1991). After experimental nerve repair on monkeys, up to nine distinct skin regions were found to drive one point in the cortex. In the noninjured, each point in the cortex interprets input from one area of skin (Wall et al., 1986). Following nerve repair, patients complain of sensory abnormalities that seem to relate to an inability to make use of spatial relationships or patterns and inaccuracy in localization of touch (Dykes, 1984). Mackinnon and Dellon (1990) reported that less than 1% of patients who had a median nerve repair recovered normal functional sensation within 5 years after repair.

Patients with complete lesions of the spinal cord show loss of sensation in the dermatomes (Fig. 8.2) below the lesion. Any sensory recovery following spinal cord injury will occur within the 1st year with the greatest recovery in the first 6 months (Waters et al., 1993).

Patients with brain lesions caused, for example, by cerebrovascular accident, head trauma, or cerebral palsy also demonstrate sensory losses. These losses vary in extent and severity, depending on the area of the lesion. **Hemianesthesia** is caused most frequently by a lesion of the thalamus and includes loss of all sensory modalities—pain, temperature, touch, and

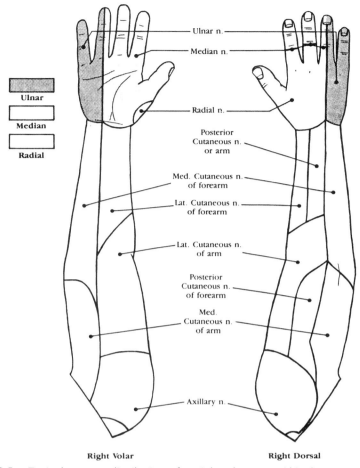

Figure 8.1. Typical sensory distribution of peripheral nerves within the upper extremity.

joint position (Cobble et al., 1991). Patients who lack awareness of a limb's position in space will not use that extremity spontaneously, if at all. Their motor control or quality of movement is impaired by absent proprioception and/or kinesthesia (Leo & Soderberg, 1981).

EVALUATION TECHNIQUES

Methods of evaluation for touch sensation are shown in Table 8.2. The following general principles apply to all sensory testing.

1. The patient needs to be comfortable and relaxed, and the temperature of the room needs to be in a comfortable range (Anthony, 1993; Waylett-Rendall, 1988).
2. Patient concentration is enhanced by reducing distractions (Anthony, 1993; Eggers, 1984; Moberg, 1990).
3. Understanding of spoken or written language is necessary for testing (Eggers, 1984). Modifications

of testing procedures are acceptable if the patient cannot give a verbal response.

4. The hand or instrument applying the stimulus needs to be stabilized as does the area of the patient being tested (Anthony, 1993; Moberg, 1990).
5. Demonstrate the test with vision, then occlude the patient's vision with a screen, a blindfold, a file folder between the patient's face and area being tested, or by asking the patient to close his eyes (Eggers, 1984; Koris et al., 1990; Moberg, 1990).
6. Eliminate auditory cues during stimulus application (Eggers, 1984).
7. Make successive applications of the stimulus as consistently as possible with each other and with the recommended methods of application (MacDermid, 1991; Nakada, 1993).
8. Apply stimuli at irregular intervals (Eggers, 1984).
9. Stimuli are generally applied to the center of each zone being tested.
10. Note any differences in skin thickness, callouses,

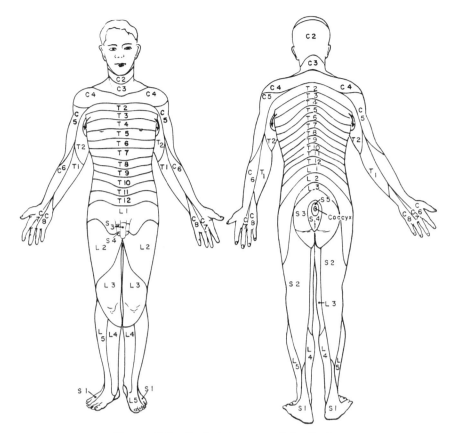

Figure 8.2. Typical dermatomal distribution.

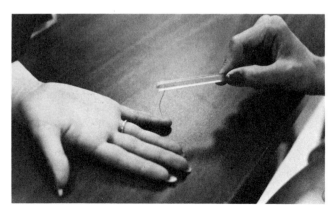

Figure 8.3. Testing the ulnar nerve distribution using Semmes-Weinstein monofilaments.

etc. Expect sensation to be slightly decreased in these areas (Moberg, 1990).

11. Demonstrate each test on an area of skin with intact sensation. Differences of opinion exist on whether to progress sensory testing in a distal to proximal or proximal to distal direction. In patients with nerve injury, it may be best to test in a distal to proximal direction to avoid influence of **Tinel's sign** on testing (Bell-Krotoski, 1990a; Tomancik, 1987; von Prince & Butler, 1967; Waylett-Rendall, 1988).

12. The therapist who completed the initial sensory evaluation should complete sensory retesting (Anthony, 1993; Bell-Krotoski & Tomancik, 1987).

MacDermid (1991) has stated that "without precision in method and interpretation, sensory examination is not an effective use of a clinician's time" (p. 174).

Selection of Sensory Evaluation Methods

Moberg (1990) pointed out some interesting comparisons between the evaluation of sensation and vision. He indicated that if one wants to know visual acuity, other visual tests (e.g., visual field, color vision, and ability to see light) are useless. In a similar way,

Table 8.2. Methods of Testing Sensation

Type of Test	What Test Measures	Test Instrument	Stimulus	Response	Scoring	Normal or Expected Score	Reference
Touch awareness	Awareness of touch input within the central nervous system	Cotton ball, cotton swab, or fingertip	Light touch to a small area of patient's skin	Patient says "yes" or makes agreed on nonverbal signal each time stimulus is felt	Number of correct responses in relation to number of stimuli applied	100%	Bickerstaff (1980)
Tactile attention	Awareness of two simultaneous inputs or presence of tactile inattention	Fingertips	Touch patient on one side of the body or on both sides simultaneously	Patient says "one" or "two" to indicate the number of stimuli he felt	Normal if patient is correct; sensory extinction is occurring if patient feels single stimuli on body part but not both stimuli presented simultaneously	100%	Barer (1990)
Touch localization	Spatial representation of sensory receptors in cortex	Pen, cotton ball, Semmes-Weinstein monofilament number 4.17	Apply touch to patient's skin, and he remembers location of stimulus	With vision no longer occluded, patient uses index finger or marking pen to point to spot just touched	Score is measured distance between location of stimulus and location of response	Expected maximal error in digit tips is 10 mm; in proximal phalanges, 11 mm; in palm, 20 mm	Nakada (1993)
Touch/pressure threshold (Fig. 8.3)	Threshold of light touch sensation	Semmes-Weinstein monofilaments	Select filament with which to begin testing based on patient's description of sensory loss (normal, 2.83; little numbness, 4.31; no feeling, 5.46); hold filament perpendicular to skin, apply in 1 to 1.5 sec, hold for 1 to 1.5 sec, remove in 1 to 1.5 sec; repeat for three applications for filaments 1.65 to 4.08; apply filaments with marking numbers above 4.08 one time to each site	Patient responds with "yes" or "touch" whenever he feels the stimulus	Score is the number of the thinnest filament felt at least once out of three trials; results usually recorded using colored pens or markers and a color key on a diagram of the hand (Fig. 8.4)	Normal touch threshold is perception of the 2.83 monofilament	Tomancik (1987)
Pain: sharp/dull awareness	Discrimination of sharp and dull stimuli	Safety pin	Randomly apply sharp and blunt end of safety pin, perpendicular to patient's skin, at constant pressure	Patient responds with "sharp" or "dull" after each stimulus	Number of correct responses out of number of stimuli	100%	Pendleton (1981)
Temperature (Fig. 8.5)	Discrimination of hot and cold stimuli	Glass test tubes filled with hot and cold water, com-	Apply cold (40°F) or hot (115° to 120°F) stimuli to patient's	Patient indicates "hot" or "cold" after each stimulus	Number of correct responses out of number of stimuli	100%	Waylett-Rendall (1988)

Table 8.2. Continued

Type of Test	What Test Measures	Test Instrument	Stimulus	Response	Scoring	Normal or Expected Score	Reference
		mercially available metal probes	skin				
Vibration awareness	Awareness of input to quickly adapting fibers	Tuning fork; 30 cycles per second or 256 cycles per second	Strike tuning fork with force to cause vibration; place prong tangentially to fingertip of injured and then noninjured hand; ask patient, "Does this feel the same or different?"	Patient responds "same" or "different" and describes difference in perception	Normal if stimuli to both hands feel the same; altered if stimuli feel different	Identical perception of stimuli to both hands	Dellon (1988)
Vibration threshold	Threshold of quickly adapting fibers	Vibrometer (BioThesiometer, BioMedical Instrument Company, Newbury, OH)	Apply vibrating head to area to be tested; gradually increase intensity of stimulus	Patient indicates when he first feels vibration	Voltage is read from vibrometer and converted into microns of displacement	Most normal scores are $\leq 0.04\ \mu$; scores $\geq 0.09\ \mu$ are considered abnormal	Szabo, Gelberman, Williamson, et al. (1984)
Proprioception (position sense)	Unknown combination of touch receptors, muscle receptors, and joint receptors	None	Hold body segment being tested on the lateral surfaces; part is moved through angles of varying degree	Patient indicates "up" or "down" or duplicates position with contralateral extremity	Proprioception is graded as intact, impaired, or absent	Nearly 100% correct duplication	Bickerstaff (1980)
Stereognosis (object identification)	Ability to interpret sensory input; intact motor function is prerequisite	A number of small objects known to the patient	Place a small object in hand to be tested	Patient may manipulate object within the hand; patient names object	Number of correct responses out of total number of objects presented	Nearly 100% correct identification	Eggers (1984)
Dellon's modification of Moberg's Picking up test	Innervation density and interpretation of sensation of the median nerve distribution	Twelve standard objects: wing nut, screw, key, nail, large nut, nickel, dime, washer, safety pin, paper clip, small hex nut, and small square nut	Tape small and ring digits to palm to prevent use. With patient using vision, have him pick up and place objects in a box as quickly as possible; time his performance on two trials; then with vision occluded, place one object at a time between three-point pinch in random order and measure speed of response; do two trials with each object	(1) Patient picks up each object and deposits it in the box as quickly as possible; (2) patient manipulates the object and names it as quickly as possible	(1) Time to pick up and place all 12 objects into a box; (2) time to recognize each object on each of two trials (up to a maximum of 30 sec)	(1) Trial 1 = 10 to 19 sec; trial 2 = 9 to 16 sec; (2) 2 sec per object	Dellon (1988)

Table 8.2. Continued

Type of Test	What Test Measures	Test Instrument	Stimulus	Response	Scoring	Normal or Expected Score	Reference
Static two-point discrimination	Innervation density of slowly adapting fibers	Bent paper clip, aesthesiometer (Fig. 8.6), DiskCriminator, Boley gauge, compass, or calipers with ends blunted	Beginning with a 5-mm separation of points, lightly (with 10 g force) apply one or two points (randomly sequenced) in a longitudinal orientation on the hand; hold until patient responds; gradually adjust distance of separation to find lowest correct level	Patient responds with "one," "two," or "I can't tell"	Smallest distance at which at least 7 out of 10 stimuli are correctly perceived	About 3 mm for distal phalanx; 4 to 5 mm for middle phalanx; 6 to 7 mm for proximal phalanx; 7 to 10 mm for palm	Callahan (1990) and Moberg (1990)
Moving two-point discrimination	Innervation density of quickly adapting fibers	Same as static two-point discrimination	Beginning with a 5- to 8-mm distance, one or two points (randomly) are moved from proximal to distal on distal phalanx, with points side by side and parallel to the long axis of the finger; use just enough pressure for patient to appreciate the stimulus	Patient responds with "one," "two," or "I can't tell"	Smallest distance at which at least 7 out of 10 stimuli are correctly perceived	About 2 mm for distal fingertip	Dellon (1988)

Figure 8.4. Results of sensory testing can be mapped on a form, such as this, that has grid lines dividing the hand into testing areas.

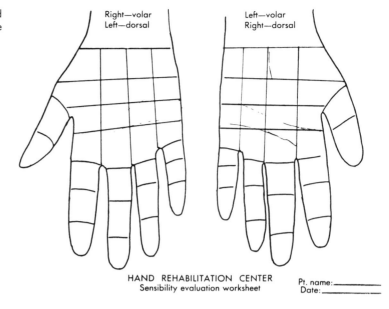

Right—volar
Left—dorsal

Left—volar
Right—dorsal

HAND REHABILITATION CENTER
Sensibility evaluation worksheet

Pt. name:_____
Date:_____

Figure 8.5. Testing ability to discriminate temperature.

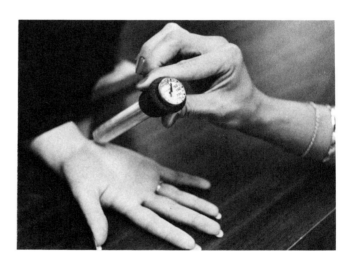

Figure 8.6. Two tools used for applying two-point discrimination stimuli: aesthesiometer and bent paper clip.

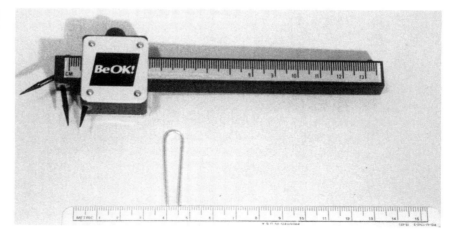

the selection of a sensory test should be based on what question is to be answered. For instance, in a patient with a complete spinal cord injury, you want to know whether sensation is present or absent in each body area. A touch awareness or pain test is common (Waters et al., 1993). To predict whether a patient with a hand injury can, in his work as a mechanic, feel for and locate automobile parts in places that cannot be seen, a stereognosis test is more appropriate than a test of touch awareness.

The following is a hierarchy of sensory capacity of the hand, according to Fess (1990b).

1. *Detection.* The ability to distinguish a single point stimulus from background stimulation.
2. *Discrimination.* The ability to distinguish the difference between stimulus A and stimulus B.
3. *Quantification.* The ability to organize tactile stimuli according to degree (i.e., roughness/smoothness or weight)
4. *Recognition.* The ability to recognize objects by touch.

This hierarchy can be used as a general guideline for selecting a sensory test. Make sure that the level of the test matches the level of information needed.

It is not necessary to test every sensory modality in every patient. Von Prince and Butler (1967) stated that if discriminative sensibility is present as indicated by the results of two-point discrimination or monofilament testing, sensation of temperature will be present, except in certain select patients such as those with a diagnosis of syringomyelia.

Select the skin areas to be assessed based on the diagnosis, the patient's description of his problem, and the question you want to answer with sensory testing (Waylett-Rendall, 1988). For instance, if you need to assess a patient with a diagnosis of nerve root involvement and a questionable peripheral nerve injury, you will need to test the entire hand and extremity and carefully map the affected sensory areas to assist in differential diagnosis. If the patient has known involvement of one peripheral nerve, detailed testing is necessary only in the areas of classic innervation by that nerve. Do a quick screening to verify that other areas are within normal limits. A general rule is to test only as proximal as the location of the injury (Werner & Omer, 1970).

Bell-Krotoski and Buford (1988) advocated testing the status of the peripheral nerves by using **Semmes-Weinstein monofilaments** at sites specific to the sensory distribution of the median and ulnar nerves as follows:

Median Nerve. Volar surface of distal and proximal phalanges of the index finger and distal phalanx of the thumb.

Ulnar Nerve. Volar surface of the distal and proximal phalanges of little finger and hypothenar eminence (Figs. 8.1 and 8.3).

To date, no single sensory evaluation has been developed that yields a complete picture of a patient's sensory status. A battery of at least three or four well-chosen tests is usually recommended (Anthony, 1993; Bell-Krotoski, 1990a; Callahan, 1990; Cooke, 1991; Eggers, 1984; Harlowe & Van Duesen, 1985; Jongbloed, Collins, & Jones, 1986).

Sensory Test Interpretation

In most sensory tests, interpretation requires comparison of involved and uninvolved areas, comparison of results with established norms, or comparison of results with expected performance based on knowledge of anatomy and pathology (Cooke, 1991).

Interpretation of **Semmes-Weinstein monofilament** testing is based on the information presented in Table 8.3. Bell-Krotoski (1990a) gave the following functional descriptions of the levels of sensation listed in Table 8.3. A patient with *normal* touch threshold has recognition of light touch and deep pressure that is within normal limits. *Diminished light touch* means that the patient will have fair use of his hand, good temperature appreciation, and stereognosis close to normal; the patient may not realize that he has a sensory loss. A patient with *diminished protective sensation* has difficulty manipulating objects and a tendency to drop them. He does have appreciation of pain and temperature. *Loss of protective sensation* indicates that the patient will have little hand usage and diminished or absent temperature appreciation, but he will feel pinprick and deep pressure. This patient has an increased risk of injury. A patient who is untestable with the **Semmes-Weinstein monofilaments** may or may not feel a pinprick but has no other level of feeling.

Table 8.3. Semmes-Weinstein Monofilaments[a]

Filament Number	Diameter (mm)	Mean Force (g)	Color Code	Interpretation
2.83	0.127	0.076	Green	Normal
3.61	0.178	0.209	Blue	Diminished light touch
4.31	0.305	2.35	Purple	Diminished protective sensation
4.56	0.356	4.55	Red	Loss of protective sensation
6.65	1.143	235.61	Red	Loss of all sensation except deep pressure

[a]Based on information in Bell-Krotoski and Tomancik (1987) and Tomancik (1987).

Testing Function Versus Testing Pathology

Moberg (1991) believed that a sensory test should yield information about function, especially for patients with hand injuries. His opinion was that the **Semmes-Weinstein monofilaments** are of little use in hand therapy but are perhaps helpful in neurology to aid in the diagnosis of lesions in the central nervous system. Bell-Krotoski (1990a), however, reported a relationship between the **Semmes-Weinstein monofilaments** and levels of functional touch and indicated that scores can be used to predict which of the other sensory modalities (e.g., pinprick and temperature) the patient can feel.

Dellon and Kallman (1983) found that the tests of sensibility that best predict hand function are the static and moving two-point discrimination tests. High correlations were found between static two-point discrimination and the time to recognize objects and between moving two-point discrimination and the number of objects identified by touch. The static version is thought to be a better predictor of functional sensation if the activity is one in which the object is held or force must be maintained on the object. The dynamic version is thought to be the best predictor of functional sensation if the activity requires moving the fingers over the object (dexterity). Van Heest, House, and Putnam (1993) also found a correlation between two-point discrimination and stereognosis.

In Dellon and Kallman's (1983) study, sensory threshold, as measured by **Semmes-Weinstein monofilaments,** did not predict scores on Dellon's modification of Moberg's picking-up test, either in number of objects identified or in mean recognition time. Dellon (1988) concluded that the **Semmes-Weinstein monofilament** score does not correlate with hand function.

Weinstein (1993) compared the results of **Semmes-Weinstein monofilament** and two-point discrimination testing in patients who were undergoing cortical surgical procedures. He applied electrical stimulation to the area of the cortex responsible for perception of touch sensation in the hand. Testing showed a complete loss of two-point discrimination while pressure threshold sensitivity showed no change. Therefore, he concluded that pressure sensitivity is most likely subsumed by subcortical structures and is more specific and appropriate in the evaluation of peripheral nerve injuries. As further evidence that two-point discrimination is a more cortical test, Weinstein demonstrated a high correlation between scores on this test and the area of the cortex serving the testing site. No such correlation exists for touch/pressure threshold testing. Transcutaneous electrical stimulation (TENS) to the median nerve altered touch/pressure sensibility but not two-point discrimination (Banner, Cautilli, & Wehbe, 1990). This research suggested that the "function" measured by **Semmes-Weinstein monofilament** testing is related to the peripheral nerves while the "function" measured by two-point discrimination is related to cortical interpretation of sensation.

Sensitivity of Sensory Tests

Weinstein (1993) advocated that clinicians ensure that their testing methods are sensitive enough to detect what they are trying to assess. Two-point discrimination was more sensitive than stereognosis testing in detecting deficits in patients with spastic cerebral palsy (Bolanos et al., 1989). **Semmes-Weinstein monofilament** testing was found to be more sensitive than two-point discrimination testing, because monofilament testing indicated a substantially greater number of abnormal results in patients who were diagnosed with carpal tunnel syndrome (Gellman et al., 1986; Szabo, Gelberman, & Dimick, 1984). **Vibrometer** testing was abnormal slightly more frequently than **Semmes-Weinstein monofilament** testing, and both the touch and vibration threshold tests were found to be more sensitive than testing with a tuning fork (Szabo, Gelberman, & Dimick, 1984).

VALIDITY AND RELIABILITY OF SENSORY TESTS

Fess (1990a) stated that while there are many methods of assessing sensibility only the reliability of the **Semmes-Weinstein monofilaments** has been statistically tested. The **Semmes-Weinstein monofilament** is the only test device in Table 8.2 that has a consistently repeatable application force. The exact level of force depends on the length and diameter of the monofilament (Bell-Krotoski & Buford, 1988). In four applications, the monofilament with a marking number of 2.83 showed less than 25 mg of difference in application force. In contrast, the variation in force of application of a tuning fork was 23 g.

Bell-Krotoski (1990b) indicated that the **Semmes-Weinstein monofilaments** give relative control of the force of application but cautioned that the force can vary with technique, time of application, and length and diameter of the filaments. Some manufacturing errors were found; therefore, it is recommended to check the length (38 mm) and diameter (Table 8.3) of the monofilaments with a micrometer (Bell-Krotoski & Tomancik, 1987).

Care must be taken with the monofilaments to maintain their consistency. Store monofilaments in an area where they will not be affected by humidity. Do not use monofilaments that are bent. Bell-Krotoski and Tomancik (1987) showed that there is some overlap in the range of forces in the kit containing 20 monofilaments and supported the use of the "mini-kit" containing 5 monofilaments (those listed in Table 8.3).

Bowen, Griener, and Jones (1990) studied the interrater reliability of the Semmes-Weinstein monofilaments and found that all testers were in agreement, based on findings of no significant differences between the mean scores in each pair of testers.

None of the currently available devices used to test two-point discrimination control the amount of force of application (Fess, 1990a). One interrater reliability study showed correlations of .917 to .961 for static two-point discrimination and .882 to .923 for moving two-point discrimination (Dellon, Mackinnon, & Crosby, 1987). Fess (1990a) noted that because this study was limited to two examiners and selected patients other studies are needed before the reliability of two-point discrimination can be accepted. Moberg (1990) reported that in 322 out of 340 normal subjects the scores by two trained raters were either equal or within 1 mm.

Moberg (1991) cautioned that the static two-point discrimination test is useful only when properly administered. He indicated that all extra motion is to be avoided by both the therapist and the patient. He believed that without appropriate technique, alterations in the speed and force of application can yield widely varying results.

Bell-Krotoski and Buford (1988), in taking strain gauge measurements of one-point versus two-point stimuli, found up to 12 g of difference in force and suggested that patients can tell the difference between a single-point and double-point application by noting the force rather than the number of points touching the skin. Moberg (1991) reported a difference in static two-point discrimination score of about 1 mm between transverse and longitudinal applications of the two points. Differences also exist in the expected normal values for static two-point discrimination (Dellon, 1988; Moberg, 1991; Werner & Omer, 1970).

Sieg and Williams (1986) reported interexaminer reliability of 0.98 for tactile localization. Test-retest reliability ranged between 0.36 and 0.71. Reliability improves as stimulus duration and intensity are increased.

Review of the literature does not yield reliability or validity information on any of the other test methods listed in Table 8.2.

RELATIONSHIPS AMONG SENSORY TESTS

Dellon (1988) stated that it is not possible to test a single type of touch receptor, because they are all mechanoreceptors and respond to any deformation of skin. It is not surprising, therefore, that relationships among tactile test scores have been found. A high correlation (0.92) was found between two-point discrimination and touch localization; however, threshold of touch correlates only weakly with two-point discrimina-

tion (0.17) and localization (0.28) (Weinstein, 1993). A deficit in vibration threshold tends to correlate with abnormal light touch and position sense (American Diabetes Association, 1988). Moberg (1991) reported that results of the static two-point discrimination test can be used to predict the presence or absence of finger proprioception, while Van Heest et al. (1993) found that two-point discrimination scores correlated with stereognosis but not with proprioception. Harlowe and Van Duesen (1985) reported correlations between perception of light touch, perception of temperature, and perception of pinprick. Although there are significant relationships among some sensory tests, no one test can predict performance on another test with 100% accuracy.

Other Tests of Sensory Function

WEINSTEIN ENHANCED SENSORY TEST (WEST)

The newest monofilament testing instrument is the Weinstein Enhanced Sensory Test (Connecticut Bioinstruments Inc., Danbury), which is considered an advancement of the Semmes-Weinstein monofilaments. It consists of five filaments mounted on levers that rotate on the handle. This smaller version can fit into a pocket and also has the advantage of being color coded. The improved tip design means that the WEST filaments have a decreased rate of slippage during application to the skin.

HYPERSENSITIVITY

Hypersensitivity is defined as a "condition of extreme discomfort or irritability in response to normally non-noxious tactile stimulation" (Yerxa et al., 1983, p. 176). The Downey Hand Center Hypersensitivity Test (Yerxa et al., 1983) requires patients to sequence, from least to most irritating, a set of 10 textures (e.g., moleskin to hook Velcro) mounted on wooden dowels and a set of 10 containers of particulate material (e.g., cotton and plastic cubes) into which patients immerse their hands. Test-retest reliability was reported by the authors to be 0.74 to 0.82. This test seems to be useful in treatment planning for the patient with hypersensitivity.

SENSORY INTEGRATION

"Sensory integration is the organization of sensation for use" (Ayres, 1979, p. 5). Several subtests of the Sensory Integration and Praxis Tests and their precursor, the Southern California Sensory Integration Test, measure sensory function. These include manual form perception, finger identification, graphesthesia, localization of tactile stimuli, and kinesthesia (Mailloux, 1990). Although these tests are designed for children ages 4 through 8, Hsu and Nelson (1981) collected normative data on adults for several of the subtests.

SUSTAINED TOUCH-PRESSURE

Sustained touch pressure sensation is thought to be necessary for all tasks involving holding an object. In patients with cortical dysfunction, there is a tendency for the depreciation of awareness of sustained touch pressure with time. Dannenbaum and Dykes (1990) developed a test specific to sustained touch pressure sensitivity for patients with cortical dysfunction. A device that gives tactile stimuli of four different weights is used. Stimuli are applied for a 20-sec duration with varying intervals between stimuli. Patients report yes or no every 2 sec to indicate whether the stimulus is touching the finger.

SUMMARY

Moberg (1991) has stated that in sensory testing real knowledge is rare and hypotheses frequent. Dellon (1988) believed that sensory function is more difficult to assess than motor function but reported progress in the investigation of sensory function within the last twenty years.

We therapists need to surrender our feeling that active motion is the only critical factor in recovery. The motor system needs adequate sensory input for function. Only with both sensory and motor function can the patient be rehabilitated (Moberg, 1990).

Acknowledgments—Appreciation is extended to Wayne Fox, Georgette Kosnosky, and Stacey Reese for their assistance with the photographs for this chapter and Chapter 23.

STUDY QUESTIONS

1. What is the importance of evaluating sensation?
2. Describe the neural pathways of sensory stimuli.
3. List several diagnostic categories of patients who need to be evaluated for sensation.
4. What are some factors that can influence reliability in evaluation of sensation?
5. For patients with brain lesions, what is the effect of a total loss of position sense on motor control?
6. Describe a few factors to consider when selecting a test of sensation for a particular patient.
7. How do you interpret the results of a sensory evaluation?

REFERENCES

American Diabetes Association. (1988). Report and recommendations of the San Antonio conference on diabetic neuropathy. *Diabetes Care, 11,* 592–597.

Anthony, M. (1993). Sensory evaluation. In G. Clark, E. S. Wilgis, B. Aiello, D. Eckhaus, & L. Eddington (Eds.), *Hand rehabilitation* (pp. 55–72). New York: Churchill Livingstone.

Ayres, A. J. (1979). *Sensory integration and the child.* Los Angeles: Western Psychological Services.

Banner, C., Cautilli, D., & Wehbe, M. (1990). Effect of TENS on sensibility of the median nerve. *Journal of Hand Therapy, 3,* 34.

Barer, D. (1990). The influence of visual and tactile inattention on predictions for recovery from acute stroke. *Quarterly Journal of Medicine, 74,* 21–32.

Bell-Krotoski, J. (1990a). Light touch-deep pressure testing with Semmes-Weinstein monofilaments. In J. Hunter, L. Schneider, E. Mackin, & A. Callahan (Eds.), *Rehabilitation of the hand* (3rd ed., pp. 585–593). St. Louis: C. V. Mosby.

Bell-Krotoski, J. (1990b). "Pocket filaments" and specifications for the Semmes-Weinstein monofilaments. *Journal of Hand Therapy, 3,* 26–31.

Bell-Krotoski, J. (1992). A study of peripheral nerve involvement underlying physical disability of the hand in Hansen's disease. *Journal of Hand Therapy, 5,* 133–142.

Bell-Krotoski, J., & Buford, W. (1988). The force/time relationship of clinically used sensory testing instruments. *Journal of Hand Therapy, 1,* 76–85.

Bell-Krotoski, J., & Tomancik, E. (1987). Repeatability of testing with Semmes-Weinstein monofilaments. *Journal of Hand Surgery, 12A,* 155–161.

Bickerstaff, E. (1980). *Neurological examination in clinical practice* (4th ed.). Boston: Blackwell Scientific Publications.

Bolanos, A., Bleck, E., Firestone, P., & Young, L. (1989). Comparison of stereognosis and two-point discrimination testing of the hands of children with cerebral palsy. *Developmental Medicine and Child Neurology, 31,* 371–376.

Bowen, V. L., Griener, J. S., & Jones, S. V. (1990). Threshold of sensation: Inter-rater reliability and establishment of normal using the Semmes-Weinstein monofilament. *Journal of Hand Therapy, 3,* 36.

Callahan, A. (1990). Sensibility testing: Clinical methods. In J. Hunter, L. Schneider, E. Mackin, & A. Callahan (Eds.), *Rehabilitation of the hand* (3rd ed., pp. 594–610). St. Louis: C. V. Mosby.

Cobble, N., Bontke, C., Brandstater, M., & Horn, L. (1991). Rehabilitation in brain disorders: 3. Intervention strategies. *Archives of Physical Medicine and Rehabilitation, 72,* S324–331.

Cooke, D. (1991). Sensibility evaluation battery for the peripheral nerve injured hand. *Australian Occupational Therapy Journal, 38,* 241–245.

Dannenbaum, R., & Dykes, R. (1990). Evaluating sustained touch-pressure in severe sensory deficits: Meeting an unanswered need. *Archives of Physical Medicine and Rehabilitation, 71,* 455–459.

Dellon, A. (1988). *Evaluation of sensibility and re-education of sensation in the hand.* Baltimore: Lucas.

Dellon, A. (1990). The sensational contributions of Erik Moberg. *Journal of Hand Surgery (Edinburgh), 15B,* 14–24.

Dellon, A., & Kallman, C. (1983). Evaluation of functional sensation in the hand. *Journal of Hand Surgery, 8,* 865–870.

Dellon, A., MacKinnon, S., & Crosby, P. (1987). Reliability of two-point discrimination measurements. *Journal of Hand Surgery, 12A,* 693–696.

Dykes, R. (1984). Central consequences of peripheral nerve injuries. *Annals of Plastic Surgery, 13,* 412–422.

Eggers, O. (1984). Occupational therapy in the treatment of adult hemiplegia. Rockville, CO: Aspen Systems.

Fess, E. (1990a). Assessment of the upper extremity: Instrumentation criteria. *Occupational Therapy Practice, 1,* 1–11.

Fess, E. (1990a). Documentation: Essential elements of an upper extremity assessment battery. In J. Hunter, L. Schneider, E.

Mackin, & A. Callahan (Eds.), *Rehabilitation of the hand* (3rd ed., pp. 53–81). St. Louis: C. V. Mosby.

Gellman, H., Gelberman, R. H., Tan, A. M., & Botte, M. J. (1986). Carpal tunnel syndrome—Evaluation of the provocative diagnostic test. *Journal of Bone and Joint Surgery, 68A*, 735–737.

Guyton, A. (1992). *Human physiology and mechanisms of disease* (5th ed.). Philadelphia: W. B. Saunders.

Harlowe, D., & Van Deusen, J. (1985). Evaluating cutaneous sensation following CVA: Relationships among touch, pain, and temperature tests. *Occupational Therapy Journal of Research, 5*, 70–72.

Hsu, Y., & Nelson, D. (1981). Adult performance on the southern California kinesthesis and tactile perception tests. *American Journal of Occupational Therapy, 35*, 788–791.

Jongbloed, L., Collins, J., & Jones, W. (1986). A sensorimotor integration test battery for CVA clients: Preliminary evidence of reliability and validity. *Occupational Therapy Journal of Research, 6*, 131–151.

Kinnealey, M. (1989). Tactile functions in learning disabled and normal children: Reliability and validity considerations. *Occupational Therapy Journal of Research, 9*, 3–15.

Koris, M., Gelberman, R., Duncan, K., Boublick, M., & Smith, B. (1990). Carpal tunnel syndrome—Evaluation of a quantitative provocative diagnostic test. *Clinical Orthopedics and Related Research, 251*, 157–161.

Leo, K. C., & Soderberg, G. L. (1981). Relationship between perception of joint position sense and limb synergies in patients with hemiplegia. *Physical Therapy, 10*, 1433–1437.

MacDermid, J. (1991). Accuracy of clinical tests used in the detection of carpal tunnel syndrome: A literature review. *Journal of Hand Therapy, 4*, 169–176.

Mackinnon, S., & Dellon, A. (1990). Clinical nerve reconstruction with a bioabsorbable polyglycolic acid tube. *Plastic and Reconstructive Surgery, 85*, 419–424.

Mailloux, Z. (1990). An overview of the Sensory Integration and Praxis Tests. *American Journal of Occupational Therapy, 44*, 589–593.

Moberg, E. (1990). Two-point discrimination test. A valuable part of hand surgical rehabilitation, e.g. in tetraplegia. *Scandinavian Journal of Rehabilitation Medicine, 22*, 127–134.

Moberg, E. (1991). The unsolved problem—How to test the functional value of hand sensibility. *Journal of Hand Therapy, 4*, 105–110.

Nakada, M. (1993). Localization of a constant-touch and moving-touch stimulus in the hand: A preliminary study. *Journal of Hand Therapy, 6*, 23–28.

Pendleton, K. (1981). *OT management of physical dysfunction—Loma Linda University*. Brookfield, IL: Sammons.

Rath, S., & Green, C. (1991). Lack of topographical specificity in sensory nerve regeneration through muscle grafts in rats. *Journal of Hand Surgery (Edinburgh), 16B*, 524–530.

Sieg, K., & Williams, W. (1986). Preliminary report of a methodology for determining tactile location in adults. *Occupational Therapy Journal of Research, 6*, 195–206.

Szabo, R., Gelberman, R., & Dimick, M. (1984). Sensibility testing in patients with carpal tunnel syndrome. *Journal of Bone and Joint Surgery, 66A*, 60–64.

Szabo, R., Gelberman, R., Williamson, R., Dellon, A., Yaru, N., & Dimick, M. (1984). Vibratory sensory testing in acute peripheral nerve compression. *Journal of Hand Surgery, 9A*, 104–109.

Tomancik, L. (1987). *Directions for using Semmes-Weinstein monofilaments*. San Jose, CA: North Coast Medical.

Van Heest, A., House, J., & Putnam, M. (1993). Sensibility deficiencies in the hands of children with spastic hemiplegia. *Journal of Hand Surgery, 18A*, 278–281.

von Prince, K., & Butler, B. (1967). Measuring sensory function of the hand in peripheral nerve injuries. *American Journal of Occupational Therapy, 21*, 385–395.

Wall, M., Kaas, J., Sur, M., Nelson, R., Felleman, D., & Merzenich, M. (1986). Functional reorganization in somatosensory cortical areas 3b and 1 of adult monkeys after median nerve repair: Possible relationships of sensory recovery in humans. *Journal of Neuroscience, 6*, 218–233.

Waters, R., Adkins, R., Yakura, J., & Sie, I. (1993). Motor and sensory recovery following complete tetraplegia. *Archives of Physical Medicine and Rehabilitation, 74*, 242–247.

Waylett-Rendall, J. (1988). Sensibility evaluation and rehabilitation. *Orthopedic Clinics of North America, 19*, 43–56.

Waylett-Rendall, J. (1989). Sequence of sensory recovery: A retrospective study. *Journal of Hand Therapy, 2*, 245–251.

Weinstein, S. (1993). Fifty years of somatosensory research: From the Semmes-Weinstein monofilaments to the Weinstein Enhanced Sensory Tests. *Journal of Hand Therapy, 6*, 11–22.

Werner, J., & Omer, G. (1970). A procedure evaluation of cutaneous pressure sensation of the hand. *American Journal of Occupational Therapy, 26*, 347–356.

Yerxa, E., Barber, L., Diaz, O., Black, W., & Azen, S. (1983). Development of a hand sensitivity test for the hypersensitive hand. *American Journal of Occupational Therapy, 37*, 176–181.

9

Evaluation of Perception and Cognition

Lee Ann Quintana

OBJECTIVES

After studying this chapter, the reader will be able to:
1. Define **cognition** and **perception.**
2. Identify and describe specific evaluation strategies to evaluate vision, body scheme, **unilateral neglect, spatial relations,** and **apraxia.**
3. Identify and describe specific evaluation strategies to evaluate **attention,** orientation, **memory,** and **problem solving.**
4. Recognize the need for evaluating the process as well as the outcome of specific cognitive and perceptual tests.
5. Value the importance of using standardized tests.

Following brain injury the patient is often left with varying degrees of cognitive and perceptual dysfunction as well as the more obvious motor and sensory deficits. The medical field has spent a great deal of time and energy understanding and developing techniques to evaluate and treat the physical and medical sequelae of brain injury. Increased and ongoing research regarding the impact of residual cognitive-perceptual deficits and development of treatment strategies to combat them is needed. Cognitive deficits and visual perceptual deficits have been found to be significantly related to eventual independence in self-care and discharge disposition (Bernspange, Vitanin, & Eriksson, 1989; Carter et al., 1988; Forer & Miller, 1980; Kaplan & Hier, 1982; Lorenze & Cancro, 1962; Sea, Henderson, & Cermak, 1993; Titus et al., 1991). Occupational therapists, therefore, need to focus attention on the evaluation and restoration of cognitive and perceptual skills as prerequisites to the overall goal of promoting achievement of optimal functional independence. The impact of cognitive and perceptual deficits on the patient's activities of daily living (ADL) skills sometimes outweigh that of physical deficits (Table 9.1).

With this increasing interest in the importance of cognitive-perceptual deficits, there has developed an overlap of services between psychologists, neuropsychologists, speech and language pathologists, and occupational therapists. The emphasis today is on a coordinated team approach with all members concerned about the total rehabilitation of the patient. These team members work together, but the occupational therapist's role in cognitive rehabilitation may vary, depending on the team with which she works.

Cognition refers to the ability of the brain to process, store, retrieve, and manipulate information (Prigatano & Fordyce, 1986). **Perception** refers to the integration of sensory impressions into psychologically meaningful information (Lezak, 1976). For a deficit in **perception** to be identified, the primary senses must be intact. For example, a person who has poor visual acuity cannot necessarily be said to have a deficit in visual **perception** when unable to match objects, whereas the patient with good acuity who is unable to match objects may be said to have a perceptual deficit. In the literature there is extensive overlap and blurring of definitions of the various cognitive and perceptual deficits seen following brain injury. For the purposes of this chapter, general evaluation guidelines will be discussed and then specific guidelines will be given for evaluation of perceptual deficits: visual foundation skills, including acuity, fields, and oculomotor function; body scheme, including right/left discrimination, body part identification, finger agnosia, and anosognosia; **unilateral neglect; spatial relations** and position in space, including topographical orientation and figure/ground discrimination; **apraxia,** including limb apraxia, constructional apraxia, and dressing apraxia;

GLOSSARY

Apraxia—Inability to carry out purposeful movement in the presence of intact sensation, movement, and coordination.

Attention—Ability to focus on a specific stimulus without being distracted.

Cognition—Ability to process, store, retrieve, and manipulate information (Prigatano & Fordyce, 1986).

Memory—Registration and encoding, consolidation and storage, and recall and retrieval of information.

Perception—Integration of sensory impressions into psychologically meaningful information (Lezak, 1976).

Problem solving—Ability to manipulate a fund of knowledge and apply the information to new or unfamiliar situations (Strub & Black, 1977).

Spatial relations—Ability to perceive self in relation to other objects or between objects.

Unilateral neglect—Failure to respond or orient to stimuli presented contralateral to a brain lesion (Helman et al., 1985).

and evaluation of cognitive deficits, including **attention,** orientation, **memory,** and **problem solving.**

Until recently, occupational therapists have tended to do only a cursory evaluation in the areas of **perception** and **cognition.** Standardized measures were not used, and there was a tendency to gather information on a subjective level (Ottenbacher, 1980). Valid and reliable standardized quantitative assessment tools must be used, when available, if treatment success is to be documented in measurable terms. When standardized tests are not available, the occupational therapist should administer and score the evaluation materials in a consistent manner.

Occupational therapists have traditionally assessed **cognition** and **perception** in adults by using a "skill-specific approach" (Abreu & Toglia, 1987). A patient who scored poorly on a test of **spatial relations** was said to have a problem with **spatial relations.** The problem with this method is that the reason for failure and how the patient went about solving the task is not considered. Failure on a task of **spatial relations** might be the result of **unilateral neglect,** decreased **attention** to detail, decreased concentration, or a problem with **spatial relations.** Test scores alone do not give a clear picture of how a given patient will perform in a functional setting. It is equally as important to note how the patient approaches a task, how he achieves the final score, and how performance changes with cuing (Lezak, 1991; Toglia, 1989; Warren, 1993b). Therefore, the occupational therapy cognitive-perceptual evaluation should emphasize quality of performance as well as test scores, and function more than dysfunction (Abreu & Toglia, 1987). It is the occupational therapist's job to determine where the patient's strengths and weaknesses are and how to use the strengths and minimize the weaknesses (Warren, 1993b).

An information-processing approach to evaluation of cognitive and perceptual deficits has been advocated (Abreu & Toglia, 1987; Toglia, 1989). Standardized tests are used whenever possible, but the tests are not terminated when the patient fails after the standard instructions are given. The patient is given additional specific standard cues to determine how they will affect his performance. These cues can provide feedback, direct **attention** to relevant features, and/or pace speed of performance. The patient's score on the test would remain the same, but now the therapist would have information on what type of cues benefit the patient and if the patient benefits from cues at all.

Toglia (1989) described a graded system of cuing for evaluation of object recognition. A repetition cue such as "Look again" subtly implies that the response was incorrect. If the patient is able to respond to this cue, he is able to self-correct his errors. With an analysis cue, the therapist asks the patient to describe different properties of the object being viewed (i.e., size, color, shape, and weight). Use of a perceptual cue emphasizes a critical feature. The therapist points out or repositions an object in a more favorable position for the patient. Semantic cues involve giving the patient a choice of three categories. These types of cues (repetition, analysis, perceptual, and semantic) can be used in the evaluation of other cognitive and perceptual deficits. For example, when evaluating **memory,** the therapist may ask the patient to remember three objects. If at the end of 5 min the patient is unable to remember any item, his performance may be improved with cues ("Think again," "It was a color," "Was it black, brown, or red?"). If the cues do not help him, the problem could be one of encoding, but if the cues do help, it could be a problem with information retrieval.

Investigative questions are used to provide insight into the underlying deficit (Toglia, 1989). For example, the therapist might ask, "Why did you think it was a book?" or "How did you know it was a book and not a tray?" Responses that appear bizarre at first may be easily explained.

Evaluation of the brain-injured patient may vary, depending on the site of lesion. There are certain general characteristics that patients have following damage to either the right or left hemisphere, which may influence the manner in which evaluation is carried out (Table 9.2).

Table 9.1. Definitions and Descriptions of Cognitive-Perceptual Deficits

Area of Deficit	Definition	Functional Description of Deficit
Body scheme	Awareness of body parts, position of body and its parts in relation to themselves and objects in the environment	May result in dressing apraxia; may not recognize body parts or relationship between them; transfers may be unsafe
Right/left discrimination	Ability to understand the concepts of right and left; with RBD deficit may be caused by a visuospatial deficit; with LBD and aphasia deficit caused by language deficit; with LBD and no aphasia deficit caused by general mental impairment	May have difficulty dressing and understanding directions that include right and left
Body part identification	Ability to identify parts on self and/or others	May respond incorrectly when told to move a specific body part
Finger agnosia	Difficulty naming or being able to name fingers touched	May have difficulty with fine dexterity
Anosognosia	Unawareness or denial of deficits	Functional activities are unsafe; unable to learn compensatory techniques
Unilateral neglect	Neglect of one side of the body or extrapersonal space; motor (output) neglect seen by impaired initiation into contralateral hemispace; perceptual (input) seen by impaired ability to attend to stimuli in contralateral hemispace	Shaves only one side of face, dresses only one side of his body; eats food from only half of his plate; reads only half of a page; deletes only half of a drawing; transfers and functional mobility are unsafe; bumps into door jambs and objects on one side
Position in space	Able to understand the concepts of over and under, above, and below, etc.	Difficulty moving through a crowded area; difficulty with dressing; difficulty following directions using these terms
Spatial relations	Ability to perceive self in relation to other objects	As above; transfers unsafe
Topographical orientation	Ability to find one's way from one place to another	Difficulty finding his way from his room to therapy or from one room to another
Figure/ground perception	Ability to distinguish foreground from background	Unable to find object in cluttered drawer, white washcloth on white sheet, brakes on wheelchair, food in the refrigerator
Limb apraxia	Inability to carry out purposeful movement in the presence of intact sensation, movement, and coordination	May experience difficulty with functional tasks involving objects, as patient does not know how to use objects or attempts to use wrong object (e.g., uses knife to eat soup); may be clumsy and have trouble with writing, knitting, etc.
Constructional apraxia	Deficit in constructional activities: graphic and assembly; with RBD drawings are complex but exhibit disorganized spatial relations and poor orientation in space (believed to be result of visuospatial deficits); with LBD drawings tend to be simplified with few details (believed to be an executive or conceptual deficit	May result in dressing apraxia; difficulty setting a table, making a dress, wrapping a gift, arranging numerical figures for mathematical processing, making a sandwich, assembling a craft project from a kit, etc.
Dressing apraxia	Inability to dress oneself	Attempts to put clothes on inside out, backwards, or in the wrong order; dresses only one-half of the body
Attention	Ability to focus on a specific stimulus without being distracted	Exhibits inability to follow directions or to learn; may appear lethargic; may have difficulty in group situations
Orientation	Oriented times three refers to knowledge of person, place, and time	Unable to answer orientation questions; may ask simple questions over and over; may be easily agitated due to disorientation
Memory	The registration and encoding, consolidation and storage, and recall and retrieval of information	Appears disoriented; will forget names, schedule, etc.; decreased ability to learn or to follow directions
Problem solving	The ability to manipulate a fund of knowledge and apply this information to new or unfamiliar situations	Difficulty with routine self-care and household chores, e.g., routine shopping, planning a meal, etc.; may be socially inappropriate; exhibit poor judgment; difficulty ordering or sequencing information, e.g., time, work, etc.

Table 9.2.   Differences Between Right and Left Hemispheres

Left Hemisphere	Right Hemisphere
Normal	
Dominant for language	Dominant for visuospatial tasks and face recognition
Analyzer, breaks down into details	Synthesizer, looks at the whole
Organizes data in conceptual similarities	Organizes data in structural similarities
Reason and attention to detail	Intuition and imagination
Verbal memory	Figural memory
Following Damage	
Aphasia	Aprosodia
Catastrophic reaction	Indifference reaction
Difficulty processing information in auditory modality; profits more from nonlanguage-related cues, pantomine, gestural demonstration, and use of visual images	Difficulty processing information in visual modality; profits more from language-related cues and verbal elaboration

EVALUATION OF PERCEPTION

Evaluation of **perception** must begin with assessment of visual foundation skills so that their influence on performance can be ruled out (Gianutsos & Matheson, 1987; Warren, 1990, 1993b). Visual foundation skills consist of visual acuity, visual fields, and oculomotor functions.

Following the completion of the evaluation of foundation skills, the therapist puts together a comprehensive perceptual evaluation with various subtests for specific deficits, which form the test battery for a specific patient. The emphasis of the evaluation will depend on such things as premorbid status, cognitive-perceptual dysfunction, discharge environment, and location or nature of the brain damage (Abreu & Toglia, 1987). The occupational therapist may do an initial screening of the various cognitive and perceptual deficits with the patient and then, depending on the patient's lifestyle and goals, might pursue a specific area in more depth.

For example, if the patient has had a stroke, is 35 years old, and works as a mechanic, the therapist might evaluate his constructional abilities in more depth, whereas if the patient is 75 years old, retired, and spends his time reading and watching television, in depth evaluation of constructional abilities may not be indicated. This idea is carried over into treatment as well. The 35-year-old mechanic will need a higher level of constructional skills than would the 75-year-old retiree. In addition, the therapist may find that the patient performs adequately on a test, but exhibits

difficulty in a functional situation. This indicates the need for further evaluation.

The *Motor-Free Visual Perception Test* (MVPT) evaluates visual perception as a whole. The MVPT was originally designed for children and measures **spatial relations,** visual discrimination, figure/ground perception, visual closure, and visual **memory.** It has been adapted for use with brain-damaged adults and standardized on a normal adult population (Bouska & Kwatny, 1983). The test was adapted by adding a time factor and interpretational guidelines designed to determine lack of compensation for visual field deficits and/or **unilateral neglect.** The score on this test gives an overall measure of visual perception and is not meant to be differentiated into the various areas tested. The adult test manual describes the specific administration instructions (Bouska & Kwatny, 1983).

Visual Foundation Skills

VISUAL ACUITY

Visual acuity should be examined in each eye for both near (16 inches or less) and far (20 feet or more) vision. Near acuity is important for any tabletop activity, and far vision is especially important for driving. Visual acuity is most often screened using conventional letter charts. Test cards are available that use symbols rather than letters for use with aphasic, non-English–speaking, and severely impaired patients. Conventional letter charts measure acuity by determining the smallest high-contrast detail a person can perceive at a given distance. Most functional settings do not provide such contrast, which may explain the patient who does well on the traditional eye chart but still complains of something wrong with his vision.

Evaluation of contrast sensitivity is now being advocated as a more functional evaluation of acuity (Gianutsos & Matheson, 1987; Warren, 1993a). A series of sinewave gratings is presented, which vary in orientation, contrast, and frequency. The patient must indicate the orientation of the grating: the poorer the acuity, the more contrast required to detect the orientation of the grating. The advantage of this test is that it provides a more comprehensive picture of the patient's visual capacity in the everyday environment (Warren, 1993a).

Evaluation of depth **perception** is important for mobility and driving (Gianutsos & Matheson, 1987). The patient who has difficulty moving through a crowded area and setting up his wheelchair for transfers may have difficulty with depth perception rather than position in space or **spatial relations.** Depth perception is generally evaluated with the therapist sitting in front of the patient, who holds up a shield at about eye level. The therapist holds up 2 identical pencils (or pens or wands) and moves them so that one or the other is closer to the patient. The patient is then asked to indicate which is closer to him. A more standardized test is part of the *DTE Porto Clinic* (Driver Testing Equipment, Inc., Scranton, PA), which is used as part of a driving evaluation. This test requires that the patient align two sticks by manipulating two strings. The patient is given three trials and allowed a total of 3 inches error.

VISUAL FIELD

Identification of visual field deficits has traditionally been determined by use of a confrontation test (Gianutsos & Matheson, 1987; Warren, 1993b). The therapist sits in front of the patient. The patient is told to fixate on the examiner's nose and asked to indicate when he detects a visual stimulus in the periphery (presented variously in the four visual quadrants). Trobe et al. (1981) found that kinetic and static finger confrontation techniques overlooked at least 50% of the hemianioptic deficits in a group of patients. They concluded that this form of testing is insensitive and only helpful with detecting gross deficits.

A more accurate method of evaluating visual fields is use of automated perimetry (Gianutsos & Matheson, 1987; Warren, 1993b). Perimetry provides an accurate description and printout of the patient's visual field deficit. Figure 9.1 shows the results of a patient with obvious visual field deficits. The results of the test

are effectively used to educate the family and patient regarding visual field losses. There are several limitations. First, the test can require up to 20 min of sustained concentration if there are significant deficits. Therefore, patients unable to maintain that level of concentration cannot be accurately tested. Second, the test requires a motor response to push a button within 1 to 3 sec of the presentation, which could exclude evaluation of patients with significantly delayed motor responses or motor planning deficits. Last, the equipment is quite expensive. The patient is generally referred to an optometrist or ophthalmologist for perimetry testing. If the automated perimetry results are not available, the therapist can use the confrontation test along with close observation of the patient during daily activities.

OCULOMOTOR FUNCTION

Control of eye movements depends on a complex interaction at cortical and subcortical levels. The role of the occupational therapist in screening oculomotor function is "not to diagnose the deficit, but to describe its functional effect and formulate the critical questions for the ophthalmologist or optometrist" (Warren, 1993b, p. 58). A screening of oculomotor function includes alignment, range of motion, convergence, saccades, and pursuits (Bouska, 1990).

Alignment is generally measured by observation of the corneal light reflex in the eyes (Bouska, 1990;

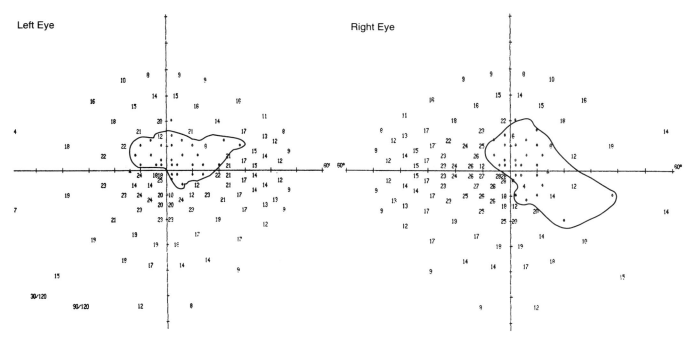

Figure 9.1. Automated perimetry results of a patient with RBD. The patient is able to see in the circled areas. She has no vision in the left inferior visual field of either eye, minimal vision in the left superior field, and even the right fields are moderately impaired.

Warren, 1993b). The therapist is seated in front of the patient and holds a penlight approximately 12 inches in front of the patient's eyes. The patient is asked to fixate on the light, and the therapist observes the reflection on the cornea of both eyes. The reflection should be in the same position in both eyes. This allows the therapist to determine if the patient is using both eyes when viewing a target, or if one eye is deviated.

Range of motion allows evaluation of the six extraocular muscles of each eye. To test this, the therapist holds up a target that is moved slowly to the extremes of gaze in a large H pattern (Bouska, 1990). The patient is tested with both eyes and with each eye separately. Double vision may be present at the extremes of gaze and should be noted.

Convergence is the closest point at which a person can fixate on a target with both eyes. Difficulty with convergence can impact a patient's ability to achieve and sustain focus on near-vision tasks. Convergence is tested by having the patient follow a target that is moved slowly toward his nose. Convergence is usually normal up to 6 to 8 inches from the nose, at which point one eye continues to follow the target and the other eye drifts outward (Bouska, 1990). Inattention and fatigue may impair convergence.

Saccades are rapid changes of fixation from one point to another in the visual field (Bouska, 1990). These are tested by holding up two targets and asking the patient to repeatedly look from one target to the other. The targets are gradually moved into all quadrants of the visual field. Note is made if the patient overshoots or undershoots the target or if he must search for the target. The patient suspected on confrontation to have a field cut, may have to search and indeed not find the target located in the suspected visual field.

Visual pursuits, often referred to as visual tracking, are those eye movements that maintain continued fixation of a moving target so as to keep it continuously on the fovea (Bouska, 1990). The therapist asks the patient to fixate on a moving target and observes if the patient is able to sustain fixation or loses it (and notes where he loses it). This test may also be influenced by fatigue and decreased **attention.**

Informal observation of the patient during functional tasks are used to augment formal evaluation. The therapist may note that the patient shuts one eye or squints during certain activities; the patient turns his head or laterally flexes his neck to one side; there is an increase in tone in the jaw, neck, shoulders; the patient complains of headaches or fatigue; and/or the patient suddenly seems agitated or is uncooperative (Warren, 1993b). Because these behaviors can be attributed to emotional or cognitive deficits, it is im-

portant for the therapist to know that oculomotor dysfunction can also elicit these responses.

Body Scheme

Body scheme is the awareness of body parts and position of the body and its parts in relation to themselves and objects in the environment. Related deficits include right/left disorientation, impaired body part identification, finger agnosia, and anosognosia. Disorders of body scheme, as measured by body part identification and right/left discrimination, are more frequently observed in patients with left brain damage (LBD) (Benton, 1985; Boone & Landes, 1968; Sauguet, Benton, & Hecaen, 1971). However, failure can be the result of several problems, including verbal, sensory, conceptual, and visuospatial deficits.

Therefore, patients may exhibit deficits in body scheme under one test condition but not under a different condition (Benton, 1985). For example, a patient with right brain damage (RBD) may have no difficulty indicating right and left or a body part on himself, but he may be unable to indicate right and left on a confronting person or to imitate right and left movements because of a visuospatial problem.

MacDonald (1960) described a test of body scheme that includes finger agnosia, right/left discrimination, body part identification, and body revisualization. Scores on this test by neurologically and nonneurologically impaired adults were significantly different at the .001 level of probability.

RIGHT/LEFT DISCRIMINATION

Right/left (R/L) discrimination denotes an ability to understand the concepts of right and left. R/L disorientation to one's own body is uncommon in nonaphasic patients (Benton et al., 1983; Sauguet et al., 1971). However, RBD patients exhibit difficulty identifying body parts of a confronting person. Nonaphasic LBD patients tend to perform adequately on R/L tasks. It appears that poor R/L discrimination in aphasic LBD patients is the result of a language problem (Boone & Landes, 1968), whereas the deficit seen in RBD patients is most likely due to visuospatial deficits (Benton, 1985). Nonaphasic patients with general mental impairment also exhibit deficits in this area, most probably because of a conceptual problem (Benton, 1985).

Tests of R/L discrimination usually include the patient's orientation to his own body (e.g., "Touch your left ear"), orientation to a confronting person (e.g.. "Touch my left hand"), or a combination of both. The complexity is increased by requiring double uncrossed tasks (e.g., "Touch your right knee with your right hand") or double crossed tasks (e.g., "Touch your right knee with your left elbow").

Benton et al. (1983) presented a standardized 20-

Table 9.3. Right/Left Orientation Test

1. Show me your *left* hand.
2. Show me your *right* eye.
3. Show me your *left* ear.
4. Show me your *right* hand.

5. Touch your *left* ear with your *left* hand.
6. Touch your *right* eye with your *left* hand.
7. Touch your *right* knee with your *right* hand.
8. Touch your *left* eye with your *left* hand.
9. Touch your *right* ear with your *left* hand.
10. Touch your *left* knee with your *right* hand.
11. Touch your *right* ear with your *right* hand.
12. Touch your *left* eye with your *right* hand.

13. Point to my *right* eye.
14. Point to my *left* leg.
15. Point to my *left* ear.
16. Point to my *right* hand.

17. Put your *right* hand on my *left* ear.
18. Put your *left* hand on my *left* eye.
19. Put your *left* hand on my *right* shoulder.
20. Put your *right* hand on my *right* eye.

item test that requires the patient to point to lateralized body parts on command. The test takes about 5 min to administer (Table 9.3). A total score of less than 17 is considered defective. Performance patterns can be classified as follows:

"Normal": score of 17–20, no more than one error on the first 12 "own body" items;

"Generalized defect": score of < 17, more than one error on the first 12 items;

"Confronting person defect": score of < 17, no more than one error on the first 12 items;

"Specific own body deficit": more than one error on the first 12 items and no more than two errors on the remaining items;

"Systematic reversal": score of 17–20 when performance is scored with rights and lefts reversed and no more than one error on the first 12 items.

BODY PART IDENTIFICATION

The ability to identify body parts on self and others is referred to as body part identification. Boone and Landes (1968) found that RBD patients perform better than LBD patients in pointing to body parts. When analyzing the errors made by both RBD and LBD patients, they found that the majority of problems were on items for which the dimensions of right and left were added. They concluded that although occasional hemiplegic patients have difficulty recognizing body parts the more prevalent disorder is a deficit in R/L discrimination.

Evaluation consists of the same items as used for R/L discrimination. Testing should include requests to

identify body parts both separately and in combination with R/L tasks; a patient with a deficit in body part identification would have difficulty on all phases of the test, whereas a patient with only R/L discrimination deficits will score well on the "pure" body part identification tasks (Boone & Landes, 1968).

FINGER AGNOSIA

Finger agnosia denotes an inability to identify one's own fingers, difficulty naming fingers, or being unable to indicate which finger was touched. This deficit is not usually seen as a single entity but in combination with either an aphasic disorder or mental impairment (Benton, 1985).

Evaluation generally consists of requiring the patient to name fingers that have been touched, to identify a finger named by the examiner, and/or to imitate the finger movements of the examiner (MacDonald, 1960; Sauguet et al., 1971). Goodglass and Kaplan (1972) described a test of finger agnosia that includes naming, finger-name comprehension, visual-visual matching, and visual-tactile matching. Further description of the test was provided (Goodglass & Kaplan, 1972).

ANOSOGNOSIA

Anosognosia refers to an unawareness of hemiplegia. The extent of this awareness of self can vary greatly among patients and can range from an unawareness of hemiparesis to lack of concern to total denial. It is most often seen in RBD patients (Critchley, 1966; Denes et al., 1982). It is usually seen immediately after an acute lesion, persisting for a few days, then ameliorating to milder forms of denial. Initially, the patient may deny that the hemiplegic limbs belong to him and insist that nothing is wrong; later, he may admit that they are his limbs, but still refer to them in the third person. Mark, Kooistra, and Heilman (1988) suggested the failure of a patient with neglect to correct spontaneously the hemispatial perseveration and motor impersistence seen with RBD may be a feature of this process of unawareness.

There are no formal tests for anosognosia. Observation should be made of how the patient positions the hemiplegic limbs, the manner in which the patient refers to his limbs (i.e., does he refer to them in the third person or indicate that they belong to someone else), and whether he spontaneously recognizes the loss of function of one side (Heilman, Watson, & Valenstein, 1985).

Unilateral Neglect

Unilateral neglect is referred to by a variety of names including hemiinattention, hemispatial neglect, and unilateral spatial agnosia. It is manifested by a failure to respond or orient to stimuli presented contralateral to a brain lesion (Heilman et al., 1985). It is observed functionally in the patient who eats the food only on half of his plate, shaves only one side of his face, and so on. It is most commonly caused by a lesion in the right hemisphere; it does occur following LBD, although the deficit is usually not as severe as it is for RBD (Denes et al., 1982; Gainotti, Messerli, & Tissot, 1972; Plourde & Sperry, 1984; Stone, Halligan, & Greenwood, 1993; Weintraub & Mesulam, 1988).

It was found that when given a task, both LBD and RBD patients were apt to scan only homolateral space and fail to attend to the whole task. However, if the task demanded active exploration, LBD patients were more able to complete the task, while the RBD patient continued to scan only homolateral space (Colombo, DeRenzi, & Faglioni, 1976). Furthermore, they found that if the patient's **attention** was directed to the fact that the task was not completed, LBD patients were able to find the errors, but the neglect persisted in the RBD patients. Functionally, tasks such as reading or eating from a tray require active exploration and would prove more difficult for the RBD patient with **unilateral neglect.**

Initially, it was believed that **unilateral neglect** was caused by defective sensory input superimposed on altered mental function (Battersby et al., 1956) or deficits in body scheme (Brain, 1941). More recently **unilateral neglect** has been attributed to a deficit in arousal and **attention** (Caplan, 1985; Heilman & Van Den Abell, 1980; Mesulam, 1981; Riddoch & Humphreys, 1983). In a study of normal individuals, it was found that the right hemisphere attends to stimuli presented on either the right or left sides, whereas the left hemisphere responds mainly to stimuli presented on the right (Heilman & Van Den Abell, 1980). It was proposed that after RBD, neglect is more severe because the left hemisphere is unable to attend to ipsilateral stimuli; after LBD the right hemisphere is able to process stimuli presented ipsilaterally to some degree. One would, therefore, expect some neglect for ipsilateral hemispace in RBD patients with neglect. In support of this hypothesis, Weintraub and Mesulam (1987) found ipsilateral neglect as well as contralateral neglect in RBD patients. Those LBD patients with neglect exhibited no ipsilateral neglect on a shape cancellation task.

It has been suggested that there exists two types of neglect: motor (or output) neglect and perceptual (or input) neglect (Bisiach et al., 1990; Coslett et al., 1990; Tegner & Levander, 1991). Motor neglect, also called directional hypokinesia, presents as impaired initiation or execution of movement into contralateral hemispace by either limb (Bisiach et al., 1990; Tegner & Levander, 1991). Perceptual neglect is similar to the attentional (Heilman et al., 1985) and representational

hypotheses (Bisiach et al., 1981). These hypotheses suggest inability to attend to stimuli in contralateral space or contralateral side of an internal representation. Neglect associated with directional hypokinesia is seen more frequently in frontal lesions, and the perceptual, attentional neglect is seen more in parietal lesions (Bisiach et al., 1990).

It has also been shown that a patient may exhibit neglect for near but not far space (Halligan & Marshall, 1991; Mennemeier, Wertman, & Heilman, 1992). On a line bisection test presented vertically rather than horizontally, the patient would bisect the line above the actual midpoint. This may be seen functionally in the patient who exhibits severe neglect at tabletop activities but is able to play darts quite well. Patients usually exhibit difficulty in both areas, but there are patients who do well at tabletop activities and then will walk into objects on their left side as well as patients who do poorly at the table but function quite well in their daily activities.

Unilateral neglect tends to be most pronounced immediately following brain damage, but may continue for a long time. Recovery tends to be slow and often incomplete (Heilman et al., 1985). **Unilateral neglect** is generally either mild or severe. In mild cases, the neglect might not be apparent during functional tasks but might be elicited in testing situations (Weinberg et al., 1977). The patient might be able to respond to unilateral stimuli, but he could exhibit difficulty with bilateral simultaneous stimulation (Heilman et al., 1985) or on tasks in which cognitive demands are more extensive (Weinberg et al., 1982). Severe neglect has been associated with functional deficits in self-care, reading, and writing (Lorenze & Cancro, 1962; Sea et al., 1993; Weinberg et al., 1977). In this case the patient presents the classic case of being able to read only one-half of the page and being unaware of, or unable to compensate for, this deficit.

Unilateral neglect is frequently seen in combination with visual field deficits, but either condition can occur independently of the other (Albert, 1973). In fact, if the neglect is severe, it may not be possible to determine accurately if there is in fact a field cut. The question remains about whether the deficit is the result of a field cut or whether the patient is just neglecting that side.

Walker et al. (1991) found that by varying the procedure for perimetry testing (the fixation point was extinguished before presentation of the target) a patient's hemianopsia was markedly reduced. They believed that the patient's reported hemianopsia was the result of neglect secondary to an inability to disengage from the fixation target to scan left.

Several studies have found that there is residual information processing in the neglected visual field

(Karnath & Hartje, 1987; Marshall & Halligan, 1988). In one study, a patient was presented with two pictures (oriented vertically): a house and a house with red flames coming out of the left side (Marshall & Halligan, 1988). She was repeatedly asked if they were the same or different and then asked in which house she would rather live. Although she said the houses were the same, she reliably chose the house that was not burning. This may be another explanation for those patients who do poorly at tabletop activities but are able to navigate through doors and around obstacles without bumping into things on the contralesional side.

Evaluating neglect can be confusing, because the patient can exhibit neglect in one situation but not in another. "Dissociations may occur between one modality and another (visual, auditory, or tactile) or between one space and another (personal, peripersonal, or extrapersonal), as well as between motor neglect and perceptual neglect" (Halligan & Marshall, 1992, p. 525).

Unilateral neglect is evaluated in a variety of ways, including drawing tasks, cancellation tasks, crossing-out tasks, and line bisection. In all such tasks the therapist looks for omissions and errors concentrated to one side.

Drawing or copying tasks could include drawing a person, clock, or flower. Observations are made of how the patient approaches the task; if his performance while copying differs from free drawing; and if one side of the drawing is missing, misformed, or complete but less sure. Figure 9.2 shows four drawings made over time by a patient who suffered a right CVA. The drawings show elements of left neglect and constructional apraxia. Picture D, which was drawn just before discharge, is fairly complete, but the lines on the left are very tentative compared with the rest of the picture.

Schenkenberg, Bradford, and Ajax (1980) designed a line bisection test that consists of 20 lines. Of these, 18 lines are organized so that 6 are primarily on the left side of the page, 6 on the right, and 6 in the middle (the top and bottom lines are used for instructions to the patient and are deleted from the score). The lines are of varying lengths and the patient is told to cut each line in half by placing a pencil mark through the center. The difference between the true center and the patient's mark is measured in millimeters. Van Deusen (1983) presented normative data based on 93 adults using this line bisection test and suggested that a standard deviation (SD) of ±1 be considered "slight neglect"; ±2 SD, "moderate neglect"; and ±3 SD, "severe neglect."

Another method of evaluation frequently used is cancellation tasks. These tests are easy to administer and score and are sensitive to milder forms of neglect (Sea et al., 1993; Stam & Bakker, 1990). Cancellation tests usually consist of a sheet of paper with several lines of typed letters or shapes. The patient is asked to mark a specific stimulus—letter or shape—that is scattered randomly throughout a structured or random array (Weintraub & Mesulam, 1988). Scoring is determined by the number of omissions (targets that are not marked), number of commissions (cancellation of items other than the target), and time (Diller et al., 1980). In addition, note is taken on what area of the page these errors are made. The greater the number of errors, the greater the visual scanning deficit. Errors on one side of the page are generally indicative of **unilateral neglect;** random errors throughout are generally the result of an **attention** problem. The patient with neglect may complete this task very rapidly because he attends to only a portion of the page and makes no attempt to compensate, or if he is aware that he has a deficit, he may take a long time because in his attempt to compensate he keeps going over the same lines gradually finding more letters on the left side (although usually not all of them).

Freidman (1992) administered the Star Cancellation subtest of the *Rivermead Behavioral Inattention Test* to 41 post-CVA patients. He used a cutoff score of less than 44/54 to indicate neglect. He also calculated a star ratio (the number of stars canceled in the left columns divided by the total number of stars canceled), which provided a measure of lateralization of neglect. It was found to be a predictor of functional outcome as measured by the Barthel ADL score at discharge.

Albert (1973) presented a test in which 40 lines were drawn in an apparently random manner on a sheet of paper, but actually the lines were drawn in six rows of six lines and one row of four lines. The examiner draws over each of the 40 lines, in a random manner, with a red pencil. The patient is asked to cross out all the lines on the page. This test was standardized on a group of normal individuals, who made no errors. Mark, Kooistra, and Heilman (1988) presented Albert's test in a novel way. In addition to having the patients draw over the 40 lines, in another condition, the patients erased the lines. They found that performance improved in the erase condition, which they believed suggested that neglect is influenced by the presence of stimuli in the ipsilateral hemispace.

Wilson, Cockburn, and Halligan (1987) developed the *Rivermead Behavioral Inattention Test* (BIT) in an attempt to assess neglect in a sample of everyday activities. Functional subtests include eating a meal (simulation), dialing a telephone, reading a menu, telling the time (both digital and analogue), setting the time, sorting coins, copying an address, and following a map. It was found to be a valid and reliable test of visuospatial neglect.

Stone, Wilson, et al. (1991) shortened the BIT and modified it for use with acute stroke patients.

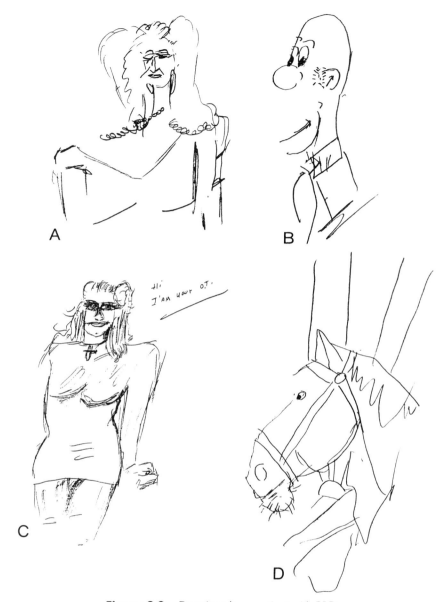

Figure 9.2. Drawings by a patient with RBD.

They validated their results against an occupational therapist's assessment of neglect behaviors during self-care. This battery of tests was also given to age-matched controls and parameters were developed to differentiate between normal and abnormal responses in the elderly (Stone, Halligan, et al., 1991). This group of researchers further developed the *Visual Neglect Recovery Index* (VNRI) based on this same battery of tests (Stone et al., 1992). The VNRI at 2 to 3 days post-onset was found to be a predictor of the degree of recovery of visual neglect.

Spatial Relations and Position in Space

A patient with a deficit in position in space has difficulty with concepts such as *over, front, back, below,* etc., whereas a patient with a deficit in **spatial relations** has difficulty perceiving himself in relation to other objects or objects in relation to himself. These two deficits are sometimes referred to as visual spatial agnosia (Brain, 1941). Functionally, a patient with a deficit in these areas might run into objects because of difficulty judging distance; may exhibit topographical disorientation, becoming easily lost; or may exhibit dressing apraxia.

The Space Visualization Test, a subtest of the *Sensory Integration and Praxis Test* (Ayres, 1987) and the Spatial Relations and Position in Space subtests of Frostig's (1966) *Developmental Test of Visual Perception* are sometimes used for evaluation. These tests are standardized for children only. Other methods of evaluation include the Bender (1946) *Visual Motor Gestalt Test*, the *Cross Test*, and *Positioning Blocks* (Zoltan, Siev, & Freishtat, 1986). The *Visual Motor Gestalt Test* consists of nine patterns, which the patient is asked to copy. Scoring depends not only on the form of the reproduced figures but on their relationship to each other. For *Positioning Blocks*, the patient is asked to describe the positions of two blocks in relation to each other (e.g., in front of, behind, on top of, etc.).

TOPOGRAPHICAL ORIENTATION

The patient with a deficit in topographical orientation exhibits difficulty finding his way from one place to another. This difficulty in route finding may have a variety of causes and is usually associated with other visual and spatial problems (Brain, 1941; McFie, Piercy, & Zangwill, 1950; Patterson & Zangwill, 1944). Left neglect of external space may be present so that the patient shows a preference for turns in one direction over another.

Topographical **memory** is the ability to visualize familiar scenes and describe familiar routes. This loss is usually independent of other forms of visual disorientation and loss of **memory** for objects (Brain, 1941).

Topographical orientation is not generally evaluated on a formal basis. Reports from staff and/or the patient himself may indicate that the patient is having difficulty finding his way to therapy or around the hospital. There are no specific tests for this deficit, although some researchers base their diagnosis on the patient's ability to draw a map of familiar places or his ability to describe familiar routes as well as on how the patient performs functionally (Brain, 1941; Patterson & Zangwill, 1944). If the patient does not exhibit topographical disorientation functionally, difficulty with map drawing may be caused by other problems such as constructional apraxia or deficits in **spatial relations**. Problems with **memory** or mental confusion must be ruled out to arrive at a diagnosis of topographical disorientation (Zoltan et al., 1986).

FIGURE/GROUND PERCEPTION

Figure/ground perception is the ability to distinguish the foreground or figure from the background. A deficit in this area can be seen functionally in the patient who is unable to find a white shirt on the bed, the brakes on his wheelchair, or eyeglasses in a cluttered drawer.

Deficits in figure/ground perception have been seen following lesions to any area of the brain. Aphasic LBD patients perform significantly worse on tests of figure/ground perception than RBD patients, and RBD patients perform significantly more poorly than non-

aphasic LBD patients (Russo & Visnolo, 1967; Teuber & Weinstein, 1956).

Evaluations most frequently used are the Figure-Ground Perception Test, a subtest of the *Sensory Integration and Praxis Test* (Ayres, 1987) and the Figure Ground Test, a subtest of the *Developmental Test of Visual Perception* (Frostig, 1966), both of which were developed for use with children. One study reported by Zoltan et al. (1986) found that the Frostig Figure Ground Test did not correlate with other figure/ground tests, although it did correlate with a constructional apraxia test. Thus it was indicated that this test may not be an appropriate test for figure/ground abilities of adult brain-damaged patients. Further research is needed.

The Figure-Ground Perception Test presents the patient with a design consisting of three overlapping objects or geometric shapes. The patient is asked to choose the correct figures from six choices, and the test is discontinued after the fifth error. This test is easy to administer, and the patient's response can be either motor (pointing) or verbal (by name of object or number of the answer). Petersen and Wikoff (1983) administered this test to 100 normal adult males aged 19 to 57. They changed the method of scoring such that points were given for each correctly identified figure through the design in which the fifth error is made (all correct responses for the design are scored, rather than immediately stopping after the subject made the fifth error). The scores they obtained had a range of 15 to 48, a mean of 29.72, and standard deviation of 8.83. They also found that the scores were not related to age, education, or socioeconomic status. Their scoring procedure should be followed when using their mean and standard deviation as norms.

Apraxia

Apraxia is the inability to carry out purposeful movement in the presence of intact sensation, movement, and coordination (DeRenzi, 1985; Goodglass & Kaplan, 1972; Poeck, 1985). **Apraxia** is generally seen in patients with LBD (Goodglass & Kaplan, 1972; Haaland, Harrington, & Yeo, 1987; Kimura & Archibald, 1974; Poeck, 1985). There are five types of **apraxia**: verbal, buccofacial, limb, constructional, and dressing. The first two are usually evaluated by a speech and language pathologist.

LIMB APRAXIA

There are two types of limb apraxia: ideomotor and ideational (Table 9.4). These are brought about by disruption of higher level motor processes, specifically in impaired selection of elements that make up a movement and impaired sequencing (Poeck, 1985). In

Table 9.4. Types of Limb Apraxia

Ideational	Ideomotor
Conceptual problem	Problem with selection, sequencing, and spatial organization of gestures
Disruption of plan	Disconnection of idea and motor plan; therefore, breakdown in motor output
Deficit in object use	Deficit in imitation, improved performance with object use
Motor output good	Clumsy
Unable to recognize correct gesture	Able to recognize correct gesture
Difficulty performing to command	Difficulty performing to command

patients who have use of both arms, the impairment can be demonstrated to be bilateral (Goodglass & Kaplan, 1972; Kimura & Archibald, 1974).

Ideomotor apraxia is generally exhibited only under testing situations, as the patient is able to carry out an activity spontaneously but fails on verbal command. For example, the patient is able to brush his teeth in the morning, but when asked, "Show me how you brush your teeth," he is unable to perform the movement adequately. The movement will be awkward but still bear a resemblance to the intended movement (DeRenzi, 1985). Heilman (1975) found that patients with ideomotor apraxia, although able to use objects, are clumsy.

Ideational apraxia is seen as difficulty with sequencing motor acts and is thought to be a disturbance in the conceptual organization of movements. This is a more serious deficit and is apparent during functional activities. For example, the patient may experience difficulty with eating, not knowing how or which utensil to use. Performance of a task may be more skillful than that of a patient with ideomotor apraxia, but it may be conceptually wrong (DeRenzi, 1985).

Although **apraxia** usually affects all modalities, there may be a disruption of gestures in one modality (visual, verbal, tactile) but not another (DeRenzi, Faglione, & Sorgato, 1982). Testing is usually done initially by verbal command. Since **apraxia** is often associated with aphasia, requests for movements presented in the visual modality might be appropriate with severe aphasics. Visual presentation can take the form of providing a model for the patient to imitate or placing the object out of reach and asking the patient to pantomime its use. Testing is carried out in the tactile modality by having the patient handle the object while blindfolded and then having him show how to use it.

Assessment has consisted of asking the patient to perform a task on command (e.g., "Show me how you comb your hair"), to imitation, and with object use.

These assessments require various types of gestures, including transitive gestures that involve object use (e.g., "Show me how a man shaves"), intransitive gestures that are meant to express ideas or feelings (e.g., "Show me how you wave good-bye"), meaningless or nonsymbolic gestures (e.g., "Put your hand under your chin"), proximal gestures (e.g., "Show me how you bounce a ball"), and distal gestures (e.g., "Show me how you would use a telegraph key"). Transitive gestures are especially sensitive to **apraxia** (Haaland, 1993). Generally patients with **apraxia** would have least difficulty with proximal, intransitive gestures away from the body (e.g., waving good-bye) and most difficulty with distal, transitive gestures on the body (e.g., putting on makeup) (Haaland, 1993; Helm-Estabrooks & Albert, 1991).

While there are no standardized evaluations for **apraxia,** there are several test batteries with subjective scoring. These tests usually consist of asking the patient to perform various gestures, and scoring is based

Table 9.5. Common Errors on Apraxia Testing

Error Type	Example
Body part as object (BPO-1)	When asked, "Show me how you brush your teeth," patient uses finger as the brush rather than pretending to hold the brush. Normal in 5- to 8-year-olds, not a mature response
Body part as object (BPO-2)	The hand position is correct but touches the target or extent of object is not taken into account; when asked to demonstrate tooth brushing, patient pretends to hold brush but rubs hand along his face. Normal in 8- to 12-year-olds, not a mature response
Orientation	Refers to position of the hand relative to the target; when asked to salute, patient positions his hand over his eye, possibly with palm forward
Hand/arm position	Refers to position of hand relative to the arm. When asked to salute, does patient have his elbow in the correct position?
Clumsiness	Are movements smooth and fluid or does the patient make awkward movements?
Perseveration	As evaluation progresses, does the patient give a response to previous command; is he still pretending to salute, when you are now asking him to show you how he combs his hair?
Target	The patient makes the correct movement, but to the wrong place
Delay/slowness	Is the patient's response timely, or does he take a while to do the motion required?

Table 9.6. Test of Apraxia

Movements to Oral Command	Movements to Imitation	Movements to Real Object
Bucco-facial		
1. Cough	If failed to command	Does not apply
2. Sniff	If failed to command	If failed to command
3. Blow out a match	If failed to command	If failed to command
4. Suck through a straw	If failed to command	If failed to command
5. Puff out cheeks	If failed to command	Does not apply
Intransitive Limb		
1. Wave good-bye	If failed to command	Does not apply
2. Beckon "come here"	If failed to command	Does not apply
3. Finger on lip for "shh"	If failed to command	Does not apply
4. Salute	If failed to command	Does not apply
5. Signal "stop"	If failed to command	Does not apply
Transitive Limb		
1. Brush teeth	If failed to command	If failed to command
2. Shave your face	If failed to command	If failed to command
3. Hammer	If failed to command	If failed to command
4. Saw board	If failed to command	If failed to command
5. Use screwdriver	If failed to command	If failed to command
Whole Body		
1. How does a boxer stand?	If failed to command	Does not apply
2. How does a golfer stand?	If failed to command	Does not apply
3. How does a soldier march in place?	If failed to command	Does not apply
4. How do you shovel snow?	If failed to command	Does not apply
5. Stand up, turn around twice and sit down	If failed to command	Does not apply

Serial Actions (with real objects only)
1. Provide paper, envelope, and stamp: "Put the paper in the envelope, seal it, and stamp it"
2. Provide candle, candlestick, and matches: "Put the candle in the holder, light it, and blow it out."

on the quality of the response. Common errors to look for are listed in Table 9.5.

Goodglass and Kaplan (1972) described a test of **apraxia** in which the patient is asked to perform common movements (Table 9.6). In this test, the patient is first asked to perform the movement on command (e.g., "Show me how you use a screwdriver"). If

unable to do this, he is asked to imitate the examiner. If unable to do this, he is then given a screwdriver. Apraxic patients frequently use body part as object when asked to perform a movement. For example, when asked, "Show me how you brush your teeth," the patient may use his index finger as the brush. If this occurs, the patient is asked to try again as if holding the object. Use of body part as object is rare in normal adults. There are no norms for this evaluation. Scoring is subjective:

"Normal": patient performed most tasks correctly on verbal request;
"Impaired": patient performed most tasks correctly only when given the actual object;
"Severely impaired": patient was unable to perform the tasks even when given the actual object (Zoltan et al., 1986).

Constructional Apraxia

Constructional apraxia "denotes an impairment in combinatory or organizing activity in which details must be clearly perceived and in which the relationships among the component parts of the entity must be apprehended if the desired synthesis of them is to be achieved" (Benton, 1967, p. 1). This deficit emerges in tasks for which individual parts must be arranged in a given spatial relationship to form a unitary structure (DeRenzi, 1982). Patients with constructional apraxia have difficulty with copying, drawing, and constructing designs in two and three dimensions. It can be seen functionally as difficulty with such activities as setting a table, making a sandwich, and making a dress and with any mechanical activity in which parts are to be combined into a whole. Constructional apraxia has been found to correlate with deficits of activities of daily living (Baum & Hall, 1981; Lorenze & Cancro, 1962; Neistadt, 1993; Warren, 1981). It is one of the causes of dressing apraxia.

Constructional apraxia can be found in both RBD and LBD patients. It has often been found to be more frequent and more severe in RBD patients (Arrigoni & DeRenzi, 1964; Benton & Fogel, 1962; Piercy, Hecaen, & Ajuriaguerra, 1960; Warrington, James, & Kinsbourne, 1966). There is some question about whether this finding may have been the result of a bias introduced by exclusion of more involved LBD patients from studies because of aphasia and their subsequent failure on intelligence tests. Other researchers, when attempting to control for these factors, have found no difference in the incidence of constructional apraxia between RBD and LBD patients (Arena & Gainotti, 1978; DeRenzi & Faglioni, 1967).

In general, drawings made by RBD patients tend to be relatively complex, show disorganized spatial

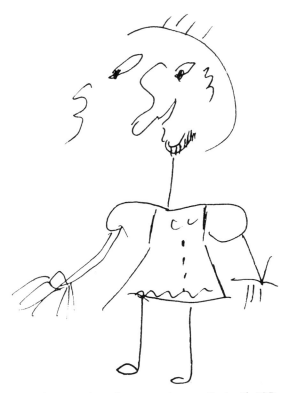

Figure 9.3. Drawing of a person by a patient with RBD.

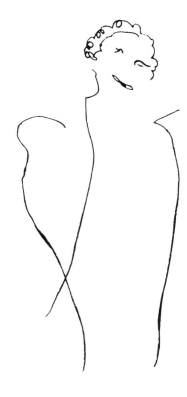

Figure 9.4. Drawing of a person by a patient with LBD.

relationships, and decreased orientation in space (Fig. 9.3). Drawings of LBD patients tend to be oversimplified and have few details (Fig. 9.4) (Gainotti & Tiacci, 1970; Piercy et al., 1960; Warrington et al., 1966). Because of these qualitative differences noted in the performance of RBD and LBD patients, some researchers feel that the basis underlying constructional apraxia differs according to the side of the lesion (Benton, 1967; Piercy et al., 1960). Constructional apraxia in RBD is believed to be the result of visuospatial deficits, while that in LBD is thought to be caused by an executive or conceptual disorder.

Benton (1967) suggested two types of constructional activities (graphic and assembly tasks) and noted that both types should be included in an evaluation of constructional apraxia. The most common example of a graphic task is copying. Copying activities include copying geometric shapes (from simple to complex) and drawing without a model (e.g., house, clock, flower).

Assembly tasks include such activities as stick arrangement and three-dimensional block designs. Common errors on stick arrangement include selecting sticks of incorrect length, failing to reproduce parts of the model (especially lateral), making lines more oblique than the model indicates, tending to remove part of the model to make the copy, and "crowding in" (the patient's copy rests on top of or touches the model) (Critchley, 1966). Assembly tasks can be varied in

numerous ways to test more subtle deficiencies by changing these aspects: copying from a model (representational or actual) may be easier than constructing from **memory** and providing the patient with the correct number and type of blocks and sticks structures the task and makes it simpler than requiring the patient to choose the correct pieces from a large number of blocks and sticks.

In general, these tasks are not standardized and rely on subjective judgment of the results. It is important to note the patient's method of completing the task; the patient's comments; any emotional display, hesitancy, indecision, and change of mind; and the type of errors made.

Benton et al. (1983) presented a standardized three-dimensional block construction task. There are two forms to allow for retesting and comparison of the patient's performance on successive occasions. This test consists of three block models, which are presented one at a time (Fig. 9.5). The patient is asked to construct an exact replica, selecting blocks from an assortment of 29 blocks. Time taken to complete each model is recorded in seconds, with a maximum of 5 min allowed. The score is obtained by crediting 1 point for each correctly placed block (29 possible points). The types of errors (omissions, additions, substitutions, and displacements) are recorded. If the total time taken to construct the three models is greater than 380 sec,

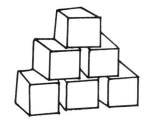

Six cubes (2.5 cm x 2.5 cm x 2.5 cm)

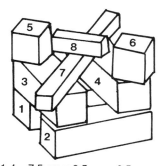

1-4 = 7.5 cm x 2.5 cm x 2.5 cm
5-6 = 2.5 cm x 2.5 cm x 2.5 cm
7 = 15 cm x 1.25 cm x 1.25 cm
8 = 3.75 cm x 1.25 cm x 1.25 cm

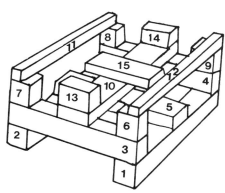

1-2 = 22.5 cm x 2.5 cm x 2.5 cm
3-4 = 15 cm x 2.5 cm x 2.5 cm
5 = 15 cm x 3.75 cm x 1.25 cm
6-9 = 2.5 cm x 2.5 cm x 2.5 cm
10 = 22.5 cm x 3.75 cm x 1.25 cm
11-12 = 22.5 cm x 1.25 cm x 1.25 cm
13-14 = 3.75 cm x 2.5 cm x 2.5 cm
15 = 7.5cm x 3.75 cm x 1.25 cm

Figure 9.5. Schematic representation of block designs.

2 points are subtracted from the score. Of the normal controls, 78% made errorless performances, 12% made one error, and 10% made three to five errors.

Goodglass and Kaplan (1972) described three tests, as part of their parietal lobe battery, for evaluation of constructional difficulties. These include drawing to command, stick construction from **memory**, and three-dimensional block designs. Drawing to command includes having the patient draw a clock, daisy, elephant, cross, cube, and house (scoring criteria are

given in Table 9.7). Stick construction from **memory** consists of 14 designs (Fig. 9.6). Each design is assembled (one at a time) by the therapist in front of the patient, who is then allowed to view it for 10 sec. The design is swept away, and the patient is asked to reproduce the design. The wood sticks are 1/4 inch square by 3 inches long. The patient receives 1 point for each correct item. Goodglass and Kaplan (1972) also described a three-dimensional block construction task that involves copying 10 block designs presented for the patient to reproduce.

The *Lowenstein Occupational Therapy Cognitive Assessment* (LOTCA) battery was standardized on brain-injured adults and contains a section on visuomotor organization (Katz et al., 1989). This section contains block design, copying, drawing, and peg-board design.

DRESSING APRAXIA

Dressing apraxia refers to an inability to dress oneself. Brain (1941) attributed it to an underlying visuospatial disorganization. It can be seen in patients with RBD or LBD and can be the result of constructional apraxia, **unilateral neglect,** and/or body scheme disorders (Critchley, 1966; McFie et al., 1950). Research has supported the link between constructional

Table 9.7. Scoring Criteria for Drawing to Command

Shape	Instruction	Scoring
Clock	"Draw the face of a clock showing the numbers and the two hands."	0 to 3: one point each for approximately circular face, symmetry of number placement, and correctness of numbers
Daisy	"Draw a daisy."	0 to 2: one point each for general shape (center with petals around it) and symmetry of petal arrangement
Elephant	"Draw an elephant."	0 to 2: one point each for general shape (legs, trunk, head, body) and relative proportions correct
Cross	"You know what the Red Cross looks like? Draw an outline of it without taking your pencil off the paper."	0 to 2: one point each for basic configuration and ability to form all corners adequately with a continuous line
Cube	"Draw a cube-shaped block in perspective, as it would look if you could see the top and two sides."	0 to 2: one point each for grossly correct attempt and correctness of perspective
House	"Draw a house in perspective, so you can see the roof and two sides."	0 to 2: one point each for grossly correct features of house and accuracy of perspective

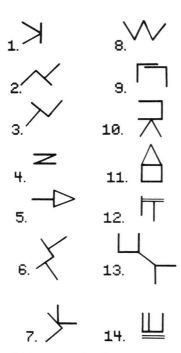

Figure 9.6. Stick construction figures.

apraxia and dressing apraxia (Baum & Hall, 1981; Bradley, 1982; Kowalski-Lundi & Mitcham, 1984; Lorenze & Cancro, 1962; Williams, 1967). In the case of constructional apraxia, the deficit "shows itself in the total disarray, whereby garments are put on in the wrong order, . . . or at the wrong end" (Critchley, 1966, p. 190). If the basis is **unilateral neglect,** the patient may put clothes on in the proper order, but leave one half of his body undressed. Other patients may exhibit problems with right and left, determining top from bottom, etc. Warren (1981) found that a test of body scheme was a better predictor of dressing performance than a constructional apraxia task, although both significantly correlated with dressing performance. She believed that both body scheme and constructional apraxia jointly contribute to dressing apraxia.

Dressing apraxia is generally evaluated functionally by observing the patient dressing himself. To better determine the cause of the dressing apraxia, the evaluation should also include evaluation of constructional apraxia, **unilateral neglect,** and body scheme.

EVALUATION OF COGNITION

"Cognitive disturbances are difficulties in information processing due to brain damage, which alter the ways in which the person experiences and responds to stimuli and interfaces with everyday life" (Ben-Yishay & Diller, 1983, p. 167). **Attention,** orienta-

tion, and **memory** are the basic processes on which are built the higher cognitive functions. Higher cognitive functions include fund of knowledge, ability to manipulate old knowledge (i.e., calculations), social awareness and judgment, and abstract thinking (Strub & Black, 1977). These higher cognitive functions are a measure of the patient's reasoning and problem-solving skills, and deficits in these areas will be exhibited by the patient's inability to function effectively in the environment. These deficits can still be a significant problem years posttrauma.

Evaluation of cognitive deficits is generally carried out by the psychologist or neuropsychologist using psychometric tests. The occupational therapist's role is to evaluate the patient's functional cognitive deficits (Zoltan et al., 1986). As the brain-injured patient often performs better in a structured testing situation used by the psychologist, his performance in a functional situation provides important information for the rehabilitation team. Therefore, while the occupational therapist specifically evaluates for various cognitive deficits, the effects of these deficits are observed during functional activities. The occupational therapist's and neuropsychologist's assessments are meant to complement each other (Morse & Morse, 1988). For example, if evaluating financial management, the neuropsychologist would assess the patient's basic math skills, arithmetic reasoning, mental arithmetic, and so on, whereas the occupational therapist would assess functional money skills by taking the patient out into the community to purchase items in a store or by testing his ability to use a checkbook.

The *Cognitive Assessment of Minnesota* (Rustad et al., 1993) is a standardized test developed by occupational therapists for use with adult patients. It consists of 17 subtests, covering cognitive skills from **attention** and orientation to **problem solving** and abstract reasoning. It is designed to evaluate patients at level 4 and above on the *Rancho Los Amigos Scale of Cognitive Functioning.*

Attention

Attention refers to the ability to focus on a specific stimulus without being distracted (Strub & Black, 1977). The patient's ability to sustain **attention** must be established before evaluation of more complex functions; if inattentive and distractible, the patient will be unable to assimilate information presented in the evaluation.

Alertness, a more basic arousal process, refers to a state in which the patient is able to respond to stimuli in the environment (Strub & Black, 1977). A patient who is attentive is alert. The opposite is not necessarily true; the patient may be alert but unable to screen out extraneous stimuli to attend to the test.

Three aspects of **attention** are vigilance, distribution, and selection (Bourne, Dominowski, & Loftus, 1979). Vigilance is the ability to sustain **attention** over a long period of time; 30 sec is required for the purposes of a mental status exam (Strub & Black, 1977). Distribution of **attention** may vary from concentrated to diffuse. For example, the patient, whose main concern is walking, may be able to focus his **attention** during gait training in physical therapy, but his **attention** may be more diffuse when presented with a perceptual task that has no functional connection to walking for him. Last, **attention** can be selective; the patient may focus on one aspect of a task while ignoring others (e.g., if being asked to scan and tell what is happening in a picture, his **attention** may focus on one detail and he'll miss the story told by the picture).

Three operations are required in moving **attention** from one stimulus to another: disengagement of **attention** from current focus, moving **attention** to another location, and engaging **attention** at the new location (Nissen, 1986; Posner & Rafal, 1987). Functionally, the patient who perseverates on an activity may have difficulty with the ability to disengage **attention**, while distractibility may reflect a failure to engage **attention** on a stimulus.

"At the present time there is little consensus about appropriate evaluation or treatment for attentional disorders" (Whyte, 1992, p. 1094). Because **attention** is the foundation of all conscious tasks, there are no pure tests of **attention**. They are all confounded by motor, perceptual, and/or cognitive performance to some degree. Frequently used tests of **attention** are discussed below, but the therapist must always be aware of other areas that may impact the evaluation and must constantly observe the patient's behavior, method of responding, etc.

Sohlberg and Mateer (1989) described a clinical model of **attention** that is multidimensional and critical to **memory**, new learning, and all other aspects of **cognition**. They addressed five levels of **attention** to focus on in evaluation and treatment: focused, sustained, selective, alternating, and divided **attention** (Table 9.8).

Attention is generally evaluated using the *Digit Repetition Test*. Numbers are presented at a rate of one per second in groups of gradually increasing lengths. When the patient fails twice at one length, the test is stopped. Normally, a person is able to repeat five to seven digits without difficulty; less than five is indicative of a deficit (Strub & Black, 1977). Reverse digit span (the patient is asked to repeat digits in reverse order) as well as serial addition and subtraction (e.g.,

Table 9.8. Attention

Type	Definition	Deficit
Focused attention	Ability to respond discretely to auditory, visual, or tactile stimuli	The patient coming out of coma is initially only able to respond to internal stimuli such as pain
Sustained attention	Ability to maintain attention during continuous and repetitive activity	Evident in the patient who is able to focus on a task only briefly or whose performance fluctuates over brief periods of time
Selective attention	Ability to focus attention in the presence of distracting stimuli	Patients who are easily distracted by external and internal stimuli
Alternating attention	Ability to shift focus of attention from one task to another	The student who experiences difficulty taking notes and listening to a lecture at the same time
Divided Attention	Ability to respond simultaneously to multiple tasks	The patient who is unable to prepare a meal and listen to the radio at the same time

"Count backwards from 100 by 3's") is used to determine the patient's ability to divide his **attention** (Mack, 1986).

The *Random Letter Test* is used as a test of vigilance or sustained **attention** (Strub & Black, 1977). This test consists of a series of letters that contain a target letter occurring with more than random frequency. The letters are read to the patient at the rate of one letter per second. The patient indicates when he hears the target letter by tapping the table with a pencil. Common errors include omissions (failure to indicate a target letter), commissions (indicating any other than the target letter), and perseveration (failure to stop tapping after presentation of a target letter). Although not standardized, the patient should be able to complete this task without error (Strub & Black, 1977).

The *Stroop Test* is often used as a test of selective **attention** (Sohlberg & Mater, 1989). The patient is asked to read a list of color names that are written in a conflicting color (e.g., the word *brown* is written in red ink). The time to read the words is compared with the time to read the color in which the words are printed.

Orientation

Following brain injury, patients are frequently disoriented in terms of person, place, and/or time. The patient may be unable to state where he is and may wander away and get lost. He may be unable to identify others or himself. One study found that RBD patients tended to be more impaired on orientation tests than LBD patients; however, patients with aphasia were excluded from this study, perhaps biasing the results (Wang, Kaplan, & Rogers, 1975). Orientation to person is determined by asking the patient such questions as: "What is your full name?" "How old are you?" and "When is your birthday?" Assessment of orientation to place usually includes questions about the name and location of the hospital/center where the patient is being tested. It might include the type of place and possibly directions between that location and his home.

Temporal orientation is generally assessed by asking the following questions: "What is today's date?" "What day of the week is it?" and "What time is it now?" Five responses are scored: the stated day of the week, day of the month, month, year, and time of day (Table 9.9) (Benton et al., 1983).

The *Test of Orientation for Rehabilitation Patients* (TORP) was designed for use in inpatient rehabilitation settings. It contains 46 items divided into five areas: person and personal situation, place, time, schedule, and temporal continuity. TORP has been found to have

Table 9.9. Test of Temporal Orientation

Administration
  What is today's date? (The patient is required to give month, day, and year.)
  What day of the week is it?
  What time is it now? (Examiner makes sure that the patient cannot look at a watch or clock.)

Scoring
  Day of week: 1 point for each day removed from the correct day up to a maximum of 3 points.
  Day of month: 1 point for each day removed from the correct day up to a maximum of 15 points.
  Month: 5 points for each month removed from the correct month with the qualification that if the stated date is within 15 days of the correct date no points are scored for the incorrect month (e.g., May 29 for June 2 = 4 points).
  Year: 10 points for each year removed from the correct year up to a maximum of 60 points with the qualification that if the stated date is within 15 days of the correct date no points are scored for the incorrect year (e.g., December 26, 1982 for January 2, 1983 = 7 points).
  Time of day: 1 point for each 30 min removed from the correct time up to a maximum of 5 points.

Interpretation
  The total number of error points constitutes the patient's obtained score.
    "Normal" = 0–2
    "Moderately defective" = 4–7
    "Borderline" = 3
    "Severely defective" = 8+

good test-retest reliability (0.83 to 0.92), except for borderline reliability for schedule (0.72) (Deitz et al., 1992) and good interrater reliability (0.94 to 0.99) (Deitz et al, 1990). This test is somewhat unusual in that items are first posed as open-ended questions (e.g., "What kind of work were you doing before your injury?"). If the patient is unable to respond, he is given three choices from which to pick. The test takes 15 to 25 min for the therapist to gather the correct answers (from the medical chart and interview with the family) and 5 to 30 min to administer, depending on level of orientation.

The *Galveston Orientation and Amnesia Test* (GOAT) is a rating scale that measures disorientation and amnesia following closed-head injury (Levin, O'Donnell, & Grossman, 1979). It evaluates orientation, posttraumatic amnesia, and retrograde amnesia. It consists of 10 questions. A perfect score is 100; the defective range is a score below 66. GOAT is designed to be used serially, on a daily basis. The serial scores have been found to be predictive of long-term outcome following acute head injury (Levin et al., 1979).

Memory

The ability to process, store, and retrieve information depends on intact **memory** systems. There are several forms of **memory,** and their definitions often overlap (Table 9.10). **Memory** processes include registration and encoding, consolidation and storage, and recall and retrieval of information. Any of these processes can be disrupted by brain damage. **Memory** deficits are common sequelae of brain injury, and their effects may continue for years posttrauma (Schacter & Crovitz, 1977).

If a patient has a decreased **attention** span and/ or poor concentration, he will have difficulty getting the information to encode to begin with; therefore, it is important to distinguish between **memory** deficits per se and problems of concentration and/or **attention.** For instance, the therapist may find that the patient does poorly on a formal **memory** test presented in a noisy and/or visually stimulating room but performs adequately in a quiet room. Functionally, the patient may have difficulty remembering a one-handed shoe-tying technique taught in a busy clinic yet remember a more complicated dressing technique taught in a quiet room.

In studies on head-injured patients, it has generally been found that although there are deficits in both short-term **memory** (STM) and long-term **memory** (LTM), LTM exhibits the major deficit (Brooks, 1975; Roth & Crosson, 1985). This may be because STM is thought to be equally represented in both hemispheres and, therefore, less affected by unilateral lesions (Wang et al., 1975).

Table 9.10. Memory Terms

Term	Definition
Memory	
Immediate	Memory held in conscious awareness, usually less than 1 min
Short term	Memory held temporarily; period of slightly longer than 1 min elapses between stimulus and recall, sometimes called primary memory
Long term	Memory that involves an interval of more than a few minutes between stimulus and recall, sometimes called secondary memory
Working	Temporary storage and manipulation of information needed to perform a task
Recent	Usually corresponds to LTM, includes memory from hours to months poststimulus presentation
Remote	Very LTM; memory for past events, as from childhood
Episodic	Memory of one's personal history (i.e., what you had for breakfast this morning, etc.)
Semantic	Personal knowledge of the world (i.e., that horses are big and ants are small, etc.)
Amnesia	
Retrograde	Loss of ability to recall events that occurred before the trauma
Anterograde	Decreased memory of events occurring posttrauma
Posttraumatic	Period following trauma during which the patient is confused, disoriented, and seems to lack the ability to store and retrieve new information

The most commonly used evaluation for **memory** is the *Wechsler Memory Scale* (Wechsler, 1945), which is generally administered by psychologists and neuropsychologists. Occupational therapists generally do a screening of **memory** skills, which includes estimation of immediate **memory,** STM, and LTM. Therapists need to know the status of **memory** to plan any relearning program for the patient. Digit repetition, discussed earlier, is generally used as an indicator for immediate **memory.**

A measure of STM and LTM is to ask the patient to remember four words (e.g., *brown, honesty, tulip,* and *eyedropper*), then test his immediate recall, recall after 5 min, 10 min, and 30 min (Strub & Black, 1977). If the patient is unable to recall any of the four words, verbal cues can be given to get an indication if there was any **memory** storage: semantic cues (i.e., "One word was a color"), phonemic cues (i.e., "Eye . . ., eyedrop . . ., eyedropper), and contextual cues (i.e., "A common flower in Holland is a . . . "). If unable to profit from these cues, the therapist may

ask the patient to choose from several examples (i.e., "Was the color red, brown, yellow, or green?"). A person should be able to remember all four words after a 10-min delay, and after 30 min, at least three of the four should be recalled (Strub & Black, 1977). This test could also be used to assess visual **memory** by pointing to four objects in the room and having the patient recall them immediately, after 5 min, and at the end of the session (Bigler, 1984).

Problem Solving

Problem solving requires both an intact fund of knowledge and the ability to manipulate and apply this information to new or unfamiliar situations (Strub & Black, 1977). **Problem solving** generally consists of three stages: preparation—understanding the problem; production—generating possible solutions; and judgment—evaluating the solutions generated (Bourne et al., 1979). When solving a problem a person may cycle repeatedly through these stages. It is closely related to executive functions of anticipation, goal selection, planning, initiation of activity, self-regulation and use of feedback (Sohlberg & Mateer, 1989). A deficit in **problem solving** will affect all phases of the patient's daily life. He may exhibit difficulty ordering or sequencing information and thus be unable to figure out what bus to take or how to plan a meal. He may experience difficulty in social situations, being unable to figure out what to do.

Problem solving is an integration of many cognitive abilities and the therapist must be aware of the effects of other cognitive functions (e.g., **attention, memory, perception,** etc.) when evaluating **problem solving.** If unable to copy a block design, the patient may lack the spatial skills or may not be able to analyze the design and figure out how to build it. Therefore, evaluation of **problem solving** begins with a comprehensive evaluation of other cognitive functions. If no deficits are noted, assessment proceeds to evaluation of **problem solving** (Goldstein & Levin, 1987).

An evaluation of **problem solving** frequently used is that of proverb interpretation. Proverbs are presented in ascending order of difficulty and scored on the basis of whether the response is concrete, semiabstract, or abstract (Table 9.11). This test is not standardized, but the average person should provide abstract interpretations to at least two proverbs and semiabstract to the remaining proverbs; any concrete response is suggestive of impairment (Strub & Black, 1977).

Social awareness is usually evaluated by responses to questions concerning environmental situations (e.g., "What should a person do if he sees smoke in a building?") (Strub & Black, 1977). Social

Table 9.11. Proverb Interpretation and Scoring

1. Rome wasn't built in a day.
   - 0 (concrete)   "It took a long time to build Rome."
     - "You can't build cities overnight."
   - 1 (semiabstract)   "Don't do things too fast."
     - "You have to be patient and careful."
     - "You can't learn everything in one day."
   - 2 (abstract)   "Great things take time to achieve."
     - "If something is worth doing, it is worth doing carefully."
     - "It takes time to do things well."

2. A drowning man will clutch at a straw.
   - 0 (concrete)   "Don't let go when you're in the water."
     - "That guy will grab anything."
   - 1 (semiabstract)   "Self-preservation is important."
     - "Nobody wants to die."
   - 2 (abstract 0   "A man in trouble tries anything to get out of it."
     - "If sufficiently desperate, a man will try anything."

3. A golden hammer breaks an iron door.
   - 0 (concrete)   "Gold can't break iron!"
     - "Hammers can break down doors."
   - 1 (semiabstract)   "Money wins everything."
     - "The harder something is, the more you have to work to get it."
   - 2 (abstract)   "Virtue conquers all."
     - "If you have sufficient knowledge, you can accomplish even the most difficult task."

4. The hot coal burns, the cold one blackens.
   - 0 (concrete)   "Hot coals will burn you and leave it black."
     - "Hot coals get black when they're cold."
   - 1 (semiabstract)   "You can get trouble from both."
     - "Getting burned and dirty are both bad."
   - 2 (abstract)   "Extremes of anything can be bad."
     - "There may be bad aspects to things that appear good."
     - "One should be careful and not impetuous in any situation."

judgment concerns the patient's actual response in real life and is, therefore, difficult to assess in a testing situation. Information from family and staff must be used to determine his performance in day-to-day events.

Verbal similarities require the patient to describe the similarity between two objects or situations. The patient is presented with the following pairs of words, one set at a time: *turnip-cauliflower, desk-bookcase, poem-novel,* and *horse-apple.* The responses are scored 0 to 2:

2 = the correct response of any abstract similarity or general classification (e.g., turnip and cauliflower are vegetables).

1 = a response that indicates specific properties of the items or only constitutes a relative similarity (e.g., turnip and cauliflower are food, grow in the ground, or are things you eat).

0 = a failure to respond or a response that reflects properties of only one of the words or generalizations not pertinent to the pair (e.g., turnip and cauliflower are bought in a store or have calories).

An average person is expected to obtain a score of at least 4; any concrete (0 points) answer or score of less than 4 is indicative of a deficit (Strub & Black, 1977).

Conceptual series completion is a test of verbal abstraction, **problem solving,** and reasoning. The patient is shown numbers, letters, and words in a series, for example,

1, 4, 7, 10, —;
AZ, BY, CX, D—;
tote to, snow on, spun up, stab —;
elephant 87654321, plant 57321, lap —.

He is then expected to provide the next item in the series. The response is either correct or incorrect, and the average person should be able to complete two of the four examples (Strub & Black, 1977).

SUMMARY

The purpose of this chapter was to serve as an introduction to the complex task of assessing the perceptual and cognitive status of the brain-injured adult. Both **perception** and **cognition** were divided into component parts and defined. Specific strategies for evaluation were presented. The importance of using standardized tests whenever possible and examining the patient's method of response as well as the results cannot be overemphasized.

STUDY QUESTIONS

1. What is the definition of perception? cognition?
2. What are the foundation visual skills? Why and how are they evaluated?
3. List two ways to evaluate each of the following: body scheme, unilateral neglect, spatial relations, and apraxia.
4. List two ways to evaluate each of the following: attention, orientation, memory, and problem solving.
5. Describe Toglia's information-processing approach.
6. Identify and describe the basic roles of the right and left hemispheres in perception and cognition.
7. List and describe common errors made by patients during apraxia testing.
8. Compare and contrast input and output neglect.

9. Discuss the need for evaluating a patient's process to complete a test in relation to his final score.

10. Why should occupational therapists use standardized tests whenever possible?

REFERENCES

Abreu, B. C., & Toglia, J. P. (1987). Cognitive rehabilitation: A model for occupational therapy. *American Journal of Occupational Therapy, 41,* 439–448.

Albert, M. L. (1973). A simple test of visual neglect. *Neurology, 23,* 658–664.

Anderson, E. K. (1971). Sensory impairments in hemiplegia. *Archives of Physical Medicine & Rehabilitation, 52,* 293–297.

Arena, R., & Gainotti, G. (1978). Constructional apraxia and visuoperceptive disabilities in relation to laterality of cerebral lesions. *Cortex, 14,* 463–473.

Arrigoni, G., & DeRenzi, E. (1964). Constructional apraxia and hemispheric locus of lesions. *Cortex, 1,* 170–197.

Ayres, A. J. (1987). *Sensory integration and praxis tests.* Los Angeles: Western Psychological Services.

Battersby, W. S., Bender, M. B., Pollack, M., & Kahn, R. L. (1956). Unilateral "spatial agnosia" ("inattention") in patients with cerebral lesions. *Brain, 79,* 68–93.

Baum, B., & Hall, K. M. (1981). Relationship between constructional praxis and dressing in the head-injured adult. *American Journal of Occupational Therapy, 35,* 438–442.

Ben-Yishay, Y., & Diller, L. (1983). Cognitive deficits. In M. Rosenthal, E. R. Griffith, M. R. Bond, & J. D. Miller (Eds.), *Rehabilitation of the head injured adult* (pp. 167–183). Philadelphia: F. A. Davis.

Bender, L. (1946). *Instructions for the use of Visual Motor Gestalt Test.* New York: American Orthopsychiatric Association.

Benton, A. L. (1967). Constructional apraxia and the minor hemisphere. *Confinia Neurologica, 29,* 1–16.

Benton, A. (1985). Body schema disturbances: Finger agnosia and right-left disorientation. In K. M. Heilman & E. Valenstein (Eds.), *Clinical neuropsychology* (pp. 115–129). New York: Oxford University Press.

Benton, A. L., & Fogel, M. L. (1962). Three-dimensional constructional praxis. *Archives of Neurology, 7,* 347–354.

Benton, A. L., Hamsher, K., Varney, N. K., & Spreen, O. (1983). *Contributions to neuropsychological assessment—A clinical manual.* New York: Oxford University Press.

Bernspang, B., Vitanin, M., & Eriksson, S. (1989). Impairments of perceptual and motor functions: Their influence on self-care ability 4 to 6 years after a stroke. *Occupational Therapy Journal of Research, 9,* 27–37.

Bigler, E. D. (1984). *Diagnostic clinical neuropsychology.* Austin, TX: University of Texas Press.

Bisiach, E., Capitani, E., Luzzatti, C., & Perani, D. (1981). Brain and conscious representation of outside reality. *Neuropsychologia, 19,* 543–551.

Bisiach, E., Geminiani, G., Berti, A. & Rusconi, M. L. (1990). Perceptual and premotor factors of unilateral neglect. *Neurology, 40,* 1278–1281.

Boone, D. R., & Landes, B. A. (1968). Left-right discrimination in hemiplegic patients. *Archives of Physical Medicine & Rehabilitation, 49,* 533–537.

Bourne, L. E., Dominowski, R. L., & Loftus, E. F. (1979). *Cognitive Processes.* Englewood Cliffs, NJ: Prentice-Hall.

Bouska, M. J. (1990, March 3–4). *Visual perceptual disorders in adults: Evaluation and treatment.* Conference of the Advanced Rehabilitation Institutes, Newton, MA.

Bouska, M. J., & Kwatny, E. (1983). *Manual for application of the Motor-Free Visual Perception Test to the adult population.* (Available from Bouska & Kwatny, P.O. Box 12246, Philadelphia, PA 19944-0346).

Bradley, K. P. (1982). The effectiveness of constructional praxis tests in predicting upper extremity dressing abilities. *Occupational Therapy Journal of Research, 2,* 184–185.

Brain, W. R. (1941). Visual disorientation with special reference to lesions of the right cerebral hemisphere. *Brain, 64,* 244–272.

Brooks, D. N. (1975). Long and short term memory in head injured patients. *Cortex, 11,* 329–340.

Caplan, B. (1985). Stimulus effects in unilateral neglect? *Cortex, 21,* 69–80.

Carter, L. T., Oliveira, D. O., Duponte, J., & Lynch, S. V. (1988). The relationship of cognitive skills performance to activities of daily living in stroke patients. *American Journal of Occupational Therapy, 42,* 449–455.

Colombo, A., DeRenzi, E., & Faglioni, P. (1976). The occurrence of visual neglect in patients with unilateral cerebral disease. *Cortex, 12,* 221–231.

Coslett, H. B., Bowers, D., Fitzpatrick, E., Haws, B., & Heilman, K. M. (1990). Directional hypokinesia and hemispatial inattention in neglect. *Brain, 113,* 475–486.

Critchley, M. (1966). *The parietal lobes.* New York: Hafner.

Deitz, J. C., Tovar, V. S., Beema, C., Thorn, D. W., & Trevisan, M. S. (1992). The Test of Orientation for Rehabilitation Patients: Test-retest reliability. *Occupational Therapy Journal of Research, 12,* 173–185.

Deitz, J. C., Tovar, V. S., Thorn, D. W., & Beeman, C. (1990). The Test of Orientation for Rehabilitation Patients: Interrater reliability. *American Journal of Occupational Therapy, 44,* 784–790.

Denes, G., Semenza, C., Stoppa, E., & Lis, A. (1982). Unilateral spatial neglect and recovery from hemiplegia. *Brain, 105,* 543–552.

DeRenzi, E. (1982). Constructional apraxia. In *Disorders of space exploration and cognition.* New York: John Wiley & Sons.

DeRenzi, E. (1985). Methods of limb apraxia examination and their bearing on the interpretation of the disorder. In E. A. Roy (Ed.), *Neuropsychological studies of apraxia and related disorders* (pp. 45–64). Amsterdam: Elsevier.

DeRenzi, E., & Faglioni, P. (1967). The relationship between visuospatial impairment and constructional apraxia. *Cortex, 3,* 325–342.

DeRenzi, E., Faglioni, P., & Sorgato, P. (1982). Modality-specific and supramodal mechanisms of apraxia. *Brain, 105,* 301–312.

Diller, L., Weinbeyer, J., Piasetsky, J. Ruckdeschel-Hubbard, M., Egelko, S., Scotzin, M. Counistakis, J., & Gordon, W. (1980). *Methods for the evaluation and treatment of the visual perceptual difficulties of right brain damaged individuals.* (Rehabilitation Monograph No. 67). New York: New York University Medical Center, Institute of Rehabilitation Medicine.

Forer, S. K., & Miller, L. S. (1980). Rehabilitation outcome: Comparative analysis of different patient types. *Archives of Physical Medicine & Rehabilitation, 61,* 359–365.

Freidman, P. J. (1992). The Star Cancellation Test in acute stroke. *Clinical Rehabilitation, 6,* 23–30.

Frostig, M. (1966). *Developmental Test of Visual Perception.* Palo Alto, CA: Consulting Psychologist.

Gainotti, G., Messerli, P., & Tissot, R. (1972). Qualitative analysis of unilateral spatial neglect in relation to laterality of cerebral lesions. *Journal of Neurology Neurosurgery and Psychiatry, 35,* 545–550.

Gainotti, G., & Tiacci, C. (1970). Patterns of drawing disability in right and left hemispheric patients. *Neuropsychologia, 8,* 379–384.

Gianutsos, R., & Matheson, P. (1987). The rehabilitation of visual perceptual disorders attributable to brain injury. In M. J. Meir, A. L. Benton, & L. Diller (Eds.), *Neuropsychological rehabilitation* (pp. 202–241). New York: Churchill Livingston.

Goldstein, F. C., & Levin, H. S. (1987). Disorders of reasoning and problem-solving ability. In M. J. Meir, A. L. Benton, & L. Diller (Eds.), *Neuropsychological rehabilitation* (pp. 327–354). New York: Churchill Livingston.

Goodglass, H., & Kaplan, E. (1972). *The assessment of aphasia and related disorders.* Philadelphia: Lea & Febiger.

Haaland, K. (1992, November). *Assessment of limb apraxia.* Paper presented at Educational Resources Conference: Apraxia in children and adults, Boston.

Haaland, K. (1993, March). *Typology and assessment of individuals with limb apraxia.* Paper presented at the AOTA Neuroscience Institute conference: Treating Adults with Apraxia, Baltimore.

Haaland, K. Y., Harrington, D. L., & Yeo, R. (1987). The effects of task complexity on motor performance in left and right CVA patients. *Neuropsychologia, 25,* 783–794.

Halligan, P. W., & Marshall, J. C. (1991). Left neglect for near but not far space in man. *Nature, 350,* 498–500.

Halligan, P. W., & Marshall, J. C. (1992). Left visuo-spatial neglect: A meaningless entity? *Cortex, 28,* 525–535.

Heilman, K. M. (1975). A tapping test in apraxia. *Cortex, 11,* 259–263.

Heilman, K. M., & Van Den Abell, T. (1980). Right hemisphere dominance for attention: The mechanism underlying hemispheric asymmetries of inattention (neglect). *Neurology, 30,* 327–330.

Heilman, K. M., Watson, R. T., & Valenstein, E. (1985). Neglect and related disorders. In K. M. Heilman & E. Valenstein (Eds.), *Clinical neuropsychology* (pp. 243–293). New York: Oxford University Press.

Helm-Estabrooks, N., & Albert, M. L. (1991). *Manual of aphasia therapy.* Austin, TX: Pro-ed.

Kaplan, J., & Hier, D. B. (1982). Visuospatial deficits after right hemisphere stroke. *American Journal of Occupational Therapy, 36,* 314–321.

Karnath, H.-O., & Hartje, W. (1987). Residual information processing in the neglected visual half-field. *Journal of Neurology, 234,* 180–184.

Katz, N., Itzkovich, M., Averbach, S., & Elazar, B. (1989). Lowenstein Occupational Therapy Cognitive Assessment (LOTCA) battery for brain injured patients: Reliability and validity. *American Journal of Occupational Therapy, 43,* 184–192.

Kimura, D., & Archibald, Y. (1974). Motor functions of the left hemisphere. *Brain, 97,* 337–350.

Kowalski-Lundi, M. H., & Mitcham, M. D. (1984). The relationship of constructional praxis to an upper extremity dressing task. *Occupational Therapy Journal of Research, 4,* 311–313.

Levin, H. S., O'Donnell, V. M., & Grossman, R. G. (1979). The Galveston Orientation and Amnesia Test: A practical scale to assess cognition after head injury. *Journal of Nervous & Mental Diseases, 167,* 675–684.

Lezak, M. D. (1976). *Neuropsychological assessment.* New York: Oxford University Press.

Lezak, M. D. (1991). Identifying neuropsychological deficits. In R. G. Lister, & H. J. Weingartner (Eds.), *Perspectives on cognitive neuroscience* (pp. 357–367). New York: Oxford University Press.

Lorenze, E. J., & Cancro, R. (1962). Dysfunction in visual perception with hemiplegia: Its relation to activities of daily living. *Archives of Physical Medicine & Rehabilitation, 43,* 514–517.

MacDonald, J. C. (1960). An investigation of body scheme in adults with cerebral vascular accidents. *American Journal of Occupational Therapy, 14,* 75–79.

Mack, J. L. (1986). Clinical assessment of disorders of attention and memory. *Journal of Head Trauma Rehabilitation, 1*(3), 22–33.

Mark, V. W., Kooistra, C. A., & Heilman, K. M. (1988). Hemispatial neglect affected by non-neglected stimuli. *Neurology, 38,* 1207–1211.

Marshall, J. C., & Halligan, P. W. (1988). Blindsight and insight into visuo-spatial neglect. *Nature, 336,* 766–767.

McFie, J., Piercy, M. F., & Zangwill, O. L. (1950). Visual-spatial agnosia associated with lesions of the right cerebral hemisphere. *Brain, 73,* 167–190.

Mennemeier, M., Wertman, E., & Heilman, K. M. (1992). Neglect of near peripersonal space: Evidence for multidirectional systems in humans. *Brain, 115,* 37–50.

Mesulam, M.-M. (1981). A cortical network for directed attention and unilateral neglect. *Annals of Neurology, 10,* 309–325.

Morse, P. A., & Morse, A. R. (1988). Functional living skills: Promoting the interaction between neuropsychology and occupational therapy. *Journal of Head Trauma Rehabilitation, 3,* 33–44.

Neistadt, M. E. (1993). The relationship between constructional and meal preparation skills. *Archives of Physical Medicine & Rehabilitation, 74,* 144–148.

Nissen, M. J. (1986). Neuropsychology of attention and memory. *Journal of Head Trauma Rehabilitation, 1*(3), 13–21.

Ottenbacher, K. (1980). Cerebral vascular accident: Some characteristics of occupational therapy evaluation forms. *American Journal of Occupational Therapy, 34,* 268–271.

Paterson, A., & Zangwill, O. L. (1944). Disorders of visual space perception associated with lesions of the right cerebral hemisphere. *Brain, 67,* 331–358.

Petersen, P., & Wikoff, R. L. (1983). The performance of adult males on the Southern California Figure-Ground Visual Perception Test. *American Journal of Occupational Therapy, 37,* 554–560.

Piercy, M., Hecaen, H., & Ajuriaguerra, J. (1960). Constructional apraxia associated with unilateral cerebral lesions—Left and right sided cases compared. *Brain, 83,* 225–242.

Plourde, G., & Sperry, R. W. (1984). Left hemisphere involvement in left spatial neglect from right-sided lesions. *Brain, 107,* 95–106.

Poeck, K. (1985). Clues to the nature of disruptions to limb praxis. In E. A. Roy (Ed.), *Neuropsychological studies of apraxia and related disorders* (pp. 99–109). Amsterdam: Elsevier.

Posner, M. I., & Rafal, R. D. (1987). Cognitive theories of attention and the rehabilitation of attentional deficits. In M. J. Meier, A. L. Benton, & L. Diller (Eds.), *Neuropsychological rehabilitation* (pp. 182–201). New York: Churchill Livingston.

Prigatano, G. P., & Fordyce, D. J. (1986). Cognitive dysfunction and psychological adjustment after brain injury. In G. P. Prigatano (Ed.), *Neuropsychological rehabilitation after brain injury* (pp. 1–17). Baltimore: Johns Hopkins University Press.

Riddoch, M. J., & Humphreys, G. W. (1983). The effects of cueing on unilateral neglect. *Neuropsychologia, 21,* 589–599.

Roth, D. L., & Crosson, B. (1985). Memory span and long term memory deficits in brain-impaired patients. *Journal of Clinical Psychology, 41,* 521–527.

Russo, M., & Vignolo, L. A. (1967). Visual figure-ground discrimination in patients with unilateral cerebral disease. *Cortex, 3,* 113–127.

Rustad, R. A., DeGroot, T. L., Jungkunz, M. L., Freeberg, K. S., Borowick, L. G., & Wanttie, A. M. (1993). *The Cognitive Assessment of Minnesota.* Tucson, AZ: Therapy Skill Builders.

Sauguet, J., Benton, A. L., & Hecaen, H. (1971). Disturbances of the body schema in relation to language impairment and hemispheric locus of lesion. *Journal of Neurology Neurosurgery and Psychiatry, 34,* 496–501.

Schacter, D. L., & Crovitz, H. F. (1977). Memory function after closed head injury: A review of the quantitative research. *Cortex, 13,* 150–176.

Schenkenberg, T., Bradford, D. C., Ajax, E. T. (1980). Line bisection and unilateral visual neglect in patients with neurologic impairment. *Neurology, 30,* 509–517.

Sea, M.-J. C., Henderson, A., & Cermak, S. A. (1993). Patterns of visual spatial inattention and their functional significance in stroke patients. *Archives of Physical Medicine & Rehabilitation, 74,* 355–360.

Sohlberg, M. M., & Mateer, C. A. (1989). *Introduction to cognitive rehabilitation.* New York: Gilford Press.

Stam, C. J., & Bakker, M. (1990). The prevalence of neglect: Superiority of neuropsychological over clinical methods of examination. *Clinical Neurology and Neurosurgery, 92,* 229–235.

Stone, S. P., Halligan, P. W., & Greenwood, R. J. (1993). The incidence of neglect phenomena and related disorders in patients with an acute right or left hemisphere stroke. *Age and Ageing, 22,* 46–52.

Stone, S. P., Halligan, P. W., Wilson, B., Greenwood, R. J., & Marshall, J. C. (1991). Performance of age-matched controls on a battery of visuo-spatial neglect tests. *Journal of Neurology, Neurosurgery, and Psychiatry, 54,* 341–344.

Stone, S. P., Patel, P., Greenwood, R. J., Halligan, P. W. (1992). Measuring visual neglect in acute stroke and predicting its recovery: the visual neglect recovery index. *Journal of Neurology, Neurosurgery, and Psychiatry, 55,* 431–436.

Stone, S. P., Wilson, B., Wroot, A., Halligan, P. W., Lange, L. S., Marshall, J. C., & Greenwood, R. J. (1991). The assessment of visuospatial neglect after acute stroke. *Journal of Neurology, Neurosurgery, and Psychiatry, 54,* 345–350.

Strub, R. L., & Black, F. W. (1977). *The mental status examination in neurology.* Philadelphia: F. A. Davis.

Tegner, R., & Levander, M. (1991). Through a looking glass: A new technique to demonstrate directional hypokinesia in unilateral neglect. *Brain, 114,* 1943–1951.

Teuber, H.-L., & Weinstein, S. (1956). Ability to discover hidden figures after cerebral lesions. *Archives of Neurology & Psychiatry, 76,* 369–379.

Titus, M. N. D., Gall, N. G., Yerxa, E. J., Robertson, T. A., & Mack, W. (1991). Correlation of perceptual performance and activities of daily living in stroke patients. *American Journal of Occupational Therapy, 45,* 410–418.

Toglia, J. P. (1989). Visual perception of objects: An approach to assessment and intervention. *American Journal of Occupational Therapy, 43,* 587–595.

Trobe, J. D., Acosta, P. C., Krischer, J. P., & Trick, G. L. (1981). Confrontation visual field techniques in the detection of anterior visual pathway lesions. *Annals of Neurology, 10,* 28–34.

Van Deusen, J. (1983). Normative data for ninety-three elderly persons on the Schenkenberg line bisection test. *Physical & Occupational Therapy in Geriatrics, 3*(2), 49–54.

Walker, R., Findlay, J. M., Young, A. W., & Welch, J. (1991). Disentangling neglect and hemianopsia. *Neuropsychologia, 29,* 1019–1027.

Wang, P. L., Kaplan, J. R., & Rogers, E. J. (1975). Memory functioning in hemiplegics: A neuropsychological analysis of the Wechsler Memory Scale. *Archives of Physical Medicine & Rehabilitation, 56,* 517–521.

Warren, M. (1981). Relationship of constructional apraxia and body scheme disorders to dressing performance in adult CVA. *American Journal Occupational Therapy, 35,* 431–437.

Warren, M. (1990). Identification of visual scanning deficits in adults after cerebrovascular accident. *American Journal of Occupational Therapy, 44,* 391–399.

Warren, M. (1993a). A hierarchical model for evaluation and treatment of visual perceptual dysfunction in adult acquired brain injury, Part 1. *American Journal of Occupational Therapy, 47,* 42–54.

Warren, M. (1993b). A hierarchical model for evaluation and treatment of visual perceptual dysfunction in adult acquired brain injury, Part 2. *American Journal of Occupational Therapy, 47,* 55–66.

Warrington, E. K., James, M., & Kinsbourne, M. (1966). Drawing disability in relation to laterality of cerebral lesion. *Brain, 89,* 53–82, 1966.

Wechsler, D. (1945). A standardized memory scale for clinical use. *Journal of Psychology, 19,* 87–95.

Weinberg, J., Diller, L., Gordon, W. A., Gerstman, L. J., Lieberman, A., Lakin, P., Hodges, G., & Ezrachi, O. (1977). Visual scanning training effect on reading-related tasks in acquired right brain damage. *Archives of Physical Medicine & Rehabilitation, 58,* 479–486.

Weinberg, J., Piasetsky, E., Diller, L., & Gordon, W. (1982). Treating perceptual organization deficits in nonneglecting RBD stroke patients. *Journal of Clinical Neuropsychology, 4,* 59–75.

Weintraub, S., & Mesulam, M. M. (1987). Right cerebral dominance in spatial attention: Further evidence based on ipsilateral neglect. *Archives of Neurology, 44,* 621–625.

Weintraub, S., & Mesulam, M. M. (1988). Visual hemispatial inattention: Stimulus parameters and exploratory strategies. *Journal of Neurology, Neurosurgery, and Psychiatry, 51,* 1481–1488.

Whyte, J. (1992). Neurologic disorders of attention and arousal: assessment and treatment. *Archives of Physical Medicine & Rehabilitation, 73,* 1094–1103.

Williams, N. (1967). Correlation between copying ability and dressing activities in hemiplegia. *American Journal of Physical Medicine, 46,* 1332–1340.

Wilson, B., Cockburn, J., & Halligan, P. (1987). Development of a Behavioral Test of Visuospatial Neglect. *Archives of Physical Medicine & Rehabilitation, 68,* 98–102.

Zoltan, B., Siev, E., & Freishtat, B. (1986). *The adult stroke patient: A manual for evaluation and treatment of perceptual and cognitive dysfunction.* Thorofare, NJ: Slack.

10
Evaluation of Emotional Adjustment to Disabilities

Hilda Powers Versluys

OBJECTIVES

After studying this chapter, the student will be able to:

1. Understand the potential for psychosocial, emotional, and behavioral reactions to **trauma,** physical impairment, and discharge.
2. Discuss the influence of **premorbid** factors such as the patient's **life stage,** psychosocial development, and **lifestyle** on rehabilitation and the adjustment process.
3. Appreciate the influence of factors such as family, sexuality and gender, and **culture** and religion on rehabilitation and the adjustment process.
4. Understand the concept of comorbidity and the psychiatric and emotional problems that coexist with physical disability, which require consideration in evaluation, treatment, and discharge planning.
5. Select appropriate evaluation instruments and methods to identify a patient's function and dysfunction.

A patient's psychologic and emotional problems will influence the outcome of rehabilitation. This chapter will help students and therapists understand and evaluate their patients' emotional responses to physical disability or illness so that a meaningful therapeutic program can be designed to integrate physical and psychosocial treatment goals that are consistent with the patients' interests and occupational performance goals.

Psychosocial sequelae that result from changes in health and loss of physical function may prevent patients from maximizing their potential or reengaging in life activities. These sequelae also present barriers to successful discharge and a good quality of life within the community. Despite excellent treatment programs, occupational therapists may encounter barriers to rehabilitation because patients may remain passive, dependent, and depressed. The patient may seem unable to accept **lifestyle** changes and fail to recognize and employ his strengths, skills, and assets.

Some psychosocial factors that influence rehabilitation are internal to the patient and some are external. The internal factors include a person's particular reaction to **trauma,** disability, and stress as well as his developmental maturity as exemplified by his breadth of interests, ability to establish and work for goals, and ability to organize and manage time. Some of the external factors are related to the patient's family and **culture** and others to the hospitalization experience. The patient's rehabilitation may also be influenced by the presence of a **comorbid** diagnosis, such as depression, a personality disorder, or alcohol abuse.

The occupational therapist has a responsibility to design treatment plans that address the physical dysfunction and those psychological and emotional factors that could hinder rehabilitation (Watson, 1986).

EVALUATION: FOCUS, PURPOSE, AND METHODS

The therapist uses **practice models** to organize and analyze evaluation data and to make clinical decisions about treatment. In some cases, the **practice model** guides the selection of an evaluation instrument; in other cases, the instrument or method of evaluation is generic to the occupational therapy domain of practice (Denton & Skinner, 1988). The purpose of a psychosocial evaluation is to gather information concerning cognitive, developmental, emotional, psychological, and social problems that are the result of reactions to the physical **trauma** or of failure to reach an age-

GLOSSARY

Comorbid—The relationship between concurrent physical and mental disorders, including coexisting physical illness, psychiatric illness, mental retardation, and hearing and visual impairments (Sabshin, 1991).

Coping skills—The ability to solve problems in a functional manner, to direct energy to overcome problems (Peloquin, 1986), to perceive the need for change, to set goals and to follow through, to test reality, to modify behavior in accordance to new environmental demands, to assume responsibility for one's own actions, and to cope with stressful events through stress reduction and anxiety management (Bruce & Borg, 1987).

Culture—Those ideas, customs, skills, and arts of a people or group that are transferred, communicated, or passed along to succeeding generations (*Webster's*, 1991).

Defense mechanisms—Unconscious mental processes used to reduce anxiety and depression and to resolve intrapsychic conflicts related to needs, wishes, reality, important people, and conscience (Kaplan & Sadock, 1991).

Life stage—"Life stages are consecutive time spans in the individual's life that provide an overarching structure for understanding development" (Bruce & Borg, 1987, p. 195). Integral to each life stage are biological, psychosocial, cognitive, and occupational tasks that must be carried out by the individual to meet his developmental needs.

Lifestyle—The consistent, integrated way of life of an individual as typified by his manner, attitudes, and possessions (*Webster's*, 1991). Lifestyle also refers to a person's preferred occupational roles, including personal and work roles, interests and hobbies, schedules, methods of carrying out activities of daily living, the use of time, and methods of socialization.

Morbidity—The rate of psychiatric disease in a physically disabled population. A coexisting psychiatric diagnosis means that the patient may require a longer hospital stay; have higher use of health services and health care resources; have increased psychiatric symptoms; and be at risk for chronic depression, failure to heal, and self-neglect (Fulop & Strain, 1991).

Practice model—Similar to a "frame of reference," based on theory and used to guide occupational therapy evaluation and interventions in clinical practice (Denton & Skinner, 1988).

Premorbid—Level of psychosocial development, medical and psychiatric illness, education, lifestyle, or occupational roles and activities that were present before the development of disease or before the traumatic event.

Trauma—A bodily injury, wound, or shock that can produce a lasting psychic effect as a result of a rapid change in physical or emotional status (*Webster's*, 1991).

appropriate developmental level. The therapist assesses a patient's functional abilities concerning his:

1. Degree of flexibility in reordering life goals and determining realistic future plans;
2. **Coping skills** (such as problem-solving skills), personal management (such as ability to manage time and organize and plan), and emotional management (including stress and frustration);
3. Understanding of the disability and how it will influence his life;
4. Ability to take personal responsibility.

Watson (1986) and Rogers (1983) encouraged occupational therapists to identify the exact psychosocial problems that may interfere with their patient's treatment and his successful discharge into the community and to analyze just how these problems may affect the patient's life, plans, and future. It is also important to identify the patient's strengths and skills so that treatment will be based on his competencies, values, and interests. The identification of strengths is motivational to the patient and can bolster self-identity and -esteem. In addition, the therapist evaluates dysfunction associated with a **comorbid** diagnosis, such as psychiatric diagnosis, mental retardation, hearing and visual impairments, and substance abuse. The evaluation data are the basis for treatment planning.

Evaluation Instruments

The therapist evaluates psychosocial areas with methods that include interviewing and skilled observation. Representative evaluation methods are discussed below.

1. The following instruments provide guidelines for observation of psychosocial and task behaviors. The *Comprehensive Occupational Therapy Evaluation* (COTE) (Brayman et al., 1976) evaluates reality orientation, responsibility, independence, interpersonal behaviors, and task behaviors. The *Social Interaction Scale* (Bloomer & Williams, 1987) provides a structure for observation of a patient's interpersonal skills. The *Task Checklist* (Lillie & Armstrong, 1982) provides an evaluation of developmental competencies to formulate educational goals.

2. Interest surveys assess a patient's interests and use of leisure time, provide information for vocational role change, and identify former or new hobby and recreational interests that are compatible with his functional limitations. Two interest evaluations are the *Interest Check List* (Matsutsuyu, 1969; Rogers,

Weinstein, & Figone, 1978), which includes a developmental personal narrative, and the *Leisure Activities Blank* (McKechnie, 1975).

3. The *Occupational Performance History Interview* (Kielhofner, Henry, & Walens, 1989) is relevant for patients who are experiencing profound **lifestyle** and role changes.

4. Role evaluations are interviews that evaluate a patient's ability to maintain, adapt, or discover new roles (Vause-Earland, 1991; Versluys, 1980b). Role evaluations include the *Role Checklist* (Barris, Oakley, & Kielhofner, 1988), the *Role Change Assessment* (Jackoway, Rogers, & Snow, 1987), and the *Adolescent Role Assessment* (Black, 1986).

5. Projective or expressive evaluations are helpful to those patients who have difficulty talking about or recognizing their fears and feelings. These instruments include a psychodynamic interview (Bruce & Borg, 1987) and projective evaluations to help patients with self-expression (Angel, 1981; Azima & Azima, 1959; Sheffer & Harlock, 1980; Watson, 1986).

Evaluation of Premorbid Conditions

A person's **premorbid** condition includes personality style, health and developmental status, preferred **lifestyle,** and occupational roles. A great variation between the **premorbid** and future **lifestyle** may not be acceptable to the patient and may reduce his motivation to identify acceptable alternative roles and retain belief in his personal competence. The therapist's understanding of the patient's **premorbid** condition results in the development of a meaningful treatment plan.

LIFE STAGE STATUS

Each **life stage** has its own schedule of developmental tasks and accompanying stresses that influence the patient's efforts to adapt to physical impairments and **lifestyle** changes. Two critical periods in the life cycle are adolescence and middle age. Adolescence is a time of identity crisis, concern with appearance, and involvement with developmental tasks of separation and individuation. During adolescence, an individual attains self- and sexual identity; age-appropriate interpersonal skills; and normal life choices, including vocational and career plans. When **trauma** and disability occur, the developmental process may be halted or prolonged, and there may be ensuing problems with development of a positive self-identity and dependency. Under these conditions, adolescent rebellions may take place around compliance with medications, health rules, and rehabilitation programs (Blazyk, 1983; Sutkin, 1984; Zager & Marquette, 1981).

The middle-aged patient may, at the time of the physical incident, be in the process of personal reappraisal, which may involve stresses associated with family responsibility, vocational disappointments, feelings of failure concerning original personal and career goals, the recognition of physical decline, and the inevitability of death. The patient at this stage of life may have economic and personal responsibilities to spouse, children, and parents. The patient may feel that it is too late to start reshaping life patterns and that the lifestyle adjustments and occupational changes are overwhelming (Block, Boyer, & Imes, 1984).

COMORBIDITY

Comorbidity refers to coexisting medical, psychiatric, or substance abuse problems (Farmer, 1987). The presence of psychosocial and occupational performance deficits related to a coexisting diagnosis influences the treatment plan. The therapist may need simply to recognize the coexisting problems or may need to evaluate and develop treatment goals for problems associated with the **comorbid** diagnosis as well as the physical disability for which the person was referred. This is important because patients with coexisting psychiatric diagnoses tend to have an increase in **morbidity** and length of hospitalization, to experience more physical symptoms such as pain and anxiety, and to have problems concentrating on the treatment program. Such patients may be at risk after discharge because they lack consistent **coping skills;** performance abilities, including self-care and problem solving; and social abilities, which leads to isolation. They also tend to neglect health care rules and fail to take advantage of outpatient treatment (Fulop & Strain, 1991). **Comorbid** psychiatric disorders include adjustment disorders, alcohol abuse, anxiety disorders (including phobias), posttraumatic stress disorders, psychogenic pain disorder, depression, dementia, and personality disorders (DSM-IIIR, 1987; Fulop & Strain, 1991). The following is a review of selected psychiatric diagnoses that coexist with physical **trauma** and medical illness.

Anxiety Disorders

The patient with agoraphobia or social phobia will have difficulty tolerating the environment of the hospital and difficulty managing relationships with the many health care providers that may be needed.

The patient with an obsessive-compulsive disorder may experience an increase in symptoms as a result of the anxiety associated with the **trauma** and the treatment. Constant cognitive obsessions and complicated rituals will distract these patients from the rehabilitation task.

The patient with a posttraumatic stress disorder may experience severe symptoms in reaction to a variety of prior traumatic experiences such as war, environmental disasters, and physical and sexual abuse as well as to the current accident. Symptoms can be severe, such as reexperiencing the **trauma,** emotional numbing, feelings of detachment and depression, problems with concentration and memory, panic attacks, hypervigilance, and substance abuse ("Post Traumatic," 1991). Hierholzer et al. (1992) encouraged therapists to inquire carefully about past traumatic experiences that may be reactivated by the stress of **trauma** and expressed in symptoms that are difficult to understand and that interfere with rehabilitation.

Depression

Depression is the most common **comorbid** psychiatric problem that requires treatment in physical rehabilitation settings (Cassem, 1991). Depression refers to a variety of primary and secondary disorders. Symptoms associated with depression include despondency, feelings of hopelessness and pessimism, indecisiveness, loss of interest in life, somatic complaints, and problems with concentration and memory as well as more severe symptoms such as recurrent thoughts of death or suicide and psychotic episodes (Grady & Sederer, 1991; Rodin & Voshart, 1986). Unrecognized and untreated depression is destructive because depressed patients require longer rehabilitation, have feelings of futility that block motivation, are often unable to make the mental effort to plan ahead, are pessimistic about the future, and may show self-neglect and a lower level of self-care at discharge (Cassem, 1991; Rodin & Voshart, 1986). Discrimination among the various types of depression ensures that the treatment approach is focused on the real problem.

Reactive depression is a normal and expected response to an identifiable loss, such as loss of autonomic body function, loss of familiar or pleasant sensations (e.g., sexual responses, physical activity, and sports), inability to meet work and family role obligations or to reach personal or career goals, and inability to live up to personal standards or to family and cultural values. Reactive depression is also linked to the length of hospitalization and lack of preparation for discharge. There is a concern that a state of reactive depression will become a chronic response and that the patient's self-concept may continue to be that of a disabled, dependent, and helpless person. Reactive depression is seen as normal at the beginning of the adjustment process and periodically as the patient becomes discouraged or overwhelmed, fails to progress in treatment, or remembers the losses in the form of an anniversary reaction (Tucker, 1980).

Personality Disorders

Patients with a personality disorder tend to be inflexible and impulsive, to lack **coping skills,** to fail to take responsibility, and to be unmotivated and noncompliant with treatment. In addition, they have difficulty tolerating the restrictions of hospitalization and the rules and procedures of medical treatment, such as casts, turning frames, or splints. They fail to exercise good judgment and often exacerbate their dysfunction by failure to comply with self-care procedures (Kaplan & Sadock, 1991; Sederer & Thorbeck, 1991). The most problematic personality disorders are borderline, antisocial, dependent, and passive-aggressive disorders. Groves (1991) illustrated some of the problems faced by staff in his description of the borderline patient as one who acts out violently, polarizes the staff, threatens suicide, and tries to leave the hospital against medical advice.

Alcohol Abuse

Alcohol may have played a significant role in the accident that culminated in the physical or cognitive injury. A patient's problems with alcohol often go unrecognized and untreated in a physical rehabilitation setting. Therapists may fail to detect symptoms of alcohol abuse because of a primary focus on the physical disability, the patient's defenses of denial and rationalization, or lack of knowledge about the signs and symptoms of addictions. Identification is important because alcoholism sabotages treatment success, increases **morbidity,** and compromises a successful discharge outcome ("Alcoholism," 1986; Brubeck, 1981, Greer, 1989; Moyers, 1988; Woosley, 1991). Impairments associated with chronic drinking can permanently affect judgment, muscle coordination, and sensory perceptions (Kaufman & McNaul, 1992; Renner, 1986; Smith, 1983).

Physically disabled persons have a greater than average risk of developing alcoholic problems caused by their personal losses, functional inability to release tension, problems coping with frustration, increased isolation, stigmatizing experiences, and stress related to **lifestyle** change. If alcohol abuse becomes a way of coping with the disability, there can be further injury, health problems, and hospitalizations (Brubeck, 1981; Gow, 1987; Hepner, Kirshbaum & Landes, 1980–1981; Woosley, 1991). If a patient has been abusing alcohol since early adolescence, crucial developmental skills may be arrested. Because the physically disabled patient must undertake tasks that require psychosocial maturity such as problem solving and replanning vocational roles, the alcoholic will be at a disadvantage (Hawthorne & Menzel, 1983; Niven, 1986; Scarth, 1990).

The occupational therapist is in an excellent position to identify the signs and symptoms of alcohol abuse. The therapist can include questions about drinking with questions about activities of daily living, interests, and time management. Evaluation of the patient's occupational functioning and performance components may also suggest a preexisting alcohol abuse problem. Guidelines for the analysis of evaluation data include the following (Moyers, 1988; Raymond, 1990; Scarth, 1990):

1. Lack of consistent performance in activities of daily living and work roles, including a history of work problems before the patient became physically disabled;
2. Inconsistent time management and inability to account for use of time or to describe the use of leisure time;
3. Lack of participation in age-appropriate roles;
4. History of frequent accidents and injuries;
5. Preoccupation with alcohol;
6. Behaviors such as missing appointments and disheveled appearance;
7. Problems with memory, concentration, and learning new material.

The therapist also should pay attention to additional clues to addiction such as withdrawal symptoms, which occur when the patient cannot obtain alcohol. Symptoms of withdrawal include irritability, mood swings, tremors and incoordination, and increased psychomotor activity (Cohen, Kern, & Hassett, 1986; Estes & Heinemann, 1986; Renner, 1986). Renner (1986) provided information on both informal and formal interview methods of establishing a diagnosis.

Behavioral Indications of Psychological Reactions

In resolution of the **trauma,** the patient may move through a sequence of emotional responses such as shock, disbelief, numbness, grief and mourning, anger, bargaining, preoccupation with the ensuing changes, and hope for recovery. Eventually, a reappraisal may take place in which the patient reorganizes his **lifestyle,** personal goals, and perception of his strengths and skills apart from the disability. This reappraisal period is significant; unless the patient can accept and integrate the disability into a framework for his life, he may fail to make adaptations and solve problems related to the disability. The patient may continue to use **defense mechanisms** such as denial and regression and behaviors such as withdrawal, or he may remain preoccupied with the disability (Lilliston, 1985; Russell, 1981). Illustrations of psychological reactions follow.

GRIEF

Grief and mourning are described as pain resulting from the physical, social, and occupational losses that are valued by the patient. Symptoms of grieving may be profound sadness and depression, anger, irritability, crying, preoccupation with the losses, personal disorganization, and somatic complaints of pain and discomfort (Rosenbaum & Groves, 1991; Stewart & Shields, 1985; Tucker, 1980).

ANXIETY

Anxiety is a normal response by the patient to the changes in his physical or medical condition. In a mild form, anxiety causes discomfort for the patient. In a more severe form, it interferes with rehabilitation, because the patient cannot concentrate and new learning does not take place. A patient who is experiencing intense anxiety may act in an unreliable and confusing manner, react to irrelevant cues, be unable to concentrate, be unrealistically fearful, and misinterpret events or develop false expectations. The staff may find that a patient has completely missed the point in discussions concerning his disability, the prognosis, or the goals of treatment. (This response may be caused by difficulty with the terminology or language or by denial.) In the former case, the patient is not deliberately trying to confuse or sabotage but is attempting to deal with considerable anxiety and fear (Russell, 1981). It is important for the therapist to understand the roots of the patient's anxiety reactions and to intervene so that the patient will be able to concentrate on learning new performance skills.

ANGER

Strong feelings of anger and hostility can be one of the patient's emotional responses to **trauma,** impairment, hospitalization, and the stress of treatment. Therapists can recognize anger in the sabotage of treatment objectives, in withdrawal, in depression-like symptoms, in verbal attacks, and in acting out and passive-aggressive behaviors (Cassem, 1991). The patient may express anger toward the occupational therapist who is present when the patient fails or struggles with seemingly unattainable tasks. Patients may deny their own residual disability and blame staff for incompetence or for not providing enough treatment time. Strong feelings of anger impede treatment, and continual expression of it causes rejection by family, staff, and other caretakers. It is important to identify the cause and to plan intervention (Gans, 1983).

DEPENDENCY

The development of dependent behaviors is an ever-present danger in the rehabilitation process. Dependency may be a predictable response to enforced helplessness and the hospital environment or may be based on a **premorbid** dependent personality that has been exacerbated by the situation. Some patients may also act in an unrealistically independent manner and may insist on impractical and impossible goals. These behaviors may be a defense against feelings of dependency and vulnerability. All factors associated with the hospitalization and the disability may feed into a patient's sense of helplessness, leading to continuation of dependent behaviors and failure to engage fully in rehabilitation or to cope successfully with community living after discharge. It is important that the behaviors be identified and intervention occur early in the rehabilitation process. At the same time, the therapist must be comfortable in meeting reasonable dependency needs.

DEFENSE MECHANISMS

Defense mechanisms are unconscious and anxiety-relieving processes that help restore a patient's psychological equilibrium and normalize emotional functioning. **Defense mechanisms** include acting out, denial, distortion, fantasy, intellectualization, projection, regression, and somatization. **Defense mechanisms** can be protective and transient forms of adaptation to the **trauma** or can be chronic and pathological adaptations to the residual disability (Caplan, 1981). Some common **defense mechanisms** are described below.

Denial

Denial is usually present in cases of severe disability and protects the patient from full recognition of the prognosis while he is still vulnerable and incapacitated. Denial allows the patient to integrate realities of the disability at an acceptable pace and prevents excessive anxiety and severe depression. For example, a state of temporary denial can be calming to a patient who has suffered a myocardial infarct and is in intensive care; denial can allow a spinal cord–injured patient time for therapeutic interventions that focus on identification of remaining competencies and potential for achievement. In other cases, a patient may appear well motivated in the initial stages of treatment until a plateau in functional progress is reached. At that point, the patient's denial concerning recovery is confronted by the reality of the situation. The patient may suddenly become anxious or depressed, insist that a cure is possible, regress, or become resistive to treatment (Cassem & Hackett, 1991; Kaplan & Sadock, 1991). The therapist needs to remember that states of denial vacillate. A patient may be insightful at times, but when threatened by overwhelming tasks of rehabilitation and awareness of the permanent barriers to life plans and satisfactions, he may again become denying (Felton & Revenson, 1984). In some cases, denial

reaches psychotic proportions and may be combined with fantasy and delusions. Psychiatric consultation may be necessary to help the patient regain a sense of control and to help him express the meaning of the loss and underlying sadness and grief.

Regression

Regression is an emotional and physical retreat from adult standards of independence to an earlier and less mature level of adaptation. Regressive behaviors include childlike behaviors, persistent dependency, lack of motivation, and passivity. Factors precipitating regressive behaviors may be the patient's inability to have personal control over his actions because of the rules of the medical regimen, loss of neurological control over autonomic bodily functions, enforced dependency common after major **trauma,** an unconscious attempt to escape from tensions and anxiety associated with treatment, or the patient's anger about the disability and its impact on his future. Regression can also be precipitated by a therapist who is too assertive and eager for results, pushes the patient too fast in treatment, and misses signs that he is becoming overwhelmed.

Acting Out

The patient who is acting out uses verbal or physical aggression to avoid conscious recognition of feelings of fear, sadness, or anxiety. For some patients, such behavior is more tolerable than feeling the disturbing emotions connected with loss of physical functions.

Somatization

Somatization occurs when the patient's emotional responses never reach the conscious level but are instead expressed through physical symptoms like pain, headaches, or back problems for which there is no discoverable organic cause (Kaplan & Sadock, 1991).

EVALUATION OF ANCILLARY FACTORS THAT AFFECT REHABILITATION

This section describes additional factors that are important in the patient's overall rehabilitation but are secondary to the physical treatment.

Sexuality

A major concern of the patient after traumatic injury or the onset of medical-neurological disease is to maintain his gender identity and continuing ability to function in sexual roles. Tardif (1989) urges therapists to improve rehabilitation by addressing the frequently overlooked and critical area of a patient's sexuality and sexual functioning. Sexuality is an essential part of a person's self-identity and self-esteem, whether a person is sexually active or not, married or unmarried, heterosexual or homosexual. Evaluation of physical and psychosocial problems related to sexuality is important (McCann, 1989; Neistadt & Freda, 1987). A patient's concerns may center around issues of body image and attractiveness, impotence and concerns about the loss of sexual interest, fears of death during intercourse, resumption of intercourse and anticipated limitations or changes in function, concerns about resumption of menstruation and fertility, alternative techniques and ways to experience sexual satisfaction, expressing affection, and dealing with the presence of a catheter or ostomy bag (Neistadt & Freda, 1987; Tardif, 1989). Intervention at some level is natural for occupational therapists because of the mandate to help the patient maintain a positive self-identity, enjoy life satisfaction in all functional areas, and compensate and adapt in all life areas. The therapist needs to obtain factual knowledge about sexual function and dysfunction for men and women and for each separate diagnostic category, since different disabilities pose different adjustment and adaptive problems (Garner & Allen, 1989; Neistadt & Freda, 1987).

Family

The support and encouragement of the family provides a foundation for successful rehabilitation. Families differ in their understanding of the patient's disability and their ability to manage caretaking roles or changes in the family **lifestyle.** Family members also experience stress and emotional reactions to the **trauma.** Some families are more emotionally and economically stable and can adjust to and deal with change, can solve problems, and can reorganize family life and activities. In other families, the ability to provide emotional support or caretaking services is impaired by severe stress reactions, lack of family unity and the ability to achieve consensus, intrafamily problems (including marital crisis), family member medical or psychiatric disease, and family deficits in coping and performance skills (Versluys, 1980a, 1993). The presence of strong emotional reactions in family members should not be viewed as leading to permanently dysfunctional behavior. Both the patient and the family need to express their grief and to mourn the health-related changes and losses. This enables them to come to terms with changes in future plans and **lifestyle** (Versluys, 1993).

Barriers to positive family involvement include some of the following situations.

1. Families may experience ongoing chronic stress with clinically significant symptoms of depression, fatigue, or anxiety and can also become ill themselves (Cella et al., 1988; Gans, 1983; Versluys, 1993).
2. If the patient has been noncompliant with medical and health care requirements, the family members may be angry and resentful and feel that the patient's problems are of his own making and that they should not have to be responsible (Gans, 1983; Versluys, 1993).
3. Separation and divorce can influence the care and placement of the patient, who may need to make new living arrangements.
4. Some family members may have psychological or medial problems or may abuse substances and are not dependable. In such a case, additional preparation for independence in the community will become a serious treatment objective (Power, 1985; Versluys, 1980a, 1986; Zisserman, 1981).
5. The threatening aspects of the patient's discharge and the possible need to care for a disabled family member can result in instinctive withdrawal and increased alienation. The family may avoid discharge planning, develop punitive behaviors toward the patient, and have difficulty making a steady commitment.

EVALUATION

The family can be a major force in the adjustment and rehabilitation of a family member. Studies have shown, however, that family members often do not receive sufficient information about the physical, emotional, and social effects of the patient's functional limitations or understand the adaptive tasks facing the patient. A family-centered interview gathers information about the following issues (Glennon & Smith, 1990):

1. The effect of the disability on the current **lifestyle** and needs of family members;
2. Family ethnic and religious background and values;
3. The psychological and physical home environment;
4. The performance skills needed by the patient for discharge to the home;
5. Family awareness of community resources such as respite care, professional follow-up services, independent living centers, and funding resources.

It is also important to identify those situations in which family dysfunction tends to exacerbate or maintain an illness in the patient, whether the patient is at risk for abuse, and if the family is noncompliant with health care rules related to the patient's well-being (Power, 1985; Versluys, 1980a, 1993).

Culture

The ethnic (cultural and religious) beliefs of a patient and family can differ in both obvious and subtle ways from Western treatment philosophies. These will influence how the patient and family interpret the cause of the disability, value and comply with the treatment methods, and accept the therapist's role in treating and advising (Fisher et al., 1992; Guendelman, 1983; Johnson et al., 1988; Low, 1984).

Historical beliefs about the sources of disease are still deeply ingrained in the folklore and religion of some cultural populations and have been integrated with current religious philosophies. Some patients believe in spiritualism and an invisible world of good and evil spirits. They see their illness as being caused by inappropriate activities or their failure to take protective measures against evil spirits. Patients may also believe in folk healing; herbal medicines; the curative powers of special foods, prayer ceremonies, and the laying on of hands; the power of symbolic artifacts, and protective acts and signs to remove evil spirits (Delgado, 1977). The therapist should feel comfortable that a patient may have a number of health care providers, including Western rehabilitation experts and spiritualists or traditional healers (Huttlinger et al., 1992). The **culture** also determines the people of authority in the patient's life. In some cases, cultural authority figures may direct decisions about rehabilitation and the opinions of lay healers, friends, and family may carry more weight than those of the physician or rehabilitation team (Meyers, 1992).

ROLE CHANGES

During the rehabilitation process it may become apparent that the patient must adapt or change his occupational and personal roles. In American and other Western **cultures,** treatment goals tend to stress the importance of being independent, having future plans, and working toward objectives. People often exclusively define themselves by their work roles with a strong emphasis on production and personal success. These goals are so internalized that not moving toward them can cause depression, self-blame, and hatred. Cross-culturally, these goals may not be seen as priorities or as having value (Kinebanian & Stomph, 1992). Roles may be limited by cultural definition, and some **cultures** have strict guidelines for male and female roles. A departure from an acceptable way of performing an adult role may be threatening. It may precipitate conflicts for the individual and among family members. This has implications for the treatment plan. Evaluation of role and performance skills must be culturally sensitive and age appropriate (Dillard et al., 1992; Fisher et al., 1992; Jackoway et al., 1987).

EVALUATION

In a cross-cultural evaluation, the therapist must understand the occupational performance norms and expectations within the patient's **culture** (Evans & Salim, 1992; Fisher et al., 1992; Westermeyer, 1987). Cultural variables must be considered in a therapist's analysis of the evaluative data, including the meaning of activities and tasks, the priorities for use of daily time, and the view of temporal orientations (i.e., the importance to the patient of past, present, and future events to his life) (Spadone, 1992). Westermeyer (1987) noted that without this understanding the therapist will not be able to evaluate accurately the patient's grooming, dress, speech, behavior, cognition, or affect.

SUMMARY

Before experiencing disability or illness, the patient, in most cases, had already developed a workable adaptation to life that required an investment of time and personal commitment. That adaptation included the development of a self-identity; **lifestyle;** and unique ways of achieving satisfaction from work, leisure, and social activities. Traumatic changes in a patient's occupational functioning can precipitate an identity crisis, because the recognizable self no longer exists. Each patient's accommodation to his physical and medical situation is highly individualistic. Each person has different **coping skills** and developmental experiences at his disposal for the battle of adjusting to the changes created by physical limitations or illness. It is important for the therapist to understand that many patients make successful **lifestyle** adjustments despite personal losses, disruptions of their lives, and the initial—sometimes severe—emotional reactions that the disability caused.

STUDY QUESTIONS

1. Why is consideration of psychosocial factors in the treatment of physically disabled patients important?
2. What are the types of psychosocial stress and the behavioral symptoms that may occur when a patient is traumatically disabled?
3. What role do defense mechanisms have in the patient's adjustment to trauma and disability?
4. How do premorbid factors influence a patient's response to trauma, adaptation, and rehabilitation?
5. Why is it important for the therapist to understand the influence of a patient's comorbid psychiatric diagnosis on the treatment of physical dysfunction?
6. What are the dangers of alcohol abuse for a patient with physical dysfunction? What is the role

of the occupational therapist in the evaluation of this problem?

7. What are the significant ancillary factors described in this chapter? How do these factors influence rehabilitation and adjustment to disability and life-style change?

8. What is the focus and purpose of psychosocial evaluation of a person referred for physical dysfunction? What are the different types of evaluation instruments and methods?

REFERENCES

Alcoholism as secondary disability: The silent saboteur in rehabilitation. (1986). *Rehab Brief, 5*, 1–4. (Available from Department of Education, National Institute of Handicapped Research, Office of Special Education and Rehabilitation, Washington, DC 20202)

Angel, S. L. (1981). The emotional identification group. *American Journal of Occupational Therapy, 35*, 256–262.

Azima, H., & Azima, F. J. (1959). Outline of a dynamic theory of occupational therapy. *American Journal of Occupational Therapy, 8*, 215–221.

Barris, R., Oakley, F., & Kielhofner, G. (1988). The Role Checklist. In B. Hemplill (Ed.), *Mental health assessment in occupational therapy* (pp. 73–91). Thorofare, NJ: Slack.

Black, M. (1986). Adolescent Role Assessment. *American Journal of Occupational Therapy, 30*, 73–79.

Blazyk, S. (1983). Developmental crisis in adolescents following severe head injury. *Social Work Health Care, 8*, 55–67.

Block, A. R., Boyer, S. L., & Imes, D. (1984). Personal impact of myocardial infarction: A model for coping with physical disability in middle age. In M. G. Eisenberg, L. C. Sutkin, & M. A. Jansen (Eds.), *Chronic illness and disability through the life span: Effect on self and family* (pp. 209–221). New York: Springer.

Bloomer, J. S., & Williams, S. K. (1987). *The Bay Area Functional Performance Evaluation* (2nd ed.). Palo Alto, CA: Consulting Psychologists Press.

Brayman, S. J., Kirby, T. F., Misenheimer, A. M. & Short, M. J. (1976). The comprehensive occupational therapy evaluation scale. *American Journal of Occupational Therapy, 30*, 94–100.

Brubeck, T. (1981). Alcoholism—The extra burden. *American Rehabilitation, 7*, 3–6.

Bruce, M. A., & Borg, B. (1987). *Frames of reference in psychosocial occupational therapy.* Thorofare, NJ: Slack.

Caplan, G. (1981). Mastery of stress: Psychosocial aspects. *American Journal of Psychiatry, 138*, 413–420.

Cassem, N. H. (1991). Depression. In N. H. Cassem (Ed.), *Massachusetts General Hospital handbook of general hospital psychiatry* (3rd ed., pp. 237–268). St. Louis: Mosby Year Book.

Cassem, N. H., & Hackett, T. P. (1991). The setting of intensive care. In N. H. Cassem (Ed.), *Massachusetts General Hospital handbook of general hospital psychiatry* (3rd ed., pp. 373–399). St. Louis: Mosby Year Book.

Cella, D. F., Perry, S. W., Kulchycky, S., & Goodwin, C. (1988). Stress and coping in relatives of burn patients: A longitudinal study. *Hospital and Community Psychiatry, 39*, 159–166.

Cohen, M., Kern, J. C., & Hassett, C. (1986). Identifying alcoholism in medical patients. *Hospital and Community Psychiatry, 37*, 398–400.

Delgado, M. (1977). Puerto Rican spiritualism and the social work professional. *Social Casework, 10*, 451–458.

Denton, P. L., & Skinner, S. T. (1988). Selecting a frame of reference/practice model. In S. C. Robertson (Ed.), *Focus: Skills for assessment and treatment* (Sec. 1, pp. 100–108). Rockville, MD: AOTA.

Diagnostic and statistical manual of mental disorders. (1987). (3rd ed. rev.) Washington DC: American Psychiatric Association.

Dillard, M., Andonian, L., Flores, O., Lai, L., MacRae, A., & Shakir, M. (1992). Culturally competent occupational therapy in a diversely populated mental health setting. *American Journal of Occupational Therapy, 46*, 721–726.

Estes, N. J., & Heinemann, M. E. (1986). Issues in identification of alcoholism. In N. J. Estes & M. E. Heinemann (Eds.), *Alcoholism: Development, consequences and interventions* (3rd ed., pp. 317–333). St. Louis: C. V. Mosby.

Evans, J., & Salim, A. A. (1992). A cross-cultural test of the validity of occupational therapy assessments with patients with schizophrenia. *American Journal of Occupational Therapy, 46*, 685–695.

Farmer, S. (1987). Medical problems of chronic patients in a community support program. *Hospital and Community Psychiatry, 38*, 745–749.

Felton, B. J., & Revenson, T. A. (1984). Coping with chronic illness: A study of illness controlment and the influences of coping strategies on psychological adjustment. *Journal of Consulting and Clinical Psychology, 52*, 343–353.

Fisher, A. G., Liu, Y., Velozo. C. A., & Pan, A. W. (1992). Cross-cultural assessment of process skills. *American Journal of Occupational Therapy, 46*, 876–885.

Fulop, G., & Strain, J. J. (1991). Diagnosis and treatment of psychiatric disorders in medically ill patients. *Hospital and Community Psychiatry, 42*, 389–400.

Gans, J. S. (1983). Hate in the rehabilitation setting. *Archives of Physical Medicine & Rehabilitation, 64*, 1775–1779.

Garner, W. E., & Allen, H. A. (1989, January–March). Sexual rehabilitation and heart disease. *Journal of Rehabilitation*, 69–73.

Glennon, T. P., & Smith, B. S. (1990). Questions asked by patients and their support groups during family conferences on inpatient rehabilitation units. *Archives of Physical Medicine & Rehabilitation, 71*, 699–702.

Gow, L. M. (1987, April 8) Substance abuse: An obstacle in the successful treatment of physical trauma. *Occupational Therapy Forum, 2*, 1–3.

Grady, T. A., & Sederer, L. I. (1991). Depression. In L. I. Sederer (Ed.), *Inpatient psychiatry: Diagnosis and treatment* (3rd ed., pp. 3–45). Baltimore: Williams & Wilkins.

Greer, B. G. (1989). Alcohol and other drug abuse by the physically impaired. *Alcohol Health and Research World, 13*, 144–149.

Groves, J. E. (1991). Patients with borderline personality disorders. In N. H. Cassem (Ed.), *Massachusetts General Hospital handbook of general hospital psychiatry* (3rd ed., pp. 191–215). St. Louis: Mosby Year Book.

Guendelman, S. (1983). Developing responsiveness to the health needs of Hispanic children and families. *Social Work Health Care, 8*, 1–15.

Hawthorne, W., & Menzel, N. (1983). Youth treatment should be a programming priority. *Alcohol Health & Research World, 7*, 46–48.

Hepner, R., Kirshbaum, H., & Landes, D. (1980–1981). Counseling substance abusers with additional disabilities: The center for independent living. *Alcohol Health and Research World, 5*, 5–10.

Hierholzer, R., Munson, J., Peabody, C., & Rosenberg, J. (1992). Clinical presentation of PTSD in World War II combat veterans. *Hospital and Community Psychiatry, 43*, 816–820.

Huttlinger, K., Krefting, L., Drevdahl, D., Tree, P., Baca, E., & Benally, A. (1992). "Doing battle": A metaphorical analysis of diabetes mellitus among Navajo people. *American Journal of Occupational Therapy, 46,* 706–712.

Jackoway, I. S., Rogers, J. C., & Snow, T. L. (1987). The Role Change Assessment: An interview tool for evaluating older adults. *Occupational Therapy in Mental Health, 7,* 17–37.

Johnson, T. M., Fenton, B. J., Kracht, B. R., Weiner, M. F., & Guggenheim, F. G. (1988). Providing culturally sensitive care: Intervention by a consultation-liaison team. *Hospital and Community Psychiatry, 39,* 200–203.

Kaplan, H. I., & Sadock, B. J. (1991). *Modern synopsis of psychiatry: Behavioral sciences clinical psychiatry* (6th ed.). Baltimore: Williams & Wilkins.

Kaufman, E., & McNaul, J. P. (1992). Recent developments in understanding and treating drug abuse and dependence. *Hospital and Community Psychiatry, 43,* 223–236.

Kielhofner, G., Henry, A. D., & Walens, D. (1989). *A user's guide to the Occupational Performance History Interview.* Rockville, MD: AOTA.

Kinebanian, A., & Stomph, M. (1922). Cross-cultural occupational therapy: A critical reflection. *American Journal of Occupational Therapy, 46,* 751–757.

Lillie, M. D. & Armstrong, H. E. (1982). Contributions to the development of psychoeducational approaches to mental health services. *American Journal of Occupational Therapy, 36,* 438–443.

Lilliston, B. A. (1985). Psychosocial responses to traumatic physical disability. *Social Work in Health Care, 10,* 1–14.

Low, S. M. (1984). The culture bias of health, illness and disease. *Social Work Health Care, 9,* 13–23.

Matsutsuyu, J. S. (1969). The Interest Check List. *American Journal of Occupational Therapy, 23,* 323–328.

McCann, M. E. (1989, September). Sexual healing after heart attack. *American Journal of Nursing,* 1133–1149.

McKechnie, G. E. (1975). *Leisure Activities Blank.* Palo Alto, CA: Consulting Psychologists Press.

Meyers, C. (1992). Hmong children and their families: Consideration of cultural influences in assessment. *American Journal of Occupational Therapy, 46,* 737–744.

Moyers, P. A. (1988). An organizational framework for occupational therapy in the treatment of alcoholism. *Occupational Therapy in Health Care, 8,* 27–46.

Neistadt, M. E., & Freda, M. (1987). *Choices: A guide to sex counseling with physically disabled adults.* Marabar, FL: R. E. Krieger.

Niven, R. G. (1986). Adolescent drug abuse. *Hospital and Community Psychiatry, 37,* 596–607.

Peloquin, S. M. (1986). Uniform terminology as a basis for goal formulation. *Occupational Therapy in Mental Health, 6,* 49–62.

Post traumatic stress. Part I: (1991, February). *Harvard Mental Health Letter, 7,* 1–4.

Power, P. W. (1985). Family coping behaviors in chronic illness: A rehabilitation perspective. *Rehabilitation Literature, 46,* 78–83.

Raymond, M. (1990, September). Life skills and substance abuse. *AOTA Mental Health Special Interest Newsletter, 13,* 1–2.

Renner, J. A. (1986). Alcoholism. In L. I. Sederer (Ed.), *Inpatient psychiatry: Diagnosis and treatment* (2nd ed., pp. 171–194). Baltimore: Williams & Wilkins.

Rodin, G., & Voshart, K. (1986). Depression in the medically ill: An overview. *American Journal of Psychiatry, 143,* 696–705.

Rogers, J. C. (1983). Clinical reasoning: The ethics, science, and art. *American Journal of Occupational Therapy, 37,* 601–616.

Rogers, J. E., Weinstein, J. M., & Figone, J. J. (1978). The Interest Check List: An empirical assessment. *Journal of Occupational Therapy, 32,* 628–630.

Rosenbaum, J. F., & Groves, J. E. (1991). Accident proneness and accident victims. In N. H. Cassem (Ed.), *Massachusetts General Hospital handbook of general hospital psychiatry* (3rd ed., pp. 431–444). St. Louis: Mosby Year Book.

Russell, R. A. (1981). Concepts of adjustment to disability: An overview. *Rehabilitation Literature, 42,* 330–338.

Sabshin, M. (1991). Comorbidity: A central concern of psychiatry in the 1990's. *Hospital and Community Psychiatry, 42,* 345.

Scarth, P. (1990, September 13). Services for chemically dependent adolescents. *AOTA Mental Health Special Interest Newsletter, 13*(3), 7–8.

Sederer, L. I., & Thorbeck J. (1991). Borderline character disorder. In L. I. Sederer (Ed.), *Inpatient psychiatry: Diagnosis and treatment* (3rd ed., pp. 108–140). Baltimore: Williams & Wilkins.

Sheffer, M., & Harlock, S. (1980). Tell us what your drawings say. *Occupational Therapy in Mental Health, 1,* 21–38.

Smith, J. W. (1983). Diagnosing alcoholism. *Hospital and Community Psychiatry, 34,* 1017–1012.

Spadone, R. A. (1992). Internal-external control and temporal orientation among southeast Asians and white Americans. *American Journal of Occupational Therapy, 46,* 713–719.

Stewart, T., & Shields, C. R. (1985). Grief in chronic illness: Assessment and management. *Archives of Physical Medicine & Rehabilitation, 66,* 447–450.

Sutkin, L. C. (1984). Introduction. In M. G. Eisenberg, L. C. Sutkin, & M. A. Jansen. (Eds.). *Chronic illness and disability through the life span: Effect on self and family* (pp. 1–19). New York: Springer.

Tardif, G. S. (1989). Sexual activity after a myocardial infarction. *Archives of Physical Medicine & Rehabilitation, 70,* 763–766.

Tucker, S. J. (1980). The psychology of spinal cord injury: Patient and staff interaction. *Rehabilitation Literature, 41,* 114–160.

Vause-Earland, T. (1991). Perceptions of role assessment tools in the physical disability setting. *American Journal of Occupational Therapy, 45,* 26–31.

Versluys, H. P. (1980a). Physical rehabilitation and family dynamics. *Rehabilitation Literature, 41,* 58–65.

Versluys, H. P. (1980b). The remediation of role disorders through focused group work. *American Journal of Occupational Therapy, 34,* 609–614.

Versluys, H. P. (1986). Thuishulpcentrale: A Dutch model for practical family assistance. *Rehabilitation Literature, 47*(3–4), 50–29.

Versluys, H. P. (1993). Family influences. In H. L. Hopkins & H. D. Smith (Eds.), *Willard & Spackman's occupational therapy* (8th ed., pp. 161–165). Philadelphia: J. B. Lippincott.

Watson, L. J. (1986). Psychiatric consultation-liaison in the acute physical disabilities setting. *American Journal of Occupational Therapy, 40,* 338–342.

Webster's New World Dictionary of American English. (1991). (3rd college ed.). New York: Prentice Hall.

Westermeyer, J. (1987). Clinical considerations: Cross-cultural diagnosis. *Hospital and Community Psychiatry, 38,* 160–165.

Woosley, E. (1991). Psycho-social aspects of substance abuse among the physically disabled. *American Archives of Rehabilitation Therapy, 29,* 1–4.

Zager, R. P., & Marquette, C. H. (1981). Developmental considerations in children and early adolescents with spinal cord injury. *Archives of Physical Medicine and Rehabilitation, 62,* 427–431.

Zisserman, L. (1981). The modern family and rehabilitation of the handicapped: A macrosociological view. *American Journal of Occupational Therapy, 35,* 13–20.

Therapeutic Mechanisms

What do occupational therapists do to cause a change in their patient's occupational functioning? Occupational therapy, as all rehabilitation services, is not done to a person. The patient is encouraged to bring about positive change in an incremental way, within his capacity, so that he gains a sense of success and efficacy. The change that occurs may be anatomical or physiological reorganization of tissue or may be behavioral adaptation. Occupational therapists facilitate ongoing recovery or change, using one or several of the therapeutic mechanisms described in this section. People change because they engage in occupation or activity that is meaningful to them; undergo a process of development by which new capacities and abilities are gained; learn and acquire new abilities and skills; and/or engage in a meaningful, positive relationship with a therapist who guides them toward success by motivating them, by creating a climate that inspires them to identify and solve problems, and by providing a genuine sense of caring and expectation of what is possible.

11
Purposeful Activity

Catherine A. Trombly

OBJECTIVES

After studying this chapter, the student will be able to:
1. Analyze activities to determine their value for remediation of sensorimotor impairments.
2. Determine whether an activity is within the capabilities of a particular person.
3. Select activities to achieve particular goals.
4. Grade activities to challenge the person's abilities to improve performance.
5. Adapt activities to increase their therapeutic value or to bring the activity within the capability of a person.

Occupation is the unique medium of occupational therapy (National Society for the Promotion of Occupational Therapy, 1917; Reilly, 1962). Occupation has been defined as "chunks of culturally and personally meaningful activity in which humans engage that can be named in the lexicon of the culture" (Clark et al., 1991, p. 301). These are the ordinary and familiar things that people do everyday (e.g., dress, garden, do puzzles, etc.). Another definition of occupation is the relationship between **occupational form** (task and context) and **occupational performance** (doing) (Nelson, 1988). The terms *occupation* and *purposeful activity* are used interchangeably by most therapists, although there is strong advocacy for *occupation* (Clark et al., 1991; Darnell & Heater, 1994; West, 1984). The Commission on Practice discriminated between occupation and purposeful activity: It defined occupation as active participation in self-maintenance, work, leisure, and play and defined purposeful activity as goal-directed behaviors or tasks that comprise occupations (American Occupational Therapy Association [AOTA], 1993). Occupation is appropriate to use when considering the integrative level of therapy where all the person's abilities, motivations, and goals come together to enable role performance. Purposeful activity

is circumscribed; it demands particular responses and is used to facilitate change in impairments and functional limitations.

The occupational therapist designs activity experiences to translate therapeutic theories and principles that apply to the particular patient's source of dysfunction into concrete tasks that will promote behavior away from dysfunction toward function (Cynkin, 1979; Tsai, 1993). Adaptations to self occur as a result of engaging in activity (Darnell & Heater, 1994; Nelson, 1988; Peloquin, 1988). Occupational therapists believe that a person develops cognitive, perceptual, psychosocial, and motor skills through engagement in activity of interest and purpose, but this assumption has hardly been researched (Ramsbey, 1993). Tables 11.1 and 11.2 suggest that the assumption might have veracity, but that much more research is needed.

To determine what the therapeutic purposes may be, the therapist analyzes activities. Based on these analyses, the therapist selects an activity expected to implement the immediate treatment goal for the particular patient. Adaptations of the activity to develop its potential value to meet the goal may be necessary. Guidelines for **activity analysis,** selection, and adaptation to remediate sensorimotor and cognitive-perceptual impairments and functional limitations are presented below. Persons with physical disabilities will not only need to develop cognitive-perceptual and motor skills but may also need to develop psychosocial skills. However, the theory of activity used for this purpose exceeds the scope of this volume and the reader is referred to textbooks concerning remediation of psychosocial components of occupational function.

ACTIVITY ANALYSIS

Activity analysis, or **task analysis,** is one of the key process skills of occupational therapists. **Activity analysis** developed from industrial time and motion study methods made famous by the Gilbreths in

GLOSSARY

Activity analysis—A process by which properties inherent in a given activity, task, or occupation may be gauged for their ability to elicit individual motivation and to fulfill patient needs in occupational performance and performance components (Llorens, 1993).

Constraints—Limitations imposed on purposeful movement or the completion of occupational performance. Extrinsic constraints include the physical and sociocultural environment and task demands. Intrinsic constraints include biomechanical and neuromuscular aspects of a person's body.

Coordinative structures—A combination of muscles (and their actions) and joints (and their stabilization or mobilization) that organize themselves so that the CNS has to control the fewest degrees of freedom necessary; then they dissolve their organization. Opposite to neuromotor synergies or pathological synergies described by Brunnstrom (see Chapter 24C) in which muscles always work together in a given pattern.

Dynamical systems theory (of motor control)—A theory of movement organization that originated from dynamical (nonlinear) systems theory developed from the study of chaotic systems. It proposes that the order and pattern of movement to accomplish a goal emerges from the interaction of multiple, nonhierarchical subsystems, e.g., biomechanical and neuromuscular constraints (coordinative structures), environmental constraints (context), and task constraints (demand) (Kamm, Thelen, & Jensen, 1990; see also Chapters 7 and 25B).

Electromyographic—Relates to the process of recording the electrical activity produced by a contracting muscle. When a muscle is at rest, no activity is recorded. As the muscle contracts, the electrical activity increases proportionately.

HRmax—Maximum heart rate. Usually calculated as 220 – age. Exercise is often limited to 65 to 85% of HRmax.

Kinematic—Relates to spatial and temporal description of movement measured by optoelectric or videographic instruments. Position data are available for every 1/100 sec (or designated time sampling). Velocity (speed) and acceleration (rate of change of speed) can be mathematically derived from positional data and allow detection of strategies for the organization of movement.

Occupational form—Environmental context in which the performance takes place (DeKuiper et al., 1993).

Occupational performance—Active response to purposeful activity developed from occupational form (DeKuiper et al., 1993).

Task analysis—Same as activity analysis; term used primarily in relation to work assessment (ergonomics) (see Chapter 17) or human factors engineering.

Table 11.1. Evidence for Effectiveness of Purposeful Activity to Remediate Physical Impairments or Disabilities

Study	Subjects	Activity	Dependent Variable	Outcome
Sietsema et al. (1993)	20 adults with brain injury	Single-purpose(rote armreach exercise) versus dual-purpose (Simon, a computer-controlled game)	Distance from hip to wrist during active reach	$t(19) = 5.77$ $P < .001$ Dual-purpose more effective

Cheaper by the Dozen (Gilbreth, 1948). The Gilbreths proposed application of these methods to rehabilitation of injured soldiers and the approach was adopted by the military occupational therapists during World War I (Creighton, 1992). The components of analysis of activity for remediation of motor impairments were put forth by Licht (1947). His "kinetic" analysis was a reaction to "craft" analysis, which focused on the craft rather than the process, which is the therapeutic aspect of activity.

Using an analytical approach, the therapist examines an activity to determine the components of the activity and the level of capability that they demand.

The analysis should occur within some conceptual framework to give it direction, coherence, and meaning (Mosey, 1981). For example, planting a tulip bulb in a plant pot can be analyzed from various frames of reference. The biomechanical approach would prompt the therapist to examine the physical aspects, such as grasp and range of motion (ROM), whereas the model of human occupation may focus the therapist's attention to examining how the patient's nurturing needs and values may be met by this activity. Some activity analyses have been published: Hi-Q game (Neistadt et al., 1993); macramé (Chandani & Hill, 1990); planting a small garden (Nelson, 1988); using a computer for skill development, education, and prevocational training (Okoye, 1988); hand activities (Trombly & Cole, 1979); and bilateral inclined sanding (Spaulding & Robinson, 1984).

Activity analysis presupposes that activities have inherent therapeutic aspects that can be reliably identified. Llorens (1986) interpreted her data "to support the concept that tasks, activities, and occupation components possess inherent factors" (p. 103). However, a recent survey of 120 experienced therapists indicated that consensus on the sensorimotor, cognitive-perceptual, or psychosocial components involved in particular activities was limited (Tsai, 1994). Neistadt et al. (1993) also reported discrepancies among therapists in identifying components of common activities. Much research on **activity analysis** and the inherent qualities of activities is necessary (Trombly & Quintana, 1983).

Analyzing for Sensorimotor Goals

Among other goals, occupational therapists who work with physically disabled persons, use purposeful activity to provide exercise to remediate physical impairments or functional limitations secondary to disruptions of voluntary movement. Organization of voluntary movement depends both on the unique problem or goal and the **constraints** operating at a given time (Granit, 1977) (Fig. 11.1).

GOAL OR OBJECTIVE

Goals are motor problems, e.g., to lift a cup, to comb the hair, to pick up a quarter. According to Jeannerod (1988), the interaction between subject and goal produces movement that is specific to the unique requirements that arise from that interaction. The purpose, goal, or objective organizes movement in terms of strategy. Strategies are general plans for movement

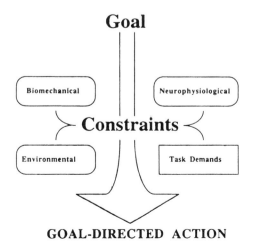

Goal

Biomechanical   Neurophysiological

Constraints

Environmental   Task Demands

GOAL-DIRECTED ACTION

Figure 11.1. Organization of goal-directed movement.

(Horak, 1991). There are two motor strategies: open loop (preplanned) and closed loop (guided).

Few studies have been done to study the effect of a goal on movement organization, and these were done outside the profession. Fisk and Goodale (1989), Adam (1992), and Marteniuk et al. (1987) showed that the objective of a movement (i.e., the performer's intent or his effort to achieve something) has important consequences on the strategy of the movement. In fact, Marteniuk et al. demonstrated that different movement strategies were used for reaches to the same object but for two different goals. One goal was to pick up a 4-cm disc and place it in a slot, and the other goal was to pick it up and throw it. Although the reach to the disc was "exactly the same" in terms of **constraints**, i.e., distance (30 cm), direction, environment, actual disc, **kinematic** analysis showed significant differences.

Recent research has also verified the effect of external **constraints** or context on motor behavior (Table 11.2). Persons of various ages and states of health who engaged in materials-based (contextually complete) activity received more benefit than those who engaged in context-free (objectless, rote) exercise. An **activity analysis** identifies or specifies the minimal necessary **constraints** that would support a given goal.

CONSTRAINTS

Constraints arise from the extrinsic limitations imposed by the environment and the task and from the intrinsic limitations imposed by the biomechanical and neurophysiological characteristics of the actor (Adam, 1992; Fisk & Goodale, 1989; Marteniuk et al., 1987). The extrinsic **constraints** constitute the context in which the goal is to be achieved, and the intrinsic **constraints** form what are called **coordinative structures,** using a term of the **dynamical systems theory of motor control.**

Environment

Environmental **constraints** refer to the physical and social surround in which the goal-directed action is being carried out. Contrast the environmental **constraints** of eating a lobster dinner in a fancy restaurant with a business associate or potential mother-in-law versus eating it at a clambake with your friends. Prior experience in an environment, including particular people, provides an individual with knowledge that serves to modify the **constraints** usually imposed by an environment. This constraint, therefore, varies between attempts at the same goal.

Task

Task **constraints** refer to the size, orientation, texture, weight, etc. of objects and tools used in ac-

Table 11.2. Evidence for Effectiveness of Purposeful Activity to Affect Physical Parameters[a]

Study	Subjects	Activity	Dependent Variables	Outcome	Comments
Kircher (1984)	26 adult females	Purposeful (jumping rope) versus nonpurposeful (jumping in place)	HR Exercise duration	$t(24) = 3.31$; $P = .001$ $t(24) = 1.90$; NS	Both groups jumped to same level of perceived exertion Concluded that S's performed harder for purposeful

Steinbeck (1986)	15 male and 15 female undergraduates	Purposeful (UE: squeeze bulb Ping-Pong ball; LE: pedaling to operate drill press) versus nonpurposeful (UE: squeeze bulb—no game or goal; LE: cycle ergometer)	HR
			  UE
			  LE
			Repetitions
			  UE
			  LE
			EMG
			  UE
			  LE
				
				$t = 2.60$; $P = .05$
				$t = -2.17$; $P = .05$
				
				$t = 2.26$; $P = .05$
				$t = 4.32$; $P < .001$
				
				$t = 2.89$; $P = .05$
				$t = -0.23$; NS
					Stopped all activities at same level of perceived exertion
					Concluded that S's performed more repetitions for purposeful because of interest
					HR and EMG showed S's performed harder for UE purposeful

Miller and Nelson (1987)	30 female college students	Single-purpose (stirring dough for exercise) versus dual-purpose (stirring dough to make cookies)	Repetitions
			Duration
			Osgood Semantic Differential
			  evaluation
			  power
			  action
				$F(1,26) = 4.1$; $P = .052$
				NS
				
				$F(1,26) = 14.3$; $P < .001$
				NS
				NS
					Grasp strength used as covariate for repetitions and duration
					S's received cookie and smelled cookies
					Concluded dual-purpose more motivating

Thibodeaux and Ludwig (1988)	15 occupational therapy students	Product-oriented (sanding a cutting board to keep) versus nonproduct-oriented (sanding for no reason)	HR Duration	NS NS	S's enjoyed product-oriented more S's who preferred product-oriented worked longer than others ($P = 0.25$)
Heck (1988)	30 male and female college students	Purposeful (mark X in a pattern on paper as much as possible before told to stop) versus purposeless (trace X repeatedly—no mark)	Duration of tolerance to pain (electrical stimulation) HR Peripheral skin temperature	$t(19) = 2.49$; $P = .02$ NS NS	S's created own diversion for purposeless activity Concluded S's tolerated pain more for purposeful
Bloch, Smith, and Nelson (1989)	30 female college students	Purposeful (jumping rope) versus nonpurposeful (jumping in place)	HR Duration Preference Osgood Semantic Differential	$t(29) = 2.72$; $P = .01$ $t(29) = -1.92$; $P = .06$ NS NS	Alarm sounded if HR exceeded 85% **HRmax** Concluded that added-purpose causes perception at higher level of exertion
Yoder, Nelson, and Smith (1989)	30 elderly nursing home residents	Single-purpose (rotary arm exercise) versus dual-purpose (same exercise to stir dough to make cookies)	Frequency of rotations Discontinuities Duration	$U = 58.5$; $P = .012$ NS not tested; correlated with frequency	Concluded purposeful more motivating Baking items were in view; S's added flavoring

Riccio, Nelson, and Bush (1990)	27 elderly nursing home residents	Imaginary goal (reach up to pick apples; reach down to pick up coins) versus exercise (reach up; bend down)	Repetitions
			  up
			  down
				
				$z = 2.25$; $P = .012$
				NS
					Outcome confounded by order effect for reaching down
					"Picking apples" motivates more than exercise

van der Weel, van der Meer, and Lee (1991)	9 children (CP-hemi) 12 matched controls	Concrete goal (bang drum) versus abstract goal (try to duplicate passive movement) versus passive	Range of motion CP controls	 $t(8) = 6.751$; $P < .0001$ $t(11) = 0.659$; NS	Concluded drum (context) helped CP children to organize movement

Table 11.2. Continued.

Study	Subjects	Activity	Dependent Variables	Outcome	Comments
Bakshi, Bhambhani, and Madill (1991)	20 female college students	Most preferred activity from eight choices versus least preferred	HR Blood pressure Perceived exertion Repetitions	$F = 8.0$; $P = .01$ NS $F = 17.5$; $P < .001$ NS	HR lower for preferred and purposeful Perceived exertion less for preferred Concluded stress greater during nonpurposeful
		Purposeful full context) versus nonpurposeful (partial context)	HR Blood pressure Perceived exertion Repetitions	$F = 16.9$; $P < .001$ NS NS NS	
Morton, Barnett, and Hale (1992)	30 middle-aged adult volunteers	Added-purpose (exercise to lift weight to ring bell as many times as possible) versus single-purpose (same, no bell)	Repetitions Task duration HR	NS NS NS	HR limited to 85% **HRmax** Inadequate purpose
Lang, Nelson, and Bush (1992)	15 elderly nursing home residents	Materials-based (kicking a balloon) versus imaginary-based (pretend to kick a balloon) versus rote exercise (kicking the leg)	Repetitions	$F(2,28) = 6.62$; $P = .004$	S's comments suggest materials-based more motivating Materials-based more than other two; imagery and exercise showed no significant difference
King (1993)	140 hand-injured clients (80 grip; 60 pinch)	Purposeful (computer game) versus nonpurposeful (exercise; same control device)	Repetitions grip pinch	$t = 3.71$; $P < .001$ $t = 1.87$; $P < .05$	Concluded purposeful more motivating
Wu (1993)	37 female college students	Materials-based (reach to pick up pen to write name) versus imagery-based (pretend to do this) versus rote exercise (reach arm forward)	Kinematics movement units movement time reaction time displacement	$F(1,62) = 11.51$; $P = .0007$ $F(1,62) = 10.93$; $P = .0008$ $F(1,62) = 14.48$; $P = .0002$ $F(1,62) = 19.05$; $P = .0003$ effect sizes: $r = 0.64–0.74$	Concluded movement better organized in materials-based condition Movement better organized for exercise than imagined goal
DeKuiper, Nelson, and White (1993)	28 elderly nursing home residents	Material-based (kick balloon) versus imagery-based (pretend to kick balloon) versus rote exercise (kick as demonstrated)	Repetitions Distance foot raised Speed (cm/sec)	$F(2,54) = 12.1$; $P < .001$ NS NS	Concluded that embedding exercise within occupation enhances performance
Yuen et al. (1994)	52 male college students	Object use (use flashlight to trace design with training prosthesis) versus no object use (practice moving in prosthesis)	Accuracy (trace maze; deviation from line = score) Speed to trace maze	$U = 225.5$; $P = .02$ NS	Concluded motor learning improved with use of object

^aHR, heart rate; NS, not significant; S's, subjects; UE, upper extremity; LE, lower extremity; CP, cerebral palsy.

complishing the goal. The distance between objects and the actor also are task **constraints.** Task **constraints** are those aspects that are considered in **activity analysis** when determining the inherent demands of an activity. They are givens and can be set up to present the same constraint to each person.

Biomechanical

Biomechanical **constraints** refer to the motion available at various joints, the torques that can be generated around each joint, the weight of the limb alone and with tools, the viscoelasticity or length-tension relationships, and the effect of gravity. These vary with time, positioning, effects of prior movement, and so forth.

Neurophysiological

Neurophysiological **constraints** include the speed that sensory information can be translated into a motor act, the activation of motor units to produce required torques, and the coactivation or reciprocal activation of muscles. There is good evidence that the same goal can be accomplished effectively by a wide variety of muscle combinations and movement patterns (Horak, 1991; Morasso & Zaccaria, 1986; Newell & Corcos, 1993). That is how the central nervous system works—it sees the goal within an environmental context, assesses the resources in relation to the demand (muscles of a given strength needed to provide the necessary forces, etc.), and activates what is necessary to achieve the goal, given the resources. Furthermore, the nervous system undergoes reorganization as the result of experience. Therefore, this constraint is highly variable.

Analysis Procedures

Whereas the process of biomechanical analysis examines joint range of motion and muscle contraction used to carry out the activity, contemporary thinking about human movement based on **electromyographic** (EMG) and **kinematic** research indicates that this may be invalid because of individual differences in muscle action and differences in movement strategies secondary to learning, maturation, and perception of goal. So the idea that doing a certain activity will always exercise a certain weak muscle may be too naive. If it is essential that a particular muscle of a particular patient be contracting to a certain level of activity, as may be the case in tendon transfer rehabilitation, then it is best to monitor the muscle directly using EMG biofeedback while the patient does the activity.

Because new concepts about human movement control are only in the beginning stage of development and because sensorimotor activity analyses has barely been researched, by default the traditional biomechanical **activity analysis** will be described here. The therapist begins the analysis by stating the goal and by establishing the exact placement of the selected tools and equipment in relation to the patient. Changes in the equipment, supplies, or placement change the task demands. The steps of an activity are identified. For example, the steps of vacuuming the carpet while standing are (1) obtain the vacuum cleaner from the closet, (2) unwind the cord, (3) plug the cord into the wall, (4) push the vacuum back and forth, (5) unplug it and wind up the cord, and (6) return the vacuum to the closet. The potential repetitions of each motion are noted. Only step 4 would be analyzed further because it is the repetitive, therapeutic aspect of this activity. The other steps occur too infrequently to be therapeutic. Each repetitive step is then subdivided into motions. For example, pushing the vacuum back and forth involves shoulder flexion with elbow extension, shoulder extension with elbow flexion, and trunk flexion and extension, although trunk movement could be eliminated depending on how the person moved in relation to the machine. Wrist stabilization (cocontraction) in extension and cylindrical grasp are also "motions" associated with vacuuming.

The range of each of the motions is estimated by observing another person or doing the activity oneself. Each motion is further analyzed to determine which muscle(s) are likely responsible, based on anatomical, kinesiological, and **electromyographic** knowledge. By examining the effect of gravity, the minimal strength necessary to do the motion can be estimated. The kind of contraction demanded for each muscle group in each motion is established by definition. Table 11.3 facilitates the analysis of activities using the traditional biomechanical approach by structuring the components to be examined. Table 11.4 illustrates activity analysis using the vacuuming example.

Other methods of analysis have been published. Cubie (1985) used the model of human occupation to analyze the inherent qualities (occupational analysis) and potential as therapeutic media (clinical occupational analysis) of activities. Gentile (1987) described analyses of movement types and environmental **constraints.** Neistadt et al. (1993) published a model for analyzing activities in relation to cognitive and perceptual demands. Davis and Burton (1991) proposed the *Ecological Task Analysis* based on Gibson's (1977) ecological theory of perception and on current theories of motor development and control. They developed the *Ecological Task Analysis* for use in adaptive physical education, but it may prove useful in the future as the task-oriented approach is developed (see Chapters 7 and 25B). Clark, Czaja, and Weber (1990) described **task analysis** used by human factor engineers. They

Table 11.3. Biomechanical Activity Analysis

1. Name the activity (goal):
2. List the steps:
3. What capacities and abilities are prerequisite to successful accomplishment of this activity?
4. Describe the external (contextual) constraints:
   a. Task constraints: how are the person and the materials positioned, especially in relation to one another?
   b. Task constraints: what utensils/tools/materials are normally used to do this activity?
   c. Environmental constraints: where is this activity usually carried out?
   d. Environmental constraints: does this activity, or how it is done, hold particular meaning for certain cultures or social roles?
5. Describe the internal constraints for step _____:

Motions	ROM	Primary Muscles	Gravity Assists/ Resists/ No Effect	Minimal Strength Required	Type of Contraction

6. What must be stabilized to enable certain patients to do this activity and how will that stabilization be provided?
7. For which ages is this activity appropriate?
8. What is the estimated MET level of this activity?[a]
9. What precautions must be considered when using this activity?
10. For which short-term goal(s) would this activity be appropriate?
11. How can this activity be graded to increase:
    a. strength?
    b. active range of motion?
    c. passive range of motion?
    d. coordination/dexterity?
    e. endurance?
    f. reduce edema?

[a]See Chapters 6 and 43.

analyzed the inherent characteristics of activities to identify those aspects of activities needing adaptation to meet limited capabilities of community-living elderly people.

The therapist who is skilled in **activity analysis** can more easily select the most appropriate activity from those that are available and are of interest to the patient. Such skill is developed through practice.

ACTIVITY SELECTION

Activities that meet each goal of the patient's program are considered. The best activity is one that intrinsically demands the exact response that has been determined to need improvement and that allows incremental gradations starting where the patient can experi-

ence success. Contrived methods of doing an ordinary activity to make it therapeutic may diminish the value of the activity in the eyes of the patient. Contrived methods also require the patient constantly to focus his attention directly on the process rather than the end purpose of the activity.

Activities selected to restore motor function must also take the person's cognitive and perceptual abilities, emotional status, and interests into consideration. Some cognitive aspects of the activity to be considered include the number and complexity of the steps involved in doing the activity, the requirements for organization and sequencing of the steps or stimuli, and the amount of concentration and memory required. Some perceptual factors to be considered are whether the activity requires the patient to distinguish figure from ground, position in space, construct a two- or three-dimensional object, or follow verbal or spatial directions. Other cognitive/perceptual considerations are found in Chapters 26 and 27. Some psychosocial aspects of an activity that may be important to patients include whether the activity must be done alone or in a group, the length of time required to complete the activity, whether fine detailed work or large expansive movements are involved, how easily errors can be corrected, the view of the activity from the person's particular cultural and social background, and the likelihood of producing a satisfying outcome.

Generally, activities should (1) have the necessary inherent characteristics to evoke the desired response, (2) allow gradation of response to progress the patient to the next higher level of function, (3) be within the patient's capabilities, (4) be meaningful to the person, and (5) be as repetitive as required to evoke the therapeutic benefit.

Characteristics of Activity and Gradation of Response

Some specific characteristics for the goals commonly addressed by occupational therapists who treat persons with physical disabilities are listed here. The dimensions along which the activity needs to be graded also are listed; when more than one dimension is listed, the therapist should be careful to grade the changes in one dimension at a time so that the patient has more of a chance at success.

TO RETRAIN SENSORY AWARENESS AND/OR DISCRIMINATION

The activity must provide components that offer a variety of textures, shapes, and sizes, graded from large, distinct, common shapes to small, less common shapes with less distinct differences between them. The texture of the various objects needs to be graded

Table 11.4.   Example of a Biomechanical Activity Analysis

1. **Name the activity (goal):** Vacuuming the hallway carpeting using a lightweight vacuum with a 25-foot cord.
2. **List the steps:**
   1. Obtain the vacuum cleaner from the closet
   2. Unwind the cord
   3. Plug cord into wall; turn vacuum on
   4. Push the vacuum back and forth
   5. Unplug it and wind the cord
   6. Return the vacuum to the closet
3. **What capacities and abilities are prerequisite to successful accomplishment of this activity?**
   1. Standing balance
   2. Ability to bend over and straighten up
   3. Ability to grasp
   4. Ability to walk forward and backward on carpeting
   5. Ability to move dominant arm against gravity and moderate resistance
   6. Vision[a]
4. **Describe the external (contextual) constraints:**
   a. **Task constraints: how are the person and the materials positioned, especially in relation to one another?**
      * The vacuum is located in a closet next to the area to be cleaned
      * The electrical plug is located halfway between the two ends of the hallway, 5 inches from the floor
      * When vacuuming, the person will be directly behind the machine
   b. **Task constraints: what utensils/tools/materials are normally used to do this activity?**
      * A lightweight vacuum
   c. **Environmental constraints: where is this activity usually carried out?**
      tb The hallway is 30 feet long, 3 feet wide
      * No furniture is in the way
      * The carpet is a flat weave
   d. **Environmental constraints: does this activity, or how it is done, hold particular meaning for certain cultures or social roles?**
      * The person takes pride in a cleanly vacuumed home
      * Not willing to switch to a nonmotorized carpet sweeper
5. **Describe the internal constraints for step _____4_:**

Motions	ROM	Primary Muscles	Gravity Assists/ Resists/ No Effect	Minimal Strength Required	Type of Contraction
shoulder flexion	0–75°	anterior deltoid corabobrachi-alis pectorals major	resists	G – to G	concentric
elbow extension	90–0°	triceps	assists	G – to G	concentric
scapular protraction	1.5 in.	serratus anterior	no effect	G – to G	concentric
shoulder extension	0–45°	posterior deltoid latissimus dorsi teres major	assists no effect resists	G – to G G – to G G – to G G – to G	concentric concentric concentric concentric
elbow flexion	90–120°	biceps brachialis	resists	G – to G G – to G	concentric concentric
scapular retraction	1.5 in.	middle trapezius	no effect	G – to G	concentric
cylindrical grasp		extensors flexors interossei	no effect	G – to G G – to G	isometric isometric
wrist stabilize		all wrist muscles	no effect	G – to G	isometric
trunk flexion	0–30°	back extensors	assists	F+ to G–	eccentric
trunk extension	30–0°	back extensors	resists	G – to G	concentric

Table 11.4. Continued

6. **What must be stabilized to enable certain patients to do this activity and how will that stabilization be provided?**
   - nothing
7. **For which ages is this activity appropriate?**
   - 18+ years primarily
   - 10–17 years secondarily
8. **What is the estimated MET level of this activity?**
   - 2–3 METs
9. **What precautions must be considered when using this activity?**
   - depends on how good the prerequisite abilities (#3) are
10. **For which short-term goal(s) would this activity be appropriate?**
    - strengthening of upper extremity musculature
    - develop functional balance
    - improve grip strength
    - improve central and peripheral endurance
    - learn proper back mechanics
11. **How can this activity be graded to increase:**
    a. **strength?**
       - heavier vacuum
       - thicker carpet
    b. **active range of motion?**
       - at limit
    c. **passive range of motion?**
       - not applicable
    d. **coordination/dexterity?**
       - place furniture in the area
    e. **endurance?**
       - increase amount of carpeting vacuumed (more rooms)
    f. **reduce edema?**
       - not applicable

ªThe blind person needs to use adaptive methods for knowing which sections of the carpet have been cleaned and which have not.

from diverse, coarse materials to similar, smooth materials. The patient and the therapist must also involve themselves in a teaching/relearning interactive experience in which the characteristics of the objects are discussed and correct identification by touch rewarded.

TO DECREASE HYPERSENSITIVITY

The activity should involve objects or media whose textures can be graded from one that the patient perceives to be least noxious to textures perceived to present increasing challenges. Another plan grades textures and objects from soft to hard to rough and the contact with the objects from touching them to rubbing them to tapping them.

TO NORMALIZE TONE

The activity must involve controlled (location, intensity, duration) sensory experiences. To facilitate hypotonic musculature, activating tactile, proprioceptive, and/or thermal facilitatory stimuli offered to the particular muscle group(s) should be a prominent feature of the activity. To inhibit hypertonic musculature, the activity should offer soothing sensory stimulation to the target muscle group(s) or to the patient as a whole.

TO REACQUIRE MATURATIONALLY BASED POSTURAL AND MOVEMENT PATTERNS

The activity should elicit righting reactions and/or increasingly challenge equilibrium reactions. Activities that require the patient to reach or use the hands bilaterally in space will evoke equilibrium reactions. To develop stability (or decrease mobility), the activity should offer resistance to axial or proximal limb musculature and/or demand weight bearing. Grading should be along a continuum of increased duration of the holding response. As stability responses are learned, activity choice or adaptation should allow increasing amounts of controlled movement of the stabilized joints. To develop mobility, the activity should offer little or no resistance and be gradable to demand increasing control of whole body movement, gross movement of the limbs, and then control of movement at specific joints.

TO REACQUIRE SKILLED VOLUNTARY MOVEMENT

The activity must have a clear goal or purpose and offer opportunity to self-monitor success (feedback). The environmental and task **constraints** should support natural responses. Grading should provide increasingly more difficult motor challenges (e.g., moving the body in various directions, moving the limbs in various directions, isolated movement of particular joints, faster movement, and more accurate movement). Opportunities for vast amounts of varied practice should be provided to enable learning to occur.

TO INCREASE COORDINATION AND DEXTERITY

The activity should allow as much range of motion as the patient can control and allow grading from slow, gross motions to the point at which the patient is able to function to more precise, faster movements. At first, if you are grading along the continuum of increasing speed, expect accuracy to suffer. A speed/accuracy trade-off is basic to the organization of the central nervous system (CNS), expressed by Fitts' law (Fitts, 1954).

TO INCREASE ACTIVE RANGE OF MOTION

The activity must require that the part of the body being treated move to its limit repeatedly and be gradable, naturally or through adaptations, to demand greater amounts of movement as the patient's limit changes.

TO INCREASE PASSIVE RANGE OF MOTION (ELONGATE SOFT TISSUE CONTRACTURE)

The activity must provide controlled stretch or traction to the part being treated for a defined period of time. See Chapter 22 for precautions.

TO INCREASE STRENGTH

Stress to muscle tissue can be graded by increasing the velocity and/or resistance needed to complete the task and by increasing the number of repetitions of an isotonic contraction or the amount of time an isometric contraction is held.

TO INCREASE CARDIOPULMONARY ENDURANCE

The metabolic demand of the activity should match the patient's current status. The demand can be graded by increasing the duration a task is done, by increasing the frequency of doing a particular task, by changing the muscles used in the task, or by increasing the intensity. The metabolic intensities (MET levels) of some activities have been measured and are listed in Chapter 43.

TO INCREASE MUSCULAR ENDURANCE

The activity must be repetitious over a controlled number of times or period of time. Resistance should be held to 50% or less of maximal strength.

TO DECREASE EDEMA

The activity should involve repetitive isotonic contractions of the muscles in the edematous part. An activity that requires repeated movement of the extremity into an elevated position would be beneficial in helping to drain the fluid out of the extremity.

TO IMPROVE PROBLEM-SOLVING STRATEGIES

The activity should involve varied practice of information processing or perceptual processing at the outside edge of the person's capability. For example, if the person has impaired figure/ground skill, practice may start with detecting one figure from a plain background and progress through finding multiple figures on a plain background or finding one figure in more complex backgrounds until the person has developed the level of functional ability he requires (e.g., able to find the scissors in the kitchen "junk" drawer). Gradation is along a continuum of increasing complexity (more stimuli). See Chapters 26 and 27 for suggestions for particular impairments.

Be Within the Patient's Capabilities

When selecting an activity, the therapist matches the particular patient's capabilities to the demand level of the activity. If an activity or task should be part of the patient's daily life, then the comparison between task demands and patient capabilities determines whether the patient will be able to do the activity independently, with adaptation, or not at all. If an activity is to be used to restore one or more abilities, then the activity must challenge that patient's present level of ability so that through effort and/or practice the patient improves.

An individual attempting a new task, analyzes the task himself according to his resources (intrinsic **constraints**). Based on this analysis, the person will either engage in the task as defined, alter the task to meet his resources, or withdraw (i.e., refuse treatment) (Higgins, 1991). The perception of self-efficacy (belief in one's personal capabilities to perform in a given situation) is a major factor in motivation to engage in therapy (Bandura, 1982; Lewthwaite, 1990). Csikszentmihalyi (1990) offered a useful guideline for therapists in his theory of flow. Flow is defined as the state that exists when an individual is engaged in (lost in) an activity that is intrinsically rewarding to him. To achieve this state, the person's skills must match the situational challenges posed by the activity and the challenge of the activity must match the person's skills. The key is to provide a task with enough interest to provoke the person into attempting it and to graduate the task demands so that they challenge, but not overwhelm, the person's estimate of his resources, and allow successful completion.

Be Meaningful

Kielhofner (1985) defined meaningfulness as "an individual's disposition to find importance, security, worthiness, and purpose in particular occupations" (p. 505). Meaningful has both overarching and immediate aspects. It is the former that is considered when discussing work activities and leisure pursuits that are valued over the years and contribute to the definition of a person's life. Choice to participate in an activity at the moment represents immediate motivation that is guided by currently perceived needs, feelings, and desires that may or may not be related to life goals. Fun is immediately motivating, but the fun aspect of activity has been reported only anecdotally. For example, Hampton (1993) reported use of pumpkin carving at Halloween to remediate wrist range of motion and grip strength. Project Magic (1985) uses magic tricks as therapy.

Although the therapist may determine what seems to be the ideal therapeutic activity to accomplish a particular goal, it would be inappropriate to assign that activity to the patient. The patient should be allowed to choose an activity from several that can be similarly effective. If he chooses the activity, it is more likely that he will be committed to doing it for therapeutic purposes.

Be Repetitive

Sensorimotor learning requires practice. The activity may provide an opportunity for practice simply through the accomplishment of the intended goal. For example, weaving requires multiple passes of the shuttle to produce the desired product and offers good practice of bilateral horizontal abduction and adduction. For other activities, the goal may quickly be achieved; and practice is sought through repetition of the whole action, e.g., ironing, polishing the silverware, and other basic activities of daily living (BADL) and instrumental activities of daily living (IADL) tasks. Variable practice will promote learning; unvaried (blocked) practice will improve performance within a session.

ACTIVITY ADAPTATION

Activity adaptation is the process of modifying a familiar craft, game, sport, or other activity to accomplish a therapeutic goal. There are two reasons to adapt an activity in the treatment of the physically disabled. One is to modify the activity to make it therapeutic when ordinarily it would not be so in the unadapted form. Many examples of this can be seen in occupa-

tional therapy clinics; two are floor loom adaptations to provide exercise to muscles not usually involved in weaving (Hultkrans & Sandeen, 1957) (Fig. 11.2) and wall checkers in which the board is mounted on the wall and has pegs at each square to hold the enlarged checkers (Fig. 11.3).

The second reason for adaptation is to graduate the exercise offered by the activity along therapeutic continua to accomplish goals. Grading of activity for this purpose is an original principle of occupational therapy (Creighton, 1993). To increase coordination, the activity must be graded along a continuum from gross, coarse movement to fine, accurate movement. Checkers and other board games lend themselves easily to such gradations; the board and pieces can be

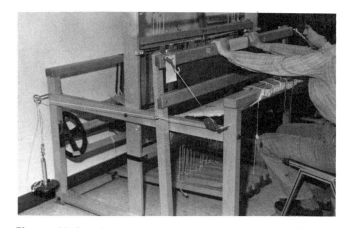

Figure 11.2. Floor loom adapted with weights and pulleys to resist elbow extension.

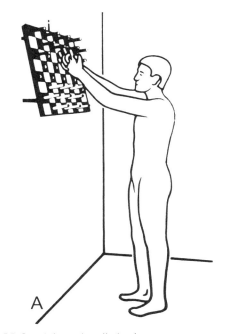

Figure 11.3. Adapted wall checkers.

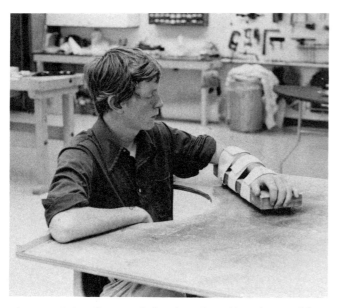

Figure 11.4. Skate and skateboard positioned at midchest level.

changed from large to small so that the checker aficionado can continue a favorite game while continuing to benefit therapeutically.

Characteristically, a good adaptation:

1. Accomplishes the specific goal;
2. Does not encourage or require odd movements or postures;
3. Is soundly constructed and is not potentially dangerous to the patient;
4. Intrinsically demands a certain response by the patient, one that he does not have to concentrate on performing; and
5. Does not demean the patient—some contrived adaptations seem ridiculous to the patient and, therefore, are embarrassing.

When adapting activities, as with all therapeutic techniques, it is vital for the patient to understand the reason that an activity will be done in an adapted manner.

Methods of Adaptation

POSITIONING THE TASK RELATIVE TO THE PERSON

The position of the person relative to the work to be done dictates the movement demanded by the activity and, therefore, which muscle groups are likely to be used (McGrain & Hague, 1987). Adaptation by positioning refers to changes in incline of work surface, height of work surface, or placement of pieces to be added to the project (Figs. 11.4–11.7).

Activities that are usually done on a flat surface, such as finger painting, board games, sanding wood, and the exercise skate, can be made more or less resistive by changing the incline of the surface. For example, if the surface is inclined down, forward, and away from the patient, resistance is given to shoulder extension and elbow flexion. If the incline is up, resistance is given to shoulder flexion and elbow extension.

The standard horizontal work surface itself can be raised or lowered to make demands on certain muscle groups or to alter the effect of gravity. For example, a table raised to axilla height allows flexion and extension of the elbow on a gravity-eliminated plane.

Placing items such as nails, mosaic tiles, pieces of yarn, beads, darts, and bean bags in various locations changes the motion required to reach them when performing the activity in an otherwise standard manner. Placement may be high enough to encourage shoulder flexion or abduction; lateral to encourage shoulder rotation, trunk rotation, or horizontal motion; or low to encourage trunk flexion, or lateral trunk flexion.

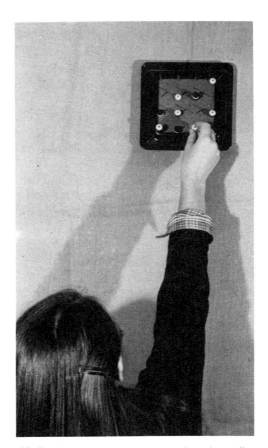

Figure 11.5. Score Four game mounted on the wall to require shoulder flexion and elbow extension.

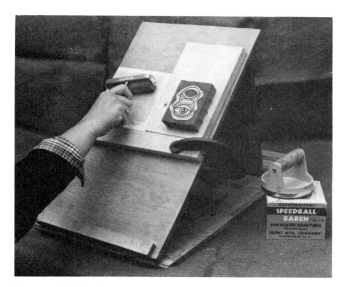

Figure 11.6. Block printing repositioned. Block is held in place by resting on nails below and to the right of the block. Height can be changed by moving the board that is held by a C-clamp to the incline board.

ARRANGEMENT OF OBJECTS RELATIVE TO EACH OTHER

To grade an activity for increasing perceptual skills (figure/ground, unilateral neglect), the arrangement of objects to be used, the printing on a page, and so on can be graded from sparse to dense.

ADDING WEIGHTS

The addition of weights adapts an activity to meet such goals as increase of strength, promotion of cocontraction, and increase of passive range of motion by stretch. Some nonresistive activities can be made resistive by adding weights to the apparatus—directly or by use of pulleys—while others may be made resistive by adding weights to the person himself. For example, to resist shoulder extension and elbow flexion, weights can be suspended from pulleys attached across from the person on a flat or inclined surface with the weight lines running from each handle of a bilateral sanding block. The line of pull can be reversed to resist shoulder flexion and elbow extension by attaching the pulleys behind the person.

Resistance can be changed on all looms; however, the floor looms lend themselves to more versatility in the application of the resistance. Weights can be added directly to the harnesses, treadles, or beater or can be added indirectly to the beater by the use of a pulley system (see Fig. 11.2).

Weights can be attached directly to the patient by means of weighted cuffs as well as by pulley line attachments. For example, when using a weighted wrist

cuff, leather lacing can become resistive to external rotation and elbow flexion. As another example, braid weaving can be made resistive to shoulder flexion by means of weights and pulleys attached over the back of the patient's chair with the lines running to a cuff fastened around his humerus.

Tools also are weights and can be selected or adjusted to offer graded resistance, for instance, hammers can be graded from lightweight tack hammers to heavy claw hammers.

ADDING SPRINGS OR RUBBER BANDS

Springs and rubber bands are means of adapting activity to increase strength or the cocontraction response through resistance, to assist a weak muscle, or to stretch muscle and other soft tissue to increase passive range of motion. When offering resistance, the spring or rubber band is positioned so that its pull is opposite to the pull of motion of the target muscle group, whereas if used for assistance, they are set to pull in the same direction as the contracting muscle group. Springs and rubber bands applied for the purpose of stretching are placed so the pull is against the tissue to be stretched (see Chapter 22 for precautions).

Springs of graduated tensions may be applied directly to the equipment. A beater of a floor loom can

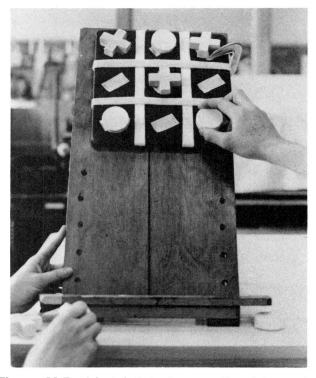

Figure 11.7. Adapted tic-tac-toe repositioned to require shoulder motions and size changed to accommodate poor coordination. The pieces are held in place with Velcro.

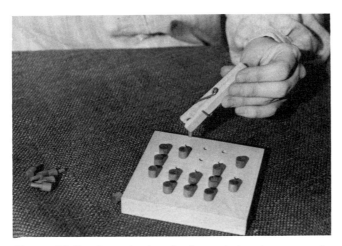

Figure 11.8. Game is played using a clothespin to move the pieces to strengthen pinch.

be made resistive to elbow extension or flexion by attaching springs either from the breast beam to the beater to resist elbow extension or from the beater to the castle (the center upright of the loom) to resist elbow flexion. Rubber bands can be added to smaller pieces of equipment and can be graded from thin and light tension to thick and heavy tension. For example, a rubber band can be wrapped around the pincer end of a spring-type clothespin to add resistance while it is used in games involving picking up small pieces (Fig. 11.8).

When rubber bands or springs are used to create a force of resistance in one direction, the return motion can involve passive stretch of the same muscle group during motion in the opposite direction, unless the person does an eccentric contraction of the resisted muscles to prevent the stretching pull. For example, if a spring is attached to a loom's beater to resist elbow flexion when the beater is pulled toward the person, on the return motion, the spring will pull into extension, thereby stretching the flexors unless the patient eccentrically contracts the flexors. Eccentric contraction would be desired as it would also exercise the weak flexors.

CHANGE OF LENGTH OF LEVER ARM

The amount of work a muscle or muscle group is doing depends on the resistance. Resistance is determined by the pull of gravity on the limb and the implements the patient is using, which together act as the resistance lever arm. The effect of a given amount of resistance can be altered by lengthening or shortening the resistance lever arm. The longer the resistance arm, the greater the force required to counterbalance it. The lever arm can be lengthened or shortened by

changing the location of the resistance on the limb, e.g., applying a weight at the end of the humerus rather than at the wrist reduces the amount of force that the shoulder flexors must generate to lift the weight. The lever arm can also be altered by "shortening or lengthening" the limb, e.g., by flexing the knee, which shortens the limb, less resistance is offered to hip extension than if the knee were extended. Another example is carrying an object close to the body, which requires less activity of back muscles than if the object were carried at arm's length. Use of a reacher to pick up an object involves more resistance and, therefore, more muscle output, than if the object were picked up directly. Use of a large paintbrush to paint a picture on the wall increases the resistance over using finger paint to make the picture.

On the other hand, increasing the length of the force lever arm decreases the muscle output needed to accomplish a task. For example, in Figure 11.8, if the clothespin were adapted to have longer handles, less pinch force would be required to open it the same distance.

Attention to lengths of lever arms is important not only in adapting an activity to make it more therapeutic but also in adapting utensils and tools used in daily life tasks to enable weak persons to use them. Furthermore, this idea can be used to guide workers in methods of lifting and handling on their jobs to avoid musculoskeletal injuries.

CHANGE OF MATERIALS OR TEXTURE OF MATERIALS

Gradation along the strengthening continuum may be accomplished by selection of material by type and also by variations of texture or density to change resistance. Coordination can be challenged by changing the material used to that of a finer, more delicate nature. Cutaneous stimulation changes as objects or surfaces that the person uses are more or less textured.

Resistance can be changed, for example, by starting a cutting project with tissue paper and then progressing to heavier materials, such as construction paper, cloth, and leather. Metal tooling can be graded for resistance by choosing materials in grades from thin aluminum to thick copper. Sandpaper is graded from extra fine to coarse, and resistance increases with the coarser grade. Mixing can be graded from making Jell-O to scrambled eggs to biscuit batter, etc. If materials are graded in the opposite direction, i.e., from heavy to light, then the activity will demand increased coordination from the patient. Weaving may begin using rug roving and be graded toward fine linen threads as the patient progresses in coordination. By making balls from yarn or terry toweling, carpeting the surfaces the person works on, padding handles with textured

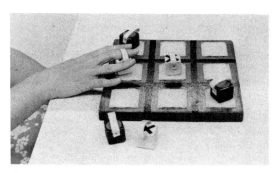

Figure 11.9. Adapted tic-tac-toe to exercise finger extensors; pieces are held by Velcro and require force to lift them.

material, etc., the therapist adapts the activity to increase sensory stimulation.

CHANGE LEVEL OF DIFFICULTY

Patterns for craft activities, game rules, extent of task (e.g., prepare instant coffee versus prepare espresso coffee), and level of creativity can be adjusted to enable the patient to experience success or to grade performance to higher levels. Changing the difficulty involves changing the number of pieces or the ideas that must be manipulated, changing the problem-solving level from concrete reasoning to abstract reasoning, changing the directions from specific to general, etc.

CHANGE OF THE SIZE OR SHAPE OF OBJECTS

Playing pieces of board games can be changed to different sizes or shapes (Figs. 11.7 and 11.9) and can, therefore, offer a therapeutic benefit that the standard objects would not. For example, checkers, which are usually flat pieces approximately 2.5 cm in diameter, can be cylinders, squares, cubes, or spheres and can range in size from tiny to as large as a person's grasp permits.

By reducing the size or changing the shape of the pieces being worked on, the goals of increased dexterity and fine coordination are facilitated. Therapists creatively change sizes of craft materials (e.g., weaving thread, tiles, paint-by-number guidelines, and ceramic pieces) and recreational materials (e.g., puzzle pieces, chess pieces, and target games) to increase coordination. Tools are adapted by changing the size or shape of their handles or adding handles to tools that do not normally have them. The actual size of the tool used can be changed to offer more or less resistance. For example, saws range in size from small coping saws and hack saws to large crosscut and rip saws. Resistance of saws can also be graded by the number of teeth per inch on the blade; the fewer the number of teeth, the greater the resistance. Wood-working planes vary in size, and the amount of exposed blade can be adjusted to provide resistance. Scissors also vary in size, and the resistance can be increased by tightening the screw.

CHANGE OF COLOR OF MULTIPLE OBJECTS

Neistadt et al. (1993) suggested grading challenge to figure-ground impairment by changing from contrasting colors of game objects to increasingly similar colors.

CHANGE OF METHOD OF DOING THE ACTIVITY

Bowling, basketball, and many other sports can be done from a seated position instead of the normal standing position. Change of rules adapts some sports, such as track and field events, to certain requirements of the physically impaired. Sewing and needlework, normally bilateral activities, can be made unilateral by adaptations that hold the material steady for the working hand. Holes can be punched in leather or packs of paper by use of a drill press in lieu of regular leather or paper punches. Block printing can be done in a hand- or foot-operated printing press rather than in a block printing press. Instead of rolling over on a therapy mat, rolling can be done in bed for more functional relevance.

Change of method is used both for exercise (Figs. 11.8 and 11.9) and for compensation (Fig. 11.10). By changing the method, an activity can be performed that would otherwise be impossible because of the person's disability. Such compensatory adaptation allows the therapist to offer an activity of interest to the patient while at the same time to accomplish certain therapeutic goals.

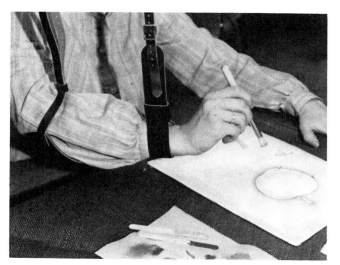

Figure 11.10. Stenciling is made possible by use of a suspension sling. Exercise to wrist extensors is obtained.

ACKNOWLEDGMENTS—I thank my students Janice Ferguson, Julie Pope, Natalia Ramsbey, Pei-Luen Tsai, Ellen Rosenberg and Ching-Yi Wu, for their library assistance, writings, graphics, and conversations about activity.

STUDY QUESTIONS

1. Why is occupation or activity used in occupational therapy?
2. What are the general characteristics required of an activity to be used to treat motor impairments?
3. How does activity analysis relate to activity selection?
4. How do goals and treatment principles relate to selection of activity for therapy?
5. What are two reasons for adapting a therapeutic activity?
6. What are the five characteristics of good adaptations?
7. What therapeutic goals can be accomplished by:
   a. Changing the position of the task relative to the person?
   b. Adding weights to tools or game pieces?
   c. Adding springs or rubber bands to craft equipment or tools?
   d. Changing the length of lever arms of tools, equipment, or the limb itself?
   e. Changing the material to be used in a project?
   f. Changing the method of doing an activity?

REFERENCES

Adam, J. J. (1992). The effects of objectives and constraints on motor control strategy in reciprocal aiming movements. *Journal of Motor Behavior, 24*(2), 173–185.

American Occupational Therapy Association. (1993). Position paper: Purposeful activity. *American Journal of Occupational Therapy, 47*(12), 1081–1082.

Bakshi, R., Bhambhani, Y., & Madill, H. (1991). The effects of task preference on performance during purposeful and nonpurposeful activities. *American Journal of Occupational Therapy, 45*(10), 912–916.

Bandura, A. (1982). Self-efficacy mechanism in human agency. *American Psychologist, 37*, 122–147.

Bloch, M. W., Smith, D. A., & Nelson, D. L. (1989). Heart rate, activity, duration, and affect in added-purpose versus single-purpose jumping activities. *American Journal of Occupational Therapy, 43*(1), 25–30.

Chandani, A., & Hill, C. (1990). What really is therapeutic activity? *British Journal of Occupational Therapy, 53*(1), 15–18.

Clark, F., Parham, D., Carlson, M. E., Frank, G., Jackson, J. Pierce, D., Wolfe, R.J., & Zemke, R. (1991). Occupational science: Academic innovation in the service of occupational therapy's future. *American Journal of Occupational Therapy, 45*(4), 300–310.

Clark, M. C., Czaja, S. J., & Weber, R. A. (1990). Older adults and daily living task profiles. *Human Factors, 32*(5), 537–549.

Creighton, C. (1992). The origin and evolution of activity analysis. *American Journal of Occupational Therapy, 46*(1), 45–48.

Creighton, C. (1993). Looking back. Graded activity: Legacy of the sanatorium. *American Journal of Occupational Therapy, 47*(8), 745–748.

Csikszentmihalyi, M. (1990). Flow: The psychology of optimal experience. New York: Harper & Row.

Cubie, S. H. (1985). Occupational analysis. In G. Kielhofner (Ed.), *A model of human occupation* (pp. 147–155). Baltimore: Williams & Wilkins.

Cynkin, S. (1979). Occupational therapy: Toward health through activity. Boston: Little, Brown.

Darnell, J. L., & Heater, S. L. (1994). The issue is: Occupational therapist or activity therapist—Which do you choose to be? *American Journal of Occupational Therapy, 48*(5), 467–486.

Davis, W. E., & Burton, A. W. (1991). Ecological Task Analysis: Translating movement behavior theory into practice. *Adapted Physical Activity Quarterly, 8*(2), 154–177.

DeKuiper, W. P., Nelson, D. L., & White, B. E. (1993). Materials-based occupation versus imagery-based occupation versus rote exercise: A replication and extension. *Occupational Therapy Journal of Research, 13*(3), 183–197.

Fisk, J. D., & Goodale, M. A. (1989). The effects of instructions to subjects on the programming of visually directed reaching movements. *Journal of Motor Behavior, 21*(1), 5–19.

Fitts, P. M. (1954). The information capacity of the human motor system in controlling the amplitude of movement. *Journal of Experimental Psychology, 47*, 381–391.

Gentile, A. (1987). Skill acquisition: Action, movement and neuromotor processes. In J. H. Carr, R. B. Shepherd, J. Gordon, A. M. Gentile, & J. M. Held (Eds.), *Movement science: Foundations for physical therapy in rehabilitation* (pp. 93–154). Rockville, MD: Aspen Systems.

Gibson, J. J. (1977). The theory of affordances. In R. E. Shaw & J. Bransford (Eds.), *Perceiving, acting, and knowing: Toward an ecological psychology* (pp. 67–82). Hillsdale, NJ: Lawrence Erlbaum.

Gilbreth, F. B. (1948). *Cheaper by the dozen.* New York: Thomas Y. Crowell.

Granit, R. (1977). *The purposive brain.* Cambridge, MA: MIT Press.

Hampton, D. S. M. (1993, October 7). Halloween tradition provides a therapeutic treat. *OT Week*, 22–23.

Heck, S. A. (1988). The effect of purposeful activity on pain tolerance. *American Journal of Occupational Therapy, 42*(9), 577–581.

Higgins, S. (1991). Motor skill acquisition. *Physical Therapy, 71*(2), 123–139.

Horak, F. B. (1991). Assumptions underlying motor control for neurologic rehabilitation. In M. Lister (Ed.), *Contemporary management of motor control problems: Proceedings of the II step conference* (pp. 11–27). Alexandria, VA: The Foundation for Physical Therapy.

Hultkrans, R., & Sandeen, A. (1957). Application of progressive resistive exercise to occupational therapy. *American Journal of Occupational Therapy, 11*(4), 238–240.

Jeannerod, M. (1988). *The neural and behavioral organization of goal-directed movements.* Oxford: Clarendon Press.

Kamm, K., Thelen, E., & Jensen, J. L. (1990). A dynamical systems approach to motor development. *Physical Therapy, 70*(12), 763–775.

Kielhofner, G. (Ed.). (1985). *A model of human occupation.* Baltimore: Williams & Wilkins.

King, T. I. (1993). Hand strengthening with a computer for purposeful activity. *American Journal of Occupational Therapy, 47*(7), 635–637.

Kircher, M. A. (1984). Motivation as a factor of perceived exertion in purposeful versus nonpurposeful activity. *American Journal of Occupational Therapy, 38*(3), 165–170.

Lang, E. M., Nelson, D. L., & Bush, M. A. (1992). Comparison of performance in materials-based occupation, imagery-based occupation, and rote exercise in nursing home residents. *American Journal of Occupational Therapy, 46*(7), 607–611.

Lewthwaite, R. (1990). Motivational considerations in physical activity involvement. *Physical Therapy, 70*(12), 808–819.

Licht, S. (1947). Kinetic analysis of crafts and occupations. *Occupational Therapy and Rehabilitation, 26*, 75–78.

Llorens, L. A. (1986). Activity analysis: Agreement among factors in a sensory processing model. *American Journal of Occupational Therapy, 40*(2), 103–110.

Llorens, L. A. (1993). Activity analysis: Agreement between participants and observers on perceived factors in occupation components. *Occupational Therapy Journal of Research, 13*(3), 198–211.

Marteniuk, R. G., MacKenzie, C. L., Jeannerod, M., Athenes, S., & Dugas, C. (1987). Constraints on human arm movement trajectories. *Canadian Journal of Psychology, 41*(3), 365–378.

McGrain, P., & Hague, M. A. (1987). An electromyographic study of the middle deltoid and middle trapezius muscles during warping. *Occupational Therapy Journal of Research, 7*(4), 225–233.

Miller, L., & Nelson, D. L. (1987). Dual-purpose activity versus single-purpose activity in terms of duration of task, exertion level, and affect. *Occupational Therapy in Mental Health, 1*, 55–67.

Morasso, P. & Zaccaria, R. (1986). Understanding human movement. *Experimental Brain Research, 15*, 145–157.

Morton, G. G., Barnett, D. W., & Hale, L. S. (1992). A comparison of performance measures of an added-purpose task versus a single-purpose task for upper extremities. *American Journal of Occupational Therapy, 46*(2), 128–133.

Mosey, A. C. (1981). *Occupational therapy: Configuration of a profession.* New York: Raven Press.

National Society for the Promotion of Occupational Therapy. (1917). *Constitution of the National Society for the Promotion of Occupational Therapy.* Baltimore: Sheppard Hospital Press.

Neistadt, M. E., McAuley, D., Zecha, D., & Shannon, R. (1993). An analysis of a board game as a treatment activity. *American Journal of Occupational Therapy, 47*(2), 154–160.

Nelson, D. L. (1988). Occupation: Form and performance. *American Journal of Occupational Therapy, 42*(10), 633–641.

Newell, K. M. & Corcos, D. M. (1993). Issues in variability and motor control. In K. M. Newell & D. M. Corcos (Eds.), *Variability and motor control* (pp. 1–12). Champaign, IL: Human Kinetics.

Okoye, R. L. (1988). Computer technology in occupational therapy. In H. L. Hopkins & H. D. Smith (Eds.), *Willard and Spackman's occupational therapy* (pp. 340–345). Philadelphia: J. B. Lippincott.

Peloquin, S. M. (1988). Linking purpose to procedure during interactions with patients. *American Journal of Occupational Therapy, 42*(12), 775–781.

Project Magic. (1985). Can magic work miracles? *Accent on Living, 30*(2), 52–55.

Ramsbey, N. (1993). Is purposeful activity effective in remediating physical impairments and/or restoring function? *Journal of Occupational Therapy Students, 7*(2), 7–14.

Reilly, M. (1962). Occupation can be one of the great ideas of 20th century medicine. *American Journal of Occupational Therapy, 16*, 1–9.

Riccio, C. M., Nelson, D. L., & Bush, M. A. (1990). Adding purpose to the repetitive exercise of elderly women through imagery. *American Journal of Occupational Therapy, 44*(8), 714–719.

Sietsema, J. M., Nelson, D. L., Mulder, R. M., Mervau-Scheidel, D., & White, B. E. (1993). The use of a game to promote arm reach in persons with traumatic brain injury. *American Journal of Occupational Therapy, 47*(1), 19–24.

Spaulding, S. J., & Robinson, K. L. (1984). Electromyographic study of the upper extremity during bilateral sanding: Unresisted and resisted conditions. *American Journal of Occupational Therapy, 38*(4), 258–262.

Steinbeck, T. M. (1986). Purposeful activity and performance. *American Journal of Occupational Therapy, 40*(8), 529–534.

Thibodeaux, C. S., & Ludwig, F. M. (1988). Intrinsic motivation in product-oriented and non-product oriented activities. *American Journal of Occupational Therapy, 42*(3), 169–175.

Trombly, C. A., & Cole, J. M. (1979). Electromyographic study of four hand muscles during selected activities. *American Journal of Occupational Therapy, 33*(7), 440–449.

Trombly, C. A., & Quintana, L. A. (1983). Activity analysis: Electromyographic and electrogonimetric verification. *Occupational Therapy Journal of Research, 3*(2), 104–120.

Tsai, P.-L. (1993). *The therapeutic value of purposeful activity.* Unpublished manuscript. Boston University, Sargent College of Allied Heath Professions, Department of Occupation Therapy, Boston.

Tsai, P.-L. (1994). *Activity analysis and activity selection among occupational therapists: A survey.* Unpublished Master's thesis, Boston University.

van der Weel, F. R., van der Meer, A. L. H., & Lee D. N. (1991). Effect of task on movement control in cerebral palsy: Implications for assessment and therapy. *Developmental Medicine and Child Neurology, 33*, 419–426.

West, W. L. (1984). A reaffirmed philosophy and practice of occupational therapy for the 1980s. *American Journal of Occupational Therapy, 38*(1), 15–23.

Wu, C.-Y. (1993). *The relationship between occupational form and occupational performance.* Unpublished Master's thesis, Boston University.

Yoder, R. M., Nelson, D. L., & Smith, D. A. (1989). Added-purpose versus rote exercise in female nursing home residents. *American Journal of Occupational Therapy, 43*(9), 581–586.

Yuen, H. K., Nelson, D. L., Peterson, C. Q., & Dickinson, A. (1994). Prosthesis training as a context for studying occupational forms and motoric adaptation. *American Journal of Occupational Therapy, 48*(1), 55–61.

12
Development

Wendy Coster

OBJECTIVES

By studying this chapter, the reader will be able to:
1. Gain understanding of how developmental theories have been incorporated into occupational therapy intervention models.
2. Recognize basic assumptions about development that are reflected in current intervention models.
3. Understand the distinction between describing and explaining development as it relates to validation of intervention models.
4. Understand the challenges posed by dynamical systems, life span, and contextualist models to current intervention approaches.
5. Identify a set of questions that can be applied in practice to evaluate the appropriateness of developmentally based therapeutic intervention for a particular individual.

Theories and models of occupational therapy intervention for adults with physical dysfunction often incorporate, either explicitly or implicitly, principles and concepts derived from theories of development. In some cases, this base may be acknowledged directly. For example, both the title and original treatment rationale of neurodevelopmental treatment (Bobath & Bobath, 1984), clearly specify that it is a treatment model based on particular developmental principles such as a stepwise, hierarchical progression from lower, primitive, stages to higher, cortical control. In other cases, the developmental basis becomes apparent when a treatment protocol incorporates a sequence modeled on typical child developmental patterns. For example, Siev, Freishtat, and Zoltan (1986) recommend a sequence of visual-perceptual remediation activities for adults that follows the sequence of typical unfolding of these skills in children, and indeed, the use of materials originally developed to facilitate these skills in children is suggested. The validity of these treatment

theories and guidelines depends to an important degree on the validity of the underlying developmental models on which they are based. If the assumptions and concepts of the models are outmoded or are being questioned, it is important for therapists to be aware of these issues and the implications that changes in the models may have for their treatment. The purpose of this chapter is to present a discussion of current developmental theory and research as it applies to intervention theories. The chapter identifies important assumptions underlying different theories, provides an overview of data that have called some of these assumptions into question, and summarizes some of the newer models of development currently receiving attention. This overview concludes with a series of questions for therapists to consider when evaluating the appropriateness of a potential intervention model for the adults they treat.

THE CONCEPT OF DEVELOPMENT

Because *development* is a commonly used word that may carry a variety of meanings, it is important to begin with an examination of terms. There is general agreement that developmental theories are those that concern themselves with changes in human behavior over time (Miller, 1989). Although development is frequently used to refer to any change in behavior over time, some researchers reserve the use of the word to changes in form, such as changes in the complexity of language or the mode of mobility, and exclude changes in quantity, such as an increased vocabulary or faster running speed (Short-DeGraff, 1988). Some theorists have also made a distinction between development and learning, particularly in reference to processes of change. Often the term development is reserved for processes thought to have a major innate or maturational impetus (e.g., walking), whereas processes that depend critically on external or environmental influences are subsumed under learning (e.g., learning to paint) (Short-DeGraff, 1988). Other times, development appears to be reserved for skills or behaviors acquired without conscious application of effort, whereas the term learning is applied to consciously directed efforts (e.g., development of grasp versus learning to ski) (Dixon & Lerner, 1991). These distinctions imply that therapists are clear about the relative role of biology (nature) and environment (nurture), or conscious versus unconscious processes, in the emergence or acquisition of new behaviors. However, as will be discussed shortly, in many domains of behavior this question is far from resolved.

One source of confusion in these definitions of development may be the failure to clarify the level of analysis being discussed. For example, motor development may be discussed and analyzed at multiple levels: at the level of synaptic connection, at the level of activation of movement synergies, and on up to the level of observable changes in quality of movement or the emergence of new patterns of mobility. Presumably, change across time (i.e., development) occurs at all of these levels. Furthermore, it is possible that changes in quantitative features at one of these levels (e.g., changes in muscle strength) may precipitate or in some way cause changes in qualitative features at another level (e.g., emergence of upright stance). Similarly, it is possible that learning a new motor skill or learning a specific movement pattern may enable the emergence of qualitatively different forms of complex motor behavior. In the latter case, development of new forms is the result of learning that has occurred at another level of behavior. Because these distinctions are unclear in many areas, this chapter adopts a broader, more inclusive definition of development, which refers to all changes across time in behavior.

Miller (1989) suggested that developmental theories have three major concerns: "(1) to describe changes over time within one or several areas of behavior, (2) to describe changes in the relationships among several areas of behavior, and (3) to explain the course of development that has been described" (p. 5). For the purposes of this chapter it is important to highlight the distinction between these tasks. The first two tasks involve describing in an organized fashion the form, timing, sequence, and relations of behavioral change. The third task involves developing and testing hypotheses about the causes or mechanisms responsible for producing change, i.e., explaining development. By and large, developmental theory and research have been descriptive, i.e., researchers have been concerned with Miller's (1989) first two tasks. For example, norms for physical, cognitive, social, and motor development have grown out of this work (Gesell, 1954; Illingworth, 1960). This type of information is used regularly by therapists to assess a patient's status rela-

tive to same-age peers, to determine the degree of loss or gain of function, and to identify areas of deficit that may require intervention.

Other researchers have focused on clarifying the relation among different aspects or domains of function. For example, Van Sant (1990) examined the relation between changes in body dimensions and movement patterns used in rising from the floor across the life span. Studies also have helped establish the relation between certain contextual factors and outcome, e.g., the relevance of socioeconomic status as a predictor of high-risk infant developmental outcome (Sameroff & Chandler, 1975) or the relation between social stress and increased risk of illness (Dohrenwend & Dohrenwend, 1984). Information of this relational type also is applied regularly by therapists. For example, when a therapist tests a poststroke patient for possible perceptual deficits, she is acting on information about the relation between damage to particular areas of the central nervous system (CNS) and the presence of specific impairments. This kind of research and theory, while quite valuable, provides a picture of individuals only at a given point in time and does not provide much insight into change over time.

When intervention must be designed, information on Miller's (1989) third question is needed. How does change happen? What processes or influences enable or inhibit development and how do they do so? What are the component processes or abilities that are necessary for change? Are there alternative means or routes to accomplish the same goal or is there only one effective means? The descriptive and relational studies and models discussed above cannot answer these questions, because they describe behavior only as it is and do not explain how the behavior came to be. Unfortunately, this distinction is frequently overlooked, with the result that inappropriate applications of developmental information may be made in treatment. This issue is considered in more detail in the next section.

(MIS)APPLICATIONS OF DEVELOPMENTAL STUDIES

In searching for theories that may provide a valid basis for intervention theory, it is important to distinguish the level of behavior or scope of different theories. Some theories, such as Piaget's (1952) theory of cognitive development, may be considered "grand" theories, in that they attempt to provide an explanation of development that applies across a large span of time and accounts for changes in major domains of human behavior. Other theories may be more modest and address change within a specific subdomain of behavior, sometimes within a narrow span of time. For example, Thelen's work has concentrated on explaining the development of infant stepping and walking (Thelen & Ulrich, 1991). Grand theories have the appeal of providing a model that can explain a variety of phenomena; however, they often lack the specificity or detail about the processes involved that may be found in the narrow theories. For example, Piaget's assimilation and accommodation constructs appear to be useful for describing adaptive processes, but just how does an individual go about making the necessary changes to accommodate to a new challenge? The theory has little to say about such specific events, and thus provides little guidance about how to assist an individual in achieving such change. In contrast, Thelen and Ulrich's (1991) detailed analysis of infant motor behavior provided some insights into the impact of specific biomechanical changes (e.g., removal of need for weight bearing) on the form of behavior seen.

Because grand theories offer models that appear to account for such a broad range of behavior, and thus to provide clarity in the face of behavioral complexity, it is easy to forget that the specifics of change are still unclear. For example, therapists may begin to use a term such as accommodation or reorganization as an explanation for the emergence of a new movement strategy and fail to recognize that they have simply relabeled the change and have not spelled out the exact mechanisms through which it happens. Other theories (Gesell, 1954) may propose that innate knowledge or prewired mechanisms are responsible for the observed unfolding of new behaviors. Once again, however, the question of how new behaviors emerge (i.e., what are the specific mechanisms) has been sidestepped rather than answered. To claim that interventions are truly guided by theory, therapists need models that specify much more precisely what mechanisms lead to change: What processes or factors are involved? How are the different factors causally related? and How might alteration of a factor lead to the specific therapeutic outcome desired? Thus, for occupational therapy practice, specific theories about development in particular domains or skill areas may provide more valid and detailed proposals about how to influence change.

A second pitfall in the application of developmental theories involves inferences about a necessary or obligatory order to the development of new competencies. When researchers see a certain sequence in development repeat itself consistently from one person to the next, it is tempting to make the assumption that the sequence is required or necessary. For example, it is observed that in normal infants the sequence of appearance of motor milestones is consistent and that manual exploration of objects almost always precedes naming and other forms of representational thought, such as symbolic play. Some theories, such as Piaget's (1952), have then gone on to propose that sensorimotor

exploration is a necessary step for further cognitive development. Similarly, Gesell (1954) maintained that development must progress through a certain sequence of motor behaviors. In a related example, when certain forms of behavior have been observed to be more prevalent in groups with good adaptive outcomes, it has often been assumed that those behaviors must be causing the outcome. Such observations form the basis of a great amount of developmental theorizing and, subsequently, intervention recommendations. However, these deductions share a common flaw: They draw causal implications from descriptive and correlational data. In other words, because change typically happens in a certain order or form, an assumption is made that it must happen that way or (at a minimum) that it is best if it happens that way. Theorists then go on to create an explanation of how these changes come about without making sure that the initial assumption about a necessary sequence is correct (see Rutter, 1989, for an excellent discussion of these issues).

The results of this assumption are seen in a number of treatment situations. For example, some treatment protocols require that a patient progress through the same sequence of steps seen in the initial development of postural and motor skills. The assumption is being made that this sequence represents a necessary hierarchy of stages required to reach the final goal of motor control (Gordon, 1987). The same assumption is being made when treatment of perceptual problems involves having the patient repeat the sequences seen in children as they first master writing or drawing (Neistadt, 1990).

This assumption is not necessarily incorrect: It may be that the typical developmental sequences do, in fact, represent a necessary set of stages that must be accomplished to reach the end skill. However, it is important for therapists to recognize that, in most areas, the correctness of these assumptions has been neither tested nor proven. In addition, there are important areas in which new research findings and revisions in theory have called into question the old developmental models from which these assumptions are derived. Some of these changes will be highlighted in the next section.

Two other important assumptions underlying many developmentally based intervention theories are (1) that the average adolescent represents the "mature" level and form of human performance and (2) that dysfunction is best understood as a regression back to a more primitive or child-typical stage. There are several problems with these assumptions. First, there is no inherent reason why behavioral changes at later ages necessarily should be considered declines or deviations in performance. The tendency to do so follows from one's particular definition of maturity and the tendency to define youth as the ideal. As an alternative, consider development as a continuous process (across the life span) of reformation and reorganization of processes and skills (Van Sant, 1990). At each stage of the life span, the individual organizes a mode of behavior that best takes into account his or her particular physical, social, motivational, and environmental realities. Instead of considering growth as being primarily a process for the young, the alternative view acknowledges the increasing evidence that both growth and decline are developmental processes that operate throughout the life span (Baltes, 1987).

There is a second problem with the assumption that dysfunction in adults reflects regression or "loss" of higher functions. The problem is that similar forms of behavior are assumed to have the same underlying explanation, and therefore, the intervention methods used with the first behavior are the most appropriate to use for the second. This assumption can be seen, for example, in the application of neurodevelopmental treatment methods both to children with cerebral palsy and to adults with brain damage from stroke. While it is quite natural to make such links between similar-appearing behaviors and to apply similar treatments in the hope of achieving positive outcomes for patients, it is important to keep in mind some weaknesses in this model. Systems-oriented theorists increasingly have argued that different processes may be employed by individuals to achieve essentially the same goals (Ford & Lerner, 1992; Horak, 1991). Thus, although the end behavior may have a similar form, there may not be one "ideal" route that is used by all individuals to achieve that form. Furthermore, dysfunctional behaviors that are similar in form may also result from different underlying mechanisms.

Researchers in motor behavior have suggested that their data are more consistent with a dynamic model in which behavior is the result of multiple influences, rather than the unfolding of a single set of hardwired plans (Heriza, 1991). In this case, the multiple differences between adults and children make it quite probable that similar behaviors may result from quite different underlying organizations. At the least, it suggests that alternative interventions that make use of some of these differences would be worthy of consideration. For example, adults have a significant accumulation of motor experience and can apply advanced reasoning and problem solving to the new challenges they face. They might place different priorities on subgoals, ranging from energy conservation to preserving self-esteem, that could affect their approach to current motor problems (Lewthwaite, 1990; Van Sant, 1991). Finally, changes in physical parameters such as body dimensions, weight, and flexibility may lend themselves to novel mobility solutions as well as constitute substantial obstacles to carrying out movement patterns more characteristic of children (Van Sant, 1990).

These questions apply not only to motor behavior but also to adult perceptual functions. As noted earlier, some intervention protocols for perceptual deficits have also adopted a model in which adult dysfunction is viewed as a regression, or loss of more mature forms, and in which experiences that facilitate development of skills in children are applied to enhance recovery of more mature skills by adults. Abreu and Toglia (1987), however, have criticized this approach. They, too, have emphasized that adults with dysfunction differ from children; adults generally have more advanced problem-solving skills and a repertoire of experiences to draw on as they work toward recovery of skills. Clearly, additional research that examines motor and cognitive-perceptual behavior from a life span perspective is needed to explore these issues and help determine whether alternative models may provide a more accurate account of adult behavior.

CONTEMPORARY THEORIES OF DEVELOPMENT AND THEIR IMPLICATIONS

As noted by Heriza (1991), in an excellent discussion of these issues, traditional, developmentally based theories of motor intervention drew strongly on the neuromaturational models proposed by McGraw (1945) and Gesell (1954), which in turn made use of current models of the central nervous system. Common to both theories is a strong emphasis on the role of the CNS in driving the motor system, i.e., the structure of behavior is seen as largely determined by the maturity of particular brain structures. Change occurs primarily as a result of change in the requisite structures, particularly from the progressive increase in cortical control, and function emerges from changes in structure, not vice versa. Motor development also is held to proceed in specific directions: cephalocaudal (head to tail) and proximal-distal (center to periphery). This model of development is hierarchical and predominantly linear. A normative sequence of steps toward a universal goal is a major feature.

Other theories of development in related domains share similar features. For example, in the cognitive domain, Piaget (1952) postulated a consistent series of stages that all children move through. Passage through the previous stage is required to provide the necessary foundation for the next stage. In particular, the child must have a period of sensorimotor engagement with the environment during the first stage to lay the proper foundation for representational thought and later forms of more advanced reasoning. Within a given stage, a particular underlying structure determines the mode of reasoning a child applies to the problems encountered. Thus a child would need to reach the stage of concrete operations before he or she could be expected to show conservation of weight or matter when reasoning about physical changes in the environment. In this theory, the form of the behavior (reasoning) is determined primarily by the cognitive structure present, not by features of the task or the environment.

Both of these examples imply models in which development is somewhat like the building of a tower from a set of graduated blocks. The most stable, or optimal, structure is one in which the largest block is on the bottom, followed by the next largest, and so on. Any variation on this design will result in a structure that is inherently less stable, and the order in which the blocks are to be placed is quite clear. By implication, if an event occurs in which the mature structure is broken (a few blocks are knocked off), the logical approach to intervention would be to try to reconstruct the tower with the blocks in the same, nested order.

In the past decade, these hierarchical and linear models of development have come into increasing question. The sources of these questions vary somewhat, depending on the domain of development under discussion. For example, in the realm of motor development, Thelen and Ulrich (1991) presented research on rhythmical movements in infants that is inconsistent with the principle of cephalocaudal direction. Rather, their data show the presence of organized movement in the lower extremities before such movement in the upper extremities. Fetters, Fernandez, and Cermak's (1989) data about infant reaching suggest a pattern of simultaneous development in both proximal and distal elements, rather than the sequential proximal to distal direction mandated by older models. Shumway-Cook and Woolacott (1985) have shown that the strategy used by young children to achieve balance in standing uses activation that moves from distal to proximal musculature. Based on a study of differences in posture and movement strategies across the life span, Van Sant (1991) suggested that the notion of linear growth toward a single ideal (the "mature" form) should be replaced with a model that views the movement of each age group as possessing a unique organization most appropriate to the individuals' physical characteristics and environmental context.

Within the field of cognitive development, Rogoff (1982) argued that theorists have ignored the critical influence of social and physical context when interpreting data on children's reasoning. She and others (Ford & Lerner, 1992; Gibson, 1988) argued forcefully that the task itself exerts a critical influence on the form and organization of the child's performance. They point out that data from a variety of research studies suggest that there is too much variability in children's problem-solving performance to be consistent with a strict stage model of development. Rather, children employ a variety of methods to achieve solutions to daily challenges. These methods reflect not only the child's intrinsic capabilities at that point (i.e., the structures present) but also the features of their physical and social environment that define, structure, and support the task (Rogoff, 1990).

The challenges raised by new developments in theory and contradictory findings in research have resulted in a search for different models to describe and explain changes in human behavior across time. In a variety of domains, this is a time of considerable discussion and reexamination of long-held assumptions about development and proposals for alternative models. This chapter focuses on two active and relevant areas: the emergence of dynamical systems theories and their application to the field of motor development and the reawakening of interest in Gibson and Gibson's theory of perception and its application to understanding action.

Dynamical Systems Models

In contrast to earlier hierarchical models that emphasized the controlling role of the CNS (particularly the cortical functions), contemporary frameworks have adopted a variety of systems models for motor behavior and development. In these systems models, the CNS is only one of several factors that contribute to movement, and a much greater role is assigned to the features of the task, biomechanical aspects of the individual, and social features of the environment. Rather than view motor behavior as the output of hardwired instructions from the central nervous system, patterns of motor coordination "instead self-organize in response to information specifying the task and the physical environment" (Thelen, 1992, p. 190). For example, instead of a maturational timetable being responsible for the progressive unfolding of skills such as walking and reaching, dynamical systems theorists propose that these skills emerge from a particular configuration of component processes and structures. This radical shift from structure to process is somewhat difficult to grasp at first. Doesn't the emergence of a new form of organized behavior require that a plan be put together? How else would the various components be assembled? In fact, theorists now argue, there are many examples in nature of the form or pattern emerging or falling out (Thelen, 1992) when the structure and energy of the system reaches a particular state. Thelen and Ulrich (1991) offer the example of a pendulum that can "keep time" without having a motor schema or internal plan. A particular rhythmic pattern emerges from the confluence of several factors, including the force of gravity, degree of friction, and height of suspension. In another example, water molecules shift among distinct states (from the calm of cool water to the turbulence of boiling) when heat is applied at a particular degree. In children, similar shifts in one of the contributing factors may result in the emergence of a distinctly new behavioral form, or what might be called a new motor milestone.

A key aspect of dynamical systems models is that change in any one of the participating parameters may dissolve (cause to disappear) the existing coordination. The system then goes through a transitional period that ends when a new pattern of stability emerges from the altered set of parameters. A particular pattern (referred to as an "attractor state") may have a high probability of occurring under those conditions, but its emergence is not guaranteed. Because individuals share certain features as a result of common genetic heritage and because there are some common problems faced by all individuals (e.g., to traverse space), it is logical to expect that individuals will show much overall similarity in their behavioral solutions, or attractor states. On the other hand, individuals also demonstrate great variation in the particular form or degree of their features such as muscle strength, processing speed, and temperament. The moment-to-moment (task goal) and larger (social, physical, and cultural) contexts also show tremendous variability among individuals as well as throughout the life span. This variability may significantly alter the dynamics of the system, resulting in different solutions, or attractor states, among individuals or within the same individual through time. Thus, although certain sequences of behavioral states may appear consistently across individuals, dynamical systems models view this consistency as reflecting the fact that certain solutions may emerge more readily than others, rather than reflecting any obligatory or necessary hierarchy (Heriza, 1991; Thelen & Ulrich, 1991).

Dynamical systems models thus provide a view of behavior that implies much more flexibility and change than was possible in older models. At any given moment, multiple components, each with its own dynamic characteristics, must be considered as potentially amenable to an alteration that will change the solutions possible for the individual. It is especially important to note that this model does not assign greater weight to central nervous system factors in precipitating the emergence of new behavior forms. For example, Thelen and Ulrich (1991) argued that early independent walking is constrained largely by lack of leg strength rather than lack of maturation of some necessary CNS structure. Nor does the model assign greater weight a priori to physical rather than cognitive, emotional, or contextual features. Instead, it is a fundamental feature of the dynamical systems model that behavioral form is a

function of organism-in-context, and thus alteration of *any* element of the organism or its context may have the potential to precipitate a change in the system and the emergence of a new attractor state. Changes in the task, context, or individual factors may lend themselves to other solutions. Thus the different stages of motor development may reflect solutions to the infant's goal of traversing space that are possible within the context of current cognitive, physical, and social parameters, rather than a set of nested, prerequisite stages. Exploration and active testing are central to the child's eventual selection of the responses that best match the functional needs and the possibilities allowed by existing conditions. Extending this argument to adults, the model implies that therapists might want to alter systematically a variety of tasks, contexts, or individual features to try to facilitate the emergence of a new solution to a motor problem.

As is apparent in this brief overview, dynamical systems models view movement as task assembled, or as Heriza (1991) noted, "It is function (task and context) that assembles behavior rather than pre-existing instructions" (p. 105). This emphasis on the importance of the task or action context is also an important feature of newer models proposed by other developmental theorists, including Ford and Lerner (1992) and Rogoff (1990). Several of these theorists have drawn ideas from the work of J. Gibson (1979) and E. Gibson (1988).

The Gibson and Gibson Model of Perceptual Development

The Gibson and Gibson ecological psychology stresses that person and environment are inextricably linked and that the actions of the person can only be understood in the context of the environment in which the actions take place. The human organism is designed for function in a particular environment, and the environment constrains the organism's possibilities for action. The term affordance is applied by Gibson (1988) to this relationship: An environment "affords" certain possibilities to a bipedal organism; it affords other possibilities to organisms that are quadruped or that are capable of flight. According to E. Gibson, perception is an active process that is motivated and directed by goals important to the individual. A major occupation of childhood, or of any individual in a new context, is to explore and discover the affordances of a given environment for the goals that have meaning to the person: Which mobility strategies are possible on a given surface, which strategies work when speed is of the essence, which features specify an object that can be grasped, and which features indicate that an object must be grasped delicately rather than roughly? Perceptual development, in the Gibson and Gibson framework, involves the increasing differentiation, or aware-ness, of these possibilities for action and thus is intimately related to the tasks that have meaning to the individual.

In Gibson's (1988) theory, perceptual development is largely a learning process. She proposes that there is structure inherent in the stimulation in the environment and the major accomplishment of develop-ment is learning to extract more and more of the information available about objects, events, and spatial arrays. This process is shaped and motivated by the individual's active engagement in meaningful tasks within a given environment. The task and its context, together with the goals and action capabilities of the person, specify which affordances are relevant. The individual's active exploration also facilitates the dis-covery of relevant affordances, the degree to which information derived from similar contexts can be gener-alized, and the increasingly efficient pickup of task- or goal-relevant information. This model contrasts with Piagetian or information-processing models, which pro-pose an additive process in which the individual gradu-ally builds up knowledge from small bits of information rather than perceiving complex relations directly (see Montgomery, 1991, for additional discussion of these theories from a rehabilitation viewpoint).

Recently, the Gibson and Gibson theory of per-ceptual development has received increasing attention by rehabilitation researchers and theorists. The theory's emphasis on the interrelation between the individual and his or her environment is highly congruent with current models of function that also emphasize the importance of looking at the individual-in-context. However, the more specific implications of the theory are just beginning to be explored. For example, it is not clear whether the developmental process described by E. Gibson also is an appropriate and useful model for thinking about loss and recovery of function in adults who have sustained neurologic damage. Fetters (1991) discussed the implications of Gibson and Gib-son's ecological psychology for pediatric physical thera-pists, e.g., how particular tasks might be used to provide motivating perceptual experiences and to elicit exploratory movements. Mayer et al. (1990) described a new way of conceptualizing and examining disorders of skilled action (apraxias) in the adult with neurologic deficits from an action theory perspective that draws directly on Gibson's (1979) theory. They proposed that the "action errors" made by a patient during the performance of a functional task may be conceptualized as disruptions in the detection of relevant affordances or as a mismatch between the goal, the affordance, and the form of response. Whether this model will yield new and more useful proposals for intervention than existing models remains to be seen. For the present

discussion, it is important to note that the model being developed by these researchers is starting from work with adults, rather than proposals based on observa-tions of children.

Implications for Intervention

One important implication of the Gibson and Gibson theory is that perceptual functions are best examined in an action context that has importance for the individual in question. Assessment of individual aspects of perception such as sensory detection, or cross-modal matching (stereognosis) may suggest hypotheses about limitations in the detection apparatus or in the initiation of effective exploratory movements. However, assessment in the task context is needed to provide a complete picture of the person's current ability to detect relevant affordances and to implement the appropriate behavioral strategies. In the treatment setting, elicitation of a desired functional response may be most effective when information specifying the affordances for the response is clear and the context is highly motivating (Fetters, 1991). Both dynamical systems theory and Gibsonian theory appear to provide valuable support for the idea that engagement in mean-ingful activity is not only an asset to treatment but an essential requirement for the reorganization of func-tional behavior. A correlate of this statement is that for the patient to regain flexible, varied responses he must be engaged in a variety of tasks or in similar tasks but in variable environments. At least during the initial phases of organization of movement patterns, practice in a single, highly controlled context will not necessar-ily result in a generalizable response.

At present, neither the data nor the emerging theory provides strong support for the practice of follow-ing the typical developmental sequence when selecting tasks and goals for the adult patient with motor impair-ment. This caution is particularly relevant for tasks that do not have current functional value and do not represent a critical element of the subsequent task. Thus, for example, achievement of upright stance is an integral element of walking, whereas creeping is not. Although creeping typically precedes walking in young children, in current system models, this temporal relation does not establish creeping as a prerequisite. Creeping may simply be a movement solution that best accommodates the typical biomechanical and strength characteristics of an infant, or it may reflect particular social practices or features of the infant environment. As described by Van Sant (1990), there are a number of differences in the musculoskeletal characteristics as well as in the relative prioritizing of goals in older adults that may contribute to different solutions to movement problems than would be seen in younger individuals. If therapists no longer insist that the solutions seen in younger children are the ideal, then they open up the possibility that different approaches may yield positive changes in adult function.

In addition, arguments have been made that even if some aspects of performance are similar in adults and children there are a number of other significant differences that caution against applying child-based models to the adult. Dynamical systems models propose that these factors, including those that are not "motor" factors at all, may critically alter the behavioral possibilities or solutions in positive and negative ways. Some of these differences include the more complex reasoning ability of adults and the availability of problem-solving strategies and information about options derived from experience (Abreu & Toglia, 1987), differences in physical and biomechanical factors influencing performance (Van Sant, 1990), differences in goals, and differences in the priority assigned to competing goals in a given task context (Lewthwaite, 1990). It is a basic tenet of transactional systems models that development transforms the person. The person is a whole that is more than a simple sum of his or her parts (skills, functions, and responses). Thus the loss of a particular capacity or skill may precipitate a readjustment and transformation, but it can never revert the person back to an earlier form. What therapists identify in their patients as dysfunction is not truly regression to an earlier state but a *new* state with its own organization and response capabilities.

SUMMARY

This is a time of reevaluation and new creative proposals in developmental theory. Many of the existing ideas that have formed the basis for intervention theories in occupational therapy are being questioned or discarded, and alternative models are being proposed for understanding changes in human behavior. The full implications of these revisions for practice are only beginning to be examined, and alternative treatment models are in the early stages of development. This state of affairs can be disconcerting to the therapist who must continue to provide treatment: The old ideas are being questioned, but a clear alternative may not yet be available. In such a situation a reflective and flexible approach to intervention is vital so that the therapist remains open to new possibilities, while examining for herself to what extent, and for whom, the current approaches appear to yield positive outcomes. Existing intervention models should be considered as a valuable starting point. Most are based not only on theory but on expert clinical observations made over the years. However, the therapist should also consider carefully her own observations, new information in the literature, and information provided by the patient that may contradict the theory. She will need to be ready to change her approach and to experiment if the positive changes predicted by the theory are not forthcoming.

The following questions provide guidelines for therapists examining the validity of a chosen intervention approach.

1. What is the basis (rationale) for the treatment sequences recommended? Is it, by analogy, to childhood sequences or based on a strict hierarchical model? Does this treatment approach acknowledge diverse pathways or solutions to functional problems, or does it insist on a strict progression of steps? If so, and if no data are available to support the efficacy of the sequence with adults, the therapist may want to consider modifying the sequence to focus on steps that are most integral to the goal or that have functional value by themselves.

The evidence to support the existence of necessary, invariant order for many functional tasks is not strong. Furthermore, the advent of technological aides has demonstrated the creative possibilities for achieving functional goals through significantly altered means, and therapists are familiar with the transforming impact of these changes on the rest of an individual's life. If change does not happen through application of typical methods, there are valid reasons to support exploration of atypical methods and alternate sequences. A therapist might consider *all* the parameters of a task situation that could be changed, including social, cognitive, and physical features. Any one of these might function as a critical stimulus for the emergence of a new solution to the functional problem.

2. Does this treatment model acknowledge differences between children and adults and make clear suggestions for how to modify treatment to take advantage of the unique characteristics of each age group? If not, the therapist may want to read and think about current information from life span studies of adult function (motor, physical, cognitive, etc.) to design adjustments to the approach. For example, the therapist might interview the patient about his history of physical activity or preferred modes of movement and may engage him in exploring different strategies for solving functional movement problems. The therapist can also take advantage of the adult's superior reasoning and problem-solving skills as they jointly try to understand the source of existing limitations and devise potential interventions.

3. Does this treatment approach engage the person in age-relevant, personally meaningful task contexts that provide the opportunity to rediscover affordances relevant to achieving his current functional goals? If not, the intervention may not be tapping into the developmental process that Gibson (1988) proposed

guides perception of information needed for adaptation. The therapist might examine the treatment setup, task selection, or physical environment to facilitate more effective action.

4. Does this treatment approach embody assumptions that remediation of components will automatically result in improved function? If so, are data provided to support these claims, and are these data sufficient to support a causal relation? In general, few studies are available to support such claims, either of the efficacy of remediation techniques focused on components or of generalized effects of such remediation. As noted earlier, much of the research in this area is from correlational studies, which describe the relation between components or between components and particular functional skills, but these data do not prove that a component skill is necessary. In the absence of solid information, the therapist should consider whether adequate provision has been made to help patients achieve desired functional goals through more direct means. Knowledge of component impairments may prove most useful in helping to guide selection of task strategies that capitalize on strengths and minimize the impact of deficits.

Although it may be disconcerting in the short term to make clinical decisions when so many questions are being raised about the basis of practice, this is a time of great creative opportunity for occupational therapy practitioners. By combining clinical expertise with new ideas generated from research and theory, therapists may discover new methods that can significantly improve the quality of life for those they assist in the recovery process.

STUDY QUESTIONS

1. What are the three major concerns of developmental theories (as outlined by Miller)? How does research directed to each of these concerns contribute to clinical practice?
2. Describe two examples of misapplications of data from developmental studies to clinical intervention. Explain what the problem is with each example.
3. What is meant by a linear hierarchical model of development? Give an example of an intervention theory that incorporates such a model.
4. How is the dynamical systems model different from the hierarchical models of behavioral development? Give an example that illustrates the contrast in the two models' explanations of the emergence of a new motor skill.
5. What is the role of the task in dynamical systems models?
6. What is meant by affordance, and what is the relation between movement and affordances in Gibson and Gibson's model?

7. What is the role of the task in the Gibson and Gibson model? Discuss how this concept relates to the use of functional activities in intervention.
8. Identify at least three factors that may significantly affect the way a child and an adult accomplish the same motor task. Discuss how these differences may be relevant to intervention.
9. Why are additional studies of performance across the full life span critical for future development of intervention theory?

REFERENCES

Abreu, B. C., & Toglia, J. P. (1987). Cognitive rehabilitation: A model for occupational therapy. *American Journal of Occupational Therapy, 41,* 439–448.

Baltes, P. B. (1987). Theoretical propositions of life-span developmental psychology: On the dynamics between growth and decline. *Developmental Psychology, 23,* 611–626.

Bobath, K., & Bobath, B. (1984). The neuro-developmental treatment. In D. Scrutton (Ed.), *Management of the motor disorders of children with cerebral palsy* (pp. 6–17). Philadelphia: J. B. Lippincott.

Dixon, R. A., & Lerner, R. M. (1991). A history of systems in developmental psychology. In M. C. Bornstein & M. E. Lamb (Eds.), *Developmental psychology: An advanced textbook* (3rd ed., pp. 3–58). Hillsdale, NJ: Lawrence Erlbaum.

Dohrenwend, B. S., & Dohrenwend, B. P. (Eds.). (1984). *Stressful life events and their contents.* New Brunswick, NJ: Rutgers University Press.

Fetters, L. (1991). Cerebral palsy: Contemporary treatment concepts. In M. Lister (Ed.), *Contemporary management of motor control problems: Proceedings of the IIStep Conference* (pp. 219–224). Alexandria, VA: Foundation for Physical Therapy.

Fetters, L., Fernandez, B., & Cermak, S. (1989). The relationship of proximal and distal components in the development of reaching. *Journal of Human Movement Studies, 17,* 283–297.

Ford, D. H., & Lerner, R. M. (1992). *Developmental systems theory.* Newbury Park, CA: Sage.

Gesell, A. (1954). The ontogenesis of infant behavior. In L. Carmichael (Ed.), *Manual of child psychology,* (2nd ed., pp. 335–373). New York: John Wiley & Sons.

Gibson, E. J. (1988). Exploratory behavior in the development of perceiving, acting, and the acquiring of knowledge. *Annual Review of Psychology, 39,* 1–41.

Gibson, J. J. (1979). *The ecological approach to visual perception.* Boston: Houghton Mifflin.

Gordon, J. (1987). Assumptions underlying physical therapy intervention: Theoretical and historical perspectives. In J. H. Carr & R. B. Shepherd (Eds.), *Movement science: Foundations for physical therapy in rehabilitation* (pp. 1–30). Rockville, MD: Aspen.

Heriza, C. (1991). Motor development: Traditional and contemporary theories. In M. Lister (Ed.), *Contemporary management of motor control problems: Proceedings of the IIStep Conference* (pp. 99–126). Alexandria, VA: Foundation for Physical Therapy.

Horak, F. B. (1991). Assumptions underlying motor control for neurologic rehabilitation. In M. Lister (Ed.), *Contemporary management of motor control problems: Proceedings of the IIStep Conference* (pp. 11–28). Alexandria, VA: Foundation for Physical Therapy.

Illingworth, R. S. (1960). *The development of the infant and young child: Normal and abnormal.* New York: Churchill Livingston.

Lewthwaite, R. (1990). Motivational considerations in physical activity involvement. *Physical Therapy, 70,* 808–819.

Mayer, N. H., Reed, E., Schwartz, M. F., Montgomery, M., & Palmer, C. (1990). Buttering a hot cup of coffee: An approach to the study of errors of action in patients with brain damage. In D. E. Tupper & K. D. Cicerone (Eds.), *The neuropsychology of everyday life: Assessment and basic competencies* (pp. 259–284). Boston: Kluwer Academic.

McGraw, M. B. (1945). *Neuromuscular maturation of the human infant.* New York: Hafner Press.

Miller, P. H. (1989). *Theories of developmental psychology* (2nd ed.). New York: W. H. Freeman.

Montgomery, P. C. (1991). Perceptual issues in motor control. In M. Lister (Ed.), *Contemporary management of motor control problems: Proceedings of the IIStep Conference* (pp. 175–184). Alexandria, VA: Foundation for Physical Therapy.

Neistadt, M. E. (1990). A critical analysis of occupational therapy approaches for perceptual deficits in adults with brain injury. *American Journal of Occupational Therapy, 44*(4), 299–304.

Piaget, J. (1952). *The origins of intelligence.* New York: International Universities Press.

Rogoff, B. (1982). Integrating context and cognitive development. In M. E. Lamb & A. L. Brown (Eds.), *Advances in developmental psychology* (Vol. 2, pp. 125–170). Hillsdale, NJ: Lawrence Erlbaum.

Rogoff, B. (1990). *Apprenticeship in thinking.* New York: Oxford University Press.

Rutter, M. (1989). Pathways from childhood to adult life. *Journal of Child Psychology and Psychiatry, 30,* 23–51.

Sameroff, A. J., & Chandler, M. J. (1975). Reproductive risk and the continuum of caretaking casualty. In F. D. Horowitz, M. Hetherington, S. Scarr-Salapatek, & G. Siegel (Eds.), *Review of child development research* (Vol. 4, pp. 187–244). Chicago: Chicago University Press.

Short-DeGraff, M. A. (1988). *Human development for occupational and physical therapists.* Baltimore: Williams & Wilkins.

Shumway-Cook, A., & Woolacott, M. H. (1985). The growth of stability: Postural control from a developmental perspective. *Journal of Motor Behavior, 17,* 131–147.

Siev, E., Freishtat, B., & Zoltan, B. (1986). *Perceptual dysfunction in the adult stroke patient.* Thorofare, NJ: Slack.

Thelen, E. (1992). Development as a dynamic system. *Current Directions in Psychological Science, 1,* 189–193.

Thelen, E., & Ulrich, B. J. (1991). Hidden skills: A dynamic analysis of treadmill stepping during the first year. *Monographs of the Society for Research in Child Development, 56*(Serial No. 223).

Van Sant, A. F. (1990). Life-span development in functional tasks. *Physical Therapy, 70,* 788–798.

Van Sant, A. F. (1991). Should the normal motor developmental sequence be used as a theoretical model to progress patients? In M. Lister (Ed.), *Contemporary management of motor control problems: Proceedings of the IIStep Conference* (pp. 95–97). Alexandria, VA: Foundation for Physical Therapy.

13
Learning

Janet L. Poole

OBJECTIVES

After studying this chapter, the reader will be able to:
1. Discuss selected motor and cognitive learning theories.
2. Understand how factors internal and external to the learner influence learning.
3. Explain how feedback and practice can be used and varied to promote learning.
4. Describe how the therapist can structure treatment sessions to better facilitate retention and **transfer of learning.**
5. Understand how to structure teaching and learning experiences.

Occupational therapy can be viewed as a learning process in which therapists assist patients to master new skills or to reacquire old skills to function independently in daily life. Therapists may teach new methods to accomplish a skill, teach the use of a piece of adapted equipment, or teach intrinsic factors such as problem solving and/or the use of memory strategies. Although individuals can and do learn naturally without formal or informal instructions, the role of the therapist is to facilitate the process.

Learning is a permanent change in behavior as a result of experience and practice (Schmidt, 1988). Learning is different from an improvement in performance, because learning is permanent and an improvement in performance may be temporary. For example, during a treatment session, a patient's ability to construct a three-dimensional block design may improve. However, if the patient cannot remember how to construct the design the next day or cannot construct a slightly different design, the task has not been learned. This chapter discusses theories related to the learning of motor tasks, explores how impairments in cognition and perception affect learning, and suggests general strategies for designing environments to facilitate reten-

tion and generalization. Generalization is the ability to apply the skills learned in therapy to a variety of similar skills in new environments.

LEARNING THEORIES

Acquiring new skills and reacquiring old skills involve both motor and cognitive learning. Motor learning theories, such as the closed-loop and schema theories, focus on the acquisition of skilled movements but not on the processing of information. Cognitive learning theories, such as information processing theory, focus on how information is stored and retrieved but not on how the individual uses information from the internal and external environment. The theories complement each other to explain how individuals learn cognitive, perceptual, and motor skills.

Adams's Closed-Loop Theory

The basis for Adams's (1971) theory is a closed-loop system that is self-regulating with mechanisms for feedback, error detection, and error correction. Error detection and correction are accomplished by comparing responses with a reference, which includes the correct response. According to Adams (1971), a memory trace exists that selects and initiates a movement response. During movement, the performer compares feedback from the ongoing movement with the memory of past movements (perceptual trace). The perceptual trace is the internal reference of correctness that was developed and strengthened by practice. If the perceptual trace determines that the movement is being performed correctly, the movement is allowed to continue. But if the trace reveals that the movement is being performed incorrectly, commands are sent from higher control centers to the muscles to make adjustments. In Adams's theory, learning and the development of the perceptual trace depend on feedback and errorless practice. If errors occur, an incorrect perceptual trace

GLOSSARY ━━━━━━━━━━━━━━━━━━━━━━━

Action plan—A strategy that is be used to solve a motor task or problem.

Chunks of information—Small, meaningful groups of information or smaller units.

Encoding—Process by which information is stored into memory using cues that later are used to retrieve information from long-term memory.

Mnemonics—Strategies to aid in recalling information from short- and long-term memory.

Oscilloscope—An instrument that displays a visual representation of an electrical wave such as a muscle contraction.

Surface characteristics—The easily observable attributes of a task such as type of stimuli, presentation mode, variable attributes, stimuli arrangement, movement requirements, environmental context, and rules or directions.

Taxonomy—A classification system.

Transfer of learning—Practice and learning of one task can influence the learning of another.

is developed. According to the theory, individuals with sensory deficits should be unable to learn motor tasks unless some other feedback, such as vision, is available. Adams's theory is limited to explaining slow limb positioning tasks, also called guided or ramp movements, such as tracing letters or using scissors to cut out a pattern.

Schmidt's Schema Theory

A schema is a set of rules developed by abstracting and combining important pieces of information from related experiences (Schmidt, 1975). For example, schemata are developed for handwriting: if an individual signs his or her name on a blackboard or with the nondominant hand, the signatures will look similar to the name written with the dominant hand on a piece of paper. When forming a schema, four pieces of information are abstracted: (1) the initial conditions of the body and environment related to the response; (2) information about the response specification related to the demands of the movement such as direction, speed, and force; (3) sensory consequences or feedback received during and after a movement; and (4) information about the response outcome in relation to the goal.

To develop a schema for moving from sitting on an object to standing, the initial conditions such as the position of the trunk, hips, and knees and the particulars of the seat are determined. For example, the trunk may be leaning against the backrest; the hips and knees may be acutely flexed, as they are when sitting in a low seat; the seat may have armrests; and the seat may be still or in motion, such as a seat on a bus. The response specifications are based on these initial conditions. If the seat is low, weight must be shifted forward, and a significant amount of force must be generated in the quadriceps and hamstrings to come to a standing position. If the seat is high, less force is needed to stand. If armrests are available, less force may be needed by the lower extremities because the arms can be used to push up. If the seat is in motion, predictions will need to be made regarding when to stand. The sensory consequences are assessed by feel-

ing and seeing an upward movement in space, whereas the outcome is determined by deciding and noting whether a standing position was achieved, given that the goal was to stand.

Once the pieces of information are synthesized, a schema is formed so that whenever a person is seated in a similar position on a bed, toilet, chair, or bench, similar movements will result in coming to a standing position, even if the individual has never before sat on that particular object. Feedback and practice help strengthen schemata. Because performers develop rules about a class of movements, they should practice variations of a skill as in the example above. Error-free practice is not critical, as responses can vary within the class of movements that make up the schema. Schmidt's schema theory applies to both slow limb positioning tasks and preplanned or rapid ballistic movements, such as a foot slamming on the brake pedal of a car.

Information Processing Memory Model

Information processing theory views humans as processors of information. Sensory input is received from the environment and processed in various ways until, eventually, output occurs as an observable motor, cognitive, or perceptual response. According to this model, information is processed within three memory buffers: sensory store, short-term memory, and long-term memory (Atkinson & Shiffrin, 1968; Shiffrin & Schneider, 1977). In the information processing model, once a goal is identified, a performer actively decides the sensory input to which attention will be directed. The sensory input includes information both internal and external to the performer. Internal information includes proprioception, touch, and vision, and external information includes where objects are in space in relation to each other and the performer and the speed of moving objects.

Information is temporarily held in sensory store until it can be attended to. Then information moves into working, or short-term, memory. Short-term memory is a temporary storage place that holds data until they are analyzed and processed. It is limited in capacity, i.e., only seven (plus or minus two) **chunks of information** can be retained at a time (Miller, 1966). The duration of temporary storage may be increased through a control process, rehearsal.

Encoding involves transforming information to be remembered into a form that can be more easily recognized later when retrieving it from long-term memory (LTM). Organizing to-be-remembered material into **mnemonics** is an example of **encoding.** For example, the mnemonic "On Old Olympic Towering Top, A Finn And German Viewed A Hop" is commonly used to remember the cranial nerves. The first letter of each word is the first letter of each of the 12 cranial nerves and thus serves as a cue to recall their names. Long-term memory contains permanent memories of past experiences that influence the attention to sensory input and decisions on how to respond in a given situation.

Control processes such as selective attention, labeling, rehearsal, organization, and retrieval are used to move information through the three buffers. Selective attention is the process by which one attends to relevant environmental cues and ignores others. Attention may be focused on one object or stimulus or divided over several objects or sets of stimuli. Labeling refers to the attachment of a verbal label to represent a stimulus or movement, e.g., assigning the word *circle* to represent the shape *O*. One must be able to label before one can rehearse (Laabs, 1973). People with aphasia may have difficulty with this aspect of processing. Rehearsal involves repeatedly attending to information in a serial fashion. Rehearsal may be physical or mental, such as mentally practicing the steps to a dance routine.

Organization involves two processes: grouping and recoding. Grouping, or chunking, occurs when information to be remembered is placed into subgroups. Phone numbers are chunked into two subgroups, the exchange number (the first three numbers) and the last four numbers. First-letter **mnemonics** and the method of loci involve chunking information to larger units in short-term memory. An example of a mnemonic device (for remembering cranial nerves) was given earlier. The method of loci involves visual imagery. For example, one might attempt to remember the names of students in a classroom by visualizing where they sit in class. Once information is in short-term memory (STM), existing information in LTM is used to encode information in more meaningful ways. Recoding involves combining items in STM based on some similarity and then reentering the new code into the long-term memory as a single item. For example, occupational therapy students learn about sock aids, reachers, long-handled shoehorns, and button hooks during their academic training. Students combine knowledge about these items and recode them in the category "devices for

dressing," which is reentered into LTM as a single item. This reduces the demands on one's memory, making it easier to recall the item.

Retrieval is searching, locating, and extracting information from memory. Retrieval of information seems to be affected by how it was encoded in the memory in the first place and the context in which it was learned. For example, students recall the steps of a wheelchair-to-toilet transfer better on a practical examination that uses the room and equipment that were used when they learned and practiced the maneuver than on an exam that uses another setting with a slightly different style of toilet.

FACTORS THAT AFFECT LEARNING

Learning is influenced by factors both internal and external to the learner. Internal factors include whether the individual has performed the task before (stage of the learner) and the individual's capabilities. A patient with cognitive and perceptual impairments may have trouble learning. Performance of an habitual motor skill, such as putting on socks, may be preserved, but learning an adapted method or how to use a sock aid, for instance, may be beyond his learning capability. Individuals must be able to receive and interpret incoming sensory information in relation to previously learned sensations. A patient with a sensory disturbance experiences a "new" sensation that may not have a learned referent. This patient, therefore, is not capable of selecting the appropriate response associated with that sensation. In formulating a response, the learner must select a plan of action from memory that will meet the demands of the task. External factors also affect learning. Complex tasks with a high level of unpredictability will demand more elaborate information processing capabilities than tasks with fewer steps and low uncertainty. If the task is too complex or too simple, motivation may decrease.

Internal Factors

STAGE OF THE LEARNER

Three sequential stages of learning were defined by Fitts and Posner (1967). In the first stage, the cognitive stage, the patient tries to understand the requirements of the task. The patient relies heavily on vision and verbal feedback from the therapist or instructor. The learner may have to think through or verbalize the steps in a task or to describe the position the body must be in. Patients may verbalize each step during a transfer or the sequence of a gait pattern. It is during this first stage that the patient must begin to learn what cues to attend to.

In the second stage, the associative or intermediate stage, the learner has determined the most effective way of doing a task and begins to make refinements in performance. The learner relies less on vision and verbal feedback and begins to use proprioceptive feedback. During this stage, practice becomes of primary importance. Whether the therapist should allow errors to occur during practice has been debated. Error-free practice has been advocated as a way for the learner to develop sensory feedback of the correct movement, or an internal reference of correctness (Adams, 1971; Kottke, 1980). It is believed that incorrect practice of a task will require unlearning. Error-free learning has been advocated for individuals with memory deficits, because these individuals tend to repeat errors (Konow & Pribram, 1970). In addition, too many errors may mean the skill is too difficult. On the other hand, learners may use error information to adjust subsequent movements (Edwards & Lee, 1985).

The third stage of learning is the autonomous stage in which the skill is under proprioceptive control and has become largely automatic or habitual. The learner can perform most of the skill without thinking about it. Performance is also less subject to interference from other ongoing activities or environmental distractions.

COGNITIVE IMPAIRMENTS

The cognitive processes that are important for learning include attention, memory processes, and problem solving. Impairments in one or more of these processes may limit the perception, organization, storage, and retrieval of information necessary for learning (Atkinson & Shiffrin, 1968). Attention is necessary to focus one's mental effort over a period of time to detect relevant stimuli and exclude other information. Indeed, Atkinson and Shiffrin (1968) consider attention to play a major role in **encoding** information to and retrieving information from memory. An individual with deficits in attention is distracted by all stimuli and is not able to differentiate relevant from irrelevant stimuli or to focus only on one part of the stimuli. For example, in copying a pegboard design, an individual may be focused on the shape and handling of the peg rather than on the task.

Memory is also necessary to store and retrieve information for learning. Memory involves a perception that has been stored and can be reproduced later. For example, to teach an adult who has sustained a stroke how to put on a shirt using essentially one upper limb, the therapist assumes that the patient once knew how to put on a shirt. However, if the patient has a memory deficit, then that perception (memory) may no longer be retrievable and the patient may have to relearn the task. Furthermore, the task now becomes a "new" task,

because the usual method of putting on a shirt can no longer be used.

Impairments in problem solving also affect learning, because control processes are not automatically used when presented with new information or are used ineffectively (Bolger, 1982). Individuals with problem-solving deficits continue to use strategies that do not work and cannot perceive their own capabilities or monitor their performance (Anderson et al., 1989; Rimel et al., 1985). Thus responses are slow and erratic because of an inability to choose a strategy. After the response is made, there is no error recognition so performance does not improve.

PERCEPTUAL IMPAIRMENTS

Perception is necessary to interpret sensory input from within the body and from the external environment. Perception relies heavily on comparing current information with past experiences. Thus memory and perception are intertwined as factors that affect learning (Sage, 1977). When perception is impaired, incoming sensory input is not accurately identified and thus not correctly matched to data in LTM. Learning is initially under visual control, so when vision or visual perception is impaired, other senses may not initially compensate for the loss (Rock & Harris, 1967). For example, a left visual field cut and hemiinattention eliminate input from the left visual field. Patients with these impairments may have difficulty learning to use their left extremity because, although they may be able to "feel" their extremity, they need more cues to effect movement.

Sensation is also thought to be necessary for learning, because it provides feedback. Individuals with sensory deficits will usually need some additional mechanism to receive input from the environment and for feedback. Rothwell et al.'s (1982) classic study demonstrated that a man with complete sensory loss could learn new motor tasks when he received extrinsic visual feedback via an **oscilloscope.** When the feedback was removed, the man continued to perform, but performance decayed over time. It appeared that sensation was needed for feedback at some point in time to inform the central nervous system about the continued success of the movements.

Individuals with deficits in figure/ground focus on the foreground or details of the environment. They cannot identify the critical features in the environment. Thus they may not be able to find objects needed for a task or do not notice objects in the environment that must be attended to until it is too late. This is a major problem for learning or performing skills with a high level of unpredictability, such as driving. To learn a skill such as driving, individuals must be able to identify cues such as turn signals from other cars, erratic behavior of other drivers, bicyclists, pedestrians, and warning signs indicating a driveway or intersection; they must also be able to predict and select correct responses based on these observations.

External Factors

External factors that affect learning are the temporal, spatial, and the social features of the environment. Different environments elicit different information-processing demands. For example, a patient who can select money for a purchase in a quiet one-to-one environment, may not select the correct amount of money in a grocery store or fast-food restaurant. In the first case, there is no competing stimuli for the patient's attention so he does not have to weed out irrelevant stimuli. In the latter, other individuals, objects, and sounds create additional demands on his attention.

The temporal and spatial features of an environment place cognitive and perceptual demands on the learner. In environments in which there is high uncertainty as to what conditions will prevail, information-processing demands are high. On the other hand, information-processing demands are low when the environment remains the same or is familiar and there are no environmental uncertainties. Gentile (1972, 1987) developed a **taxonomy,** or classification, of motor tasks based on environmental conditions and the demands placed on the performer (Table 13.1). Environments are considered to be on a continuum from stable or stationary to unpredictable or constant motion. As the predictability decreases, the need to attend to and quickly process information from the environment increases.

Tasks for which the critical features of the environment—such as objects, people, and the terrain—are stationary and do not change from trial to trial are called closed tasks. Walking up the stairs in one's own home, dart games, putting together a particular puzzle, gymnastics routines, getting on and off the toilet in one's own bathroom are examples of closed tasks. In all of these tasks, the performer's movements are constrained by the spatial features of the environment. There are no temporal constraints, as the movements are self-paced. The performer controls the start, stop, and duration of the task. In closed tasks, all the relevant information is immediately available in the environment. Because the environment stays the same over repeated trials, movements become more consistent, automatic, and fixed. The movement seems to be stored in memory and then reproduced. There are no uncertainties in terms of what the environment will be like. Therefore, the information-processing demands are low and the need to monitor the environment to

Table 13.1. Gentile's Taxonomy

Temporal Features	Variability in Spatial Features	
	Absent	Present
Stationary	Closed (brushing teeth, typing, climbing stairs at home)	Variable motionless (putting on different styles of shirts, transfers to different surface heights)
Motion	Consistent motion (step on a escalator, lift baggage from conveyor belt, assembly line work)	Open (driving, catching a fly ball, propelling a wheelchair in a crowded mall)

pick up information decreases. The familiarity of the environment provides additional cues to help select and organize a response (Kelso & Tuller, 1981).

There are other tasks for which the spatial features of the environment vary from trial to trial but are stationary or motionless during performance. The temporal features remain the same. These are called variable motionless tasks. Examples of variable motionless tasks include arising from different pieces of furniture, constructing several different block designs, putting on different styles of shoes or shirts, walking on different surfaces, and grasping different styles of drinking containers. A group task in which individuals share materials and tools would be a variable motionless task because the location of materials and equipment would change after each individual used them. Because variable motionless tasks are also self-paced, there are no predictive demands on the performer. Movement patterns begin to be diversified because the conditions in the environment change. An individual cannot always use just any movement pattern from memory but may have to generate a novel movement based on the current environmental conditions. Thus information-processing demands are higher than for closed tasks.

At the other end of the continuum are tasks in which the temporal features change. The environment is in motion. In one type of task, consistent motion tasks, the environment is in motion but moves at a constant rate from trial to trial. Stepping on an escalator, lifting boxes or luggage from conveyer belts, and working at an assembly line are examples of consistent motion tasks. One must predict when to step on and off the escalator or lift the suitcase or boxes from the conveyer belt.

Open tasks are those tasks in which the supporting surfaces, objects, or people in the environment are in motion and or change from one trial to the next. The performer's movements must match both the spatial and the temporal features of the environment. Examples of open tasks are driving a car, catching a fly ball, and walking or propelling a wheelchair down a crowded path. Open tasks force the performer to predict events in the environment and learn where to pick up advance information. Skilled performers know where to look in a complex environment to pick up critical information. They know what the advanced cues are and where to look for them. What is stored in memory is probably strategies on how to vary movements to fit a number of environmental situations. For open tasks, the performer develops probability functions as to the likelihood certain conditions will occur. There are uncertainties as to what conditions will prevail. Information demands are high, because the learner must continually attend to the environment.

Along with environmental demands, certain characteristics of the tasks themselves can alter information-processing demands: amount of stimuli, speed of response, amount of sensory integration, and familiarity with the task (Barth & Boll, 1981; Hart & Hayden, 1986). Block designs can be simple or complex, depending on the number of blocks and number of different colors in the design. The rate or speed of a conveyer belt in an assembly line job could be increased, which increases processing demands on the performer. The amount of sensory integration during a catching activity can be increased by playing catch in the context of a baseball game; now the performer must determine what to do with the ball once it is caught. Familiarity can be manipulated by changing the environment in which the task is performed such as cooking in the occupational therapy kitchen versus in one's own kitchen.

TEACHING AND LEARNING SKILLS
Role of Feedback

Feedback is information about the outcome of a response or what caused the outcome (Magill, 1989). Feedback can be intrinsic and/or extrinsic to the learner. Intrinsic feedback is inherent sensory feedback such as feedback from the visual, auditory, tactile, vestibular, and proprioceptive systems. Individuals feel that their weight is distributed evenly over both lower extremities or see that their fingers are flexing. Individuals with cognitive and perceptual deficits may need to be especially encouraged to use intrinsic feedback to check their work to recognize and correct errors (Ben-Yishay et al., 1970).

Extrinsic feedback comes from an external source such as a therapist, a device (e.g., a biofeedback machine), or the observation of an effect on the environment. Extrinsic feedback augments intrinsic feedback and can be especially important if sensory receptors are impaired. A therapist can provide two types of extrinsic feedback: knowledge of results and knowledge of performance. Knowledge of results (KR) provides information about how well the performance met the goal and helps the patient recognize and correct errors. For example, the therapist may say, "You did not comb the hair on the left side of your head," "The collar of your shirt is turned under," or "Your block design does not look like the one in the picture." KR may or may not overlap with intrinsic feedback. Patients may also see that their block designs do not look like the picture. However, KR may need to be more explicit for those with cognitive and perceptual deficits. The therapist may have to point to the blocks that are incorrect and describe the error, saying, for example, "This block is the wrong color" or "This block is turned in the wrong direction." Knowledge of performance (KP) is verbal feedback about the nature of a response. It is usually not redundant with intrinsic feedback so it provides information that the learner may not be aware of. For example the therapist would say, "You are not standing up straight" or "You did not move your eyes while looking for your fork."

Feedback can also be used for motivational purposes. It can help keep the patient alert and encourage him to continue to participate in a long, boring, or difficult task. Feedback can also be used to reward effort rather than accuracy. This is especially important when teaching patients tasks that are more challenging. However, the use of words such as *good* should be used judiciously. *Good* should be used as a reward for accomplishing some specific desired behavior. If patients are not successful but try hard, the therapist should use other words or gestures for encouragement, such as making a suggestion on how to improve performance next time or commenting that the task is certainly difficult.

Feedback helps accelerate the learning process. Visual and verbal feedback seem to be especially important in acquiring skills (Keele & Posner, 1968; Zelaznik, Hawkins, & Kisselbaugh, 1983). In one study, when visual and verbal feedback were eliminated although proprioceptive feedback continued, accuracy of movements in the early stage of learning was impaired (Williams & Stelmach, 1968).

When to give feedback is also important in teaching. Feedback can be given after every attempt at a task or at the end of several trials. Feedback after every trial does improve performance but does not seem to affect learning and retaining of information (Winstein & Schmidt, 1990). The learner begins to depend on it. The feedback acts as a crutch, so the learner may not be processing important task-related information. On the other hand, feedback given at random intervals may assist with processing relevant information and developing error-detection capabilities.

Role of Practice

Practice involves more than mere repetition of a task. It involves an effort to improve. Practice should consist of developing new solutions or retrieving a solution from a repertoire of solutions to cognitive, perceptual, or motor problems that were successful in the past (Bernstein, 1967; Whiting, 1980). Practice is essential to skill acquisition. Although it has been estimated that millions of repetitions are necessary to develop skilled movement (Kottke, 1980), the practice of motor skills in therapy is often limited to several times per session. Therapy sessions should be structured to promote learning.

There are certain practice schedules that seem to improve task performance but do not affect retention or transfer. For example, a therapist may have a patient practice three bed-to-wheelchair transfers during a treatment session or the therapist may have the patient practice a bed transfer, a chair transfer, and a toilet transfer. Which practice session would be better for learning? Transferring to the bed three times is blocked practice, in which a single task is practiced before proceeding to the next task. Blocked practice improves performance but results in poor retention. Practicing three different transfers is random practice. In random practice, several variations of a task are practiced during skill acquisition. Random practice results in retention and transfer to a novel skill (Magill, 1989; Shea & Morgan, 1979). Blocked practice may be more effective at the beginning of the first stage of learning. However, Schmidt (1988) recommends starting random practice once the movement can be performed at all.

The difference in the effects of blocked and random practice may be due to contextual interference (Battig, 1979). Contextual interference refers to the detrimental effect that practice of one task may have on another. Low contextual interference is created by blocked practice, because the situation remains constant; high contextual interference is created by random practice. When tasks are presented in an unpredictable fashion, as with random practice, the learner is forced to engage in more active processing during practice, because the solution developed for the first task must be modified to be totally successful for the second task (Lee & Magill, 1983). Thus the **action plan** must be reconstructed. During this process of constructing and reconstructing a plan for action, patients are developing problem-solving strategies that will help them transfer the skill to a novel task. Thus contextual interference seems to facilitate cognitive processes necessary for the memory of schemata.

Transfer of learning may also be affected by how much of a task is practiced. A task may be practiced in isolation or as part of a whole activity (Stammers, 1982; Wightman & Lintern, 1985). Using simulators for work-related activities, buttoning buttons on a button board, and making one part of a meal such as a dessert are examples of part practice. Generally, part practice does not transfer or generalize unless the subskills designated as parts are natural subunits (Newell, Carton, & Fish, 1989). For example, Winstein et al. (1989) noted that isolated lower extremity weight-bearing exercises did not result in equal weight distribution during gait. Thus weight shifting did not appear to be a natural subunit of locomotion.

A part-whole technique called chaining has been used in memory rehabilitation and with profoundly brain-damaged patients. Chaining involves breaking a skill down into a series of steps. Only one step is taught at a time. Eventually, each step acts as a stimulus or trigger for the next step. In backward chaining, the therapist guides or assists the patient up to the last step. When the patient can do that step, the therapist guides up until the preceding step and so on until the patient can do the whole task from start to finish.

It is assumed that the processing skills practiced during remedial activities for learning cognitive and perceptual skills (such as puzzle construction and computer activities) will transfer to different activities (Neistadt, 1990). There is evidence that remedial activities transfer to dissimilar tasks (Lincoln et al., 1985; Sivak et al., 1984), but other evidence that they transfer to very similar tasks only (Glisky, Schacter, & Tulving, 1986; Neistadt, 1992).

Generally, the more two skills or situations are perceived as similar, the greater the likelihood transfer will occur (Oxendine, 1968; Stallings, 1982). Toglia (1991) classified degrees of transfer on a continuum based on the **surface characteristics** of the tasks. **Surface characteristics** are the easily observed attributes of a task such as type of stimuli, presentation mode, variable attributes, stimuli arrangement, movement requirements, environmental context, and rules or directions (see Table 27.3). According to Toglia's (1991) system, near transfer occurs when one to two **surface characteristics** are different from each other, intermediate transfer occurs when some **surface characteristics** are similar but less readily identified, far transfer occurs when tasks are conceptually similar but the **surface characteristics** are completely different or share only one similar characteristic, and very far transfer, or generalization, occurs when the task can be applied spontaneously to everyday life.

To illustrate how the **surface characteristics** can be changed for near, intermediate, far, and very far transfers, consider teaching self-care skills to a patient who has had a total hip replacement. For near transfer, the single **surface characteristic** of size could be changed: the patient could apply principles of using a reacher to put on his underpants to the task of putting on his slacks. In intermediate transfer, the **surface characteristics** of type of clothing, texture of material, and movement requirements could be changed, such as using a sock aid to put on a sock. In far transfer, the **surface characteristics** are different but the task is conceptually the same, for example, washing and drying the leg and foot on the side of the total hip replacement. Finally, far transfer involves application of information: the patient applies hip precautions when he puts his legs into the bathtub at home.

It is assumed that the cognitive, perceptual, and motor skills patients master in therapy will transfer to the home or work environments. To facilitate this process, practice conditions must simulate the real-life environment as much as possible. Ideally, therapy should be done in the home or work environment. Because this is not always possible, random practice schedules of whole tasks while systematically varying **surface characteristics** of a task should help facilitate transfer. For some individuals with brain damage, the skills learned in therapy may not transfer. These individuals may need a blocked practice schedule within the actual context, and they may not be independent outside a sheltered or familiar environment.

Role of the Therapist

The therapist is a facilitator in the patient's learning or reacquiring of motor, cognitive, and perceptual skills. The learner's capability, the environment, and type of task all influence the ability to process information and must be considered when teaching motor, cognitive, or perceptual skills. The following strategies can be used by therapists to facilitate skill acquisition (Table 13.2).

1. Clarify the goal of the task and the critical features to which attention should be focused. In the early stages of learning, the learner must understand the goal whether it be to put on a shirt, copy a block design, or protract a shoulder to operate a below-elbow prosthesis. The therapist can give verbal instructions or manual guidance, demonstrate how to do the task, or show a video of the task being performed by an expert. The therapist should direct the learner's atten-

Table 13.2. Strategies for Skill Acquisition

1. Clarify the goal and critical features of the skill.
2. Set up learning environment relative to the patient's capabilities.
3. Teach the patient use of strategies.
4. Provide feedback.
5. Structure practice for retention and generalization.

tion to critical environmental cues and the essential aspects of the task. In teaching a patient to put on a pair of pants, the therapist may remind the patient that the label is on the back of the garment and the opening is on the front. The patient with a visual field deficit may need to be cued to turn his or her head to the side before eating a meal.

The critical features of the environment can be highlighted using color, some other marking, or contrasting backgrounds. The keys on a typewriter or computer can be color coded according to which finger is assigned to which key. A red piece of tape or line can be placed on the side of a page in a book (called anchoring by Diller and Weinberg, 1977). Contrasting color for top and bottom bed sheets can help the patient with deficits in figure/ground make a bed. For tasks in which the environment is in motion, the learner could learn which cues are relevant and observe them (Gentile, 1987; Spaeth-Arnold, 1981). To help a confused individual or one with limited attention or decreased figure/ground discrimination ability learn, the environment may need to be uncluttered and void of people and noise.

2. Design the learning environment to present the activity according to the patient's information-processing capabilities. Start with tasks that are already within the patient's information-processing capabilities and behavioral repertoire. Gradually increase the processing demands. Increase the rate, duration, and amount of information presented before increasing the complexity of information and the amount of sensory integration required (Abreu & Toglia, 1987; Hagan, 1982).

3. Teach strategies that the patient can use when presented with oncoming information. Strategies may include teaching a patient to plan ahead, control speed of response, check self, or generate an alternative response (Fertherlin & Kurland 1989; Lawson & Rice, 1989). Other strategies may involve cuing the patient to use control processes such as rehearsal and grouping. The use of a particular strategy will need to be applied in several situations for generalization to occur. The learner also must learn when the strategy does not apply (Gagne, 1985). For example, rehearsal may be effective to remember the steps to operate a microwave oven but would not be appropriate for completing a cooking task or operating a car.

4. Provide feedback. In early learning, cuing and feedback should be given frequently so that the learner understands what is considered correct performance for a task and what is an error (Adams, 1971; Gentile, 1972; Kottke, 1980). Feedback should be delayed for a few seconds after the task is completed so that the patient can use those few moments to process intrinsic feedback (Gentile, 1987). In the associative stage of learning, feedback should be precise but start to be gradually withdrawn so that the learner depends less on external and more on intrinsic feedback (Glisky & Schacter, 1988; Salmoni, Schmidt, & Walter, 1984). For habitual, closed, and consistent motion tasks, knowledge of performance is more appropriate because the patient is trying to achieve a consistent response. For a perceptual or cognitive task, KR is appropriate, because the patient needs information about how to correct the error. Feedback for variable motionless and open tasks should emphasize how well the patient predicted the events in the environment and selected a correct response.

5. Structure practice for retention and transfer (generalization). In initial learning, or the cognitive stage, in which the learner is trying to understand the requirements of the task, constant and blocked practice schedules may be more appropriate than random practice to improve performance. Patients may need to practice the same movements several times before they get the idea. Transfers to the same chair can be practiced before proceeding to different heights or types of surfaces. As soon as the patient has the idea of the transfer, the therapist should vary the surface (bed, toilet), and then vary the height, e.g., kitchen chair and low armchair. The patient may practice using an external memory aid such as a notebook to help remember his or her daily schedule. However, for generalization to occur, the patient must practice using the aid in other situations as well. Teaching a confused patient requires a constant practice schedule (Shea, Kohl, & Indermill, 1990).

Practice in the associative and autonomous stages of learning is more task specific. Although a constant practice format has been advocated for tasks for which the environment is stable and predictable, motor-learning research shows that a variable practice schedule is superior in improving learning and transfer (McCracken & Stelmach, 1977; Shapiro & Schmidt, 1982). In later stages of learning open and variable motionless tasks, practice should be done under diverse environmental conditions (Siegel & Davis, 1980). The learner must develop flexibility and a repertoire of strategies for responding to changing and novel environmental conditions. The therapist should systematically change environmental conditions during practice to encompass all possibilities (Spaeth-Arnold, 1981). For example, a work-retraining program for a food service worker should be done in both empty and crowded and noisy environments. Patients learning to dress should practice dressing with all styles of clothing they normally wear. Patients redeveloping hand skills should practice grasping objects that vary in size, shape, and weight.

Structuring and Implementing a Teaching/Learning Experience

Occupational therapists educate patients and often their families in some aspects of care. For example, the therapist may inform patients with arthritis about the principles of protecting their joints, may teach stress reduction techniques to patients with cardiac dysfunction, and may teach family members how to transfer a patient to the car. In these examples, the teaching may take place in only one to two sessions with the patient and family. The strategies discussed earlier for facilitating skill acquisition also apply to any teaching/learning situation. More specific guidelines to help a therapist structure a patient education session are discussed next (Table 13.3).

1. Explain why the material or techniques being taught will be helpful to the patient. For example, the therapist could inform the patient that using the principles of joint protection helps minimize inflammation and the deforming forces that can damage joints.

2. Establish both the learning and the teaching goals with the patient. This process is especially important when educating a patient to make a behavioral change. In that case, the goals may need to be stated as small and behaviorally measurable, e.g., "Relax in an easy chair for 15 min after arriving home from work."

3. Use a presentation style relevant to the patient's information-processing capabilities and preferences. Oral, written, and/or visual materials can all be used. When teaching a patient with aphasia, a demonstration or visual materials are more appropriate than verbal instructions. If the patient has problems with spatial orientation, the therapist must sit next to the patient and demonstrate the task in the same plane in which the patient is expected to perform. When teaching an older patient, instructions should be given slowly, and written instructions may need to be in large, bold print. When teaching joint protection to a patient with arthritis or stress reduction to a patient with cardiac or pulmonary involvement, written instructions that supplement the oral directions reinforce what is being

Table 13.3. Structuring and Implementing a Teaching/Learning Experience

1. Explain why the material is important to the patient.
2. Establish the teaching and learning goals with the patient.
3. Teach the material according to the patient's capabilities.
4. Use examples relevant to the patient's lifestyle and needs.
5. When specific techniques are taught, practice is necessary.
6. Assess whether the material and technique have been learned correctly.

taught. The written instruction can be referred to when the patient is in the home environment.

4. *Use examples relevant to the patient's lifestyle and needs.* For example, patients with arthritis do not need to be told to eliminate ironing to save energy and protect their joints if they never iron. The principles for joint protection should relate to the patient. Thus, patients who are secretaries and receptionists need information about how to protect their joints when writing, typing, holding a telephone, sitting, and so on.

If the therapist is helping a patient with a behavioral change, such as joint protection or stress management, the therapist should find out how the patient performs different activities or has been managing stress. The patient's own method may be acceptable. If it is not, then the therapist can provide more relevant feedback.

5. *When specific techniques are being taught, the patient and/or family must practice them.* Besides hearing and reading about ways to protect the joints, the patient must actually practice correct alignment and methods to decrease joint stress. This is important to ensure that the principles will continue to be practiced at home. A patient who is learning to reduce stress by listening to relaxation tapes in therapy should be provided with the means to listen to the tapes in his hospital room at night or over the weekend. Family members may be hesitant about physically transferring the patient from the wheelchair to the car. They must be able to practice the transfer in the presence of the therapist to gain the skill and confidence necessary to do the transfer on their own.

6. *Evaluate whether the patient and/or family member has learned the material correctly.* The therapist can ask the patient or family member to explain or demonstrate the principle or technique. This provides an opportunity for feedback and error correction. If the patient and/or family member does not perform or explain the material correctly, then the therapist will need to repeat the teaching/learning process. Another way to assess whether the material has been learned is to ask the patient to apply the material to other problems or situations. For example, to evaluate whether a patient has learned principles of joint protection and work simplification, the therapist might have the patient prepare a meal and do the cleanup.

SUMMARY

Learning implies a permanent change in behavior. To assess learning, the therapist notes whether the patient can perform a skill or explain material that was learned earlier or within a different context. Ideally, the skills patients learn in therapy should generalize to real-life situations. Although this may not be possible for all patients, therapy should be structured to facilitate generalization. For learning to occur, the skill must be relevant and patients must understand the goal of the skill. The skill should be taught using a presentation mode relevant to the patients' capabilities. Patients must be taught strategies to use when presented with information pertinent to the skill. Therapists can manipulate feedback and practice schedules to enhance the learning of a skill. Feedback is provided frequently in early learning. In later learning, feedback is gradually withdrawn, and that which is given is precise. When structuring the practice schedule and context, the therapist should set as random a schedule as possible, because a random schedule facilitates retention and generalization to real-life situations.

STUDY QUESTIONS

1. Compare and contrast Adams's closed loop, Schmidt's schema, and the information processing theories.
2. How can a therapist structure a treatment program to increase independence in typing skills for a secretary with a high spinal cord injury versus another patient with a high spinal cord injury who has never typed but now needs to use a computer?
3. How can transfer of learning be facilitated?
4. Discuss how cognitive and perceptual impairments affect learning.
5. Describe Gentile's four types of tasks, and give an example of each.
6. How would practice be structured for a closed task versus an open task?
7. Discuss the two types of extrinsic feedback and give an example of each.
8. Think about an activity you might have to teach a patient's family. Describe how you would go about teaching the family the activity.
9. Describe the three stages of learning.
10. What is learning? How can a therapist decide whether a patient has learned an activity or not?

REFERENCES

Adams, J. A. (1971). A closed-loop theory of motor learning. *Journal of Motor Behavior, 3,* 111–149.

Anderson, S. W., Damasio, R. A., Damasio, H., & Tranel, D. (1989). Impaired awareness of disease states following right hemisphere damage. *Neurology, 39*(suppl. 1), 232.

Abreu, B. C., & Toglia, J. P. (1987). Cognitive rehabilitation: A model for occupational therapy. *American Journal of Occupational Therapy, 41,* 439–448.

Atkinson, R. C., & Shiffrin, R. M. (1968). Human memory: A proposed system and its control processes. In K. W. Spence & J. T. Spence (Eds.), *The psychology of learning and motivation: Advances in research and theory* (Vol. 2, pp. 89–197). New York: Academic Press.

Barth, J., & Boll, F. (1981). Rehabilitation and treatment of central nervous system dysfunction: A behavioral medicine perspective. In C. Prokop & L. Bradley (Eds.), *Medical psychology: Contributions to behavioral medicine* (pp. 241–265). New York: Academic Press.

Battig, W. F. (1979). The flexibility of human memory. In L. S. Cermak & F. I. M. Craik (Eds.), *Levels of processing and human memory* (pp. 23–44). Hillsdale, NJ: Lawrence Erlbaum.

Ben-Yishay, Y., Diller, L., Gerstman, L. J., Gordon, W. (1970). Relationship between initial competencies and abilities to profit from cues in brain-damaged adults. *Journal of Abnormal Psychology, 75*, 248–259.

Bernstein, N. (1967). *The coordination and regulation of movements.* Elmsford, NY: Pergamon Press.

Bolger, J. P. (1982). Cognitive retraining: A developmental approach. *Clinical Neuropsychology, 4*, 66–70.

Diller, L., & Weinberg, J. (1977). Hemi-attention in rehabilitation: The evolution of a rational remediation program. In E. A. Weinstein & R. P. Friedland (Eds.), *Advances in neurology* (pp. 63–82). New York: Raven Press.

Edwards, R. V., & Lee, A. M. (1985). The relationship of cognitive style and instructional strategy to learning and transfer of motor skills. *Research Quarterly for Exercise and Sport, 56*, 286–290.

Fertherlin, J. M., & Kurland, L. (1989). Self-instruction: A compensatory strategy to increase functional independence with brain injured adults. *Occupational Therapy Practice, 1*, 75–88.

Fitts, P. M., & Posner, M. I. (1967). *Learning and skilled performance in human performance.* Belmont, CA: Brooks/Cole Publishers.

Gagne, E. (1985). *The cognitive psychology of school learning.* Boston: Little, Brown & Co.

Gentile, A. M. (1987). Skill acquisition: Action, movement, and neuromotor processes. In J. H. Carr, R. B. Shepherd, J. Gordon, A. M. Gentile, & J. M. Held (Eds.), *Movement science: Foundations for physical therapy in rehabilitation* (pp. 93–154). Rockville, MD: Aspen Systems.

Gentile, A. M. (1972). A working model of skill acquisition with applications to teaching. *Quest, 17*, 3–23.

Glisky, E. L., & Schacter, D. L. (1988). Acquisition of domain-specific knowledge in patients with organic memory disorders. *Journal of Learning Disabilities, 21*, 333–339.

Glisky, E. L., Schacter, D. L., & Tulving, E. (1986). Computer learning by memory-impaired patients: Acquisition and retention of complex knowledge. *Neuropsychologia, 24*, 313–328.

Goldstein, L. H., & Oakley, D. A. (1985). Expected and actual behavioral capacity after diffuse reduction in cerebral cortex: A review and suggestions for rehabilitation techniques with the mentally handicapped and head injured. *British Journal of Clinical Psychology, 24*, 13–24.

Hagen, C. (1982). Language cognitive disorientation following closed head injury: A conceptualization. In L. Trexler (Ed.), *Cognitive rehabilitation conceptualization and intervention* (pp. 131–151). New York: Plenum Press.

Hart, T., & Hayden, M. E. (1986). The ecological validity of neuropsychological assessment and remediation. In B. P. Uzzell & Y. Gross (Eds.), *Clinical neuropsychology of intervention* (pp. 257–282). Boston: Martinus Nijhoff Publishers.

Keele, S. W., & Posner, M. I. (1968). Processing of visual feedback in rapid movements. *Journal of Experimental Psychology, 77*, 155–158.

Kelso, J. A. S., & Tuller, B. (1981). Towards a theory of apractic syndromes. *Brain and Language, 12*, 224–245.

Konow, A., & Pribram, K. (1970). Error recognition and utilization produced by injury to the frontal cortex. *Neuropsychologia, 8*, 489.

Kottke, F. J. (1980). From reflex to skill: The training of coordination. *Archives of Physical Medicine & Rehabilitation, 61*, 551–561.

Laabs, G. J. (1973). Retention characteristics of different reproduction cues in motor short-memory. *Journal of Experimental Psychology, 100*, 168–177.

Lawson, M. J., & Rice, D. N. (1989). Effects of training in used of executive strategies on a verbal memory problem resulting from closed head injury. *Journal of Clinical and Experimental Neuropsychology, 11*, 842–854.

Lee, T. D., & Magill, R. A. (1983). The locus of contextual interference in motor-skill acquisition. *Journal of Experimental Psychology, 9*, 730–746.

Lincoln, N. B., Whiting, S. E., Cockburn, J., Bhavnani, G. (1985). An evaluation of perceptual training. *International Rehabilitation Medicine, 7*, 99–110.

Magill, R. A. (1989). *Motor learning: Concepts and application.* Dubuque, IA: W. C. Brown Publishers.

McCracken, H. D., & Stelmach, G. E. (1977). A test of the schema theory of discrete motor learning. *Journal of Motor Behavior, 9*, 193–201.

Miller, G. A. (1966). The magical number seven, plus or minus two: Some limits on our capacity for processing information. *Psychological Review, 63*, 81–97.

Neistadt, M. E. (1990). A critical analysis of occupational therapy approaches for perceptual deficits in adults with brain injury. *American Journal of Occupational Therapy, 44*, 299–304.

Neistadt, M. E. (1992). Occupational therapy treatments for constructional deficits. *American Journal of Occupational Therapy, 46*, 141–148.

Newell, K. M., Carlton, M. J., & Fisher, A. T. (1989). Whole-part training strategies for learning the response dynamics of microprocessor driven simulator. *Acta Psychologica, 71*, 197–216.

Oxendine, J. B. (1968). *Psychology of motor learning.* Englewood Cliffs, NJ: Prentice-Hall.

Rimel, R. W., Giordani, B., Barth, J. T., Boll, T. J., & Jane, J. A. (1985). Disability caused by minor head injury. *Neurosurgery, 9*, 221–228.

Rock, I., & Harris, C. S. (1967). Vision and touch. *Scientific American, 216*, 96–104.

Rothwell, J. C., Traub, M. M., Day, B. L., Obeso, J. A., Thomas, P. K., & Marsden, C. D. (1982). Motor performance in a deafferented man. *Brain, 105*, 515–542.

Sage, G. H. (1977). *Introduction to motor behavior: A neuropsychological approach.* Reading, MA: Addison-Wesley.

Salmoni, A. W., Schmidt, R. A., & Walter, C. B. (1984). Knowledge of results and motor learning: A review and critical reappraisal. *Psychological Bulletin, 95*, 355–386.

Schmidt, R. A. (1975). A schema theory of discrete motor skill learning. *Psychological Review, 82*, 225–260.

Schmidt, R. A. (1988). *Motor control and learning: A behavioral emphasis.* Champaign, IL: Human Kinetics Publishers.

Shapiro, D. C., & Schmidt, R. A. (1982). The schema theory: Recent evidence and developmental implication. In J. A. S. Kelso & J. E. Clark (Eds.), *The development of movement control and coordination* (pp. 113–150). New York: John Wiley & Sons.

Shea, C. H., Kohl, R., & Indermill, C. (1990). Contextual interference: Contributions of practice. *Acta Psychologia, 73*, 145–157.

Shea, J. B., & Morgan, R. L. (1979). Contextual interference effect on the acquisition, retention, and transfer of motor skill. *Journal of Experimental Psychology, 5*, 179–187.

Shiffrin, R. M., & Schneider, W. (1977). Controlled and automatic human information processing: II Perceptual learning, automatic attending, and a general theory. *Psychological Reviews, 84*, 127–190.

Siegel, D., & Davis, C. (1980). Transfer effects of learning at specific speeds on performance over a range of speeds. *Perceptual and Motor Skills, 50*, 83–89.

Sivak, M., Hill, C. S., Henson, D. L., Butler, B. P., Silber, S. M., & Olson, P. L. (1984). Improved driving performance following perceptual training in persons with brain damage. *Archives of Physical Medicine & Rehabilitation, 65*, 163–167.

Spaeth-Arnold, R. K. (1981). Developing sport skills: A dynamic interplay of task, learner, and teacher. *Motor Skills, 2*, 3–81.

Stallings, L. M. (1982). Retention and transfer. In L. M. Stallings (Ed.), *Motor learning: From theory to practice* (pp. 197–218). St. Louis: C. V. Mosby.

Stammers, R. B. (1982). Part and whole practice in training for procedural skills. *Human Learning, 2*, 185–207.

Toglia, J. P. (1991). Generalization of treatment: A multicontext approach to cognitive perceptual impairment in adults with brain injury. *American Journal of Occupational Therapy, 45*, 505–516.

Whiting, H. T. A. (1980). Dimensions of control in motor learning.

In G. E. Stelmach & J. Requin (Eds.), *Tutorials in motor behavior* (pp. 537–550). New York: Elsevier.

Wightman, D. C., & Lintern, G. (1985). Part-task training for tracking and manual control. *Human Factors, 27*, 279–296.

Williams, I. D., & Stelmach, G. E. (1968). The accuracy of reproducing target positions under various tensions. *Psychonomic Science, 13*, 287–293.

Winstein, C. J., Gardner, E. R., McNeal, D. R., Barto, P. S., & Nicholson, D. E. (1989). Standing balance training: Effect on balance and locomotion in hemiparetic adults. *Archives of Physical Medicine & Rehabilitation, 70*, 755–762.

Winstein, C. J., & Schmidt, R. A. (1990). Reduced frequency of knowledge of results enhances motor skill learning. *Journal of Experimental Psychology, 16*, 677–691.

Zelaznik, H. N., Hawkins, B., & Kisselburgh, L. (1983). Rapid visual feedback processing in single-aiming movements. *Journal of Motor Behavior, 18*, 353–372.

Therapeutic Rapport

Linda Tickle-Degnen

The origins of the term *rapport* reflect an emphasis on communication and connection between individuals (Oxford English Dictionary, 1971). Individuals who are finely tuned to one another's actions and ideas, such that they respond to one another "immediately, spontaneously, and sympathetically" (Park & Burgess, 1924, p. 893), are said to be in rapport with one another. Although rapport can occur in any social situation, the type of rapport developed in therapy has its own special characteristics.

DEFINITION OF HIGH THERAPEUTIC RAPPORT

The definition of high **therapeutic rapport** offered here involves the experience and behavior of the patient and therapist during their interaction with each other as well as the outcome of the interaction for the patient:

1. It is an optimal interpersonal *experience* for both the patient and the therapist that involves concentra-

tion, masterful communication, and enjoyment (Csikszentmihalyi, 1990).
2. It occurs with *behavior* that reflects high levels of mutual attentiveness, interpersonal coordination, and mutual positivity (Tickle-Degnen & Rosenthal, 1990, 1992).
3. It has a *beneficial effect* on patient performance and follow-through with treatment plans (Dixey, Haslerud, & Brown, 1956; Feinberg, 1992; Hall, Roter, & Katz, 1988; Porszt-Miron, Florian, & Burton, 1988; Rosendahl & Ross, 1982; Rosenthal, 1966).

Table 14.1 provides a more detailed definition of high **therapeutic rapport.** It is important to note that rapport involves the *mutual* experience and behavior of the patient and therapist, but for rapport to be therapeutic it must have beneficial effects for the patient. The therapist holds an ethical responsibility to make sure that the fulfillment of her own personal needs is not the primary goal of the therapeutic relationship. Rather, the primary goal is to help the patient. Table 14.1 lists two outcomes that serve as measures of whether high rapport is truly therapeutic or not.

MUTUALITY AND THERAPEUTIC RAPPORT

Mutuality in the relationship between patient and therapist is relatively new in the philosophy of occupational therapy. In the first half of this century, occupational therapists were expected to be friendly and cheerful, but not intimate (Aitken, 1948), with patients. For example, therapists were not to discuss a patient's illness with the patient (American Occupational Therapy Association, 1948). It was expected that therapists and patients would not affect each other through their personal attributes. Starting at mid-century, the "therapeutic use of self" (Frank, 1958) became the prevailing philosophical position guiding the

277

GLOSSARY

Mutuality—Interaction between the patient and therapist in which they influence one another.

Nonverbal communication—The process of interpreting another's nonverbal behavior and expressing one's own thoughts and emotions through nonverbal behavior. Nonverbal behavior includes positions and movements of the face and body as well as qual-

ities of the voice, such as vocal tone, intensity, and speed.

Therapeutic rapport—The qualities of patient and therapist experience and behavior during interaction with one another that affect patient performance and involvement in therapy.

Verbal communication—The process of interpreting another's words and expressing one's own thoughts and emotions through words.

Table 14.1. Definition of High Therapeutic Rapport

Qualities of Experience	
Concentration	The patient and therapist experience a deep and effortless concentration on the interaction. Distractions, worries, and self-concern disappear.
Masterful communication	They are challenged by the interaction yet feel skillful in meeting the challenge. The goals of the interaction are experienced as clear and shared by both. Each understands immediately how well these goals are being met.
Enjoyment	They experience the interaction with deep satisfaction.
Qualities of Verbal and Nonverbal Behavior	
Attentiveness	The patient and therapist demonstrate verbally and nonverbally that their attention is focused on the other.
Interpersonal coordination	They demonstrate a highly tuned responsiveness to each other such that behavior and emotional expression are highly coordinated between the two.
Positivity	They demonstrate verbally and nonverbally that their feelings are positive toward one another and the interaction.
Beneficial Effects for the Patient	
Enhanced patient performance	Qualities of the patient-therapist interaction are beneficial if they improve patient performance during evaluation and treatment.
Patient follow-through with therapeutic activities	Qualities of the patient-therapist interaction are beneficial if they support patients' continued involvement in activities that enable them to make progress toward their goals.

therapeutic relationship. Therapists recognized that not only modalities but their own selves could be agents of therapeutic change in their patients. By being role models to their patients and by behaving in certain ways, they could help patients change. Although therapists could influence patients, therapists were to remain somewhat professionally detached to ensure that they themselves were not unduly affected by patients.

Starting in the late 1960s, with the inception of the human rights, human potential, and consumer movements, and continuing into the early 1990s, occupational therapy's view of the therapeutic relationship has been undergoing a major transformation. The profound shift has been toward viewing the relationship as a mutual and collaborative exchange between equals, a perspective exemplified by Yerxa's (1973) work:

> The therapist allows himself to feel real emotion as he enters into mutual relation with the client. . . . The authentic occupational therapist is involved in the process of caring and to care means to be affected just as surely as it means to affect (p. 8).

Currently, the philosophy of the therapeutic relationship has advanced the **mutuality** perspective to the image of friendship (Peloquin, 1990). This image is revolutionary in that it conveys that the patient and therapist *together* engage in mutually satisfying occupation and interaction, just as friends do (e.g., Clark, 1993). Although the friendship imagery is useful for conveying the depth of respect that a patient and therapist can hold for one another, it would be misleading to think that the patient-therapist relationship is equivalent to typical social friendships. Unlike typical friendships, a patient and an occupational therapist usually meet and grow to know one another because the therapist is expected to provide a service to the patient. This service relationship may arise when it is difficult for the patient, because of suffering or impairment, to experience or communicate feelings that contribute to the development of rapport (Gans, 1983; Tickle-Degnen & Rosenthal, 1992). Finally, the therapist usually is paid for the services, often not by the patient directly, and is accountable to institutional and professional systems that are charged with monitoring therapy and tracking patient response to therapy.

It may be misleading to think of the therapeutic relationship as a typical friendship, but the view of the relationship being one in which the patient and therapist mutually influence one another is quite consistent with theory and research about how practitioners and patients actually interact with one another in the clinic (Buller & Street, 1992; Fleming, 1991; Gans, 1983; Kleinman, 1988; Tickle-Degnen & Rosenthal, 1992).

This work suggests that if either the patient or the therapist is not attentive, responsive, or positive—or perceived as such by the other—then the interaction will not be one of high **therapeutic rapport.**

EXPERIENTIAL AND BEHAVIORAL QUALITIES OF HIGH THERAPEUTIC RAPPORT

Health care research findings and patient autobiographical accounts demonstrate that both the therapist and the patient contribute to the development of a relationship. The following sections first discuss the therapist's rapport qualities and then the patient's.

Therapist's Concentration and Attentiveness

A person who is paying attention to another will tend to orient his or her body and eyes toward the other (Rosenfeld & Hancks, 1980; Scheflen, 1964). In therapy, this type of behavior enables the therapist to watch the patient and to pick up cues from the patient's face and body, sources of much expression of emotion. Therapists also show that they are paying attention to patients by taking the time to sit down and talk with them. Verbal and nonverbal attentiveness has been found to be positively associated with patient satisfaction (Hall et al., 1988), test performance (Rosendahl & Ross, 1982), and successful performance of occupational therapy activities (Dixey et al., 1956).

Paying attention to a patient goes beyond sitting down with him and conducting a standardized evaluation, and it goes beyond physical attention. It requires listening carefully to what the patient has to say about his life, the illness, and the experience of treatment (Crepeau, 1991; Kautzmann, 1993; Kleinman, 1988; Peloquin, 1990). Without this kind of attentiveness, the therapist may well apply a "cookbook" treatment that is not individualized to the needs of the patient, as happened to the elderly woman narrating this poem (Maclay, 1977):

> I want to relive a day in July
> When Sam and I went berrying. . .
> Oh, here she comes, the therapist, with scissors and
> 　　paste.
> Would I like to try decoupage?
> "No," I say, "I haven't got time."
> "Nonsense," she says, "you're going to live a long, long
> 　　time."
> That's not what I mean.
> I mean that all my life I've been doing things
> For people, with people, I have to catch up
> On my thinking and feeling.
> About Sam's death, for one thing (pp. 46–47).

The therapist in this poem clearly had an agenda—using crafts—that prevented her from accurately perceiving the needs of this particular patient. Craft activities in and of themselves are not at fault here. They can be exactly what a particular patient needs. However, in this case, they were not. Practitioners, as the therapist in the poem, usually are well intentioned, but unless these intentions are consistent with what the patient perceives to be important, they may be less than beneficial. As a child with spina bifida, Saxton (1987) needed someone to listen to her:

> In all my hospital experiences, the saddest part was always the same. All those people trying so hard to help me. . . . All of them hoping for me to get better and do well, all wanting to be kind and useful, all feeling how important helping me was, yet never did any one of them ask me what it was like for me. They never asked me what I wanted for myself. They never asked me if I wanted their help. . . . I just wish all disabled children would say to their helpers: "Before you do anything else, just listen to me" (p. 55).

Craig (1991) described how powerful the right kind of attention can be to a patient. She wrote of her husband's nurse:

> Every Tuesday and every Friday when she came, she began by listening. And anything Ed wanted to tell her was relevant. She let him tell her, in his own way and in his own time, about everything that was happening to his body. And in that way, she came to know his soul (p. 241).

Patient's Concentration and Attentiveness

Therapists need attention from their patients as well. A patient who does not attend to the therapist cannot give or get important information from her. Many pathological conditions (e.g., traumatic brain damage or attention deficit disorders) affect the ability to concentrate and, therefore, interfere with the patient's ability to pay attention to others, including the therapist. In addition, people who feel embarrassed (Exline, Gray, & Schuette, 1965) or highly anxious (Waxer, 1977) make less eye contact with others. Patients may not be able to engage attentively with a therapist when they are in situations of potential embarrassment or anxiety.

Patients may be more involved and attentive when they value their therapy than when they do not value it (Kielhofner & Nelson, 1983). The elderly woman in the poem quoted above wanted the therapist to leave her alone, because she did not perceive the therapy as valuable for meeting her need to rethink her past. Unfortunately, it has been my experience that such patients—ones who refuse to become involved in therapy—may be labeled by the therapist as "unmotivated" (Tickle & Yerxa, 1981), when it is highly probable that the patient merely has needs and goals inconsistent with those of the therapist.

Therapist's Communication and Interpersonal Coordination

It is impossible for even the most attentive therapist to apprehend and feel exactly what the patient feels about his own illness and life. Likewise, the patient cannot fully comprehend the personal experience and role obligations of the therapist. Each is a unique individual with a unique life history and perspective. Despite these differences, the therapist and patient can teach each other their personal perspectives through **verbal** and **nonverbal communication** (Crepeau, 1991). When there is high rapport, the behaviors of the therapist and patient will be highly coordinated, a phenomenon called interactional synchrony (Bernieri, 1988; Kritzer & Valenti, 1990).

The fundamental condition for the therapist to communicate effectively with the patient is for the therapist to direct her attention toward the patient, as discussed above. The next step is for the therapist to *interpret* accurately the patient's verbal and nonverbal behavior (Tickle-Degnen & Rosenthal, 1992). This interpretation process involves first the observation that another person has behaved, and then the translation of this observation into an inference about the other's thoughts and emotions. Svidén and Säljö (1993) found that over a 1.5-year period the impressions by occupational therapy students of patients became increasingly complex. In the example below, note the difference between a new student's impression of a videotaped patient's nonverbal behavior and that same student's impression 1.5 years after beginning her training:

First viewing: It was rather difficult for her psychologically.

Second viewing: She looks away and only speaks when she is directly questioned/ I think she feels she is in a difficult situation/ she has given up hope/ as if she doesn't know what to do and where to start/ perhaps she doesn't want to talk about it as she doesn't feel able to cope/ she doesn't look as if she was happy/ although she laughs/ but perhaps she is embarrassed/ or hesitant (Svidén & Säljö, 1992, p. 494).

In the second viewing, the student had a better articulated and more complex impression of the patient and, as a result, would have been able to engage in a more effective dialogue with the patient to confirm or disconfirm elements of the impression.

After accurate interpretation of a patient's message, the next step in effective communication is for the therapist to *express* her own emotions and thoughts in a manner that is beneficial for the patient and clearly interpreted by the patient (Tickle-Degnen & Rosenthal, 1992). Patients have more positive impressions (Reade & Smouse, 1980), are more satisfied, and do not cancel their appointments as much (DiMatteo, Prince, & Hays, 1986) when their practitioners express their emotions in a generally positive, consistent, and unambiguous manner.

The manner that the therapist uses to express her feelings and attitudes toward the patient can be profoundly moving for the patient. A woman with multiple sclerosis (Brack & Collins, 1981) describes how her physical therapist conveyed a sense of compassion and hopefulness after a long period of little progress in therapy:

Weeks passed and there was no sign of improvement. One afternoon I rolled into my place in the line of wheelchairs, bone-tired and beaten. Doreen, in charge of physiotherapy, strode briskly down the line like a sergeant on inspection. She had a curt or kind word for everyone. . . . I lowered my head. Tears of despair rolled down my cheeks and I was so ashamed. She passed me without comment. . . . Suddenly she whisked my chair out of the line and into her office.

I couldn't speak. I felt no self-pity, just the emptiness of total defeat. I tried to explain—and broke into tears. Then, suddenly, the invincible Miss Moore wept with me. We had both tried so hard and so long. Was it all for nothing?

Our eyes met. "Do you want to quit?" she said. "I know it's tough and you know you may never get any better. But shall we try a little longer?"

Right away I knew I had to. I smiled damply and dried my eyes. What a friend!

We went to the parallel bars. . . . I didn't make the step that day but we didn't give up. . . . And I did walk again (pp. 71–72).

The therapist in this example does not simply say "Keep trying, I know you can do it." Because she has worked with this patient for a long period of time, she can express her understanding of the patient's feelings in an heartfelt and intimate manner. This example demonstrates that effective communication occurs not only through verbal and nonverbal behavior but also through the types of activities in which the therapist and patient engage. The act of engaging in therapy and walking, even when it seems that hope is lost, is a message to the patient that hope is *not* lost.

Likewise, messages are conveyed through the tools that occupational therapists offer their patients. When an occupational therapist gives a buttonhook to a patient, several messages are offered, among them, that the patient is capable of using a buttonhook and that dressing independently is a valued goal of the patient. In high rapport interactions, the patient is aware of the goals of the interaction and feels control during the interaction. Thus the performance of activities that are clearly consistent with the patient's goals communicate that the therapist understands the patient's perspective. For example, Hanlan (1979), who had amyotrophic lateral sclerosis, found that his occupational therapists provided him with tools that were completely in line with his needs:

> Of increasing importance to me is the help of occupational therapists, who can provide me with a variety of aids and appliances to keep me physically mobile. Simple, practical help becomes of enormous importance in maintaining some degree of my daily functioning. My first O.T., a man with a direct and kind manner, provided me with a buttonhook, so I could button and unbutton my clothing. I had an almost childlike, happy response to discovering this little tool (p. 40).

When practitioners have assessed accurately the needs of their patients and have responded effectively, either verbally, nonverbally, or through therapeutic media, patients respond with renewed energy and engagement in therapy.

Patient's Communication and Interpersonal Coordination

Some patients may not be able accurately to interpret a therapist's social behavior. Individuals with brain damage, particularly in the right hemisphere, have difficulty perceiving and interpreting social nonverbal cues (Rosenthal & Benowitz, 1986). Among individuals with left hemispheric damage, those with a receptive form of aphasia may be unable to understand the therapist's speech. It is difficult for patients with these types of problems to make sense of the therapist's social overtures and respond appropriately to them.

Likewise, problems of expression could interfere with the development of rapport. Right brain damage and Parkinson's disease have been found to interfere with an individual's ability to express interpretable emotions to others (Borod, Koff, & Buck, 1986; Buck & Duffy, 1980). Patients with an expressive aphasia have difficulty communicating their thoughts and needs.

Therapist's Enjoyment and Positivity

Patients who are liked by their practitioners have better therapeutic outcomes (Ehrlich & Bauer, 1967; Gelso, Mills, & Spiegel, 1983). Practitioners express their warmth and liking through nonverbal behaviors such as leaning forward and smiling (Hill et al., 1981). Patients interpret positively these and other types of friendly verbal and nonverbal behavior (Hall et al., 1988; Tickle-Degnen & Rosenthal, 1992) and respond with reduced anxiety (Ben-Sira, 1988), increased follow-through with treatment regimens (Feinberg, 1992), and more successful performance (Harris & Rosenthal, 1985; Rosenthal, 1966).

Beisser (1989), a man with polio, described how the mood of his hospital attendants affected his own mood: "Everything that affected them affected me. If I was cared for willingly and without reluctance, I felt good and the world was sunny. If my care was given grudgingly or irritably, in a callous way, powerful feelings of degradation swept over me" (p. 34). Beisser went on to talk about how his most effective helpers were ones who enjoyed their work and were nurtured by their relationships with patients. With these helpers, Beisser felt human again, able to reciprocate their warmth and concern.

What may be most critical in therapists' expression of positivity toward patients is the genuine feeling and communication of concern and caring (King, 1980; Yerxa, 1980). For example, research findings (Milmoe et al., 1967; Rosenthal, Blanck, & Vannicelli, 1984) suggest that the tone of voice of a caring therapist is not necessarily uniformly positive and cheerful. Rather, there is an element of anxiousness conveyed.

Patient's Enjoyment and Positivity

Patients who are very anxious or depressed demonstrate less warmth nonverbally (Waxer, 1976, 1977). For example, they smile less and make less eye contact. This lack of warmth by some patients may be taken personally by practitioners, especially those who are more inexperienced and less likely to interpret this behavior as either a normal response to illness or a sign of disease (Tickle-Degnen & Rosenthal, 1992).

Misery from illness may encompass the patient's life, reducing his ability to respond warmly toward others (Gans, 1983). As Brack, suffering from multiple sclerosis, noted: " 'Thanks' is a near-forgotten word among us patients as we wallow in our private miseries" (Brack & Collins, 1981, p. 47). From an ethical and professional standpoint, practitioners are expected to rise above petty responses to unpleasant behavior in patients, but unfortunately, they may begin to resent and hate some of those that they are supposed to help (Gans, 1983). For example, Beisser (1989) found that his helpers on the polio ward had a powerful form of retribution for patients who were thought to be difficult: "You cannot get mad in hospitals. If you do, you may be in trouble. . . . Angry patients come last. So I quickly learned to smile patiently. . . . I had to be careful, for they were more in control of my body than I was" (p. 19). Even practitioners who do not engage in this form of retribution may find it hard to work with a patient who lacks warmth and happiness.

In occupational therapy, patients may have strong and negative reactions to the frustrations involved in trying to perform what they perceive to be simple tasks:

> In Shaughnessey's domain [physical therapy] we did hard, demanding work that left us sore and exhausted, while in

OT the tasks were often less physically demanding, but equally frustrating. It was grueling to try to lift the increasingly heavy weights that Shaughnessey added as my weight lifting progressed, but there were times in OT when I felt like screaming as I tried to learn how to button clothes or to thread a needle (Puller, 1991, p. 181).

Such frustration is bound to impinge on the patient's view of therapy and the therapist, and should not be ignored. The therapist may have to reevaluate the balance of the emotional costs and physical benefits of particular forms of activity and to confirm that these activities are in fact in line with the patient's own goals.

Evidence suggests that practitioners must be careful not to view all expressions of frustration, sadness, or anger as confirmation of pathology (Langer & Abelson, 1974; Rosenhan, 1973). For example, Widome (1989) described how a nurse responded to his social outburst, an outburst that apparently was his expression of anger at being in the horrible predicament of having cancer:

> One morning, as I walked along the hallway pushing the IV stand, a young nurse passed by and then came back to talk to me. She asked how I was feeling. It was the wrong question at the wrong time, and I let loose with a tirade of words. I wasn't going to make it back to a full life, I told her. . . . Would she, the young pretty nurse, want to be a vegetable, a burden to her family? Wouldn't she rather have a choice, a say in the matter? Wouldn't she prefer no life to a thread of existence?
>
> I might as well have shown up in the hallway with a noose hanging around my neck.
>
> The nurse made a notation on my chart that I had made a decision to end my life, that I was considering self-destruction. I was now a marked man—suicidal (pp. 99–100).

Some expressions of frustration and anger may be indeed signs of a pathological process that requires diagnosis. However, other expressions of this sort are simply normal responses to the experience of illness and treatment. In this latter case, I believe the therapist must determine how to ease the burden and suffering of the patient while supporting his continued involvement in treatment.

BENEFICIAL EFFECT AND HIGH THERAPEUTIC RAPPORT

There are several reasons why attentive, coordinated, and positive patient-therapist interactions may have a beneficial effect on the patient's performance and follow-through with treatment. Listed below are three of the possible explanations.

1. The interaction provides the external "scaffolding" necessary for skill development, by directing attention to important aspects of a task problem, by communicating the information necessary to solve the problem, and by giving motivational support for pursuing problem solution (Wood, Bruner, & Ross, 1976).

2. The interaction reduces disabling anxiety. As the patient learns—by communicating with a warm, supportive therapist—to trust the therapist, anxiety is reduced (Ben-Sira, 1988). Anxiety may interfere with therapeutic progress by engulfing the patient's attention, leaving limited capacity for focused involvement in therapeutic tasks or by increasing physical tension and interfering with the physical performance of these tasks.

3. The interaction creates a self-fulfilling prophecy of improved performance (Harris & Rosenthal, 1985). Through **verbal** and **nonverbal communication** a therapist conveys her expectations for the progress of a patient, with the effect being that the patient's actual performance conforms to those expectations. Informative, warm, and respectful behavior may affirm to the patient that he is a capable and valued human being, thus mobilizing the patient's psychological, intellectual, and physical resources toward fulfillment of the implications of those labels.

DEVELOPMENT OF A HIGH THERAPEUTIC RAPPORT RELATIONSHIP

All relationships take time to develop. Theoretical literature (Altman & Taylor, 1973; Duck, 1977) on the development of relationships holds clues as to how the patient-therapist relationship would most likely unfold. During the first meeting, the patient may convey private information to the therapist, but the depth of intimacy and **mutuality** will continue to grow over subsequent interactions, if all goes well. This increasing depth of knowledge about each other has been called the social penetration process (Altman & Taylor, 1973), a process by which each penetrates farther and farther into the core of the other's personality and personal experience.

First meetings tend to be somewhat superficial and rigidly constrained by role expectations. The therapist will most likely perform an evaluation, and the patient will most likely try to answer the questions or perform the activities involved in the evaluation. In addition, during first meetings, individuals often actively try to control the image that they are conveying, while simultaneously forming positive or negative impressions of the other (Duck, 1977). It is at this time of initial impression formation that the therapist's attentiveness and positivity may be most critical for the development of high **therapeutic rapport** (Tickle-Degnen & Rosenthal, 1990). Early on, the patient and therapist may accept awkwardness during interaction, but as they get to know one another their expectations for more effective and coordinated communication may grow. If after a few interactions, it becomes clear that communication is not effective, no amount of warmth or attentiveness on the therapist's part will be able to sustain rapport. After the patient and therapist are less concerned with the impressions they are conveying to each other, have stable impressions of the other, and have experienced consistently high rapport, they will most likely be able exchange praise and criticism more freely (Altman & Taylor, 1973) and engage in a flexible, less rigidly role-constrained interaction.

Therapist and patient characteristics, as well as conditions in the therapy setting, can facilitate or inhibit the development of high rapport. Based on the evidence presented here, Table 14.2 gives guidelines

Table 14.2. Therapist Guidelines for Facilitating the Development of High Therapeutic Rapport

Create conditions that maximize therapist and patient concentration and attention
• Set aside time to listen to patient
• Reduce distractions in therapy setting
• Reduce potential for patient embarrassment or anxiety
• Position own body to see and hear patient clearly
• Position patient so that patient can see and hear therapist clearly
• Listen for issues that are most important to patient

Create conditions that maximize therapist and patient masterful communication and interpersonal coordination
• Remain open and sensitive to verbal and nonverbal messages from the patient
• Provide assistance as needed for the patient to express emotions and thoughts
• Check with the patient to see if therapist interpretation of patient messages is accurate
• Clearly express emotions and thoughts that are consistent with the needs and goals of the patient
• Check with the patient to see if the patient is interpreting therapist messages accurately
• Create a challenging and interesting interaction, but one in which the patient can interact skillfully
• Engage patient in activities and interaction that are consistent with patient goals

Create conditions that maximize therapist and patient enjoyment and positivity
• Find a satisfying, fulfilling aspect to every interaction with a patient
• Express genuine concern and caring for the patient through verbal and nonverbal behavior
• Resolve own personal problems and fulfill personal social needs outside of the patient-therapist interaction
• Determine whether patient sadness or anger is normal or of pathological origin and respond appropriately to alleviate suffering
• Engage patient in activities and interaction that are inherently enjoyable for the patient

for enhancing the development of rapport. It is not the patient's responsibility to try to change himself to enhance the rapport, rather it is the therapist's. Therefore, the guidelines are directed at actions that the therapist can take. As a last resort, if the patient and therapist cannot get along with one another, the therapist may want to consider referring the patient to a new therapist.

Once high rapport is obtained with a patient, the therapist must adhere to strong ethical standards. First of all, the therapist must never use the relationship to meet personal needs or goals that are inconsistent with or overshadow the needs of the patient. Second, the therapist must recognize that a relationship of **mutuality** makes the therapist and patient emotionally interdependent (Martin & Schurtman, 1985). As discharge approaches, the therapist should work actively with the patient to transform their relationship appropriately so that the patient does not feel abandoned (e.g., Clark, 1993). The form that this transformation takes will depend on the setting. For example, the therapist may help the patient to develop other fulfilling relationships in the community or may keep in contact with the patient through the phone or occasional clinic visits. Because a relationship of high **therapeutic rapport** affects both the therapist and patient, the therapist must use careful and ethical judgment throughout its course.

Acknowledgments——The ideas in this chapter evolved during a Mary Switzer Research Fellowship supported by the National Institutes for Disability and Rehabilitation Research. Although innumerable students and therapists have contributed to these ideas through involvement either as subjects or assistants in my research, a special thanks to Irene Zombek who carefully searched a large number of patient autobiographies for excerpts related to rapport.

STUDY QUESTIONS

1. What are the elements involved in a definition of high therapeutic rapport?
2. What are two benefits that the patient should gain from having a high rapport with the therapist?
3. How has the view of the patient-therapist relationship in occupational therapy changed during this century?
4. How are the therapist's experience and behavior related to high therapeutic rapport?
5. How are the patient's experience and behavior related to high therapeutic rapport?
6. What are three reasons why high rapport may be beneficial for patients?
7. How can the therapist facilitate the development of high therapeutic rapport?
8. What are two of the ethical responsibilities that a therapist holds in a relationship of high therapeutic rapport with a patient?

REFERENCES

Aitken, A. N. (1948). Values of occupational therapy in the rehabilitation of the tuberculosis patient. *American Journal of Occupational Therapy, 2,* 219–222.

Altman, I., & Taylor, D. A. (1973). *Social penetration: The development of interpersonal relationships.* New York: Holt, Rinehart, & Winston.

American Occupational Therapy Association. (1948). Professional attitudes. *American Journal of Occupational Therapy, 2,* 97–98.

Beisser, A. R. (1989). *Flying without wings: Personal reflections on being disabled.* New York: Doubleday.

Ben-Sira, Z. (1988). Affective behavior and perceptions of health professionals. In D. S. Gochman (Ed.), *Health Behavior* (pp. 305–317). New York: Plenum Press.

Bernieri, F. (1988). Coordinated movement and rapport in teacher-student interactions. *Journal of Nonverbal Behavior, 12,* 120–138.

Borod, J. C., Koff, E., & Buck, R. (1986). The neuropsychology of facial expression: Data from normal and brain-damaged adults. In P. D. Blanck, R. Buck, & R. Rosenthal (Eds.), *Nonverbal communication in the clinical context* (pp. 196–222). University Park: Pennsylvania State University Press.

Brack, J., & Collins, R. (1981). *One thing for tomorrow: A woman's personal struggle with MS.* Saskatoon, Sask., Canada: Western Producer Prairie.

Buck, R., & Duffy, R. J. (1980). Nonverbal communication of affect in brain-damaged patients. *Cortex, 16,* 351–362.

Buller, D. B., & Street, R. L. Jr. (1992). Physician-patient relationships. In R. S. Feldman (Ed.), *Applications of nonverbal behavioral theories and research* (pp. 119–141). Hillsdale, NJ: Erlbaum.

Clark, F. (1993, June). *Occupation embedded in real life: Interweaving occupational science and occupational therapy.* Paper presented at the annual meeting of the American Occupational Therapy Association, Seattle, WA.

Craig, J. (1991). *Between hello and goodbye.* Los Angeles: Tarcher.

Crepeau, E. B. (1991). Achieving intersubjective understanding: Examples from an occupational therapy treatment session. *American Journal of Occupational Therapy, 45,* 1016–1025.

Csikszentmihalyi, M. (1990). *Flow: The psychology of optimal experience.* New York: HarperCollins.

DiMatteo, M. R., Prince, L. M., & Hays, R. (1986). Nonverbal communication in the medical context: The physician-patient relationship. In P. D. Blanck, R. Buck, & R. Rosenthal (Eds.), *Nonverbal communication in the clinical context* (pp. 74–98). University Park: Pennsylvania State University Press.

Dixey, E., Haslerud, G. M., & Brown, N. C. (1956). The effect of the professional activity of occupational therapists on the behavior of mental patients. *American Journal of Occupational Therapy, 10,* 298–303.

Duck, S. (1977). *The study of acquaintance.* Westmead, UK: Saxon House.

Ehrlich, H. J., & Bauer, M. L. (1967). Therapists' feelings toward patients and patient treatment outcome. *Social Science and Medicine, 1,* 283–292.

Exline, R., Gray, D., & Schuette, D. (1965). Visual behavior in a dyad as affected by interview content and sex of respondent. *Journal of Personality and Social Psychology, 1,* 201–209.

Feinberg, J. (1992). Effect of the arthritis health professional on compliance with use of resting hand splints by patients with rheumatoid arthritis. *Arthritis Care and Research, 5,* 17–23.

Fleming, M. H. (1991). The therapist with the three track mind. *American Journal of Occupational Therapy, 45,* 1007–1014.

Frank, J. D. (1958). The therapeutic use of self. *American Journal of Occupational Therapy, 12,* 215–225.

Gans, J. S. (1983). Hate in the rehabilitation setting. *Archives of Physical Medicine & Rehabilitation, 64,* 176–179.

Gelso, C. J., Mills, D. H., & Spiegel, S. B. (1983). Client and therapist factors influencing the outcome of time-limited counseling one and 18 months after treatment. In C. J. Gelso & D. H. Johnson (Eds.), *Explorations in time-limited counseling and psychotherapy* (pp. 87–115). New York: Teachers College.

Hall, J. A., Roter, D. L., & Katz, N. R. (1988). Meta-analysis of correlates of provider behavior in medical encounters. *Medical Care, 26,* 657–675.

Hanlan, A. J. (1979). *Autobiography of dying.* New York: Doubleday.

Harris, M. J., & Rosenthal, R. (1985). Mediation of interpersonal expectancy effects: 31 meta-analyses. *Psychological Bulletin, 97,* 363–386.

Hill, C. E., Siegelman, L., Gronsky, B. R., Sturniolo, F., & Fretz, B. R. (1981). Nonverbal communication and counseling outcome. *Journal of Counseling Psychology, 28,* 203–212.

Kautzmann, L. N. (1993). Linking patient and family stories to caregivers' use of clinical reasoning. *American Journal of Occupational Therapy, 47,* 169–173.

Kielhofner, G., & Nelson, C. (1983). A study of patient motivation and cooperation/participation in occupational therapy. *Occupational Therapy Journal of Research, 3,* 35–46.

King, L. J. (1980). Creative caring. *American Journal of Occupational Therapy, 34,* 522–528.

Kleinman, A. (1988). *The illness narratives.* New York: Basic Books.

Kritzer, R., & Valenti, S. S. (1990). *Rapport in therapist-client interactions: An ecological analysis of the effects of nonverbal sensitivity and interactional synchrony.* Paper presented at the 61st annual meeting of the Eastern Psychological Association, Philadelphia.

Langer, E. J., & Abelson, R. P. (1974). A patient by any other name . . . : Clinician group differences in labeling bias. *Journal of Consulting and Clinical Psychology, 42,* 4–9.

Maclay, E. (1977). Occupational therapy. In E. Maclay (Ed.), *Green winter: Celebrations of old age* (pp. 46–48). New York: Readers Digest.

Martin, E. S., & Schurtman, R. (1985). Termination anxiety as it affects the therapist. *Psychotherapy, 22,* 92–96.

Milmoe, S., Rosenthal, R., Blane, H. T., Chafetz, M. E., & Wolf, I. (1967). The doctor's voice: Postdictor of successful referral of alcoholic patients. *Journal of Abnormal Psychology, 72,* 78–84.

Oxford English Dictionary (compact edition). (1971). Oxford, UK: Oxford University Press.

Park, R. E., & Burgess, E. W. (1924). *Introduction to the science of sociology.* Chicago: University of Chicago Press.

Peloquin, S. M. (1990). The patient-therapist relationship in occupational therapy: Understanding visions and images. *American Journal of Occupational Therapy, 44,* 13–21.

Porszt-Miron, L., Florian, M., & Burton, J. (1988). A pilot study on the effect of rapport on the task performance of an elderly confused population. *Canadian Journal of Occupational Therapy, 55,* 255–258.

Puller, L. B. (1991). *Fortunate Son.* New York: Grove Weidenfeld.

Reade, M., & Smouse, A. D. (1980). Effect of inconsistent verbal-nonverbal communication and counselor response mode on client estimate of counselor regard and effectiveness. *Journal of Counseling Psychology, 27,* 546–553.

Rosendahl, P. P., & Ross, V. (1982). Does your behavior affect your patient's response? *Journal of Gerontological Nursing, 8,* 572–575.

Rosenfeld, H. M., & Hancks, M. (1980). The nonverbal context of verbal listener responses. In M. R. Key (Ed.), *The relationship of verbal and nonverbal communication* (pp. 193–206). The Hague: Mouton.

Rosenhan, D. L. (1973). On being sane in insane places. *Science, 179*, 250–258.

Rosenthal, R. (1966). *Experimenter effects in behavioral research.* New York: Appleton-Century-Crofts.

Rosenthal, R., & Benowitz, L. I. (1986). Sensitivity to nonverbal communication in normal, psychiatric, and brain-damaged samples. In P. D. Blanck, R. Buck, & R. Rosenthal (Eds.), *Nonverbal communication in the clinical context* (pp. 223–257). University Park: Pennsylvania State University Press.

Rosenthal, R., Blanck, P. D., & Vannicelli, M. (1984). Speaking to and about patients: Predicting therapist's tone of voice. *Journal of Consulting and Clinical Psychology, 52*, 679–686.

Saxton, M. (1987). The something that happened before I was born. In M. Saxton & F. Howe (Eds.), *With wings: An anthology of literature by and about women with disabilities* (pp. 51–55). New York: Feminist.

Scheflen, A. E. (1964). The significance of posture in communication systems. *Psychiatry, 26*, 126–136.

Svidén, G., & Säljö, R. (1993). Perceiving patients and their nonverbal reactions. *American Journal of Occupational Therapy, 47*, 491–497.

Tickle, L. S., & Yerxa, E. J. (1981). Need satisfaction of older persons living in the community and in institutions, Part 1. The environment. *American Journal of Occupational Therapy, 35*, 644–649.

Tickle-Degnen, L., & Rosenthal, R. (1990). The nonverbal correlates of rapport. *Psychological Inquiry, 1*, 285–293.

Tickle-Degnen, L., & Rosenthal, R. (1992). Nonverbal aspects of therapeutic rapport. In R. S. Feldman (Ed.), *Applications of nonverbal behavioral theories and research* (pp. 143–164). Hillsdale, NJ: Erlbaum.

Waxer, P. H. (1976). Nonverbal cues for depth of depression: Set versus no set. *Journal of Consulting and Clinical Psychology, 44*, 493.

Waxer, P. H. (1977). Nonverbal cues for anxiety: An examination of emotional leakage. *Journal of Abnormal Psychology, 86*, 306–314.

Widome, A. (1989). *The doctor/the patient.* Miami: Editech.

Wood, D., Bruner, J. S., & Ross, G. (1976). The role of tutoring in problem solving. *Journal of Child Psychology and Psychiatry, 17*, 89–100.

Yerxa, E. J. (1973). Authentic occupational therapy: The 1966 Eleanor Clarke Slagle Lecture. In American Occupational Therapy Association (Ed.), *The Eleanor Clarke Slagle Lectures: 1955–1972* (pp. 155–173). Dubuque, IA: Kendall/Hunt.

Yerxa, E. J. (1980). Occupational therapy's role in creating a future climate of caring. *American Journal of Occupational Therapy, 34*, 529–534.

Treatment Principles and Practices

This section includes the treatment of deficits of occupational performance. There are two approaches. One is to remediate impairments of the sensory, perceptual cognitive and motor components of occupational performance to enable the person to perform the tasks and activities of his roles as nearly "normal" as possible. The other is to restore the person's ability to carry these out using adapted equipment and/or methods. The remediational approach encompasses two frames of reference: the biomechanical and the neurodevelopmental-motor learning. The restorative approach has also been termed the *rehabilitative approach*. Treatments relative to this approach are described in Chapters 15 through 21.

The *biomechanical approach* deals with increasing strength, endurance, range of joint motion in patients who have an intact central nervous system (and according to new, as yet incomplete, information probably also for patients with central nervous system dysfunction). This frame of reference applies mechanical principles of kinetics and kinematics to movement of the human body. Treatments related to the biomechanical approach are described in Chapter 22.

The *neurodevelopmental-motor learning approach* deals primarily with improving motor control and performance as described in Chapters 24 and 25. It is used for persons with impairments or functional limitations of movement secondary to a dysfunctional central nervous system. The patient's movement may be dominated by immature patterns or reflect lack of sensorimotor integration needed to produce coordinated, goal-directed movement. This approach formerly focused on the use of sensory input and developmental sequences to facilitate change in the sensorimotor organization of the central nervous system, i.e., neurological recovery. These older treatment regimens (Chapter 24) used procedures that were based on early neurophysiological research. Because of technological advances that enable study of central nervous system mechanisms in living, awake animals and people, new treatment is developing that focuses on the acquisition of motor control and motor performance through learning, i.e., behavioral recovery (Chapter 25).

Sensorimotor recalibration and cognitive-perceptual processing are involved in learning to improve motor performance. Chapter 23 describes treatments used to reeducate sensory awareness and interpretation and to redevelop sensory tolerance for patients with peripheral or central sensory impairment and to teach adaptations necessary for those with sensory loss. Chapters 26 and 27 describe therapy to improve cortical functions of perception and cognition, not only in relation to motor performance but also in relation to higher functions needed for successful, everyday interaction with the environment.

Retraining Basic and Instrumental Activities of Daily Living

Catherine A. Trombly

OBJECTIVES

After studying this chapter, the student will be able to:
1. Distinguish between BADL and IADL.
2. State principles to restore adapted function to persons with various functional limitations.
3. Modify tasks and/or the environment to promote independence.
4. Prescribe and evaluate the use of adaptive equipment to promote safe independence.
5. Guide problem solving and implementation of solutions to unique situations for persons with a variety of functional limitations.

Activities of daily living (ADL) are a major performance area within the domain of practice of occupational therapy. The assumption is that people want to direct their own lives and care for themselves to the best of their ability. This may include directing and/or delegating tasks that are beyond the person's capabilities to others. ADL includes those tasks that a person regularly does to prepare for, or as an adjunct to, participating in his or her social and work roles. The term *basic activities of daily living* (BADL) is synonymous with self-care. BADL includes mobility, which refers to being able to turn over in bed, come to a sitting position, and move to and transfer from place to place; feeding; grooming; dressing; bathing; and personal hygiene and toileting. These tasks are necessary to maintain health and are universal. While every human does these to some degree, the way that each is done and the importance attached to each differ culturally.

Stating that a person is independent based only on these activities underestimates those who will need assistance once the environment is taken into consideration (Spector et al., 1987). The term *instrumental activities of daily living* (IADL) refers to tasks, beyond caring for oneself, that involve interaction with the physical and social environment. IADL include such tasks as putting things away and getting things out of closets, drawers, and cupboards; telephoning; written communication and handling mail; using paper money, checks, coins, ATMs, and vending machines; using books, newspapers, and entertainment equipment; using public or private transportation; obtaining needed objects and services from stores, businesses, or governmental agencies; caring for wheelchair, orthosis, or ambulatory aids; emergency procedures for fire (Schroeder & Benedict, 1984; Strawn, 1989), weather emergency, automobile breakdown, sudden illness; and other like tasks. Homemaking, home maintenance tasks, and leisure activities are also considered IADL; they are covered in other chapters of this text. There is no order in developing ability to perform IADL in contrast to BADL, which follow an ontogenetic sequence from feeding to toileting (Katz et al., 1963; Norström & Thorslund, 1991).

The occupational therapist is the rehabilitation specialist responsible for teaching the patient to accomplish these tasks, except for ambulation, which is the responsibility of the physical therapist. The occupational therapist and physical therapist may share the responsibility for functional mobility training.

If remedial therapy is able to correct impairments, no special therapy will be needed to teach ADL; the patient will be doing the tasks important to him as he becomes able. For those persons who do not regain full capabilities, intervention must occur.

The extent of services offered to a particular patient depends on the person's motivation and need for various levels of independence. Independence in BADL may be sufficient for a person returning to a sheltered and supportive living situation in which his

GLOSSARY

Adaptation—The process of modifying a task, the method of accomplishing the task, and/or the environment to promote independence in occupational functioning.

Blocked practice—Practice that consists of drills of many repetitions of the same task in the same way (Schmidt, 1991).

Dressing stick—A long rod with a clothes hook attached to one end used to pull on clothing that cannot be reached with the hands.

Random practice—Practice of several related tasks within one session; the sequence of the tasks varies randomly (Schmidt, 1991).

IADL needs are few and willingly assumed by others. It is never enough for a person who expects to reintegrate into community life. This person not only needs to learn solutions to BADL and common IADL tasks but also must learn how to identify and solve problems that prevent accomplishment of unique tasks. On the other hand, independence in one task, e.g., transferring or toileting, may make the difference between discharge to home or institution and full effort would concentrate on achievement of this goal for the person of otherwise limited potential for full independence.

Based on the person's goals and values, the occupational therapist helps the patient determine whether tasks can be eliminated or reassigned and teaches him to modify tasks, to use adapted methods of doing tasks, or prescribes adapted equipment that will enable him to be independent of another person for the task or a major aspect of the task. The therapist suggests environmental **adaptations** to promote independence.

Compensatory intervention, or a rehabilitative frame of reference, uses education and **adaptation** to enable patients to live with a disability on a permanent or temporary basis.

EDUCATION

The rehabilitative approach involves the therapist as teacher and patient and family as learner(s). Teaching and learning are active processes for both the learner and the teacher. The patient must be motivated to learn and must be able to learn. Motivation is sparked by values; values guide actions and efforts (Chiou & Burnett, 1985). Therefore, the therapist must plan which particular aspects of ADL to concentrate on, guided not only by knowledge of the tasks that will be within the person's capabilities but also by the patient's goals.

There are some patients who are unable to learn. Learning is prevented by loss of recent (or short-term) memory, severe receptive aphasia, disorientation to person and place, or ideational apraxia (see Chapter 9). A person who cannot follow directions imparted to him through his most receptive channels or who cannot remember will not be a candidate for ADL training.

The family should be taught how to care for the patient and told to seek reevaluation if the patient's cognitive status improves. High anxiety also blocks learning. Therapy to reduce anxiety (Chapters 10 and 20) and that includes low-challenge activities at first may allow learning to take place. Those patients who speak a language not known to the therapist and who do not understand demonstration will need to be taught through the help of an interpreter.

To teach effectively (Table 15.1), the therapist needs to do the following activities.

1. Determine what tasks the learner can do and whether he does them safely. Determine whether the learner figures out adapted methods on his or her own.

2. Find out what the learner needs to know—his goals. These become learning objectives. A learning objective is a goal expressed in behavioral terms (Margolis & Savino, 1992), e.g., "The patient will be able to don his shirt, without assistance or supervision, in less than 10 minutes."

3. Present the material in a way that is congruent with the objective. If the patient needs to learn some principles of energy conservation, the teaching method will involve auditory and visual methods, such as discussion perhaps with slides or videotaped examples, problem solving, and application of ideas to the patient's own situations. If the patient needs to learn a motor task, such as putting on a shirt when one arm is paralyzed, the teaching will be guided by the four stages of motor learning (see Chapter 13) in which the person first gains an understanding of the task, then

Table 15.1. Effective Teaching

1. Determine what the learner knows.
2. Establish the learning objective.
3. Choose teaching techniques congruent with what is to be taught.
4. Adapt the presentation to the learner's capabilities.
5. Provide opportunities for practice, considering context and schedule.
6. Offer useful feedback at the right time.
7. Test the learner in the appropriate context(s) to confirm learning.

visually pays attention to the steps of the task, then begins to pay attention to the proprioceptive feedback as he does the task, and finally does the task skillfully.

When first learning an activity, the challenge should be kept low to avoid anxiety and to promote success (Law, 1991). The learning situation should be structured so that the patient experiences success. For example, if the patient must learn to feed himself using adapted utensils, the training starts with sticky foods that will not easily slide off of the spoon and progresses to difficult foods such as spaghetti and sliced peaches.

4. Adapt the presentation to the particular learner, given his abilities and deficits. Break down complex tasks into segments that the learner is able to comprehend and remember.

For those patients without brain damage and of average intelligence, the teaching methods can be discussion, demonstration, or simply describing methods that others have found helpful. Non–brain-damaged persons should be taught in such a way that they become independent problem solvers. They need to learn to identify the problem, to understand the principle involved, and to be able to match a solution from a repertoire of solutions that have been found helpful in the past or that others have used. The patient may have suggestions about how a task might be accomplished, and his ideas should be respected and encouraged. Many techniques commonly in use have been developed by therapist-patient collaboration.

Patients with brain damage require more attention to the actual teaching process, which will be guided by the patient's particular learning problem. If the patient is unable to do the task automatically using old habit programs, he will be learning a new skill. Therefore, organization of the sequence of the steps and much repetition is necessary (Diller, Buxbaum, & Chiotelis, 1972). The learning may or may not transfer to other familiar tasks or other contexts; therefore, he will need to practice each task until it is learned and in the contexts in which it will be required. Brain-damaged patients may not become problem solvers, and their prognosis for independence outside of a sheltered or familiar environment may be limited. ADL tasks that could result in injury if precautions are not practiced by the person (e.g., cutting with a sharp knife or standing to pull up trousers) require supervision for as long as judgment is impaired.

Brain-damaged patients often have difficulty processing abstract information or large chunks of information at a time and need the instructions reduced to one- or two-word concrete cues. Given consistently over the course of practice sessions, these key word cues help the patient chain the task from beginning to end. It may be necessary to practice one step at a time;

steps may be combined as learning progresses. Some patients, however, can only do a task if the whole chain is completed (Brodal, 1973).

Some profoundly brain-damaged, yet teachable, patients benefit from backward chaining. Backward chaining is an adaptation of Skinner's (1938) Law of Chaining in which one step acts as the stimulus for another. In backward chaining of dressing skills, for example, assistance is given to do the task until the last step of the process is reached. The patient performs this one step independently with the satisfaction of having completed the task. Once the patient has mastered the final step, the therapist assists only to the next to the last step and the patient completes the two remaining steps. This process continues until the patient can do the entire task from start to finish independently. Progress in learning ADL for those with brain damage is slow, with regressions (Diller et al., 1972).

Patients who suffer damage to their dominant hemispheres usually have difficulty processing verbal or written language but are able to benefit from demonstrated or pictorial instruction (Diller et al., 1972). Those who suffer damage to their nondominant hemispheres may have difficulty with spatial relationships (pictures and demonstrations) but be able to process step-by-step verbal instruction.

5. Arrange appropriate practice schedules. Motor skills are learned only through practice. Mental practice (rehearsing the step-by-step process and trying to imagine the feel of the motor task) has some minor benefit for athletes, but actual, physical practice is necessary to perfect the skill. Practice within contexts that are natural for the task facilitates performance. Performance is enhanced through a practice schedule of **blocked practice**, whereas **random practice** has been found to facilitate motor learning (Schmidt, 1991). Motor learning is defined as a more or less permanent change in motor behavior (Schmidt, 1988, 1991). Motor performance refers to the quality of the outcome of any one particular trial.

6. Provide appropriate feedback. Motivational feedback ("Great!" "Looks good!" "Keep trying!") does have some benefit, but specific feedback about what was correct and what was not correct during a particular trial has more definitive benefit for motor learning for athletes learning their sport so it stands to reason it probably does for patients learning a new motor skill also. Occasional feedback concerning the performance ("your elbow needs to be straighter next time" offered immediately after a trial is helpful. If the person is not aware of the outcome of his efforts, his attention should be called to it so that he gains knowledge of the results, a requirement for learning (Schmidt, 1988).

7. Test to see if the learner has acquired the knowledge or skill by requiring him to do it on his own at the appropriate time and place.

ADAPTATION

Adaptation refers to modifying the task, the method of accomplishing the task, and/or the environment to promote independence in occupational functioning. Examples of modifying the task are to switch to loafer-type shoes instead of tie shoes or to order from catalogs instead of going to the shops. Adapted methods of dressing for persons with loss of the use of one side of the body or for weakness of all four extremities (discussed below) are examples of modifying the method of accomplishing a task. Installation of grab bars in the bathroom to enable safe transfers or changing storage location of often used items to within easy reach are examples of modifying the physical environment. Teaching a wheelchair user to maneuver within typical physical environments and situations and ways of interacting with nondisabled individuals so that he presents himself as a self-assured, capable person is an example of modifying the social environment.

Adaptation of objects, tools, and utensils used in accomplishing a task or introduction of equipment to enable accomplishment of a task is a primary function of occupational therapy relative to improving occupational functioning in the physically disabled. Examples are adding extensions to keys or door handles to extend the force arm and reduce the force required to turn the key or knob (Fig. 40.8), use of a buttonhook to button a shirt, and development of jigs to enable work tasks (Chase, 1989).

Grasp is a common problem for many patients, which can be helped by using enlarged handles. A therapist may begin considering **adaptations** to utensils by temporarily enlarging handles by wrapping a washcloth, foam rubber, or other material around the handle and securing it with a rubber band. If enlarging the handle improved performance, permanent **adaptation** will be prescribed and purchased commercially or built if the handle needs to be customized. Low-temperature thermoplastic materials that bond to themselves can be used for this purpose.

The process of **adaptation** involves the following seven aspects (Table 15.2).

1. *Task analysis.* Determine the essential demands of the task. The task demands are a combination of the performance requirements of a task (e.g., lifting, reaching, bending, and pulling) and the environmental requirements (e.g., counter height, location of faucets in the bathtub, and type of carpeting). Performance requirements need to be quantified: What is the weight to be lifted? How high must it be lifted? and so on.

Table 15.2. Adaptation Process

1. Analyze task demands.
2. Identify functional limitation and problem.
3. Know principles of compensation.
4. Creatively apply principles of compensation to solve the problem.
5. Know sources for implementing the solution.
6. Check out the modification.
7. Train in safe use.

Instruments used in job task analysis (described in Chapter 17) are applicable to determining these requirements. Examination of these objective dimensions of the tasks will suggest how the environment and equipment can be adapted to meet the capabilities of the person (Clark, Czaja, & Weber, 1990). Studies are beginning to appear that evaluate specific performance requirements of particular ADL tasks, e.g., the minimal wrist ranges of motion needed to accomplish ADL (Ryu et al., 1991).

2. *Identification of the problem.* Why can't the person accomplish the task demands? The reason will identify his functional limitation(s), e.g., inability to reach above shoulder height.

3. *Knowledge of the principles of compensation.* Some of the principles of compensation are listed below for each functional limitation. Examples are add extensions to utensils or implements that need to be used higher or at a distance greater than the person can reach, such as a comb (Fig. 15.1), or relocate objects to within easy reach.

4. *Propose solutions.* Creatively consider ways that the principles of compensation can be applied to a particular task to enable the particular person to do it. Collaboration with the patient, or a group of similarly involved patients, often generates potential solutions.

5. *Knowledge of resources for implementing the solution.* For example, it is important to know what reliable and safe equipment is available to accomplish the **adaptation.** The therapist must know construction techniques needed to implement the solution, if it is not commercially available. What contractors reliably provide quality home modifications?

Sources of equipment are rehabilitation supply stores, catalog mail-order businesses, and gadget stores. The annual *Accent on Living Buyer's Guide* (see "Resources") lists sources for all types of equipment. Although there are many pieces of adaptive equipment available for purchase, the occupational therapist needs to know and evaluate each piece of equipment before recommending it to the patient. Just because a piece of equipment is sold does not mean that it is effective or safe (Conine & Hershler, 1991). *Consumer Reports* has a project under way to include the point of view of

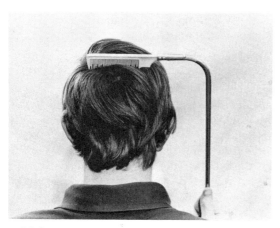

Figure 15.1. Long-handled comb.

disabled consumers in the evaluation of equipment it reviews ("Program for Consumers," 1991).

6. *Check out.* The adapted device or environmental modification needs to be checked out for reliability (i.e., always works as it should), durability (i.e., can withstand repeated use at the force levels the person will apply to it), and safety.

7. *Training.* The person must be trained in the safe use of the adapted device, environment, or method.

It is important to some people that adapted devices be "transparent" (McCuaig & Frank, 1991). That is, not call attention to the person as a disabled person or reveal how disabled he actually is. Use of conventional devices or gadgets that are sold to the general public qualify as transparent. Examples are felt-tipped pens, slip-on shoes, lightweight pots and pans, and magnifying makeup mirrors. They become adaptive because of their specific application. This perception of transparency and its importance is unique to the individual. Beyond this issue of transparency, is the issue of gadget tolerance. Transparent or not, some people do not want to use special tools to do a task most people do without such a tool. However, if the task is important and cannot be done any other way, the device will be valued (Bynum & Rogers, 1987; Parker & Thorslund, 1991; Rogers & Holm, 1992; Tyson & Strong, 1990). The number of devices prescribed should be reasonable and should enable important tasks. Otherwise the device will end up in the closet.

ADL METHODS

The remainder of this chapter will describe methods and devices suggested by therapists and former patients to enable independence in mobility, transfers, and driving as well as basic and instrumental activities of daily living. These suggestions will be presented

according to problem that has to be overcome. Patients often have more than one problem. For example, persons with rheumatoid arthritis have weakness as well as limited range of motion. Persons with spinal cord injury have decreased sensation as well as weakness. The therapist will have to use information from both sections for a patient with particular combinations of impairments. Mobility, transfers, and driving will be considered first. Next, procedures to enable key basic activities of daily living will be presented. The need to do these activities and the task demands of each are fairly universal among people. Representative instrumental activities of daily living will be included as examples of solutions for a particular problem. Each person will have unique constellations of IADL that describe their roles (Trombly, 1993).

Mobility and Transfers

Mobility refers to movements on one surface that involves change of position or location. Bed mobility refers to rolling side to side, going from supine to sit, etc. Wheelchair mobility refers to propelling the wheelchair on various surfaces as well as managing its parts. Functional ambulation refers to walking with some aid (e.g., crutches) to accomplish some task such as moving a coffee cup from the counter to the table or getting clothes out of the closet.

Transfers refer to movement from one surface to another. For example, movements from the bed to the wheelchair or from the wheelchair to the car seat. The type of transfer used depends on the degree of disability. If the patient is unable to move at all, a lift is required to carry him from one surface to another. If the patient is unable to bear weight on his lower extremities and has weak upper extremities, an assisted or independent sliding transfer is taught. If the patient is unable to bear weight on his lower extremities but has strong upper extremities enabling him to depress his scapulae to lift his buttocks off of the surface, a depression transfer is the appropriate choice. If weight bearing on the lower extremities is possible and permitted, a pivot transfer is used. When standing balance is a problem, this transfer is assisted.

Transfers are described here going in one direction. Reversing the process will accomplish the transfer in the other direction. **Note that the wheelchair must be locked for all transfers.** Transfers are most easily accomplished when the heights of the two surfaces involved in the transfer are the same.

When lifting or assisting a patient to transfer, the therapist must protect her own back by using proper body mechanics. The strong leg muscles are used by keeping the back straight and bending or straightening at the knees to lower or lift the patient. The therapist should not attempt a transfer that seems unmanageable because of the discrepancy between the patient's size and her own or because of the patient's level of dependency. If the therapist should overestimate and find, after the transfer has started, that the patient is slipping from her control, the therapist should ease the patient to the floor and cushion the fall.

LIMITED RANGE OF MOTION

For patients with limited range of motion of the hips and knees combined with muscle weakness, coming to a standing position is facilitated by use of raised seating. Some examples are (1) a raised toilet seat that can be attached to the rim of the toilet, (2) high or adjustable-height chairs such as executive office chairs, (3) an electric or spring-loaded lift for existing chairs that tilts the chair seat forward to assist standing, (4) an additional cushion placed in existing chairs to raise the seat height to the required level, (5) a wheelchair fitted with an hydraulically controlled elevating seat that raises the seat when the patient is preparing to transfer.

Persons with arthritis need to use their joints correctly and avoid deforming forces. This includes avoidance of twisting the joints and use of the larger, stronger joints instead of the smaller joints whenever possible. In transferring from one place to another, the person will stand up and then change the position of the feet, rather than twisting at the knees, to orient himself to the other place.

WEAKNESS

Bed Mobility

The ability to roll over and to sit up in bed are necessary prerequisites to being able to dress and transfer. To roll over, the person with weakness in all four extremities holds the bedside rail or the arm of the wheelchair, which has been placed beside the bed and locked. He holds by grasping with the hand closest to that side of the bed or, if he lacks grasp, by hooking the distal forearm or extended wrist around the rail or the wheelchair handle. To gain the momentum necessary for rolling the upper trunk over, he then flings the other arm across the body using proximal musculature. He may then need to reach down and hook his extended wrist under his distal thigh to pull the leg over.

One method a weak person can use to sit up is to use a rope ladder, which is tied to the foot of the bed. It has webbing bars attached between two webbing strips to form the "ladder." He loops his arms first in the near loop and then each next one to pull up to sitting. A sitting position beyond 90° of hip flexion must be achieved to maintain balance. To avoid the

necessity for equipment, the patient can learn to come to a sitting position as follows:

1. Roll to one side (e.g., the right).
2. Fling the top arm (left) backward to rest the elbow on the bed.
3. Roll onto the left elbow and quickly fling the right arm back to rest the palm of the hand or fist on the bed.
4. Roll to the right and quickly move the left arm to rest the hand on the bed.
5. Having achieved a semisitting position resting on both hands, with the elbows extended or locked, the patient "walks" his hands forward to come to a forward-leaning position of greater than 90° of hip flexion to maintain balance.

Wheelchair Mobility

A powered wheelchair is required for persons too weak to propel a standard wheelchair (see Chapter 30). For the patient who is confined to a wheelchair but has adequate upper extremity strength to propel a standard wheelchair, mobility training is important. A graded program toward independent wheelchair mobility proceeds from level, smooth indoor surfaces to inclined, rough outdoor surfaces, to ascending and descending one step. Basic wheelchair mobility is the responsibility of the physical therapist. Functional wheelchair mobility is a shared responsibility.

Although the Americans with Disabilities Act of 1990 (ADA) requires wheelchair access in public buildings and in private buildings that are open to the public (e.g., movie theaters) and requires cities and towns to have curb cuts in sidewalks, there are still times when a person in a wheelchair must go up and down some steps.

Ascending and descending several stairs requires the assistance of two people. To take a person in a wheelchair up a flight of stairs, approach the stairs backward. One person stands behind the chair and tips it backward into its balanced position. The second person stands in front of the chair and holds on to the leg rest upright (making sure she is holding on to part of the frame of the chair, not a detachable part). While maintaining the chair at its point of balance on the back wheel, the person behind the chair pulls it up each step in succession while the person at the foot assists in lifting and maintaining the point of balance. To take a person in a wheelchair down a flight of stairs, approach the stairs forward with the wheelchair in a tipped, balanced position. The two people reverse the process for ascending stairs to lower the chair down each step in succession.

If the person can do an independent floor to

wheelchair transfer, it would be possible for him to "bump" himself up and down the stairs in an emergency and pull his wheelchair after him.

To assist a person in a wheelchair up and down a curb or one step, the helper approaches the curb with the front of the wheelchair and depresses the foot projection on the back of the wheelchair frame while pulling back on the handles to put the casters over the curb. To assist a wheelchair down a curb, the helper approaches the curb backward, lets the large back wheels down first and then the casters. An alternative method of assisting a wheelchair down a curb uses a forward approach: Tip the wheelchair back onto the large back wheels to the point of balance where the center of gravity is over the rear axle and then let the large wheels gently down the curb.

Good upper extremity strength and the ability to do a "wheelie" are needed to maneuver curbs independently. A wheelie is done by giving a quick forward push on the hand rims while simultaneously throwing the trunk back against the seat back; this tips the chair backward to its point of balance and raises the casters off the floor. The person then must hold the wheelchair at its point of balance over the rear axle. The patient approaches the curb forward. As the casters near the curb, he does the wheelie which lifts the casters onto the curb. Then, while leaning far forward to redistribute the weight, he propels the large back wheels onto the curb. To go down a curb the patient approaches the curb backward, leans forward in the chair, and rolls down the curb. An alternative method for going down a curb uses a forward approach: The patient does a wheelie and rolls off the curb using the back wheels.

Learning to do a wheelie takes practice and courage. Training aids have been developed to allow the patient to practice without a staff member present to guard (Dutton et al., 1979; Hinrichsen, Nordström, & Law, 1984). These catch the patient and prevent him from going over backward when he fails to find the balance point.

Transfers

Persons who are very weak in all four extremities will be dependent in transfers. In that case, they will be lifted or rolled into place by another person.

Two-Person Carry

To transfer a person who can be placed in a sitting position, one lifter positions herself at the patient's head. After lifting the patient toward the edge of the bed and into a partial sitting position, the lifter flexes the patient's elbows so that his forearms rest across his body. The lifter pushes her hands in under the axillae from back to front to grasp both of the patient's forearms just distal to the elbows. The other lifter assists by moving the patient's hips over to the edge of the bed by holding the patient securely under the knees. On signal from the person supporting the upper body, both lifters move the patient from the bed to the waiting wheelchair.

Logroll Transfer

A logroll transfer can be done by one person. The wheelchair is locked in position, facing the foot of the bed; the seat is near the patient's hips, the detachable arm is removed, and a pillow is placed over the wheel. The patient is rolled onto his side with his back toward the chair. His hips are near the chair seat at the edge of the bed and his arms and legs are flexed, which distributes the weight to prevent rolling out of bed. The hips are moved onto the chair seat while the upper trunk and legs remain on the bed. Then the upper trunk is moved to an upright position in the chair, and finally, the feet are moved from the bed to the footrests of the wheelchair.

Mechanically Assisted Transfer

If the person who is to do the lift is not strong enough to move the patient, and the patient is allowed to sit, a mechanical lifter can be used. The nylon seat and back support is slid under the patient. The support is then hooked to the hydraulic lifting mechanism, which, when pumped, will lift the patient off the surface. The device is wheeled to the other surface, and slow release of the hydraulic mechanism lowers the patient to the surface. Similar devices include one adapted from a garage door opener (Alexander, 1979) and a battery-operated winch (Petersen, 1984) to allow "independent dependent" transfer from one specific place to another other, e.g., bed or wheelchair to commode. The use of a mechanical lift may mean the difference between discharge home or discharge to nursing home.

Persons with some strength in the upper extremities may be able to transfer independently or with the assistance of a device or one person.

Assisted Trapeze Transfer

A swivel trapeze bar attached to an orthopedic frame at the head of the bed can be used if the patient has upper extremity strength equal to lifting half his body weight. The wheelchair is positioned next to the bed, with the armrest removed and the brakes locked. The patient holds on to the trapeze by hooking his extended wrists around the bar and pulls to sitting. Then he puts both forearms across the bar, assisted, if necessary. The patient then contracts his elbow flexors to support the weight of his upper trunk. The therapist holds the patient's legs and pulls him off of the bed surface toward the foot of the bed and swings his lower body over to the chair; the trapeze swivels with the motions. Once seated, the patient releases his arms from the trapeze and positions his trunk in the chair.

Assisted Wheelchair Positioning

A patient may also need assistance positioning himself in the wheelchair. This may be accomplished by one person standing behind the wheelchair, which is locked and tipped backward to its point of balance. Shaking the chair assists gravity in sliding the patient's hips back into the chair. **Caution:** Do not shake the chair if the patient has spasticity. If the patient needs more assistance than this, his elbows are flexed so that his forearms rest across his body. With the wheelchair still tipped and resting against the therapist's thighs, the therapist pushes her arms in between the patient's arms and chest wall under the axillae from behind to grasp each forearm just distal to the elbow. Force is applied upward to pull the patient into an upright posture.

Independent Trapeze Transfer

The swivel trapeze bar transfer, previously described, can be done independently if upper extremity strength permits. The patient would lift his legs from the bed to the wheelchair footrests himself after he was in the wheelchair. If the person is unable to bear weight on the legs and has weak arms, a sliding depression transfer is chosen. This transfer can be assisted or independent, depending on the extent of the person's disability.

Assisted Sliding Transfer

For an assisted sliding transfer, a transfer board is used to bridge the space between the transfer surfaces. A long sliding board may be necessary for bridging the space between a wheelchair and the car, whereas a short board would be more appropriate for toilet transfers. The sliding board is positioned with one end well under the patient's hips and the other end on the surface to which the patient is transferring. Assistance is provided by holding the patient around the rib cage, waist, or waistband of trousers and sliding him along the board. The patient can place his arms around the therapist's neck or waist during the transfer. After the patient is safely onto the new surface, the legs are carried into place by the patient, if possible, or by the therapist, if necessary.

Independent Sliding Transfer

The person does a series of minidepression transfers as he slides along the sliding board from one surface to the next (Fig. 15.2).

Independent Depression Transfer

For patients with paralyzed lower extremities but strong scapular depression and elbow extension, an independent depression transfer is done in this way: The wheelchair is positioned as close to the surface being transferred to as possible, and the brakes are locked. The feet are lifted off the footrests and placed on the floor one by one. Each footrest is raised out of the way. If the patient has poor trunk balance, he can hook one of his arms around the wheelchair upright while leaning to pull up the footrests with the other. The arm of the wheelchair on the side to which the transfer is to be done is removed. The patient slides forward on the seat of the wheelchair. He places one hand at a distance onto the surface he is transferring to and the other under his hip. He pushes down using scapular depression and elbow extension to lift the buttocks clear of the wheelchair and swings over to the other surface in one quick, smooth action. For the weaker person, the transfer can be done by a series of minidepressions, but the two surfaces have to be contiguous and of the same height.

Sometimes, it is not possible to get the wheelchair close enough to the transfer surface. This most often occurs in toilet or bathtub transfers. In this case, a sliding board or a sturdy straight-backed chair can be

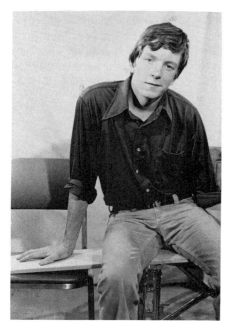

Figure 15.2. Transferring using a sliding board.

used to bridge the gap between the wheelchair and the toilet or tub seat.

Car Transfer

One method a person with bilateral lower extremity weakness could use to transfer into a two-door car and bring the wheelchair in is as follows. He would approach the car on the passenger side, move the power seat all the way back, and transfer into the car using either a depression transfer or a sliding board transfer. Once transferred into the car, the person secures his trunk balance, and then leans to remove the wheelchair cushion. He folds the chair and puts the casters on the edge of the car near the entrance to the backseat. He moves to the driver's seat and then moves the entire seat forward. He tips the seat back on the passenger side forward and leans to reach the front casters of the wheelchair to pull the wheelchair into the space behind the passenger seat. A board that levels the back floor makes it easier. Then he tips the passenger seat back into place and adjusts the entire seat to a comfortable driving position. He reaches across to close the passenger door. A stick with a hook may be helpful to extend the reach. If spasm is a problem or a possibility, the legs are positioned so that spasm would not send the feet against the brake or accelerator.

LOSS OF THE USE OF ONE SIDE OF THE BODY

Bed Mobility

The person who has suffered a stroke and lost the strength of one side of the body must relearn how to roll over and come to a sitting position in bed. The hemiplegic patient is generally able to roll toward the affected side, but experiences difficulty rolling toward the unaffected side. In one method of rolling to the unaffected side from a supine position, the hemiplegic patient puts his unaffected foot under the affected ankle, carries his affected arm across his body, and then pulls himself over onto his unaffected side by holding the side of the bed. Another method is for the patient to clasp his hands with the thumb of the affected hand above the sound one (see Chapter 24), the elbows extended, and the shoulder flexed above 90°. Then he quickly swings his arms from one side to the other side, building momentum. Finally, the momentum carries him onto his side (Bobath, 1990).

One method of coming to a sitting position on the edge of the bed is to put the unaffected foot under the affected ankle and carry the legs to the edge of the bed. Next, the affected arm is carried across the body. While the head is simultaneously thrust forward, the uninvolved arm pushes against the bed to come to a

sitting position. The patient continues the upward thrust of his upper body while swinging his legs over the side of the bed. The important thing to remember is that the person should roll all the way onto his side before pushing to sit up. This puts the arm in a better position to push up and puts less strain on the back. He should be guarded until the therapist is satisfied that he can do this procedure independently and safely. A hard mattress reduces the danger of falling. If the mattress at home is soft, a bed board can be suggested.

Another method of coming to a sitting position was advocated by Bobath (1990). The patient starts by clasping his hands with shoulders flexed and elbows extended. He then rolls over onto the sound side. With the arms still clasped together, he bends his sound elbow and pushes it against the bed to lift the upper trunk off the bed. Simultaneously, he brings his sound leg over the edge of the bed, which brings him to a semisitting position. He then pushes against the mattress with both arms (hands still clasped), while flexing the head toward the affected side, to bring himself upright. The therapist may need to assist with the head lateral flexion and swinging the affected leg off the bed until the patient learns the technique and gains sufficient strength.

Wheelchair Mobility

Hemiplegic patients who are confined to a wheelchair, either temporarily or permanently, learn to propel a standard wheelchair. The person uses the unaffected arm on the wheelchair rim to provide power and the unaffected leg to provide both power and compensatory steering by "walking" forward on the floor. One-arm drive wheelchairs (Chapter 30) are available for those whose combination of disabilities warrant their use.

Transfers

A patient who is able to accept weight on one or both lower extremities is a candidate for an assisted or independent pivot transfer. In the case of a hemiplegic patient, he initially always transfers with his strong side leading, or toward the noninvolved side. Later, the patient must learn to transfer in both directions if he is to be independent.

Assisted Pivot Transfers

For a pivot transfer from wheelchair to chair, the locked wheelchair is positioned next to the surface to be transferred to, located on the noninvolved side. The front of the wheelchair seat should be perpendicular to (at 90°), or at an acute angle to, the front of the seating surface to be transferred to. First, the patient must scoot forward in the wheelchair. The therapist assists

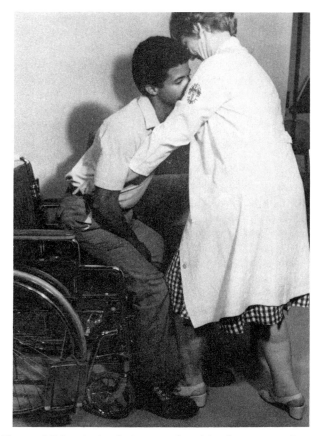

Figure 15.3. Assisted pivot transfer: rising from one surface.

by having the patient lean to one side and then gently pulls the opposite hip forward in the chair; the patient leans to the other side and the other hip is pulled forward. This is repeated until the patient is near the front edge of the chair. Then the therapist faces the patient, who is sitting with his feet on the floor approximately 20 to 30 cm apart, and bends her knees to meet and support the patient's knees. She reaches under the patient's affected arm to position her hands on the scapula of the involved side or takes hold of the waistband of the patient's trousers. As the patient leans forward and pushes down on the wheelchair armrest with the noninvolved arm to assist standing, the therapist supports one of the patient's knees and assists it into extension while lifting from the scapula or trousers (Fig. 15.3). The important thing is to get the patient to lean forward enough to get his center of gravity over the feet when coming to standing. Patients are often afraid to lean forward enough, but if they do not, the therapist ends up doing more work than she needs to do. The therapist may place one hand on the patient's upper back/neck area to assist and guide the patient to bend forward enough.

After the patient is standing and balanced, the

therapist pivots with the patient to turn so that the patient now stands in front of the chair. The therapist helps to lower the patient into the chair slowly by bending her knees as the patient sits. The patient puts his noninvolved hand on the armrest to assist in lowering himself slowly into the chair (Fig. 15.4). The patient must bend forward during sitting to keep the center of gravity over the feet; if he does not, sitting will be uncontrolled, and he will flop down into the chair.

Before the student therapist does this transfer with a patient, she needs to experiment and practice with a nondisabled person to learn to do it smoothly and to avoid tripping the other person.

Independent Pivot Transfers

The process of independent pivot transfers is the same as for the assisted pivot transfer, except that it is done without help. Again, the wheelchair is locked in position and the patient lifts the footrests and slides forward. The feet are located directly below the knees and are flat on the floor. Bending forward and using a rocking motion to gain momentum, the patient then presses with the noninvolved foot to extend that leg

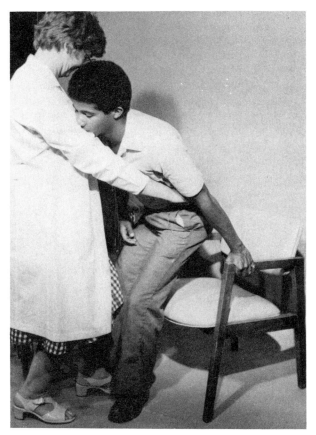

Figure 15.4. Assisted pivot transfer: lowering onto the other surface.

while pushing down on the arm of the wheelchair with the noninvolved arm to come to a standing position. Pausing to balance in a fully standing position, he then reaches to the surface to which he is transferring, pivots, and lowers himself to the surface.

The 180° independent pivot transfer is done similarly to the 90° pivot but requires the patient to turn fully around after standing to reach the surface to which he is transferring. This transfer may be required by circumstances such as in a bathroom or other areas where the wheelchair cannot be positioned for the 90° pivot. Grab bars assist in doing a 180° pivot safely.

INCOORDINATION

Wheelchair Mobility

Persons with upper extremity incoordination find it easier to propel a standard wheelchair by using their feet. Pushing backward is easiest, but a rearview mirror is needed to prevent accidents! Incoordination of all limbs may require a powered wheelchair with adapted controls (see Chapters 30 and 31).

Transfers

Persons with incoordination can use any of the types of transfers described above or a nonadapted method if strong enough in both lower extremities. With these patients, however, the problem of safety arises, and they must pay particular attention to such factors. If judgment is poor, the patient must depend on others for supervision during transfer.

Driving

The ability to drive provides the greatest freedom of mobility. For those persons who do not have brain damage, the potential for driving is good. Those with limited range of motion may require special seating, extensions to controls, and smaller-diameter steering wheels but may otherwise be able to drive. Those with severely limited lower extremity range can use hand controls. Many persons with decreased strength can be safe drivers with the proper selection of the car, necessary **adaptations,** and training in the use of hand or foot controls as appropriate to the disability (Kent, 1986). Tetraplegic patients with a level of injury at C6 or below are considered potential candidates for driver training.

Car Selection

If a wheelchair-bound person is to drive independently, the car must be a two-door sedan that is large enough to allow access for the wheelchair to be stored behind the front seat, with high enough door opening to accommodate the wheelchair handles, and with a large enough door to allow ease of transfer (Short, 1991).

If it is not possible for a person who uses a wheelchair to get it into the car independently, hydraulic lifts are available that attach to the car and lift the wheelchair up and into the car. When parking the car, it is important for the wheelchair user to remember that a 1.3-m (4-foot) space on the passenger side is required for transfer. Parking spaces designated for handicapped drivers are marked to allow for transfer space.

Persons with weak lower extremities need to control brake and accelerator functions manually. There are many different types of hand controls. Most require at least moderate strength (4 to 6 kg) to push or pull the levers. Finger controls are similar to hand controls but are more sensitive to smaller movements. Foot controls can be used to steer by those with no upper extremity function (Rosenkoetter, 1980). A swivel steering wheel knob or cuff allows the steering wheel to be operated with one hand while the other controls the hand-operated accelerator and brake. The keys can be built up to provide leverage for turning.

An automatic transmission is needed if hand or foot controls are used. Power seats, power steering, power brakes, power windows, remote-controlled mirrors, cruise control, and a cellular telephone are recommended (Short, 1991). A seat belt and shoulder harness are essential. Chrysler and General Motors, recognizing this market, are currently offering financial assistance for installing hand controls into their automobiles. Governmental standards have been set for acceptable safety and quality of automobile driving aids. Disabled drivers would be wise to adhere to the standards.

Incoordinated persons may or may not be able to drive safely, depending on the severity of their disability. Persons with the loss of use of one side of the body due to stroke may, with medical clearance, drive with few **adaptations.** Medical clearance is needed not so much for physical health problems, but rather the sequelae of the stroke. Whether or not the patient has hemianopsia; impaired perception, thought processes, or judgment; or slow automatic reactions must be taken into account before the patient is cleared for driving training.

The car of a person with loss of one upper extremity ought to have automatic transmission and power steering. A swivel steering wheel knob is needed to steer safely. If the patient has lost the use of his right arm, the gear shift lever and turn indicator will need to be remounted on the left of the steering column. A left-foot accelerator may also be indicated; these can be ordered as options on a new car.

An evaluation with a simulator is recommended for all patients with brain damage or probable brain damage, such as chronic obstructive pulmonary disease (COPD) patients, because judgment deficits and slow reactions are sometimes not apparent during other evaluations but would definitely interfere with safe driving abilities.

Driver Evaluation

A driving simulator is used to evaluate defensive driving skills, hazard perception, and emergency procedures (Cimolino & Balkovec, 1988; Quigley & De-Lise, 1983). The patient sits in a mock-up car module with standard (or adapted) driving devices mounted as in a car. He watches a movie, steers, and reacts to the driving situations as they appear on the screen. His timing and responses are electronically recorded. If these aspects of driving are all right, an actual driving test or driver-training course is then appropriate. Most states require disabled drivers to be tested before receiving their driver's license; some require newly disabled drivers to be reeducated before examining them for a license.

Activities of Daily Living

All tasks that the patient expects to perform independently once discharged must be practiced in a manner similar to the way they will be done. For example, if a patient will bathe in a tub at home, it is inadequate to practice only sponge bathing while hospitalized. It is also inadequate to eliminate from practice the details of self-care such as nail care, ear care, menstrual care, handling catheters, hair care, and contact lens care and use or to assume that all self-care tasks that a particular person may need to learn are listed on the evaluation checklist.

Techniques and equipment for self-care presented in this chapter are not the only methods of accomplishing these particular tasks. This presentation is meant to provide the student therapist with a repertoire of basic skills with which she can approach the patient with confidence. The principles of compensation for each problem are key pieces of information that allow the student to evaluate other techniques or equipment to meet the needs of the patient. Many tasks not mentioned here either do not require **adaptation** or the **adaptation** can be extrapolated from the examples cited.

As each task is taught, all potentially needed equipment should be close at hand. For early training in dressing, clothing that is a size too large should be used, because it can be managed more easily. The patient's attention should be called to design details of clothing as some designs are more easily donned by persons with certain disabilities. The details to be considered are the cut of the garment, the sleeve style,

type of closure or fasteners, and type of fabric (Dallas & White, 1982; Levitan-Rheingold, Hatte, & Mandel, 1980). Clothing especially designed for the handicapped can be purchased or made from patterns published by commercial pattern makers (Joe, 1992).

WEAKNESS
Principles

1. Use lightweight objects, utensils, and tools.
2. Let gravity assist.
3. Use adapted equipment or methods to replace lost functions such as grasp.
4. Use powered tools and utensils.
5. Use biomechanical principles of
   a. Levers (e.g., force arm > resistance arm);
   b. Application of force (e.g., apply force closer or farther from the fulcrum to change length of lever arms);
   c. Friction (e.g., increased friction decreases power required for pinch or grasp).
6. Use two hands.

Suggestions for BADL

When muscle weakness involves all four extremities, the techniques and devices are extensive; therefore, this section will focus on compensation for involvement of all four extremities. Many equipment suggestions have been listed in Chapter 39. When weakness is extensive, personal care attendants (PCAs) will be needed to carry out basic activities of daily living. The patient will need to learn how to hire, supervise, instruct, compensate, set limits for, and terminate personnel (DeGraff, 1989; Rush, 1987). If the patient is weak in his lower extremities with normal upper extremities, many of the techniques or devices will be unnecessary. The principles apply as well to limited weakness such as weak pinch secondary to osteoarthritis of the carpometacarpal (CMC) joint.

Feeding

The problem with feeding is the inability to grasp and/or bring the hand to the mouth. A universal cuff can be used to hold the utensil if grasp is absent (Fig. 15.5) or the handle can be "woven" through the fingers (i.e., index and ring fingers on top and middle and little fingers under) and held in place passively. A "spork," a utensil that combines the bowl of a spoon with the tines of a fork, is used with the cuff to eliminate the need to change utensils. Some of these have a swivel feature to substitute for the inability to supinate. Gravity and weight of the food keep the bowl level on the way to the mouth; sporks with enlarged handles can be purchased (Fig. 15.6). If the patient

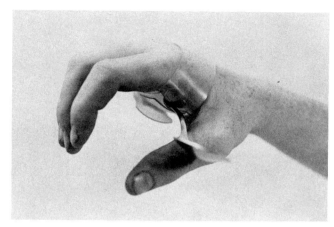

Figure 15.5. Universal cuff.

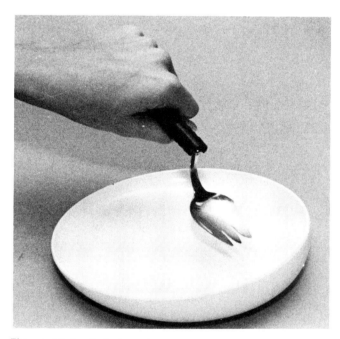

Figure 15.6. Swivel spork.

axilla height offers support for the arm and eliminates gravity, allowing the patient to bring the food to his mouth. As strength increases, the surface can be lowered.

Grooming

The inability to grasp and pinch needs to be dealt with to enable the patient to groom himself or herself. **Adaptations** for makeup jars, tubes, and applicators have been suggested (Hage, 1988). A universal cuff or a splint can be used to hold a rattail comb, toothbrush, lipstick tube, or safety razor if grasp is absent. A handcuff can be constructed to hold an electric razor. If grasp is present but weak, lightweight, enlarged handles may be enough. Added assistance could be obtained by applying friction material to the utensil or tool. A small plastic brush with or without a cuff attachment may be used to assist in shampooing hair.

Toileting

Transfers, the handling of the body to lower and raise the clothing, and weak pinch and grasp are problems. For patients with spinal cord injury, concomitant loss of bowel and bladder control requires special procedures, including bladder irrigation and use of a catheter (Jetter, 1988; Lewis, 1993). Pants can be generally pushed down while in the wheelchair by the patient leaning to one side and then the other. If the patient has precarious standing balance, it may be necessary to transfer back to the wheelchair before raising the clothing after toileting. If the patient uses an indwelling catheter or external drainage device, the collection bag can be emptied into the toilet without the need to transfer or remove clothing.

has weak grasp, lightweight, enlarged handles can be used. The patient may use a flexor hinge hand splint to increase the strength of grasp (Chapter 28).

For cutting, a sharp, serrated knife is used, because less force is needed and it is less likely to slip.

An attachable, open-bottomed handle can be added to a glass or soft drink can to permit picking it up in the absence of grasp. A mug with a T-shaped handle (Fig. 15.7) or a handle that allows all four fingers to be inserted provides leverage and stabilizes the fingers around the mug, allowing pick up with tenodesis grasp. A foam can insulator can be used with glasses to provide friction to assist weak grasp. Mobile arm supports or suspension slings (see Chapter 28) may be required to allow reaching. A table placed at

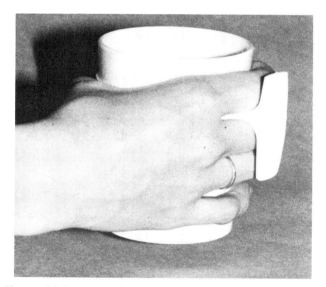

Figure 15.7. Cup with T-shaped handle assists drinking when one has a weak grasp.

A raised toilet seat is used by tetraplegic individuals to create a space between the seat and toilet bowl rim to allow for insertion of a suppository. Suppository inserters are commercially available for those with weak or absent pinch. Cuffs are attached to these devices so that patients who lack good grasp can manipulate them using leverage. They may have a spring ejector that releases the suppository after it is properly positioned in the rectum. An inspection mirror is needed if the patient lacks anal sensation. Digit stimulators may be the method of choice (see Chapter 39). For those patients with weak grasp and pinch, toilet tissue can be wrapped around the hand for use. Menstrual needs can be met by **adaptations** to positioning, pants, pad versus tampons, and aids such as mirrors or knee spreaders (Duckworth, 1986).

Dressing

Dressing in less than 1 hr is considered functional for tetraplegics (Weingarden & Martin, 1989). Problems include moving the paralyzed limbs to dress them as well as the need to compensate for the lack of pinch and grasp. While in bed and by using the wrist extensors and elbow flexors, patients with spinal cord injuries at C6 and below can pull the knees up to dress the lower extremities. A **dressing stick** with a loop that goes around the wrist attached to the end opposite the hook can help. The person pulls against the loop, using wrist extension and leverage, to stabilize tenodesis grasp of the stick. The sock aid and long-handled shoehorn, described later in this chapter, may be useful. Loops of twill tape can be added to the cuffs of socks to facilitate pulling them on by hooking the thumb in the loop.

A buttonhook, attached to a cuff or with a built-up handle, is used when fingers are unable to manipulate buttons. The hook is inserted through the buttonhole to hook the button and pull it through the buttonhole. The other hand is used to hold the garment near the buttonhole (Fig. 15.8). A loop of string or leather lacing may be attached to the zipper pull of trousers or other garments, so that in the absence of pinch, the thumb can be hooked in the loop to close the zipper. A hook can also be used.

Primarily, the following methods of tetraplegic dressing were described by Runge (1967).

Trousers (and undershorts). While the patient is sitting in bed with side rails up, the trousers are positioned with the front up and legs over the bottom of the bed. The trousers are positioned by tossing them or using a **dressing stick** with a wrist loop. One leg is lifted by hooking the opposite wrist or forearm under the knee, and the foot is put into the pants leg. The thumb of the other hand hooks a belt loop or pocket to hold the trousers open. Working in a

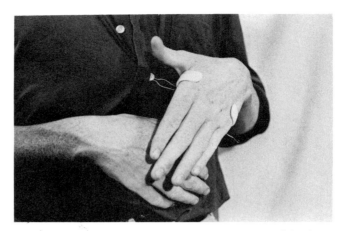

Figure 15.8. Buttonhook on a cuff. Note zipper pull hook on the other end.

cross-body position aids stability for those with poor balance. The other foot is inserted. The palms of the hands are used to pat and slide the trousers onto the calves, attempting to get the trouser cuffs over the feet. The wrist(s) is hooked under the waistband or in the pockets to pull the trousers up over the knees. The patient continues to pull on the waistband or pockets while returning to supine position to pull the trousers up onto the thighs. This may need to be repeated. Hooking the wrist or thumbs in the crotch helps pull up the trousers. In a side-lying position, the thumb of the top arm is hooked in the back belt loop, and the pants are pulled over the buttocks. Then the patient rolls to the other side and repeats the process until the trousers are on. In a supine position, the trousers can be fastened using a zipper pull loop and Velcro tab closing or buttonhook. Removing the trousers is accomplished essentially by reversing the procedures and pushing the pants off.

Socks. While sitting in the wheelchair, the patient crosses one leg over the other and uses tenodesis grasp to put on the sock and the palms of the hands to help pull it on. If the patient is unable to cross his legs, the foot can be placed on a stool or chair. If trunk balance is poor, one arm can be hooked around the wheelchair upright while reaching with the other hand, or the socks can be put on in a sitting position in bed by crossing first one leg and then the other. A sock cone or aid may be helpful in getting the sock over the toes if the patient is unable to reach his feet. Socks are removed by pushing them off with a **dressing stick,** long shoehorn, or the thumb hooked in the sock edge.

Long leg braces for paraplegics (or knee-ankle-foot orthosis; KAFO). While the patient is sitting in bed the brace is positioned beside the leg, and then the patient lifts his leg over into the brace. If the shoe is attached to the brace, the foot is first put into the shoe. It is helpful to unlock and flex the knee of the brace to press the shoe against the bed and pull on the uprights to get the heel into the shoe. Then, with the knee still flexed, the shoe can be tied. Next, the knee is straightened, the knee pad is fastened, and then the thigh band is fastened. For a brace to be worn under trousers, the brace must be attached to the shoe with removable calipers. In this instance, the patient first puts on his socks, the brace, his trousers, then his shoes, and finally attaches the brace to the shoe. Once the patient is in the wheelchair, other garments are put on.

Shoes. Loafer-type shoes are most practical for nonambulatory patients. Shoes are put on by crossing one leg at a time as for putting on socks. The shoe is pulled onto the foot by holding the sole of the shoe in the palm of the hand. With the foot on the floor, or on the foot pedal of the wheelchair, the foot is pushed down into the shoe by pushing on the knee. A long shoehorn may be helpful for getting the heel into the shoe. Shoes can be removed by pushing them off with the shoehorn.

Cardigan garments (shirts or blouses). The shirt is positioned with the brand label of the shirt facing down and the collar toward the knees. The patient puts his arms under the shirt and into the sleeves. The shirt is pushed on until the sleeves are over the elbows. The shirt is gathered up by using wrist extension and by hooking the thumbs under the shirt back. Then the shirt is placed over the head. The patient shrugs his shoulders to get the shirt down across the shoulders. He hooks his wrists into the sleeves to free the axillae. The patient then leans forward and reaches back with one hand to rub on the shirt back to pull it down. The shirt fronts are lined up, and buttoning begins from the bottom button up, using a buttonhook.

A cardigan garment is removed by pushing first one side and then the other off the shoulders and then alternately elevating and depressing the shoulders to allow gravity to assist in lowering the shirt down the arms. Then one thumb is hooked into the opposite sleeve to pull the shirt over the elbow, and the arm is removed from the shirt.

With the exception of buttons, an overhead garment is put on in a similar manner and removed by hooking one thumb in the back of the neckline and pulling the shirt over the head. The sleeves are then pushed off each arm.

Bra. Either a front- or back-closure bra can be used. Velcro can replace hooks for fastening, but many patients can manage the standard hook fastener if it is hooked in front at waist level. After the bra is hooked, it is positioned with the cups in front, and the arms are placed through the shoulder straps. Then, by hook-

ing the opposite thumb under a strap, one strap at a time is pulled over the shoulder.

Bathing

The problems with bathing include the transfer, sitting equilibrium, lack of lower extremity movement (Shillam, Beeman, & Loshin, 1983), and lack of pinch and grasp. A padded board placed across one end of the tub provides a level transfer surface. The padding helps to prevent decubiti. The back of the wall of the tub enclosure can be used for trunk support. Bath seats are available with and without back support or padding. Transfer tub seats, which have two legs in the tub and two legs outside the tub, provide a safe means to transfer from the wheelchair to tub. Each patient's requirements need to be evaluated and a seat selected to fit him. Grab bars secured to the studs of the wall help during the transfer and while seated. A suction cup–backed bath mat is used in the bottom of the tub. The bath seat must be placed so that the faucets are within reach. The faucets must have flat handles for ease in tapping them off and on using the fist. A hand-held shower is used; it can be adapted as suggested for cups, above. If the shower does not have a mixer valve, water temperature is adjusted by turning on the cold water first and then adding the hot, which prevents scalding desensitized skin. No-scald faucets and shower heads are now available and easily installed. Soap on a string or dispenser soap is helpful. A bath mitt is used if grasp is weak or absent. The person dries off before transferring back to the wheelchair. Bathing and drying the feet and legs are particular problems for patients with poor trunk balance; such patients may prefer to do foot hygiene while in bed (Shillam et al., 1983).

A custom-made shower stall provides the best solution for a patient confined to a wheelchair. The shower area should have a raised slope to prevent the water from running out, but allow the person to enter the shower on a special shower wheelchair. Plans for such bath enclosures have been published in the popular press.

Suggestions for Selected IADL

For the severely paralyzed, high-tech **adaptations,** as described in Chapter 31, offer opportunities to engage in communication, leisure, and work activities. Some low-tech **adaptations** are suggested here.

Handling a Book

The tetraplegic patient will encounter problems with holding a book and turning the pages, with writing or recording notes in business or school, and possibly in telephoning. Book holders are available. Some support a book on a table, whereas others are designed to hold a book when reading supine in bed. If a person is reading while supine and the book is not held directly above, prism glasses are needed to direct the vision to a 90° angle so that the book may be seen.

To turn pages, some solutions are as follows: (1) when wearing a splint, the patient can use a rubber thimble or finger cot on the posted thumb; (2) a pencil with the eraser end down can be used in a universal cuff (typing stick) or hand splint; (3) a mouthstick with a friction tip end can be used; and (4) electric page turners, which automatically turn pages when activated by a microswitch or other means of control, can be used. An alternative to turning pages of a book is "talking books," or books on tape. Tape recordings of popular books can be obtained from libraries and bookstores. The Library of Congress has a large collection of tapes, including many current issues of magazines, and tape players that are available to the blind and the physically disabled. They are free and can be ordered from the Library of Congress through local libraries. Particular books needed by students or professionals will be recorded on request.

Writing

Extensive writing is usually done using computerized word processing with typing sticks or a mouthstick for hitting the keys. A mouthstick preferably has a molded mouthpiece that conforms to the patient's dentition (Smith, 1989). To the mouthpiece is added a lightweight wooden, plastic, or aluminum rod with an eraser or other type of end piece. Directions have been published for a custom-made, dentally correct one (Puckett, 1990). Mouthsticks with flat mouth pieces but that have various interchangeable tips such as pencil, pen, and brush can be purchased commercially. If speed of recording is important, as in taking notes in the classroom, a tape recorder can be used.

Handwriting is important for legal documents and personalizing cards and typed notes. Splints that provide pinch can be used to hold a writing instrument. If pinch is absent, and the patient does not use a splint, a pencil holder (Fig. 15.9) that encircles the pencil as well as the thumb and index finger can be made of thermoplastic materials (Barsamian, 1983). If the arms cannot be used, a mouthstick with pencil attached can, with practice, become an effective writing tool. Pens with textured grip provide friction to make a weak grip more effective. Felt-tipped pens require little pressure and are, therefore, easier to use than other types of pens.

Telephoning

A person whose spinal cord was injured at C6 can pick up a telephone receiver and bring it to his

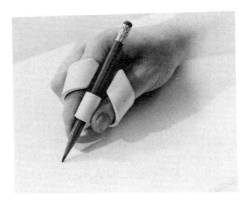

Figure 15.9. A pencil holder made from thermoplastic material.

ear. An executive shoulder rest attached to the receiver holds it there until the conversation is finished. Push-buttons can be depressed using a mouthstick or typing stick. Phones that automatically dial when one button is pressed are very useful. For persons with greater paralysis, automatic telephone dialers are available (see Chapter 31). These persons will find use of a headset instead of a handset more convenient.

LOW ENDURANCE

Principles

1. Use energy-conservation methods.
2. Pace work to prevent fatigue.
3. Use principles listed for weakness that reduce workload, such as lightweight utensils and powered equipment.
4. Match activity demands to ability.
5. Avoid stressful positions and environmental stressors.

Suggestions for BADL

Patients of various diagnoses and circumstances (e.g., bed rest) experience low endurance at least temporarily. Patients with cardiac or pulmonary disease have a more or less permanent reduction of endurance to which they must adapt. These patients have reduced ability to use oxygen needed for muscle (including cardiac muscle) and brain functions. If oxygen deprivation is severe enough, neuropsychological changes involving memory, perception, and information processing occur. These would affect the effectiveness of the teaching and learning process as well as performance.

Adaptations for basic and instrumental activities of daily living involve awareness and reduction of the metabolic cost of activiiies and working within limits of cardiac and pulmonary capacity. Cardiac patients are cautioned to stop activity when they experience angina or shortness of breath (SOB). Patients with COPD are taught to work slowly, pacing themselves and taking "resting pauses" during tasks (Barstow, 1974). Both types of patients are taught to intersperse rest periods throughout the day and use other energy-conserving techniques. Energy-conservation methods are listed in Table 15.3 and elaborated on in Chapter 16.

Some activities require higher levels of energy than do others. One way to guide activity selection is to use metabolic equivalent tables (MET) (see Table 43.3). Most self-care activities require less than three METs; however, showering, tub bathing, toileting, and washing and setting hair require higher levels (Huntley & Mullivan, 1978). It should be remembered that MET charts are averages and do not account for particular circumstances and cannot, therefore, be used without also monitoring the patient's breathing or heart rate. Dyspnea (SOB) signals the patient that the activity he is doing is beyond his capacity. Angina or excessive increase in heart rate (20 beats over resting rate) signals the cardiac patient that he has reached his limit. Stressful positions and circumstances are to be avoided, including the following (Barstow, 1974; Berzins, 1970; Cristy & Sarafconn, 1990; Pomerantz, Flannery, & Findling, 1975):

1. *Bending over.* Slip-on shoes, sock aids, reachers, and long-handled sponges can be used to assist ADL independence without bending over.
2. *Reaching overhead.* Store clothes and utensils within easy reach; rest arms on something when reaching or repeatedly lower arms to rest if reaching up is necessary.
3. *Isometric contractions, including pushing, pulling, and maintained grasp.* Patients are taught to exhale or count while they do these actions, if such actions cannot be avoided.
4. *Hot, humid environment.* Such conditions increase SOB and reduce the patient's aerobic capacity.
5. *Overexertion.*

Suggestions offered for persons with low endurance are the following (Cristy & Sarafconn, 1990):

Table 15.3.   Energy-Conservation Methods

1. Plan ahead. Organize work.
2. Eliminate unnecessary tasks.
3. Sit to work.
4. Have all required equipment ready before starting a task.
5. Combine tasks to eliminate extra work.
6. Use electrical appliances to conserve personal energy.
7. Use lightweight utensils and tools.
8. Work with gravity assisting, not resisting.
9. Rest before fatiguing.

1. *Get sufficient sleep.* If the patient is having trouble sleeping, some strategies that the therapist can suggest include developing a bedtime routine and schedule, practicing relaxation techniques (visualization, listening to soothing music, progressive relaxation technique, and meditation), and avoiding upsetting or exciting activities just before bedtime.
2. *Consider your energy budget.* Identify essential tasks and eliminate nonessential ones. Spread the performance of tasks that must be done throughout the day or week and delegate the rest to others.
3. *Do preventative maintenance and cleaning.* A small chore, left undone, becomes an energy-consuming one later on.
4. *Organize working space.* Organize to allow sitting while working without reaching, stretching, or bending.
5. *Use labor-saving products and techniques.* Examples of ways to save energy include soaking dishes before washing them and using a computer program that writes checks and maintains household accounts simultaneously.
6. *Organize work and errands.* Organize to eliminate backtracking, extra steps or trips, and to allow planned rest periods. Keep commitments within manageable limits.
7. *Emotions—good or bad—use energy, too.* Consider the emotions when budgeting energy.

LIMITED OR RESTRICTED RANGE OF MOTION

Principles

1. Use **adaptations** to increase reach.
2. Use **adaptations** to eliminate the need to bend over.
3. Use **adaptations** to compensate for limited grasp.
4. Store frequently used things within easy reach.
5. Use joint protection techniques for rheumatoid arthritis.

Suggestions for BADL

Feeding

The problem with feeding may be one of inability to close the hand enough to grasp the utensil or the inability to bring the hand to the mouth. Enlarged or elongated handles can be added to spoons or forks. The elongated handle may need to be angled to enable the patient to reach his mouth. Remember that the longer the handle (resistance arm), the heavier and less stable the device; therefore, the handle should be only as long as is absolutely necessary and made from lightweight material.

A universal cuff, or utensil holder, can be used

when grasp is not possible. This cuff fits around the palm and has a pocket for insertion of the handle of a utensil (Fig. 15.5).

Grooming

The problems with grooming are the same as for feeding. Enlarged or extended handles can be attached to a comb (Fig. 15.1), brush, toothbrush, shampoo brush, lipstick tube, or safety razor. Aerosol deodorant, hair spray, powder, and perfume can be used by those with limited range. Another person may be needed to wash thoroughly and style a woman's hair; if the person can reach the head to do it herself, a simple hairstyle is recommended. A person with chronic back pain should sit rather than bend over the lavatory to brush teeth and shave.

Toileting

The problem with toileting is the inability to reach. The toilet tissue dispenser should be located within reach. Wiping tongs can extend reach when using toilet tissue. If grasp is poor, the tissue can be wrapped around the hand to eliminate the need for grasping it. A bidet eliminates the need for wiping by hand. A bidet accessory is available to retrofit regular toilets. Gravity will assist in pulling clothes down; larger clothes slide off more easily. A **dressing stick** can be used to pull up the clothing. A folding **dressing stick** for use away from home can be made from a folding cane used by blind people for mobility (Lykouretzos & Thompson-Rangel, 1990). Sanitary napkins with adhesive strips can be used more easily than tampons; the protective paper can be removed using the teeth. If the patient is not be able to sit and arise from a low commode, a raised toilet seat may solve the problem.

Dressing

Lack of ability to reach and grasp and limited shoulder, back, hip, or knee range of motion are possible problems encountered in dressing. For 3 months following hip replacement, patients are restricted from flexing the hip past 90°, adducting the leg past midline, externally rotating the leg, or bearing full weight on the leg (Seeger & Fisher, 1982); therefore they need to use the suggestions in this section temporarily (see also Chapter 37).

A **dressing stick** can be used to pull clothing over the feet or to reach hangers in the closet. Reachers can be used to remove clothes from shelves, to start clothes over parts of the body, or to pick up objects from the floor (Fig. 15.10).

Dressing the lower extremities is a particular problem. People who are unable to reach their feet or

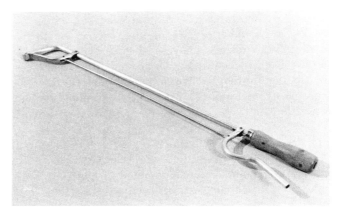

Figure 15.10. Voluntary opening reacher that remains closed to hold objects without exerting the patient.

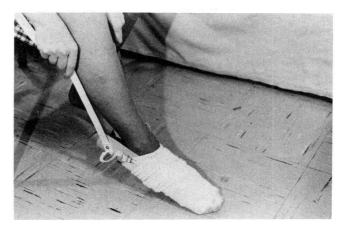

Figure 15.11. One type of stocking aid.

who are not allowed to flex the hip can dress the lower extremities as follows. For them, a sock or stocking aid (Fig. 15.11) is a valuable piece of adapted equipment. To use, the cone is inserted into the foot of the stocking; the top of the stocking is pushed down below the top edge of the cone. While the strings are held, the stocking aid with stocking in place is tossed over the toes, and the person's foot is moved into the foot of the stocking. The cone is then removed by pulling the strings, bringing it out of the stocking behind the heel. The stocking will now be within reach and can be pulled up onto the leg.

An alternative method is to place a piece of foam rubber on the floor to help get the stocking onto the foot after it is placed on the toe with a reacher. This method consists of pushing the foot forward across the foam rubber, which provides friction and holds the stocking as the foot slides into the stocking. As this method can be done standing up or sitting on a high stool, it may be particularly helpful to post–hip replacement patients who are not allowed to flex the hip.

Another solution is to sew a garter to each end of a long piece of webbing. The garters are attached to either side of a sock or stocking to pull them up to a point on the leg where they may be reached.

A long shoehorn assists in putting on shoes when the feet cannot be reached (Seeger & Fisher, 1982). Some long shoehorns have a hook on the opposite end that may be used as a **dressing stick.** Slip-on shoes and elastic shoelaces avoid the need to tie shoelaces. Garters attached to webbing straps may be used to pull up slacks.

Dressing the upper body can be accomplished by using cardigan-type garments instead of slipover garments. A **dressing stick** or reacher is used to bring the garment around the shoulders. Fasteners are particularly difficult, especially if the range of motion limitation is accompanied by weakness. In a study of ability of 97 arthritic women to use clothing fasteners, zippers—especially easy sliding, large-toothed plastic ones—were found to be the easiest. Snaps and buttons were rated as difficult, although vertical buttonholes made buttoning easier (Dallas & White, 1982). Velcro tabs can replace buttons, snaps, or hooks if limited mobility in the fingers prevents buttoning or fastening. Because few clothes come with this type of fastener, the patient's clothing must be adapted. To preserve the look of a buttoned garment, the buttonhole is sewn closed, and the button is attached over the hole. The hook and pile Velcro tabs are sewn to replace the buttons (Reich & Otten, 1980).

Bathing

The transfer into the tub is facilitated by grab bars securely mounted to the studs in the wall beside the bathtub or attached to the side of the bathtub. A securely fastened rubber mat should be placed in the tub, even if the tub has a nonskid surface, and another should be placed outside the tub, unless the bathroom is carpeted. A tub seat is used when the patient is unable, or not allowed, to get down into or up from the bottom of the tub (Seeger & Fisher, 1982). Different heights and styles of tub benches are available and need to be evaluated for each patient in terms of stability and ease of transfer. A hand-held shower hose is used for rinsing if a tub seat is required. Flat handles on faucets do not require grasp and allow better leverage for turning on and off. It is helpful if the soap is on a string. It can be purchased that way or made by drilling a hole through a cake of soap and attaching a cord. The soap is either worn around the neck or hung within easy reach.

The same problems of reach and grasp encountered in dressing are seen to interfere with bathing. When grasp is limited, a sponge or terry cloth bath mitt works well. A long-handled bath sponge can be used to reach the feet or back; some are designed to hold the soap inside of the sponge and others are designed especially for cleaning feet. A terry cloth bathrobe is effective for drying.

Suggestions for Selected IADL

Writing

If pinch is limited, the size of the writing instrument can be increased by using sponge rubber, passing it through the holes in a practice golf ball, or using commercially available grips that slip on the instrument.

Telephoning

If the person cannot raise the telephone receiver to the ear and hold it there, an extended arm that permanently clamps onto the table holds the receiver at a convenient height. A lever is attached to the phone to depress the activator buttons, and the phone is answered by raising this lever. A speaker phone is another solution.

Shopping

Shop at off-hours so that clerks are available to get out-of-reach items too heavy to be obtained by use of a reacher.

INCOORDINATION AND/OR POOR DEXTERITY

Principles

1. Stabilize the object being worked on.
2. Stabilize proximal body parts so that need to control is reduced to just the distal body parts.
3. Use adapted equipment that reduces slipperiness or provides stability.
4. Use heavy utensils, cooking equipment, tools, etc.
5. Use **adaptations** that substitute for lack of fine skill.

Suggestions for BADL

The patient is taught to use his body in as stable a posture as is possible, to sit when possible, and to stabilize the upper extremities by bearing weight on them against a surface or by holding the upper arms close to the body, or both. Stabilizing the head may improve a person's ability to control his upper extremities. Friction surfaces, weighted utensils, or weighted cuffs added to the distal segments of the extremities, and the use of larger and/or less precise fasteners, all contribute to increasing independence by lessening the effects of the incoordination.

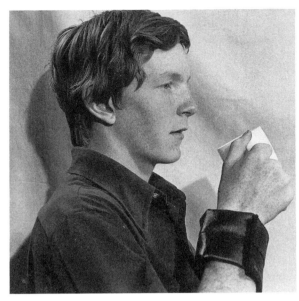

Figure 15.12. Weight cuff used to damp intention tremor or other incoordinated movements.

Feeding

The plate is stabilized on a friction surface (wet towel, wet sponge cloth, nonskid mat, etc.). A plate guard or scoop dish can be used to prevent the food from being pushed off the plate. The utensil may be weighted for stability, may have an enlarged handle to facilitate grasp, and may be plastisol-coated to protect the person's teeth. Sharp utensils are to be avoided. A weight cuff on the wrist is often chosen rather than a weighted utensil because the cuff can be heavier; also the cuff makes it unnecessary to weight each item that the patient will use (Fig. 15.12). The person may successfully drink from a covered glass or cup that has a sipping spout. A cup can be so adapted by using plastic food wrap as a cover, with a straw poked through it. Some may use a long plastic straw that is held in place by a straw holder attachment; the patient moves his head to the straw, but he does not touch it with his hand.

Grooming

Weighted cuffs on the wrists may help some patients gain greater accuracy while grooming. Large lipstick tubes are easier to use than small ones. The arms will need to be stabilized to use lipstick. A simple hairstyle that does not need setting or arrangement is the best choice. For a patient who has difficulty holding a large comb, a military-style brush with a strap can be used. Roll-on or stick deodorant is preferred to spray because these types eliminate the risk of accidentally spraying the substance into the eyes. An electric razor

is preferred to a safety razor both because it is more easily held and because a safety razor can cause a cut if it is involuntarily moved sideways over the skin. Patients with fairly good head control improve their accuracy by holding the electric razor steady and moving their face over the cutting surface. An electric toothbrush is also useful both because it is heavier and because it can be held steady while the head is moved. This same principle can be employed when filing the nails: fasten the emery board to a flat surface and move each nail over the emery board. Cutting the nails may be an unsafe procedure for incoordinated patients; therefore, filing is recommended. Sanitary napkins with adhesive strips to hold them in place may be easier to use than tampons.

Dressing

Clothes that facilitate independent dressing are front-opening, loosely fitting garments with large buttons, Velcro tape closures, or zippers. Wrinkle-resistant and stain-shedding materials enable the person to look well groomed throughout the day. To overcome difficulty with buttoning, a buttonhook with an enlarged and/or weighted handle, if necessary, can be used. A loop of ribbon, leather, or chain can be attached to the zipper pull so that the person can hook it with a finger instead of pinching the zipper pull. Velcro can be substituted to eliminate the need to fasten hooks on a bra. To don the bra, it is easier for the patient to put it around her waist, which is thinner and puts less tension on the garment, then fasten it in front where she can see what she is doing, turn it around, put her arms in, and pull it up into place. Elastic straps make this a relatively easy procedure.

Shoe style should eliminate tying. Tie shoes can be adapted using zipper shoelaces or elastic shoelaces. If a man wears a tie, he may choose to slide the knot down and pull the tie off over his head without undoing the knot or to use clip ties if his degree of coordination allows that.

Bathing

The patient may independently bathe, but must adhere closely to safety precautions. A bath mat with rubber suction cups is placed outside the tub to stand on while transferring and another is placed in the tub. It is important to be certain that the mats are securely stuck. Safety grab bars should be placed where they would be most useful to the particular person's needs: one mounted into the studs of the wall at the side of the tub and one mounted on the rim of the tub may be necessary. A bath seat can eliminate the difficulty of trying to stand up from a sitting position at the bottom of the tub and provides a stable position for the patient when trying to wash his feet. If a seat is used, a hand-held shower spray needs to be available.

If the patient chooses to shower instead of bathe, the mats, safety bars, and seat also must be provided. In either case, the water should be drawn once the patient has transferred in and is seated; a mixer tap is ideal, but if unavailable, the cool water should be turned on first and the hot water added to prevent scalding. Soap on a string keeps the soap retrievable, or a bath mitt with a pocket to hold the soap is useful. The water should be drained before the person attempts to stand to transfer out of the tub. An extra large towel or large terry wrap-around robe facilitates the drying process.

Suggestions for Selected IADL

Communication

Writing and sometimes speech are problems for some incoordinated persons. See Chapter 31 for the many alternate communication systems and **adaptations** for computers that are appropriate for incoordinated patients.

Playing Games

Board game pieces can be weighted or turned into pegs for stability. Game boards can be reproduced to enlarge the size of the squares. Card holders and card shufflers are useful. Computer games that use keyboarding or switches to select choices, rather than a mouse or joystick, are appropriate.

LOSS OF THE USE OF ONE SIDE OF THE BODY

Principles

1. Provide substitution for the stabilizing or holding function of the involved upper extremity.
2. Adapt the few truly bilateral activities so they can be done unilaterally.

Suggestions for BADL

The methods described below pertain to the hemiplegic patient who has lost the use of one side of his body. Stroke patients can be independent in their BADL; however, cognitive-perceptual impairments may prevent developing independence, especially of the less automatic tasks such as upper extremity dressing (Edmans & Lincoln, 1990; Walker & Lincoln, 1991).

The methods and equipment may also be used by the unilateral upper extremity amputee if necessary. However, the amputee will need less **adaptation** because he has normal trunk and lower extremity function as well as normal perception and cognition. Persons with temporary casts or restrictions of use of one upper extremity can also benefit from these ideas.

Feeding

Feeding is essentially a one-handed task, except for cutting meat and spreading bread. These tasks can be done by use of adapted equipment. Meat can be simultaneously stabilized and cut by use of a rocker knife, a knife with a sharp curved blade that cuts when rocked over the meat (Fig. 15.13). Bread can be spread if stabilized on a nonslip surface or trapped in the corner of a spike board and spread toward the corner (Fig. 15.14). Soft spreads facilitate this process.

Grooming

The problem with grooming is the care of the unaffected extremity and to find substitutions for two-handed activities. Spray deodorant for the unaffected arm is easier to use than other types of applicators. Fingernails of the unaffected hand are cleaned by

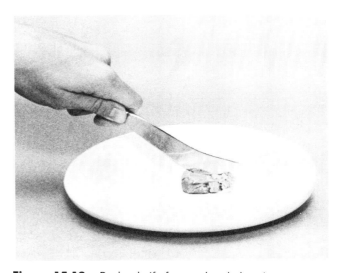

Figure 15.13. Rocker knife for one-handed cutting.

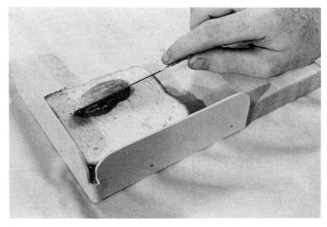

Figure 15.14. Spreading one handed by trapping bread in the corner of a spike board.

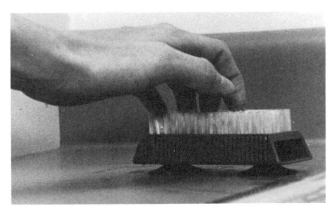

Figure 15.15. Suction cup brush for cleaning nails or dentures one handed.

rubbing them on a small suction cup brush attached to the basin (Fig. 15.15); they are filed by rubbing the nails over an emery board secured to a table or other flat surface. The nails of the affected hand can be cleaned and trimmed using the person's habitual methods. Using another suction cup brush, fastened to the inside of the basin, the person can scrub his dentures by rubbing them over the brush. Partially filling the basin with water and laying a face cloth in the bottom cushions the dentures if they are dropped accidentally. An electric razor is recommended for shaving for a poststroke patient because accidents are possible with a safety razor.

Toileting

The problem with toileting is arranging the clothing, which is normally a two-handed activity. There should be a grab bar mounted on the wall beside the toilet or a frame mounted on the toilet to assist transfers. Once standing, anyone wearing trousers unfastens them and gravity takes them down. If the patient's balance is precarious and will interfere with retrieving them after using the toilet, the person can put the affected hand in the pocket, which prevents the trousers from sliding below the knees. A woman with a dress can lean her affected side against the adjacent wall, if available, for balance; she can then raise her dress on the affected side and tuck it between her body and the affected arm. Then she lowers her underpants to knee level and pulls the dress up on the unaffected side. A dress or skirt that wraps around facilitates this process by allowing the woman to reach across the front of herself and pull the material forward to anchor it between her body and the affected arm; then she lowers her underpants and holds the remaining material aside while seating herself using the grab bar. The toilet tissue should be mounted conveniently to the unaffected side. The patient will be able to manage men-

strual needs by use of tampons or adhesive-type sanitary napkins.

Dressing

Certain prerequisite abilities are considered important for successful dressing. These are ability to reach each foot, stand unsupported for 10 sec, and achieve sitting balance when reaching down. The most difficult tasks for both men and women were found to be pulling trousers up, putting the shoe on the affected foot, and lacing shoes (Walker & Lincoln, 1991).

The following methods are taken from material prepared by the occupational therapy staff of the former Highland View Cuyahoga County Hospital (Cleveland, Ohio) and from Brett (1960). As a general rule, the affected limb is dressed first and undressed last.

Shirt or cardigan garment. Overhead method. The overhead method for putting on and removing cardigan-style tops is least confusing for a patient with sensory and perceptual impairment. But this method is cumbersome for dresses and is not used for coats.

1. To keep the shirt from twisting, hold the collar and shake.
2. Put the shirt on the lap, label facing up, and the collar next to the abdomen; drape the shirttail over the knees.
3. Open the sleeve for the affected arm from the armhole to the cuff.
4. Pick up the affected hand and put it into the sleeve.
5. Pull the sleeve up over the elbow; if not pulled past the elbow, the hand will fall out when continuing.
6. Put the unaffected hand into the armhole. Raise the arm out and push it through the sleeve.
7. Gather the back of the shirt from tail to collar.
8. Hold the gathered shirt up, lean forward, duck the head, and put the shirt over the head.
9. To straighten the shirt, lean forward, work the shirt down over the shoulders (often the shirt gets caught on the affected shoulder and must first be pushed back over the shoulder), and reach back and pull the tail down.
10. To button, line up the shirt fronts and match each button with the correct buttonhole, starting with the bottom button.

To remove the shirt, the patient unbuttons it, leans forward, and uses the unaffected hand to gather the shirt up in back of the neck. He ducks the head, pulls the shirt over the head, then takes the shirt off the unaffected arm first.

Over-the-shoulder method. Some patients may do better with the over-the-shoulder method, especially if they have some voluntary control of the affected extremity and can place it into the garment, because it is similar to the customary method. This method is also used for coats.

1. To keep the shirt from twisting, hold the collar and shake.
2. Put the shirt on the lap, label facing up, and the collar next to the abdomen, with the shirttail draped over the knees.
3. Put the affected hand into one sleeve.
4. Pull the sleeve up over the elbow.
5. Grasp the collar at the point closest to the unaffected side.
6. Hold tightly to the collar, lean forward, and bring the collar and shirt around the affected side and behind the neck to the unaffected side.
7. Put the unaffected hand into the other armhole. Raise the arm out and up to push it through the sleeve.
8. To straighten the shirt, lean forward, work the shirt down over the shoulders, reach back and pull the tail down, and then straighten the sleeve under the affected axilla.
9. To button, line up shirt fronts and match each button with the correct buttonhole, starting with the bottom button.

To remove the shirt, unbutton it and use the unaffected hand to throw the shirt back off the unaffected shoulder. Work the shirtsleeve off the unaffected arm. Press the shirt cuff against the leg and pull the arm out. Lean forward. Use the unaffected hand to pull the shirt across the back. Take the shirt off of the affected arm.

Pullover garment.   The following steps are used for putting on a pullover garment.

1. Garment is positioned on the lap, bottom toward chest and label facing down.
2. Using the unaffected hand, roll up the bottom edge of the shirt back, all the way up to the sleeve on the affected side.
3. Spread the armhole opening as large as possible. Using the unaffected hand, place the affected arm into the armhole and pull the sleeve up onto the arm past the elbow.
4. Insert the unaffected arm into the other sleeve.
5. Gather the shirt back from bottom edge to neck, lean forward, duck the head, and pass the shirt over the head.
6. Adjust the shirt on the involved side up and onto the shoulder and remove twists.

To remove, starting at top back, gather the shirt up, lean forward, duck the head, and pull the shirt forward over the head. Remove the unaffected arm and then the affected arm.

Trousers.   The following steps describe how to put on trousers. Modifications of the following method are used for men's and women's underclothing and pantyhose.

1. Sit. **Note:** If a wheelchair is used, the brakes should be locked and the footrests should be in the up position and/or swung out of the way. Move the unaffected leg beyond the midline of the body for balance.
2. Grasp the ankle or calf of the affected leg. Lift and cross the affected leg over the unaffected leg.
3. Pull the trousers onto the affected leg up to, but not above, the knee.
4. Uncross the legs.
5. Put the unaffected leg into the other pant leg.
6. Remain sitting. Pull the pants up above the knees.
7. To prevent the pants from dropping when standing, put the affected hand into the pant pocket, or the thumb into a belt loop.
8. Stand up. Pull the pants up over the hips; button and zip pants while standing. Persons with poor balance should remain seated and pull the pants up over the hips by shifting from side to side; they should button and zip the pants from a seated position.

To remove, unfasten the trousers and work them down on the hips as far as possible. Stand. Let the trousers drop past the knees. Sit. Remove the trousers from the unaffected leg. Cross the affected leg over the unaffected leg. Remove the trousers from the affected leg. Uncross the legs. Persons with poor balance should use this method: Place locked wheelchair or chair against a wall. Sit. Unfasten the trousers. Work the trousers down on the hips as far as possible. Put the wheelchair footrests in the up position and/or swing them out of the way. Lean back against the chair and press down with the unaffected leg to raise the buttocks slightly. Lean from side to side in the chair. Use the noninvolved arm to work the trousers down past the hips. Remove the trousers from the unaffected leg. Cross the affected leg over the unaffected leg. Remove the trousers from the affected leg. Uncross the legs.

Socks or stockings.   The following method is used to put on socks or stockings.

1. The person sits in a straight chair (with arms if balance is questionable) or in a locked wheelchair with footrests in the up position.
2. The unaffected leg is placed slightly beyond midline of body toward the affected side, and the affected leg is crossed over it by grasping the ankle. If the person has difficulty in maintaining the leg in this position, a small stool under the unaffected leg will increase hip flexion angle and hold the affected leg

more securely. If the patient cannot cross his legs, the heel is rested on a small stool, and a reacher is used to put the sock onto the toe and pull it up.

3. The top of the sock is opened by inserting the fist into the cuff area and then opening the fist and spreading the fingers.
4. The sock is put on the foot by slipping the toes into the cuff opening made under the spread hand. The sock is then pulled into place, and wrinkles are eliminated.

To remove, the leg is positioned as it is when putting the sock on. The sock is then pushed off with the unaffected hand.

Shoes. A loafer-type shoe is put on the affected foot with the shoe on the floor. The foot is started into the shoe, and a shoehorn is used to help ease the foot into the shoe. A tie shoe is put onto the affected foot after the leg is crossed over the unaffected one to bring the foot closer. If the laces have been thoroughly loosened, the person is often able to work the shoe on while the leg is crossed over by grasping the heel of the shoe with the unaffected hand and working it back and forth over the heel until it goes on completely. Sometimes it is necessary to insert a shoehorn while the leg is crossed over and then carefully lower the foot with the shoe half on and finish getting the shoe on the foot by repeatedly pushing down on the knee and adjusting the shoehorn.

Tying the shoes is a problem. It is possible to tie a conventional bow one-handed, but it requires fine dexterity and normal perception. The amputee may prefer to do this or use loafer-style shoes. The hemiplegic patient can use adapted shoe closures or he can learn a simplified, effective one-handed shoe tie as illustrated in Figure 15.16. By putting the lace through the last hole from the outside of the shoe toward the tongue of the shoe, the tension of the foot against the shoe will hold the lace tight while the bow is being tied. One-hand shoe tying is especially difficult for patients with cognitive-perceptual deficits.

Short leg brace (or ankle-foot orthosis; AFO). The posterior shell or molded AFO is put on the leg, and the strap is fastened before the shoe is put on. It may be necessary to add a temporary strap near the ankle to hold the brace onto the foot while attempting to put on the shoe. The shoe is put on as mentioned above for the unaffected foot. It is difficult to put the shoe on with the posterior shell in place. Plans for a shoe donner for those who wear an AFO have been published (Bobco, 1988). If all else fails (as this method could bend or break the brace—check with your orthotist first), the plastic AFO can be placed into the shoe first and then the patient puts his foot in. The important thing to remember is to have the laces

very, very loose to allow the maximum room possible for getting the foot into the brace and shoe.

Bra. To put on a bra, it is placed around the back at waist level and turned to hook in front where the patient can see what she is doing. It is then rotated to proper position, the affected arm is placed through the shoulder strap, and then the unaffected arm is placed through the other shoulder strap. The bra is pulled up into place. It is removed by reversing the process. In some cases, the patient is able to leave the bra closures hooked and don the bra by putting it over her head in a manner similar to donning a pullover garment.

A plump patient may need an adapted front-closing bra if she cannot approximate the two edges of the bra to fasten it. The bra is adapted by using belt keepers attached on the side of the bra opening that is on the involved side and cotton twill straps opposite these keepers on the other side of the bra opening. After the bra is on, the straps are threaded through the keepers and pulled to bring the two ends of the bra together. The straps are secured with Velcro closures. These bras are now commercially available.

Bathing

The bathing arrangements described for patients with incoordination apply to hemiplegic persons also. In addition, these patients find a long-handled bath sponge that has a pocket to hold the soap useful to allow bathing of the unaffected upper arm and the back. The lower arm of the unaffected side is bathed by putting the soapy washcloth across the knees and rubbing the arm back and forth over it, unless the patient has some return of function and can use a bath mitt on the affected hand.

If sensory impairment exists, extra precautions should be taken to be certain of water temperature. The hemiplegic patient should dry himself as much as possible while still seated on the bath seat before transferring out of the tub. The water should be completely drained from the tub before the transfer is attempted. The patient may need assistance with the transfer if there is not enough room near the tub to position the wheelchair so that his noninvolved side leads.

A unilateral amputee can bathe as usual, but a rubber mat or nonskid strips in the tub, a grab bar, and letting the water drain before exiting are worthwhile safety measures.

Suggestions for Selected IADL

Writing

Persons with only one functional arm need to stabilize the paper when writing. The paper can be

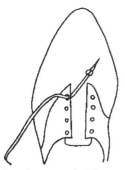

1. Tie a knot in one end of the shoelace.

   Thread the unknotted end up through the hole nearest the toe of the shoe, on the left

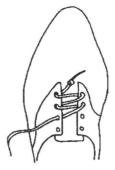

2. Take the lace across the tongue of the shoe and up under the flap on the opposite side of the shoe.

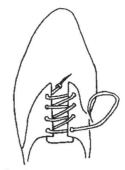

3. Continue to go across the tongue and up under the flap on the next highest hole on the opposite side untill you reach the top (or go down through the last hole so the tension will be maintained for tying.)

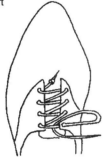

4. Circle around toward the toe of the shoe and go under the part of the lace that is going across the tongue to the last hole.

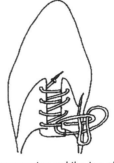

5. Circle arouang toward the top of the shoe. Pull free lace through the loop down toward the ankle and out to the left side.

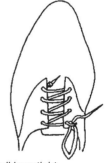

6. Pull loop tight

Figure 15.16. One-handed shoe tie—left hemiplegic.

secured using masking tape, a clipboard, a weight, the affected extremity, or other similar means.

Leisure Activities

Devices can be made to allow two-handed tasks to be done unilaterally. Some examples are a frame that holds cloth for embroidering (Fig. 15.17), an upended scrub brush, a slotted piece of wood, and a commercial card holder to hold a hand of cards.

LIMITED VISION

Principles

1. Organize so that there is a place for everything and everything is kept in its place.
2. Use Braille labels to distinguish canned goods, clothing colors, etc.
3. Use techniques and devices that magnify type or images or provide high contrast.
4. Use adapted equipment that provides auditory, tactile, or kinesthetic feedback to compensate for low vision or blindness.

Suggestions for BADL

The suggestions listed here pertain primarily to blindness. The person with low vision may find some of these useful and others unnecessary. Organization and consistency in the placement of objects is necessary for the blind person to be able to locate things efficiently. Memory training may be necessary for the newly blinded individual. He will need to develop increased awareness of the information that he receives from his senses of smell, touch, hearing, and taste. This awareness does not automatically occur but must be developed through training. Orientation to the environment is achieved through these senses, although a verbal description of the surroundings by someone else is extremely valuable. The American Foundation of the Blind is a major source of obtaining information and adapted devices for blind persons.

Feeding

The patient explores the placement of dishes, glasses, and utensils at his place. If dining alone, he

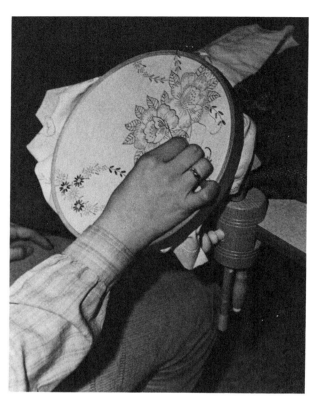

Figure 15.17. Frame for one-handed embroidery and sewing.

explores the location and identifies the food by feel, using his fork and taste. If dining with a companion, the companion can tell him the locations using a clock method of description, e.g., meat is located at 3 o'clock. When pouring liquid, the correct amount is determined by the weight of the cup when it is full. Salt is distinguished from pepper by taste or use of differently shaped shakers. Food is cut by finding the edge of the food with the fork, moving the fork a bite-size amount onto the meat, and then cutting the food, keeping the knife in contact with the fork.

Grooming

A major problem is identification of objects. This can be done through the use of taste, touch (size, shape, and texture), location, or Braille labels. The application of cosmetics or toiletries is another problem; fingers of the assistive hand can be guides, e.g., when shaving sideburns or applying eyebrow pencil. Aerosol sprays are a poor choice because the blind person cannot determine the extent of the spray.

Dressing

The blind person has no difficulty with the physical aspects of dressing. The only problems that arise relate to appearance and appropriateness. The blind person needs a system to coordinate colors of clothes and compatibility of style. One system of identification is to use French knots in certain patterns to designate color or identify all components of a total costume. Another system is to store clothes of like color together. Hems, buttons, seams, and socks should be checked for mending. Colorless wax polishes can be used to shine shoes. Clothes should always be hung properly to prevent wrinkles. Wrinkle-free, stain-resistant, no-iron fabrics are preferred. Listening to the weather report guides the person's selection of appropriate clothing, as for anyone. Clothing selection should be done with the assistance of a sighted person who can describe colors and style. Purchase of garments of the same style in different colors should be avoided because color identification is often done by remembering which style is a certain color.

Suggestions for Selected IADL

Writing and Reading

The blind person can use a signature or writing guide to stay within boundaries while writing in longhand. The person with low vision can use a black felt-tipped pen for good contrast. Braille can be written by hand using a stylus and plate or on a Braille writer. Besides Braille and talking books, technological advances are providing the means for the blind to "read" regular print. Computerized optical scanning devices convert the printed word into spoken word and Braille displays (see Chapter 31). For those with low vision, books, popular magazines, and *The New York Times* come in large-print versions.

Telephoning

Using a telephone is no problem for the blind person as soon as he memorizes the dial or location of touch buttons. A phone with one-button automatic dialing is very useful.

Time

The person can tell time using a Braille watch. Sounds of the day, the radio, or television can provide a general orientation to time. Clocks that announce the time are sold in gadget catalogs.

Handling Money

Tactile discrimination enables the person to identify coins. Paper money is discriminated by the way it is folded after its denomination has been identified previously by someone else. Consistency is important here as in all aspects of the blind person's life. Some countries use paper money of different sizes for different denominations, but unfortunately that is not so in the United States yet.

Playing Games

Braille versions of popular games, such as Monopoly, Bingo, and playing cards, are available.

DECREASED SENSATION

Principles

1. Protect the anesthetic part from abrasions, bruises, cuts, burns, and decubiti.
2. Substitute vision for poor awareness of limbs and limb movement or to detect texture.
3. Develop habits of directing attention to the affected part.

Suggestions for BADL

Problems of absent, decreased, or disturbed sensation affect performance of ADL whenever a potentially harmful situation is encountered and because the automatic knowledge of the performance of limbs may be missing.

Transferring

In transferring, there is danger of skin abrasion due to friction between the skin and the bedclothing or clothing if the person drags across surfaces instead of lifting over them.

Wheelchair Mobility and Driving

The person must remember, or use a device that reminds him, to do pressure relief every 15 to 20 min to prevent development of decubiti (see Chapter 39). Wheelchair cushions of various types are available to help in the prevention of decubiti, but they do not substitute for pressure-relief maneuvers. Alternating air pressure mattresses and chair pads are effective in preventing pressure sores in persons unable to do the maneuvers.

Dressing

Wrinkles and pressure are potential problems. Wrinkled socks pressed against the skin inside the shoe and tight elastic cuffs and waists can cause decubitus ulcers within a short time. Persons with insensitive skin must be careful to dress warmly in cold weather to prevent frostbite.

Bathing

With bathing, there is a danger of scalding the skin. When turning water on, the cold is turned on first then the hot added gradually. Mixer valves should be installed to compensate for a permanent condition.

Suggestions for Selected IADL

Cooking

With cooking, burns are a consideration. Full attention should be directed toward the activity and pot holders and insulated utensils and equipment should be used.

Use of Tools and Utensils

Poor sensation does not allow graduated pinch and grip on tools and utensils to meet the demands of the task. The person grips with excess pressure (Johansson & Westling, 1984). Prolonged, excessive grip or pinch can cause bruising and decubiti. Poor sensation also results in letting go, when the attention is directed away from the object being held. The person's attention will need to be directed to maintain the grip of an object.

Use of Riding Mowers and Snow Blowers

A patient using a riding mower or snow blower must use caution, because the lower extremities can be burned if allowed to rest against the hot engine cover.

Continued Independence

Studies have reported that patients lose some of their independence when discharged home (Andrews & Stewart, 1979; Egan et al., 1992; Strub & Levine, 1987; Weingarden & Martin, 1989). There are no studies that identify the reasons for this. I will suggest a few hypotheses and propose counteractions.

1. Adjustment to living on a day-to-day basis with a permanent disability is overwhelming and confusing. Full education of the patient and family in preparation for the return home, including weekend passes and community reintegration preparation, may help (Strub & Levine, 1987). Home care follow-up to facilitate the adjustment may prove to be very helpful. Rehabilitation done in the home may prevent this reaction.

2. The patient who expects that "everything will be okay" when he gets home encounters reality and undergoes reactive depression and reduced activity. Attention to the emotional aspects of disability during inpatient rehabilitation (Chapters 10 and 20), community reintegration practice, community follow-up, and support groups may be effective interventions.

3. The family provides more care than they did before the disability and more than they need to. Family education about the person's abilities and the importance of activity for health may prevent this.

Community follow-up and support groups may also be beneficial. Family dynamics and family values may resist a change toward independence for the former patient.

4. "Too much time and too much work." Persons with new or severe disabilities have limited energy. They may choose to use their time and energy for activities of greater value to them than BADL. That may be a healthy choice for them. They still need to learn the techniques because they have to instruct PCAs.

STUDY QUESTIONS

1. What conditions interfere with the patient's ability to benefit from instruction concerning ADL methods?
2. How is the type of transfer to be used for a particular patient decided on?
3. State the steps of an assisted 90° pivot transfer.
4. What principle of compensation is being implemented when a patient with limited or restricted range of motion uses a stocking aid?
5. What device can be used to enable use of utensils when a patient lacks grasp?
6. Describe the steps a C6 tetraplegic will use to come to a sitting position in bed.
7. Describe how a C6 tetraplegic college student will be able to do tasks required of his role.
8. What are the principles of compensation used for problems of incoordination?
9. State the steps a stroke patient can use to put on and remove a cardigan-type garment.
10. Name five energy-conservation techniques and give an example of each that could be used by a cardiac patient.
11. What automobile **adaptations** will be required to enable a right below-elbow amputee to drive safely?

REFERENCES

Alexander, L. (1979). Bed to commode lift increases independence. *Accent on Living, 23*(4), 108–109.

Andrews, K., & Stewart, J. (1979). Stroke recovery: He can but does he? *Rheumatology and Rehabilitation, 18,* 43–48.

Barsamian, P. (1983). *More splinting with Aquaplast.* (Available from WRF/Aquaplast Corp., P.O. Box 635, Wycoff, NJ 07481)

Barstow, R. E. (1974). Coping with emphysema. *Nursing Clinics of North America, 9*(1), 137–145.

Berzins, G. F. (1970). An occupational therapy program for the chronic obstructive pulmonary disease patient. *American Journal of Occupational Therapy, 24,* 181–186.

Bobath, B. (1990). *Adult hemiplegia: Evaluation and treatment* (3rd ed.). London: William Heinemann Medical Books.

Bobco, J. M. (1988). Shoe donner. *American Journal of Occupational Therapy, 42*(12), 811–813.

Brett, G. (1960). Dressing techniques for the severely involved hemiplegic patient. *American Journal of Occupational Therapy, 14,* 262–264.

Brodal, A. (1973). Self-observations and neuro-anatomical considerations after a stroke. *Brain, 96,* 675–694.

Bynum, H. S., & Rogers, J. C. (1987). The use and effectiveness of assistive devices possessed by patients seen in home care. *Occupational Therapy Journal of Research, 7*(3), 181–191.

Chase, J. (1989). Case Report. Equipment adaptations to improve workshop performance. *American Journal of Occupational Therapy, 43*(8), 545–548.

Chiou, I.-I. L., & Burnett, C. N. (1985). Values of activities of daily living: A survey of stroke patients and their home therapists. *American Journal of Occupational Therapy, 65*(6), 901–906.

Christy, D., & Sarafconn, C. A. (1990). *Pacing yourself: Steps to help save your energy.* Bloomington, IL: Accent Special Publications.

Cimolino, N., & Balkovec, D. (1988). The contribution of a driving simulator in the driving evaluation of stroke and disabled adolescent clients. *Canadian Journal of Occupational Therapy, 55*(3), 119–125.

Clark, M. C., Czaja, S. J., & Weber, R. A. (1990). Older adults and daily living task profiles. *Human Factors, 32*(5), 537–549.

Conine, T. A., & Hershler, C. (1991). Effectiveness: A neglected dimension in the assessment of rehabilitation devices and equipment. *International Journal of Rehabilitation Research, 14,* 117–122.

Dallas, M. J., & White, L. W. (1982). Clothing fasteners for women with arthritis. *American Journal of Occupational Therapy, 36,* 515–518.

DeGraff, A. H. (1989). Managing your own care. *Accent on Living, 34*(2), 42–47.

Diller, L., Buxbaum, J., & Chiotelis, S. (1972). Relearning motor skills in hemiplegia: Error analysis. *Genetic Psychology Monographs, 85,* 249–286.

Duckworth, B. (1986). Overview of menstrual management for disabled women. *Canadian Journal of Occupational Therapy, 53,* 25–29.

Dutton, N., Davis, K., Lupo, S., & Wepman, S. (1979). "Wheelie" aide. *Physical Therapy, 59*(1), 35–36.

Edmans, J. A., & Lincoln, N. B. (1990). The relationship between perceptual deficits after stroke and independence in activities of daily living. *British Journal of Occupational Therapy, 33*(4), 139–142.

Egan, M., Warren, S. A., Hessel, R. A., & Gilewich, G. (1992). Activities of daily living after hip fracture: Pre- and post-discharge. *Occupational Therapy Journal of Research, 12*(6), 342–356.

Hage, G. (1988). Makeup board for women with quadriplegia. *American Journal of Occupational Therapy, 42*(4), 253–255.

Hinrichsen, L. C., Nordström, C., & Law, D. F. (1984). Device to assist training in balancing on the rear wheels of a wheelchair. *Physical Therapy, 64*(5), 672–673.

Huntley, N., & Mullivan, M. A. (Eds.). (1978). *Basics of cardiac rehabilitation.* Minneapolis: Minnesota Occupational Therapy Association

Jetter, K. F. (1988). Incontinence. *Accent on Living, 32*(4), 76–82.

Joe, B. E. (1992, February 6). Design book offers accessible fashions. *OT WEEK,* 17.

Johansson, R. S., & Westling, G. (1984). Roles of glabrous skin receptors and sensorimotor memory in automatic control of precision grip when lifting rougher or more slippery objects. *Experimental Brain Research, 56,* 550–564.

Katz, S., Ford, A. B., Moskowitz, R. W., Jackson, B. A., & Jaffee, M. W. (1963). Studies of illness in the aged—The Index of ADL: A standardized measure of biological and psychosocial function. *Journal of the American Medical Association, 185,* 914–919.

Kent, H. (1986). Automobile modifications for the disabled. In

J. B. Redford (Ed.), *Orthotics etcetera* (3rd ed., pp. 595–622). Baltimore: Williams & Wilkins.

Law, M. (1991). Muriel Driver Lecture: The environment: A focus for occupational therapy. *Canadian Journal of Occupational Therapy, 58*(4), 171–180.

Levitan-Rheingold, N., Hotte, E. B., & Mandel, D. R. (1980). Learning to dress: A fundamental skill toward independence for the disabled. *Rehabilitation Literature, 41*(3–4), 72–75.

Lewis, R. I. (1993). Catheter choice if needed. *Accent on Living, 38*(1), 44–48.

Lykouretzos, J., & Thompson-Rangel, T. (1990). A folding dressing stick. *American Journal of Occupational Therapy, 44*(1), 77.

Margolis, D. L., & Savino, L. A. (1992). Effective education programs for geriatric patients. *The American Occupational Therapy Association Gerontology Special Interest Section Newsletter, 15*(4), 1–3.

McCuaig, M., & Frank, G. (1991). The able self: Adaptive patterns and choices in independent living for a person with cerebral palsy. *American Journal of Occupational Therapy, 45*(3), 224–234.

Nordström, T.. & Thorslund, M. (1991). The structure of IADL and ADL measures: Some findings from a Swedish study. *Age and Ageing, 20*, 23–28.

Parker, M. G., & Thorslund, M. (1991). Use of technical aids among community-based elderly. *American Journal of Occupational Therapy, 45*(8), 712–718.

Petersen, R. (1984). Electric lift. *Accent on Living, 28*(4), 100–102.

Pomerantz, P., Flannery, E. L., & Findling, P. K. (1975). Occupational therapy for chronic obstructive lung disease. *American Journal of Occupational Therapy, 29*, 407–411.

Program for consumers with disabilities. (1991, September 5). *OT WEEK*, 10.

Puckett, A. (1990). New mouthpiece is durable and easy to fit. *Accent on Living, 35*(3), 86–88.

Quigley, F. L., & DeLise, J. A. (1983). Assessing the driving potential of cerebral vascular accident patients. *American Journal of Occupational Therapy, 37*, 474–478.

Reich, N., & Otten, P. (1980). Are buttons and zippers confidence trippers? *Accent on Living, 25*(3), 98–99.

Rogers, J. C., & Holm, M. B. (1992). Assistive technology device use in patients with rheumatic disease: A literature review. *American Journal of Occupational Therapy, 46*(2), 120–127.

Rosenkoetter, R. (1980). Valerie drives with her bare feet. *Accent on Living, 25*(1), 100–102.

Runge, M. (1967). Self dressing techniques for patients with spinal cord injury. *American Journal of Occupational Therapy, 21*, 367–375.

Rush, W. L. (1987). PCA's. *Accent on Living, 32*(1), 76–80.

Ryu, J., Cooney, W. P., Askew, L. J., An, K.-N., & Chao, E. Y. S. (1991). Functional ranges of motion of the wrist joint. *Journal of Hand Surgery, 16A*, 409–419.

Schmidt, R. A. (1988). *Motor control & learning: A behavioral emphasis* (2nd. ed.). Champaign, IL: Human Kinetics.

Schmidt, R. A. (1991). Motor learning principles for physical therapy. In M. Lister (Ed.), *Contemporary management of motor control problems: Proceedings of II Step conference* (pp. 49–63). Alexandria, VA: Foundation for Physical Therapy.

Schroeder, C., & Benedict, P. (1984). Egress during fire—wheelchair exiting in an emergency. *American Journal of Occupational Therapy, 38*, 541–542.

Seeger, M. S., & Fisher, L. A. (1982). Adaptive equipment used in the rehabilitation of hip arthroplasty patients. *American Journal of Occupational Therapy, 36*, 515–518.

Shillam, L. L., Beeman, C., & Loshin, P. M. (1983). Effect of occupational therapy intervention on bathing independence of disabled persons. *American Journal of Occupational Therapy, 37*, 766–768.

Short, L. E. (1991). What's your criteria when buying a car? *Accent on Living, 36*(2), 54–56.

Skinner, B. F. (1938). *The behavior of organisms*. New York: Appleton-Century-Crofts.

Smith, R. (1989). Mouthstick design for the client with spinal cord injury. *American Journal of Occupational Therapy, 43*(4), 251–255.

Spector, W. D., Katz, S., Murphy, J. B., & Fulton, J. P. (1987). The hierarchical relationship between activities of daily living and instrumental activities of daily living. *Journal of Chronic Disease, 40*(6), 481–489.

Strawn, L. P. (1989). Staying alive. *Accent on Living, 33*(4), 74–78.

Strub, N., & Levine, R. E. (1987). Self care: A comparison of patients' institutional and home performance. *Occupational Therapy Journal of Research, 7*(1), 53–56.

Trombly, C. A. (1993). Anticipating the future: Assessment of occupational function. *American Journal of Occupational Therapy, 47*(3), 253–259.

Tyson, R., & Strong, J. (1990). Adaptive equipment: Its effectiveness for people with chronic lower back pain. *Occupational Therapy Journal of Research, 10*(2), 111–121.

Walker, M. F., & Lincoln, N. B. (1991). Factors influencing performance after stroke. *Journal of Neurology, Neurosurgery, and Psychiatry, 54*, 699–701.

Weingarden, S. I., & Martin, C. (1989). Independent dressing after spinal cord injury: A functional time evaluation. *Archives of Physical Medicine & Rehabilitation, 70*(7), 518–519.

SUPPLEMENTARY RESOURCES

Suggested Readings

American Occupational Therapy Association. (yearly). AOTA's Occupational Therapy Buyer's Guide. *American Journal of Occupational Therapy*, supplement.

Clearinghouse on Disability Information. Office of Special Education and Rehabilitative Services. (1993). *Pocket guide to federal help for individuals with disabilities* (ED/OSERS 93-3). Washington, DC: U.S. Government Printing Office.

Garee, B. (Ed.). (yearly). *Accent on Living buyer's guide*. (Available from *Accent on Living*, P.O. Box 700, Bloomington, IL 61710)

Garee, B. (1988). *Single-handed: Devices and aids for one handers and sources of these devices*. Bloomington, IL: Cheever Publishing Inc. (Available from P.O. Box 700, Bloomington, IL 61702)

Kennedy, E. (n.d.) *Dressing with pride*. (Available from P.R.I.D.E. Foundation, 71 Plaza Court, Groton, CT 06340; 203-445-1448)

Richardson, N. K. (n.d.) *Type with one hand*. (Available from Wadsworth, 7625 Empire Drive, Florence, KY 41042)

Resources

ABLEDATA. Database funded by the U.S. Department of Education National Institute on Disability and Rehabilitation Research. (National Rehabilitation Information System Center, 4407 Eighth Street NE, Washington, DC 20017; 202-635-6090)

American Foundation for the Blind. (15 West 16th Street, New York, NY 10011)

Automobiles. Chrysler (800-255-9877) and General Motors (800-323-9935) offer financial assistance for installing hand controls into their automobiles.

Canine Companions for Independence. There are five regional centers in the United States; they supply service dogs (to perform helpful tasks), signal dogs (to alert owners), social dogs (to provide pet-facilitated therapy for persons with developmental disability), specialty dogs (for persons with multiple handicaps and who have unique needs). (P.O. Box 446, Santa Rosa, CA 95402-0446)

Comfortably Yours: Aids for Easier Living. Catalog. (52 West Hunter Avenue, Maywood, NJ 07607)

Doron Precision Systems, Inc. Driving simulator. (174 Court Street P.O. Box 400, Binghamton, NY 13902-0400)

DOS—ABLEDATA (IBM version) and *Hyper-ABLEDATA* (Mac version). Computer database of 17,000 + rehabilitation products, including pictures of devices; available on CD-ROM or computer disk. (Trace R&D Center, University of Wisconsin at Madison, S-151 Waisman Center, 1500 Highland Avenue, Madison, WI 53705)

Easy Street Environments. Customized, real-life settings for evaluation and training in IADL. (6908 East Thomas Road, Suite 201, Scottsdale, AZ 85251)

FashionABLE. Clothing for the disabled; catalog. (5 Crescent Avenue, Box S, Rocky Hill, NJ 08553)

National Library Service for the Blind and Physically Handicapped. (800-424-9100)

North Coast Medical, Inc. *ADL—Products for the activities of daily living.* Professional catalog. (187 Stauffer Boulevard, San Jose, CA 95125-1042)

Quinn, M. D., & Chase, R. W. (n.d.). *Design without limits.* Suggestions for adaptations and alterations of ready-made clothing to achieve aesthetic and functional goals of persons with various disabilities. Includes many other clothing resources. A joint project of Drexel University and Simplicity Pattern Co.

(Available from Simplicity Pattern Co., Box 2102, Niles, MI 49120-8102)

REHABDATA. A bibliographic database on rehabilitation that includes journals, unpublished documents, commercial publications, and government reports. (Available from NARIC, 4407 Eighth Street, Washington, DC 20017; 800-34-NARIC)

Sammons—A Bissell Healthcare Company. *Orthopedic and ADL Products.* Professional catalog. (P.O. Box 386, Western Springs, IL 60558-0386)

Techni-Flair. Adapted clothing catalog. (P.O. Box 40, Cotter, AR 72626)

The Left Hand. Catalog. (140 West 22nd Street, New York, NY 10011)

Lighthouse Low Vision Products. (36-02 Northern Boulevard, Long Island City, NY 11101)

Reliable SOURCE, The (formerly *OT SOURCE*). On-line information system of the American Occupational Therapy Association, Inc. It can be accessed from a IBM (or compatible) or Macintosh computer using a Hayes-compatible modem. Includes databases (e.g., *DOS—ABLEDATA* and a professional resource list of names and addresses of experts in various practice areas), occupational therapy literature citations (e.g., OT BibSys), conferences on particular subjects and for each special interest section, and E-mail. (800-729-AOTA)

Retraining Housekeeping and Child Care Skills

Cara Stewart

OBJECTIVES _____

After studying this chapter the student should be able to:
1. Understand the principles of work simplification and energy conservation.
2. Recognize two levels of home management training.
3. Discuss the principles of compensation for six categories of disability.
4. Understand adaptive methods and equipment for home management and child care skills.

Training in adapted methods of home management and child care begins when the patient's function has been restored to the expected near-maximum level. This training, therefore, usually takes place close to the time of discharge. Some housekeeping activities can appropriately be used as therapeutic media in restorative therapy.

WORK SIMPLIFICATION

Home management and child care are energy consuming for anyone, but for the person with a disability, techniques to conserve personal energy become indispensable (Gilbert, 1965).

The principles of energy conservation or work simplification listed here apply in general to all disabilities presented and to all aspects of occupational performance tasks.

Limit the Amount of Work

Eliminate steps of a job or entire jobs that are not essential to one's lifestyle. Analyze the task to determine why the job is necessary, if it is worth the energy required, and what would happen if the job were left undone. Specific examples of reducing the amount of work will be discussed later on in this chapter.

Plan Ahead

Plan activities so that heavy tasks can be distributed evenly throughout the week. Each day's activity should be carefully planned to alternate active jobs with quiet ones and to incorporate periods of rest between periods of work. To improve efficiency, tasks should be prioritized so that important jobs are accomplished before running out of time and energy. If a task doesn't seem to be getting done day after day because of its low priority, perhaps it is not important and should be eliminated. All necessary supplies and equipment need to be gathered before doing the job. The equipment should be put away before starting the next task so that if energy fails, the home is still neat. The contribution of other family members should be included in the weekly plan.

Use Correct Body Mechanics

Use of correct body mechanics is absolutely necessary for those with chronic low back pain, but it is also recommended for all persons engaged in physical work inside or outside the home. The principles of good body mechanics elaborate on the ideas of joint alignment, use of large muscles, and working in harmony with gravity. Specific principles of correct body mechanics are listed below (Frederick, 1979).

1. Keep the head aligned with the trunk and tuck the chin.
2. Keep the shoulders and hips parallel and do not twist the trunk.

3. Maintain pelvic tilt by tucking in the buttocks or keeping one foot raised on a low stool while standing.
4. Maintain good balance by positioning the feet shoulder-distance apart with one foot forward.
5. Keep the back straight, bending at the hips and knees simultaneously rather than bending over at the waist.
6. Push before pulling and pull before lifting.
7. While lifting or carrying, keep the object close to the body.

Use Efficient Methods

Arrange work areas so that implements are within easy reach of the posture normally assumed for the task. Sit while working, because it requires less energy than standing. Use both arms in symmetrical, smooth motions when possible, using the force available from proximal muscles rather than distal muscles. Work should be performed using gravity and leverage to assist. Contiguous counter space—especially between the sink, stove, and refrigerator—is very important. Use a wheeled service cart or laundry basket when possible to transport items. Avoid prolonged holding by stabilizing items, using nonskid mats, wet towels, or suction cup bases. Be sure lighting is good.

Use Correct Equipment

Energy is conserved if the tools fit the job and are in good condition. Lightweight utensils and electrically powered equipment can also minimize fatigue. Many of these appliances will be discussed later on in this chapter. It is strongly recommended that equipment be tested in the store before purchase.

Rest

Fatigue leads to poor body mechanics and decreased safety awareness. Regular rest periods should be incorporated into the day's work plan. Mothers of young children are advised to rest when the child sleeps, even though it is tempting to use that time for doing a task uninterrupted. To conserve energy, it is strongly recommended that heavy tasks such as cleaning the oven, washing walls, vacuuming wall to wall carpet, etc. be assigned to other family members or a hired cleaning service.

HOME MANAGEMENT TRAINING

Home management takes place on two levels: managerial and participative performance of tasks. The therapist should assess the patient's physical ability and discuss what activities the individual can reasonably expect to perform.

Although people with severe disabilities may not be able to perform many household tasks, they can be effective home managers. They can direct the efforts of other family members or paid household help, manage the finances, and oversee the shopping. Training for this level may not be necessary for an experienced homemaker. An inexperienced homemaker may need practice in financial management, planning a weekly schedule, and directing others effectively. Homemaker services, home health aides, and Meals on Wheels are programs available in many communities that enable a person with limited abilities to remain in the home because they provide essential services that the homemaker is unable to perform.

To train the participative homemaker using adapted methods or equipment, the therapist should demonstrate the technique, sitting or standing beside the individual to eliminate right-left confusion. For mothers of infants, a life-size doll that is weighted to simulate a real baby may be used to practice child care methods.

Principles of Compensation and Home Management Adaptations

The following sections describe principles of compensation as well as adapted methods for home management and child care. The therapist must first determine what activities are important to the patient and then discuss how those activities can be accomplished. To determine what adaptations are most useful, the therapist and patient should understand the compensation principles. Training must emphasize problem solving so the person with the disability can develop true independence. It is important to remember that each person is unique and each situation may have a different solution.

LIMITED RANGE OF MOTION

Increase the person's reach via extended handles and confine the work to a compact area.

CHRONIC BACK PAIN

Use principles of body mechanics when performing physical tasks.

WEAKNESS AND LOW ENDURANCE

Use lightweight and/or powered equipment and allow gravity to assist. Perform activities using energy conservation techniques.

INCOORDINATION

Use weight to minimize distal movement of limbs while stabilizing proximal segments.

LOSS OF ONE UPPER EXTREMITY OR ONE SIDE OF THE BODY

Use adapted methods and/or equipment to perform bilateral activities with one hand.

VISUAL IMPAIRMENT

Use senses of smell, touch, and hearing to substitute for vision. Develop systems of organization and adhere to an established routine (Caldwell, 1983).

Grocery Shopping

To make the most efficient use of time it is important to have a shopping list. To conserve energy, shop during nonpeak hours, when the store is not crowded and the service is best (Hale, 1979).

CARTS

Many grocery stores have special carts that attach to the wheelchair. Although these attachments eliminate the need to push the cart, some individuals find it limits their ability to reach items off the shelf. Motorized carts are also available in some stores. These carts are especially useful for individuals with limited endurance, but their use requires transferring for those who use a wheelchair. The baskets in these carts are smaller than regular carts, which may be a problem if the person is shopping for a large family.

Some individuals with normal upper body strength who use a wheelchair prefer to use a regular cart. The person can leave the cart at the top of each aisle, wheel down the aisle placing needed items in a small lap basket, and then place those items in the cart.

A heavy grocery cart can be used by a person with hemiplegia for support while walking, but he must not rely on it for support when bending to reach items. A lightweight cart is unsafe to lean on while walking. The person should give the cart a push, then walk using his cane or walker to meet the cart.

RETRIEVING ITEMS

Reaching items on high shelves can be very difficult for individuals using wheelchairs or those with limited upper body range of motion. A reacher can be used to retrieve lightweight, nonbreakable items, but assistance may be needed for heavier items.

It is important that individuals with chronic back pain use proper body mechanics while shopping. To reach low-placed items, the person should kneel on one knee (keeping the back straight), hold the item close to the body, and then stand to lift. If prolonged standing is necessary, the person should place one foot on a low object such as the bottom of the grocery cart

(this causes the pelvis to tilt anteriorly into proper alignment).

Some individuals with hemiplegia have visual perceptual problems that may interfere with the efficiency of their shopping, e.g., hemianopsia, impairment of figure/ground discrimination, or discrimination of depth perception. A person with severe visual impairments will probably need a companion for shopping.

BAGGING

Generally, plastic grocery bags with handles are easiest to manage. Items should be bagged as light as possible. Most stores will provide assistance for placing bags in the car, but instruction should be given to place the bags in the car within easy reach. At home, a wheeled cart can be used to transport the bags into the house.

Although shopping by telephone or mail is useful, the social aspects of going to the store can be beneficial and should not be underestimated.

Meal Preparation, Service, and Cleanup

Although remodeling can be expensive, there are certain large items that may need to be replaced or modified to enable a person with a disability to be independent in the kitchen. This section describes features of major kitchen appliances that allow for greater independence.

REFRIGERATOR

The most convenient refrigerator for any disability is a double-door model, which has the refrigerated section located next to the freezer. Placing turntables on the lowest and highest shelves will make items more accessible. Heavy items should be stored on a shelf that is level with a lapboard or a wheeled cart so items can be slid in and out more easily. An automatic ice dispenser, with a through-the-door feature is very useful.

OVEN

The conventional 36-inch-high, freestanding oven is not recommended because lifting heavy dishes in and out of the low oven shelf can be dangerous. A built-in wall oven with the oven base approximately 30 inches from the floor is safer and more accessible. A heat-resistant counter surface or a wheeled cart that is equal in height to the oven shelf should be next to the oven for transferring dishes in and out. A 15-inch flat wooden stick with notched edges can be used to pull out or push in oven racks (Strebel, 1980) (Fig. 16.1). Countertop appliances such as microwave ovens

Figure 16.1. Oven push/pull stick.

(Whiteman, 1989), portable ovens, and electric skillets may be a useful alternative to the conventional oven.

STOVE

An electric stove with push-button controls at the front of the appliance is safer than a gas model. A handheld mirror can be used to see into pots sitting on the burners. A mounted mirror is a problem, because it steams up easily and requires frequent cleaning (Hale, 1979). A tabletop range with two burners can be an alternative to the conventional stove.

SINK

For wheelchair users, the sink should be modified so it is open underneath with a minimum clearance of 27 inches. Any exposed piping should be insulated to protect from potential burns. A single lever handle and a retractable hose spray are useful for easy rinsing.

STORAGE

The forward reach range for a person using a wheelchair is 15 inches (low reach) to 48 inches (high reach) from the floor. For individuals who are ambulatory but have difficulty bending, the forward reach range is generally 30 inches (low reach) to 60 inches (high reach) from the floor, depending on the person's height (Anderson, 1981). Pull-out shelves, pull-out drawers, and turntables for cabinets will maximize usable storage space. Reachers are helpful but should only be used for retrieving lightweight, unbreakable items. Pans, dishes, etc. should be stored vertically to alleviate the need to lift off items stored on top of one another. Pegboards with hooks can hold pots, pans, and utensils for easy access. Duplicate sets of equipment in different locations are useful, i.e., vacuums should be located on the first and second floors.

WORK AREA AND TRANSPORTING ITEMS

For the wheelchair user, there should be one well-lit counter, approximately 32 inches in height, that is open underneath. Carrying should be eliminated as much as possible by sliding items across countertops between appliances or by use of a wheeled cart with large, 3-inch swivel, ball-bearing casters (Hale, 1979).

A lap apron is useful for the homemaker using a wheelchair, because it provides a firm surface with a lip to prevent items being knocked off in transit (Fig. 16.2). The apron, however, should not be used to carry hot items, especially liquids. Transporting items can also be done using a basket or an apron with large pockets.

KITCHEN EQUIPMENT

Lightweight utensils and dishes and pots and pans with nonstick finishes are easiest to handle (individuals with incoordination may find that heavy equipment and utensils provide more stability). Casseroles, pots, and pans with double handles offer greater stability by anchoring the distal parts of both upper extremities or by allowing one extremity to help the other. Electric equipment such as food processors, blenders, can openers, and electric knives conserve energy. Equipment should be kept on the counter or work area and plugged into an outlet to eliminate moving items in and out of storage. Specially adapted equipment for those who are one-handed is commercially available, including an electric or cordless can opener (Fig. 16.3), jar opener, egg slicer, grapefruit sectioner, and a garlic press.

Knives and peelers should be sharp so the tool does the job easily. The point of the knife blade should be kept on the board when cutting to reduce excess motion. A serrated knife is less likely to slip than a straight-edged knife (Klinger, Freiden, & Sullivan, 1970). A rocker knife or pizza-cutting wheel can be used by those who are one handed for cutting nonstabilized food, because the push force is downward. If

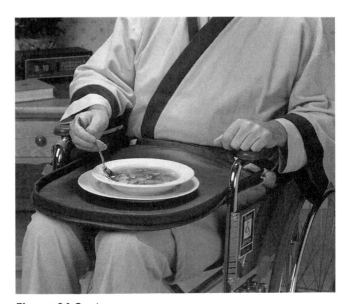

Figure 16.2. Lap apron.

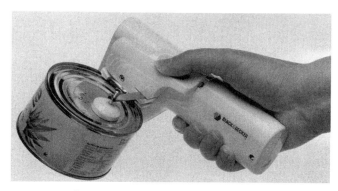

Figure 16.3. One-handed cordless can opener.

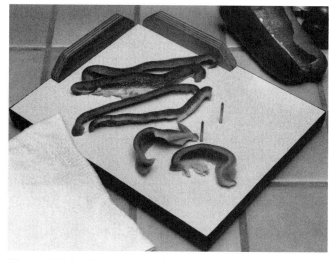

Figure 16.4. Spiked cutting board with corner guards.

grasp is limited, built-up or looped handles on these utensils may be needed (Burkhardt, 1975).

A spike board with suction feet may be necessary to anchor meat, fruit, or vegetables while peeling or cutting. A raised edge on one corner of the board is useful for stabilizing a slice of bread (Fig. 16.4).

FOOD PREPARATION

Nonslip mats or sponge cloths can be used under most items to provide stability. There are also commercially available mixing bowls with suction cup bases. A slide-out cutting board can be adapted by cutting out a circular hole to fit the size of bowls usually used. An anchoring device to hold the handle of a pot on the stove is commercially available. A wire whisk, pastry blender, or a wall-mounted cordless beater can be used for simple mixing, but a heavy countertop mixer provides more stability, especially for individuals with incoordination.

To conserve energy, use leverage to pour by resting the container on the edge of a stabilized bowl

while slowly pouring contents. To drain, use a slotted spoon or a french fry basket placed in the pot before cooking. Another method for draining is to place a freestanding strainer in the sink, then with an oven mitt, slide the pot off the stove and across the counter; tip the pot so the food falls into the strainer. There are also commercially available adjustable strainers that clamp onto the top of a pot or pan.

There are several methods for cracking eggs. Individuals with weak grasp can grossly hold the egg, throw it sharply into the bottom of an empty bowl (where it will split in two), and then remove the shell. Individuals with the use of only one hand can use the chef's method. Hold the egg in the palm with one end held by the index and middle fingers, and the other end by the thumb to form a **C** around the egg. Sharply crack the egg on the side of the bowl, then in one motion, pull the thumb down and the fingers up to pull the two halves apart.

Scissors, especially the heavy-duty loop handle type, are very useful for many tasks in the kitchen, including opening plastic or cellophane bags (Fig. 16.5). Milk jugs with plastic lids are easier than cartons, though the cartons can usually be opened by prying the edges with a table knife. There are also commercially available carton openers. Boxes that open at the top, such as cereal boxes, can be pried open with a knife. Other boxes can be opened by stabilizing the box on its long edge and cutting the top with a sharp serrated knife. Individuals with weakness may find small containers easier to handle than large ones.

DISH WASHING

If an individual uses a wheelchair, the sink should be shallow, approximately 5.5 inches deep. A removable wooden rack can be used on the bottom of a standard sink to reduce its depth. A rubber mat in the bottom of the sink is useful for reducing breakage. It is important to eliminate unnecessary cleaning. Use

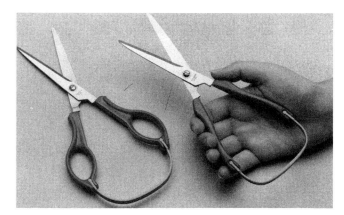

Figure 16.5. Long-handled looped scissors.

oven-to-table ware or serve directly from the pot. Line pans with foil when cooking meat or fish to reduce washing. Clean up as the meal is prepared or at least soak the dishes to reduce the likelihood of stuck-on soil.

Plan washing in a logical flow from one direction to the other—dirty dishes, wash water, rinse water, drying rack or dishwasher (Hale, 1979). Air drying can conserve energy and is more hygienic. If an individual can only use one hand, the rinse water and dish rack should be next to the working hand. The step of returning clean dishes to the cupboards can be eliminated by reusing them directly from the dish drainer or dishwasher. Suction bottlebrushes and suction scrub brushes attached to the bottom of the sink can be used to clean glasses and dishes with one hand. Individuals with limited grasp can use a terry cloth (Vorburger, 1980) or sponge mitt when washing dishes. An electric dishwasher is convenient, especially for large loads. The dishwasher should be front loading, with the controls on the front panel. Some dishwashers require little rinsing, which can conserve energy.

Household Maintenance

EQUIPMENT

Test household equipment in the store before purchasing to determine what features are most useful or manageable. Equipment should be lightweight and require little lifting or bending (heavier work tools may provide more stability for those with incoordination).

A dolly with large casters can eliminate carrying heavy items such as a pail of water for mopping. Cleaning supplies should be stored together in a bin or canvas bag with a shoulder strap. A wheeled cart can be helpful for moving equipment and supplies from room to room and an apron with large pockets can be useful for carrying small items. Individuals with upper extremity weakness may need a cuff for maintaining grasp on handles, such as brooms and mops. Working one room at a time can eliminate carrying equipment and supplies back and forth.

FLOOR CARE

Although it is easier to clean under furniture with a canister-style vacuum cleaner, an upright vacuum is generally easier to handle and requires less bending (Hale, 1979). A self-propelled vacuum with an automatic cord rewinder is useful, but the pull of the vacuum should be considered, because it might cause a problem with balance. Attachments should hook on the side of the vacuum. A lightweight carpet sweeper can be useful because it is more maneuverable, less expensive, and does not require an electrical outlet

(Fig. 16.6). Although the carpet sweeper is easier to push, it has to be pushed for a longer time to cover the same area (Hale, 1979). A cordless handheld vacuum cleaner is a good tool for touch-ups or small messes. If the individual is working from a wheelchair, it is best to start at the farthest corner and work backward out of the room. Furniture should be fitted with casters if moved regularly.

Lightweight brooms with an angle cut, a long-handled dustpan that balances open (Fig. 16.7), and a sponge mop with the squeeze lever on the handle are all helpful items, because they minimize bending and can be used with one hand.

DUSTING

Although there are long-handled dusters commercially available, a dust cloth secured with a rubber band over a toy broom can be used instead. The attachments on the vacuum cleaner or a reacher holding a dust rag can also be used for dusting out-of-reach places. For individuals with limited grasp, a duster mitten can be used. Furniture sprays may need an adaptive device to help the individual depress the button.

BED MAKING

When changing a bed, blankets and spreads can be placed on a chair located at the foot of the bed (Hale, 1979). The bottom sheet should be fitted, but it should not be too tight. Fitted sheets can be adapted by opening the two fitted corners at the bottom edge and sewing touch fasteners, so when the bed is made, the bottom corners can be secured tightly (Fastow,

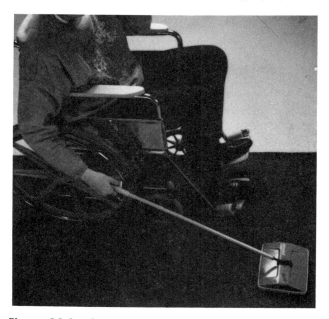

Figure 16.6. Carpet sweeper.

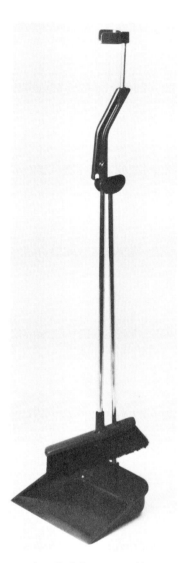

Figure 16.7. Long-handled dustpan and broom.

OVEN CLEANING

Oven cleaning is an energy-consuming task that requires a good deal of mobility. A piece of aluminum foil placed at the bottom of the oven can catch spills and keep the oven cleaner. Self-cleaning ovens can make the job much easier. A handheld cordless vacuum can be used to clean up crumbs.

Clothing Care

EQUIPMENT AND LOCATION

The laundry room should be well lit and located on the same floor as the bedrooms to minimize transporting the clothes. For a person who is ambulatory, a top-loading automatic washer and a raised dryer would eliminate bending. The table for folding clothes should be waist level and convenient to the dryer.

If the person uses a wheelchair, a front-loading washer and dryer with side-hinged doors would be best. Unfortunately, it is now very hard to find a front-loading washer. To use a top-loading washer, the wheelchair user can hold a hand-held mirror to see into the tub and a reacher can be used to pull out clothes. A wheelchair-accessible table for sorting and folding should be available.

Push-button controls or large knobs that are easy to turn are most manageable. Maytag washer and dryer controls can be optionally fitted with larger four-pronged knobs. There are turning handles available that will adapt to any knob and provide leverage and a secure grip (Fig. 16.8).

An adjustable clothes rod (42 to 72 inches) with hangers should be available for immediate hanging of permanent-press items as they are removed from the dryer (Wylde & Baron-Robbins, 1990).

1980). For daily bed making, complete one corner at a time, starting with the head of the bed. If the person is working from a wheelchair, the bed must be placed so the individual can work from both sides.

If a person has a figure/ground deficit, contrasting top and bottom sheets can be helpful. Individuals with visual impairment can discriminate the top from the bottom of sheets by feeling the hem. The bedclothes can be centered on the bed by matching the center fold to the center of the bed frame.

Lightweight blankets and spreads are easier to handle and satin pillow cases can be easier to get off and on. A duvet, or quilt cover, makes a neat bed without having to tuck in sheets. The covering opens entirely on one side to insert a quilt. Because the covering takes the place of a sheet, it should be laundered as frequently as regular sheets.

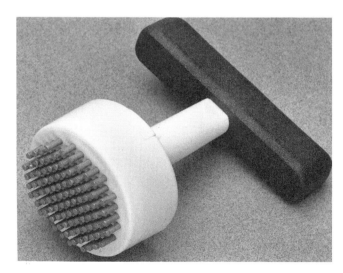

Figure 16.8. T turning handle.

COLLECTING AND TRANSPORTING SOILED CLOTHING

Soiled clothing can be placed in a hamper lined with a plastic bag with handles. To transport clothes to the washer, the bag can be lifted out of the hamper and the drawstrings hooked onto the wheelchair handles. If the person is ambulatory but has difficulty bending, the clothes baskets should be kept on a table or shelf that is waist level and a wheeled cart can be used to transport clothing to the laundry area.

WASHING AND FOLDING

Laundry detergents and bleaches should be kept within easy reach of the washing machine. Individuals with weakness, incoordination, or visual impairment may find premeasured packages of soap and bleach easier to handle. Hand washing can be eliminated by using a net laundry bag in the washing machine. Individuals with visual impairments should fasten paired items together with pins when they are taken off. If a person only has the use of one hand, a clip attached to the wall is helpful for holding a corner while folding large items such as sheets (Anderson, 1981).

IRONING

For individuals who use a wheelchair, an ironing board can be mounted to the wall or door at 28 to 32 inches high, as appropriate for the user. A cord holder can reduce effort and keep the cord from being entangled in the wheelchair. A heat-resistant pad can be used on the end of the ironing board to eliminate the need to stand the iron up.

SEWING

Individuals with the use of only one hand can sew by using an electric machine with foot or knee controls. To sew by hand, the material can be placed in an embroidery hoop, mounted at a convenient place. The needle can be threaded while it is held in a pin cushion or a bar of soap. For those individuals who do not have use of their lower extremities, an electric sewing machine with a foot pedal can be used. The individual can place the pedal up on the table next to the machine and depress it with one hand or elbow.

Child Care

Two of the most important aspects to independent child care are organization and proper selection of equipment. It is important that the parent with the disability test baby furniture or equipment before purchase.

EQUIPMENT

A standard drop-side crib can be adapted several ways, depending on the parent's disability. For the parent who is ambulatory but has difficulty bending, the crib's height can be modified by raising the crib legs. The mattress height should be adjustable. To raise the mattress height further for the very young infant, two mattresses can be used. For parents using wheelchairs, the crib sides can be adapted to form two gates by cutting the middle of the crib side and then attaching two hinges at each end with a latch at the center. Another design is to adapt the crib side so it slides along horizontal channels (Dunn, 1978) (Fig. 16.9). Whatever crib design is used, the parent should be able to manipulate the release mechanism for the crib side with one hand (be sure it is child resistant).

There are several options for bathing an infant. The kitchen sink, modified for a wheelchair, can be an ideal location, because it is easy to fill and drain and there is counter space available for supplies. The ambulatory parent may also find the kitchen a good bathing location, because the site is stable and the height of the sink minimizes bending. If the kitchen sink is not suitable, a portable plastic tub can be placed on an accessible table near a sink. A hose attachment can be used to fill the tub, but emptying may be difficult. To help support and protect the infant,

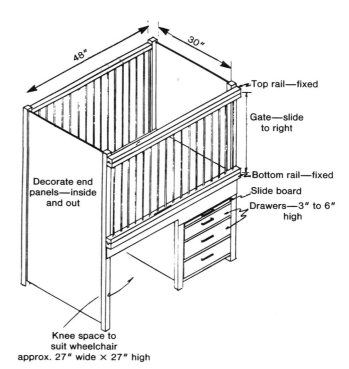

Figure 16.9. Crib with storage area, sliding gate side rails, and knee space to accommodate a wheelchair.

a foam rubber pad or a semireclining plastic baby seat should be placed in the tub. The older child can be placed in a regular tub with a suction-based bath seat for support. All necessary equipment and clothes should be assembled before bathing. The tub should be filled before putting the child in and drained before lifting him out. A terry cloth apron can be worn by the parent during bathing to protect the parent's clothing and for drying the baby.

Playpens are useful for confining the baby in a safe environment. Raising the legs of a conventional playpen, or using a portable crib are several ways to minimize bending. The side of the portable crib may need to be adapted so that the parent in a wheelchair can lift the baby in and out.

DIAPERING/DRESSING

Using disposable diapers is the easiest method of diapering, but it can be expensive. There are prefolded diapers with touch fastener closures that are commercially available. Clothing should have full-length openings with closures the parent can manage.

The changing table, positioned at the proper height (31 inches for wheelchairs), should have a strap with touch fasteners to secure the infant during dressing and diapering. The safest place to handle the baby for dressing and other activities is the floor, but the parent must be able to get up and down safely with the child.

FEEDING

Breast feeding is generally easier than bottle feeding, because it eliminates the chore of formula preparation. A pillow can be used to support the holding arm and the infant or the mother can breast-feed while lying in bed positioned on her side. If the mother is on medication, it is important that she check with her physician before deciding to breast-feed, as some medications can be transmitted to the infant through the milk (Hale, 1979).

Some mothers find bottle feeding easier and more convenient. Lightweight plastic bottles with screw-on lids are the easiest to manage. Disposable liners eliminate the need for sterilization, but individuals with limited strength or coordination may find them difficult to manage. Using premeasured formula is ideal but expensive. The infant can be held in a similar manner to breast feeding or he can be placed in a plastic infant seat, which is held or set on a table.

The highchair should be sturdy and have a swing-away tray with a one-handed release mechanism and a safety strap. An electric baby dish can keep the food warm throughout the meal. The parent can wear a plastic apron and the child can wear a plastic bib with pockets to minimize cleaning the floor. Bibs should have touch fastener closures instead of ties. A parent with minimal incoordination should use a rubber-coated spoon to protect the baby's gums and teeth. The parent who is severely incoordinated will need assistance feeding the infant.

LIFTING AND CARRYING

It is important that the disabled parent have a safe method of carrying the baby. If the parent is ambulatory, the infant can be transported using a bassinet on wheels or even a reclining stroller. Many parents find a cloth infant carrier useful, especially outside the home. If the parent has back pain, the choice of a front or back carrier depends on the individual's particular problem. A front-style carrier requires the back muscles to contract against the load, whereas a back-style carrier compresses the vertebrae.

If the parent uses a wheelchair, the infant can be placed on the parent's lap supported by a soft pillow. The sides of the pillow can be attached to the armrests by touch fastener straps to keep it from slipping. As the baby gains sitting balance, he can be placed on the parent's lap, secured by a touch fastener strap attached to the wheelchair.

SAFETY

A parent with a disability must be consistent in requiring obedience to verbal commands, especially when the child is told to stop or come. A harness can be useful when outside the home to keep a child from running or wandering away. Because modifications for a parent using a wheelchair may put equipment, supplies, or appliance controls within the reach of children, safety devices should be installed to protect the child from accidents.

As long as the parent doesn't expect perfection, a child can become self-reliant at a young age (Stewart, 1989). He can be taught to dress, wash, and even help with the dishes, if the parent arranges the tasks so they are accessible to the child.

SUMMARY

Home management and child care training are important areas of occupational performance. Many women measure their success or failure to be independent in accordance with their ability to engage in household management and caretaking activities (Crist, 1991). Although complete independence may not always be possible, the therapist should emphasize the abilities and potential of the patient. Current research on occupational therapy's role in home management and parenting is limited. Although many patients can attest to the valuable role of occupational therapy, documentation in the literature is needed.

STUDY QUESTIONS _____

1. What are the principles of work simplification? Briefly describe each principle.
2. What are three responsibilities of the managerial homemaker?
3. How would a person with chronic back pain use the principles of body mechanics to do the laundry?
4. What adaptive methods or equipment would a person with hemiplegia use to make a cheese omelet?
5. Using the principles of energy conservation, what adaptive methods would a person with rheumatoid arthritis use while grocery shopping?
6. Describe two methods that a person with paraplegia would use to bathe an infant.
7. Develop a weekly house-cleaning plan for a person with multiple sclerosis.
8. How would a person with severe visual impairment make the bed?
9. What adaptive methods or equipment would a person with cerebral palsy use to wash dishes?

REFERENCES

Anderson, H. (1981). *The disabled homemaker.* Springfield, IL: Charles C. Thomas.

Burkhardt, B. (1975). Loop-handled utensils. *American Journal of Occupational Therapy, 29,* 423.

Caldwell, J. (1983, January 12). Her special touch. *The Boston Globe,* pp. 25, 38.

Crist, P. (1991). Motherhood revisited: Balancing parenthood and disability. *Journal of Occupational Therapy Practice, 2*(4), 34–47.

Dunn, V. M. (1978). Tips on raising children from a wheelchair. *Accent on Living, 22*(4), 78–83.

Fastow, K. (1977). Adapted fitted bed sheets. *American Journal of Occupational Therapy, 31*(6), 63.

Frederick, B. B. (1979). *Body mechanics instruction manual: A guide for therapists.* Redmond, WA: Express.

Gilbert, D. W. (1965). Energy expenditures for the disabled homemaker: Review of studies. *American Journal of Occupational Therapy, 19,* 321–328.

Hale, G. (Ed.). (1979). *The source book for the disabled.* New York: Paddington.

Klinger, J., Freiden, F., & Sullivan, R. (1970). *Mealtime manual for the aged and handicapped.* New York: Simon & Schuster.

Stewart, C. (1989). Raising children from a wheelchair. *AOTA Physical Disabilities Special Interest Newsletter, 12*(2), 5–7.

Strebel, M. B. (1980). *Adaptations and techniques for the disabled homemaker* (5th ed.). Minneapolis: Sister Kenny Institute.

Vorburger, L. (1980). Wash up. *Accent on Living, 25*(2), 125.

Whiteman, E. (1989). Microwave cookers: Their value for people with disabilities. *British Journal of Occupational Therapy, 52*(2), 55–58.

Wylde, M., & Baron-Robbins, A. (1990). *Residential access.* Unpublished manuscript, Institute for Technology Development. Oxford, MS.

SUPPLEMENTARY RESOURCES

Suggested Readings

Cochrane, G. M., & Wilshere, E. (Eds.). (1984). *Equipment for the disabled: Disabled mother.* Oxford, UK: Oxfordshire Health Authority.

Garee, B. (Ed.). (1989a). *Parenting: Tips from parents (who happen to have a disability) on raising children.* Bloomington, IL: Cheever.

Garee, B. (Ed.). (1989b). *Single-handed: Devices and aids for one-handers and sources of these devices.* Bloomington, IL: Cheever.

Resources

American Foundation for the Blind, Inc. (15 West 16th Street, New York, NY 10011)

Buyer's guide (yearly). (Available from *Accent on Living,* P.O. Box 700, Bloomington, IL 61701)

Through the Looking Glass. An organization for assisting parents with a disability. (801 Peralta Avenue, Berkeley, CA 94707)

17
Preparing for Return to Work

Karen Jacobs

OBJECTIVES _____

Upon completion of this chapter the reader will be able to:
1. Define the occupational performance area called work.
2. List four types of work evaluations.
3. Define **work hardening.**
4. Discuss the role of the occupational therapist in a typical return to work program.

The focus of this chapter is preparing to return to work. It begins with an overview of the concept of work and its meaning and a discussion of unemployment and employment issues, including the Americans with Disabilities Act (ADA). Prevention, work site health promotion, assessment, and intervention strategies are some of the services provided by occupational therapists. The roles and responsibilities of occupational therapists in work disability prevention and management are discussed in this chapter separately, although they are integrated.

The concept of work is fundamental to the occupational therapy profession. However, the definition of work and interest for this area of practice has varied over the extent of the profession's history (Harvey-Krefting, 1985). Work is an occupational performance area that encompasses vocational and educational activities, care of others, and home management (American Occupational Therapy Association [AOTA], 1989). In 1992, the American Occupational Therapy Association (AOTA) published its definitive document on this area of practice (Jacobs et al., 1992). According to this document, "any activity that contributes to the goals and services of a society, whether paid or unpaid, is considered a work activity. Engaging in work is a productive activity and a medium and goal of occupational therapy" (p. 1086). **Work behaviors** and skills

and physical capacities are performance components that constitute important elements of work. **Work behaviors,** also termed prevocational readiness or personal skills, refer to those behaviors that are necessary for successful participation in a job or independent living, e.g., the ability to behave appropriately; to have a sense of time and responsibility; to read, write, and handle money; to engage in acceptable personal hygiene; to accept and use supervision; to make friends and get along with others; and to be able to do other similar developmental tasks (Jacobs, 1993; Ryan, 1979).

Frequently referred to as vocational skills, work skills and physical capacities, are required to perform the tasks of an actual job. Work skills are capabilities that the worker has learned or has the potential to learn, e.g., typing. Physical capacities are abilities that are, to one degree or another, possessed by nearly all workers. They are described by the U.S. Department of Labor in terms of the **physical demands** needed to perform a job. Standing, walking, sitting, lifting, carrying, pushing, and pulling are **physical demands** that are classified in terms of five work levels of strength: sedentary, light, medium, heavy, and very heavy (Table 17.1). These ratings are determined by the amount of weight lifted or carried, frequency of the lift, and the amount of standing or walking required (Matheson, 1982). Other **physical demands** are climbing, balancing, stooping, kneeling, crouching, crawling, reaching, handling, fingering, feeling, talking, hearing, visual acuity (far and near), depth perception, visual accommodation, color vision, and field of vision (U.S. Department of Labor, 1991a). Additional criteria used in assessing **physical demands** of particular jobs include duration of static or dynamic posture; the nature of the posture itself; repetitive motion over time; force required to, e.g., adjust a knob or engage a press, distance of reach, carry, and push and pull; shape, size, and contour of object and tools; weight of

GLOSSARY

Ergonomics—Refers to the characteristics of people that need to be considered in arranging things that they use so that the people and things will interact most effectively and safely.

Essential functions—Fundamental, not marginal, job duties.

Physical demands—As defined in the *Dictionary of Occupational Titles*, there are 20 demands: lifting, standing, walking, sitting, carrying, pushing, pulling, climbing, balancing, stooping, kneeling, crouching, crawling, reaching, handling, fingering, feeling, talking, hearing, and seeing.

Reasonable accommodations—Any modification in the work environment or in the way work is customarily performed that enables an individual with a disability to enjoy equal employment opportunity.

Work behaviors—Also termed prevocational readiness or personal skills. Those behaviors that are necessary for successful participation in a job or independent living, e.g., the ability to behave appropriately.

Work capacity evaluation—Defined as a comprehensive process that systematically uses work, real or simulated, to assess and measure an individual's physical abilities to work.

Work hardening—A work-oriented treatment program, the outcome of which is measured in terms of improvement in the client's productivity.

Work tolerance—Defined as the ability to sustain a work effort for a prolonged period of time, to maintain a steady flow of production at an acceptable pace and an acceptable level of quality, and to handle a certain amount of pressure.

Table 17.1. Classification of Work Level

Sedentary work	Requires a maximum lift of 10 pounds infrequently and occasional lifting or carrying of papers, small tools, or file folders; sedentary work may require occasional walking or standing
Light work	Requires a maximum lift of 20 pounds with frequent lifting or carrying of up to 10-pound objects; if a great deal of walking, standing, or pushing and pulling of arm or leg controls is required by the job, the job is classified at the light level even though the lifting requirements do not exceed 10 pounds
Medium work	Requires a maximum lift of up to 50 pounds with frequent lifting or carrying of weights up to 25 pounds
Heavy work	Requires a maximum lift of 100 pounds with frequent lifting or carrying of objects weighing up to 50 pounds
Very heavy work	Requires lifting objects greater than 100 pounds with frequent lifting or carrying of objects weighing 50 pounds or more

parts and tools; heights and direction of placement; number of repetitions and/or production quotas (in terms of work or speed); and variations in routine (Heck, 1987).

To achieve the outcome of returning to work, the client may need to address specific performance components such as strength, endurance, and time management. In addition, the meaning of work to the client needs to be understood by the therapist.

THE MEANING OF WORK

For some people, work (i.e., employment) is one of the most important social roles a person fulfills in a lifetime. Work provides economic security, intellectual or physical challenge, and friendships; helps promote life satisfaction; and helps in self-definition and estimating self-worth (Kemp & Kleinplatz, 1985). Others value work simply as a means to earn money to participate in other aspects of life that they find more meaningful. There are also those who find no value whatever in work, and see it as an interruption of their true lives. People in this latter category easily accept the limitations of an injury relative to work and prefer to receive compensation from insurance companies or federal social security.

Clients who value work for whatever reason are typically eager to participate in work intervention. Some clients who do value work are not ready at the time of discharge from rehabilitation to consider return to work or to work through the process of determining abilities for work, because they are still in a period of mourning for their loss. Such clients need to know where to go for these services when they are ready. There are some people with disabilities for whom work is no longer possible, despite its positive value to them. Those with frequent concurrent illnesses that would result in absenteeism are not good candidates unless their illnesses can be controlled. For example, a client with a spinal cord injury prone to urinary tract infections needs to have that condition corrected before seeking employment. People with head injuries that severely interfere with learning or appropriate social behavior would also not be ideal candidates. When it is determined that a client is indeed unemployable, he must be taught satisfying avocational pursuits, if possible, to enhance his quality of life.

The level of motivation of the individual is probably the greatest determining factor concerning return to work after injury. Motivation refers to a person's determination or persistence in pursuing a goal. When no motivation exists or can be generated, the rehabilitation specialists must realize that work planning, evaluation, and training will be unsuccessful. For those clients motivated by earning power and/or personal satisfaction, more opportunities than ever exist for employment. Ongoing technological advances are providing significant employment opportunities for people with disabilities, including those individuals with severely limited physical abilities.

The job should fit a person's realistic self-image and values regarding work. Discussions during early phases of work rehabilitation concerning work-related issues—e.g., job versus career, pay versus personal satisfaction, office work versus physical work, and small company or large—help the person not only to clarify his values but also to develop realistic attitudes and self-perceptions. The *Worker Role Interview*, an instrument in its early phases of development, may be a useful tool in assisting occupational therapists in identifying psychosocial and environmental variables associated with return to work (Velozo, Kielhofner, & Fisher, 1990).

UNEMPLOYMENT/EMPLOYMENT

Unemployment is common among people with disabilities. According to the President's Committee on Employment of People with Disabilities (1993), there was a 70% unemployment rate for people with disabilities in 1993. This is approximately 10% higher than the rate indicated in the 1990 census data. According to the 1990 survey, the 39.3% who were working either full or part time earned 35% less than their able-bodied coworkers. There are probably many reasons for the underemployment of people with disabilities. One reason may be that people with disabilities are unwilling to jeopardize their Social Security Supplemental Security Income benefits, although the 1980 Social Security Amendments were meant to enable people with disabilities to have a trial at gainful employment without loss of such benefits (Greenberg, 1981). Another problem may be the lack of knowledge on the part of able-bodied employers about the capabilities of workers with disabilities. The unwillingness of some insurance companies to insure small private industries who hire workers with disabilities is another problem. Furthermore, many people with disabilities have a lower level of education and training than many types of available jobs require. This problem is not limited to people with disabilities; however, the job market is even more competitive for them ("Job Market," 1976).

Perhaps the greatest barrier to employment of people with disabilities is attitude. Sensitivity training is needed to assist coworkers and employers to overcome negative stereotypes of people with disabilities. Although over the last 20 years there has been little

progress in increasing labor force participation rates of people with disabilities, the U.S. government continues to be a committed advocate for people with disabilities. Two important strides forward were the establishment of the President's Committee on Employment of People with Disabilities and the enactment of the ADA. The committee is an independent federal agency whose mission is to facilitate the communication, coordination, and promotion of public and private efforts to empower Americans with disabilities through employment. The committee provides information, training, and technical assistance to American business leaders, organized labor, rehabilitation and service providers, advocacy organizations, and families and individuals with disabilities. The committee's information programs include publications dealing with the Americans with Disabilities Act, employment issues, job accommodation, data related to people with disabilities, the promotion of the National Disability Employment Awareness Month, and a national conference on issues related to the employment and empowerment of people with disabilities. The committee also sponsors the Job Accommodation Network (JAN), a free service that provides information and consultation on accommodating people with disabilities in the workplace (President's Committee, 1993).

In 1990, the Americans with Disabilities Act was passed. Under this landmark legislation, persons with disabilities are protected from discrimination in employment, transportation, public accommodations, telecommunications, and activities of state and local governments (Golden, 1991). Table 17.2 provides an overview of the five titles composing the ADA. Title I, Employment, is of interest to the individual with a disability returning to work. Nondisabled workers are not entitled to the benefits covered under the law. First, the ADA clearly delineates who is an individual with a disability; such a person

1. Has a permanent or temporary physical or mental impairment that substantially limits one or more major life activities (e.g., walking, speaking, breathing, seeing, hearing, learning, caring for oneself or working); *substantially limits* refers to the nature and severity of the disability, how long it will, or is expected to, last; and its permanent or long-term impact;
2. Has a record of such an impairment, e.g., a history of cancer or heart disease (even if cured, controlled, or in remission);
3. Is regarded as having such an impairment, e.g., a person who is treated as if he or she had AIDS.

Title I prohibits discrimination against any *qualified* individual with a disability in regard to job application procedures; the hiring, advancement, or discharge

Table 17.2. Americans with Disabilities Act, A Summary

Title	Law's Effective Date	Regulations by Federal Agency	Enforcement
Title I Employment	July 26, 1992, for employers with 25 or more employees; July 26, 1994, for employers with 15 or more employees	July 26, 1991, all regulations from Equal Employment Opportunity Commission (EEOC)	Remedies identical to those under Title VII of the Civil Rights Act of 1964, which are private right of action, injunctive relief, i.e., job reinstatement, back pay, and EEOC enforcement
Title II Public Services All activities of local and state governments	January 26, 1992	July 26, 1991, all regulations from attorney general	Remedies identical to those under the Rehabilitation Act of 1973 §505, which include private right of action, injunctive relief, and some damages
(Part I) Public transportation (buses, light and rapid rail including fixed-route systems, paratransit, demand response systems and transportation)	August 26, 1990, all orders for purchases or leases of new vehicles must be for accessible vehicles; one-car-per-train must be accessible as soon as practicable, but no later than July 26, 1995; paratransit services must be provided after January 26, 1992; new stations built after January 26, 1992, must be accessible; key stations must be retrofitted by July 26, 1993, with some extensions allowed up to July 26, 2020	July 26, 1991, all regulations from secretary of transportation	Same as above
(Part II) Public transportation by intercity Amtrak and commuter rail (including transportation facilities)	By July 26, 2020, Amtrak passenger coaches must have same number of accessible seats as would have been available if every car were built accessible; half of such seats must be available by July 26, 1995; same one-car-per-train rule and new stations rule as above; all existing Amtrak stations must be retrofitted by July 26, 2020; key commuter stations must be retrofitted by July 26, 1993, with some extensions allowed up to 20 years	July 26, 1991, all regulations from secretary of transportation	Same as above
Title III Public accommodations operated by private entities A. Public accommodations (all business and service providers)	In general, January 26, 1992, except no lawsuits may be filed before July 26, 1992, against businesses with 25 or fewer employees and revenues of $1 million or less, or before January 26, 1993, for businesses with 10 or	July 26, 1992, regulations from attorney general; standards must be consistent with the Architectural and Transportation Barriers Compliance Board (ATBCB) guidelines	For individuals, remedies identical to Title II of the Civil Rights Act of 1964, which are private right of action, injunctive relief; for attorney general enforcement in pattern or practice cases or cases of general importance with

Table 17.2. Continued

Title	Law's Effective Date	Regulations by Federal Agency	Enforcement
B. New construction or alteration to public accommodations and commercial facilities	fewer employees and revenues of $500,000 or less January 26, 1992, for alterations; January 26, 1993, for new construction	Same as above	civil penalties and compensatory damages Same as above
C. Public transportation provided by private entities	In general, January 26, 1992, but by August 26, 1990, all orders for purchases or leases of new vehicles must be for accessible vehicles; calls for a 3-year study of over-the-road buses to determine access needs with requirements effective July 26, 1996, to July 26, 1997	July 26, 1991, regulations from secretary of transportation; regulations will be based on standards issued by the Architectural and Transportation Barriers Compliance Board (ATBCB)	Same as above
Title IV Telecommunication	July 26, 1993, telecommunications relay services to operate 24 hours per day	July 26, 1991, all regulations by the Federal Communications Commission	Private right of action and Federal Communications Commission
Title V Miscellaneous	Effective dates of Title V are those determined by most of the analogous sections in Titles I through IV	In general, this title depicts the ADA's relationship to other laws, explains insurance issues, prohibits state immunity, provides congressional inclusion, sets regulations by ATBCB, explains implementation of each title and notes amendments to the Rehabilitation Act of 1973	

of employees; employee compensation; job training; social or recreational programs that are sponsored by the employer; and other terms, conditions, and privileges of employment. A qualified individual with a disability is one who satisfies the requisite skill, experience, education, and other job-related requirements of the position and who, with or without **reasonable accommodation,** can perform the **essential functions** of the position. Two key terms within this definition are **reasonable accommodation** and **essential functions** of the job. **Essential functions** of a job are fundamental, not marginal, job duties. In deciding whether a function is essential, the following questions are considered:

1. Are employees in the position required to perform the function?
2. Will removing that function fundamentally change the job?

Further, a function is essential if:

1. The position exists to perform that function, e.g., a person is hired to proofread documents, thus the ability to proofread accurately is an **essential function** because this is the reason that the position exists.
2. There are a limited number of other employees available to perform the function or among whom the function can be distributed.
3. It is highly specialized and the person in the position was hired for special expertise or ability to perform it, e.g., communicating fluently in Spanish.

The factors considered in determining whether a function is essential are employer's judgment, job descriptions written before advertising or interviewing, and the amount of time an employee would spend performing the function. For example, if the individual is supposed to spend the majority of his or her time operating one machine, this would constitute evidence that operating the machine was an **essential function.** Another factor to be considered includes the consequences of not requiring the worker to perform a particular function. For example, a firefighter may only occasionally have to carry a person from a burning building, but being able to perform this function would be essential to the firefighter's job. The terms of a collective bargaining agreement, particularly if they list duties and the work experience of people who have performed the job in the past or present, are also factors considered when determining the importance of a particular function to a given job (American with Disabilities Act of 1990).

Determining **essential functions** of a job is a task that occupational therapists may perform. If this is the case, it is important to keep in mind that in identifying an **essential function,** therapists should focus on the purpose of the function and the result to be accomplished rather than the manner in which the function presently is performed. For example, for a job that requires use of a computer, the **essential function** would be the ability to input, access, and retrieve information from a computer not necessarily the ability to finger the keyboard or to see the monitor.

Reasonable accommodations include any modifications in the work environment or in the way work is customarily performed that enable an individual with a disability to enjoy equal employment opportunity. For example, a **reasonable accommodation** might be restructuring the job, adjusting a work schedule to meet an individual's needs, adapting equipment, or providing a reader or interpreter. However, the employer does not have to make an accommodation if it causes the business undue hardship. An undue hardship is an action requiring significant difficulty or expense (American with Disabilities Act of 1990). As of May 1993, the second most common employment discrimination issue cited by people with disabilities (21.5%, or 2136 alleged violations) is related to employers' failure to provide a **reasonable accommodation** (Equal Employment Opportunity Commission [EEOC], 1993).

Occupational therapists have an important role in the implementation of the ADA (Shamberg, 1993). For example, to improve hiring practices, the occupational therapist might structure employee job descriptions in terms of functional performance of specific tasks, aid in the development of effective employee evaluations based on performing the essential tasks of a job, or recommend and/or oversee installation of adaptive equipment or modification of the environment or tools to accommodate an employee with a disability (AOTA, 1993b).

THE ROLES OF OCCUPATIONAL THERAPY PRACTITIONERS IN WORK PRACTICE

Occupational therapists offer services to people with disabilities who need to establish or reestablish salable skills and abilities and to the injured worker to restore function and to recover capacities needed to return to the job. Occupational therapists also offer services to nondisabled workers to prevent injury (or illness) at the workplace and to help those clients who are displaced or retired early from work to reestablish their sense of productivity and worth.

To plan and direct efficiently the return to work of a client, the occupational therapy practitioner needs to be current on local, state, and federal rules and regulations and the expectations of the workers' compensation system (Bear-Lehman & McCormick, 1986). The roles and responsibilities of the occupational therapist in work disability prevention and management can be described as follows:

> Obtain a comprehensive history of the individual's occupational performance related to activities of daily living, work, and play/leisure, and identify the individual's work-related behaviors, interests, abilities, needs, and goals. Assess the sensorimotor, cognitive, and psychological skills and deficits of the worker and potential worker while considering his or her future goals. Analyze resources, constraints, demands, and expectations in the home, school, worksite, or community environment of the worker or potential worker to facilitate progress toward identified goals (Jacobs et al., 1992, p. 1086).

The ideal goal is injury or disability prevention. When this goal is not attainable and the client sustains an injury or becomes disabled, therapists focus their attention on assessing individual needs and follow that with any form of intervention deemed appropriate (Jacobs, 1990). These occupational therapy roles will be discussed separately, although they are actually integrated.

Prevention

By the 21st century, 50% of the workforce will suffer some type of occupational disorder unless preventative measures are taken (Schwartz, 1991). The annual cost to society will be billions of dollars. Clearly, work site injury prevention and health promotion are more viable alternatives to injury management (Jacobs, 1992). Prevention programs focus on the prevention of work-related injuries and the early return to work of injured employees.

The majority of workers seen are those at risk for back injury or cumulative trauma disorders of the hand and wrist. Musculoskeletal diseases are exceedingly common in industry. Low back pain accounts for millions of days lost from work and billions of dollars of lost productivity as well as workers' compensation claims (Schwartz, 1993). Most clients with back disease are involved in materials handling and lifting (Hadler, 1977).

Tenosynovitis, seen increasingly in industry, seems precipitated by the initiation of intense repetitive stereotyped usage. One type of tenosynovitis, De Quervain, is associated with performance of repetitive manual tasks involving a firm grip together with a deviated wrist (Chandani, 1986; Hadler, 1977). Carpal tunnel syndrome is associated with tight pinching in combination with wrist flexion or maintained wrist flexion.

Studies have identified relationships between specific injuries and the work that produced them. This enables development of primary prevention screening programs to prevent the injury-producing event from occurring and secondary prevention programs to detect disease, deficit, deviation, dysfunction, and disability early. This program is followed by appropriate interventions to prevent progression to a more serious or chronic condition (Bear-Lehman & McCormick, 1986). Services offered are tailored to the needs of the particular company. One service offered is a comprehensive work site analysis in which the occupational therapist analyzes tasks from an **ergonomic** perspective. For companies whose workers are primarily engaged in assembly tasks, the analysis focuses on the stressful positions of the hand and wrist, the forces required, the number of repetitions required, and the tool design. From information gathered from the work site analysis, the therapist recommends job or tool modification and/or the minimal worker capacities required of those assigned to a particular job. This type of recommendation guides decisions regarding return of a worker to that job (Holman & Becker, 1987). Ergonomic work site analysis and education and training are two types of prevention services provided by occupational therapists.

ERGONOMIC WORK SITE ANALYSIS

Ergonomic work site analyses are performed to classify jobs according to the qualifications and **physical demands** that they require to determine whether or not an individual is capable of safely doing the job. Ergonomic work site analyses are performed to determine whether a person with a disability can return to his former job or can apply for a specific new job and to prevent workplace injuries, such as biomechanical cumulative trauma disorders of employed workers. The term **ergonomics** or human factors refers to the characteristics of people that must be considered when arranging tools and equipment so that the job can be performed effectively and safely (Mish, 1984; Rohmert, 1987).

The science and techniques of **ergonomics** are used to determine whether or not certain work activity causes an observed incidence of cumulative trauma disorders. The procedure has three facets: (1) a structured oral interview to identify the worker's perceptions of hazards and sources of physical discomfort; (2)

screening for impairments and functional limitations—including measures of sensation, strength, and range of motion—to obtain a clearer picture of the nature and severity of the health complaints (this is especially helpful when the worker's complaints suggest preclinical stages of disease and when there are still few documented cases of musculoskeletal injuries related to a certain job within a company); and (3) an ergonomic work site analysis to determine the relationship between work patterns and musculoskeletal impairment.

Many ergonomic work site analysis forms are available for use by the occupational therapist. Figure 17.1 provides an example of a comprehensive format developed by the Occupational Safety and Health Administration (OSHA). Suggested equipment for conducting work site evaluations include a portable video camera that operates well in low light to record worker performance and to allow detailed study of the job tasks, a camera for still pictures, a retractable steel tape measure to determine lift and reach distances, a wheeled measuring device to determine carry distances, a push-pull gauge capable of measuring 250 pounds to determine forces that need to be exerted, and a 2-foot welded chain with a locking link at one end and a minimum pull strength of 250 pounds to use with the push-pull scale. Also recommended are a 3-foot steel cable with formed loops at each end, a scale for weighing, one pair each of wide- and narrow-jaw locking pliers, heavy-duty work gloves, hand towel, clipboard, pencil, graph paper, stopwatch, and a case to transport these items (Heck, 1987).

The ergonomic analyses are confined to three major areas: work methods, workstation design and worker posture, and handle and tool design. Work method analysis is concerned with determining what the worker must do to perform the task successfully, which requires direct observation or videotaping of the worker, counting the number of repetitive movements in a given work cycle, and measuring or estimating the forces required by the job. In the case of hand and wrist injuries, suspected problematic postures are noted and documented. These postures are simultaneous full extension of the fingers and wrist, simultaneous full flexion of the wrist with grasp, forceful pinch, or ulnar or radial deviation. The amount of time that the extremity is maintained in a certain stressful posture is important to note because the stress on the structure accumulates. Also considered are the speed, intensity, and pace at which the worker must perform repetitive movements to meet production standards.

Analysis of the workstation examines the relationship of the worker and workstation features as they relate to postures required, especially stressful ones. Proper workstation design has been extensively studied to relieve musculoskeletal problems of video display

Industrial Ergonomic Analysis Checklist (data may be gathered during and after the on-site inspection and the checklist may be tailored to suit your needs)

Worker's job title: _____ Worker's Age: _____

Worker's name: _____ Height/weight: _____ (in./lb.)

Department: _____ Shift hours: _____

Hours/week: _____ Breaks: (A.M.) _____ (Lunch) _____ (P.M.) _____

Describe task(s) performed by worker (in sequence):

Does the employee rotate to other jobs?   Y   N

If so, how often? _____ Describe the other jobs _____

_____

How often does the employee work overtime? _____ How long? _____

Is overtime voluntary? _____

Number of employees on this same job: _____

Number of items produced per hour: _____

Workstation features (delete questions that do not apply):

1. Are there sharp edges that press on the worker's hand _____
   fingers _____ wrist _____ forearm _____ thighs _____ other _____
2. How long does the employee stand? _____ (hours/day)
   Floor type? _____
3. Is antifatigue matting used? _____ Type? _____
4. What type of chair is used? Model _____ Mfr. _____
5. Indicate on the illustration below where the workpieces and tools are located with respect to the worker (provide distances in inches).

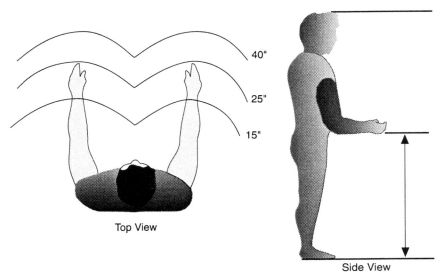

Figure 17.1. OSHA ergonomic work site analysis survey form.

terminal (VDT) operators (Arndt, 1983). The American National Standards Institute (1988), in collaboration with the Human Factors Society, published a comprehensive technical standard for the design of VDTs. The standards present good suggestions related to chair height, back support, head angle, viewing distance, document holder placement, display angle, arm support, leg room, footrests, display height, keyboard location, and working height, which can be used by therapists for evaluation of other types of work sites as well (Arndt, 1983).

On city and state levels, there is a movement for the establishment of guidelines or standards for some jobs. For example, New York City employees receive frequent breaks, regular eye examinations, ergonomically designed furniture, and training to reduce disorders associated with VDT use (Bloswick, 1993; "What's on the Books," 1992). On the federal level, the U.S.

Department of Labor (1991b) has published guidelines for the meatpacking industry. Although these guidelines are specific to meatpacking, they are useful for an overall **ergonomic** program for other work sites. Presently, OSHA is in the process of developing **ergonomic** program management guidelines for general industry. Occupational therapists interested in consulting to industry, must develop an understanding of these guidelines and keep current with new standards.

Analysis of handle and tool design is important, because poor design is the most common cause of hand and wrist disability. The most common problem is that the handle of the tool is too short for the worker's hand (Habes & Putz-Anderson, 1985; Putz-Anderson, 1988; Tichauer, 1966, 1978). Tichauer (1966, 1978) has redesigned many tool handles used by electronic assembly workers; the new designs prevent stress that results in cumulative trauma disorders. As a general rule, tools or tasks should be designed so that the wrist is maintained in the neutral position (Habes & Putz-Anderson, 1985; Tichauer, 1966). A combination of flexed wrist with significant grip force and repetitive movement requirements are biomechanical stresses commonly associated with cumulative trauma disorders (Habes & Putz-Anderson, 1985).

Instructing clients in good body mechanics and **ergonomic** principles helps them manage their symptoms. Clients can be taught, e.g., that decreasing the horizontal distance to lift, enlarging a tool handle so only the distal phalanges of the fingers and thumb overlap, and lowering work surfaces so elbows are not abducted more than 30° from the torso can prevent injury (Heck, 1987). For hand tasks it has been suggested that dynamic work forces should not exceed 50% of the maximum dynamic strength for short durations or more than 30% of the maximum dynamic strength for long periods. Dynamic strength is determined by measurement of forces throughout a range of motion (Morris & Anderson, 1988). Required static forces should not be greater than 15% of the maximum static strength. If job demands exceed these limits, the chance for trauma (or deterioration) is increased. Static forces of the hand are considered to be a significant **physical demand** if a high level of effort is sustained for 10 sec or more, a moderate demand if effort is required for 60 sec or more (Heck, 1987).

Although the quantification of risk factors has been particularly difficult for researchers, and "hard data" on the hazardous levels of exposure relating to repetition rates, force levels, and postures are presently unavailable, the ANSI has established the following general recommendations to reduce work site risk factors:

1. Design the workstation so that the worker can maintain an upright, neutral posture;
2. Minimize contact stress by spreading out the force through tool shape or padding;
3. Arrange the work site to reduce the number of hand-arm directional changes required; and
4. Reduce hand-arm vibration by tool selection and appropriate tool grips and/or gloves (Bloswick, 1993).

For companies whose workers are required to handle materials, the work site analysis concentrates primarily on lifting tasks; the analyst uses the National Institute for Occupational Safety and Health's *Work Practices Guide for Manual Lifting* (WPG) (Habes & Putz-Anderson, 1985; Putz-Anderson, 1988) to determine if the lifting task places the worker at risk for injury. The National Institute for Occupational Safety and Health (NIOSH) manual lifting equation for calculating a recommended weight for lifting tasks has been used extensively for identifying manual lifting tasks that might pose a risk of low back injury. However, during the decade the lifting equation has been in use positive and negative feedback from practitioners has indicated that the equation needs to be revised.

The revised NIOSH manual lifting equation is *not* a governmental standard but rather a recommendation or guideline. Table 17.3 lists the revised equation that calculates the recommended weight limit (RWL). Table 17.4 presents the frequency multiplier and Table 17.5 shows the coupling multiplier that are used in the

Table 17.3. Equation for Calculating the Recommended Weight Limit

$$RWL = LC \cdot HM \cdot VM \cdot DM \cdot AM \cdot FM \cdot CM$$

Symbol	Meaning	U.S. Customary
LC	Load Constant	51 pounds
HM	Horizontal Multiplier	$10/H$
VM	Vertical Multiplier	$1 - (.0075V - 30)$
DM	Distance Multiplier	$0.82 + (1.8/D)$
AM	Asymmetric Multiplier	$1 - (0.0032A)$
FM	Frequency Multiplier	See Table 17.4
CM	Coupling Multiplier	See Table 17.5
RWL	Recommended weight limit	
H	Horizontal location of the hands from midpoint between the ankles	
V	Vertical location of the hands from the floor	
D	Vertical travel distance between the origin and the destination of the lift	
A	Angle of asymmetry, the angular displacement of the load from the sagittal plane	

Table 17.4. Frequency Multiplier

Frequency (lifts/min)	≤8 hr		≤2 hr		≤1 hr	
	V[a]<30	V≥30	V<30	V≥30	V<30	V≥30
0.2	0.85	0.85	0.95	0.95	1.00	1.00
0.5	0.81	0.81	0.92	0.92	0.97	0.97
1	0.75	0.75	0.88	0.88	0.94	0.94
2	0.65	0.65	0.84	0.84	0.91	0.91
3	0.55	0.55	0.79	0.79	0.88	0.88
4	0.45	0.45	0.72	0.72	0.84	0.84
5	0.35	0.35	0.60	0.60	0.80	0.80
6	0.27	0.27	0.50	0.50	0.75	0.75
7	0.22	0.22	0.42	0.42	0.70	0.70
8	0.18	0.18	0.35	0.35	0.60	0.60
9	0.00	0.15	0.30	0.30	0.52	0.52
10	0.00	0.13	0.26	0.26	0.45	0.45
11	0.00	0.00	0.00	0.23	0.41	0.41
12	0.00	0.00	0.00	0.21	0.37	0.37
13	0.00	0.00	0.00	0.00	0.00	0.34
14	0.00	0.00	0.00	0.00	0.00	0.31
15	0.00	0.00	0.00	0.00	0.00	0.28
>15	0.00	0.00	0.00	0.00	0.00	0.00

[a]Vertical height, in inches.

Table 17.5. Coupling Multiplier

Couplings	V[a]<30 inches	V≥30 inches
Good	1.00	1.00
Fair	0.95	1.00
Poor	0.90	0.90

[a]Vertical height.

equation (Putz-Anderson & Waters, 1991). Once the RWL is calculated and the weight of the object being lifted is obtained (load weight), a simple estimate of the hazard of overexertion injury for a specific manual lifting task can be computed, using the following lifting index (LI) equation:

$$LI = L/RWL$$

where L is the load weight. If LI is > 1.0, an overexertion injury is likely, because job demands exceed the recommended weight limit; if LI < 1.0, then the job represents a nominal risk of an overexertion injury. Although the revised equation is much better than the original, the reader should note that limitations remain. According to Aja (1994), the 1991 lifting formula is applicable only to lifting tasks that fit the following conditions:

1. Favorable temperature conditions of the work environment, e.g., temperatures between 65° and 80°F and no more than 50% humidity;
2. Other work tasks do not require high energy expenditure;

3. The lifting task is two-handed and is not performed in a high-speed, jerky manner; and
4. There is friction between the worker and the floor surface that is equivalent to that between a smooth, dry floor and a clean, dry leather boot sole (Aja, 1994).

EDUCATION AND TRAINING

Occupational therapists usually provide education and training programs that are job specific rather than generalized principles. Carlton (1987) tested the effectiveness of a presentation format on changing the practices of food service workers. Results indicated that the group that received instruction in proper body mechanics performed significantly better on a novel lifting task, but there was no carryover of the information to the actual work site. The instruction was via a 1-hr body mechanics course that emphasized high-risk work-style factors and the importance of maintaining a straight back during lifting and lowering of objects. The teaching methods included lecture, use of a visual aid (model of the back), actual practice of the principle during a lift, a videotape of the lift, and group critique of the tape. Ideally, education and training should occur in the actual environments and under the actual work conditions in which the worker will be expected to use such learning (Schwartz, 1991). Studies by Snook (1988), Dortch and Trombly (1990), Boffetti (1990), Schwartz and Jacobs (1991), and Fitzler and Berger (1983) demonstrated that educational programs resulted in significant improvement in knowledge and productivity and reduction in days lost because of injury.

Many educational and training programs provided by occupational therapists involve demonstration and practice of biomechanically correct techniques that were first presented to the workers via lecture and discussion (Boffetti, 1990; Dortch & Trombly, 1990). Such programs may also include feedback to the workers at the work site and positive reinforcement regarding the use of body mechanics and safe work postures. This coaching is typically done a few weeks after the classroom presentation to give the worker time to practice the new methods. Follow-up to the on-site coaching by providing training sessions to managers and supervisors is needed so that safe work habits are continually reinforced (Holman & Becker, 1987). This type of education is more effective than presentation alone.

Work Site Health Promotion

Work site health promotion is another service provided by occupational therapy practitioners. Wellness is perceived as a dynamic way of life in which good health habits are incorporated into one's lifestyle to improve both health and the quality of life (Johnson, 1986).

Not only do the scope and nature of work site health promotion programs vary, but the professional who is responsible for development and provision of services also varies. An accurate figure for the number of occupational therapy practitioners presently involved in work site health promotion is unavailable. However, the number of practitioners hired directly by business is small. The area of work site health promotion appears to be a window of opportunity for occupational therapists because of their knowledge of biomechanics, prevention, pathology, and working with an aging population. However, to be effective, it is paramount that therapists have a strong foundation in exercise physiology and fitness. Occupational therapists can make major contributions to this area by providing assessment of daily living skills for maintenance of productivity; leisure, home, and family management; assessment of and recommendations for adapting work and home environments to improve health and well-being; task analysis and instruction in work simplification to reduce stress and strain on body parts; and conservation of energy and time to improve job performance. Other areas of service for occupational therapists are identification of architectural barriers; instruction in the use of adaptive devices; promotion of a milieu supportive of occupational role performance through interpersonal skill development; and development of support groups and activities for health and fitness promotion, stress reduction, and retirement and leisure planning (Maynard, 1986).

Work Assessments

Work assessment begins the rehabilitation process for individuals injured on the job and should provide the foundation for the development and provision of comprehensive intervention. Presently, there are numerous work assessments available (Velozo, 1993); however, their quality varies greatly and few evaluate the worker in the actual work environment. The occupational therapist as an evaluator must be an educated consumer when deciding which assessment is most appropriate for a client's individual needs. The therapist should look for reliability, validity, sensitivity, and objectivity in measurement tools and should strive for timely, clear, and logical report formats (Miller, 1991).

Maki et al. (1979) described work assessment as a four-step process based on a systems approach:

1. Formulation of objectives of the assessment (e.g., whether the client will be able return to work);
2. Definition of content to be addressed (e.g., what the client's existing physical capacities are following injury);
3. Selection of appropriate strategies, inventories, checklists, and standardized measurement instruments (e.g., WEST 7—Bus Bench for a client who has a low back injury); and
4. Analysis and interpretation of data to formulate recommendations for intervention (e.g., recommending a **work hardening** program for a client who has carpal tunnel syndrome) (McCracken, 1991).

Typically, once the objectives and content have been determined, a work assessment consists of a series of standardized evaluations or job simulation activities. This assessment can have a duration ranging from 2 hr to 1 week. Functional capacity evaluation (FCE), physical capacity evaluation (PCE), **work capacity evaluation** (WCE), and functional capacity assessment (FCA) are terms that have been used interchangeably with work assessment in return-to-work programs. However, clarification is needed in the usage of these terms. Functional capacity evaluation is the broad umbrella term applied to work assessment and can be delineated into physical capacity evaluation and **work capacity evaluation.**

FUNCTIONAL CAPACITY EVALUATION

Broadly, a functional capacity evaluation may include tests of manual material handling capabilities, aerobic capacity, posture and mobility tolerance, anthropometric measurements, activities of daily living (ADLs), energy conservation techniques, and need for adaptive methods or technology (Lechner, Roth, &

Straaton, 1991; Scheer, 1990). The results of a study of 66 clients with chronic back pain indicated that quantitative functional capacity evaluation can give objective evidence of clients' physical abilities and degree of effort and can significantly guide treatment programs (Mayer et al., 1985). According to Lechner et al. (1991) one way of judging comprehensiveness of the FCE is to examine how many of the U.S. Department of Labor's 20 **physical demands** of work are addressed and how each is being evaluated (either pass/fail or with more specific performance parameters). A total of 10 functional capacity evaluations have been comprehensively reviewed by these authors according to this standard.

The *EPIC Functional Capacity Evaluation System* is an example of a commercially available functional capacity evaluation. It provides six modules that evaluate lift capacity, motor coordination, finger and hand dexterity, standing whole body range of motion, balance while walking, carrying and climbing, and industrial pushing and pulling (Fig. 17.2). Formalized training and a certification process are required for users.

PHYSICAL CAPACITY EVALUATION

A physical capacity evaluation typically assesses isolated parts of the body or functional units, e.g., lumbar region (Velozo, 1993). In some return to work programs, high-tech instrumentation is used, e.g., the Cybex Sagittal Strength Device.

The *Smith Physical Capacity Evaluation* is used by many occupational therapists. It has 154 performance items and was found to be 86.5% accurate in predicting reemployment of workers with physical disabilities (Smith, Cunningham, & Weinberg, 1983, 1986). This result must be accepted with caution because the respondents represented only 41% of the invited sample, but it does model one type of research that should be done concerning work assessments. Figure 17.3 is an example of a physical capacity evaluation.

WORK CAPACITY EVALUATION

Residual physical disability requires the person to either change his type of employment or to resume previous employment using adapted tools or methods. In either case, the person's ability to work safely and efficiently must be determined. **Work capacity evaluation** is defined as a comprehensive process that systematically uses work, real or simulated, to assess and measure an individual's physical abilities to work (AOTA, 1985; Holmes, 1985). Practical, reality-based assessments are used to evaluate work abilities related to specific job tasks.

Historically, **work capacity evaluation** consid-

ers aptitudes, interests, and vocational skills as secondary factors (Matheson, 1982; Matheson et al., 1985). Primary evaluation factors are those that comprise general "work-ability", i.e., employment feasibility and **work tolerance.** Feasibility is concerned with those basic factors that affect work acceptability to an employer in the labor market: worker productivity, safety, and interpersonal behavior. It functions as a gatekeeper to triage clients into those who are able and unable to benefit from the vocational rehabilitation process. Those who are unable to benefit may be able to profit after using prevocational services designed to optimize their potential. The **work capacity evaluation** certifies that the person possesses those basic attributes necessary for employment somewhere in the labor mar-

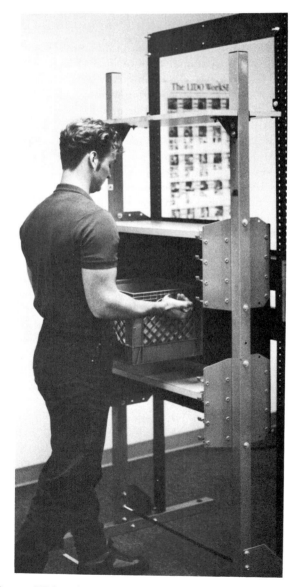

Figure 17.2. The EPIC Lift Capacity Module.

1. Number of hours capable of work:

2. Given the workday, the client can: Comments:

    Sit: 1/2 1   2   3   4   5   6   7   8 (hours)
    Stand: 1/2 1   2   3   4   5   6   7   8 (hours)
    Walk: 1/2 1   2   3   4   5   6   7   8 (hours)

3. Physical Demands:

LIFTING STRENGTH: (position)	(0) Never	(1-10) Occasional	(11-20) Frequent	(40-over) Continuous
Sedentary 0-10 lbs.				
Light 11-20 lbs.				
Moderate 21-50 lbs.				
Heavy 51-65 lbs.				
Very Heavy 66-100 lbs.				
CLIMB (stairs or ladders)				
BALANCE				
CROUCH				
SQUAT				
REACH - at shoulder height				
REACH - below shoulder height				
PUSHING				
PULLING				

4. Client can use feet for repetitive movements: Right_____   Left_____   Both_____

5. Client can use hands for repetitive movements:
   Simple grasping: Yes_____ No_____   Fine Manipulation: Yes_____ No_____

6. Client is restricted by the following environmental factors:
   _____hot/cold   _____dust   _____height   _____noise

7. Client will be required to use the following assistive devices or braces: _____
   _____
   _____

Additional Comments:_____
   _____

DATE:_____   THERAPIST:_____

Figure 17.3. Example of a physical capacity evaluation form.

ket, which can buoy spirits during subsequent repeated unsuccessful attempts to secure employment. Initial **work tolerances** are evaluated after feasibility has been determined. These include the general factors that affect the worker's physical competence to perform basic work tasks, i.e., strength, energy reserve, flexibility, and the effect of pain and other limiting factors on task performance.

Results of client's performance on the functional **work capacity evaluation** are compared with the demands of the job, which are found in the *Dictionary of Occupational Titles* (U.S. Department of Labor, 1991a). If there is a deficit that affects performance of the job, then an action plan is formed. This plan can involve placement of the worker in a modified **work hardening** or work conditioning program.

The following discussion provides an overview of some commonly used work evaluation tools that can be used independently or as part of a work assessment. There are four categories of work evaluation tools:

1. On-the-job, or work site, evaluations
2. Situational assessments
3. Psychometric instruments
4. Work samples

On-the-Job, or Work Site, Evaluations

Work site evaluations are done to determine whether a person with a disability can return to his old job or can apply for a particular new job. During the evaluation, a clinical assessment of the client's abilities and physical status are compared with the **physical demands** of the job. For efficiency's sake, the analysis should be limited to critical work demands of a particular job as they may be affected by the client's diagnosis and limiting symptoms (Heck, 1987; U.S. Department of Labor, 1991a).

Situational Assessments

A situational assessment involves placing an individual into a realistic work situation and systematically altering variables, such as **physical demands** or stress factors, to ascertain the person's performance under each circumstance (Jacobs, 1993; Marshall, 1983). For example, how will a client's performance be affected by increasing the distance a box must be transported?

Psychometric Instruments

Psychometric instruments include numerous pencil-and-paper and apparatus instruments used for measuring general intelligence, achievement, abilities, and related characteristics (Botterbusch, 1987). Examples of psychometric tests include the *Kuder Occupational Interest Survey* (Kuder, 1960) and the *General Aptitude Test Battery* (U.S. Department of Labor, 1970).

Work Samples

The primary technique of work evaluation is use of work samples. A work sample is a "well-defined work activity involving tasks, materials, and tools that are identical or similar to those in an actual job or cluster of jobs. Work samples are used to assess an individual's vocational aptitude, worker characteristics, and vocational interests" (Hursh & Kerns, 1988, p. 119).

The *Testing, Orientation, and Work Evaluation in Rehabilitation* (TOWER) system is the oldest complete work evaluation system. It was originally developed for use with people with physical disabilities, but it is now also used with other types of clients, such as people with mental illness. The system contains 110 work samples organized into 14 job training areas: clerical, drafting, drawing, electronics assembly, jewelry manufacturing, leather goods, machine shop, lettering, mail clerk, optical mechanics, pantograph engraving, sewing machine operating, welding, and workshop assembly. Within each major area, the work samples are graded in complexity. The recommendations that can be derived from the results are limited to jobs that relate to the work samples and do not relate to *Dictionary of Occupational Titles* classifications. The system was normed on people with disabilities, and no industrial norms are available. It is a useful system for thorough evaluation in limited areas. Each facility must build its own work samples, following the instructions in the

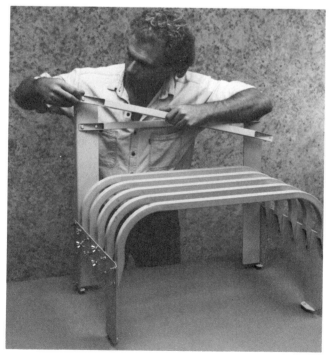

Figure 17.4. WEST 7—Bus Bench.

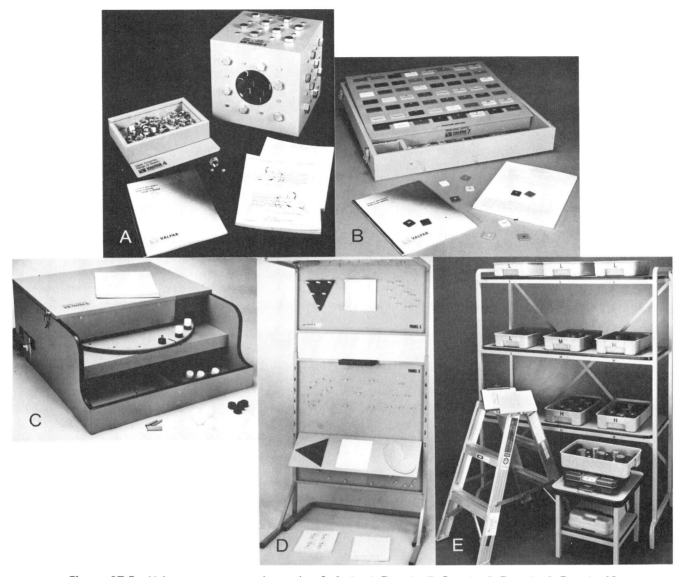

Figure 17.5. Valpar component work samples. **A,** Series 4; **B,** series 7; **C,** series 8; **D,** series 9; **E,** series 19.

manual, which is available from the Institute for Crippled and Disabled (see the Supplementary Resources for this chapter). The assembly of work samples is at the evaluator's discretion; usually, not all samples are administered to each client because not all are appropriate and the completion of the entire TOWER system takes 3 weeks.

Some of the more common work samples used by occupational therapists are WEST 2A, 3, 4A, and 7 (Jacobs, 1991b) (Fig. 17.4) and the Valpar component work samples 1, 4, 7, 8, 9, and 11 (Fig. 17.5). Each of these work samples is briefly described below.

Work Evaluation Systems Technology (WEST)

The WEST system has a series of work samples that are increasingly popular in return-to-work pro-

grams. These include the WEST 2A—Whole Body Range of Motion Work Sample, the WEST 3—Comprehensive Weight System, WEST 4A—Upper Extremity Strength and Fatigue Tolerance Work Sample, and WEST 7—Bus Bench. They all include norms for healthy male college students or methods-time measurements (MTMs) identified by the *Dictionary of Occupational Titles.*

Valpar Component Work Samples

The Valpar system consists of subtests to measure those worker characteristics that have been found to be basic indicators of success within numerous job families (Valpar International Corp., 1986). The work samples are intended for use as individual components, are packaged separately, and have minimal expendable materials. They are keyed to the worker traits listed in *Dictionary of Occupational Titles* and include MTMs and norms derived from various groups of employed workers and special disability groups. All the Valpar component work samples (VCWSs) are described below. The components with stars are the samples most commonly used by occupational therapists. Note that component 13 is no longer used.

1. * Small Tools (mechanical) measures the person's ability to understand and work with small tools. This task is related to jobs in small appliance repair, bicycle and auto repair, jewelry making, and assembly tasks in a wide variety of manufacturing settings.

2. Size Discrimination measures a person's ability to perform work tasks requiring visual size discrimination, such as grading and sorting jobs; performing work with close supervision using gauges, calipers, and other tools; and working within prescribed standards and tolerances.

3. Numerical Sorting measures a person's ability to perform work tasks using numbers or numerical series; the tests are sorting, filing, and categorizing. This test relates to occupations dealing with data and things such as examining, grading and sorting, keeping records and receipts, recording or transmitting verbal or coded information, and posting verbal or numerical data on stock lists.

4. * Upper Extremity Range of Motion measures **work tolerance** related to the upper torso. It is meant to isolate the client's pain and fatigue as related to the physical requirements that a worker must meet in the completion of particular work tasks. It is closely related to the following job task factors: reaching, handling, fingering, feeling, and seeing.

5. Clerical Comprehension and Aptitude measures both the person's ability to do and ability to learn these types of tasks. The areas measured include telephone answering, alphabetical filing, bookkeeping, and typing. This sample best relates to those occupations dealing with data, people, and things.

6. Independent Problem Solving measures a person's ability to do tasks requiring visual comparison and proper selection of a series of abstract designs. This sample best relates to jobs such as verifying computations, checking items for accuracy and consistency, and record keeping.

7. * Multilevel Sorting measures a person's ability to make decisions while performing tasks requiring physical manipulation and visual discrimination of colors, numbers, letters, and a combination of these. Jobs that this sample best relate to include

laboratory tester, insurance sales agent, hair stylist, and sales route driver.

8. * Simulated Assembly measures a person's ability to do a task requiring repetitive physical manipulation and bilateral use of the upper extremities. Jobs related to this sample include operating and monitoring automatic assembly machines.

9. * Whole Body Range of Motion measures the agility of a person's gross body movements as they relate to the functional ability to perform job tasks. It is a fatiguing sample that estimates the person's **work tolerance.** It measures the person's ability to stoop, kneel, crouch, reach, handle material, and finger material, which are basic abilities required by many occupations.

10. Tri-Level Measurement measures the person's ability to perform very simple to very precise inspection and measurement tasks. Jobs related to this sample include machinist, metal fabrications inspector, press operator, plumber, and glazier.

11. * Eye-Hand-Foot Coordination measures, in addition to these factors, the person's ability to concentrate, his reaction time, and his planning and learning capacity as these relate to the task. Work activities related to this sample include starting, stopping, and observing the functions of machines, perceiving relationships between moving objects, fixtures, and surfaces; and planning the order of successive operations. Jobs related to this sample include shoe repairer, heavy-equipment operator, milling-machine operator, and offset-press operator.

12. Soldering and Inspection-Electronic measures the person's ability to acquire and apply basic skills necessary to perform soldering tasks that vary in difficulty. Observation of the client also allows judgments concerning his ability to follow directions, eye-hand coordination, dexterity, ability to measure accurately, visual acuity, frustration tolerance, attentiveness, and judgment. Jobs related to this sample include jewelry solderer, electronic assembler, and tester.

14. Integrated Peer Performance has been designed to allow evaluation of worker interaction during assembly tasks.

15. Electrical Circuitry and Print Reading measures a person's ability to understand and apply principles of electrical circuits and to use pictorial materials such as blueprints, schematics, and drawings. Jobs related to this sample include electrical appliance repairer, electrician, and electronics mechanic.

16. Drafting measures ability from minimal expertise to sophisticated, high-level performance.

17. Prevocational Readiness Battery assesses a per-

son's ability to function in a vocational, educational, sheltered, or independent living setting.

18. Conceptual Understanding Through Blind Evaluation (CUBE) measures perceptual abilities that help a person compensate for visual difficulties.

19. * Dynamic Physical Capacities is composed of 28 individual tasks that are similar to those of a shipping and receiving clerk or parts-order clerk (e.g., lifting, climbing, stooping, and balancing).

The Baltimore Therapeutic Work Simulator

The *Baltimore Therapeutic* (BTE) *Work Simulator* is a computerized measuring device that allows measurement of repetitive upper limb motions against measurable resistance over a specified amount of time. It quantitatively documents the work output of the user (Bear-Lehman & McCormick, 1986). It can be used to estimate **work tolerance** and cardiac and pulmonary stress and for **work hardening** with feedback. The interchangeable handles simulate the **physical demands** of most jobs, such as grip, pinching, lifting, carrying, and reaching.

Intervention

Once assessment is completed, the client enters into the intervention phase. The occupational therapist, in cooperation with team members (e.g., physical therapist, vocational specialist, and psychologist), uses planned interventions to achieve the desired outcome of returning the client to work. When developing a program, the therapist tries to prevent the client from losing his identity as a worker, to encourage further healing following injury, to prevent secondary deficits, to prevent reinjury, and to minimize losses to the worker and to employer (Schwartz, 1993).

The preparation for work starts from the beginning of the work process with training to improve function. Independence in self-care and mobility are generally prerequisites to being able to work outside of the home. Therapy to improve strength, range of motion, coordination, perception, etc. that is done to improve the person's independence in self-care and mobility also improves the person's work-related skills. Ability to manipulate objects in the environment and/or problem solve are other prerequisite skills addressed in occupational therapy. Self-care training, therapeutic activity and sports, group discussions, and group projects all generate pieces of information concerning the person's readiness for employment. Special situations may need to be devised, however, to gather information or to allow the client to practice basic skills such as promptness, thoroughness, neatness, safety, accuracy, use of supervision without dependence or resentfulness, acceptance of responsibility, and tolerance for working

a full day. The nature of occupational therapy provides an ideal laboratory experience for such learning to take place.

Therapy to address the emotional issues of returning to work with a physical disability may be considered a part of intervention also. To facilitate the client's emotional adjustment, group therapy is used (see Chapter 20). Goals are to assist the client to accept himself as a worthy person, though changed; to value his working ability, although skills that may have been a source of pride to him are now impossible; to develop realistic expectations of himself and the working community; to redevelop his former level of motivation for work; and to explore new career possibilities. The group discussions could be organized around information presented by former clients with similar diagnoses, by group interviews of experts in the fields of interest to find out what the job requirements actually are, or by discussion of published information. The group discussions should help the person realize that work for people with disabilities is no longer stereotyped, e.g., watchmaking for paraplegics and broom making for the blind, but encompasses a large variety of jobs that are being done successfully by even the most severely disabled, limited only by drive and imagination.

The client who has never worked before may need assistance in learning job acquisition skills. All persons seeking a job for the first time after disability need to learn that in addition to the usual behavior of any job applicant (good grooming, knowledge about the particular business, a definite job goal, evidence of dependability, and a well-composed résumé or reference list), he needs to take the initiative to put the interviewer at ease regarding what **reasonable accommodation** (if any) will be needed to perform the **essential functions** of the job ("Your Job Interview," 1978; Hopkins-Best, 1987). This would prevent a naive interviewer from refusing the job on the basis of preconceived ideas. The person needs to act confidently and let the interviewer know what skills he expects to bring to the company. Role playing in occupational therapy can provide the opportunity to learn good job interview skills.

Three types of intervention used with clients with the goal of returning to work are **work hardening,** work conditioning, and vocational training.

WORK HARDENING

Work hardening is a work-oriented treatment program, the outcome of which is measured in terms of improvement in the client's productivity (Matheson et al., 1985; Ogden-Niemeyer & Jacobs, 1989). The ultimate goal is to help the person achieve a level of productivity that is acceptable in the competitive labor market. It is a comprehensive interdisciplinary approach (team members include an occupational therapist, physical therapist, psychologist, and vocational specialist) that uses graded work simulation to address the biomedical and psychosocial problems of the injured worker. The clients who benefit from this type of programming are those who are seriously deconditioned after an impairment caused by an injury or disease and those people who have major discrepancies between their symptoms and objective findings (Matheson et al., 1985).

Improvement in productivity is achieved through graded activity designed to increase **work tolerances,** improve work rate, master pain, improve work habits, increase confidence and proficiency with work adaptations or assistive devices. It involves the client in highly structured, simulated work tasks in an environment in which expectations for basic worker behaviors (timeliness, attendance, and dress) are in keeping with workplace standards. Program duration varies from 2 to 12 weeks with daily participation ranging from 2 to 8 hr (Bettencourt, 1991).

Work hardening programs use a variety of tools, equipment, work samples and **work capacity evaluation** devices (WCEDs). WCEDs allow presentation of tasks that simulate job tasks and that can be graded in difficulty or length of time involved. Most of the devices in use are homemade, although many are commercially available. Some therapists use traditional craft activities in treatment of industrial injuries to simulate job requirements and to develop **work tolerance.** The reader is referred to Ogden-Niemeyer and Jacobs (1989) for a thorough listing of **work hardening** tools and equipment.

The present form of **work hardening** originated at Rancho Los Amigos Hospital in Downey, California, in the late 1970s. By 1988, more than 500 programs identified themselves as **work hardening** programs. These programs were established in hospitals, as freestanding units affiliated with a hospital or rehabilitation facility, and as independent or within industry organizations (Ogden-Niemeyer & Jacobs, 1989). The large majority of these programs were established by occupational therapists. In 1988, the Commission of Accreditation for Rehabilitation Facilities (CARF) developed **work hardening** guidelines, which were later incorporated into its standards manual. These guidelines have attempted to ensure quality of program structure and content.

One of the classic **work hardening** programs is at the Liberty Mutual Medical Service Center in Boston, Massachusetts (Bettencourt et al., 1986; Jones et al., 1991). Occupational therapy at this center offers clients with chronic low back injuries a favorable environment where they can practice and improve the execution of work-related activities needed to perform their jobs while learning to live with, or control, symptoms. Monitors and workstations have been especially designed and developed to evaluate and develop **work tolerances.** Treatment includes client education through discussion, demonstration, active participation, and visual aids. Topics include anatomy of the spine, body mechanics, energy conservation, relaxation techniques, and weight reduction, if appropriate. Relaxation techniques include progressive relaxation techniques, meditation, increased body awareness, and control of breathing and muscle tension.

The client begins with activities that simulate his work. Treatment time is gradually increased to equal the person's premorbid work schedule. Modalities used include a balance monitor that provides feedback on weight bearing and symmetry of posture. A multi-workstation simulates construction jobs. The truck simulator uses a truck cab along with a computerized video road screen to simulate and measure the driving process. A computerized pneumatic lift has been designed to simulate the lifting process. An upper extremity work simulator, similar to the BTE, is used to simulate various upper extremity work tasks. Clients maintain an activity log to develop a sense of responsibility for their own rehabilitation and pain control (Bettencourt et al., 1986; see also Chapters 37 and 38).

Research on the effectiveness of **work hardening** programs has been systematically gathered since the mid-1980s. Return to work statistics obtained from individual programs range from 50–60% to 85–88% (Ogden-Niemeyer & Jacobs, 1989; Wyrick et al., 1991). By far the strongest variable related to return to work in clients entering **work hardening** programs was length of disability, whether measured as time since date of injury or last date worked (Niemeyer et al., 1994). In a program for 292 clients in a hand rehabilitation center, 80% of the clients returned to work within 6 weeks after entering the **work hardening** program (Baxter-Petralia & Beaulieu, 1986).

WORK CONDITIONING

When a client has an uncomplicated injury but physical limitations preclude return to work, work conditioning may be an appropriate intervention (Darphin, Smith, & Green, 1992). Work conditioning is typically provided as a unidisciplinary or bidisciplinary (occupational and/or physical therapy) half-day program that uses exercise, aerobic conditioning, education, and limited work tasks to restore an individual's systemic and neuromusculoskeletal function (strength, endurance, movement, flexibility, and motor control) so that the client can return to work or become physically reconditioned so vocational services can commence (Darphin et al., 1992).

VOCATIONAL TRAINING

Vocational training refers to the actual training program that the worker will undergo to learn the trade or profession that he has decided on. The training prepares the person for competitive job seeking and is done by persons expert in the trade or profession. The cost of training may be funded by the Rehabilitation Services Administration, as finances permit. The vocational specialist finds the training program to suit the client's need and may help place the client in a job, once trained.

One role the occupational therapist would have at this stage of vocational rehabilitation is to evaluate the client's need for, or design the necessary **reasonable accommodations** that the person will need to have to do, the job for which he is training.

Ideally, once the client has completed either a **work hardening** or conditioning program or received vocational training, he will be able to return to work and resume his role as a productive member of society.

STUDY QUESTIONS

1. What are the roles of occupational therapists in work practice?
2. Define work.
3. What is an ergonomic work site analysis?
4. Define reasonable accommodations.
5. Name 10 physical demand characteristics as described in the U.S. Department of Labor's *Dictionary of Occupational Titles* and its supplements.
6. List the four commonly used categories for work evaluations.
7. Define work capacity evaluation.
8. What is work hardening?
9. Describe the *Work Practice Guide for Manual Lifting.*
10. List three work behaviors.

REFERENCES

Aja, D. (1994). Revision of the 1991 NIOSH lift formula. In K. Jacobs & C. Bettencourt (Eds.), *Ergonomics for therapists.* Newton, MA: Butterworth-Heinemann.

American National Standards Institute. (1988). *American National Standards for Human Factors Engineering of Visual Display Terminal Workstations* (ANSI/HFS Standard No. 100-1988). Santa Monica, CA: Human Factors Society, Inc.

American Occupational Therapy Association. (1989). Uniform terminology for occupational therapy—Second edition. *American Journal of Occupational Therapy, 43,* 808–815.

American Occupational Therapy Association. (1993a). *1993 membership data survey.* Rockville, MD: Author.

American Occupational Therapy Association. (1993b). *Why worry about the ADA?* Rockville, MD: Author.

American Occupational Therapy Association Practice Division. (1985, April). I'm glad you asked. *Occupational Therapy Newspaper,* p. 6.

Americans with Disabilities Act of 1990, PL 101-336.

Arndt, R. (1983). Working posture and musculoskeletal problems of video display terminal operators: Review and reappraisal. *Journal of Industrial Hygiene Association, 44,* 437–446.

Baxter-Petralia, P., & Beaulieu, D. (1986). Therapeutic activity in treatment of industrial injuries. *AOTA Physical Disabilities Special Interest Newsletter, 9,* 3, 6.

Bear-Lehman, J., & McCormick, E. (1986). The expanding role of occupational therapy in the treatment of industrial hand injuries. *Occupational Therapy in Health Care, 2,* 79–88.

Bettencourt, C. (1991). Chronic back pain, disability, and rehabilitation of the injured worker. In Jacobs, K. *Occupational therapy: Work-related programs and assessments* (pp. 257–273) Boston: Little, Brown & Co.

Bettencourt, C., Carlstrom, P., Hargreaves, S., Lindau, K., Long, C. (1986). Using work simulation to treat adults with back injuries. *American Journal of Occupational Therapy, 40,* 12–18.

Bloswick, D. (1993). *Developing ergonomics programs in industry: A practical guide.* Salt Lake City: University of Utah.

Boffetti, H. (1990). *The influence of an education program upon industrial workers' habits as a possible preventative measure in cumulative trauma disorders of the hand and wrist.* Unpublished Master's thesis, Boston University.

Botterbusch, K. (1987). *Vocational assessment and evaluation systems: A comparison.* Menomonie, WI: Materials Development Center.

Carlton, R. (1987). The effects of body mechanics instruction on work performance. *American Journal of Occupational Therapy, 41,* 16–20.

Chandani, A. (1986). Tenosynovitis of hand and wrist: A literature review. *British Journal of Occupational Therapy, 49,* 288–292.

Darphin, L., Smith, R., & Green, E. (1992). Work conditioning and work hardening. *Orthopaedic Physical Therapy Clinics, 1,* 105–124.

Dortch, H., & Trombly, C. (1990). The effects of education on hand use with industrial workers in repetitive jobs. *American Journal of Occupational Therapy, 44,* 777–782.

Equal Employment Opportunity Commission. (1993). Personal communication.

Fitzler, S. & Berger, R. (1983). Chelsea back program: One year later. *Occupational Health & Safety, 52,* 52–54.

Golden, M. (1991). The Americans with disabilities act of 1990. *Journal of Vocational Rehabilitation, 1,* 13–20.

Greenberg, R., (1981). Amendments support SSI recipient's efforts to be self-supporting. *Accent on Living, 26,* 50–52.

Habes, D., & Putz-Anderson, V. (1985). The NIOSH program for evaluating biomechanical hazards in the workplace. *Journal of Safety Research, 16,* 49–60.

Hadler, N. (1977). Industrial rheumatology: Clinical investigations into the influence of the pattern of usage on the pattern of regional musculoskeletal disease. *Arthritis Rheumoid, 20,* 1019–1025.

Harvey-Krefting, L. (1985). The concept of work in occupational therapy: A historical review. *American Journal of Occupational Therapy, 39,* 301–307.

Heck, C. (1987). Job-site analysis for work capacity programming. *AOTA Physical Disabilities Special Interest Newsletter, 10,* 2–3.

Holman, C. , & Becker, V. (1987). Occupational therapists design work injury programs. *OT WEEK, 1,* 8–9.

Holmes, D. (1985). The role of the occupational therapist—Work evaluator. *American Journal of Occupational Therapy, 39,* 308–313.

Hopkins-Best, M. (1987). How to answer the unasked questions. *Accent on Living, 32,* 32–35.

Hursh, N., & Kerns, A. (1988). *Vocational assessment and evaluation systems: A comparison.* Boston: College-Hill Press.

Jacobs, K. (1990). From the Editor. *WORK, 1,* 5.

Jacobs, K. (1991a). From the Editor. *WORK, 1,* 6.

Jacobs, K. (1991b). *Occupational therapy: Work-related programs & assessments.* Boston: Little, Brown & Co.

Jacobs, K. (1992). From the Editor. *WORK, 2,* 1.

Jacobs, K. (1993). Work assessments and programming. In H. Hopkins & H. Smith (Eds.), *Willard and Spackman's occupational therapy* (8th ed., pp. 226–248). Philadelphia: J. B. Lippincott.

Jacobs, K., Bettencourt, C., Ellsworth, P., Lang, S., Levitan, C., Niemeyer, L., Place-Hayes, J., Ratcliffe, D., Reynolds-Lynch, K., & Sutherland, R. (1992). Statement: Occupational therapy service in work practice. *American Journal of Occupational Therapy, 46,* 1086–1088.

Job market for diabled: Good and bad news. (1976). *Accent of Living, 21*(2), 63.

Johnson, J. (1986). Wellness and occupational therapy. *American Journal of Occupational Therapy, 40,* 753–758.

Jones, V., Gagnon-Stryke, P., Fenton, S., & McGauley, P. (1991). Liberty mutual medical service center. In K. Jacobs (Ed.), *Occupational therapy: Work-related programs & assessments* (pp. 293–300). Boston: Little, Brown & Co.

Kemp, B., & Kleinplatz, F. (1985). Vocational rehabilitation of the older worker. *American Journal of Occupational Therapy, 39,* 322–326.

Kuder, F. (1960). *Kuder Occupational Interest Survey—Form dd.* Chicago: Science Research Associates.

Lechner, D., Roth, D., & Straaton, K., (1991). Functional capacity evaluation in work disability. *WORK, 1,* 37–47.

Maki, D., McCracken, H., Pape, D., & Scofield, M. (1979). A systems approach to vocational assessment. *Journal of Rehabilitation, 10,* 48–51.

Marshall, E. (1983). *Notes on situational assessment.* Unpublished manuscript. Loma Linda Department of Occupational Therapy, Loma Linda, CA.

Matheson, L. (1982). *Work capacity evaluation: A training manual for occupational therapists.* Trabuco Canyon: Rehabilitation Institute of Southern California.

Matheson, L., Ogden, L., Violette, K., & Schultz, K. (1985). Work hardening: Occupational therapy in industrial rehabilitation. *American Journal of Occupational Therapy, 39,* 314–321.

Mayer, T., Gatchel, R. J., Kishino, N., Keeley, J., Capra, P., Mayer H., Barnett, J., & Mooney, V. (1985). Objective assessment of spine function following industrial injury. *Industrial Injury, 10,* 481–493.

Maynard, M. (1986). Health promotion through employee assistance programs: A role for occupational therapists. *American Journal of Occupational Therapy, 40,* 771–776.

McCracken, N. (1991). Conceptualizing occupational therapy's role within vocational assessment: The cornerstone of effective program planning and marketing. *WORK, 1,* 77–83.

Miller, M. (1991). Functional assessments: A vital component of work injury management. *WORK, 1,* 6–10.

Morris, A. & Anderson, C. (1988). Pre-employment screening: The physical perspective. In S. Iserhagen (Ed.), *Work injury* (pp. 92105). Rockville, MD: Aspen Systems.

Niemeyer, L., Jacobs, K, Reynolds-Lynch, K., Bettencourt, C., & Lang, S. (1994). Outcome study. *American Journal of Occupational Therapy, 48,* 327–339.

Ogden-Niemeyer, L., & Jacobs, K. (1989). *Work hardening: State of the art.* Thorofare, NJ: Slack.

President's Committee on Employment of People with Disabilities. (1993). *ADA Brochure.* (Available from 1331 F Street NW, Washington, DC 20004)

Putz-Anderson, V. (Ed.). (1988). *Cumulative trauma disorders: A manual for musculoskeletal diseases of the upper limbs.* Bristol, PA: Taylor & Francis.

Putz-Anderson, V., & Waters, T. (1991, April). *Revisions in NIOSH guide to manual lifting.* Paper presented at the conference National Strategy for Occupational Musculoskeletal Injury Prevention—Implementation Issues and Research Needs, Ann Arbor, MI.

Rohmert, W. (1987). Physiological and psychological work load measurement and analysis. In G. Salvendy (Ed.), *Handbook of human factors* (pp. 402–452). New York: John Wiley & Sons.

Ryan, P. A. (1979). Widening their horizons: A model career development program for severely physically disabled youth. *Rehabilitation Literature,* 72–74.

Scheer, S. (1990). *Multidisciplinary perspectives in vocational assessment of impaired workers.* Rockville, MD: Aspen Systems.

Schwartz, R. (1991). Prevention of work-related injuries. In K. Jacobs (Ed.), *Occupational therapy: Work-related programs & assessments* (pp. 365–381). Boston: Little, Brown & Co.

Schwartz, R. (1993). Return-to-work programs. *WORK, 3,* 2–8.

Schwartz, R., & Jacobs, K. (1991). Body basics: A cognitive approach to body mechanics training in elementary school back pain prevention programs. *WORK, 2,* 53–60.

Shamberg, S. (1993). The accessibility consultant: A new role for occupational therapists under the Americans with Disabilities Act. *Occupational Therapy Practice, 4,* 14–23.

Smith, S., Cunningham, S., & Weinberg, R. (1983). Predicting reemployment of the physically disabled worker. *Occupational Therapy Journal of Research, 3,* 178–179.

Smith, S., Cunningham, S., & Weinberg, R. (1986). The predictive validity of the functional capacities evaluation. *American Journal of Occupational Therapy, 40,* 564–567.

Snook, S. (1988). Approaches to the control of back pain in industry: Job design, job placement and education/training. *State of the Art in Occupational Medicine. 3,* 45–59.

Tichauer, E. (1966). Some aspects of stress on forearm and hand in industry. *Journal of Occupational Medicine, 8,* 63–71.

Tichauer, E. (1978). *The biomechanical basis of ergonomics.* New York: John Wiley & Sons.

U.S. Department of Labor. (1970). *Manual for the uses General Aptitude Test Battery.* Washington, DC: U.S. Government Printing Office.

U.S. Department of Labor. (1991a). *Dictionary of occupational titles: The classification of jobs according to worker trait factors* (4th ed.). Washington, DC: U.S. Government Printing Office.

U.S. Department of Labor. (1991b). *Ergonomics program management guidelines for meatpacking plants.* Washington, DC: Occupational Safety and Health Administration.

Valpar International Corp. (1986). *Valpar component work samples.* (Available from 3801 East 34th Street, Tucson, AZ 85713)

Velozo, C. (1993). Work evaluations: Critique of the state of the art of functional assessment of work. *American Journal of Occupational Therapy, 47,* 203–209.

Velozo, C., Kielhofner, G., & Fisher, G. (1990). *A user's guide to the worker role interview.* Unpublished manuscript. Chicago: University of Illinois at Chicago.

Webster's Ninth New Collegiate Dictionary. (1984). Springfield, MA: Merriam-Webster.

What's on the books in your state? (1992). *CTD News, 1,* 2.

Wyrick, J., Niemeyer, L., Ellexson, M., Jacobs, K., & Taylor, S. (1991). Occupational therapy work-hardening programs: A demographic study. *American Journal of Occupational Therapy, 45,* 109–112.

Your job interview. (1978). *Accent on Living 23,* 40–43.

Supplementary Resources

American Fitness in Business. (342 Massachusetts Avenue, Indianapolis, IN 46204; phone: 317-636-6621, fax: 317-638-0539).

Baltimore Therapeutic Equipment Co. (7455-L New Ridge Road, Hanover, MD 21076)

Cybex. (2100 Smithtown Avenue, Ronkonkoma, NY 11779)

EPIC-WEST. (600 South Grand Avenue, Suite 101, Santa Ana, CA 92705)

Institute for Crippled and Disabled (ICD). (340 East 24th Street, New York, NY 10010; 212-679-0100)

Regaining Participation in Leisure-Time Activities

Lyn Jongbloed and Marilyn Ernest-Conibear

OBJECTIVES

After studying this chapter, the reader will be able to:
1. Understand the relation of **leisure** to **work** and **self-care.**
2. Justify **leisure** intervention as part of any occupational therapy program.
3. Identify the purposes of a variety of **leisure** assessments.
4. Identify major categories of occupational therapy intervention related to **leisure** participation of adults with physical disabilities.

The concept of **leisure** as part of the triune of human **occupational performance (self-care, work,** and **leisure)** is broadly accepted in the occupational therapy literature (Katz & Sachs, 1991). However, it has yet to assume an equal importance in occupational therapy practice compared with **self-care** and **work.** Bundy (1993) noted the paradox of play, or **leisure,** activities by pointing out that in our Western society **leisure** is not taken seriously because it is not considered to be productive. If therapists do not view **leisure** as important, then it is difficult to justify the time and costs of assessment and intervention of **leisure** activities to others, such as administrators and third-party payers. As occupational therapists, we acknowledge the importance of **leisure** and yet slide quickly over it in practice or make apologies for attempts to intervene in **leisure** activities by referring to **leisure** as a form of **work.** Bundy (1993) defined this paradox clearly:

> We recognize that play is a powerful tool through which we can diminish the consequences of real life and promote our clients' abilities to express themselves, yet we fear the repercussions of being thought less than serious about

the real-life difficulties confronting our clients. We want to take play seriously, but if we do, we may not be taken seriously ourselves. The use and promotion of play presents us with a paradox (p. 218).

It appears, then, that to justify our philosophical belief in the value of **leisure** we must educate ourselves regarding the importance of **leisure** in the lives of our clients. Only then can we be comfortable in justifying the time and effort we should spend on occupational therapy intervention related to **leisure.** As Reed (1984) pointed out, "The challenge is to explain the role of leisure as an occupational area, a changing social phenomenon and a means of developing competence and increasing satisfaction for individuals" (p. 273).

DEFINITIONS OF LEISURE

One of the difficulties in defining **leisure** is that it is not easy to approach the topic objectively. The definition of **leisure** tends to be determined by the therapist's view of what it ought to be, which is, in turn, influenced by society and culture. Reed (1984) emphasized that **leisure** is a concept that is strongly influenced by culture and that as culture changes so does the concept of **leisure.** In contrast, the concept of **work** has continued to have a consistent meaning over time. Traditionally, **leisure** has been viewed as time free from **work** and daily living/**self-care** tasks or participation in nonpaying, and thus unproductive, tasks.

Although there is no one universally recognized definition of **leisure,** researchers have identified some of its basic characteristics: enjoyment, relaxation, freedom of choice, intrinsic motivation, commitment, control, and challenge (Iso-Ahola, 1979; Shaw, 1985). Given these elements, **leisure** may be defined as "experience associated with self-determined participation in any activity which is characterized by pleasure,

GLOSSARY _____

Environment—(1) Cultural environment: The ethos and value system of a particular people or group. (2) Physical environment: The natural or man-made surroundings of an individual and structural living space boundaries. (3) Social environment: The patterns of relationships of people living in an organized community.

Integration—Measures and practices that maximize a person's potential participation in the mainstream of his culture.

Leisure—Components of life free from work and self-care activities.

Normalization—Making available to people with disabilities patterns and conditions of everyday life that are as close as possible to the norms and patterns of the mainstream of society.

Occupational performance—Activities carried out by the client in the areas of self-care, work, and leisure influenced by environment.

Self-care—Activities or tasks done routinely to maintain the client's health and well-being, considering the environment and social factors.

Work—Activities or tasks done to provide meaning and support to the self, family, and society.

enjoyment, fulfillment, competence, and control" (Caldwell & Smith, 1988, p. S45). In occupational therapy intervention, activities that are pursued voluntarily (alone or with others), that allow the person with a disability to feel in control of the situation, that match the individual's skills with a challenge, and that are enjoyable are **leisure** experiences (Caldwell & Smith, 1988). When considering the client, one might indeed place qualifying emphasis on the words *self-determined* and *control*.

THE MEANING OF LEISURE

Leisure is idiosyncratic and personal. Thus one individual may value daydreaming, reading, and walking with friends in a park, while another may gain satisfaction from running, planting a garden, acting as a volunteer, or going on a pub crawl with friends (Hutchinson, 1984).

Leisure participation is also affected by the developmental stage of one's life. During early and middle adulthood, **work** represents the major path toward achievement, while **leisure** allows the opportunity to explore and develop competence without fear of failure. Some people may not have the chance to achieve at **work** and seek, instead, to achieve in the sphere of **leisure** (e.g., music and athletics). Thus **leisure** may act as a source of meaning that complements **work** or compensates for a lack of meaning at **work** (Barris & Kielhofner, 1985).

Leisure interests may also serve to structure the unobligated time of older adults. Older persons tend to spend more time than younger individuals in activities that are solitary and sedentary (Rogers & Snow, 1985).

THE PURPOSE OF LEISURE

Leisure experiences are often vehicles for:

1. Acquiring personal skills such as learning to play the guitar, physical skills such as learning to ski, and social skills such as learning to dance.

2. Developing self-awareness and confidence, e.g., joining a Toastmasters Club to gain confidence and skills in public speaking.
3. Sharing with friends and developing close relationships, e.g., taking cooking lessons so that one can feel comfortable inviting friends in for an evening of food, conversation, and company.
4. Participating in the community and feeling part of one's neighborhood such as joining a neighborhood special-interest group or attending city council meetings to become aware of community problems and plans.

For an individual with a disability, these four dimensions are especially important, because a disability can be either a cause of or a reason for social isolation and loss of previously acquired personal skills (Hutchinson, 1984).

Normalization, Integration, and Community Participation

Over the last decade, there has been considerable emphasis on the rights of persons with disabilities to live and participate in the community. This includes persons with disabilities having the right to, and opportunities for, the range of **leisure** experiences to which other citizens are entitled. One of the most significant changes that occurred was the realization that community agencies were responsible for providing services for all citizens, including persons with disabilities. Thus a shift occurred from voluntary associations and specialized agencies to community agencies (Hutchinson, 1984).

The emphasis on **normalization** and integration has influenced the development and planning of recreation programs that formerly focused solely on the needs of persons with disabilities. For example, the Special Olympics and the games for the physically disabled now offer more integrated programs (Hutchinson, 1984).

OCCUPATIONAL THERAPY STUDIES ON LEISURE

Although **leisure** is considered to be a part of human **occupational performance**, occupational therapists have contributed relatively little to the theoretical and practical knowledge about **leisure** (Bundy, 1993). They have conducted much more research on **self-care** and **work** than on **leisure**.

Studies on **leisure** in the occupational therapy literature vary in focus. Marino-Schorn (1986) showed a significant relationship between morale and the balance of time spent in **work**, rest, and **leisure** in a retired population. Levine (1984) demonstrated the strength of culture as a filter through which clients determine the direction and degree of their involvement in **self-care, work,** and **leisure** activities. Morgan and Jongbloed (1990) examined the factors that influenced **leisure** activities following a stroke and used Kielhofner's model of human occupation to organize the data.

Kautzmann (1984) formulated and categorized a list of **leisure** activities to be used as an instrument for assessing the **leisure** activities of adults with arthritis or degenerative joint disease. Other studies examined **leisure** activities of persons with tetraplegia (Rogers & Figone, 1978), with Parkinson's disease (Manson & Caird, 1985), and with cardiac pathology (Fitts & Howe, 1987).

In addition to examining **leisure** patterns with specific client populations, therapists have looked at the meaning of specific activities that could be applied to **leisure** activities (Katz, 1991; Nelson, Thompson, & Moore, 1982), the meaning of *time* in relation to **leisure** (Peloquin, 1991; Rosenthal & Howe, 1984; Yerxa & Locker, 1990), and the relationship of motivation to activity participation (Doble, 1988; Ray & Heppe, 1986). Although the study by Ray and Heppe (1986) was carried out in relation to older adults (retired or near retirement), the findings are relevant for therapists who work with those who, temporarily or permanently, are not engaged in paid employment, i.e., the physically disabled. For example, Ray and Heppe found that commitment to a few activities was a more important indicator of happiness than the number of activities pursued and that activities with worklike qualities were more satisfying than any other activities. Doble's (1988) study identified four determinants of intrinsic motivation: orientation of the task **environment,** the meaningfulness of the activity, the opportunity the activity affords for personal control, and the ability of the activity to generate feelings of competence.

To date only one study has examined efficacy of occupational therapy intervention related to **leisure** participation. Jongbloed and Morgan (1991) randomly assigned 40 discharged stroke clients either to an experimental group that received occupational therapy intervention related to **leisure** activities or to a control group that received no intervention related to **leisure.** Results showed no statistically significant differences between the experimental and control groups in activity involvement or satisfaction with that involvement. The authors stated that there are likely several reasons for these findings. First, the intervention was limited in scope (i.e., only five therapy visits). Second, many environmental factors strongly influence activity participation and satisfaction. Third, the instruments used to measure outcome—Level of Free-Time Activities and Level of Satisfaction with Free-Time Activities from the Katz Adjustment Index (Katz & Lyerly, 1963)—did not adequately take into account the clients' roles and **environments.**

BARRIERS TO PARTICIPATION IN LEISURE ACTIVITIES

Various studies have identified barriers that prevent individuals from achieving an optimal level of **leisure** participation (Costilow et al., 1982; Witt & Goodale, 1981). Costilow et al. (1982) identified the following types of barriers. A barrier in the area of social skills or communication is demonstrated by people who avoid experiences that require social interaction. A barrier in the area of motivation or decision making is demonstrated by people who require others to initiate involvement. Rigid schedules and lack of time for intrinsically satisfying experiences are evidence of a time barrier. Monetary barriers are shown by people who do not feel they have the financial resources to participate in activities of their choice. The lack of opportunities barrier is evident when people make choices but perceive that they have few alternatives from which to choose. Individuals may also lack the ability to participate in **leisure** activities at their desired level. Closely related to lack of abilities is the barrier caused by poor health or disability. Health directly affects individuals' levels of involvement, opportunities, and abilities and consequently influences their ability to attain a satisfying **leisure** lifestyle. The final barrier is environmental. Resources that are physically inaccessible are not usable and, therefore, reduce the number of **leisure** opportunities for individuals with mobility impairments.

The Effect of Physical Disability on Participation in Leisure-Time Activities

The impact of disability on people is a complex and individual matter. Physical disabilities are disturbances to neurologic and/or musculoskeletal components of skill. The disability may reduce the client's ability to perform and erode his belief in his skill. People with physical disabilities frequently encounter a wider variety of barriers and are inhibited to a greater extent in their **leisure** involvement than people without disabilities, but barriers *within* the individual who has a disability are not necessarily the most important barriers to be overcome. Hutchinson (1980) asked people with disabilities to identify barriers to community involvement. The most significant barriers were the following.

1. Financial (low pensions and unemployment combined with high costs), e.g., a person with a disability may wish to join a special-interest club that has a minimal membership fee, but the only way he can attend meetings is by taking an expensive taxi ride that he cannot afford.
2. (a) Lack of legislation to ensure equal rights and access to community facilities and resources, e.g., the person may wish to go swimming in the local swimming pool but finds he cannot be admitted because the managers of the pool feel there are not enough lifeguards to take special note of people with disabilities and not enough staff to help such individuals maneuver in and out of the pool. (b) Inconvenient and inaccessible facilities, e.g., a person with a physical disability may wish to visit the local public library but finds the building is inaccessible to wheelchairs, because there has been no local legislation requiring public buildings to be accessible to all citizens.
3. Lack of a continuum of services that would enable participation at a variety of levels, e.g., a person with a disability may wish to join a keep-fit club only to find that the program is aimed at young, able-bodied individuals and the club is unwilling to add a program for lower-functioning individuals.

Much lower on the list came items that reflected individual skills, such as lack of self-confidence and low social skills—areas in which most occupational therapists feel confident assisting clients to improve.

The relatively recent emphasis on the rights of people with disabilities has reduced some of these barriers. However, occupational therapists need to be aware that factors in the social, political, and economic **environment** may be barriers to **leisure** participation of people with disabilities and that focusing primarily on individual skill development may not be sufficient to alleviate the larger barriers.

ASSESSMENT

The occupational areas of **self-care**/daily living, **work,** and **leisure** overlap and are integrated into the occupational schema of an individual (Reed, 1984). The basic purpose of occupational therapy is to enable the client to engage in roles, tasks, and activities that are important to him, i.e., that are related to his quality of life. Occupational therapy assessment, therefore, cannot focus solely on the client's **leisure** activities. Occupational therapy assessment should explore the client's view of all aspects of his **occupational performance,** with **leisure** being emphasized equally with **work** and **self-care.** Therapy should determine what roles, tasks, and activities are important in the client's life and the context in which he functions (McKenna, 1993).

According to Dunn (1987), **leisure** assessment procedures can be classified into three categories: (1) published activity inventories; (2) behavioral performance measures; and (3) locally constructed instruments. Activity inventories measure participation in **leisure** activities as indications of **leisure** interests (McKechnie, 1975). The major focus of these inventories is on the structure of activities. This is based on the assumption that participation in activities with similar structures will provide the individual with similar levels of satisfaction.

Another group of assessments emphasizes the performance of **leisure** activity skills (Berryman & Lefebvre, 1981). These instruments have been designed to measure behavioral skills needed for participating in various **leisure** activities. The underlying assumption behind these procedures is that specific cognitive, perceptual, and motor skills can be identified as problematic and improved through individual treatment. Thus, once the particular skill is improved, participation in **leisure** activities will be improved (Dunn, 1987). Locally constructed instruments, designed for use in a particular setting, usually lack information regarding reliability and validity. The types of assessments identified above have demonstrated a lack of sophistication in conceptualization. They have been found to be unidimensional, focusing on a single aspect of **leisure** activity and ignoring the individual element of participation in leisure-time activities. Researchers have published evidence that discounts the validity of the theoretical structure on which many existing assessment procedures are based (Dunn, 1987).

Trombly (1993) believed that there should be a universal occupational therapy assessment procedure and that, because length of stays with the health care system are generally short, assessments should be quick and easy to administer. The *Canadian Occupational Performance Measure* (COPM) is intended to be universal and quick (Law et al., 1991, 1994; Pollock, 1993). It was designed to assess all spheres of **occupational performance—self-care,** productivity (**work**), and **leisure**—for a client within his **environment.** Based on a semistructured interview, COPM is a five-step process that measures individual, client-identified problem areas in daily function. Two scores, one for performance and one for satisfaction with performance, are obtained. The measure takes into account the client's roles and role expectations and, in focusing on the client's own **environment,** ensures the relevance of the problem to the client (Law et al., 1990). Studies documenting the reliability and validity of COPM are in progress.

The following case study illustrates the use of COPM as an assessment.

CASE 1

Mr. C was a 62-year-old janitor unable to return to **work** following a right cardiovascular accident (CVA). His previous activities had involved **work,** home maintenance, church, and occasional visits with family and friends. Following the CVA, Mr. C's son assumed responsibility for home maintenance, and Mr. C did not attend church, as he was afraid of embarrassing himself because of his incontinence. In addition, he was unable to resume driving, so visiting was limited to times when his son was available to drive. Mr. C expressed his acceptance of not returning to **work** but was frustrated by his inactivity. He had no knowledge of **leisure** opportunities in his neighborhood and, in fact, had very few ideas about activities he might enjoy, whether at home or in the community. He also had no knowledge of incontinence control systems that would have relieved his fears and allowed him to enjoy longer outings.

CASE STUDY

Administering and Scoring of COPM

Step 1: Problem Identification

During the course of the interview, the therapist and client discussed the kinds of activities the client needed to, wanted to, or was expected to perform. The client then rated his ability to carry out these activities on a scale of 1 to 10 and his satisfaction with the way in which he could carry them out, also on a scale of 1 to 10. This discussion of the following areas led to the creation of the client-identified problem list.
Self-care:
  Personal care;
  Functional mobility;
  Community management, e.g., transportation, shopping;

Productivity:
  Paid/unpaid work;
  Household management;
Leisure:
  Quiet recreation, e.g., hobbies, crafts, reading, watching television;
  Active recreation, e.g., sports, outings, travel, club activities;
  Socialization, e.g., visiting, phone calls, correspondence.
  Job cost
Client-identified problems:
  Transportation—cannot drive and unsure if he is able to use a bus;
  Home maintenance;
  Unsure what quiet activities he would enjoy or could manage with the use of one hand.;
  Visiting;
  Going to church.

Step 2: Problem Weighing

The client was then asked to rate the importance of each problem activity on a 1 to 10 scale, with a 10 being the most important. These scores acted as weighing factors in the scoring of the client's performance and satisfaction for each activity.

Step 3: Scoring

After the client had rated the importance of these activities, the five most urgent problems were identified and included in COPM form (Table 18.1) along with his performance and satisfaction ratings. Both the ability and satisfaction ratings are multiplied by the importance rating to determine a baseline score. The baseline scores can range from 1 to 100, with 100 indicating a high degree of importance, ability, and satisfaction. Obviously, then, a **leisure** problem with two baseline scores of 100 is not a problem at all and should be removed from the problem list. On the other hand, a **leisure** problem with baseline scores considerably below 100 requires intervention.

These two scores, one for performance and one for satisfaction, are divided by the number of rated activities to provide scores that can be used for comparisons across time.

Step 4: Reassessment Following Intervention

The time interval depends on the judgment of the client and therapist. The therapist again requests the client to rate his performance and satisfaction with the activities that were identified as problems in Step 1. To calculate the change in the client over time, these ratings are multiplied by the original importance ratings, summed, and divided.

Step 5: Follow-Up Phase

The purpose of the follow-up step is to plan for discharge or for treatment continuation. Using a new COPM form, the therapist repeats the process described in Step 1 to determine if any

Table 18.1. COPM Scores

Problems	Importance	Performance	Satisfaction	Importance × Performance[a]	Importance × Satisfaction[a]
Transportation	10	1	1	10	10
Home maintenance	5	5	4	25	20
Quiet recreation	5	2	3	10	15
Active recreation	9	2	1	18	9
Socialization	7	2	3	14	21

[a]Totals: (1) Total importance × performance/number of problems = 77/5 = 15.4. (2) Total importance × satisfaction/number of problems = 70/5 = 14.

occupational performance problems remain or if new difficulties have developed.

This case study showed how COPM could be used to identify what the client views as his most significant problems in the area of **occupational performance.** There are two major benefits to using this assessment process. First, the client's priorities may be found to be different from the therapist's priorities. Second, the assessment process may help the client gain or clarify insight into his own abilities and difficulties in his **occupational performance.**

Whatever assessment is used, it is essential that the therapist ask the client to identify problems related to **leisure** participation and decide how important these are in relation to **work** and **self-care** roles and activities.

The timing of assessments and intervention related to **leisure** must also be considered. It may be prudent to establish a positive relationship with the client before administering an assessment (Law et al., 1990). Furthermore, it may be premature to expect a client to pursue leisure-time activities until his medical, **work,** financial, and living situations are under control. However, as motivation has a great bearing on the client's cooperation, the therapist may be able to incorporate the client's existing **leisure** interests into various parts of the treatment program.

INTERVENTION STRATEGIES FOR LEISURE ACTIVITIES

According to Christiansen (1991), the major intervention categories in occupational therapy are

1. Use of occupation as a therapeutic medium;
2. Education and training strategies;
3. Strategies for sensory and neuromotor remediation;
4. Application of technological aids and devices;
5. Modification of the physical **environment.**

Each of these intervention categories is examined below in relation to **leisure** participation.

Use of Occupation as a Therapeutic Medium

The use of occupation as a therapeutic medium includes strategies in which occupation as activity, task, or role is planned with therapeutic intent.

CASE 2

Mrs. Green was a 50-year-old widow with multiple sclerosis. A primary goal in occupational therapy was to increase arm strength and coordination. The therapist initially thought of using various checker games that could be played at various heights and with light to heavy weighted checkers. However, on reviewing Mrs. Green's **leisure** interests, it was found that although she watched television, read, and phoned friends and family, she was not satisfied with the way she was able to use all the **leisure** time she had. She had always been interested in creative arts involving color and design but had never had the time or opportunity to develop this interest. Therefore, the therapist introduced a number of possible activities to Mrs. Green that could be adapted to fulfill the primary goal and also lead to a long-lasting and satisfying **leisure** activity that she could continue at home. Mrs. Green chose to learn macramé. She first learned the basic steps, using a coarse cord while sitting at a table, and then progressed to working with the macramé suspended higher and higher on a frame. She moved from working with no resistance to working with weights on her wrists, from working with a coarse cord to working with finer cords, and from working for brief periods of time to working for longer periods of time as her strength and coordination increased and her interest and skills with design, texture, and color possibilities increased.

CASE 3

Carlos was a 27-year-old architect who sustained a traumatic head injury in a car accident. A primary goal in occupational therapy was to stimulate higher cognitive functioning and increase attention, concentration, memory, and problem-solving skills. On first meeting Carlos, the therapist found him to be depressed, confused, and uncooperative. The therapist first thought of using various memory games and quizzes to attain the primary goal, but on examining Carlos's assessment, she found he was injured while traveling to another city to attend a duplicate bridge tournament. The therapist found that, outside of his **work,** Carlos's sole **leisure** interest had been duplicate bridge. The therapist then planned to use card games of varying degrees of cognitive complexity, memory requirements, and difficulty to attain the primary goals. After showing Carlos a list of the games they could use that would help him progress from simple games such as fish and hearts to more complex games such as whist and, finally, bridge, Carlos was a more enthusiastic client.

Education and Training Strategies

Education and training strategies include those in which the therapist uses education or training to enable the client to acquire skills needed for performing **leisure** activities or roles, or to use remaining abilities to compensate for skill deficits.

CASE 4

Mrs. Lee was a 60-year-old cancer client undergoing intensive radiation and chemotherapy, which results in generalized fatigue. She was able to accept the need to have someone come into her home to assist with cooking, cleaning, and shopping, but she felt a particular loss in her inability to continue with her volunteer work with a group of seniors at her church. The therapist obtained information for Mrs. Lee on various volunteer agencies in her community. After checking on the requirements and needs of the various agencies, Mrs. Lee found that, despite her fatigue, she could still volunteer as a phone friend to a number of elderly house-bound persons. Her need to serve others was satisfied by accepting the responsibility to telephone three people every day to check on their well-being.

CASE 5

Mr. Reed was admitted to hospital following a myocardial infarction. He was the owner of a large engineering firm and was married with two sons and a daughter who no longer live at home. He had diabetes mellitus and a family history of coronary problems. He spent an excessive amount of time at **work** because he was driven by a desire for business success. He had never valued **leisure** activities and was consequently unaware of what activities he might enjoy, apart from watching television. Occupational therapy intervention included a graded activities program and the monitoring of his cardiac capacity. The therapist also provided education regarding relaxation skills and stress management techniques and helped Mr. Reed reexamine his values related to **work,** family, and **leisure.** He began to recognize the importance of including more **leisure** activities in his life and of doing more activities with his wife. His wife was included in some of these education sessions. Mr. Reed realized that he needed to change his lifestyle and that this would be a difficult, slow process that would require the support of his wife.

Strategies for Sensory and Neuromotor Remediation

Strategies for sensory and neuromotor remediation frequently use principles of reflex maturation and neurophysiology.

CASE 6

Mr. dos Santos was a 70-year-old retired teacher with left-sided paralysis following a stroke. His arm was more severely affected than his leg. The therapist started a neurodevelopmental treatment program involving active, resisted movements against the therapist's hand, but Mr. dos Santos expressed obvious frustration with the treatment, as he could not "see the sense in all this—I just want to go home." The therapist discovered that his hobby since his retirement was woodworking, particularly making name and address signs for his friends and relatives. The therapist then designed a simple woodworking project for which the wood was positioned so that attempts by Mr. dos Santos to sand it with fine to coarse grades of sandpaper attached to a sanding block resulted in the appropriate resisted movements of the affected limb and greater participation in, and enthusiasm for, treatment.

CASE 7

Joanne was a 16-year-old high school student who acquired a closed head injury and right hemiparalysis as a result of a motor vehicle accident. She was transferred to a rehabilitation unit after 13 weeks in acute care. Before her accident, her **leisure** interests were cooking, gymnastics, and socializing with friends. Her friends were very supportive and visited her frequently. One of the treatment goals was to facilitate voluntary movement in her right upper extremity using Bobath techniques. Rolling cookie dough accomplished this objective, and Joanne enjoyed this activity because it produced a tangible product she could share with the staff and other clients on her ward as well as her friends.

Application of Technical Aids and Devices

Intervention that includes both high- and low-technology aids and equipment may enable a person to carry out activities or roles despite limitations in abilities or skills.

CASE 8

John was an 18-year-old high school student who sustained a C_{5-6} tetraplegia in a diving accident. Although he had some use of his shoulders and elbows, he had very little use of his hands. Once his medical situation had stabilized, the therapist approached him to show him various aids he could use to feed himself, comb his hair, and brush his teeth. John felt that the devices were, in his words "weird and ugly" and refused even to try them, despite the therapist's efforts to convince him of their usefulness. The therapist thought that if John could be happy with one device, he might well be willing to try others. The therapist noted that, according to John's initial assessment, he had intended to attend a university to study computer sciences. During their discussions, John said that he and a number of his friends had formed their own computer hackers club and communicated with other hackers all over the world via computer bulletin boards. The therapist took John to the department computer, but after one clumsy poke at the keyboard, John asked to be taken back to his room. Once there, the therapist described a mouth stick that would enable John to continue using his computer. John's friends, who were visiting him at the time, encouraged him to try the device so that they could communicate with each other over the department computer. They also said they could bring John's own computer to the hospital so he could use it there. With such enthusiastic support, John tried the mouth stick with the computer. He was immediately successful in making contact with his friends through the modem hookup and, shortly after, offered to try the other **self-care** devices the therapist had suggested.

Modification of the Physical Environment

Modification of the **environment** may include changing the physical, social, or arousal properties of the **environment.**

CASE 9

Mrs. Jones was a 63-year-old widow who lived alone in a small, single-level cottage. She had diabetes and, over time, had lost much of her vision. She was in the hospital because of circulation problems and had undergone a below-knee amputation. Because of her obesity, age, poor vision, and circulation problems, it was felt that she would not be a successful candidate for an artificial leg. It was decided that, with some home modifications, she would be able to continue to care for herself in her own home. However, Mrs. Jones was not completely happy because she had been known in her neighborhood for her small but beautiful flower gardens, and she felt that she would no longer be able to manage the gardens—her pride and joy. Mrs. Jones was financially comfortable, and the therapist described how the garden beds could be built up so that she could reach everything from her wheelchair. In this way, all the flowers would be even closer to her and she could identify each flower both by smell and by the Braille tags she had previously stuck by each plant.

SUMMARY

The purpose of this chapter is to introduce the reader to **leisure** as an area of **occupational performance.** The chapter describes the meaning and purpose of **leisure.** It outlines some occupational therapy assessment and intervention strategies related to **leisure** participation of adults with physical disabilities. The chapter is not intended either as an exhaustive treatment of occupational therapy interventions or as an indication of all possible physical disabilities that could influence ability to participate in leisure-time activities. The various recommended treatment strategies require examination in research to validate their effectiveness.

STUDY QUESTIONS

1. Why are leisure-time pursuits important in a person's life?
2. Why has there been so little emphasis on occupational therapy intervention in leisure in the past?
3. How would you justify the time and effort you feel should be spent on leisure intervention in occupational therapy?
4. What are some barriers to leisure participation in your own life?
5. What can you do, if anything, to overcome some of those barriers?
6. How do the barriers to leisure participation in your life differ from the barriers to leisure participation for a 20-year-old individual with high-level tetraplegia?
7. Do you think that assigning a leisure activity to all clients (e.g., deciding that all the clients will be taken to play bingo) would be an effective intervention? Justify your answer.
8. What could you do if a client with two new upper extremity prostheses expressed a strong desire to play chess and you did not know how to play chess?
9. Think of an example of a leisure activity that you are familiar with and describe its structure and the skills required to carry out the activity. What are the inherent difficulties in selecting leisure activities for a client based on (1) the structure of the activity or (2) the skills required to carry out an activity?

REFERENCES

Barris, R., & Kielhofner, G. (1985). Early and middle adulthood. In G. Kielhofner (Ed.), *A model of human occupation. Theory and application* (pp. 112–122). Baltimore: Williams & Wilkins.

Berryman, K., & Lefebvre, C. (1981). *The recreation behavior inventory.* Denton, TX: Leisure Learning.

Bundy, A. (1993). Assessment of play and leisure: Delineation of the problem. *American Journal of Occupational Therapy, 47,* 217–222.

Caldwell, L., & Smith, E. (1988). Leisure: An overlooked component of health promotion. *Canadian Journal of Public Health, 79,* S44–48.

Christiansen, C. (1991). Occupational therapy: Intervention for life performance. In C. Christiansen & C. Baum (Eds.), *Occupational therapy: Overcoming human performance deficits* (pp. 3–43). Thorofare, NJ: Slack.

Costilow, A., Ellis, G., Forsyth, P., & Witt, P. (1982). Barriers to leisure opportunities. In P. A Witt, G. Ellis, T. Aguilar, S. Niles, A. Costilow, P. Forsyth, N. Carnes, N. Silva, & D. Compton (Eds.), *The leisure diagnostic battery user's guide.* Denton: North Texas State University Press.

Doble, S. (1988). Intrinsic motivation and clinical practice: The key to understanding. *Canadian Journal of Occupational Therapy, 55,* 75–81.

Dunn, J. (1987). *Generalizability of the leisure diagnostic battery.* Unpublished doctoral dissertation, University of Illinois at Urbana-Champaign.

Fitts, H., & Howe, M. (1987). Use of leisure time by cardiac patients. *American Journal of Occupational Therapy, 41,* 583–589.

Hutchinson, P. (1980). Perceptions of disabled persons regarding barriers to community participation. *Journal of Leisurability, 7*(3), 4–16.

Hutchinson, P. (1984), Social, recreation and leisure opportunities. In N. J. Marlett, R. Gall, & A. Wight-Felske (Eds.), *Dialogue on disability: A Canadian perspective: Vol. 1. The service system* (pp. 47–60). Calgary, Alta., Canada: University of Calgary Press.

Iso-Ahola, S. (1979). Basic dimensions of definitions of leisure. *Journal of Leisure Research, 15,* 15–26.

Jongbloed, L., & Morgan, D. (1991). An investigation of involvement in leisure activities. *American Journal of Occupational Therapy, 45,* 420–427.

Katz, M., & Lyerly, S. (1963). Methods for measuring adjustment and social behavior in the community: Rationale, description, discriminative validity and scale development. *Psychological Reports, 13,* 503–535.

Katz, N. (1991). Meanings ascribed to four craft activities before and after extensive learning. *Occupational Therapy Journal of Research, 11,* 24–39.

Katz, N., & Sachs, D. (1991). Meaning ascribed to major professional concepts: A comparison of occupational therapy students and practitioners in the United States and Israel. *American Journal of Occupational Therapy, 45,* 137–145.

Kautzmann, L. (1984). Identifying leisure interests: A self-assessment approach for adults with arthritis. *Occupational Therapy in Health Care, 1*(2), 45–52.

Law, M., Baptiste, S., Carswell-Opzoomer, A., McColl, M., Polatajko, H., & Pollock, N. (1991). *The Canadian Occupational Performance Measure.* Toronto, Ont.: Canadian Association of Occupational Therapists.

Law, M., Baptiste, S., Carswell-Opzoomer, A., McColl, M., Polatajko, H., & Pollock, N. (1994). *The Canadian Occupational Performance Measure* (2nd ed.). Toronto, Ont.: Canadian Association of Occupational Therapists.

Law, M., Baptiste, S., McColl, M., Opzoomer, A., Polatajko, H., & Pollock, N. (1990). The Canadian Occupational Performance Measure: An outcome measure for occupational therapy. *Canadian Journal of Occupational Therapy, 57,* 82–87.

Levine, R. (1984). The cultural aspect of home care delivery. *American Journal of Occupational Therapy, 38,* 734–738.

Manson, L., & Caird, F. (1985). Survey of the hobbies and transport of patients with Parkinson's disease. *British Journal of Occupational Therapy, 48,* 199–200.

Marino-Schorn, J. (1986). Morale, work and leisure in retirement. *Physical and Occupational Therapy in Geriatrics, 4,* 49–59.

McKechnie, G. (1975). *Manual for the leisure activities blank.* Palo Alto, CA: Consulting Psychologists.

McKenna, K. (1993). Quality of life: A question of functional outcomes or the fulfillment of life plans. *Australian Occupational Therapy Journal, 40,* 33–35.

Morgan, D., & Jongbloed, L. (1990). Factors influencing leisure activities following a stroke: An exploratory study. *Canadian Journal of Occupational Therapy, 57,* 223–229.

Nelson, C., Thompson, G., & Moore, J. (1982). Identification of factors of affective meaning in four selected activities. *American Journal of Occupational Therapy, 36,* 381–387.

Peloquin, S. (1991). Time as a commodity: Reflections and implications. *American Journal of Occupational Therapy, 45,* 147–154.

Pollock, N. (1993). Client-centered assessment. *American Journal of Occupational Therapy, 47,* 298–301.

Ray, R., & Heppe, G. (1986). Older adult happiness: Contributions of activity breadth and intensity. *Physical and Occupational Therapy in Geriatrics, 4*(4), 31–43.

Reed, K. (1984). *Models of practice in occupational therapy.* Baltimore: Williams & Wilkins.

Rogers, J., & Figone, J. (1978). The avocational pursuits of rehabilitants with traumatic quadriplegia. *American Journal of Occupational Therapy, 32,* 571–576.

Rogers, J., & Snow, T. (1985). Later adulthood. In G. Kielhofner (Ed.), *A model of human occupation. Theory and application* (pp. 123–133).Baltimore: Williams & Wilkins.

Rosenthal, L., & Howe, M. (1984). Activity patterns and leisure concepts: A comparison of temporal adaptation among day versus night shift workers. *Occupational Therapy in Mental Health, 4*(2), 59–78.

Shaw, S. (1985). The meaning of leisure in everyday life. *Leisure Sciences, 7,* 1–24.

Trombly, C. (1993). Anticipating the future: Assessment of occupational function. *American Journal of Occupational Therapy, 47,* 253–257.

Witt, P. A., & Goodale, T. (1981). Barriers to leisure and stage of family lifestyle. *Leisure Sciences, 4*(1), 29–50.

Yerxa, E., & Locker, S. (1990). Quality of time use by adults with spinal cord injuries. *American Journal of Occupational Therapy, 44,* 318–326.

SUPPLEMENTARY RESOURCES

Suggested Readings

Accent on living. Quarterly journal that includes many ideas for leisure activities for the physically disabled. (Available from Cheever Publishing, Inc., Gillum Road and High Drive, P.O. Box 700, Bloomington, IL 61702)

Bauer, J. *Riding for rehabilitation: A guide for handicapped riders and their instructors.* (Available from Can Ride, 209 Deloraine Avenue, Toronto, Ont. M5M 2B2 Canada)

Handicapped Boater's Association Magazine. (Available from P.O. Box 1134, Ansonia Station, NY 10023)

Hedley, E. *Boating for the handicapped: Guidelines for the physically disabled.* (Available from Products Manager, Human Resources Center, I. U. Willets Road, Albertson, NY 11507)

National Spinal Cord Injury Association. *Spinal cord injury life.* (Available from the National Spinal Cord Injury Association, 545 Concord Avenue, Suite 29, Cambridge, MA 02138)

Resources

American Wheelchair Bowling Association. (N54W15858 Larkspur Lane, Menomonee Falls, WI 53051)

Blind Outdoor Leisure Development (BOLD). (533 East Main Street, Aspen, CO 81611)

Breckenridge Outdoor Education Center. (P.O. Box 697, Breckenridge, CO 80424)

Disabled Artists' Network. (P.O. Box 20781, New York, NY 10025)

Mobility International (P.O. Box 3551, Eugene, OR 97403)

National Association of Sports for Cerebral Palsy. (66 East 34th Street, New York, NY 10016)

National Foundation of Wheelchair Tennis. (4000 MacArthur Boulevard, Newport Beach, CA 92660)

National Handicapped Sports and Recreation Association. (Capitol Hill Station, P.O. Box 18664, Denver, CO 80218)

National Inconvenienced Sportsmen's Association (NISA). (3738 Walnut Avenue, Carmichael, CA 95608)

National Wheelchair Athletic Association. (40-24 62nd Street, Woodside, NY 11377)

New England Handicapped Sportmen's Association. (26 McFarlin Road, Chelmsford, MA 01824)

North American Riding for the Handicapped Association (NARHA). (Thistlecroft, Park Street, Mendon, MA 01756)

Project Magic. (c/o Julie DeJean, Box 100, Inglewood, CA 90306)

Senior Olympics. (5670 Wilshire Boulevard, Los Angeles, CA 90036)

Society for the Advancement of Travel for the Handicapped (SATH). (26 Court Street, Suite 1110, Brooklyn, NY 11242)

Therapeutic Horsemanship, Inc. (c/o Sandy Rafferty, Director, Route 1, Valley Road, Pacific, MO 63069)

U.S. Association for Blind Athletes. (55 West California Avenue, Beach Haven Park, NJ 08008)

Achieving Access to Home, Community, and Workplace

Mary Law, Debra Stewart, and Susan Strong

OBJECTIVES _____

The information in this chapter will help the reader to:
1. Understand the societal and legislative context in which persons with disabilities live, work, and play.
2. Gain knowledge about the diverse environmental factors affecting community living for persons with disabilities.
3. Understand the role of an occupational therapist in enabling community living.
4. Gain knowledge about methods to ensure clients' access to home, work, and community.

Occupational therapists believe that the individual has a right to achieve maximum potential and to control his own life through educated choices in interaction with the environment. Occupational therapists join with other rehabilitation service providers and with consumers to facilitate a continuum of services that support independent living. To ensure that individuals have successful reintegration into communities, rehabilitation must be viewed as a long-term process that may continue well past discharge from an acute hospital or rehabilitation setting (Wright, 1985). Occupational therapists have been involved in assisting individuals with disabilities to achieve access in different environments throughout the history of the profession. Recently, occupational therapists have emphasized the importance of the transactional relationship between persons and the environment in which they live and the potential focus on changing environments to enable community living (Law, 1991). Current occupational therapy frameworks support the profession's role in environmental access (Barris, 1982; Canadian Association of Occupational Therapists [CAOT], 1991; Kielhofner & Burke, 1980; Yerxa et al., 1990).

This chapter focuses on transitions from institutional to community living and on methods of environmental change that occupational therapists use to enable individuals to achieve access to home, work, and community activities. Using a **client-centered approach** to occupational therapy, the occupational therapist gains information about the client's current or former roles and the environment in which he lives. This, together with a knowledge of the individual's occupational performance, informs the occupational therapist about the congruence or fit between the individual and the environment in which he lives. Information about societal environmental issues, such as consumer movements and legislation, sets the context in which environmental change is facilitated. Environmental change is discussed, using a matrix format and focusing on the environmental locations of home, community, and work and on environmental supports or barriers, such as cultural, institutional, physical, and social factors (Table 19.1).

SOCIETAL ENVIRONMENTAL ISSUES

There have been significant changes over the past decade in consumer movements of people with disabilities and in legislation pertaining to disability. These changes have caused rehabilitation services to focus increasingly on community living and reintegration. Three particularly important historical developments have been the rise of the independent living movement, adoption of national building standards for accessibility, and the passage of the Americans with Disabilities Act of 1990.

Independent Living Movement

Independent living is defined as noninstitutional living in which individuals have primary responsibility

GLOSSARY

Client-centered approach—An approach to therapy that emphasizes the client's right to autonomy and choice and that focuses intervention on client-defined needs.

Clustered independent living arrangements—Apartment clusters or other types of housing in close proximity to each other, in which groups of residents with disabilities share services such as attendants and transportation (Spencer, 1991).

Contact broker—A person who serves as a linkage between a smaller (local) system and a larger (regional) system. In independent living arrangements, the contact broker is used by residents with disabilities as role model, consultant, and teacher to assist the residents in learning independent living skills (Spencer, 1991).

Cradle-to-grave homes—Homes that are designed with consideration of accessibility at the time of construction (e.g., wider door for wheelchair access). The design allows a person potentially to remain in the same home throughout his life.

Day Programs—Structured health and/or rehabilitation programs that are provided on an outpatient basis in a facility (often a hospital or rehabilitation setting) during the day for clients who live in the community. Transportation may or may not be provided as part of the program.

Easy Street—A commercially available simulated environment that can be purchased and installed in rehabilitation centers. It includes full-size market, banking, street, and other community environments and props.

Energy conservation techniques—"Skill and performance in applying energy-saving procedures, activity restriction, work simplification, time management, and/or organization of the environment to minimize output" (Reed & Sanderson, 1992, p. 338); see also Chapter 16.

Graded work hardening programs—A treatment program that uses highly structured, simulated work tasks in an environment based on work place standards to improve clients' productivity and employability. Clients are involved in graded work tasks that progress in stages of increasing levels of difficulty, complexity, or length of time (Matheson et al., 1985); see also Chapter 17.

Home Health Program—Health and/or rehabilitation services (including occupational therapy) are provided in a client's own home.

Transitional living centers—Facilities that provide temporary living arrangements for individuals who are in a transitional phase between hospital or institution and independent community living. Professional staff, including occupational therapists, assist the residents in gradually assuming responsibility for self-maintenance.

Table 19.1.   Environmental Matrix—Examples of Environmental Supports or Barriers[a]

Environment	Home	Work	Community
Cultural	Ethnicity Roles Community involvement	Ethnicity Diversity	Cultural norms Diversity Organizations
Institutional	Education Socioeconomic status	Work patterns Work milieu Bureaucracy	Service availability Economic state Funding Service continuum
Physical	Equipment Accessibility Size/design	Equipment Accessibility Physical design Legislation	Transportation Location Weather Physical design Housing Legislation
Social	Social contacts Self-reliance Family cohesion Knowledge of resources	Social support Attitudes Integration	Support networks Attitudes Community cohesion Interagency cooperation

[a]This table provides some examples; it is not meant to be exhaustive.

for their own choices, decision making, and performance of self-care and home-community activities within the limits of their physical, emotional, social, mental, and economic capabilities (Cooper & Hasselkus, 1992). Based on the Comprehensive Rehabilitation Services Amendment of the Rehabilitation Act of 1973, Title VII Public Law 95-602, services to increase the quality of life for citizens with disabilities were established. This marked the beginning of the independent living movement (ILM) (Ross, 1978). The goal of the ILM, which modeled itself on the civil rights movement, was to facilitate independent living through independent living centers, which were established to provide referral and direct services relating to housing, attendant care, transportation, sports and recreational resources, and social-vocational counseling. These centers are important because modern family life is changing. Families are smaller and more mobile, both spouses work, people live longer and may live a distance from their grown children, and the divorce rate is high. The family is often ill-equipped to deal with members with permanent handicaps (Zisserman, 1981). Centers for independent living are unique, community-based, nonprofit, nonresidential programs that are consumer oriented and are substantially controlled by consumers with disabilities (Johnson, 1986).

Environmental Standards

The American National Standards Institute (ANSI) (Accreditation Standards Committee, 1986) outlined specifications that must be met for accessibility of buildings for people with disabilities (see Appendix to this chapter). Cooper and Hasselkus (1992), in a survey of the literature, found that the ANSI standards have been adopted by many jurisdictions as the basis for barrier-free design. Examples of barrier-free design include ramping stairs, widening doorways, and installing grab bars in a bathroom. Acquisition of the ANSI standards document and knowledge of its contents is essential for occupational therapists in designing and adapting environments for maximum accessibility.

Americans with Disabilities Act

The Americans with Disabilities Act of 1990 (ADA) (Public Law 101-336) is a civil rights law designed to increase the integration and successful community living of people with disabilities in American society. Comprehensive civil rights protection is particularly focused in five areas: employment, public accommodations (i.e., places frequented by the general public), state and local government, public transportation, and telecommunications (Tables 19.2 and 17.2). For example, the ADA (1990) mandates that a qualified person with a disability cannot be discriminated against when seeking or participating in employment. The intent behind the law is to create equal opportunity and mandate reasonable accommodations so that persons with disabilities can achieve equal access to public environments, services, and transportation. It is also hoped that these changes will over time eliminate social barriers that are present in society against persons with disabilities (Kalscheur, 1991). The ADA focuses on achieving integration and independent living through societal change. The American Occupational Therapy Association stated that it supports the mandates of the ADA and encouraged occupational therapists to pursue opportunities to help with implementation of ADA standards (Kornblau, 1991).

The key phrase in the Americans with Disabilities Act is the obligation to provide reasonable accommodation to ensure that employment, public services, facilities, transportation, accommodations, and telecommunications are accessible. Reasonable accommodation in terms of employment refers to whatever adaptations are necessary—without imposing undue hardship on the employer—to enable an otherwise qualified person to perform the work. Changing hours of work or making changes in nonessential duties of the job would be

Table 19.2.   Americans with Disabilities Act (ADA)

Section	Area	Applicability	Effective Dates
Title I	Employment	25+ employees 15–24 employees	July 1992 July 1994
Title II	Public services, programs and facilities under state and local government	Existing facilities New facilities	January 1992 January 1993
	Public transportation	New vehicles General accessibility	August 1990 January 1992
Title III	Public accommodations and services under private control	New facilities	January 1993
Title IV	Telecommunications	24 hr per day	July 1993

considered reasonable accommodations. Reasonable accommodations in accessibility requirements to services, facilities, and transportation include such things as training bus drivers to be able to meet the needs of persons with a disability, availability of paratransit services when mainline public facilities are unavailable (and with a comparable response time), curb cuts in all new construction, seating in recreational and cultural facilities to permit people with wheelchairs to sit with family or friends, adjustment of store layout to improve accessibility, and availability of telecommunications devices for the deaf (TDD) in public facilities (Bartels & Earsy, 1992). A number of guides are available to enable occupational therapists, businesses, and others to assess compliance with the Americans with Disabilities Act (Adaptive Environments Center, 1992; Goldman, 1991; Texas Governor's Committee, 1992).

Although the ADA does not mandate professional involvement in achievement of the criteria set forth in the Americans with Disabilities Act, occupational therapists, with their skill in activity analysis and environmental accommodation, are well suited to assist people with disabilities, employers, and public and private officials in achieving compliance with the provisions of the ADA. Kalscheur (1991) pointed out that to do this, occupational therapists will have to shift from a deficit model of intervention that focuses on changing the person to a model that focuses on changing environments. Occupational therapists can assist services, organizations, companies, and individuals to self-evaluate their ability to fulfill the provisions of the Americans with Disabilities Act. For example, occupational therapists can analyze both the requirements of a job and the physical capabilities of an individual to determine what accommodations are required to do the essential functions of that job. Suggestions about reasonable accommodations, including adaptive equipment, modifications to schedules, modifications to job sites, and training, are all areas in which occupational therapists can work to enable implementation of the ADA (see Chapter 17).

EVOLVING ROLES AND FUNCTIONS OF OCCUPATIONAL THERAPISTS

Traditionally, occupational therapists have separated the physical environment from the social and cultural environments in which their clients live. The physical environment has been the domain of those therapists working in the area of physical dysfunction with previous emphasis on barrier-free design, mobility, adaptive aids, and equipment (Cooper, Cohen, & Hasselkus, 1991). Accessibility issues were primarily situation specific with the home as the key intervention focus.

The importance of early intervention, health promotion, prevention, and client-centered practice have led occupational therapists to focus on client-identified needs in many environments. With the expansion of health care into the community, occupational therapists have broadened their roles to include consultation, advocacy, and education in relation to accessibility. There is a greater focus on an individual's ability to participate and function in society within his "occupational environment" (Schkade & Schultz, 1992), rather than a focus on individual skill development.

The multifaceted nature of the environment requires the roles and functions of occupational therapists today to continue to expand to meet client needs. The use of an environmental "matrix" helps occupational therapists systematically to identify various levels of the environment with which the client may need to interact.

When addressing accessibility issues, the occupational therapist must first identify who the client is, as this will direct the therapist's roles and functions. Traditionally, the client was a person with a disability. Today, the therapist may also provide services to a system and may have two or more clients, including the individual, school board, employer, insurance company, law firm, and community agency. Each client has his set of priorities that need to be addressed. In addition, there may be several other key players involved: other health care professionals, architects, union representatives, and occupational health personnel. A key role for occupational therapists is to coordinate communication and gain cooperation of all players.

The evaluation function of the occupational therapist includes assessment of environmental barriers and supports as they relate to the client's ability to access and participate in daily activities (see Chapter 5). Assessment findings will guide the occupational therapist's intervention in developing strategies to promote supports and reduce barriers, with the goal of maximizing a client's access to different environments. The therapist and client must work together to seek creative methods to match the client's skills with environmental demands. For example, a client with an increasing visual impairment from the complications of diabetes may require a modified office design and a large-display computer system to enable him to continue his current employment.

The therapist often works directly with the individual. For example, the therapist may teach skills for independent living and support the client to take control of his daily activities through improving self-advocacy skills by providing information, options, and a structure for dealing with bureaucratic systems. At the same time, the therapist focuses intervention on environmental accessibility. For example, to reduce barriers, the occupational therapist identifies appropriate assistive technology to meet the individual's needs and then helps integrate that technology into the client's everyday life. The process may involve exploring technical options with the individual, facilitating acquisition of funding, overseeing installation of equipment, and training in its safe and effective use. An example follows.

CASE STUDY

Nancy is a 20-year-old woman with cerebral palsy who lived with her parents until a year ago, when she entered a **transitional living center.** When she was ready to move out into her own apartment, her occupational therapist provided help and support. She was to have a personal care attendant for basic activities of daily living (ADL) needs. Nancy and the occupational therapist began to explore her needs for assistive technology to support independent living.

The occupational therapist first assessed Nancy's ability to perform a variety of functional activities as well as her needs and preferences for assistance. The environment of the apartment and community were also addressed for inherent barriers and supports. The technology alternatives were then evaluated to determine an appropriate match of technology to Nancy and her living environment. An environmental control system using human voice frequency as the method of control for lights, television, radio, and drapes was selected. Funding sources were then explored and several written requests were submitted. Upon approval of funding from one agency, the occupational therapist prescribed the device and arranged for setup in the **transitional living center** for training. By the time Nancy moved into her apartment, she was proficient in the use of the environmental control unit. The occupational therapist assisted Nancy in setting up the system in the apartment, monitored its use, and made minor revisions to the system, as Nancy required, to facilitate her independence.

In the role of consultant, the occupational therapist interacts with influential people at each level of the environment. At the level of the individual and family, the therapist enables individuals to become informed consumers and to advocate for change. Healthy, supportive family interactions are facilitated (Jongbloed, Stanton, & Fansek, 1993). The occupational therapist can also link clients with appropriate self-help groups to develop community social supports. To reduce attitudinal barriers, occupational therapists educate community members about disability and accessibility issues. Occupational therapists work with clients in advocating for changes in the physical, social and institutional environments to facilitate access and inclusion. Advocacy takes place at many different levels, from government officials and business people to public forums, conferences, and professional associations.

TRANSITION FROM INSTITUTION TO COMMUNITY

The first time many individuals with disabilities confront accessibility issues occurs when they move from an institution to the community. Various transition programs have been established to help bridge this gap. Occupational therapists are actively involved in many of these programs, which currently operate in both institutions and the community.

Transitional programs prepare individuals for community living by providing opportunities to practice overcoming barriers (physical, social, cultural, and institutional), developing supports, and identifying strategies to deal with daily problems and issues. In various environments, realistic activities are used to integrate skills, develop solutions to problems and barriers, and diffuse fear of community integration through rehearsals and anticipatory guidance. In contextually relevant practice sessions, the individual is presented with problem situations that are within his capabilities to learn to anticipate and to solve. Examples of such bridging activities include shopping alone or with others, attending community programs and activities, job interviewing, or visiting independent living centers.

At the institutional level, examples of transition programs include family group programs to improve communication and provide an opportunity to express feelings related to discharge; presentations about law, finances, vocational exploration, housing, and emergency procedures; and activities in simulated environments such as **Easy Street.** People with disabilities who are living successfully in the community can speak to patients to provide valuable information about architectural barriers, transportation, adapting homes, adapted equipment, and recreational possibilities.

Transition programs in the community provide a continuum of services, ranging from **home health programs** and **day programs** to **clustered independent living arrangements.** Programs oriented to return to work also vary in the amount of support and types of services provided, from prevocational assessment to job retraining. In determining the most suitable transition program for an individual client, the occupational therapist often acts as a "broker," matching the client's abilities and needs to available services. Important factors to consider in community placement include not only the physical accessibility of living or working settings but also the availability of role models or **contact brokers** and social supports (Spencer, 1991).

Transitional living centers exist in many communities for adults with physical disabilities. In some centers, the individual becomes a resident for varying lengths of stay and works with a multidisciplinary team, including an occupational therapist, to reach his discharge goals. Family members are active participants in the program. Vocational rehabilitation programs and supported employment in the community are often offered. At the other end of the continuum are cooperative apartments, run by the residents, where attendant support services are available on request. Because some form of transportation is provided, most residents attend school or are employed. An occupational therapist may offer consultation and advice at a resident's request.

Accessing Home

Occupational therapists working with people with physical disabilities face two main issues related to home accessibility. The first is housing. The occupational therapist is concerned with matching an individual's abilities and needs with the environmental demands of different types of housing. The second issue relates to adaptations and modification of the home environment and the provision of equipment to facilitate accessibility. The roles and functions of the occupational therapist may include evaluation of both client needs and the dwelling, prescription of necessary modifications and equipment, and training of the individual and family in the use of the equipment and modifications (Colvin & Korn, 1984).

The range of housing choices available to people with physical disabilities has grown in the past decade (Canada Mortgage and Housing Corporation [CMHC], 1992). Increasing consumer demands for the right to live in home communities have led governments and builders to develop new housing arrangements. For example, the awareness of the demographics of an increasing number of elderly people in the North American population has led builders to develop **cradle-to-grave homes** (Samson, 1992), which are fashioned after the concept of life-span houses in Norway and Sweden. This design concept enables many people with disabilities to live independently in the same home throughout their life, and thus reduce the demand on relatives and government to provide care (CMHC, 1992).

Some examples of housing options available to people with physical disabilities demonstrate the available range of options. For some clients, a transitional living arrangement will be the most suitable, as skills and strategies for independent living still need to be developed. For those individuals who are able to live independently but require attendant care for specific activities (personal care and homemaking tasks), there are **clustered independent living apartments,** or

housing complexes, in many communities. The amount of attendant care and support services vary greatly and must be investigated carefully before a choice is made. For elderly people with acquired disabilities, a new concept of "eldercare" is developing, which provides a full range of health and social services to seniors wishing to live independently in a clustered setting (Egan, 1992).

Most individuals with disabilities wish to return to, or move into, their own homes. In many cases, some environmental modifications or equipment will be necessary to facilitate safe and easy access. As with any accessibility issue, the occupational therapist first needs to assess the individual's skills and resources in relation to the home environment. Home visits with the client and weekend trials at home before discharge are highly recommended to evaluate occupational performance in this environment and to work out problems ahead of time. An environmental evaluation of the home setting is also required to determine the barriers and supports available. The physical environment is of primary concern to the occupational therapist working with clients with physical disabilities, but consideration must also be made of the social, cultural, and institutional demands. A current example of an occupational therapy program designed to help clients remain in their homes is a computer-based system called *EASE* (developed by Christensen). This system enables occupational therapists to evaluate the client and the home environment together, including physical factors such as lighting and carpeting as well as options in assistive technology (Joe, 1992). Through environmental assessment (see Chapter 5), the occupational therapist can identify the individual's needs for access and match them with environmental resources.

Occupational therapy intervention for home accessibility usually involves both direct and indirect care. Direct intervention with a client may include programs to develop skills in occupational performance—ADL, homemaking, and leisure activities. Adapting activities to enable an individual to perform them independently is often a key function of occupational therapy. For example, advising a client recovering from a stroke to purchase comfortable loose clothing with no buttons or zippers, and training the individual in one-handed dressing techniques may allow the client to dress himself every morning. In other situations, the occupational therapist will teach an individual to direct an attendant to assist with his personal care when required. The occupational therapist can also help a client develop strategies to deal with physical and social barriers in the home or neighborhood.

Indirect intervention focuses on the elimination of barriers and facilitation of supports in the home for freedom of access. Often the occupational therapist will work with architects, builders, and/or contractors to design a barrier-free environment for a particular client. Many companies now exist to provide specific housing design advice to people with disabilities, and some employ occupational therapists. Publications are also available with detailed design information that is based on ANSI standards (see Appendix to this chapter) and specific municipal and state building codes.

The process of barrier-free design is straightforward, but requires attention to many details. Environmental barriers and supports—physical, social, cultural, and institutional—that affect home renovations must be considered early to ensure success. The use of a matrix (Table 19.1) to identify systematically the barriers and supports involved will help the occupational therapist cover all areas. For example, at home, personal design preferences and cultural meaning attached to certain rooms in a house or to equipment may be important. Municipal bylaws and building codes at the community level will also influence design. Funding of any modifications or equipment may involve the individual, his family, the community, and institutions. All possible funding sources for renovations must be investigated, as costs can be high.

Two basic points are usually considered in barrier-free home design: access to and within the home and the provision of accessible outdoor space (Kelly & Snell, 1987). Access to the outdoors and to community life is essential for successful integration. Some basic elements to consider in the design of the outdoor space of a home include smooth, hard, even surfaces that are wide enough for a wheelchair to turn around; raised gardens to allow easy access from a wheelchair; and curb ramps on sidewalks and paths. The occupational therapist may provide consultation about outdoor space design to the client or family and may also advocate on the client's behalf for changes in the physical environment of the neighborhood.

On the home site, the main entrance and exit is often the first area considered in barrier-free design. The occupational therapist may recommend a ramp or lift to replace stairs and doors that are easy to open and wide enough for a wheelchair. An effective fire evacuation route, with primary and secondary exits, must be determined.

Inside a home, the occupational therapist considers access throughout the house and between rooms. The width of corridors and doors and, most important, stairs are key elements of accessibility. A wide variety of stair lifts and elevating devices are now available to allow a person with a physical disability to access all levels of the home.

The main rooms in a home that are considered in any design process are the bathroom, the kitchen, the bedroom, and living spaces. When an occupational therapist views each room in terms of the activity patterns related to a particular space, the needs of the client for access and participation in daily activities become the focus. Environmental modifications and equipment can then be designed to match a client's needs for participation in activities.

The bathroom is a primary space for personal care and hygiene activities. Privacy and respect of an individual are paramount in this space. It is also a prime area for accidents—mostly falls—and safety considerations are important in design. An emergency call system to alert someone elsewhere in the house or in the community is often a simple safety solution. Many adaptive aids and equipment are available to facilitate independence in bathing, showering, toileting, and personal hygiene. They range from a simple grab bar to a custom-made curbless shower stall accessible by shower chair.

In the kitchen, eating and related household activities are performed. The design of a kitchen must consider the individual's interests and personal needs to complete kitchen tasks as well as ergonomic factors such as **energy conservation techniques.** Environmental modifications and equipment are determined by analyzing the activity requirements for key kitchen tasks, i.e., food preparation, cooking, eating, and cleanup.

Eating and meal preparation have many social and cultural meanings and rituals attached to them, and these elements must be accommodated in kitchen design. For example, some cultures involve the whole family in meal preparation so space is an important issue, while others view this activity to be the sole domain of a woman of the household. Role expectations may need to be explored and modified (Jongbloed et al., 1993).

The bedroom is a private area for most individuals. It is where many personal care activities and quiet leisure pursuits are carried out. Environmental modifications to allow ease of transfers and movement in bed will support an individual's personal sense of comfort and safety. An emergency call system from the bed enhances safety and security. Environmental controls to access the television, radio, and telephone from the bed are common aids in a bedroom. If attendant care is required, a bedside call system is required.

The living room or family room usually serves as a space for socialization and leisure activities. It is, therefore, important before recommending any changes in design to identify the client's interests and needs for social and leisure activities. Matching client needs to environmental resources and the needs of other family members may involve discussion about such issues as designing furniture layouts for wheelchair access and/or environmental controls for appliances such as television and stereo, touch lamps, and adaptive leisure aids such as page turners and hands-free telephone systems.

Accessing Community

In the past, occupational therapists have not been extensively involved in changing environments to enable access at the community level. The impact of occupational therapy consultation and intervention, however, can be much greater in ensuring accessibility and participation when changes are made at the community level. In working to enable access at the community level, occupational therapists work with clients and other agencies as facilitators. Therapists act as supports in enabling clients and others to break down environmental barriers that hinder clients from achieving their desired community roles.

At the individual and family levels, therapists provide knowledge of and access to community resources that will help clients to participate in the daily activities that they wish to accomplish. For example, an occupational therapist's knowledge of community resources can be particularly helpful in linking persons with disabilities with self-help or support groups for social networking, with municipalities and YMCAs for recreational opportunities, and with municipalities for access to transportation. Some municipalities have recreational access programs through which they work with volunteers and persons with disabilities to facilitate access to recreational programs (Richardson et al., 1987).

Research has shown that community attitudes play an important role in determining the reintegration of people with disabilities. Persons with disabilities face many social barriers and stigmata within communities (West, 1984; Zola, 1982). Occupational therapists, along with other rehabilitation team members, can work with persons with long-term or new disabilities to develop coping strategies to enable them to access and maintain involvement in their communities. On an individual level as well, occupational therapists provide information about physical accessibility and driving assessment and training programs to ensure physical access to the community.

In changing community environmental barriers, a systems approach to removing barriers has been shown to be most effective (West, 1986). Using a systems approach, an occupational therapist assesses all of the barriers (social, cultural, physical, or institutional) that are limiting access to programs or community environments. Once all barriers are identified, clients and therapists work together to change these limitations. Partial removal of barriers is unlikely to be successful in ensuring access to community services. For example,

there is little point in providing ramped access to a building when the bathrooms within the building are not accessible to a person in a wheelchair. Likewise, providing ramped access to a building in which the services are bureaucratically difficult to access is not helpful enough.

Accessing Work

The Americans with Disabilities Act significantly affects the occupational therapist's role in the work place. Occupational therapists act as consultants to reduce barriers for persons with disabilities by suggesting methods of reasonable accommodation for each stage of the employment process. The therapist performs job-site analysis to assist employers to specify a job's essential functions and qualifications (e.g., lifting x number of pounds or kilograms). The occupational therapist can assist in the interview and hiring process by suggesting reasonable accommodations to enable a qualified applicant to proceed with the interview (e.g., adapted keyboard). By conducting training sessions with interviewers, the occupational therapist can sensitize staff about dealing with disability issues and enable effective interactions.

Whether dealing with a new employee or a returning employee who is newly disabled, the occupational therapist aids employers to match qualified staff with the demands of the work place by ensuring suitability of the job to the person's abilities and by determining what reasonable accommodations may be required. This is accomplished by the occupational therapist performing an analysis of the cognitive, social, psychological, and physical demands of the job (see Chapter 17). The occupational therapist then conducts a functional assessment of the individual's occupational performance capacity within the context of cultural and family values, and predisability functioning. Based on these assessments, the therapist provides options and/or strategies to reduce barriers to enable employment participation. Suggestions may include installation of adaptive equipment (e.g., adaptive computer software and a talking calculator for an employee with visual impairment) or modifications of the physical environment (e.g., a raised desk and bathroom modifications to enable wheelchair access). Job restructuring, which involves changing nonessential job duties so the worker with a disability can perform other essential tasks, is another option. For example, a clerk with a hearing impairment may change a weekly rotational lunch hour coverage for a receptionist to an hour's filing. Another strategy involves a modified work schedule. For example, scheduled work hours are adjusted to accommodate transportation system restraints for a worker with mobility impairments (Bartels & Earsy,

1992). The occupational therapist is often involved in the training and follow-up of accommodations to ensure success.

The occupational therapist is confronted with several important issues when trying to improve access to work at different levels of the system. At the level of the individual, the therapist challenges the person with a disability to overcome his fear and facilitates the client's self-understanding of capabilities (Holmes, 1985). By establishing a therapeutic relationship and providing relevant work experiences, the therapist assists the client to generalize what has been learned in therapy (e.g., interviewing skills, strength through activity) to the work place. To act as a bridge from the clinic to the real world, the occupational therapist uses strategies such as **graded work hardening programs, energy conservation techniques,** cognitive retraining, and training in simulated environments. Intervention works best when it occurs before dysfunctional roles are incorporated into a person's lifestyle. At the level of the organization (i.e., supervisors, managers, and peers), there is often a lack of understanding and knowledge of what a worker with a disability can do and the possibilities for simple, often inexpensive environmental modifications. Changes in attitudes are possible through a process of educating others about disability issues and solving problems through collaborative negotiation. Communication barriers easily arise when the community of people with a vested interest in whether a person returns to work is made up of many different perspectives or agendas. The occupational therapist often assumes the role of a case manager to facilitate coordination of information and gain cooperation of all key players. Funding issues can be alleviated by the client negotiating funding that is facilitory rather than adversarial to the reentry process. For example, increases in funding could depend on changes such as increased work hours.

SUMMARY

Occupational therapists in the past have focused most often on changing physical barriers at a community level. However, it has been shown social and institutional barriers are often the greatest limiting factors in accessing activities at a community level (West, 1984). Persons with disabilities have found that they live in two worlds: a regular and a disabled world. It is they who must adapt to these worlds (Law, 1993). Occupational therapists can work with social, planning, and cultural groups to provide education about the need to celebrate our diversity. In working with clients, occupational therapists can facilitate and support consumers as they develop advocacy skills to ensure that community accessibility is a reality for them.

STUDY QUESTIONS

1. Identify barriers and supports in cultural, physical, social, and economic areas that either hinder or help people with disabilities to achieve independent living.
2. Define independent living.
3. What did the Americans with Disabilities Act provide for people with disabilities?
4. What services do independent living centers offer consumers?
5. Why are transitional community reintegration programs needed?
6. What are some methods that occupational therapists use in community reintegration?
7. What is the value of the American National Standards specifications?
8. What are key issues that an occupational therapist needs to consider in facilitating a client to achieve access to work?
9. What are key issues that an occupational therapist needs to consider in facilitating a client to achieve access to home?
10. What are key issues that an occupational therapist needs to consider in facilitating a client to achieve access to community?

REFERENCES

Accreditation Standards Committee on Architectural Features and Site Design of Public Buildings and Residential Structures for Persons with Handicaps. (1986). *American national standard for buildings and facilities—providing accessibility and usability for physically handicapped people.* New York: American National Standards Institute.

Adaptive Environments Center. (1992). *The Americans with Disabilities Act checklist for readily achievable barrier removal.* Washington, DC: National Institute on Disability and Rehabilitation Research.

Americans with Disabilities Act. (1990). Public Law 101-336, 42 U.S.C. §12101.

Barris, R. (1982). Environmental interactions: An extension of the model of occupation. *American Journal of Occupational Therapy, 36,* 637–644.

Bartels, E. C., & Earsy, N. F. (1992). *Americans with Disabilities Act: Examples of reasonable accommodation.* Boston: Massachusetts Rehabilitation Commission, Legal Department.

Canada Mortgage and Housing Corporation. (1992). *Housing choices for Canadians with disabilities.* Ottawa, Ont., Canada: Author.

Canadian Association of Occupational Therapists. (1991). *Guidelines for the client-centred practice of occupational therapy.* Toronto, Ont., Canada: Author.

Colvin, M. E., & Korn, T. L. (1984). Eliminating barriers to the disabled. *American Journal of Occupational Therapy, 38,* 748–753.

Cooper, B., Cohen, U., & Hasselkus, B. R. (1991). Barrier-free design: A review and critique of the occupational therapy perspective. *American Journal of Occupational Therapy, 45,* 344–350.

Cooper, B., & Hasselkus, B. R. (1992). Independent living and the physical environment: Aspects that matter to residents. *Canadian Journal of Occupational Therapy, 59,* 6–15.

Egan, M. (1992, June 18). Planning for the future: Designing communities of all-inclusive care for the elderly. *OT Week*, 44–45.

Goldman, C. D. (1991). *Disability rights guide: Practical solutions to problems affecting people with disabilities.* Lincoln, NE: Media Publishing.

Holmes, D. (1985). The role of the occupational therapist—Work evaluator. *American Journal of Occupational Therapy, 39,* 308–313.

Joe, B. E. (1992, October 22). Software provides independence with EASE. *OT Week,* 14–15.

Johnson, J. (1986). Centers for independent living: A new concept in promoting independence. *AOTA Physical Disabilities Special Interest Newsletter, 9*(3), 4–5.

Jongbloed, L., Stanton, S., & Fansek, B. (1993). Family adaptation to altered roles following a stroke. *Canadian Journal of Occupational Therapy, 60,* 70–77.

Kalscheur, J. A. (1991). Benefits of the Americans with Disabilities Act of 1990 for children and adolescents with disabilities. *American Journal of Occupational Therapy, 46,* 419–426.

Kelly, C., & Snell, K. (1987). *The source book: Architectural guidelines for barrier-free design.* Toronto, Ont., Canada: Barrier-Free Design Center.

Kielhofner, G., & Burke, J. P. (1980). A model of human occupation, Part 1. Conceptual framework and content. *American Journal of Occupational Therapy, 34,* 572–581.

Kornblau, B. L. (1991). The American Association of Occupational Therapists—White paper: Occupational therapy and the Americans with Disabilities Act. *American Journal of Occupational Therapy, 46*(5), 470–471.

Law, M. (1991). The environment: A focus for occupational therapy. *Canadian Journal of Occupational Therapy, 58,* 171–179.

Law, M. (1993). *Changing disabling environments for children with physical disabilities: A research study completed with participating families—Cambridge* (Working Paper Series No. 31). University of Waterloo, School of Urban and Regional Planning, Waterloo, Ont., Canada.

Matheson, L. N., Ogden, L., Violette, K., & Schultz, K. (1985). Work hardening: Occupational therapy in industrial rehabilitation. *American Journal of Occupational Therapy, 39*(5), 314–321.

Reed, K. L., & Sanderson, S. N. (1992). *Concepts of occupational therapy.* Baltimore: Williams & Wilkins.

Richardson, D., Wilson, B., Wetherald, L., & Peters, J. (1987). Mainstreaming initiative: An innovative approach to recreation and leisure services in a community setting. *Therapeutic Recreation Journal, 24,* 9–19.

Ross, E. C. (1978). New rehabilitation law. *Accent on Living, 23*(3), 23.

Samson, L. (1992). Consultancy issues concerning accessibility. In E. Jaffe & C. Epstein (Eds.), *Occupational therapy consultation: Theory, principles and practice* (pp. 385–394). St. Louis: C. V. Mosby.

Schkade, J. K., & Schultz, S. (1992). Occupational adaptation: Toward a holistic approach for contemporary practice, Part 1. *American Journal of Occupational Therapy, 46,* 829–837.

Spencer, J. C. (1991). An ethnographic study of independent living alternatives. *American Journal of Occupational Therapy, 45,* 243–249.

Texas Governor's Committee for Disabled Persons. (1992). *ADA self-evaluation guide.* Houston.

West, P. C. (1984). Social stigma and community recreation participation by the mentally and physically disabled. *Therapeutic Recreation Journal, 18,* 1.

West, P. C. (1986). Environment and the handicapped. *Environments, 18*(3), 89–106.

Wright, B. A. (1985). Value-laden beliefs and principles for rehabilitation. In S. J. Regnier & M. Petkovsek (Eds.), *Rehabilitation: 25 years of concepts, principles, perspectives.* Chicago: National Easter Seals Society.

Yerxa, E. J., Clark, F., Frank, G., Jackson, J., Parham, D., Pierce, D., Stein, C., & Zemke, R. (1990). An introduction to occupational science, a foundation for occupational therapy in the 21st century. *Occupational Therapy in Health Care, 6,* 1–17.

Zisserman, L. (1981). The modern family and rehabilitation of the handicapped. *American Journal of Occupational Therapy, 35,* 13–20.

Zola, I. K. (1982). Social and cultural disincentives to independent living. *Archives of Physical Medicine & Rehabilitation, 63,* 394–397.

Supplementary Resources

Suggested Readings

Airports Council International—North America. (1993). *A guide to accessibility of terminals. Access travel: Airports.* Pueblo, CO: Consumer Information Center.

American Occupational Therapy Association. (1993). *Readily achievable checklist: A survey for accessibility.* Rockville, MD: Author.

Office of Special Education and Rehabilitative Services. (1993). *Pocket guide to federal help for individuals with disabilities* (DOE Publication No. ED/OSERS 93-3). Washington, DC: U.S. Government Printing Office.

U.S. Equal Employment Opportunity Commission and U.S. Department of Justice Civil Rights Division. (1991). *The Americans with Disabilities Act questions and answers* (Publication No. GPO: 1991-299-558). Washington, DC: U.S. Government Printing Office.

Resources

ANSI. (American National Standards Institute, Inc., 11 West 42nd Street, New York NY 10036)

EASE. (Lifease, Inc., 2550 University Avenue W, Suite 317 North, St. Paul, MN 55114)

Easy Street. (Guynes Design, David Guynes or Patricia Moore, 1201 East Jefferson Street, Suite B125, Phoenix, AZ 85034)

APPENDIX: ANSI DESIGN EXAMPLES

The American National Standards Institute (ANSI) publishes the document *American National Standard for Buildings and Facilities—Providing Accessibility and Usability for Physically Handicapped People.* It details specifications to make any building or facility accessible to and usable by people with a variety of physical disabilities.

Brief examples of the ANSI document are printed here to provide the occupational therapist with a sense of the range of standards and the detailed specifications. Although the use of ANSI standards is completely voluntary, it is recommended that any person working with people with physical disabilities in their daily environments be familiar with the standards and use them when designing, constructing, or renovating buildings and facilities.

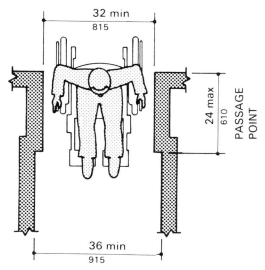

Figure 19A.1. Minimum clear width for single wheelchair.

Accessible Elements and Spaces

1. BASIC COMPONENTS

Accessible sites, facilities, and buildings, including public-use, employee-use, and common-use spaces in housing facilities, shall provide accessible elements and spaces as identified in Table 19A.1. Application by adopting authorities shall be in accordance with Section 2.

2. SPACE ALLOWANCES AND REACH RANGES

2.1 Wheelchair Passage Width

The minimum clear width for single wheelchair passage shall be 32 in (815 mm) at a point and 36 in (915 mm) continuously (see Fig 19A.1)

2.2 Width for Wheelchair Passing

The minimum width for two wheelchairs to pass is 60 in (1525 mm) (see Fig. 19A.2)

2.3 Wheelchair Turning Space

The space required for a wheelchair to make a 180-degree turn is a clear space of 60 in (1525 mm) diameter or a T-shaped space.

2.4 Clear Floor or Ground Space for Wheelchairs

2.4.1 Size and Approach

The minimum clear floor or ground space required to accommodate a single, stationary wheelchair and occupant is 30 in by 48 in (760 mm by 1220 mm). The minimum clear floor or ground space for wheelchairs may be positioned for forward or parallel approach to an object. Clear floor or ground space for wheelchairs may be part of the knee space required under some objects.

2.4.2 Relationship of Maneuvering Clearances to Wheelchair Spaces

One full unobstructed side of the clear floor or ground space for a wheelchair shall adjoin or overlap an accessible route or adjoin another wheelchair clear floor space. If a clear floor space is located in an alcove or otherwise confined on all or part of three sides, additional maneuvering clearances shall be provided.

2.4.3 Surfaces of Wheelchair Spaces

Clear floor or ground spaces for wheelchairs shall comply with [section] 4.5 [not reprinted here]. . . .

32 DWELLING UNITS

32.1 General

Accessible dwelling units shall comply with 4.32.

32.2 Adaptability

Subsections 4.32.4, Bathrooms, and 32.5, Kitchens, specify a range of heights and clearances within which certain fixtures may be installed (for example, grab bars at bathtubs and toilets, and work surfaces and sink heights in kitchens). In the case of grab bars, provision can be made for later installation within the specified height range, as requested by the occupant

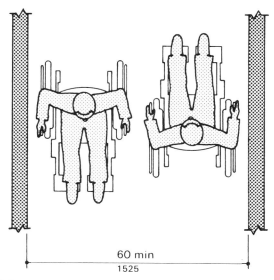

19A.2. Minimum clear width for two wheelchairs.

Table 19A.1. Basic Components for Accessible Sites, Facilities, and Buildings

Accessible Element or Space	Section	Application (to the Extent Specified by the Adopting Authority)
1. Accessible route(s)	4.3	Within the boundary of the site: (a) From public transportation stops, accessible parking spaces, accessible passenger loading zones, and public streets or sidewalks to accessible building entrances (b) Connecting accessible buildings, facilities, elements and spaces that are on the same site (c) Connecting accessible building or facility entrances with accessible spaces and elements within the building or facility
2. Protruding objects	4.4	Accessible routes or maneuvering space including, but not limited to, halls, corridors, passageways or aisles
3. Ground and floor surface treatments	4.5	Accessible routes, rooms, and spaces, including floors, walks, ramps, stairs, and curb ramps
4. Parking and passenger-loading zones	4.6	If provided at the site
5. Curb ramps	4.7	Accessible routes crossing curbs
6. Ramps	4.8	Accessible routes with slopes greater than 1:20
7. Stairs	4.9	Stairs on accessible routes connecting levels not connected by an elevator
8. Elevator	4.10	Accessible routes connecting different accessible levels
9. Platform lift	4.11	May be used in lieu of an elevator or ramp under certain conditions
10. Windows	4.12	If windows are intended to be operated by the occupant
11. Doors	4.13	Accessible entrances, accessible spaces, accessible routes, egress
12. Entrances	4.14	When part of accessible routes. Generally, one or more accessible entrances will serve transportation facilities, passenger loading zones, parking facilities, taxi stands, public streets and sidewalks, and interior vertical access
13. Drinking fountains and water coolers	4.15	If provided in the facility or at the site
14. Toilet rooms and bathing facilities including water closets, toilet rooms and stalls, urinals, lavatories and mirrors, bathtubs, shower stalls, and sinks	4.22	Public-use and common-use facilities
15. Storage facilities including cabinets, shelves, closets and drawers	4.23	If provided in accessible spaces
16. Grab bars, tub and shower seats	4.24	Accessible toilet and bathing facilities
17. Controls and operating mechanisms	4.25	Accessible spaces, accessible routes, or as parts of accessible elements
18. Emergency warning systems	4.26	If provided in the facility or at the site
19. Tactile warnings	4.27	Doors to hazardous areas
20. Signs	4.28	Rooms and spaces
21. Public telephones	4.29	If provided in the facility or at the site
22. Seating, tables, or work surfaces	4.30	If provided in accessible spaces
23. Places of assembly	4.31	If provided in the facility or at the site
24. Public-use spaces	4.1–4.30	Buildings and facilities, including housing
25. Employee-use spaces and facilities	4.1–4.30	Buildings and facilities, including housing
26. Common-use spaces and facilities. Including, swimming pools, playgrounds, entrances, rental offices, lobbies, elevators, mailbox areas, lounges, halls, corridors, and the like	4.1–4.30	Buildings and facilities, including housing

Table 19A.2. Basic Components for Accessible and Adaptable Dwelling Units

Accessible Element or Space	Section	Application (to the Extent Specified by the Adopting Authority)
1. Space allowances	4.2	All rooms and spaces
2. Accessible routes	4.3	(a) Within dwelling unit to all rooms and spaces (b) Connecting accessible dwelling unit(s) to accessible entrance(s) and to common-use spaces and facilities (c) From public transportation stops, accessible parking spaces, accessible passenger-loading zones, and public streets or sidewalks to accessible building entrance(s) (d) Connecting accessible buildings, facilities, elements, and spaces that are on the same site (e) Connecting accessible building or facility entrances with accessible spaces and elements within the building or facility
3. Floor surfaces	4.5	Accessible routes, rooms, and spaces
4. Parking and passenger-loading zones	4.6	If provided at facility
5. Windows	4.12	If operable windows are provided within dwelling units
6. Doors	4.13	At entrance, to and in accessible spaces
7. Entrances	4.14	To dwelling unit
8. Storage	4.23	If provided in accessible spaces
9. Controls	4.25	Within dwelling units, including heating, ventilating and air conditioning equipment (other than air distribution registers) requiring regular, periodic maintenance and adjustment by the occupant of the dwelling unit
10. Emergency alarms	4.26	If provided within the dwelling unit
11. Bathrooms	4.32.4	Design for fixed installation of grab bars within specified range of heights, or with provision for subsequent addition of grab bars within the range
12. Kitchens	4.32.5	Work surfaces and sinks may be designed for fixed installation within specified range of heights or for adjustable heights within the range
13. Laundry facilities	4.32.6	If provided in dwelling unit or if common-use facility serving accessible dwelling unit
14. Common-use spaces and facilities	4.2–4.32	If provided at facility and serving accessible dwelling unit
15. Patios, terraces, balconies, carports, and garages	4.2–4.32	If provided with accessible dwelling unit

of the dwelling unit. Other fixtures may be permanently installed at a height within these ranges, or the fixtures may be adjustable within the ranges. A unit in which fixtures may be added or adjusted in height is an adaptable unit. Both adaptable units and units in which fixtures are permanently installed within the heights specified in 32 are accessible dwelling units.

32.3 Basic Components

Accessible dwelling units shall provide accessible elements and spaces as identified in Table 19A.2. In establishing administrative provisions as described in Section 2, adopting authorities shall specify the number of dwelling units to be accessible, or procedures for determining the number to be accessible, for different types of construction (i.e., new construction or remodeling/alterations). In addition, adopting authorities may specify whether those fixtures for which height ranges are provided in 32.4 and 32.5 are to be permanently

installed at a specific height or whether they are to be designed for adaptability. Table 19A.2 identifies spaces where fixtures are subject to these requirements.

32.4 Bathrooms

Accessible bathrooms shall be on an accessible route and shall comply with the requirements of 32.4.

32.4.1 Doors

Doors may swing into the clear floor space required for any fixture only when the bathroom provides sufficient maneuvering space within the bathroom for a person using a wheelchair to enter and close the door, use the fixtures, reopen the door, and exit.

32.4.2 Water Closets

1. Clear floor space at the water closet shall be as shown in Figure 19A.3a. The water closet may be

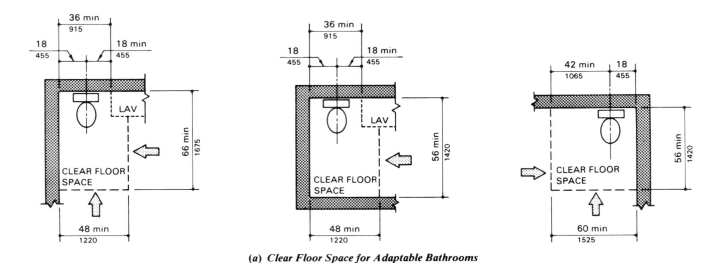

(a) Clear Floor Space for Adaptable Bathrooms

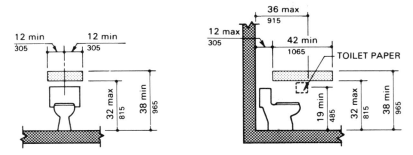

NOTE: The lightly shaded areas are reinforced to receive grab bars.

B

Figure 19A.3. Water closets in adaptable bathrooms. **A,** Clear floor space for adaptable bathrooms. **B,** Reinforced areas for installation of grab bars. Note: The lightly shaded areas are reinforced to receive grab bars.

located with the clear area at either the right or left side of the toilet.

2. The height of the water closet shall be at least 15 in (380 mm) and no more than 19 in (485 mm), measured to the top of the toilet seat.

3. Grab bars shall be installed and shall comply with 24, or structural reinforcement or other provisions shall be made that will allow installation of grab bars in the locations shown in Figure 19A.3b.

4. The toilet paper dispenser shall be installed within reach as shown in Figure 19A.3b.

32.4.3 Lavatory, Mirrors, Medicine Cabinets

1. The lavatory and mirrors shall comply with 19.

2. If a cabinet is provided under the lavatory, it shall provide, or shall be removable to provide, the clearances specified in 19.2

3. If a medicine cabinet is provided above the lavatory,

then the bottom of the medicine cabinet shall be located with a usable shelf no higher than 44 in (1120 mm) above the floor.

32.4.4 Bathtubs

If a bathtub is provided, it shall have the following features:

1. *Floor Space.* Clear floor space at bathtubs shall be as shown.

2. *Seat.* An in-tub seat or a seat at the head end of the tub shall be provided as shown. The structural strength of seats and their attachments shall comply with 24.3. Seats shall be mounted securely and shall not slip during use.

3. *Grab Bars.* Grab bars shall be installed within the [specified] range of heights and shall comply with 24, or structural reinforcement or other provisions

shall be made that will allow installation of grab bars meeting these requirements.

4. *Controls.* Faucets and other controls shall be located as shown [earlier] and shall comply with 4.25.4.
5. *Shower Unit.* A shower spray unit shall be provided with a hose at least 60 in (1525 mm) long that can be used as a fixed shower head or as a hand-held shower. If an adjustable-height shower head mounted on a vertical bar is used, the bar shall be installed so as not to obstruct the use of grab bars.

4.32.4.5 Showers

If a shower is provided, it shall have the following features:

1. *Size and Clearances.* Showers stall size and clear floor space shall comply with [standards shown earlier]. The shower stall shall be 36 in by 36 in (915 mm by 915 mm) [or] the shower stall will fit into the same space as a standard bathtub, 60 in (1525 mm) long.
2. *Seat.* A seat shall be provided in the shower stall. The seat shall be 17 in to 19 in (430 mm to 485 mm) high measured from the bathroom floor and shall extend the full depth of the stall. The seat shall be on the wall opposite the controls. The structural strength of seats and their attachments shall comply with 24.3. Seats shall be mounted securely and shall not slip during use.

3. *Grab Bars.* Grab bars shall be installed within the range of heights shown [earlier] and shall comply with 24, or structural reinforcement or other provisions shall be made that will allow installation of grab bars meeting these requirements.
4. *Controls.* Faucets and other controls shall be located as shown [earlier] and shall comply with 4.25.4. In the shower stall all controls, faucets, and the shower unit shall be mounted on the side wall opposite the seat.
5. *Shower Unit.* A shower spray unit shall be provided with a hose a least 60 in (1525 mm) long that can be used as a fixed shower head at various heights or as a hand-held shower. If an adjustable-height shower head mounted on a vertical bar is used, the bar shall be installed so as not to obstruct the use of grab bars.

32.4.6 Bathtub and Shower Enclosures

Enclosures for bathtubs or shower stalls shall not obstruct controls or transfer from wheelchairs onto shower or bathtub seats. Enclosures on bathtubs shall not have tracks mounted on their rims.

32.4.7 Clear Floor Space

Clear floor space at fixtures may overlap.

20
Facilitating Psychosocial Adjustment to Disability

Hilda Powers Versluys

OBJECTIVES

After studying this chapter, the student will have had the opportunity to:
1. Understand why psychosocial treatment improves the success of a patient's physical rehabilitation program and future occupational functioning.
2. Appreciate how the quality of the treatment environment, the patient's methods of adaptation, and the therapist's role in the treatment of the patient influence rehabilitation.
3. Recognize the occupational therapy role in the treatment of a patient's comorbid psychiatric problems and emotional and psychological reactions to the disability.
4. Compare occupational therapy psychosocial practice models and understand the need to use these models in individualizing treatment for each patient.
5. Discuss the typical psychosocial problems of representative disabilities, the psychosocial goals for those disabilities, and what treatment methods might be applicable.

The purpose of treatment is to work with the patient to restore occupational performance by minimizing physical and psychosocial dysfunctions when possible or finding satisfactory alternative solutions when necessary. Throughout the treatment continuum, the objective is to promote the patient's positive self-identity by discovering and reinforcing the patient's strengths, skills, and competencies.

TREATMENT CONTINUUM

The identification and treatment of psychosocial impairments help motivate the patient, reduce morbidity, encourage the patient to participate in his rehabilitation program, and create a more successful transition to the community. The therapist analyzes the evaluation data and selects an occupational therapy practice model that guides the choice of psychosocial goals. These goals are ones that the patient is able to achieve and that are important to him personally and to his lifestyle in the community (Rogers, 1983).

The following example illustrates how the therapist integrates several goals within one treatment plan. The patient's treatment program includes a recreation and sports activity group. Treatment goals include increasing physical components of performance such as strength and mobility, practicing the use of adaptive equipment, and learning compensatory techniques. Psychosocial goals include increasing feelings of personal control, self-esteem, and mastery; developing social and communication skills within an interactive team experience; developing of recreational and hobby interests; and decreasing depression and dependency.

OCCUPATIONAL THERAPY MODELS OF PRACTICE

A practice model guides the occupational therapist in the selection of primary treatment goals for the individual patient's array of psychosocial problems. It is the responsibility of the therapist to recognize that patients have different rehabilitation needs, to analyze the evaluation data, and to select one or more practice models that have principles relevant to the needs of the individual so that treatment options will not be limited (Bruce & Borg, 1987; Denton & Skinner, 1988).

This chapter provides an abridgment of practice models congruent with psychosocial treatment of patients with physical impairments. The student is encouraged to study of the referenced literature.

377

GLOSSARY

Behavioral rehearsals—A structured learning experience that provides an opportunity to experiment with new performance skills and behavior and to practice solving problems before entering the community. Learning objectives are graded according to the patient's level of function. The behavioral rehearsal provides the opportunity for role modeling, role playing, and positive social feedback. The active-doing experiences are motivational (Bruce & Borg, 1987).

Home work assignments—The assignment is structured with specific learning objectives, and the tasks are carried out independently by the patient. The use of a record-keeping system such as a checklist or self-report encourages responsibility and helps the patient learn and remember. The assignment is then discussed with the therapist. This learning method may be part of a treatment group (Crist, 1986; O'Neill & Gardner, 1983).

Modeling—A person learns by observing the behaviors and actions of a role model and then by imitating and practicing that behavior. Models can include the therapist, other patients, or a person with similar problems who has been successfully discharged. Observational learning can also help the patient to improve social behaviors and be more effective in solving problems and making decisions (Bruce & Borg, 1987; Maslan, 1982).

Perseverate—The person continues to focus on and to talk about an idea, concern, or experience without the ability to shift his focus to another topic. The persistent repetition of a verbal or motor response often seen in organic brain disease and schizophrenia (*Webster's*, 1991).

Role play—Role play experiences take place individually or as part of a group experience. The activity is usually planned around a simulated situation such as being appropriately assertive or learning work behaviors. The patient may identify problems he is anticipating at home or at work. The therapist assists him in acting out and practicing new behaviors or skills (Bruce & Borg, 1987; Maslan, 1982).

Shaping—The therapist analyzes the behavior or skills the patient needs and develops successive, graded goals. The patient reaches the end behavior by achieving sequential learning on a step-by-step basis. The therapist reinforces behaviors or skills that are preliminary to the desired target behavior, and the patient receives a preplanned reinforcement as he reaches each subgoal (Bruce & Borg, 1987; Stein 1982).

Social reinforcement—The therapist provides positive supportive feedback, such as praise and attention, in response to the patient's efforts and progress in treatment. Social reinforcement can be verbal or nonverbal and group members may be taught how to reinforce each other. This behavioral method is motivational and helps a patient know how his behaviors are perceived by others (Bruce & Borg, 1987; Stein, 1982).

Values clarification—A person's willingness to accept a disability, to retain a positive self-identity and to endure lifestyle changes is contingent on a change within that person's value system. This process can be facilitated by examining what has not changed, determining the significance of what has changed, discovering what is still available that is valued, enlarging the scope of valued items, and realigning the priority of values (Wright, 1983).

Model of Human Occupation

The model of human occupation focuses on a patient's ability to function in occupational and personal roles and illustrates how a physical impairment can influence a patient's psychosocial functioning. A treatment plan addresses all areas that enable a patient to interact successfully within his environment. These include the patient's values and cultural standards; belief in his own skills; occupational and leisure interests; and problem solving, social skills, and communication skills. For example, the inability to drive can prevent independence in transportation that can preclude maintenance of a favorite leisure interest or require a change in career plans, which could lead to problems with self-identity. The resulting inability to maintain one's own standards and reduced feelings of control over the environment can lead to depression and failure to carry out medical and self-care activities (Kielhofner et al., 1985).

Behavioral Theories

Treatment methods associated with the behavioral approach enable a patient to change noncompliant or maladaptive behaviors that may endanger his rehabilitation success and to learn new behaviors and skills that will make transition into the community more successful. Examples of problem areas include difficulty following a schedule of medical care and self-care, difficulty remembering travel safety precautions, and lack of social-assertive skills necessary for community living. The patient's participation is enhanced by use of individualized self-report inventories and self-monitoring instruments (Bruce & Borg, 1987; O'Neill & Gardner, 1983). Behaviorally stated, treatment goals are precise and describe exactly what the patient needs to accomplish to succeed in the treatment program. Behavioral treatment methods are based on learning theory principles and include **social reinforcement, modeling, shaping** of adaptive behavior, feedback, teaching, demonstration and education, contracting, **role play** and **behavioral rehearsals,** and **home work assignments.** Examples of training programs also include social and assertion skills training, stress and relaxation training, and use of educational modules (Bruce & Borg, 1987; Crist, 1986; Johnston, 1987; Neistadt, 1993b; O'Neill & Gardner, 1983; Stein, 1982).

Psychodynamic Practice Model

The psychodynamic approach assists the patient in recognizing, understanding, and resolving his unconscious or repressed emotional responses to the trauma and the outcomes of the physical disability. A patient, through the use of expressive modalities, can begin to understand the reality of his repressed anxiety, anger, loss of self-esteem and/or intense fears concerning safety and personal security. Both evaluation and treatment occur by the use of expressive modalities and activities. The therapist guides the patient in gaining more personal control over daily events and in expressing his feelings appropriately.

FACTORS THAT INFLUENCE TREATMENT

Methods of Adjustment

The patient's subjective understanding of the cause of his disability or disease influences his acceptance of a treatment plan. It is important that the therapist understand the patient's viewpoints that may influence acceptance of treatment, such as:

1. The injury is seen as confirmation of lack of self-worth, which reduces the patient's motivation for treatment.
2. The injury is viewed as punishment, relieving the patient of guilt for some real or imagined past act and leading to a sense of well-being or relief.
3. Physical illness and disability satisfy security and dependency needs without stigmatizing the patient, because an invalid role is accepted by society and provides justification for dependent behavior.
4. The patient wishes to continue receiving financial support (insurance or family assistance).
5. The patient experiences deep feelings of guilt and holds onto painful symptoms as a form of self-punishment (Safilios-Rothschild, 1970; Versluys, 1980a).

Safilios-Rothschild (1970) described three modes of accommodation to physical disability. Some patients are committed to preventing the breakdown of their denial. They desperately attempt to retain all their usual activities and act surprised and grieved when they cannot do everything that a nondisabled individual can. They tend to refuse the company of other disabled people and prefer to develop a group of nondisabled friends. This group of patients remains unaccepting and frustrated. Another group of patients seem eager to accept the limitations, even those that could be overcome. When treatment is successful for these patients and the physical limitations or effects of the disease are ameliorated, they continue to demonstrate impairments in the psychological and social spheres. Patients also may ignore their intact skills and abilities and become preoccupied with their losses. Other disabled patients are able to accept the fact that they are still worthwhile and build a life on their unchanged assets, both physical and nonphysical. Such patients eventually accept the limitations of the disease and make the most of their lives.

Therapist's Role

The therapist's role differs during each phase of rehabilitation. At one point the patient may need to have his regression understood and supported, and at another stage, the therapist needs to encourage autonomy and personal decision making. The therapist's management of the therapeutic relationship is learned through experience and supervision (see also Chapter 14).

THERAPEUTIC RELATIONSHIP

The patient is assisted in adaptation and rehabilitation by a steady, understanding, and accepting therapeutic relationship. The relationship between the patient and the therapist is motivational when the therapist is consistent; maintains daily contact, at least initially; acts as the patient's advocate; deals with concrete, real issues that are important to the patient; and identifies those areas in which the patient can be proficient. Such a therapist shows respect for the patient and validates his individuality, but she can also be firm and clear about important intervention objectives. The therapist tests reality with understanding and can help and guide without being too authoritarian (Rogers & Figone, 1979b; Versluys, 1984).

What is important to a patient is that the therapist understand his unique case, provide an opportunity to discuss concerns, communicate helpful information about the implications of the injury, encourage experimentation and development of the patient's own ideas, and demonstrate concern about the quality of the patient's future life. It is important to remember that the principal investment is the patient's. The therapist can provide treatment, education, and guidance, but the motivation and effort must come from the patient (Power, 1985; Versluys, 1980a).

TERMINATION OF THE THERAPEUTIC RELATIONSHIP

Courtney (1993) stated that therapists advocate a working relationship with a patient that spans the length of treatment. Although in psychiatric practice the sensitive termination of the therapist-patient relationship is a crucial part of therapy, termination of the therapist-patient relationship in physical rehabilitation practice has received minimal attention. It is important, however, that both the patient and the therapist have an opportunity to acknowledge the quality and the meaning of their relationship and the significance of the termination phase of treatment. Methods of easing termination include home visits, out trips, family involvement, and encouragement to seek support networks and reengagement in role responsibilities. Predischarge discussions emphasize the therapist's interest in the patient's success in the community. Topics of discussion are the patient's achievements in physical, adaptive, and psychosocial areas as well as the patient's plans for management of physical, emotional, and social challenges after discharge, including engaging in hobbies and recreational interests (Courtney, 1993).

PROBLEM AREAS

Some individuals choose a helping profession because of personal interest or special skills, while others are partly influenced by unconscious motivation. The therapist may unconsciously want to relieve others' suffering and thus expurgate her own, or the therapist may have an excessive need to nurture or to be in an authoritative role with respect to others. Without conscious intent, therapists may encourage unrealistic treatment goals based on the need to feel successful professionally (therapeutic ambitiousness) and to be liked by the patients and their families. When patients do not improve, some therapists have difficulty maintaining an objective point of view and may express anger and rejection toward the patient. Therapists may also feel overwhelmed with the severity of the patient's disability and feel guilty over good personal health. They may thus deny the extent of the patient's disability and his right to a period of reactive mourning of losses. Support groups for therapists are helpful in retaining perspective (Tucker, 1980).

Premorbid Conditions

The following psychosocial and emotional problems are also reviewed in Chapter 10.

AGE

Zemke and Grantz (1982) described developmental treatment goals, based on Erikson's psychoso-cial developmental principles. The treatment approach for patients with a physical dysfunction and premorbid life-stage difficulties should include activities to facilitate age-appropriate developmental tasks and to enhance normal psychosocial development, e.g., an adolescent patient may need age-appropriate skills to separate from an overprotective family, to develop a sense of his own identity and interests, to learn performance components for the occupational role of student, and to develop social and communication skills to relate to his peer group. A middle-aged patient may benefit from assistance with planning for career and vocation, developing recreational outlets to compensate for loss of an active career, exploring new interests, and/or reassessing and reengaging in past interests. This focus encourages continued maturation and remotivation toward a satisfactory lifestyle rather than stagnation and regression.

PSYCHIATRIC ISSUES

The patient with a comorbid psychiatric diagnosis faces added adjustments and a more difficult rehabilitation. The occupational therapy approach includes identifying treatment priorities for each condition, collaborating with other treatment providers, grading difficult learning and rehabilitation tasks associated with both the primary and the comorbid diagnosis, problem solving to help the patient manage engagement in treatment, and planning for a safe discharge.

Treatment for conditions of depression, whether reactive or primary major depression, includes assisting the patient to:

1. Identify strengths and skills for a positive self-identity;
2. Establish short-term goals so he can see results;
3. Find alternative ways to fulfill significant adult roles;
4. Establish feelings of personal control over events;
5. Express the sadness and loss; and
6. Test the actual boundaries and influence of the disability.

Therapists working with a depressed patient should inform others of the patient's interests and accomplishments so that they can use this information during treatment sessions. Therapists must guard against the tendency to identify with such patients' moods, becoming depressed themselves.

ALCOHOLISM

Treatment of alcohol addiction is complicated, as patients may not be willing to recognize their problems or to participate in curative actions. Specialists differ in their opinions about how to approach a patient who is abusing alcohol; however, it is agreed that a patient cannot make use of education and skill training until he has been substance free for at least 2 weeks, and preferably longer (Renner, 1986). Cassidy (1988) reported that to be effective, the therapist must understand the difficulties associated with abstinence, provide empathetic education, and hold out optimistic encouragement about potential for recovery. After the symptoms of alcohol abuse have been identified and documented, the focus is to help a patient to explore the relationship between alcohol and his medical, psychosocial, and occupational problems; to encourage the patient to join appropriate self-help groups such as Alcoholics Anonymous; to participate in alcohol or drug education groups within the hospital; and to seek counseling from specialists in alcoholism treatment (Moyers, 1988; Renner, 1986). The occupational therapy approach includes an emphasis on treatment to provide skills for living with physical impairment as well as for sobriety and long-term recovery from alcohol abuse. Treatment goals that may be addressed in occupational therapy include the following (Cassidy, 1988; Kaufman & McNaul, 1992; Raymond, 1990; Scarth, 1990):

1. Develop effective coping strategies to prevent self-medication with substances.
2. Help patients communicate needs and feelings appropriately and in a timely way.
3. Instill a philosophy of solving daily problems one step at a time.
4. Teach appropriate self-assertion to improve social and communication skills, which will increase feelings of control and reduce feelings of vulnerability.
5. Teach relaxation and stress management techniques to enable coping with excessive anxiety and to maintain recovery.
6. Develop leisure interests and time management to help fill the time previously spent drinking.

During preparation for discharge it is important that therapists remain aware of the personal stress and anxiety that independence and responsibility within the community may pose for the patient who is a recovering alcoholic or has current problems with alcohol. The therapists should suggest a sequenced and moderate approach to adaptation in all areas of occupational functioning.

Psychological and Emotional Reactions to Disability

Severe emotional reactions are usually reversible in formerly healthy patients as the medical status improves, the hospital milieu becomes less threatening, and trust is established in the personnel. Management of grief, anxiety, and anger is facilitated when the patient can acknowledge the normal feelings of anger, sadness, and loss and at the same time recognize and build on those aspects of life that are not affected by the disease (Stewart & Shields, 1985; Tucker, 1980; Versluys, 1984).

Occupational therapy treatment approach includes helping patients understand the real boundaries of the disability, why they feel anxious, that they have some control over the direction of their treatment, that there are alternative ways to achieve satisfaction, and that planning for the future is possible. It is important to help the patient identify situations that are especially stressful for him and to teach him stress management techniques (Engel, 1992; Gage, 1992; Lysaght & Bodenhamer, 1990; Neistadt, 1993b). To reduce anxiety and anger, the therapist should provide the opportunity for clarification of feelings, help the patient feel more in control, encourage safe avenues of both verbal and nonverbal expression of feelings, and create outlets through activities and recreation. This is important for severely injured patients who may have difficulty with expression of angry feelings because they cannot use physical activity as a medium and because they may fear alienating family, caretakers, and other support systems. The therapist can also indicate that it is important to express such strong feelings and that such feelings are normal.

DEPENDENCY

Dependency can be a problem in the rehabilitation of the disabled patient. Rehabilitation personnel should dissuade the development of dependent and passive behaviors through a consistent staff approach. The therapists also need to assist the patient in understanding and accepting appropriate aspects of a dependent role when necessary. In such cases, dependency should be understood as a positive rather than a negative factor. For example, the occupational therapist can help the patient to recognize that assistance with time-consuming skills relating to activities of daily living will free energy for involvement in more interesting and creative activities. The occupational therapist can also help the patient to maintain responsibilities in personal and family roles and provide the patient with opportunities to make choices and decisions. Treatment is planned to assist patients to deal with personal feelings concerning accepting necessary help, to retain a positive self-view, to accent competencies, to develop communication and interactive skills that help them tactfully direct others, and to engage in problem solving for maximum independence (Safilios-Rothschild, 1970).

DENIAL

The patient's denial of the nature of his disability may curtail rehabilitation. During rehabilitation, patients may hold on to the belief that when they are discharged the physical impairments will have lessened, and they will again be able to function in their usual manner. When the patient rejects the need for treatment on this basis, the therapist can suggest that, while waiting for return, the patient learn performance skills for use now. Sometimes a weekend pass, or a planned out trip, or other reality experience may influence the patient to accept the need to engage in treatment that focuses on development of functional skills. As the patient progresses toward clear, observable treatment goals, reality may be less threatening. Time and experience in the community may allow the patient to be more realistic, but he may wish to hold on to the hope of future functional return (Felton & Revenson, 1984). A state of entrenched denial that prevents rehabilitation and places the patient at risk in the community requires psychiatric intervention. Patients at risk for regression may need time out from therapy; protection from an internal sense of failure; or an alternative therapeutic approach such as group work, adaptive play, or recreational experience.

Sexuality

Other important factors in rehabilitation are issues relative to sexuality. A vital part of psychosocial rehabilitation is to eradicate myths and misinformation and to educate the patient about his sexual functioning (Block, Boyer, & Imes, 1984; Garner & Allen, 1989; Neistadt, 1993a; Neistadt & Freda, 1987). Occupational therapists should help patients find ways to overcome physical limitations that constrain sexual activity, explore value conflicts about alternate ways to achieve sexual satisfaction, solve environmental problems that make socializing difficult, and develop the confidence to overcome negative societal attitudes (Goldman, 1978). Sexual education is most successful within a comprehensive educational and counseling program and should be offered to all patients and their partners before discharge (Neistadt, 1993a; Tardif, 1989). In a study reported by Cushman (1988) patients reported that they would like more formal education, including both verbal and written approaches. The preferred method involved greater staff initiative and private discussions about sexual matters rather than group meetings.

Ancillary Factors

The role of the family in the rehabilitation process is vital, and studies reveal that patients look first to their families for support and then to the professional staff (Power, 1985). Therapists are increasingly involving the family in goal setting and treatment decisions. However, it is important that the therapist recognize that the current life demands on each family member are sometimes incompatible with the patient's need for services within the home and community. It is clear that some families who are urged to take on major caretaker roles are not able to do so while simultaneously meeting other important obligations and retaining family stability (Power, 1985; Versluys, 1980a, 1993; Zisserman, 1981). The occupational therapy treatment approach to including the patient's family involves (Versluys, 1980a, 1993) the following:

1. Help the family to understand the role of the occupational therapist and the purpose of the treatment procedures.
2. Explain the realities of therapeutic outcome to offset family disappointment and discouragement.
3. Help the family understand and integrate information about the patient's care and physical limitations and potential as well as how to plan for discharge.
4. Support and guide the family while it makes necessary arrangements, including adaptation of the home, seeking out community resources, and ordering necessary equipment.
5. Educate the family about the effect of the patient's residual impairment on his work, family, and social roles.
6. Guide family members to adapt hobby and recreational equipment so that the patient and the family continue common interests.
7. Help the family recognize the patient's continuing abilities and degree of independence in self-care and other occupational performance areas (Frey, 1984).
8. Encourage the family to use community resources.

A patient's cultural background can influence attitudes toward acceptance of therapy. The patient's noncompliance with treatment may be the result of different cultural values. Expecting all patients to adhere to the values of the major population is often a barrier to effective treatment. A patient's beliefs and ceremonies should be accepted as part of the treatment regimen when possible. The therapist needs to select culturally relevant activities that will be accepted by the patient as meaningful and that will aid the patient in developing performance components for occupational performance areas consistent with his cultural values. Some activities may not be considered purposeful, germane, or even respectable within a social and cultural context (Dillard et al., 1992; Kinebanian & Stomph, 1992).

TREATMENT OF DISEASE-SPECIFIC PSYCHOSOCIAL REACTIONS

This section provides examples of the psychosocial adjustment requirements of different physical disabilities treated by occupational therapists. Illustrative examples include permanent functional disabilities such as cerebral vascular accident (CVA), rheumatoid arthritis (RA), and spinal cord injury (SCI) as well as the complicated psychosocial effects of invisible disabilities such as diabetes, renal disease, cardiac disease, and traumatic brain injury.

Cerebral Vascular Accident

At one time, psychosocial sequelae were considered irreversible and a result of neurologic damage. A more current view recognizes psychosocial dysfunction as an outcome of the residual effects of the stroke and changes in occupational, personal, social and leisure roles. Researchers indicate that even when patients attain independence in most daily living skills, they may not resume premorbid social activities (Belcher, Clowers, & Cabanayan, 1978; Feibel & Springer, 1982; Labi, Phillips, & Gresham, 1980).

EMOTIONAL REACTIONS

Common emotional reactions after stroke are anxiety, denial, and depression. These responses are compounded by perceptual and visual impairments and by cognitive and language impairments that affect the ability to plan and to use logic, memory, and judgment. Behavioral outcomes can include impatience, irritability, extreme frustration, overdependence, insensitivity to others, rigid and inflexible thinking, and paranoid delusional thinking. Poor social perception, caused by the effects of the stroke, can lead to misinterpretations of others' behavior or intent that result in angry outbursts. Difficulties with communication can result in a buildup of annoyances and angry feelings. These behavioral reactions and misinterpretations of environmental events can lead to a breakdown in social and family relationships (Binder, 1983; Labi et al., 1980).

Anxiety

Anxiety is a common problem caused, e.g., by brain damage, cognitive impairments, and psychologic concerns such as fear of abandonment and feelings of helplessness. Other causes of anxiety are the patient's inability to externalize concerns, his fear of a second stroke, obsessive thinking, and cognitive confusion. Anxiety may be fixed on somatic preoccupation such as paralysis of the arm. Or it may be experienced by the patient as a general uneasiness or a series of catastrophes that never end (Diller, 1973).

Denial

In the stroke patient, the origins of denial can be organic, psychological, or a combination of both. The following are examples of denial in the stroke patient: (1) the presence of the disability (paralyzed limb) is denied or is neglected; (2) the disabling condition is acknowledged, but the patient fails to accommodate to his condition, (3) the slightest change in function or spasm is interpreted as evidence that complete return will occur, (4) the patient insists that he can read but rationalizes his failure to do so (i.e., too small print or lack of glasses). In addition, the patient may deny the need for treatment. He may want to do things no longer possible such as drive a car or go immediately back to work. Or the patient may continue to work obsessively toward goals that are no longer possible. Years after the initial insult, some stroke patients still appear bewildered about the presence of the disabling condition and still insist that they can carry out tasks and activities that are no longer possible. While these descriptions are illustrative of the stroke patient, the information also pertains to patients with other kinds of cerebral trauma or neurologic disease (Binder, 1983; Diller, 1973).

Depression

Up to 50% of stroke patients experience clinically significant depression, including major depressive disorders and reactive depression (Binder, 1983; Starkstein et al., 1990). Depression in stroke survivors is the result of a combination of functional and psychosocial losses. Some of the symptoms may also be neurologically based, may occur as a reaction to medication, or may be the result of easy fatigue or confusion and disorientation. Treatment of the patient's depression is complicated by the unique neurologic impairments. Some stroke patients tend to **perseverate** both mood and affect and thus remain preoccupied with the somatic losses and changes in activities and lifestyle. The patient may be unable to shift his attention from the physical impairment and loss of competencies. He appears unable to focus on his remaining skills or positive rehabilitation gains (Binder, 1983; Labi et al., 1980).

PSYCHOSOCIAL DYSFUNCTIONS

The patient experiences significant social and personal loss and is at risk for depression when he can no longer function in those activities and roles that supported a sense of identity, belonging, and status. It is thought that stroke patients, even after a good recovery, may still remain isolated and may be unable to initiate resumption of social, leisure, recreational, or community activities outside the home. Some patients become especially anxious during, or even when thinking about, social interaction within the community because of changes in body image, difficulty in communication and eating, cognitive disorientation, fatigue, or visual-perceptual problems (Feibel & Springer, 1982; Labi et al., 1980; Malec et al., 1990). These problems, when possible, should be counteracted by an integrated treatment plan that encourages graduated social and community experiences, provides education, and encourages family participation.

TREATMENT

A comprehensive approach to the treatment of stroke patients should include not only treatment of neurologic impairments but also treatment for psychosocial dysfunction. Psychosocial goals to be integrated into the treatment plan include (Feibel & Springer, 1982; Kielhofner et al., 1985) the following:

1. Preserving a sense of mastery through maintenance of role performance skills when possible;
2. Increasing a positive self-concept by helping the patient resume social group activities;
3. Training to generalize activities of daily living and leisure activities into the community, because of the patient's difficulty in transferring skills from one environment to another;
4. Adapting those leisure activities (one-handed if necessary) that are possible within the limitations of the disability; and
5. Recommending self-help groups for continuing education and support.

The therapist should be aware that some patients do not want to return to activities if previous standards of performance cannot be met (Jongbloed & Morgan, 1991). It is important to remember that even though neurologic recovery may occur soon after the medical incident, many stroke patients can continue to develop and refine performance skills after discharge, but they require postdischarge treatment to do so. The therapist should suggest community resources such as recreational opportunities for persons with disabilities and self-help groups, which are important sources of continued psychological, social, and educational support (Evans & Northwood, 1983; Feibel & Springer, 1982). The occupational therapist's role with the family of the stroke patient in education, training, support, and counseling is considered valuable.

Rheumatoid Arthritis

PSYCHOSOCIAL PROBLEMS

Researchers currently believe that the difficulties with affective, behavioral, and social functioning that most patients with RA experience are reactions to the chronic pain, fatigue, and the variable and unpredictable course of the disease. A person with RA is at risk for significant levels of anxiety and depression. He must cope with a disease process that is to some degree invisible and must maintain a consistent regimen of health care that includes rest and joint protection. Education and reality testing are important to offset a person's tendency toward denial during symptom-free remissions (Anderson et al., 1985). A patient with RA is concerned about making long-range plans because he never knows if physical function will be possible on a particular day or when social plans or activities will have to be abandoned. The effort to complete just the basic daily activities often diverts time and energy from more enjoyable pursuits. In addition, it is difficult to maintain personal standards, which leads to a reduction in life satisfaction. Over time, the exacerbations and remissions of painful symptoms and lack of control over health and activities lead to secondary behavioral responses such as overreaction to events, rigidity, conformity, perfectionism, and difficulty in expressing or dealing with hostile and aggressive feelings. The reduction of involvement in life activities, including social events and interests, leads to boredom that precipitates discouragement and depression (Anderson et al., 1985; Baum, 1982; Locker, 1983; Melvin, 1989).

Dependency may also be a reaction to the constellation of physical and psychosocial problems of the RA patient. Although dependency may not have been a personal characteristic of the patient before the onset of RA, it can become a way of life as the patient becomes more disabled and has difficulty in consistent functioning regarding responsibilities and activities. Under these conditions, the family may become overprotective and assume some or all of the patient's responsibilities (Anderson et al., 1985). Self-devaluation accompanies the reduction in those roles and activities that provided a self-identity, e.g., changes in work involvement with resultant reduction in income (Anderson et al., 1985; Kielhofner et al., 1985; Melvin, 1989).

TREATMENT

Psychosocial goals include development of problem-solving strategies and coping skills to help maintain functional abilities and interests, **values clarification** to aid in a lowering of expectations for consistent performance, and identification of alternative methods to engage in occupational performance areas. Baum (1982) suggested training in self-control interventions such as relaxation, pain management, stress reduction, and biofeedback to increase pain tolerance and to foster a sense of personal control and mastery (Achterberg-Lawlis, 1982; Brown, 1983; Kielhofner et al., 1985).

Educational models of treatment are more successful than mental health models for both the patient and the family. Educational approaches include discovering problem-solving and energy-conservation techniques for adaptation of hobbies and favorite activities, telling family members and the patient about the effects of RA, and encouraging intrafamily communication. The therapist should be aware that the patient's participation in therapy is influenced by the degree of pain and discomfort present at a given time. In addition, his anxiety over the variability of the disease and its effect on his body may decrease his ability to listen to the therapist and to cooperate in the treatment session (Melvin, 1989). It is important that verbal education be accompanied by written and illustrated materials that can be referred to when the need arises.

Spinal Cord Injury

PSYCHOSOCIAL CONSEQUENCES

A spinal cord–injured patient's physical limitations in function cause him to feel vulnerable to attack from others, place him at a disadvantage when insisting on his rights during interpersonal encounters, and require him to deal with nondisabled individuals from a seated position. In addition, dysfunction and mobility problems alter the patient's ability to use familiar behaviors and actions to release tension, to externalize anger through physical action, to escape from unpleasant situations by moving away, or to gain pleasure from intrinsically satisfying action activities. To the SCI patient, the losses and changes experienced are not only continually frustrating but also threatening to his developmental maturation and his sense of mastery and personal control over life events and the environment (Kielhofner et al., 1985; Tucker, 1980).

The severely disabled patient tends to internalize hostility and negative feelings because the expression of these feelings may damage social relationships and prevent access to needed caretakers. This continual repression may find an outlet through passive-aggressive behavior (procrastination or sabotage) or result in regression, depression, verbal explosions, or acting-out behaviors that others do not understand. The long-term nature of the physical impairments may reduce the patient's involvement in work, school, social, and community activities. The patient's total expenditure of available mental and physical energy and daily time may be required to carry out basic activities of daily living. This limits activities of interest and choice.

TREATMENT FOCUS

The patient's psychosocial adjustment is an important long-term treatment goal. Patients may experi-

ence difficulty in accepting the need to be dependent in some living-skill areas and in retaining, at the same time, a sense of personal causation, mastery, and competence. Successful treatment outcomes depend on the patient's ability to (Kanellos, 1985; Kielhofner et al., 1985):

1. Reappraise his values and life goals;
2. Analyze and solve problems;
3. Plan and execute personal, social, and vocational plans; and
4. Apply adapted performance skills and components successfully for engagement within the physical and social environment.

The therapist must also consider the patient's life stage position and address relevant, important developmental tasks (Mulcahey, 1992). Thus treatment goals for adolescents with spinal cord injuries might include achievement of age-appropriate tasks, such as returning to the student role; engagement in social activities within the hospital or community; and mobility and recreational interests (Frieden & Cole, 1985; Mulcahey, 1992).

Rogers and Figone (1979a) described the critical nature of helping the SCI patient develop leisure skills. Treatment goals should include the identification and practice of hobbies and recreational or sports interests (Decker & Schulz, 1985; Versluys, 1984). The development of vocational skills is important for those patients with work-oriented values and helps to reduce a diminished sense of self-worth. Vocational planning should start early in the restorative phase of treatment. Treatment can include **behavioral rehearsals** to increase confidence, guided planning of balanced daily schedule, and problem solving around challenges to accessibility (Kanellos, 1985).

Invisible Disability

Certain medical and neurologic conditions (e.g., cardiac disease, diabetes mellitus, asthma, traumatic brain injury, and the initial and remission stages of multiple sclerosis) do not present visual evidence that clues others to the medical or neurologic problems of the patient. Thus the expectations of others are not adjusted to accommodate to the presence of a disability. The patient with a physical disability reality tests daily, because of his limitations in the performance of activities. The responses of others, based on their observation of the disabling condition, provide social validation of the presence of the disability. The dynamics of adjustment for the person with an invisible disability are different, because when he is symptom free, it is easy to deny the presence of a disease and to forget essential rules of health care. When a person with an invisible disability does not participate in organized activities at school or in the community, his lack of participation may be viewed as malingering, passivity, lack of interest, noncompliant behavior, or rejection of activities planned by others. Medical requirements such as rest periods, special diets, and refraining from strenuous activity may be viewed as personal weakness, rigidity, or hypochondriacal behavior, which may limit social acceptance and cause rejection. Misunderstandings can also occur when others interpret the symptoms of grieving and depression that are precipitated by the illness as neurotic (Flavo, Allen, & Maki, 1982; Lilliston, 1985). It becomes the patient's responsibility to explain his hidden health problem in a way that his audience can understand. The patient with an invisible disability must continually let others know about his disease and lifestyle requirements. This requires self-confidence and good social and communication skills.

TREATMENT

A psychosocial treatment focus for the patient with an invisible disability includes examining and understanding how the disease alters and influences his lifestyle, occupational performance, personal standards, interests, and future plans. Treatment should include the identification of alternative occupational roles, development of interests consistent with the restrictions of the disability, discovery of lifestyle management techniques; and practice of social and communication skills to increase involvement and to feel confident in informing others concerning the limitations posed by the disability. Treatment programs that include exercise, sports, and recreational experiences help dispel the myth of invalidism (Flavo et al., 1982; Lilliston, 1985).

TREATMENT METHODS

Education

Educational curricula and teaching techniques are important components of occupational therapy treatment programming (see Chapter 13). Educational methods include the following (Crist, 1986; Lillie & Armstrong, 1982; Schmitt, 1982):

1. Development of an educational plan consistent with the patient's learning style and previous knowledge;
2. Pursuit of individualized, reachable learning goals;
3. Selection and assignment of learning tasks;
4. Dissemination of information to the patient and family about the tasks the patient needs to perform; and
5. Identification of the patient as an adult learner.

Education programs are designed to increase knowledge and skills in such areas as daily living skills, health and safety, time management, transportation, management of self-care attendants, repair of equipment, social assertiveness, stress reduction, and survival skills for discharge (Crist, 1986). Educational methods include building knowledge through reading; using films and video tapes; using behavioral techniques such as **modeling,** role playing, and **behavioral rehearsals;** taking field trips; listening to guest speakers; and providing active help in transferring skills to the expected environment (Bruce & Borg, 1987; Crist, 1986; Johnston, 1987; Lillie & Armstrong, 1982; Maslan, 1982).

Group Treatment

Group treatment is an effective way of providing integrated treatment for a patient's psychosocial and physical impairments. A well-designed group provides a therapeutic environment wherein the patient's psychosocial dysfunction can be identified and treated. Evaluation within a group format highlights not only the patient's psychosocial problems but also his positive qualities such as initiative, persistence, originality, and altruism. Group methods contribute to treatment for some of the following reasons (Democker & Zimpfer, 1981; Falk-Kessler, Momich, & Perel, 1991; Howe & Schwartzberg, 1986; Janosik & Miller, 1982; Schmitt, 1982; Versluys, 1980b, 1984; Vinogradov & Yalom, 1989):

1. The group offers peer support and education to assist the patient in adjusting to hospitalization and to treatment regimens.
2. The group activity and group treatment plan can be adjusted and sequenced to allow the patient's participation at his current level of functioning.
3. Therapist and peer feedback prevent entrenchment of feelings or behaviors that are the result of the disability, such as feelings of disfigurement or passivity.
4. The patient who becomes actively involved with other group members feels more confident, more in control, and more positive about his own ability to handle change.
5. Group membership reduces social isolation and strengthens personal identity, counters the tendency to brood, and provides an opportunity to develop new friendships that may evolve into a community support network.
6. Intermember problem solving promotes a useful exchange of ideas and a breadth of alternatives to encourage lifestyle changes.
7. Group member support assists the patient in reducing denial and confronting reality in a supportive environment.

8. Patient and family groups maintain family relationships and encourage open communication.
9. Peer support and interaction are motivational, and the group expands the patient's support system within the rehabilitation setting.
10. The group experience provides feelings of support and belonging, develops social abilities, restructures a more hopeful view of the future, and reveals that others also have problems.

There are a wide range of group themes in physical rehabilitation, including the following:

1. Groups designed for physical treatment only such as range of motion and exercise groups (Reichel, Fee, & Wilkerson, 1988: Trahey, 1991);
2. Groups that combine physical treatments with psychosocial goals such as discharge planning groups, problem solving for community living and planning accessibility, and recreational and hobby groups (Adamczyk, 1989; Gauthier, Dalziel, & Gauthier, 1987; Versluys, 1984).
3. Groups that have primary psychosocial goals such as stress management groups; remotivation groups to help members deal with depression, grieving and loss; groups to develop skills of assertion for community interaction; role change groups; and groups for learning new coping mechanisms (Versluys, 1980b, 1984; Vinogradov & Yalom, 1989).
4. Peer groups to help patients adjust successfully after discharge and provide active help, social support, and education (Schmitt, 1982).

SUMMARY

It is important that the rehabilitation effort not ultimately fail because of unrecognized and untreated psychosocial dysfunctions. Prevention includes expanding the patient's potential for independence and satisfaction by the integration of physical and psychosocial goals into a comprehensive treatment program. Treating patients with psychosocial dysfunction depends on knowledge and experience but also on the therapist's perception, warmth, sincerity, and responsiveness. Therapists need to recognize when to support the patient, when to give more responsibility, when to be the patient's advocate, and when to encourage the patient to solve his own problems and initiate his own planning.

STUDY QUESTIONS

1. What are the major psychosocial problems that a patient may experience after physical trauma? How would you state these psychosocial problems in terms of treatment goals?

2. What are some of the most important psychosocial areas and problems related to successful discharge and to independent occupational functioning in the community?
3. What is a therapeutic relationship? What are the characteristics of a quality relationship? What are the therapist's objectives in termination of the therapeutic relationship, and why is this important?
4. Why is consideration of ancillary or secondary factors associated with the patient so important in treatment planning?
5. Why are practice models important, and what are the principles of selecting a practice model for treatment?
6. Describe the treatment methods and how each method can contribute to achievement of a patient's psychosocial treatment goals.
7. What are some primary psychosocial treatment goals and treatment methods you would choose for each of the diagnoses described in this chapter?

REFERENCES

Achterberg-Lawlis, J. (1982). The psychological dimensions of arthritis. *Journal of Consulting and Clinical Psychology, 50,* 984–992.

Adamczyk, H. (1989, February 2). Interdisciplinary efforts ease group interaction for clients recovering from head injury. *OT WEEK, 2,* 6–7.

Anderson, K. O., Bradley, L. A., Young, L. D., & McDaniel, L. K. (1985). Rheumatoid arthritis: Review of psychological factors related to etiology, effects, and treatment. *Psychological Bulletin, 98,* 358–387.

Baum, J. (1982). A review of the psychological aspects of rheumatoid arthritis. *Seminar of Arthritis and Rheumatism, 11,* 352–360.

Belcher, S. A., Clowers, M. R., & Cabanayan, A. C. (1978). Independent living rehabilitation needs of postdischarge stroke persons: A pilot study. *Archives of Physical Medicine & Rehabilitation, 59,* 404–409.

Binder, L. M. (1983). Current concepts of cerebrovascular disease. *Stroke, 18*(4), 17–21.

Block, A. R., Boyer, S. L., & Imes, D. (1984). Personal impact of myocardial infarction: A model for coping with physical disability in middle age. In M. G. Eisenberg, L. C. Sutkin, & M. A. Jansen (Eds.), *Chronic illness and disability through the life span: Effect on self and family* (pp. 209–221). New York: Springer.

Brown, D. (1983). A community model for arthritis rehabilitation. *Canadian Journal of Occupational Therapy, 50,* 115–118.

Bruce, M. A., & Borg, B. (1987). *Frames of reference in psychosocial occupational therapy.* Thorofare, NJ: Slack.

Cassidy, C. L. (1988). Occupational therapy intervention in the treatment of alcoholics. *Occupational Therapy in Mental Health, 8,* 17–26.

Courtney, E. A. (1993). *Termination of the therapeutic relationship: Themes and techniques in occupational therapy.* Unpublished master's thesis, Tufts University, Medford, MA.

Crist, P. H. (1986). Community living skills: A psychoeducational community based program. *Occupational Therapy in Mental Health, 6,* 51–64.

Cushman, L. A. (1988, April–June). Sexual counseling in a rehabilitation program: A patient perspective. *Journal of Rehabilitation, 65–69.*

Decker, S. D., & Schulz, R. (1985). Correlates of life satisfaction and depression in middle-aged and elderly spinal cord injured persons. *American Journal of Occupational Therapy, 39,* 740–745.

Democker, J. E., & Zimpfer, D. G. (1981). Group approaches to psychosocial intervention in medical care: A synthesis. *International Journal of Group Psychotherapy, 31*(2), 247–259.

Denton, P. L., & Skinner, S. T. (1988). Selecting a frame of reference/practice model. In S. C. Robertson (Ed.), *Focus: Skills for assessment and treatment. Section 1* (pp. 100–108). Rockville, MD: American Occupational Therapy Association.

Dillard, M., Andonian, L., Flores, O., Lai, L., MacRae, A., & Shakir, M. (1992). Culturally competent occupational therapy in a diversely populated mental health setting. *American Journal of Occupational Therapy, 46,* 721–726.

Diller, L. (1973). Hemiplegia. In J. F. B. Garrett & E. S. Levine (Eds.), *Rehabilitation practices with the physically disabled* (pp. 294–328). New York: Columbia University Press.

Engel, J. M. (1992). Relaxation training: A self-help approach for children with headaches. *American Journal of Occupational Therapy, 46,* 591–596.

Evans, R. L., & Northwood, L. K. (1983). Social support needs in adjustment to stroke. *Archives of Physical Medicine & Rehabilitation, 64,* 61–64.

Falk-Kessler, J., Momich, C., & Perel, S. (1991). Therapeutic factors in occupational therapy groups. *American Journal of Occupational Therapy, 45,* 59–66.

Feibel, J. H., & Springer, C. J. (1982). Depression and failure to resume social activities after a stroke. *Archives of Physical Medicine & Rehabilitation, 63,* 276–278.

Felton, B. J., & Revenson, T. A. (1984). Coping with chronic illness: A study of illness controlment and the influences of coping strategies on psychological adjustment. *Journal of Consulting and Clinical Psychology, 52,* 343–353.

Flavo, D. R., Allen, H., & Maki, D. R. (1982). Psychosocial aspects of invisible disability. *Rehabilitation Literature, 43,* 2–6.

Frey, J. (1984). A family systems approach to illness-maintaining behaviors in chronically ill adolescents. *The Family Process, 23,* 251–260.

Frieden, L., & Cole, J. A. (1985). Independence: The ultimate goal of rehabilitation for spinal cord-injured persons. *American Journal of Occupational Therapy, 39,* 734–739.

Gage, M. (1992). The appraisal model of coping: An assessment and intervention model for occupational therapy. *American Journal of Occupational Therapy, 46,* 353–362.

Garner, W. E., & Allen, H. A. (1989, January–March). Sexual rehabilitation and heart disease. *Journal of Rehabilitation, 69–*73.

Gauthier, L., Dalziel, S., & Gauthier S. (1987). The benefits of group occupational therapy for patients with Parkinson's disease. *American Journal of Occupational Therapy, 41,* 360.

Goldman, F. (1978). Environmental barriers to sociosexual integration: The insiders' perspectives. *Rehabilitation Literature, 39,* 185–189.

Howe, M. C., & Schwartzberg, S. L. (1986). *A functional approach to group work in occupational therapy.* Philadelphia: J. B. Lippincott.

Janosik, E. H., & Miller, J. R. (1982). Group work with the elderly. In E. H. Janosik & L. B. Phipps (Eds.), *Life cycle group work in nursing* (pp. 248–265). Monterey, CA: Wadsworth.

Johnston, M. T. (1987). Occupational therapists and the teaching of cognitive behavioral skills. *Occupational Therapy in Mental Health, 7*(3), 69–81.

Jongbloed, L., & Morgan D. (1991). An investigation of involvement in leisure activities after a stroke. *American Journal of Occupational Therapy, 45,* 420–427.

Kanellos, M. C. (1985). Enhancing vocational outcomes of spinal cord-injured persons: The occupational therapist's role. *American Journal of Occupational Therapy, 39,* 726–733.

Kaufman, E., & McNaul, J. P. (1992). Recent developments in understanding and treating drug abuse and dependence. *Hospital and Community Psychiatry, 43,* 223–236.

Kielhofner, G., Shepherd, J., Stabenow, C. A., Beledsoe, N., Furst, G., Green, J., Harlan, B. H., McLellan, C. L., & Owens, J. (1985). Physical disabilities. In G. S. Kielhofner (Ed.), *A model of human occupation: Theory and application* (pp. 170–247). Baltimore: Williams & Wilkins.

Kinebanian, A., & Stomph, M. (1992). Cross-cultural occupational therapy: A critical reflection. *American Journal of Occupational Therapy, 46,* 751–757.

Labi, M. L. C., Phillips, T. F., & Gresham, G. E. (1980). Psychosocial disability in physically restored long-term stroke survivors. *Archives of Physical Medicine & Rehabilitation, 61,* 561–565.

Lillie, M. D., & Armstrong, H. E. (1982). Contributions to the development of psychoeducational approaches to mental health services. *American Journal of Occupational Therapy, 36,* 438–443.

Lilliston, B. A. (1985). Psychosocial responses to traumatic physical disability. *Social Work in Health Care, 10,* 1–14.

Locker, D. (1983). Disability and disadvantage: The consequences of chronic illness. New York: Ravistock.

Lysaght, R., & Bodenhamer, E. (1990). The use of relaxation training to enhance functional outcomes in adults with traumatic head injury. *American Journal of Occupational Therapy, 44,* 797–802.

Malec, J. F., Richardson, J. W., Sinake, M., & O'Brien, M. W. (1990). Types of affective responses to stroke. *Archives of Physical Medicine & Rehabilitation, 71,* 279–284.

Maslan, D. (1982). Rehabilitation training for community living skills: Concepts and techniques. *Occupational Therapy in Mental Health, 2,* 33–49.

Melvin, J. L. (1989). *Rheumatic disease in the adult and child: Occupational therapy and rehabilitation* (3rd ed.). Philadelphia: F. A. Davis.

Moyers, P. A. (1988). An organizational framework for occupational therapy in the treatment of alcoholism. *Occupational Therapy in Health Care, 8,* 27–46.

Mulcahey, M. J. (1992). Returning to school after a spinal cord injury: Perspectives from four adolescents. *American Journal of Occupational Therapy, 46,* 305–312.

Neistadt, M. E. (1993a). Human sexuality and counseling. In H. L. Hopkins & H. D. Smith (Eds.), *Willard & Spackman's occupational therapy* (8th ed., pp. 148–154). Philadelphia: J. B. Lippincott.

Neistadt, M. E. (1993b). Stress management. In H. L. Hopkins & H. D. Smith (Eds.), *Willard & Spackman's occupational therapy* (8th ed., pp. 588–596). Philadelphia: J. B. Lippincott.

Neistadt, M. E., & Freda, M. (1987). *Choices: A guide to sex counseling with physically disabled adults.* Melbourne, FL: R. E. Krieger.

O'Neill, G. W., & Gardner, R. (1983). Behavior therapy: An overview. *Hospital and Community Psychiatry, 34,* 709–715.

Power, P. W. (1985). Family coping behaviors in chronic illness: A rehabilitation perspective. *Rehabilitation Literature, 46,* 78–83.

Raymond, M. (1990, September). Life skills and substance abuse. *AOTA Mental Health Special Interest Newsletter, 13,* 1–2.

Reichel, D. A., Fee, P., & Wilkerson, J. (1988, July). Breakfast club helps OT clients achieve independence in feeding skills. *OT WEEK, 14,* 1–3.

Renner, J. A. (1986). Alcoholism. In L. I. Sederer (Ed.), *Inpatient psychiatry: Diagnosis and treatment* (2nd ed., pp. 171–194). Baltimore: Williams & Wilkins.

Rogers, J. C. (1983). Clinical reasoning: The ethics, science, and art. *American Journal of Occupational Therapy, 37,* 601–616.

Rogers, J. D., & Figone, J. J. (1979a). The avocational pursuits of rehabilitants with traumatic quadriplegia. *American Journal of Occupational Therapy. 32,* 571–576.

Rogers, J. D., & Figone, J. J. (1979b). Psychosocial parameters in treating the person with quadriplegia. *American Journal of Occupational Therapy, 33,* 432–439.

Safilios-Rothschild, C. (1970). *The sociology and social psychology of disability and rehabilitation.* New York: Random House.

Scarth, P. (1990). Services for chemically dependent adolescents. *AOTA Mental Health Special Interest Newsletter, 13,* 7–8.

Schmitt, M. H. (1982). Groups for the chronically ill. In E. H. Janosik & L. B. Phipps (Eds.), *Life cycle group work in nursing* (pp. 266–290). Monterey, CA: Wadsworth.

Starkstein, S. E., Cohen, B. S., Fedoroff, P., Parikh, R. M., Price, T. R., & Robinson, R. G. (1990). Relationship between anxiety disorder and depressive disorders in patients with cerebrovascular injury. *Archives of General Psychiatry, 47,* 246–251.

Stein, F. (1982). A current review of the behavioral frame of reference and its application to occupational therapy. *Occupational Therapy in Mental Health, 2,* 35-61.

Stewart, T., & Shields, C. R. (1985). Grief in chronic illness: Assessment and management. *Archives of Physical Medicine & Rehabilitation, 66,* 447–450.

Tardif, G. S. (1989). Sexual activity after a myocardial infarction. *Archives of Physical Medicine & Rehabilitation, 70,* 763–766.

Trahey, P. J. (1991). A comparison of the cost-effectiveness of two types of occupational therapy services. *American Journal of Occupational Therapy, 45,* 397–400.

Tucker, S. J. (1980). The psychology of spinal cord injury: Patient and staff interaction. *Rehabilitation Literature, 41,* 114–160.

Versluys, H. P. (1980a). Physical rehabilitation and family dynamics. *Rehabilitation Literature, 41,* 58–65.

Versluys, H. P. (1980b). The remediation of role disorders through focused group work. *American Journal of Occupational Therapy, 34,* 609–614.

Versluys, H. P. (1984). Community reintegration. The value of educational-action-training models. *Rehabilitation Literature, 45,* 138–145.

Versluys, H. P. (1993). Family influences. In H. L. Hopkins & H. D. Smith (Eds.), *Willard & Spackman's occupational therapy* (8th ed., pp. 161–165). Philadelphia: J. B. Lippincott.

Vinogradov, S., & Yalom, I. D. (1989). *A concise guide to group psychotherapy.* Washington, DC: American Psychiatric Press.

Webster's New World Dictionary of American English. (1991). 3rd college edition. New York: Prentice-Hall.

Wright, B. A. (1983). *Physical disability: A psychological approach* (2nd ed.). New York: Harper & Row.

Zemke, R., & Grantz, R. R. (1982). The role of theory: Erikson and occupational therapy. *American Journal of Occupational Therapy, 2,* 45–63.

Zisserman, L. (1981). The modern family and rehabilitation of the handicapped: A macrosociological view. *American Journal of Occupational Therapy, 35,* 13–20.

Preventing Occupational Dysfunction Secondary to Aging

Bette R. Bonder and Glenn Goodman

OBJECTIVES

After studying this chapter, the reader will be able to:
1. Describe normal age-related changes in sensation, neuromuscular function, cognition, and psychosocial factors.
2. Discuss activity patterns of older adults as related to self-care, work, and leisure.
3. Describe considerations in assessing the function of older adults.
4. Discuss preventive interventions through which occupational therapists can facilitate function in older adults.
5. Describe the factors that make intervention following illness or injury for older adults different from that for younger adults.

Life expectancy has increased markedly with the advent of antibiotics, vaccinations for disease, improvement in trauma care, and other medical technology. Presently, 12% of U.S. citizens are over the age of 65. By the year 2020, the proportion will increase to 21% (Lewis, 1990). The most rapid growth is and will continue to be among the old-old, those over age 85. Most older adults reside in the community. Only 5% of American citizen over the age of 65 are in institutions such as nursing homes (U.S. Congress, 1991). However, most older adults experience some physiological changes that impact performance; and older individuals, regardless of living situation, have an average of two to three chronic diseases (Cutler, 1994).

Among the **old-old** (over age 85), 50% of individuals have substantial disability (U.S. Congress, 1991). Thus, although most older adults remain in their homes, almost all will experience some difficulty in performing desired or necessary activities, and many will experience periods of significant disability during later life (Cutler, 1994)

The figures have considerable import for health care providers, particularly occupational therapists, who are concerned with assisting individuals to maintain or regain ability to perform daily activities. Enhancing functional performance of older adults in the areas of self-care, work, and leisure can have economic, social, and personal benefits for these individuals, their families, and society as a whole.

These concerns are becoming more salient as society focuses attention on health care costs and the rights of individuals. Approximately 30% of health care expenditures are for individuals aged 65 or over (Davis & Kirkland, 1988), and costs are increasing rapidly. One way to address cost issues is by focusing on functional outcomes rather than cure of disease. Thus occupational therapists are in a vital position to contribute to both health care policy and the individual well-being of elders.

This chapter provides an overview of the neuromuscular, sensory, cognitive, and psychosocial changes that accompany normal aging. It then considers the activity patterns of older adults and the meaning of those activities to them. Finally, it discusses the ways in which health care providers can intervene to maximize function and enhance quality of life for older individuals, both those who are residing in the community and those who have experienced debilitating illness or injury.

This chapter focuses on adults aged 65 and older. It should be noted, however, that definitions of old age are changing rapidly. Because of the increase in longevity, the improved health of older individuals, and societal changes, some gerontologists have adopted terminology first introduced by Neugarten (1975): The *young-old* are those aged 60 to 74; the *middle-old*, 75

GLOSSARY

Advance directives—Instructions provided by an individual before onset of a disabling or life-threatening condition that outline his or her wish for treatment (or cessation of treatment) in the event that such a situation occurs.

Crystallized intelligence—Recall of stored memories.

Dementia—A symptom caused by a number of conditions, characterized by loss of memory, language functions, ability to think abstractly, and ability to care for oneself.

Excess disability—Inability to perform tasks as a result of environmental, rather than intrapersonal, factors.

Fluid intelligence—Ability to use new information.

Instrumental activities of daily living—Self-care activities that are more complex and less directly personal than basic activities of daily living, e.g., cooking, housekeeping, shopping, and money management.

Old-old—The most rapidly growing segment of the population, which is made up of individuals who are over age 85.

Presbycusis—Age-related sensorineural hearing loss, especially for high-frequency sounds.

Presbyopia—Age-related vision changes, caused by loss of flexibility of the lens, which leads to poor near vision.

Productivity—Activities that make an economic contribution to society, including, but not limited to, paid employment, volunteer work, child care, and homemaking.

to 84; and the *old-old*, 85 and older. There is great individual variation, so that none of these categories necessarily defines the circumstances of individual clients.

The emphasis here is on the normal aging process. Older adults are obviously subject to all the illnesses and injuries that affect younger individuals as well as some that are far more likely to occur in older individuals (e.g., cerebrovascular accidents, dementing illnesses, and cancer). Other chapters in this volume address mechanisms by which therapists can provide effective intervention for these conditions. When illness or injury occurs, however, the therapist must put the consequences in the context of the individual's life stage, making understanding of normal aging essential. There are some special considerations in intervening with older adults who experience acute illness or injury, and those will be considered in this chapter as well.

NORMAL AGING

Changes that accompany normal aging occur in every sphere, both internal to the individual—including neuromuscular, sensory, cognitive, and psychological abilities—and external to the individual—as in social situations. It is essential to remember, however, the wide range of variability among individuals. Any generalization must be considered just that. All of us know individuals who at age 55 have wrinkled, leathery skin; stooped shoulders; shuffling gait; and poor vision and hearing and whose favorite activity is napping. We also know individuals who at age 80 are still relatively unwrinkled, have a vigorous stride, and engage in activities that would exhaust many a younger individual.

Similarly, it is essential that assumptions not be

made about the impact of these changes on performance. In the early years of research on Alzheimer's disease (AD), it was believed that AD resulted from loss of cortical tissue and expansion of the ventricles, because these changes were seen on many brain x-rays of individuals with AD. This theory was discarded when it was found that many individuals who were completely intact cognitively also had these cortical changes (Tomlinson, Blessed, & Roth, 1968, 1970). Thus the existence of a change cannot be assumed to lead to a commensurate decrement in function.

This section considers typical neuromuscular, sensory, cognitive, and psychosocial changes that accompany aging. These changes occur to varying degrees in different older adults, with varying impact on performance.

Sensory Changes

Some sensory changes normally occur with aging, whereas others result from disease processes that are more common among older adults (Cunningham et al., 1987). One role of the occupational therapist is to evaluate the level of disability caused by sensory differences and to determine strategies to compensate for problems that interfere with ability to complete desired or needed tasks in work, leisure, and self-care.

Changes typically occur in all sensory spheres, including vision, hearing, gustation, smell, touch, and vestibular sensation. Changes in multiple sensory channels require careful intervention to optimize function. Furthermore, decrements may occur at the level of reception or at the level of interpretation or integration (Ayres, 1985), i.e., either peripherally or centrally in the nervous system.

VISION

More than 11 million people in the United States have severely reduced vision, more than 2 million have visual deficits that impair function, and more than 1 million are totally blind. A total of 70% of these individuals are age 65 or older (U.S. Public Health Service, 1983; Weinreb, Freeman, & Selezinka, 1990).

Around the age of 40, most individuals experience a deterioration of near vision, called **presbyopia** ("old vision"). The lens loses its elasticity and becomes less able to focus because of weakness in the ciliary body; thus visual acuity diminishes (Davis & Kirkland, 1988). This is among the most common changes that accompany aging; however, it is relatively easily accommodated through the use of a well-known assistive device: eyeglasses. Because both near and far vision are affected, bifocal or trifocal lenses are often required.

Another common change is development of degenerative opacities (cataracts) of the lenses, which lead to decreased sensitivity to colors, increased sensitivity to glare, and diminished acuity (Hooper, 1994).

Several diseases can affect the retina at any age, including diabetic retinopathy and retinitis pigmentosa. The effects of these diseases, both of which may lead to total blindness, are most pronounced in the elderly population, because both are progressive degenerative diseases (Hooper, 1994). Macular degeneration is a disorder most common among older individuals. For unexplained reasons, the macula deteriorates, causing loss of central vision. For most older individuals with macular degeneration, sufficient peripheral vision is retained to assist in mobility, but not enough for activities such as reading and watching television (Hooper, 1994).

Musculature that controls eye movement tends to lose strength and tone (Sullivan, 1984). This can decrease upward gaze, focusing, and convergence. There may be a reduction in tear secretion (Furukawa & Polse, 1978) as well as degenerative changes in the sclera, pupil, and iris (Kasper, 1978). Results of such changes include excessive dryness, loss of light/dark accommodation, and poor night vision.

HEARING

Hearing loss, especially for high frequencies, accompanying aging is well documented (Kiernat, 1991). Conductive hearing loss may be the result of problems in the external or middle ear, such as wax buildup, eustachian tube blockage, or increased stiffness of the ossicles and membranes. These are all common age-related changes.

Age-related sensorineural hearing loss, known as **presbycusis,** results from dysfunction of the sensory hair cells of the cochlea, neural connections from the cochlea to the cerebral cortex and brainstem, or vascular changes in the auditory system (Corso, 1977; Davis & Kirkland, 1988; Lewis, 1990).

Functional consequences of these changes include difficulty hearing high-frequency sounds, distinguishing consonants during conversation, and filtering background noise during conversation.

TASTE AND SMELL

Thresholds for taste and smell increase with age (Baum, 1985; Davis & Kirkland, 1988; Kiernat, 1991). This has several functional implications. First, the ability to appreciate food flavor is closely related to olfaction. Because ability to detect smells diminishes with age, the potential for various nutritional problems arises, as food that cannot be smelled may seem tasteless or unappealing. Second, safety may become a concern; individuals may not be able to detect harmful odors such as natural gas, spoiled food, or smoke (Davis & Kirkland, 1988). Factors such as smoking or environmental exposures may exacerbate age-related changes in taste and olfaction (Baum, 1985).

TACTILE

Studies of tactile changes related to aging are sparse and inconclusive (Davis & Kirkland, 1988; Kenney, 1982; Kiernat, 1991). Complicating factors in studying this question include disease processes that may coincide with or contribute to sensory loss, the subjective nature of many tests of sensation, and the absence of longitudinal data. From the existing data, researchers have concluded that older adults are more susceptible to hypothermia and hyperthermia (Kiernat, 1991), losses in vibratory and touch sensitivity are minimal to moderate and occur in less than 50% of subjects over age 50 (Kenshalo, 1977), and loss of position sense is more likely to occur in the lower extremities (Davis & Kirkland, 1988). It appears that all these changes are related to central nervous system dysfunction rather than to aging per se.

VESTIBULAR

Vestibular changes are particularly significant because of the importance of falls as a health risk for older adults. Approximately 33% of older adults fall each year (Perry, 1982), and 15% of these individuals experience serious health consequences such as broken hips (Tinetti, Speechley, & Ginter, 1988). In fact, falls are the leading cause of accidental death in persons over age 65 (Baker, O'Neil, & Kark, 1984).

Older adults have more postural sway than

younger adults (Kalish, 1975), a condition that is exacerbated when vision is impaired. Vestibular righting response diminishes with age (Cape, 1978), which can lead to problems in maintaining balance. This combination of changes appears to contribute substantially to falls.

Neuromuscular Changes

The central nervous system, peripheral nervous system, and musculoskeletal system all appear to alter with age.

CENTRAL NERVOUS SYSTEM

With age, the cerebrum atrophies (Takeda & Matsuzawa, 1984), and cerebrospinal fluid space increases. There is a loss and atrophy of neurons, particularly in the precentral gyrus, postcentral gyrus, superior temporal gyrus, and Purkinje cells of the cerebellum (Dayan & Lewis, 1985; Rosser, 1985). The number of synapses is reduced, and neurotransmitter systems are altered (Brizzee, 1985; Hoyer, 1990). In addition, plaques and fibrillary tangles (Dayan, 1970a, 1970b) and other cellular abnormalities (Dayan & Lewis, 1985) have been found in the brains of functionally normal older adults. Neurons are lost from the spinal cord (Rosser, 1985), and there is a slowing of responsiveness to stimuli, as measured by electroencephalogram (Keller et al., 1985).

PERIPHERAL NERVOUS SYSTEM

Two major age-related changes in the peripheral nervous system have been identified. Nerve conduction velocity decreases (Norris, Shock, & Wagman, 1953; Potvin, 1980), and motor nerve fibers reduce in number (O'Sullivan & Swallow, 1968; Swallow, 1966).

MUSCULOSKELETAL SYSTEM

The number of muscle fibers decreases with age (Grimby, 1990; Swallow, 1966). There is also loss of muscle mass (Grimby, 1990; Swallow, 1966); an increase in fatty and connective tissue (Swallow, 1966); decreased strength (Fiatarone et al., 1990); and loss of type II, fast-twitch anaerobic muscle fibers that are responsible for phasic movement (Grimby, 1990).

Functionally, these changes may impact such abilities as rising from a chair and gait speed (Fiatarone et al., 1990). Weakness in ankle dorsiflexion and knee extension has also been correlated with falls in older individuals (Jebsen et al., 1969).

Loss of dexterity and coordination with aging is well documented. Scores on the *Jebsen Hand Function Test* (Jebsen et al., 1969), the *Nine-Hole Peg Test* (Mathiowetz, Weber, et al., 1985), the *Box and Block Test* of manual dexterity (Mathiowetz, Volland, et al., 1985), and the *Pennsylvania Bimanual Work Sample* (Roberts, 1945) all decline with age. These appear to impact some self-care activities, such as placing a plug into a wall socket and cutting with a knife (Potvin, 1980).

Age-related changes in static balance (Potvin, 1980), dynamic balance (Hageman & Blanke, 1986), and gait (Winter, Patla, Frank, & Walt, 1990) have been documented. These appear to increase the probability of falls.

Cognitive Changes

Age-related changes occur in intelligence, problem solving, abstract reasoning, memory, memory processing, and attention. In all these functions, changes are most noticeable after age 70, although they have been documented in younger individuals (Cunningham, 1987; Woods & Britton, 1985).

As measured by the *Weschler Adult Intelligence Scale* (WAIS), intelligence quotient (IQ) decreases with advancing age, a finding that is quite consistent among studies. This is largely the result of decreases in the performance rather than verbal subscales. Performance subscales may depend on **fluid intelligence** (the ability to use new information), whereas verbal subscales may use **crystallized intelligence** (recall of stored memories) (Cattell, 1963; Horn & Cattell, 1967). It may be that the decline in IQ is most reflective of a general slowing of information processing.

Like intelligence, problem-solving skills seem to become less efficient (Albert & Heaton, 1988; Woods & Britton, 1985). This may be the result of poor selection of problem-solving strategies or organization of information.

Older adults also seem to be less efficient in abstract reasoning. Flexibility in reasoning tasks, in particular, seems to decline (Horn & Cattell, 1967).

Memory is perhaps the best-studied cognitive process in older adults (Riley, 1994). This may be because of concerns about **dementia**, which is becoming increasingly common as the population ages. However, **dementia** is clearly a symptom of disorder, rather than a normal part of aging.

Several factors contribute to memory. To remember, one must first attend to the matter to be recalled and be able to receive information through sensory channels. Then the information must be processed (interpreted) and stored. Initial storage may be relatively short term. In all these abilities, older adults show few decrements (Arenberg, 1982; Cattell, 1963). Some adults experience sensory decrements, as described above, and some adults have difficulty encoding large amounts of information at once (Arenberg, 1982).

Overall, however, well older adults do not experience memory loss in processing and short-term storage of information.

There are noticeable decrements, however, in long-term memory and encoding (Cattell, 1963). Older adults have more trouble than younger individuals recalling information (Rabbitt, 1982; Woods & Britton, 1985), although retrieval difficulty is not as noticeable for recognition. For example, on seeing a name, an older person might remember the face and personality of an acquaintance, although it might be difficult for the elder to retrieve the name without help. This difficulty is much less pronounced when the information to be stored for later retrieval has practical significance. Remote or very long-term memory appears not to decline. However, this finding is more anecdotal than data based, and must be accepted with caution (Riley, 1994).

Overall memory loss is most pronounced in the area of long-term memory. This condition is sometimes labeled age-associated memory impairment (AAMI) (Albert, 1988). AAMI seems to begin in late middle age, when individuals begin to complain of difficulty remembering names or finding items in the house. By definition, this occurs only in healthy older adults. For some individuals, memory training has helped minimize associated functional decrements (Riley, 1994).

Psychosocial Changes

Changes in psychosocial status must be separated into those that are psychological and those that are social in nature. In a well elderly individual, the former relate to developmental tasks of later life. The latter relate to external factors, including major life changes such as retirement and the probability of loss of social contacts through moves, retirement, or death of family and friends.

A number of theorists have attempted to identify the normal psychological processes that accompany aging. Among the theories are disengagement, activity, continuity, and life span models. The principal characteristics of these theories are noted in Table 21.1. Although each theory has appeal, each also has limitations in explaining the psychological functioning of older individuals, and all remain to be carefully tested.

Social changes are also less than entirely clear. It is well established that older individuals will experience significant losses of social contacts (Smyth, 1994). However, it is less clear how or whether individuals will compensate for those losses. For example, loss of a spouse is devastating for most older individuals (Smyth, 1994). Some individuals, however, seem to compensate for the loss within a year or so, while others never recover.

Psychosocial status may well be a more significant predictor of functional ability than any other factor. Highly motivated, enthusiastic individuals tend to fare well, often in spite of what appear to be substantial physical limitations. The example of Miss Q. is instructive.

Miss Q. was a 73-year-old retired teacher. She lived alone in a third-floor apartment. Miss Q. had a bilateral congenital upper extremity deformity that left her with flipper-like appendages at the shoulders rather than arms. She had, through her life, adapted her environment so that she could function with almost no

Table 21.1.   Activities of Older Adults Summary of Theories

Theory	Constructs	References
Disengagement	1. Elders withdraw from activity 2. Elders disengage emotionally from people and events	Cummings and Henry (1961)
Activity	1. Elders strive to maintain activity 2. High levels of activity correlate with well-being	Havighurst (1963)
Continuity	1. Elders attempt to continue activities that were always important to them 2. Elders perceive activities as continuous 3. Elders adapt activity to compensate for change 4. Successful aging is characterized by degree of continuity achieved	Atchley (1976)
Life span	1. Old age is a continuation of the developmental process, representing a new developmental stage 2. Tasks specific to the stage can be identified 3. Successful aging results from accomplishing tasks	Neugarten (1975), Erikson (1963)
Model of human occupation	1. The individual is an open system 2. Subsystems are volition habituation, and performance 3. Effectiveness of the development of each subsystem reflects successful performance	Kielhofner and Burke (1985)

assistance. Her main limitation was an inability to drive, but with the help of friends and public transportation she got around to her volunteer job with children in the inner city, the lectures she enjoyed, and exhibits at the local art museum.

Then Miss Q. slipped on the ice outside her building and broke her hip. During surgical repair of the hip a significant amount of bone loss due to osteoporosis was discovered. The physicians and therapists working with her were pessimistic about prospects for her return to her home. Miss Q., however, was not at all gloomy, and within 1 month was back home, and within 2 months was engaged again in all the activities she had enjoyed before.

When questioned about her recovery, she acknowledged that she was in a great deal of pain, but indicated that she was "not about to let a little thing like pain interfere with my fun."

What is significant about this story is the level of physical impairment and the absence of accompanying functional deficit. Unfortunately, the reverse story is all too common, one in which the individual, following an injury or illness, becomes depressed, loses motivation, and becomes increasingly disabled.

ACTIVITY PATTERNS OF OLDER ADULTS

The changes that have been discussed are common among older adults, although highly variable for individuals. To consider providing support for performance of older adults, these changes must be appreciated in the context of the roles and activity patterns of older individuals, i.e., the activities that they need and want to accomplish.

In recent years, there have been increasing attempts by researchers to understand the activities in which older adults engage (Bonder & Fisher, 1990; Herzog & House, 1991; Rapkin & Fischer, 1992; Smith, Kielhofner, & Watts, 1986). In particular, researchers are interested in knowing what is important to elders and how their activities contribute to life satisfaction, defined as a positive evaluation of one's life (Rapkin & Fischer, 1992), both present and past.

Occupational therapists theorize that individuals are most satisfied with their lives when they are engaged in a variety of activities that balance self-care, work, and leisure (Kielhofner & Burke, 1985). Existing research suggests that this is true for older adults as well as younger individuals (Bonder & Fisher, 1990; Elliott & Barris, 1987; Longino & Kart, 1982; Ogilvie, 1987). Ogilvie (1987) found that individuals who were able to express their identities through activity were more

satisfied with their lives than those who experienced limitations.

As with physiological change, activity patterns are highly variable (Bonder & Fisher, 1990). Some older adults engage in many activities related to self-care, work, and leisure, whereas others focus on one or two activities. For example, some older adults report activities that are related primarily to family, while others may be active in volunteer work, several hobbies, social relationships, and care of all their personal needs. This section considers some issues related to particular areas of activity and the ways in which these activities for older individuals are different from those of younger ones.

Self-Care

The most significant issue for older adults has to do with level of independence in self-care and availability and acceptability of assistance. Most older adults have difficulty with at least one or two self-care activities. Bonder and Fisher (1990) found that among 98 community-living individuals, every one reported difficulty cutting toenails. Most had solved this problem by having their toenails cut during a pedicure or by visiting a podiatrist. Similarly, heavy housework, such as mopping floors and washing windows, was difficult for many of the subjects in the study. These activities were often hired out or accomplished by family members.

These forms of assistance seem relatively acceptable. Many older adults also make use of other forms of help as activities become more difficult for them and accommodate quite well to changes in status. Trouble may arise when there is a sudden situational or physical change. For example, when a spouse dies, the surviving spouse may be forced to manage finances, or drive, or cook, when he or she had never done so before. Similarly, an individual who experiences a cerebrovascular accident with accompanying hemiplegia may have difficulty with cooking, bathing, and driving. In either case, the individual may experience a level of dependency that is unacceptable, even though help received before the life change was not unacceptable. One possible explanation for the difference is the perception that in the new situation, such assistance is not solicited voluntarily.

Several summary statements can be made about self-care of older adults. First, most older adults require some assistance with some self-care (Cutler, 1994), particularly what are known as **instrumental activities of daily living** (IADL), activities that relate to self-care but are not of an intimate, personal nature (e.g., shopping, budgeting, housekeeping, and cooking). It is likely that assistance will be required for at least some activities of daily living (ADL) as well.

Second, most older adults accommodate to these needs well, both in terms of locating and accepting assistance. This is especially true when the activity is one for which it is socially acceptable to receive help. No one expects any adult to be competent in all self-care activities, so help with driving, cooking, or managing finances is unlikely to be viewed negatively.

Third, older individuals have very different wishes and perceptions about independence in these activities. Some are adamant that they must do for themselves, while others are accepting, even relieved, when they rely on others to take care of them.

Fourth, substantial disability in self-care is most likely to be perceived when there is a sudden change in status, rather than the gradual ones experienced by most well elders. The sudden change may be either related to personal factors (e.g., health) or to external factors (e.g., social or environmental changes). If the difference is loss related, emotional reactions that typically accompany loss must be addressed. It is important to remember, however, that changes perceived as positive (e.g., a move to a long-desired retirement location) can also cause unanticipated emotional difficulties.

Work

Issues related to work and retirement are undergoing significant change for older adults. New patterns are emerging that, as with other spheres of function, reflect increasing diversity in the older population (Sterns, Laier, & Dorsett, 1994). For example, there is a trend for earlier retirement for some older adults, followed by second careers in different areas or return to part-time work or a move to volunteer work.

There is a substantial body of literature about abilities of older workers (Sterns et al., 1994) that suggests that physiological changes do not interfere with work. One area of particular concern is in continuing or expanding competency, and it is clear that elders require somewhat different kinds of in-service training. For example, they may require slightly more time than younger adults to learn new skills and will respond best to learning that is based on practical examples. If these special needs are accommodated, however, they are as capable as younger individuals of maintaining their skills.

There is also substantial evidence that retirement, popular perception notwithstanding, is not viewed as a negative event if an older adult chooses to retire (Ekerdt, 1987). It is when retirement is involuntary, either as a result of a personal situation (e.g., failing health) or external events (e.g., lay-offs) that individuals are likely to be dissatisfied with their postwork experiences.

Retirement often does not mean the cessation of productive activity (Herzog & House, 1991). The concept of **productivity** as encompassing a broad range of activities that are of value to society appears to clarify the reasons that some older adults who highly value "making a contribution" are not unhappy when they retire from paid employment. Herzog and House (1991) noted that individuals who engage in volunteer work, child care or other service for family members, or other forms of unpaid service are likely to report that these have value both to them and to others. A substantial majority agree that contributing to the well-being of others gives meaning to life. At the same time, older adults feel that they have earned the right to rest and enjoy retirement and leisure.

Leisure

Leisure activities among older adults are not well explained or documented. A number of studies have examined informal social activities (Okun et al., 1984) and have concluded that these are important to older adults' well-being. It is also apparent that older adults engage in a wide range of leisure activities, including sports, arts and crafts, and attending concerts and lectures (Bonder & Fisher, 1990).

There is a general belief, consistent with activity theory, that maintaining a high level of activity is positive. However, this theory has been challenged by some who believe that an important component of later life is reflection and life review (Ekerdt, 1986; Rowles, 1991).

FACILITATING PERFORMANCE

Assessment of Performance

As with younger individuals, careful assessment is vital to successful intervention focused on supporting functional performance of older adults. Perhaps most attention has been given to assessment of self-care (Rogers & Holm, 1994). This may be based on an assumption that it is of vital importance to older adults to maintain independence in this performance sphere or on health care finance issues, because individuals with self-care deficits are most likely to require ongoing assistance.

However, it is most important in assessing older adults to be cognizant of the goals of that individual (Rapkin & Fischer, 1992). Assessment should begin with identification of the individual's valued goals and then proceed to determination of factors that interfere with accomplishment of those goals.

Several instruments may be helpful in determining those goals. The *Canadian Occupational Performance Measure* (Pollack, 1993) involves interview of the client and joint identification of goals for therapy. These goals then become the measures of outcome (see Chapters 4 and 18). Other instruments that may be helpful include the *Role Change Assessment* (Jackoway, Rogers, & Snow, 1987) and *Interest Checklist* (Matsutsuyu, 1963). The point of all these assessments is to determine what matters to the client.

Assessment of the environment is also essential (Davidson, 1991) (see Chapter 5). The environment can be particularly supportive (Rowles, 1991) or may lead to so-called **excess disability** by presenting significant barriers to performance.

In general, a combination of observational and interview measures will be most helpful. It is beneficial to obtain information from potential caregivers as well as the client, because caregiver willingness to provide assistance may be a crucial factor in outcomes of intervention. Specific advantages and disadvantages of various methods of assessment can be found in Rogers and Holm (1994). Once careful assessment is complete, the therapist can focus on factors that interfere with performance, i.e., specific skill areas, such as mobility and sensation, which contribute to disability.

Intervention

An important role for occupational therapists working with older adults is prevention of functional disability. Intervention may include prevention, screening, environmental modifications, modification or substitution of activities, educational interventions, and acceptance of individual needs and wishes by health care providers.

PREVENTION

The wellness movement (Dunn, 1961) is based on the principle of maximizing both health and performance. Activities such as stress management, exercise to increase physical fitness, maintenance of adequate nutrition, safe driving habits, avoidance of alcohol and drugs, and cessation of smoking as well as activities to increase safety in the home, community, and work environments are associated with this model (Lewis, 1990).

In prevention programs, occupational therapists work with health educators, nurses, social workers, and other health care providers to maximize the individual's physical and functional well-being. The occupational therapist may emphasize activities that encourage socialization and physical fitness, modification of the environment to reduce the possibility of accidents, and

identification of roles and activities that are satisfying to the individual.

For example, one therapist offered a preretirement workshop at a large company. She assisted individuals in identifying their personal goals, activities that were important to them, and ways to continue those activities. When one participant voiced a concern about no longer being valued for his contributions to the workforce, the therapist helped him locate the local Retired Senior Volunteers Program (RSVP). He found a number of volunteer positions that appealed to his need to make a contribution and to feel valued by others.

SCREENING

During the course of prevention activities, occupational therapists should be alert to potential problems and make efforts to intervene before serious difficulty arises (Rogers & Holm, 1994). If individuals who are nutritionally compromised or who have experienced a recent life-changing loss receive early intervention, disability may be minimized or avoided. For example, if a client becomes unable to drive because of increasing visual impairment, the therapist may acquaint him with the services of Community Responsive Transit, help him make contact with friends and relatives who can provide occasional transportation, or encourage him to contact his church to ensure that a member of the congregation will provide rides to services and other activities. Such an intervention helps reduce the likelihood of social isolation, which can lead to depression and perhaps to significant disability.

ENVIRONMENTAL MODIFICATIONS

If it is not feasible to increase the individual's performance ability, another highly effective intervention is to reduce some demands through alteration of the environment. Recent legislation, particularly the Omnibus Budget Reconciliation Act (OBRA) (Glantz & Richman, 1991), requires that environmental assessment be done in nursing home settings, but such assessment should be done in community settings as well. A number of good environmental assessment instruments are available (Davidson, 1991) (see Chapter 5). It is important to evaluate both the physical and the social environment to understand fully the individual's situation.

Some environmental alterations are preventive in nature. For example, improved lighting may reduce the probability of falls. Among the interventions that may be helpful are the following. To enhance cognitive function:

1. Reduce clutter;
2. Label drawers and cabinets by their contents; for

individuals who have **dementia** or other serious cognitive deficits, pictures may be easier to understand than words;

3. Use color, texture, and lighting changes to provide location cues, e.g., changes from carpet to tile may signal the move from dining area to hallway;
4. Use timers as reminders for specific functions;
5. Put safety turn-off switches on stoves and furnaces.

To enhance visual function the following interventions may help:

1. High tone colors and low gloss finishes may improve visual acuity and depth perception (Tiedeksaar, 1994);
2. Devices to increase magnification or enlarge print, the use of contrasting colors, and dependence on other sensory systems such as touch can be of help;
3. Maintenance of a consistent environment allows the visually impaired individual to function more effectively;
4. Writing with felt-tipped pens and in bold print helps improve visibility (Mann, 1994);
5. Optometrists, ophthalmologists, and staff at sight centers or the Society for the Blind can provide helpful input.;
6. As a rule, provide high-intensity, low-glare light; avoid fluorescent lights; and put glare-reducing screens over televisions and windows (Tiedeksaar, 1994);
7. Teach compensatory techniques to individuals who have reduced peripheral vision or who have only peripheral vision (Kasper, 1978).

For hearing and communication problems:

1. Obtain a thorough evaluation from a speech pathologist, audiologist, or otolaryngologist;
2. Speak slowly and clearly and use a lower tone of voice with someone who has high-frequency loss; do not shout;
3. Make sure the individual can see you when you speak (Lewis, 1990);
4. Write messages if necessary;
5. Select activities for which verbal interaction may not be essential, such as bowling, swimming, checkers, and walks;
6. Check that hearing aids are fitted and used properly and that batteries are fresh; remember that these aids do not restore normal hearing and may not be helpful to all individuals with hearing impairments;
7. Use visual cues such as flashing lights to get the client's attention.

For neuromuscular, motor, or mobility problems try some of these interventions:

1. Make sure that the environment is free of hazards such as slippery floors, poorly marked stairs, and architectural barriers;
2. Adjust the height of chairs, beds, dressers, clothes, and toilet seats, and provide bath chairs if needed; ensure that grab bars are within easy reach;
3. Provide task-oriented treatment in the individual's environment; remember that numerous repetitions enhance learning and that simulated activities may not be easily transferred to real situations;
4. In institutional settings, keep in mind OBRA regulations that mandate reduced use of restraints; careful evaluation of seating can eliminate the need for restraints, e.g., a chair that is higher in front than in back can make it more difficult to rise and well-fitted chairs can enhance balance.

TECHNOLOGICAL AIDS TO FUNCTION

Numerous technological assists can maximize function. Some are simple (e.g., an alarm on the doorknob to warn family members that an individual is wandering away and automatic turn-off switches on stoves to reduce fire hazard). Others, such as the computer-operated "smart house" are highly sophisticated and expensive. Some applications of technology for problems associated with aging include the following:

1. Telephones with amplifiers, large-print numbers, one-touch dialing, cordless features, and external speakers;
2. Screen magnification, print enlargers, and voice synthesizers for screen reading;
3. Assistive listening devices, telecommunication devices (TDDs), and closed captioning for television as well as devices to convert auditory output into flashing lights for smoke detectors, telephones, and doorbells;
4. Life call systems that provide a link with emergency services;
5. Advances in cataract and other optical surgery, including lens implants;
6. Advances in technology for mobility such as wheelchair seating systems, power carts that are easy to disassemble, lightweight wheelchairs, wheeled walkers with brakes and built-in seating systems, and adaptive controls for cars.

There are limits to the application of technology with older clients. Some clients may resist learning how to use the new technologies. Devices can break down and may be expensive to repair. Acquiring the devices in the first place may be expensive and not covered by insurance. It is difficult to keep up with advances, and sometimes a new and better device appears on the market as soon as a client has purchased an expensive piece of equipment.

However, many older adults enjoy technological devices, learn to use them quickly, and gain considerable independence through their use. For example, one 77-year-old woman was extremely discouraged when a polyneuropathy greatly reduced her upper extremity strength. She resisted the use of adaptive devices because of the stigma she thought was associated with them, but she did not reject a computer, which she felt was a more common piece of equipment. With the help of an overhead sling, she was able to use the computer to express her feelings and enjoyed learning about advances such as "cut and paste" and "spell checking" that the computer offered. Both she and her husband reported being much happier once she was able to undertake this activity.

MODIFICATION AND SUBSTITUTION OF ACTIVITY

Activity analysis is a cornerstone of occupational therapy and can be particularly helpful in assisting older clients. The process involves matching present skills, interests, and motivation with activities that are stimulating, challenging, enjoyable, goal directed, and purposeful. Some specific considerations include the following:

1. Older adults will persist for longer periods of time with activities that are purposeful (Kircher, 1984; Nelson et al., 1988; Steinbeck, 1986).
2. Reminiscence is particularly important to older clients; activities such as telling a life history may encourage clients to go to the senior center or occupational therapy department, enhancing mobility, or may encourage them to use a typewriter, increasing hand strength and mobility.
3. Repetitive activities are often rejected.
4. Activity inventories can stimulate an older client to think about what he values.
5. When an activity becomes too difficult for a client, the therapist may adapt the activity or help him identify an activity that meets similar needs; it is important to ascertain what component of the activity is meaningful, e.g., if he likes to cook because it is a way to socialize, substituting an activity that is not social will not be satisfying.

EDUCATIONAL INTERVENTIONS

Sometimes instruction is an effective intervention either by itself or in combination with other forms of treatment. Energy conservation, stress reduction, and information about the aging process or community resources can all be helpful to older adults. As noted earlier, most older adults cope independently with normal age-related decrements in ability quite well; educational interventions can reduce the need for trial-and-error learning. For example, Miss Q., described above, had managed to construct an environment in which she could function quite adequately. She indicated, however, that it was only through years of experimentation that she had learned how to alter her apartment satisfactorily. If a therapist had referred her to the Services for Independent Living for advice about modifying her environment, Miss Q. would have been saved considerable difficulty and frustration.

ACCEPTANCE OF INDIVIDUAL NEEDS AND WISHES

Acceptance of individual needs and wishes is targeted to the family and the health care provider rather than the client. Often, an older client is quite satisfied with his situation, but family members or well-meaning therapists are not. Family members worry about the individual being insufficiently active (Ekerdt, 1986); therapists are concerned that inactivity may signify impending depression. Obviously, distinctions must be made between problems such as depression and personal choices such as a wish to enjoy sitting in the garden on a sunny day. Numerous theoreticians (Ekerdt, 1986; Havighurst & Albrecht, 1953; Rowles, 1991) have noted that life review is an important part of later life, and individuals must be afforded the opportunity for such reflection.

Perhaps the most troubling aspect of such acceptance comes in the form of **advance directives** (U.S. Office of Technology Assessment [OTA], 1987). Increasingly, older adults are instructing their families and health care providers about their wishes for cessation of intervention or about circumstances in which they prefer that intervention not be started. The ethical issues around such decisions are far from resolved, but increasingly, clearly documented instructions are followed.

INTERVENTION FOLLOWING DISEASE OR INJURY: SPECIAL CONSIDERATIONS FOR OLDER CLIENTS

Almost all older adults will eventually experience an illness or injury that may call for secondary or tertiary preventive interventions, i.e., minimizing consequences early in treatment or enhancing rehabilitation once severe disability has occurred. Some special characteristics of older adults must be considered in planning intervention.

Differential Severity of Condition

Some conditions that are relatively innocuous in younger individuals can have severe consequences for older individuals. One example is influenza, which, while unpleasant for younger adults, may be lethal for older individuals. On the other hand, cancers that may be terminal in younger adults are often quite slow growing in older individuals, thus leading to much less severe outcomes.

Multiple Conditions

"Well" older adults are likely to have two to three chronic conditions (Cutler, 1994), each of which may require a different intervention. A common example is a client who has both rheumatoid arthritis and osteoporosis. Although moderately strenuous weight-bearing exercise may be the treatment of choice for prevention of bone loss, such activity may exacerbate the arthritis.

Duration of Intervention

Older adults generally have slower recuperative abilities than younger individuals. Even if the eventual outcome may be every bit as good, it may take the older individual longer to arrive at that point. Treatment often ends too soon for older individuals.

Attitudes of Care Providers

Health care professionals may tend to be less aggressive in their rehabilitation of older adults than younger individuals. In one study, a group of health care providers presented with case descriptions that were identical except for the age of the client developed much more aggressive goals for the client described as young (Barta-Kvitek et al., 1986). This may be appropriate in some circumstances, but professionals must exercise considerable caution in assuming bad outcomes. For example, consider Mrs. P.

Mrs. P. was a 73-year-old woman who had been in declining health for many years. She lived alone and had a part-time job, but she had few other activities and few friends. When she was found collapsed on the floor, she was taken by ambulance to the hospital, where physicians found a severe systemic infection (source unknown), a severe heart murmur (discovered to be caused by two defective heart valves), and an enlarged heart. She was delirious and in extremely poor condition. After much discussion, the physicians decided to operate to repair the defective heart valves and remove growths on the heart wall caused by the infection.

All the health care professionals who worked with Mrs. P. were quite pessimistic about the probable outcome and were extremely surprised when she responded very well to treatment. Within 2 months she was living independently, working, and engaging in

many more leisure activities than before. It became apparent that the condition that had caused her problems had developed over a long period of time, leading her to limit her activities because she felt bad. All the individuals involved took this as a lesson about avoiding assumptions when working with older individuals.

Policy Considerations

The complex conditions often found in older individuals are cause for concern when examined in the light of current trends in health care policy. Shorter treatment, as a way to reduce costs, is the rule. Diagnostic related groups (DRG) reimbursement is based on identification of a primary diagnosis that determines payment in the absence of consideration of coexisting conditions. There is increasing concern about employing expensive, high-technology interventions (like Mrs. P.'s surgery) when the potential benefit appears limited. Current debates about health care policy will not lead to positive outcomes unless these issues are resolved.

A Special Note about Dementia

Dementing illnesses are extremely common among older adults. Some epidemiologists suggest that as many as 50% of individuals over 85 experience some **dementia** (OTA, 1987). **Dementia,** characterized by forgetfulness, difficulty finding words, and other cognitive loss, is not a normal condition of aging, in spite of the high rate at which it occurs in older adults.

Rather, **dementia** is the result of disease processes (Berilla, 1994), some of which are reversible, such as depression, sensory deprivation syndrome, malnutrition, and drug toxicity (often the result of incompatible or excessive medication by multiple physicians being seen for multiple conditions). Other dementias are not reversible, most notable is AD. AD, the most common form of **dementia,** is a progressive disorder that eventually leads to total disability and death.

It is beyond the scope of this chapter to deal with the methods for intervening with individuals with dementing disorders. However, health care professionals should be familiar with the early symptoms of cognitive disorder, such as difficulty finding words, forgetfulness about everyday events and procedures, lack of recollection of familiar individuals. When noted, these symptoms should be carefully evaluated by a geriatrician, a physician trained in working with older individuals. Reversible causes may be treated relatively easily, often by treating a depression or by reducing medications. If the individual has an irreversible dementing illness, a variety of management strategies can help informal and formal caregivers to cope more effectively with resulting problems. This will enhance quality of life for the individual as well. One excellent source of information about management is *The 36-Hour Day* (Mace & Rabins, 1981). **Dementia** can have obvious impact on the outcome of all interventions, so health care professionals should be alert to signs that it is present.

SUMMARY

Intervention with older adults requires understanding of the normal developmental processes that affect performance as well as the special life circumstances of older adults. Intervention must address all spheres of function—physical, cognitive, sensory, and psychosocial—to be most effective. The special factors that alter intervention with older adults must be taken into account, in terms of identifying goals, selecting types of intervention, determining duration of intervention, and measuring outcomes. With older adults, the goal of perfect health is likely to be elusive. However, the goal of good quality of life, as measured by satisfying activities is in reach in many situations. Thoughtful intervention by occupational therapists can ensure that this occurs.

STUDY QUESTIONS

1. In a well elderly individual, what are the most typical changes in sensation? How might these affect function?
2. How will normal neuromuscular changes that accompany aging affect mobility?
3. An older client complains of occasionally losing keys and of sometimes having difficulty remembering names of acquaintances he has not seen for a while. What age-related condition would you suspect?
4. If the same older client complained of being unable to balance his checkbook, of having difficulty finding his way home from the corner grocery store, and of not remembering his wife's name, would you suspect a different condition? If so, what might the condition be?
5. In general, what impact does retirement have on an older individual who has planned for the event?
6. What is the first step an occupational therapist should take in assessing the status of an older individual?
7. What factors are important in selecting substitute activities for an older adult?
8. In deciding about technological interventions, what factors must be considered to ensure acceptance of the device?
9. What factors complicate intervention with an older adult who experiences an illness or injury?

REFERENCES

Albert, M. S. (1988). Cognitive function. In M. S. Albert & M. B. Moss (Eds.), *Geriatric neuropsychology* (pp. 33–53). New York: Guilford Press.

Albert, M. S., & Heaton, R. K. (1988). Intelligence testing. In M. S. Albert & M. B. Moss (Eds.), *Geriatric neuropsychology* (pp. 13–32). New York: Guilford Press.

Arenberg, D. (1982). Changes with age in problem solving. In F. I. Craik & S. Trehub (Eds.), *Aging and cognitive processes* (pp. 221–235). New York: Plenum.

Atchley, R. C. (1989). Continuity theory of normal aging. *Gerontologist, 29,* 183–190.

Ayres, A. J. (1985). *Developmental dyspraxia and adult-onset apraxia.* Paper presented at Sensory Integration International, Torrance, CA.

Baker, S., O'Neil, B., & Kark, R. (1984). *The injury fact book.* Lexington, MA: Lexington Books.

Barta-Kvitek, S. D., Shaver, B., Blood, H., & Shephard, K. (1986). Age bias: Physical therapists and older patients. *Journal of Gerontology, 41,* 706–709.

Baum, B. J. (1985). Alterations in oral function. In R. Andres, E. Bierman, & W. Hazzard (Eds.), *Principles of geriatric medicine* (pp. 288–296). New York: McGraw-Hill.

Berilla, R. A. (1994). Dementia. In B. R. Bonder & M. Wagner (Eds.), *Functional performance of older adults* (pp. 240–255). Philadelphia: F. A. Davis.

Bonder, B. R., & Fisher, A. G. (1990). *Roles and activities of older adults.* Paper presented at the annual meeting of the Gerontological Society of America, San Francisco, CA.

Brizzee, K. (1985). Neuron aging and neuron pathology. In H. Johnson (Ed.), *Relations between normal aging and disease* (pp. 191–224). New York: Raven Press.

Cape, R. (1978). *Aging: Its complex management.* New York: Harper & Row.

Cattell, R. B. (1963). The theory of fluid and crystalline intelligence. *Journal of Educational Psychology, 54,* 1–22.

Corso, J. (1977). Auditory perception and communication. In J. Birren & K. Schaie (Eds.), *Handbook of the psychology of aging* (pp. 535–553). New York: Van Nostrand, Reinhold.

Cumming, E. M., & Henry, W. E. (1961). *Growing old: The process of disengagement.* New York: Basic Books.

Cunningham, D., Rechnitzer, P., Howard, J., & Donner, A. (1987). Exercise training of men at retirement: A clinical trial. *Journal of Gerontology, 42,* 17–23.

Cunningham, W. R. (1987). Intellectual abilities and age. In K. W. Schaie & C. Eisdorfer (Eds.), *Annual review of gerontology and geriatrics* (Vol. 7, pp. 117–134). New York: Springer.

Cutler, N. E. (1994). Functional limitations and the need for personal care. In B. R. Bonder & M. Wagner (Eds.), *Functional performance in older adults* (pp. 210–222). Philadelphia: F. A. Davis.

Davidson, H. (1991). Assessing environmental factors. In C. Christiansen & C. Baum (Eds.), *Occupational therapy: Overcoming human performance deficits* (pp. 426–452). Thorofare, NJ: Slack.

Davis, L., & Kirkland M. (Eds.). (1988). *The role of occupational therapy with the elderly.* Rockville, MD: American Occupational Therapy Association.

Dayan, A. (1970a). Quantitative histological studies on the aged human brain. I. Senile plaques and neurofibrillary tangles in "normal" patients. *Acta Neuropathologica, 16,* 85–94.

Dayan, A. (1970b). Quantitative histological studies on the aged human brain. II. Senile plaques and neurofibrillary tangles in senile dementia. *Acta Neuropathologica, 16,* 95–104.

Dayan, A., & Lewis, P. (1985). The central nervous system:

Neuropathology of aging. In J. Brocklehurst (Ed.), *Textbook of geriatric medicine and gerontology* (pp. 268–293). London: Churchill-Livingstone.

Dunn, H. (1961). *High level wellness.* Arlington, VA: Beatty Press.

Ekerdt, D. J. (1986). The busy ethic: Moral continuity between work and retirement. *Gerontologist, 26,* 239–244.

Ekerdt, D. J. (1987). Why the notion persists that retirement harms health. *Gerontologist, 27,* 454–457.

Elliott, M. S., & Barris, R. (1987). Occupational role performance and life satisfaction in elderly persons. *Occupational Therapy Journal of Research, 7,* 215–224.

Erikson, E. H. (1963). *Childhood and society.* New York: W. W. Norton.

Fiatarone, M., Marks, E., Ryan, N., Merideth, C., Lipsitz, L., & Evans, W. (1990). High intensity strength training in nonagenarians. *Journal of the American Medical Association, 263,* 3029–3034.

Furukawa, R., & Polse, K. (1978). Changes in tearflow accompanying aging. *American Journal of Optometric Physiology and Optometry, 55,* 69–74.

Glantz, C., & Richman, N. (1991). *Occupational therapy: A vital link to implementation of OBRA.* Rockville, MD: American Occupational Therapy Association.

Grimby, G. (1990). Muscle changes and trainability in the elderly. *Topics in Geriatric Rehabilitation, 5,* 54–62.

Hageman, P., & Blanke, D. (1986). Comparison of gait of young women and elderly women. *Physical Therapy, 66,* 1382–1387.

Havighurst, R. J. (1963). Successful aging. In R. H. Williams, C. Tibbitts, & W. Donahue (Eds.), *Processes of aging* (Vol. 1, pp. 299–320). New York: Atherton.

Havighurst, R. J., & Albrecht, F. (1953). *Older people.* New York: Longmans Green.

Henderson, G., Tomlinson, B., & Gipson, P. (1985). Cell counts in human cerebral cortex in normal adults throughout life using an image analyzing computer. *Journal of the Neurological Sciences, 46,* 113–119.

Herzog, A. R., & House, J. S. (1991, Winter). Productive activities and aging well. *Generations,* 49–54.

Hooper, C. R. (1994). Sensory and sensory integrative development. In B. R. Bonder & M. Wagner (Eds.), *Functional performance in older adults* (pp. 93–106). Philadelphia: F. A. Davis.

Horn, J. L., & Cattell, R. B. (1967). Age differences in fluid and crystallized intelligence. *Acta Psychologica, 26,* 107–129.

Hoyer, S. (1990). Brain glucose and energy metabolism during normal aging. *Aging, 37,* 245–267.

Jackoway, I. S., Rogers, J. C., & Snow, T. L. (1987). The Role Change Assessment: An interview tool for evaluating older adults. *Occupational Therapy in Mental Health, 7,* 17–37.

Jebsen, R., Taylor, N., Trieschmann, R., Trotter, M., & Howard, L. (1969). An objective and standardized test of hand function. *Archives of Physical Medicine and Rehabilitation, 50,* 311–319.

Kalish, R. (1975). Basic processes. In R. Kalish (Ed.), *Late adulthood: Perspectives on human development* (pp. 156–174). Monterey, CA: Brooks/Cole.

Kasper, R. (1978). Eye problems of the aged. In W. Reichel (Ed.), *Clinical aspects of aging* (pp. 393–402). Baltimore: Williams & Wilkins.

Keller, W., Largen, J., Burch, N., & Maulsby, R. (1985). Physiology of the aging brain: Normal and abnormal states. In H. Johnson (Ed.), *Relations between normal aging and disease* (pp. 165–190). New York: Raven Press.

Kenney, R. (1982). *Physiology of aging.* Chicago: Year Book.

Kenshalo, D. (1977). Age changes in touch, vibration, temperature, kinesthesis, and pain sensitivity. In J. Birren, & K. Schaie (Eds.), *Handbook of the psychology of aging* (pp. 562–579). New York: Van Nostrand, Reinhold.

Kielhofner, G., & Burke, J. P. (1985). Components and determinants of human occupation. In G. Kielhofner (Ed.), *A model of human occupation: Theory and application* (pp. 12–36). Baltimore: Williams & Wilkins.

Kiernat, J. (1991). *Occupational therapy and the older adult.* Rockville, MD: Aspen Systems.

Kircher, M. (1984). Motivation as a factor of perceived exertion in purposeful versus nonpurposeful activity. *American Journal of Occupational Therapy, 38,* 165–170.

Lewis, C. (1990). *Aging: The health care challenge.* Philadelphia: F. A. Davis.

Longino, C. F., & Kart, C. S. (1982). Explicating activity theory: A formal replication. *Journal of Gerontology, 37,* 713–722.

Mace, N. L., & Rabins, P. V. (1981). *The 36-hour day.* Baltimore: Johns Hopkins University Press.

Mann, W. C. (1994). Tecnology. In B. Bonder & M. Wagner (Eds.), *Functional performance in older adults* (pp. 323–338). Philadelphia: F. A. Davis.

Mathiowetz, V., Volland, G., Kashman, N., & Weber K. (1985). Adult norms for the Box and Block Test of manual dexterity. *American Journal of Occupational Therapy, 39,* 386–391.

Mathiowetz, V., Weber, K., Kashman, N., & Volland G. (1985). Adult norms for the Nine Hole Peg Test of finger dexterity. *Occupational Therapy Journal of Research, 5,* 24–38.

Matsutsuyu, J. (1963). The Interest Checklist. *American Journal of Occupational Therapy, 32,* 628–630.

Nelson, D. Peterson, C., Smith, D., Boughton, J., & Whalen, G. (1988). Effects of project versus parallel groups on social interaction and affective responses in senior citizens. *American Journal of Occupational Therapy, 42,* 23–29.

Neugarten, B. L. (1975). *Middle age and aging.* Chicago: University of Chicago Press.

Norris, A., Shock, N., & Wagman, I. (1953). Age change in the maximum conduction velocity of motor fibers of human ulnar nerves. *Journal of Applied Physiology, 5,* 587–593.

Ogilvie, D. M. (1987). Life satisfaction and identity structure in late middle-aged men and women. *Psychology and Aging, 2,* 217–224.

Okun, M. S., Stock, W. A., Haring, M. J., & Witter, R. A. (1984). The social activity/subjective well-being relation: A quantitative synthesis. *Research on Aging, 6,* 45–66.

O'Sullivan, D., & Swallow, M. (1968). Fiber size and content of the radial and sural nerves. *Journal of Neurology, Neurosurgery and Psychiatry, 31,* 464–470.

Perry, B. (1982). Falls among the elderly living in high rise apartments. *Journal of Family Practice, 14,* 1069–1073.

Pollack, N. (1993). Client-centered assessment. *American Journal of Occupational Therapy, 47,* 298–301.

Potvin, A. (1980). Human neurologic function and the aging process. *Journal of the American Geriatric Society, 28,* 1–9.

Rabbitt, P. (1982). How do old people know what to do next? In F. I. Craik & S. Trehub (Eds.), *Aging and cognitive processes* (pp. 79–97). New York: Plenum.

Rapkin, B. D., & Fischer, K. (1992). Framing the construct of life satisfaction in term of older adults' personal goals. *Psychology and Aging, 7,* 138–149.

Riley, K. (1994). Cognitive development in later life. In B. R. Bonder & M. Wagner (Eds.), *Functional performance in older adults.* Philadelphia: F. A. Davis.

Roberts, J. (1945). *Manual for the Pennsylvania Bi-manual Worksample.* Circle Pines, MN: American Guidance Service.

Rogers, J. C., & Holm, M. (1994). Assessment of self-care. In B. R. Bonder & M. Wagner (Eds.), *Functional performance in older adults* (pp. 181–202). Philadelphia: F. A. Davis.

Rosser, M. (1985). The central nervous system: Neurochemistry of the aging brain and dementia. In J. Brocklehurst (Ed.), *Textbook of geriatric medicine and gerontology* (pp. 294-308). London: Churchill-Livingstone.

Rowles, G. D. (1991). Beyond performance: Being in place as a component of occupational therapy. *American Journal of Occupational Therapy, 45,* 265–271.

Smith, N. R., Kielhofner, G., & Watts, J. H. (1986). The relationships between volition, activity pattern, and life satisfaction in the elderly. *American Journal of Occupational Therapy, 40,* 278–283.

Smyth, K. (1994). Activity and loss. In B. R. Bonder & M. Wagner (Eds.), *Functional performance in older adults* (pp. 366–377). Philadelphia: F. A. Davis.

Steinbeck, T. (1986). Purposeful activity and performance. *American Journal of Occupational Therapy, 38,* 165–170.

Sterns, H., Laier, M. P., & Dorsett, J. G. (1994). Work and retirement. In B. R. Bonder & M. Wagner (Eds.), *Functional performance in older adults* (pp. 148–164). Philadelphia: F. A. Davis.

Sullivan, N. (1984). Vision in the elderly. In E. Stilwell (Ed.), *Handbook of patient care for gerontological nurses* (pp. 2–9). Thorofare NJ: Slack.

Swallow, M. (1966). Fiber size and content of the anterior tibial nerve of the foot. *Journal of Neurology, Neurosurgery and Psychiatry, 29,* 205–212.

Takeda, S., & Matsuzawa, T. (1984). Brain atrophy during aging: A quantitative study using computed tomography. *Journal of the American Geriatrics Society, 32,* 520–524.

Tiedeksaar, R. (1994). Falls. In B. R. Bonder & M. Wagner (Eds.), *Functional performance of older adults* (pp. 224–239). Philadelphia: F. A. Davis.

Tinetti, M., Speechley, M., & Ginter, S. (1988). Risk factors for falls among elderly persons living in the community. *New England Journal of Medicine, 319,* 1701–1707.

Tomlinson, B. E., Blessed, G., & Roth, M. (1968). Observations on the brains of non-demented old people. *Journal of Neurological Sciences, 7,* 331–336.

Tomlinson, B. E., Blessed, G., & Roth, M. (1970). Observations on the brains of demented old people. *Journal of Neurological Sciences, 11,* 205–270.

U.S. Congress. House of Representatives, Committee on Ways and Means, Subcommittee on Health. (1991, March 4). *Long term care: Proposals to improve Medicare's skilled nursing facility and health care benefits.* Washington, DC: U.S. Government Printing Office.

U.S. Office of Technology Assessment. (1987). *Losing a million minds.* Washington, DC: U.S. Government Printing Office.

U.S. Public Health Service. (1983). *Vision research, a national plan* (Publication No. 83-2471). Washington, DC: Author.

Weinreb, R., Freeman, W., & Selezinka, W. (1990). Vision impairment in geriatrics. In B. Kemp, K. Brummel-Smith, & J. Ramsdell (Eds), *Geriatric rehabilitation* (pp. 223–225). Boston: Little, Brown & Co.

Winter, D., Patla, A., Frank J., & Walt, S. (1990). Biomechanical walking pattern changes in the fit and healthy elderly. *Physical Therapy, 70,* 340–347.

Woods, R. T., & Britton, P. G. (1985). Clinical psychology with the elderly. Rockville, MD: Aspen Systems.

22

Remediating Biomechanical and Physiological Impairments of Motor Performance

Ruth Zemke

OBJECTIVES

After studying this chapter, the reader will be able to:
1. Understand the biomechanical and physiological factors contributing to musculoskeletal function.
2. Understand the application of principles to prevent limitation of range of motion, including movement, positioning, and compression.
3. Understand the application of principles to increase passive range of motion, including active and passive stretch.
4. Understand the application of the principle to increase strength through increased stress to the muscles, using the intensity, type or level, duration, rate, and frequency of contraction or exercise activity.
5. Understand the application of the principle to increase endurance through increased duration of activity of moderate rate and intensity.

A goal of occupational therapy is to assist people in engaging in a satisfying round of daily activities. When desired or necessary activity is threatened because of potential or actual limited range of motion (ROM), strength, or endurance, preventative or restorative treatment may be appropriate. The biomechanical approach is used to treat impairments secondary to sudden or cumulative trauma or disease affecting the musculoskeletal system, spinal cord, or peripheral nervous system, integumentary (skin) system, or cardiopulmonary system. Based on evaluations, problems are identified and treatment goals are established.

The evaluations and treatment goals are based on principles of biomechanical and physiological function and change. The biomechanical aspects of the human body are considered in terms of the (1) **kinematics,** or form of motion, and (2) **kinetics,** or forces, both static forces (i.e., forces acting to balance or stabilize) and dynamic forces that mobilize.

MUSCULOSKELETAL SYSTEM

Biomechanical Aspects

Kinematic characteristics describe three-dimensional time-space movement trajectories, or paths, in terms of the amount and direction of displacement (meters); velocity, or speed (m/sec); and acceleration, or rate of change of speed (m/sec^2), of body segments. Joint angles and the velocity and acceleration of joint angle changes in a given direction are also kinematic characteristics. Researchers have used these quantitative kinematic descriptors to describe movement of infants (Fetters & Todd, 1987), motor-impaired children (Downing, Martin, & Stern, 1991), adults with cerebral palsy (McPherson et al., 1991), and adults with stroke (Trombly, 1992). These descriptions allow a better understanding of the motor impairment than do qualitative descriptors of motion such as "fast," "smooth," or "athetoid."

Kinetics considers the forces acting in and on the body to produce stability or mobility. Forces that commonly affect the human body are sometimes discussed in terms of weight in pounds, which is a measure of the mass of an object or body segment relative to gravity (Roberts & Falkenburg, 1992). These forces may be external forces (such as the resistance of objects to be moved or the weight of a body segment such as the upper extremity) or internal forces (such as active

GLOSSARY

Concentric contraction—The isotonic muscle contraction that moves a limb segment in the direction of the muscle pull.

Contractures—Static shortening of muscle and connective tissue that limits range of motion at a joint.

Cross-bridges—ATP segments that move and connect actin and myosin fibrils during muscle contraction.

Decubitus ulcers—Also called bedsores; open sores in skin and tissue, usually related to decreased circulation to the area secondary to maintained pressure on the tissue.

Eccentric contraction—The isotonic muscle contraction that applies a braking force to a movement produced by an opposing force or resistance because the direction of the muscle pull is opposite to the actual movement.

Electrogoniometer—Electronic device used to measure range of motion; by measuring electrical potential as motion occurs or at static positions, a digital readout can be produced representing joint angles.

Isometric contraction—Contraction of a muscle that does not produce joint motion.

Isotonic contraction—Muscle contraction that produces joint motion.

Kinematics—Study of the form of motion, describing movement paths in terms of the amount and direction of displacement (in meters), velocity or speed m/sec), and acceleration or rate of change of speed (m/sec^2) of body segments. Joint angles and the velocity and acceleration of joint angle changes in a given direction are also kinematic characteristics.

Kinetics—Study of forces, including static forces, which balance or stabilize, and dynamic forces, which mobilize.

Newtons—Units of force (kg × m/sec^2) in which 1 N is the force that accelerates a 1-kg mass 9.8 m/sec^2; 1 N = 9.8 kg (Roberts & Falkenburg, 1992).

Torque—The product of the rotary component of force and the length of the force arm ($F \times FA$) or of resistance and the resistance arm ($R \times RA$).

Training effect—As a result of exercise, HR and blood pressure are less than previously required for the same amount of work (Fletcher & Cantwell, 1979).

muscle contraction or elasticity of structural and connective tissue).

The human body has many mechanical characteristics subject to the laws of physics. The weight of the body against the resistance of a wheelchair seat compresses tissue, restricts blood flow, and over time, encourages **decubitus ulcers.** The tensile forces of connective tissue bind the skeleton together, promoting joint stability. Limbs can act as springs or pendulums based on the inherent elasticity of muscle and connective tissue (Thelen et al., 1993).

In addition, of interest in **kinetics,** muscle contractions act as forces on bony levers. Motion occurs about the bony lever's axis of rotation, the joint. Most simple single joint movement is of this type, rotary motion, in which each point on the limb segment moves through an arc at the same time, at a constant radius or distance from the axis. The arc formed by the rotary movement is called the range of motion of that joint.

Effective muscles provide forces able to overcome the resistance of body weight and added resistance of objects being manipulated, used as tools, or moved. Force is defined as mass times acceleration. Forces that commonly affect the human body are sometimes discussed in terms of weight in pounds times the acceleration of gravity (32 ft/sec^2) or in **Newtons** (kg × m/sec^2) (Roberts & Falkenburg, 1992). An estimate of the amount of resistance force against which muscles are effective is referred to as strength. In manual muscle testing, the resistance of the body segment's

weight and/or the resistance added by the tester determines strength described as a muscle grade. Mechanical devices provide resistance and offer estimates of strength in pounds or metric quantities. For example, grip or pinch strength is measured as the force developed against the resistance of the dynamometer or pinchmeter.

In lever systems, there are force arms (defined as the distance between the point of application of the force and the axis of motion) and resistance arms (defined as the distance between the point of application of the resistance and the axis). **Torque** reflects the product of the rotary component of force and the length of the force arm ($F \times FA$) or of resistance and the resistance arm ($R \times RA$). A **torque** provides a tendency toward rotation around the axis of the lever. Equilibrium or stability at a joint results when the algebraic sum of the **torque** of all forces (resistance is a force) is zero ([$F \times FA$] − [$R \times RA$] = 0) or, in an alternate form, when the **torques** of opposing forces are equal ($F \times FA = R \times RA$). Movement results when the opposing **torques** are unequal. Lever systems illustrate the application of this concept.

In a first-class lever, such as a seesaw, the force arm and the resistance arm are on opposite sides of the axis, meaning that forces of effort and resistance can easily produce equilibrium. The erector spinae muscles of the back act with the first-class lever systems of spinal segments such that, in balanced standing, small muscle components lying close to the axis balance small amounts of resistance also located close to the axis, primarily resulting in small adjustments to maintain postural stability.

Second-class lever systems, such as a crowbar or wheelbarrow, in which the resistance is between the axis and the force, will always have longer force arms than resistance arms. Thus equal amounts of force and resistance produce greater force **torques** (force × moment arm) than similar forces and resistances would produce in a first-class lever system. Therefore, they have a mechanical advantage, i.e., they allow a greater amount of resistance to be overcome by a lesser force than do the other lever systems, facilitating the task performance. This system is more commonly found in the tools that are functional extensions of our body than in our muscle functions.

Usually, the insertions of muscles (the point at which the force is assumed to act on the bony lever) lie between the joint axis and the center of gravity of the limb (which is the point at which the resistance of the weight of the limb is assumed to act), illustrating a third-class lever. In this case, the force arm will always be shorter than the resistance arm, and the **torque** is effective only with less resistance than can be generated by the muscle's rotary force. In contrast to the stability of first-class levers and the mechanical advantage of second-class levers, third-class levers are able to move the distal end of the limb a greater distance with more speed than the proximal end.

Thus the mechanical aspects of our musculoskeletal system promote both proximal stability (in the first-class lever systems of some muscles of the trunk and neck) and distal mobility (through the third-class levers characteristic of much of the limb musculature). Together, stability and mobility provide the basis for our action in occupation.

When a force acts (on an object) for a distance, e.g., when a muscle's **isotonic contraction** moves a limb segment, work occurs. Work is the force times the distance times repetitions and is measured in foot-pounds or **Newtons** per meter (Joules). Positive work occurs when the resultant motion is in the same direction as the force. A **concentric contraction** performs positive work, moving a limb segment in the direction of the muscle pull. When an **eccentric contraction** applies a braking force to a movement produced by an opposing force or resistance, the muscle is performing negative work, because the direction of the muscle pull is opposite to the actual movement. With equal energy expenditure, more force can be generated by a muscle's isotonic **eccentric contraction** during negative work, and the benefit of this effect will be discussed later in this chapter. Muscles in the human body are often required to contract without doing work, for example during an **isometric contraction,** when there is no movement at the joint, as in holding something still.

The potential work capacity of the various muscles of the body depends on the force they can generate and the distance over which they can shorten. The resulting work capacity depends not only on biomechanical factors but also on physiological factors such as the amount of tension a muscle is able to produce. Physiological factors will be discussed in relation to some of the principles of change that affect the work capacity of the musculoskeletal system.

Biomechanical concepts provide a basis for normal function and guidelines for promoting the characteristics of interest, namely range of motion, strength, and endurance. These concepts provide a basis for occupational therapy roles in prevention programs such as those described by Jaffe (1986). In primary prevention activities undertaken before the onset of disease, biomechanical concepts are used for industrial back injury prevention, cumulative stress trauma prevention, and other work-related prevention programs (Ellexson, 1986; Smith, 1989; see also Chapters 17 and 38). Secondary prevention programs refer to early treatment to prevent a condition from worsening or becoming permanently disabling. Biomechanical concepts are extended to include joint protection principles (Cordery, 1965), energy conservation, positioning, and splinting (Fess & Philips, 1987). Tertiary prevention refers to reducing disability as an aftereffect of a disease or condition through remediation, prevention of further loss, and compensation for chronic impairment. This level of program incorporates not only the physics-based mechanical aspects of biomechanics, but the physiological aspects as well.

Physiological Aspects

A muscle is composed of thousands of muscle fibers bound together in fascicles. Segal and Wolf (1990) described each fiber as a large cell filled with sarcoplasm, which principally has the metabolic function of storing glycogen and enzymes used during contraction. Within each fiber are myofibrils, the contractile portion of skeletal muscle. Myofibrils are composed of overlapping layers of actin filaments and myosin filaments. The myosin filaments have tiny adenosine 5'triphosphate (ATP) projections at the ends that form **cross-bridges** extending toward the actin filaments.

According to the sliding filament theory, the sequence of muscle contraction begins when the ATP **cross-bridges** connect the actin and myosin fibrils (Murray & Weber, 1974). Next, ATP is broken down, and the released energy swivels the **cross-bridges,** which pulls the actin over the myosin, producing tension and shortening in the muscle. Following contraction, the ATP must be regenerated. Regeneration occurs either by the highly efficient aerobic process in which aerobic enzymes use oxidation of fatty acids and glucose to synthesize ATP or by the less efficient anaerobic process in which anaerobic enzymes break down glucose to produce smaller quantities of ATP along with lactic acid as a by-product. Recycling of actin and myosin follows, in preparation for another contraction sequence.

The sliding filament theory of muscle contraction offers potential explanations for two documented muscle characteristic relationships: the length-tension and force-velocity curves (Spielholz, 1990). These curves demonstrate that the greatest amount of contraction tension occurs at the resting length of the muscle (length-tension) and that force decreases as the velocity of the shortening motion increases (force-velocity). At resting length, there is optimum overlap of actin-myosin binding sites, and if the joint is not moving (no velocity), maximum tension in contraction and thus maximum force could be generated. This is why standardized muscle testing positions approximate resting positions of muscles and why the tests are isometric.

Muscle units, the muscle fibers innervated by one motor unit, have been differentiated in terms of their speed of contraction and fatigability. The most common fiber types are fast-contracting fatigable (FF); fast-contracting, fatigue-resistant (FR); and slow-contracting, low fatigability (S) (Stuart, Binder, & Enoka, 1984). These also have been called, respectively, fast glycolytic (FG), fast oxidative glycolytic (FOG), and slow oxidative (SO) units, based on their primary enzyme source for ATP synthesis (Peter, Barnard, & Edgerton, 1972). That is, they tend to depend either on anaerobic enzymes for metabolism (FG) or on oxygen delivered by the cardiovascular system (SO) or on both (FOG). Aerobic fibers tend to have more capillaries in their vicinity to deliver the needed oxygen (Spielholz, 1990). As the result of these characteristics, the FG fibers are also called "white, fast-twitch fibers" and the SO "red, slow-twitch fibers" (Peter et al., 1972).

The all-or-none principle of neural propagation states that a neuron will propagate the impulse completely or not at all, regardless of the incremental size of the stimulus. This holds true in muscle innervation, not for the muscle as a whole but for individual motor units. The order of recruitment of additional motor units has been described as occurring according to Henneman's (1957) size principle in which smaller motor neurons are usually activated before larger ones. Smaller motor neurons tend to have lower thresholds and innervate the slow, tonic (S or SO) muscle fibers and the faster, fatigue-resistant ones (FR or FOG) (Sypert & Munson, 1981; Ulfhake & Kellerth, 1982). This suggests that minimum muscle tension will utilize tonic, fatigue-resistant muscle fibers, producing milder contractions that could be sustained for a longer time.

When great force or speed is required however, the more phasic, fast-contracting fibers will be recruited to assist in increasing muscle tension. Recruitment order is not absolute, however; it can be affected by many factors, including resistance to movement, cocontraction, and higher-level neural influences such as voluntary movement goal changes (Segal & Wolf, 1990).

Muscle fatigue can be defined internally as a reduction in the force-generating capacity of the system and seen externally as inability to maintain the expected force (Porter & Whelan, 1981). Fatigue can occur as the result of buildup of by-products of contraction (e.g., lactic acid) or secondary to insufficient energy supply (e.g., insufficient oxygen delivery or glycogen depletion).

In contrast to the mechanical aspects of the musculoskeletal system, the physiological aspects reflect an open adaptable system that can alter some characteristics of muscle to better enable it to perform as needed for function (Salmons, 1980). Other elements of the system, including blood flow to deliver oxygen and nutrients, lymph fluid movement, and connective tissue elasticity adapt both to activity demands and to inactivity.

A muscle's strength and endurance depend on multiple factors. Muscle strength changes are related to muscle size through myofibrillar changes. Myosin and actin filaments are added to the myofibrils when activity stresses the muscle's ability to produce sufficient tension and force. (From lack of use, myosin and actin filaments can also be lost.) Additional neural changes relating to synchrony of activation of motor units accompany these fiber changes (Segal & Wolf, 1990). The strength of a muscle has been shown to be a function not only of muscle size and synchrony of motor unit firing but also of psychological factors such as motivation. However, training (and, the alternative, immobility) have been shown to affect these factors as well as the physiological ones (Spielholz, 1990).

For improved muscle endurance, more oxygen must become available. The exent to which muscle can improve endurance with increased amounts of repetitive, mild activity is one of the most dramatic examples of adaptability (Haggmark, Eriksson, & Jansson, 1986). Because of these adaptations to exercise and inactivity, muscle fatigue occurs less readily after training and more readily after immobilization. These changes are related to changes in the cardiopulmonary system.

As an immediate effect of exercise, heart rate (HR) and stroke volume (the amount of blood pumped per heartbeat) increase (Ellestad, 1986). Heart rate increases to deliver the required amount of oxygenated blood to the active muscles. Stroke volume increases because of increased venous flow into the heart during diastole (the period of muscle relaxation when the chambers fill) (Ellestad, 1986; Thomas, 1973). The mechanical response of the ventricle is based on Starling's Law: the force of the contraction is a function of the degree of stretch of the muscle fibers during diastole. Over time, a **training effect** is seen, which means that HR and blood pressure are lower than what was once required for the same amount of work (Fletcher & Cantwell, 1979).

As heart rate changes, so does the amount of oxygen that the person can take in (in a given amount of time) and dispense to the muscles ($\dot{V}O_2$), up to about 80 to 90% of maximum capacity (Ellestad, 1986). Aerobic exercise programs frequently set goals for participants at a given percent of maximum heart rate (HRmax) to encourage the **training effect** on maximum oxygen consumption ($\dot{V}O_2$max), HR, and blood pressure. HRmax for an individual is calculated by subtracting the person's age from 220. When the heart rate during exercise reaches a stable level, it means that enough oxygen is being supplied to meet the demand (Ellestad, 1986).

Based on this physiological information, programs can be developed to remediate problems affecting range of motion, strength, and endurance.

BIOMECHANICAL APPROACH TO TREATMENT

Goal: To Prevent Limitation of Range of Motion

Many range of motion limitations can and should be prevented. Patients who are unable to move their own joints, and for whom motion is not contraindicated, should receive passive range of motion exercises. The part should be properly positioned between treatments.

If edema exists, range of motion will be limited and **contractures,** due to both the lack of movement and to the developing viscosity of the fluid, are a possibility. A subgoal would be to reduce edema, using principles of dynamic muscle contraction, positioning, and compression.

PRINCIPLE: MOVEMENT THROUGH FULL RANGE OF MOTION

The methods used for ranging (movement through full range of motion) are teaching the patient to move actively the joints that are involved in, or adjacent to, an injury and passively moving the joints if the patient is paralyzed. In the case of edema, active ranging is preferred because the contraction of the muscles will help pump the fluid out of the extremity. However, if active range of motion (AROM) is not possible, passive range of motion (PROM) must be done.

The ranging technique is the same for AROM and PROM. Each involved joint is slowly and gently moved three times, twice daily from one limit of motion to the other (Kottke, 1990; Tookey & Larson, 1968). **Exception:** The hands of tetraplegic persons who will rely on tenodesis action for grasp must be ranged in the following manner to allow finger flexor tendons to develop necessary tightness for function. When flexing the fingers, the wrist must be fully extended, and when extending the fingers, the wrist must be fully flexed.

Battery-operated continuous passive motion (CPM) machines are commercially available orthoses used to maintain ROM and prevent postoperative swelling by continually moving the part from one limit of motion to the other. CPM is a well-tolerated, painless procedure that stimulates healing and remodeling of tissue (Salter, 1983; Salter et al., 1984). There are CPM units for large joints and hands. In the hand units, one to five digits can be exercised simultaneously. The limits of motion are adjustable to fit the patient's requirements, and the speed of each full cycle can be set. CPM used postoperatively is prescribed by the physician, who should specify the safe limits of motion and duration of daily treatment. CPM is contraindicated in cases of unstable fractures or joints or lacerations of nerves or arteries. Continuous passive motion instituted immediately postoperatively and continued for at least 1 week has been found to prevent loss of range of joint motion gained at surgery (Salter, 1983). It was also found to be successful in correcting knee flexion **contractures** in one patient who continued to worsen despite treatment with manual passive ranging and stretching (Stap & Woodfin, 1986).

PRINCIPLE: POSITIONING

Positioning of joints too weak to resist the force of gravity is essential to avoid development of deformities. All potentially nonfunctional positions are avoided throughout the day and night. Positioning can be accomplished by the use of orthoses, pillows, rolled towels, positioning boards, etc. For example, when the patient is in bed, orthoses may be used to prevent foot drop, and sandbags or trochanter rolls can be placed along the lateral aspect of the thigh to prevent hip external rotation (Bergstrom & Coles, 1971; Feinberg & Andree, 1980). Elevating a patient's edematous hand by use of a suspension sling or pillow will allow the fluid to drain back to the body.

Sometimes **contractures** and subsequent ankylosis are unavoidable, because of the disease process. In these instances positioning, splinting, and bracing are used to ensure that ankylosis occurs in as nearly a functional position as possible. Functional positions are those that if fixed will still allow the person to manage his self-care and other functional tasks. For example, the functional position of the hand and wrist is slight (10° to 30°) extension of the wrist, opposition and abduction of the thumb, and semiflexion of the finger joints. If the hand contracted in that position, the person would be able to use it to hold objects. If, however, the hand were to contract in a fully flexed position, it would not only be useless but would also present a hygiene problem. If it contracted in full extension, it would have no holding capability and be equally useless. Whenever positioning a patient, the occupational therapist must be vigilant in anticipating eventual outcomes of prolonged immobilization that could compromise function.

PRINCIPLE: COMPRESSION

Edema can be controlled by compression with elastic strip bandages or tubular bandages. Care must be exercised so that these are applied correctly and do not constrict circulation in the more distal part of the extremity. Skin color is observed regularly to confirm that circulation is preserved. Coban (3M Co., St. Paul), a self-adherent elastic wrap bandage, is wrapped around the part spirally in a distal to proximal direction; the edges are overlapped by at least 25% of the width of the material so that the fluid can flow evenly back toward the body and not be trapped in pockets of unwrapped tissues (Enos, Lane, & MacDougal, 1984). Tubigrip (Mark One Health Care Products, Inc., Philadelphia) is a tubular elastic support bandage that provides graduated constant pressure support when the correct size is applied.

Goal: To Increase Passive Range of Motion

If the results of evaluation of PROM indicate that limitations in joint motions are significant, i.e., if they impair the patient's ability to function independently in life tasks or are likely to lead to deformity, then treatment may be indicated. Whereas some significant limitations of ROM can be ameliorated or corrected by activity or exercise, some cannot. Problems that can be changed include **contractures** of soft tissue, i.e., skin, muscle, tendon, and ligament. Problems that cannot be changed include bony ankylosis or arthrodesis, long-standing **contractures** in which there are extensive fibrotic changes in soft tissue, and severe joint destruction with subluxation. Occupational therapy for limited ROM problems that cannot be treated restoratively is compensatory in nature and focuses on providing techniques and/or equipment to reduce the disability from the impaired range of motion.

PRINCIPLE: STRETCH

Stretch produces change only if done to the point of maximal stretch, defined as a few degrees beyond

the point of discomfort, and held there for a few seconds. The stretching may be active or passive, depending on the source of the force. The patient controls the amount of stretch and force in active stretching, while the setup of the activity or exercise equipment controls the direction of force. By using activities that combine active stretch and minimal resistance to the contracting muscle, the patient can make instantaneous adjustments in the force of the stretch in response to pain by relaxing the contraction and moving away from the stretched position. On the other hand, in passive stretch, the force applied by an external source cannot be immediately adjusted to accommodate pain experienced by the patient. Nonetheless, passive stretch is usually more effective than active stretch, because the therapist carefully ensures that each limited joint is stretched to the point of maximal stretch. When precautions are in effect even greater caution must be used in doing passive stretch, and active stretch is preferable. Precautions are noted below.

Use of an **electrogoniometer** that provides feedback to the patient at the desired limit of motion may increase the effectiveness of active stretching (see Fig. 6.56). A simple **electrogoniometer** that can be constructed by an occupational therapist has been described (Brown, DeBacher, & Basmajian 1979; Fig. 22.1).

Active Stretching

At the limited joint, the patient contracts the muscles antagonistic to the contracture, providing a force against the resistance of the contracture. For

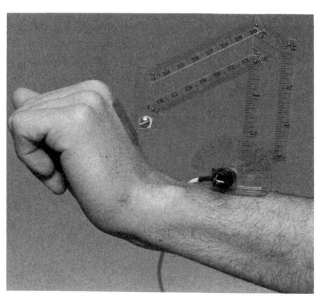

Figure 22.1. A wrist electrogoniometer constructed by Gary DeBacher according to the instructions given in Brown, DeBacher, and Basmajian (1979).

example, if there is a flexion contracture, the extensors must contract to pull against it. Patients control the force, speed, extent, and direction of the stretch within their own tolerance for pain. It is the therapist's role to instruct and encourage the patient to stretch the part frequently and correctly throughout the day.

Passive Stretching

An external force stretches the contracture at the limited joint. It is used when the patient does not have sufficient strength in the antagonist to do active stretching.

METHODS

Ways to provide passive stretching include orthoses that provide traction, manual stretching, joint mobilization techniques, exercise, and/or activities. All methods stretch the tissue beyond its customary limit of motion.

The force, speed, direction, and extent of stretch must be controlled. The force must be enough to put tension on the tissue but not enough to rupture it. Different tissues tolerate stretch differently; tight muscles can be stretched more vigorously than tight joints (Kottke, 1990). The speed should be slow to allow the tissue to adjust gradually. The direction of stretch is exactly opposite to the tightness. The extent of stretch is to the point of maximal stretch, defined above.

Orthotic devices that provide a continuous, gentle stretch (traction) are used to supplement gains made by means of exercise or activity as well as to provide a form of continuous, controlled passive stretching. One such device is the glove flexion mitt used to put a constant stretch on extensor **contractures** of the metacarpophalangeal and interphalangeal joints (Heurich & Polansky, 1978; see also Chapter 28).

Manual stretching, a form of passive stretching, is done by the therapist. Ideally, the environment and the therapist are quiet and relaxed to encourage relaxation of the patient. The therapist describes the process of manual stretching, noting that it involves tolerable pain.

The therapist holds the extremity in such a way that the part proximal to the joint is stabilized and the part distal to the joint is moved. The motions used in stretching are identical to those described in Chapter 6 for range of motion evaluation. The patient is encouraged to assist in moving the part if possible. The therapist moves the part smoothly, slowly, and gently to the point of mild discomfort, which the patient indicates verbally or by facial expression (Kisner & Colby, 1990). The therapist then holds the part at that point of maximal stretch. There should be relief of discomfort immediately following release of stretch.

Residual pain after stretching indicates that the stretch was too forceful and caused tearing of soft tissues or blood vessels (Kottke, 1990).

Gentle stretching that achieves small increments of gain over a period of time is more effective than vigorous stretching aimed at large gains quickly. As a protective mechanism, connective tissue resists quick, vigorous stretching, which is thus ineffective or injurious (Kottke, 1990). The method of moving gently to the point of maximal stretch and holding that position allows connective tissue, which has plasticity, to adapt to new requirements and adjust its length gradually over time. It is clinically recognized that maintained stretching is most effective; however, gains are also noted using briefly held stretch, usually 15 to 30 sec (Kisner & Colby, 1990). A study of healthy subjects found that 15 sec of passive stretch was as effective as 2 min (Hallum & Medeiros, 1987). A stretch of 20 sec has been recommended for athletes who stretch their muscles before strenuous activity (Agre, 1978).

During each treatment session, each joint with limitation of PROM is gently stretched in the described manner several times to ensure achieving maximal stretch at least once. To maximize gains achieved by stretching, it is necessary to stretch daily, because microscopic examination of connective tissue has determined that the process involved in contracture formation begins in 1 day (Kottke, 1990).

In ligament or tendon tightness resulting from weakness of the shoulder musculature, it has been clinically demonstrated that pain, caused by the weight of the arm pulling on the rotator cuff muscles, can be reduced by approximating the head of the humerus into the glenoid fossa, while simultaneously ranging or stretching this joint (Fig 22.2). In ligament, muscle, or tendon tightness of the wrist, thumb, and fingers, it has been clinically demonstrated that pain associated with stretching can be reduced by traction applied to each joint to separate the articular surfaces during stretching (Kottke, 1971).

Joint mobilization techniques are primarily used in physical therapy; however, the occupational therapist may find the techniques useful to increase range of motion in stiff hands and wrists. Maitland (1977) described methods of joint manipulation and joint mobilization. *Manipulation* is defined as either a sudden thrusting movement of small amplitude or a steady controlled stretch strong enough to break adhesions. Manipulation is usually done under anesthesia and is never used without extensive special training. Mobilization is defined as passive movements done at such a speed that the patient could prevent them if he chose. Two types of movement are included: (1) oscillatory movement (two to three per second) of small or large amplitude applied anywhere within the range of motion

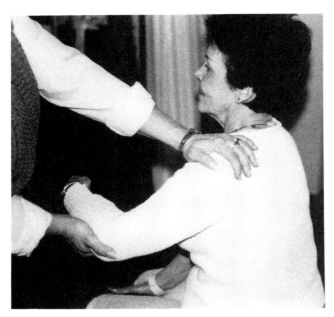

Figure 22.2. Method of doing range of motion of a hemiplegic shoulder to avoid rotator cuff tears.

or (2) sustained stretching with tiny amplitude oscillations done at the limit of range. The oscillatory movements may be of the physiologic movements or accessory movements (also called "joint play," i.e., movement possible within a joint but not under voluntary control). Details of this treatment are provided by Maitland (1977).

An exercise that has been found to be effective in increasing the PROM of shortened tissue is the proprioceptive neuromuscular facilitation (PNF) technique called "hold/relax" (Tanigawa, 1972). The hold/relax procedure involves a brief (4 to 6 sec) and maximal **isometric contraction** performed at the point of limitation (Moller et al., 1985). The tight muscle is contracted maximally and then relaxed for 2 sec. During the relaxation phase, the therapist moves the part in the direction opposite to the contraction into the new maximal range and holds it for 8 sec. The effect in the lower extremities has been found to last up to 90 min. The hold/relax procedure may be repeated at each succeeding limit of range until a large gain in range is made. For example, if there were a contracture of elbow flexors, the elbow would be extended to its limit. The patient would be instructed to contract his flexors isometrically and maximally, then relax, at which moment the therapist would smoothly extend the elbow into greater range until resistance was felt. The hold/relax procedure would be repeated until as many increments of gain as possible are achieved.

The comparative effectiveness of passive stretch and hold/relax has been studied on normal young adult males. One study (Tanigawa, 1972) found hold/relax

to be the more effective procedure, and another study (Medeiros et al., 1977) found no statistically significant difference between the two. Both treatments produced improved range of motion. In a study of 30 young adult females, "contract/relax," an **isotonic contraction** against maximal resistance, was found to be superior to hold/relax in increasing ROM; both, however, did improve ROM (Markos, 1977).

Activity used for increasing PROM must provide a gentle active stretch by use of slow, repetitive **isotonic contraction** of the muscles opposite the contracture or by use of a prolonged passive stretched position of the tissue producing limitation. In both types of activity, the requirement is that the range be increased slightly beyond the patient's limitation. The use of activity for stretching is empirically based on the idea that a person involved in an interesting and purposeful activity will gain greater range, because he is relaxed, is not anticipating pain, is motivated to complete the task, and will be more likely to move as the activity demands. The *ROM Dance Program,* devised by Harlowe and Yu as a home program for rheumatoid arthritic patients, is an example of use of purposeful, meaningful activity to achieve physical goals. The program is made up of expressive dance techniques and relaxation techniques used during rest periods (Harlowe, 1982; Van Deusen & Harlowe, 1987). The 7-min dance, modeled after tai chi chuan, incorporates joint motion in all ranges recommended for patients with rheumatoid arthritis. The dance is done while listening to or reciting a poem that is meant to evoke pleasurable images of warmth and friendship. An outcome study indicated that significant gains in ROM were made by the experimental subjects compared with control subjects who did a "traditional home program" (Van Deusen & Harlowe, 1987). Another example is the use of *Simon,* an electronic game device that produces sound and light patterns, to increase range of shoulder motion of posttraumatic brain-injured patients (Sietsema et al., 1993). When compared with arm reach exercise, the use of the game elicited significantly greater range of motion for 20 adult subjects.

The selected activity must be interesting to the patient and must intrinsically demand the correct motion without requiring the patient to concentrate on the movement instead of the goal. Reasonable adaptations of the activity may be necessary to elicit the desired motion. An example of an adaptation of an activity to provide active stretch of an elbow flexion contracture of a jigsaw puzzle enthusiast could be to position the puzzle pieces just beyond the comfortable range, requiring elbow extension to reach for them. One point to remember is that if the contracture existed when the limb was not immobilized in some way then active stretch will not be effective, i.e., if the patient was free to move and did not during daily activities then it is unlikely gains will be made using activity to correct the contracture.

Adaptations can be made through the tools or equipment used in doing the activity. Equipment used in activities can provide traction (passive stretch) if resistance is provided by means of springs, weights, elastic material, or the weight of the tool. For example, weights can be used when sanding long boards like those used to make a bookcase. Each of the shelf boards are clamped in turn to an inclined sanding frame. The patient tries to push the sander to the end of the board. Weights fixed to the sander are attached to a line suspended through a pulley at the top of the incline, creating a force greater than that of the contracted tissue, thus stretching the shoulder extensors and elbow flexor.

Adaptations made to adjust the size or location of handles of craft or recreational equipment can require the patient to move further into range actively. The size or location is gradually changed by the therapist as the patient improves (Maughan, 1962). One cannot prescribe activity for specific purposes similar to the way a physician prescribes medication, because people move in individually characteristic ways. The therapist must carefully monitor the patient's method of doing an activity and not assume that the activity per se will evoke the desired result in all persons. An example illustrates this. Pressing the weft of finger weaving using a passive hand and the force of shoulder extensors provides stretch to the finger flexors because the resultant force of the motion and the resistance acts in the direction of finger extension. Actively pressing the weft into place using finger flexion, however, stretches the finger extensors, because the flexors contract forcefully against the extensors' resistance. Both methods accomplish the same activity goal.

It is best to avoid the use of an activity that requires a motion that is habitual for the patient if the habitual manner of movement does not meet the therapy goal. Otherwise, the patient must concentrate on the new movement to maintain it, and often when the patient begins focusing on the activity, the motion will revert back to the habitual method of moving.

PRECAUTIONS

Inflammation, sensory loss, and consequences of immobilization require modifications of procedure. Inflammation weakens the structure of collagen tissues (i.e., bone, cartilage, tendon, ligament, artery, fascia, dermis, and other connective tissues) (Downey & Darling, 1971). Inflamed tissue must be stretched cautiously with slow, gentle motion (Kottke, 1990). If steroids are used to treat the inflammation, they may cause side effects such as osteoporosis that would also require modified procedures.

Sensory loss prevents the patient from monitoring pain, thus permitting overstretching to occur unless the therapist pays particular attention to the tension of the tissues being stretched. Overstretching causes internal bleeding with subsequent scar formation that may eventually ossify (Kottke, 1990). An unfortunate common example of such calcification, heterotrophic ossification, occurs in hip and elbow flexor musculature of spinal cord–injured patients because of the cumulative effects of overstretching inherent in their performance of daily life tasks.

Stretching tissue after it has been immobilized must be done carefully because prolonged immobilization or bed rest produces many side effects, including osteoporosis. Bone loses calcium because there has been no compression forces on the bone to maintain its integrity, and it can be more easily fractured by tension or shear forces applied during stretching (Downey & Darling, 1971). Tendons and ligaments also change biochemically and lose tensile strength in the absence of motion and stress. With immobilization, muscle filaments lose their ability to slide, which is necessary for muscle contraction. The resultant adhesions may be torn when stretched. Bed rest causes a decrease in blood pressure in the extremities, which reduces the stress necessary for maintaining the strength of the collagen fibers of the vessel walls; consequently, blood vessels are weakened. To reduce the effects of immobilization and bed rest, the physician may prescribe weight bearing, isometric muscle contraction, or CPM during this period.

Goal: To Increase Strength

If evaluation of the patient's strength reveals a significant limitation, one that prevents the person from carrying out his life tasks or that may lead to deformity, then treatment is aimed at gradually increasing the patient's strength. Weakness is potentially deforming if muscles on one side of a joint are weaker than their antagonists.

Strength of contraction is gained when more motor units are recruited, which occurs when a muscle is stressed by increasing the load or speed requirements of a movement or when the muscle begins to tire. Muscle fibers of repeatedly recruited motor units hypertrophy in response to increased resistance or load, thereby increasing strength (Downey & Darling, 1971; MacDougall et al., 1977; Moritani & deVries, 1979).

PRINCIPLE: INCREASE STRESS TO MUSCLE

Stress is applied to the muscle or muscle group to the point of fatigue (DeLateur, Lehmann, Stonebridge, et al., 1972). Parameters that may be manipulated to alter the stress on a muscle include intensity or load (resistance), duration of a contraction or exercise activity, type of contraction, rate or velocity of contraction (number of repetitions per period of time), and the frequency of exercise (exercise periods/day). Each parameter may be manipulated independently. There may be precautionary reasons why the load should not be increased for a given patient. In that case, the therapist has the option of increasing one of the other parameters, e.g., increasing the frequency of exercise to increase the stress on the muscle, leading to increased strength.

The intensity of exercise refers to the amount of resistance offered. Although research is limited, it seems that intensities as low as 50 to 67% of maximum capability increase strength (Dons et al., 1979; Hislop, 1963). Resistance is graded by the type of exercise chosen, by adding a load to the extremity, by changing the length of the resistance arm by changing the point where the load is applied to the limb, or by changing the plane of movement. It must be remembered that the weight of the extremity itself is a load as are the weights of tools and the resistiveness of work materials.

Increasing the duration of a contraction causes fatigue of the active muscles. As fatigue progresses more motor units are recruited to maintain the goal posture. The muscle fibers recruited later thus have the opportunity to hypertrophy, which would not occur if they were not activated. It should be noted that a weak muscle activates more motor units to exert a given force than a strong muscle does (Fuglsang-Frederiksen, 1981; Trombly & Quintana, 1983).

Another factor that should be considered in designing a strengthening program is the type of muscle contraction to be required. Exercise to increase muscle strength can be accomplished by means of **isotonic** or **isometric contraction. Isotonic contraction** has two forms. In an isotonic **concentric contraction,** the internal force produced by the muscle exceeds the external force of the resistance, and the muscle shortens (Gowitzke & Milner, 1980). In an isotonic **eccentric contraction,** a lengthening contraction occurs when an external force slightly greater than the internal force acts on an already shortened muscle. The internal force of the contracting muscle allows a controlled and gradual lengthening of the muscle against the external force. In an **isometric contraction** the internal and external forces are in equilibrium and the length of the muscle remains the same. The three types of contraction are illustrated in these examples. Raising a mug of coffee to your mouth requires **concentric contraction** of the elbow flexors, whereas carefully lowering the mug requires **eccentric contraction** of the same muscle group. Maintaining the grasp on the handle of

the mug exemplifies **isometric contraction.** Lifting a 10-lb bag of flour from a countertop to a storage shelf uses **concentric contraction** of shoulder flexors, and lowering it back to the counter eccentrically contracts these muscles. Holding it out to read a recipe from the bag requires **isometric contraction** of these muscles.

If **isotonic contraction** is required in a person's important daily life tasks, then treatment should use **isotonic contraction,** because transfer of the effects of training is poor between isometric and isotonic training programs (Carlson, 1970; DeLateur, Lehmann, Stonebridge, et al., 1972; Dons et al., 1979; Lindh, 1979). When no movement of the joint is permitted or possible because of a cast, **isometric contraction** is the only choice. **Isometric contraction** at resting length can produce the most forceful contraction. However, when the patient has hypertension or cardiovascular problems, **isometric contraction** should be avoided, because **isometric contraction** of either small or large muscles increases blood pressure and heart rate (Riendl et al., 1977; Smith & Lukens, 1983). Grasp and pinch, grasp in combination with pushing using total body force, and manual muscle testing of upper extremity musculature were studied in 40 normal subjects aged 19 to 30. Significant increases in systolic and diastolic blood pressure and heart rate were found, which increased with duration of contraction. Approximately 25% of the subjects had to be eliminated from the study when their values exceeded safe limits (Smith & Lukens, 1983).

The effectiveness of concentric (DeLateur, Lehmann, Warren, et al., 1972; DeLorme & Watkins, 1948; McGovern & Luscombe, 1953) and isometric (Carlson, 1970; Hislop, 1963, 1964; Lawrence, 1960) exercise to increase strength has been documented. However, isometric training does not effectively strengthen a muscle much beyond the length (or joint angle) at which it was exercised, nor does isotonic exercise stress the muscle at maximum through the entire range (Lindh, 1979). Because of changing force and resistance **torques** as the muscle moves the joint through its range, the muscle must produce more force in some positions of the range of motion than others. The speed of the motion may also vary, affecting the muscle's ability to provide equal tension throughout the motion (as demonstrated by the force-velocity curve).

In isotonic function, more weight can be lowered by a given muscle during an **eccentric contraction** than can be lifted concentrically or held at any one point. A corollary is that less effort is exerted when lowering a given weight than when lifting it. For very weak muscles, it may be advantageous to start with **eccentric contraction,** because less tension is required for the same load (Rasch, 1974). The **eccentric contraction** should be a slow, *controlled* lengthening in the direction of the pull of gravity. **Eccentric contraction** is less stressful cardiovascularly (Downey & Darling, 1971; Gowitzke & Milner, 1980) and thus would be a more appropriate exercise for patients with cardiac or pulmonary conditions. Eccentric exercise has been found to be helpful in treatment of patients with chronic tendinitis (Stanish, Rubinovic, & Curwin, 1986).

When an agonist muscle is significantly weaker than its antagonist, an exercise or activity that requires the weaker muscle to contract concentrically and then eccentrically for the return motion may be more effective than one that requires reciprocal contraction of the agonist and antagonist. Assistance may be provided for the **concentric contraction** that would not be necessary for the eccentric return.

By choosing a certain type of exercise, intensity can be graded from full assistance to full resistance. The choice, based on the measured strength of the muscle(s), should require effort. The appropriate level of exercise for a patient who cannot move at all is passive exercise to maintain range of motion. If he is able to, the patient should contract the contralateral muscle or muscle group, because it has been demonstrated that a 30 to 50% increase in strength of the nonexercised muscle group can occur as a result of cross-education (Hellebrandt & Waterland, 1962; Stromberg, 1986).

For muscles graded "trace" (*T*) strength, the force of contraction is not sufficient for movement of the joint. Passive exercise, in which the part is moved by an outside agent, does not stress muscles to increase strength, but does maintain range of motion. Isometric exercise and activity is used to increase strength.

Muscles graded "poor minus" (*P* −), "poor" (*P*), and "poor plus" (*P* +) are exercised in a gravity-eliminated plane. Active assistive exercise, in which the patient moves the part as much as possible by force of muscle contraction and is then assisted by an external force (provided by therapist or equipment), is appropriate at the *P* − grade. Active exercise, in which the patient moves the part through the entire gravity-eliminated range of motion without external assistance or additional resistance, is used for muscles graded *P*. Active resistive exercise, in which external resistance to the movement is added, is appropriate for muscles graded *P* + when the resistance is less than gravity and the movement is still in a gravity-eliminated plane.

Muscles graded "fair minus" (*F* −), "fair" (*F*), and "fair plus" (*F* +) are, by definition, exercised against the force of gravity. Once again, the sequence of active assistive (for *F* − muscles), active (for *F*), and active resistive (for *F* +) exercise is used to grade the effort to produce strengthening effects. Muscle grades "good minus" (*G* −), "good" (*G*), and "good

plus" (*G*) indicate the need for further increases in resistance.

Great intrasubject and intersubject differences have been seen electromyographically in the patterns of muscle contraction people use to accomplish the same goal (Hinson & Rosentswieg, 1973; Newell & Corcos, 1993; Trombly & Quintana, 1983). For a particular treatment program to be effective for a particular person, careful monitoring, preferably using electromyographic biofeedback (see Chapter 32), should be done.

METHODS

Exercise, other purposeful activity, or a combination of both can be used to increase strength. The use of non−product-producing exercise in occupational therapy was a source of controversy (Hollis, 1986; Trombly, 1982). Exercise has been considered an example of an adjunctive method (Pedretti et al., 1992) and can fit the definition of purposeful activity proposed by the American Occupational Therapy Association (1993), depending on its meaning in a specific context. Exercise allows greater control over the parameters (such as resistance type, and rate of contraction) than do other activities. Using exercise, the therapist can manipulate any or all of these parameters more exactly to alter the stress on a muscle. Changes can be graphed so that improvement can be understood easily by the patient and others. Other purposeful activities, however, may provide greater interest and may better motivate some patients to endure the ordeal necessary to make gains. Those activities that can be adapted to provide some control over the parameters are chosen.

Isometric Exercise and Activity

Lawrence (1956) reported successful case outcomes using two kinds of isometric exercise programs: the *Progressive Prolonged Isometric Tension Method* and *Progressive Weighted Isometric Exercise Method*. The prolonged method is defined as holding the **isometric contraction,** at whatever level the patient is capable, for as long as possible. This is repeated 10 times. The duration of maximal contraction is determined by trial and error during day 1 of treatment. The time is increased as the patient improves so that maximal effort is exerted to hold the contraction for 10 repetitions, with rest periods between each contraction. The weighted method requires the patient to hold a contraction against weight—determined by the DeLorme method (described below)—for a given period of time (30 or 45 sec), with 15-sec rest periods between each of the 10 repetitions.

Brief (6-sec) maximal **isometric contraction** once per day has been found to be effective in increasing strength (Rose, Radzyminski, & Beatty, 1957). Hislop (1963) found that holding the contraction for 15 sec twice a day was more effective than for less amounts of time.

Isometric contraction is achieved in activity by grasp of handles (the force of grasp increases with increasingly resistive material that the tool is used against), stabilization of materials being used, or by positioning projects so that the limbs must maintain antigravity positions during the activity. Isometric activity should be characterized by a requirement to hold the contraction for increased periods of time and/or against increased loads.

Isotonic Assistive Exercise and Activity

Active assistive exercise can be accomplished manually. The patient moves the part as far as he can actively, and he, or the therapist, completes the motion manually. This is the method of choice for movements not easily exercised using equipment or activity. In progressive assistive exercise (PAE), equipment is used to provide the minimal amount of weight required to complete the motion after the patient has moved as far as possible by means of muscle contraction. As strength increases, the task is made more difficult by reducing the amount of weight, i.e., the amount of assistance (DeLorme & Watkins, 1948).

The schedule for weight reduction is based on the repetition minimum, which is determined by trial and error on day 1 of treatment. The repetition minimum is the least amount of weight necessary to assist the limb to full range, 10 times. On day 2 of treatment, the program begins using this schedule:

10 repetitions with 200% of repetition minimum, rest 2–4 min;

10 repetitions with 150% of repetition minimum, rest 2–4 min;

10 repetitions with 100% of repetition minimum.

In other words, if 12 lb are required to assist the patient to flex the shoulder through full range 10 times, the program would start out using 24 lb and then go to 18 and then 12. The muscle is assisted by some apparatus, such as a counterbalanced sling or skate with weights and pulley attached. The antagonistic muscles must be strong enough to return the apparatus to the starting position, pulling against the weight that assisted the completion of motion by the weak muscles.

The therapeutic skate has free-moving ball bearings on the bottom to assist the patient to move more easily on a flat, smooth surface in a gravity-eliminated plane. The motions that can best be exercised by using this apparatus are shoulder-horizontal abduction and adduction and elbow flexion and extension. Assistance

is achieved by use of weights hanging on a rope that passes through a pulley. Location of the pulley on the board provides guidance for the correct direction of movement (Fig. 22.3). The overhead counterbalanced sling suspension (Fig. 22.4) suspends the extremity from straps or lines that extend from the elbow and wrist cuffs to the overhead bar and finally to weights at the back of the apparatus. Antigravity motions of the proximal extremity, such as shoulder abduction, flexion, and external rotation, can be assisted. Dynamic orthoses that assist motion provide active assistive exercise (see Chapter 28).

Overhead slings are quite useful in providing assistance during activity. However, few opportunities exist to provide assistive exercise within the activity itself. Although a strong extremity can assist a weak one to do the gross, repetitious motions of an activity, the resistance offered by the activity itself must be low. Rolling dough or sanding using a bilateral sander would be too resistive for muscles requiring active assistive exercise, whereas polishing a smooth surface would be possible, but limited in scope.

Isotonic Active Exercise and Activity

Active exercise requires the patient to complete the range of motion without assistance or resistance. Activities are selected that allow these criteria to be met. For example, eating finger food offers no appreciable resistance, and the active motion can be done by F elbow flexors. Contraction of the biceps in this

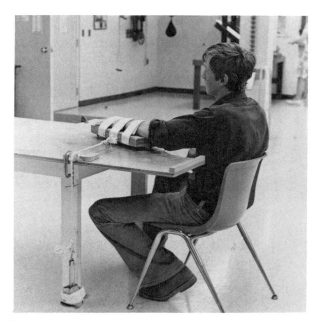

Figure 22.3. Skate with pulley and weight attached to resist horizontal adduction or assist horizontal abduction.

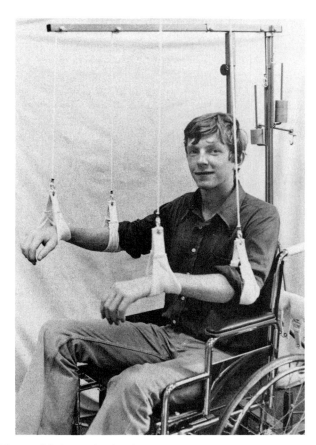

Figure 22.4. Deltoid aid counterbalanced sling.

Isotonic Active Resistive Exercise and Activity

Progressive Resistive Exercise

DeLorme (1945) organized an elaborate system of gradation of resistance to achieve maximal strength quickly. The rationale for progressive resistive exercise (PRE) was to provide a warmup exercise period so that a greater maximal strength could be achieved.

The amount of weight the patient can carry through range of motion using maximal effort for 10 repetitions is designated the 10 repetition maximum (10 RM). Determination of 10 RM is done by trial and error: A load is selected that is anticipated to be maximal, and then weight is added or subtracted until 10 RM is established (DeLateur & Lehmann, 1990). Jones (1962) found that the trial-and-error method of determining the 10 RM is extremely reliable, even if the subject must lift a load 70 times before the correct weight is discovered.

In the original technique, the resistance was increased in increments of 10% of 10 RM up to 100%, with 10 repetitions at each increment. Between each set of repetitions the patient rested 2 to 4 min. This was a time-consuming process, and two modifications have been found to be equally effective. The DeLorme and Watkins (1948) modification consists of 10 repetitions at 50% of 10 RM, 10 repetitions at 75% of 10 RM, and 10 repetitions at 100% of 10 RM. In other words, if the 10 RM is 12 lb, the patient does 10 repetitions using 6 lb. After a rest period, the patient would do 10 repetitions with 9 lb and (after a rest) then 10 repetitions with 12 lb. The McGovern and Luscombe (1953) modification requires 5 repetitions at 50% of 10 RM and 10 repetitions at 100% of 10 RM. In either modification, between each set of repetitions, the patient rests for 2 to 4 min. This sequence is repeated daily. The weight is increased as strength improves.

Regressive Resistive Exercise

McGovern and Luscombe (1953) reported a modified sequence of Zinovieff's (1951) *Oxford Technique* in which strength was as effectively increased using regressive resistive exercise (RRE) as it was using PRE. The modification sequence is

10 repetitions at 100% of 10 RM;
10 repetitions at 75% of 10 RM;
10 repetitions at 50% of 10 RM.

The 10 RM is determined as described above for PRE. These researchers based this plan on the rationale that resistance should decrease as the muscle fatigues and contracts less effectively.

case is alternately concentric and eccentric: The force against which the muscle acts in both cases is that offered by the force of gravity on the forearm and hand. An activity that demands contraction of the same muscle during both phases of a movement offers greater exercise potential than one in which return motion is accomplished by the antagonist muscles or by an outside force.

Tools or utensils of some sort are usually required to use activity in therapy. Therefore, muscles must be able to take the resistance of the tool and the material being used. An *F* graded muscle operating against gravity cannot take resistance. However, if this motion were changed to a gravity-eliminated plane, a light tool could be used (Trombly & Scott, 1989). For example, an *F* biceps on a gravity-eliminated plane could take enough resistance to function in a game of chess. In this example, when moving in a gravity-eliminated plane, the biceps contract concentrically. Grading of this type of exercise could be accomplished by changing the rate of contraction, the duration, and/or the frequency of the exercise bouts or by using game pieces that are increasingly weighted.

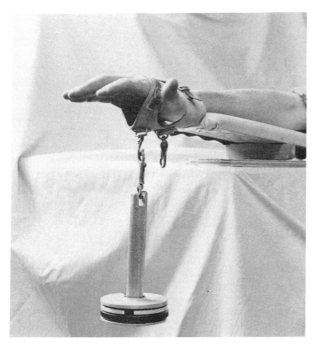

Figure 22.5. Progressive resistive exercise for wrist extension.

The overhead counterbalanced sling suspension (see Fig 22.4) is a means of providing active assistive exercise for antigravity motions of the shoulder. It can also provide active resistive exercise to motions working against the pull of the weights. The motions that can be resisted by this device are scapular depression, shoulder adduction, shoulder extension, and shoulder internal rotation. The overhead suspension can be positioned for use with patients in a semireclined position and is consequently often selected in the initial strengthening program for patients with tetraplegia and other conditions with proximal weakness for whom treatment begins before the patient has gained full sitting tolerance. The counterbalanced weights provide direct and easily gradable resistance through a large range of motion. The skate can be set up to provide resistance to horizontal abduction or adduction or elbow flexion or extension through weights on a pulley or by use of a motor that puts a preselected amount of tension on the cable attached to the skate (Roemer, Culler, & Swartt, 1978).

Exercise of the wrist extensors of a C_6 tetraplegic person who will rely on tenodesis grasp may be done by supporting the forearm on an inclined board set at the edge of the table. The hand and wrist are free. A cuff is placed on the hand around the metacarpals to hold the weights (Fig. 22.5). To exercise a weak extensor digitorum, the forearm and hand can be similarly supported on a table with the fingers hanging free. Finger loops, to which weights are attached, are placed on each finger over the proximal phalanx (Fig. 22.6)

and the patient repeatedly extends the metacarpophalangeal (MP) joints.

Isotonic activity should be characterized by repetition, movement to full range, and a means to increase resistance in small increments. One example is woodworking, in which the weight of the sanding block or other tools can be graded (Fig. 22.7). Another example is a game in which the equipment or playing pieces can be changed to increase the resistance, such as grading balls from balloons to medicine balls or grading checkers from foam rubber pieces to lead pieces.

Weakness rarely exists in only one motion. If one activity involving several motions provided the correct amount of resistance for each of the motions needing strengthening, this activity would be ideal. Usually, however, the therapist must plan different activities within a given treatment period to provide exercise to all the weak muscles of a patient. The therapist should plan several activities that provide exercise to each motion to be strengthened and then allow the patient to select the activities of interest.

Goal: To Increase Endurance

PRINCIPLE: INCREASED DURATION AT LESS THAN 50% MAXIMAL INTENSITY AND RATE

In ordinary daily activities that are lightly resistive, motor units are activated asynchronously. After a motor unit ceases activity, the muscle fibers recover to some degree while fellow units take their turn. Fatigue occurs more slowly with these movements than with maximal contraction, in which many more units

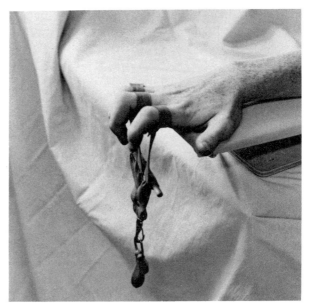

Figure 22.6. Progressive resistive exercise for extensor digitorum.

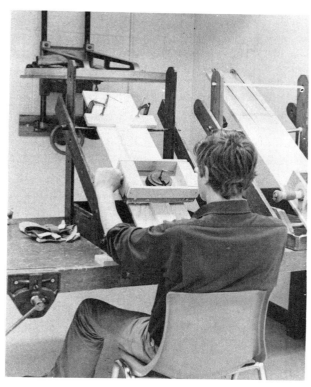

Figure 22.7. Sanding on an inclined plane, using a bilateral sander with weights for resistance.

must contract simultaneously without the opportunity to recover. Exercise to increase endurance, therefore, uses moderately fatiguing activity for progressively longer periods of time with intervals of rest to allow metabolic recovery (DeLateur & Lehman, 1990).

Doing **isotonic contractions** against less-than-maximal resistance repetitively results in increased endurance through less glycogen depletion and improved oxidative capacity of SO and FOG muscle fibers. Dickinson et al. (1983) showed that endurance-type training was more effective when done before heavy resistance exercise, perhaps because muscles, joints, and connective tissues were able to adapt before being presented with major stresses.

Activity or exercise used to build endurance is graded by increasing the exercise period, which is done by raising the number of repetitions of an **isotonic contraction** or lengthening the time an **isometric contraction** is held. An interim method of upgrading the output of the patient who is not ready to increase the duration is to increase the frequency of exercise or activity.

Occupational therapy provides the patient with interest-sustaining activities that are gradable along the dimension of time or repetition. In normal subjects, activity increases the effort and time to fatigue significantly more than do comparable exercises (Kircher, 1984; Steinbeck, 1986). As an example, a patient with

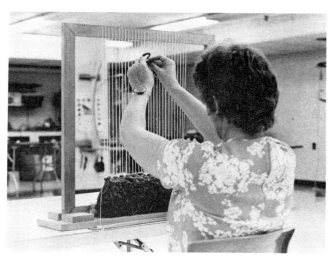

Figure 22.8. Turkish knot weaving.

severely low endurance can do light activities such as mosaic tiles or Turkish knotting (Fig. 22.8). The pieces completed each day can be counted, and progress can be easily measured by the therapist and the patient.

With the current emphasis on physical fitness in the United States, some people prefer exercise to crafts. In that case, the patient may want to continue beyond the PRE or RRE regime required to increase strength. The resistance can be reduced to less than 50% of 10 RM and the activity continued for a longer period of time. When the objective of treatment is to increase endurance, less than maximal effort is required, but strengthening will also occur if the activity is repeated to the point of fatigue (DeLateur, Lehmann, Stonebridge, et al., 1972). Programming for increasing endurance in patients with cardiopulmonary problems is discussed in Chapter 43.

STUDY QUESTIONS

1. How do the mechanical aspects of the musculoskeletal system promote stability and mobility?
2. What mechanical qualities of muscle are reflected in the standard muscle test method?
3. How are the physiology of muscle contraction, fiber type, recruitment order, and the physiology of muscle fatigue related in normal musculoskeletal function?
4. How does the physiological training effect relate to decreased muscle fatigue?
5. For whom is treatment using the biomechanical approach appropriate?
6. What treatments are appropriate to prevent development of range of motion limitations?
7. What treatments are appropriate to correct range of motion limitations?
8. How should passive stretching treatment be modi-

STUDY QUESTIONS (continued)

fied if the patient acknowledges residual pain after treatment?

9. What are the two mechanisms by which strength of contraction increases?

10. What are the five parameters that can be manipulated to alter stress on muscle to increase strength?

11. What are the characteristics that isometric activity should have to promote strengthening? Isotonic?

12. What are the necessary characteristics of exercise, or activity, used to increase endurance?

REFERENCES

Agre, J. C. (1978). Static stretching for athletes [Abstract]. *Archives of Physical Medicine & Rehabilitation, 59,* 561.

American Occupational Therapy Association. (1993). Position paper: Purposeful activity. *American Journal of Occupational Therapy, 47,* 1081–1082.

Bergstrom, D., & Coles, C. (1980). *Basic positioning procedures.* Minneapolis: Kenny Rehabilitation Institute.

Brown, D. M., DeBacher, G., & Basmajian, J. V. (1979). Feedback goniometers for hand rehabilitation. *American Journal of Occupational Therapy, 33,* 458–463.

Carlson, B. R. (1970). Relationship between isometric and isotonic strength. *Archives of Physical Medicine & Rehabilitation, 51,* 176–179.

Cordery, J. (1965). Joint protection: A responsibility of the occupational therapist. *American Journal of Occupational Therapy, 19,* 285–293.

DeLateur, B. J., & Lehmann, J. F. (1990). Therapeutic exercise to develop strength and endurance. In F. J. Kottke & J. F. Lehmann (Eds.), *Krusen's handbook of physical medicine and rehabilitation* (4th ed., pp. 480–519). Philadelphia: W. B. Saunders.

DeLateur, B., Lehmann, J., Stonebridge, J., & Warren, C. G. (1972). Isotonic versus isometric exercises: A double-shift transfer-of-training study. *Archives of Physical Medicine & Rehabilitation, 53,* 212–216.

DeLateur, B., Lehmann, J. F., Warren, C. G., Stonebridge, J., Funita, G., Cokelet, K., & Egbert, H. (1972). Comparison of effectiveness of isokinetic and isotonic exercise in quadriceps strengthening. *Archives of Physical Medicine & Rehabilitation, 53,* 60–64.

DeLorme, T. (1945). Restoration of muscle power by heavy resistance exercises. *Journal of Bone and Joint Surgery, 27,* 645–667.

DeLorme, T. L., & Watkins, A. L. (1948). Technics of progressive resistance exercise. *Archives of Physical Medicine & Rehabilitation, 29,* 263–273.

Dickinson, A. L., Jackson, C. G., Layne, D. L., & Ringel, S. P. (1983). The effect of different sequences of high and low intensity resistance exercises on muscular performance and cellular change. *Medicine and Science in Sports and Exercise, 15,* 154–155.

Dons, B., Bollerup, K., Bonde-Petersen, F., & Hancke, S. (1979). The effect of weight-lifting exercise related to muscle fiber composition and muscle cross-sectional area in humans. *European Journal of Applied Physiology, 40,* 95–106.

Downey, J., & Darling, R. (1971). *Physiological basis of rehabilitation medicine.* Philadelphia: W. B. Saunders.

Downing, A., Martin, B., & Stern, L. (1991). Methods for measuring the characteristics of movements of motor-impaired children. *Assistive Technology, 2,* 131–141.

Ellestad, M. H. (1986). *Stress testing: Principles and practice* (3rd ed.). Philadelphia: F. A. Davis.

Ellexson, M. T. (1986). The unique role of OT in industry. *Occupational Therapy in Health Care, 2*(4), 35–46.

Enos, L., Lane, R., & MacDougal, B. A. (1984). Brief or new: The use of self-adherent wrap in hand rehabilitation. *American Journal of Occupational Therapy, 38,* 265–266.

Feinberg, J., & Andree, M. (1980). Dynamic foot splint for the Hoffman apparatus. *American Journal of Occupational Therapy, 34,* 45.

Fess, E. E., & Philips, C. A. (1987). *Hand splinting: Principles and methods.* St. Louis: C. V. Mosby.

Fetters, L., & Todd, J. (1987). Quantitative assessment of infant reaching movements. *Journal of Motor Behavior, 19,* 147–166.

Fletcher, G. F., & Cantwell, J. D. (1979). *Exercise and coronary heart disease: Role in prevention, diagnosis and treatment* (2nd ed.). Springfield, IL: Charles C. Thomas.

Fuglsang-Frederiksen, A. (1981). Electrical activity and force during voluntary contraction of normal and diseased muscle. *Acta Neurologica Scandinavica, 63*(Suppl. 83), 22–23.

Gowitzke, B. A., & Milner, M. (1980). *Understanding the scientific bases of human movement* (2nd ed.). Baltimore: Williams & Wilkins.

Haggmark, T., Eriksson, E., & Jansson, E. (1986). Muscle fiber type changes in human skeletal muscle after injuries and immobilization. *Orthopedics, 9,* 181–185.

Hallum, A., & Medeiros, J. M. (1987). Effect of duration of passive stretch on hip abduction range of motion. *Journal of Orthopedic and Sports Physical Therapy, 18,* 408–415.

Harlowe, D. (1982). The ROM Dance Program. *AOTA Physical Disabilities Special Interest Newsletter, 5*(4), 1, 4.

Hellebrandt, F. A., & Waterland, J. C. (1962). Indirect learning: The influence of unimanual exercise on related muscle groups of the same and opposite side. *American Journal of Physical Medicine, 41,* 45–55.

Henneman, E. (1957). Relation between size of neurons and their susceptibility to discharge. *Science, 126,* 1345–1347.

Heurich, M., & Polansky, S. (1978). An adaptation of the glove flexion mitt. *American Journal of Occupational Therapy, 32,* 110–111.

Hinson, M., & Rosentswieg, J. (1973). Comparative electromyographic values of isometric, isotonic, and isokinetic contraction. *Research Quarterly, 44*(1), 71–78.

Hislop, H. (1963). Quantitative changes in human muscular strength during isometric exercise. *Physical Therapy, 43,* 21–38.

Hislop, H. (1964). Response of immobilized muscle to isometric exercise. *Physical Therapy, 44,* 339–347.

Hollis, L. I. (1986). Identifying occupational therapy: The use of purposeful activities. *AOTA Physical Disabilities Special Interest Newsletter, 9*(4), 2–3.

Jaffe, E. (1986). Nationally speaking: The role of occupational therapy in disease prevention and health promotion. *American Journal of Occupational Therapy, 40,* 749–752.

Jones, R. E. (1962). Reliability of the ten repetition maximum for assessing progressive resistance exercise. *Journal of the American Physical Therapy Association, 42,* 661–662.

Kircher, M. A. (1984). Motivation as a factor of perceived exertion in purposeful versus nonpurposeful activity. *American Journal of Occupational Therapy, 38,* 165–170.

Kisner, C., & Colby, L. A. (1990). *Therapeutic exercise: Foundations and techniques* (2nd ed.). Philadelphia: F.A. Davis.

Kottke, F. J. (1971). Therapeutic exercise. In F. H. Krusen, F. J. Kottke, & P. M. Ellwood (Eds.), *Handbook of physical medicine and rehabilitation* (2nd ed.). Philadelphia: W. B. Saunders.

Kottke, F. J. (1990). Therapeutic exercise to maintain mobility. In F. J. Kottke & J. F. Lehmann (Eds.), *Krusen's handbook of physical medicine and rehabilitation* (4th ed., pp. 436–451). Philadelphia: W. B. Saunders.

Lawrence, M. S. (1956). Strengthening the quadriceps: Progressively Prolonged Isometric Tension Method. *Physical Therapy Review, 36,* 658–661.

Lawrence, M. S. (1960). Strengthening the quadriceps femoris: Progressive Weighted Isometric Exercise Method. *Physical Therapy Review, 40,* 577–584.

Lindh, M. (1979). Increase of muscle strength from isometric quadriceps exercises at different knee angles. *Scandinavian Journal of Rehabilitation Medicine, 11,* 33–36.

MacDougall, J. D., Ward, G. R., Sale, D. G., & Sutton, J. R. (1977). Biochemical adaptation of human skeletal muscle to heavy resistance training and immobilization. *Journal of Applied Physiology, 43,* 700–703.

Maitland, G. D. (1977). *Peripheral manipulation* (2nd ed.). Stoneham, MA: Butterworth.

Markos, P. (1977). *Comparison of hold-relax and contract-relax and contralateral effects.* Unpublished master's thesis, Boston University.

Maughan, I. V. (1962). Graduated supination-pronation attachments for table and floor looms. *American Journal of Occupational Therapy, 16,* 285–286.

McGovern, R. E., & Luscombe, H. B. (1953). Useful modifications of progressive resistive exercise technique. *Archives of Physical Medicine & Rehabilitation, 34,* 475–477.

McPherson, J., Schild, R., Spaulding, S., Barsamian, P., Transon, C., & White, S. C. (1991). Analysis of upper extremity movement in four sitting positions: A comparison of persons with and without cerebral palsy. *American Journal of Occupational Therapy, 45,* 123–129.

Medeiros, J. M., Smidt, G. L., Burmeister, L. F., & Soderberg, G. L. (1977). The influence of isometric exercise and passive stretch on hip joint motion. *Physical Therapy, 57,* 518–523.

Moller, M., Ekstrand, J., Oberg, B., & Gillquist, J. (1985). Duration of stretching effect on range of motion in lower extremities. *Archives of Physical Medicine & Rehabilitation, 66,* 171–173.

Moritani, T., & deVries, H. A. (1979). Neural factors versus hypertrophy in the time course of muscle strength gain. *American Journal of Physical Medicine, 58,* 115–130.

Murray, J. M., & Weber, A. (1974). The cooperative action of muscle proteins. *Scientific American, 230*(2), 58–71.

Newell, K. M., & Corcos, D. M. (Eds.). (1993). *Variability and motor control.* Champaign, IL: Human Kinetics.

Pedretti, L. W., Smite R. O., Hammel, J., Rein, J., Anson, D., McGuire, M. J. (1992). Use of adjunctive modalities in occupational therapy. *American Journal of Occupational Therapy, 46,* 1075–1081.

Peter, J. B., Barnard, R. J., & Edgerton, V. R. (1972). Metabolic profiles of three fiber types of skeletal muscle in guinea pigs and rabbits. *Biochemistry, 11,* 2627–2633.

Porter, R., & Whelan, J. (Eds.). (1981). *Human muscle fatigue: Physiological mechanisms* (CIBA Foundation symposium 82). London: Pitman Medical.

Rasch, P. J. (1974). The present status of negative (eccentric) exercise: A review. *American Corrective Therapy Journal, 28*(3), 77–94.

Riendl, A. M., Gotshall, R. W., Reinke, J. A., & Smith, J. J. (1977). Cardiovascular response of human subjects to isometric contraction of large and small muscle groups. *Proceedings of the Society for Experimental Biology and Medicine, 154,* 171–174.

Roberts, S. L., & Falkenburg, S. A. (1992). *Biomechanics: Problem solving for functional activity.* St. Louis: C. V. Mosby.

Roemer, R. B., Culler, M. A., & Swartt, T. (1978). Automated upper extremity progressive resistance exercise system. *American Journal of Occupational Therapy, 32,* 105–108.

Rose, D. L., Radzyminski, S. F., & Beatty, R. R. (1957). Effects of brief maximal exercise on the strength of the quadriceps femoris. *Archives of Physical Medicine & Rehabilitation, 38,* 157–164.

Salmons, S. (1980). Functional adaptation in skeletal muscle. *Trends in Neurosciences, 6,* 134–137.

Salter, R. B. (1983). *Textbook of disorders and injuries of the musculoskeletal system* (2nd ed.). Baltimore: Williams & Wilkins.

Salter, R. B., Hamilton, H. W., Wedge, J. H., Tile, M., Torode, I. P., O'Driscoll, S. W., Murnaghan, J. J., & Saringer, J. H. (1984). Clinical application of basic research on continuous passive motion for disorders and injuries of synovial joints: A preliminary report of a feasibility study. *Journal of Orthopaedic Research, 1,* 325–342.

Segal, R. S., & Wolf, S. L. (1990). Morphological and functional considerations for therapeutic exercise. In J. V. Basmajian & S. L. Wolf (Eds.), *Therapeutic exercise* (5th ed., pp. 1–48). Baltimore: Williams & Wilkins.

Sietsema, J. M., Nelson, D. L., Mulder, R. M., Mervau-Scheidel, D., & White, B. E. (1993). The use of a game to promote arm reach in persons with traumatic brain injury. *American Journal of Occupational Therapy, 47,* 19–24.

Smith, D. A., & Lukens, S. A. (1983). Stress effects of isometric contraction in occupational therapy. *Occupational Therapy Journal of Research, 3,* 222–239.

Smith, E. R. (1989). Ergonomics and the occupational therapist. In S. Hertfelder & C. Gwin (Eds.), *Work in progress: Occupational therapy in work programs* (pp. 127–156). Rockville, MD: American Occupational Therapy Association.

Spielholz, N. I. (1990). Scientific basis of exercise programs. In J. V. Basmajian & S. L. Wolf (Eds.), *Therapeutic exercise* (5th ed., pp. 49–76). Baltimore: Williams & Wilkins.

Stanish, W. D., Rubinovic, R. M., & Curwin, S. (1986). Eccentric exercise in chronic tendinitis. *Clinical Orthopaedics and Related Research, 208,* 65–68.

Stap, L. J., & Woodfin, P. M. (1986). Continuous passive motion in the treatment of knee flexion contracture. *Physical Therapy, 66,* 1720–1722.

Steinbeck, T. M. (1986). Purposeful activity and performance. *American Journal of Occupational Therapy, 40,* 529–534.

Stromberg, B. V. (1986). Contralateral therapy in upper extremity rehabilitation. *American Journal of Physical Medicine, 65,* 135–143.

Stuart, D. G., Binder, M. D., & Enoka, R. M. (1984). Motor unit organization: Application of the quadripartite scheme to human muscles. In P. J. Dyck (Ed.), *Peripheral neuropathy* (2nd ed., pp. 1067–1090). Philadelphia: W. B. Saunders.

Sypert, G. W., & Munson, J. B. (1981). Basis of segmental motor control: Motoneuron size or motor unit type? *Neurosurgery, 8,* 608–621.

Tanigawa, M. (1972). Comparison of the hold-relax procedure and passive mobilization on increasing muscle length. *Physical Therapy, 52,* 725–735.

Thelen, E., Corbetta, D., Kamm, K., Spencer, J. P., Schneider, K., & Zernicke, R. F. (1993). The transition to reaching: Mapping intention and intrinsic dynamics. *Child Development, 64,* 1058–1098.

Thomas, C. L. (Ed.). (1973). *Taber's cyclopedic medical dictionary* (12th ed.). Philadelphia: F. A. Davis.

Tookey, P., & Larson, C. (1968). *Range of motion exercise: Key to joint mobility.* Minneapolis: American Rehabilitation Foundation.

Trombly, C. A. (1982). Include exercise in purposeful activity. *American Journal of Occupational Therapy, 36,* 467–468.

Trombly, C. (1992). Deficits of reaching in subjects with left hemiparesis: A pilot study. *American Journal of Occupational Therapy, 46*(10), 887–897.

Trombly, C. A., & Quintana, L. A. (1983). Activity analysis: Electromyographic and electrogoniometric verification. *Occupational Therapy Journal of Research, 3,* 104–120.

Trombly, C. A., & Scott, A. D., (1989). Activity adaptation. In C. A Trombly (Ed.), *Occupational therapy for physical dysfunction* (3rd ed., pp. 311–315). Baltimore: Williams & Wilkins.

Ulfhake, B., & Kellerth, J. O. (1982). Does alpha-motoneurone size correlate with motor unit type in cat triceps surea? *Brain Research, 251,* 201–209.

Van Deusen, J., & Harlowe, D. (1987). The efficacy of the ROM Dance Program for adults with rheumatoid arthritis. *American Journal of Occupational Therapy, 41,* 90–95.

Zinovieff, A. N. (1951). Heavy-resistance exercises: The "Oxford" Technique. *British Journal of Physical Medicine, 14,* 129–132.

Remediating Sensory Impairment

Karen Bentzel

A hand with severe sensory loss is guided by visual feedback. Therefore, it cannot be used successfully for activities that do not allow for visual control such as getting an object out of a pocket or closing clothing fasteners behind the back. Lack of sensation in the upper extremity can lead to neglect, or to a pattern of nonuse, because of an accumulation of failure experiences, including knocking things over, dropping objects, bumping into objects, or generally uncoordinated use (Eggers, 1984). The force with which a person grips an object varies with the weight of the object and the amount of friction of the surface material. Determination of the amount of force in the grip depends on sensory afferent signals from the skin areas in contact with the object (Johansson & Westling, 1984).

The importance of sensation in performance of daily tasks has led to the development of techniques aimed at remediating sensory impairment. One technique is called sensory reeducation and teaches the patient to attend to and interpret sensory stimuli. Sensory reeducation is provided for patients who have impaired but not absent sensation (Callahan, 1990). A second technique for sensory impairment is called desensitization and is provided for patients who demon-

strate hypersensitivity, which is a condition of extreme discomfort or irritability in response to normally nonnoxious stimuli (Barber, 1990). A third type of treatment for sensory impairment is designed to teach the patient to compensate for the absence of protective sensation and is used with patients in whom sensation of pinprick, touch/pressure, and temperature are absent or severely decreased (Callahan, 1990).

SENSORY REEDUCATION

Sensory reeducation is defined as "a method or combination of techniques that help the patient with a sensory impairment learn to re-interpret the altered profile of neural impulses reaching his conscious level" (Dellon, 1988, p. 210). Dellon (1988) related his experience with patients following nerve injury who would respond to fingertip stroking, pinprick, and pressure but were unable to identify correctly a nickel and a quarter using only touch sensation. These patients stated that they could feel a difference between the coins, but that they could not identify them and that the coins did not feel the same as a nickel and quarter used to feel before the injury. Dellon concluded that the sensibility was recovered but that there was a mismatch of the new sensory profile with past profiles in the association cortex. Within a few minutes, he could train patients to tell the difference between the two coins. He gave the patient a nickel, told him what it was, and explained that it did not feel the way a nickel used to feel but that what the patient was currently feeling should thereafter be called a nickel. After repeating the process with a quarter, the patient could correctly identify them. The sensation had been reeducated.

Sensory reeducation is appropriate for patients following nerve injuries, replantations, toe-to-thumb transfers, skin grafts, and cerebral vascular accidents (CVA) (Dellon, 1988). Cutaneous information from the fingers, palm, and toes are most important in rehabilita-

GLOSSARY

Autolysis—Disintegration of cells by self-digestion (*Dorland's*, 1988).

Friction massage—Massage applied with pressure, usually in a circular motion.

Kinesthesia—The perception of the direction and excursion of joint movement (American Occupational Therapy Association [AOTA], 1989).

Proprioception—The perception of the position of a body part in space or in relationship to another body part (AOTA, 1989).

Semmes-Weinstein monofilaments—Set of nylon filaments of various diameters but constant length set at a right angle in acrylic handles and used for testing of the threshold of touch sensation.

Somatotropic boundaries—Areas or regions within the brain that are related to certain areas of the body (*Dorland's*, 1988)

Tactile gnosis—Ability to perceive and interpret tactile stimuli in a meaningful way (Dellon, 1990), often tested by asking a patient to identify an object by touching it (with vision occluded).

Two-point discrimination—The ability to identify whether a tactile stimulus consists of a single application point or two separate points of application.

Vibrometer—Device designed to test the threshold of vibration sensation, consisting of a vibrating head that is applied to the patient's skin and a control unit that allows for gradual changes in the amplitude of vibration.

tion, because it is generally these skin surfaces that interact with the external environment (Dannenbaum & Dykes, 1988).

Rationale

Cortical maps have been found to respond to peripheral nerve injuries (Dykes, 1984). Loss of sensory input causes cortical areas to begin to serve sensory inputs from adjacent areas. These changes are restricted to similar modalities (i.e., cutaneous versus muscular) and cannot cross certain **somatotropic boundaries** within the brain. Dykes believed that if a lesion in the central nervous system causes the loss of a portion of the cortex serving a certain class and area of receptors, then the remaining intact portion of the brain will reorganize. If, for instance, half of the area of representation of touch sensation of the hand is lost as a result of a CVA, the cortical map of the hand will reorganize so that the entire hand is represented, but by a smaller volume of cortical tissue. Therefore, there will be decreased acuity of tactile sensation.

The rationale for sensory reeducation following CVA is based on the belief that functional use of a body part is possible with reduced sensation but that, without training, a learned disuse phenomenon occurs that leads to loss of motor abilities. Often, the patient will be able to perceive at least a portion of the information from the cutaneous receptors. Therapists may alter the cortical map by directing the sensory experiences of the patient. Therefore, the goal of sensory reeducation following CVA is to gain a larger cortical representation for those areas of skin from which sensory feedback is crucial to performance of daily tasks. Treatment includes repeated sensory stimuli to those skin areas of sufficient intensity so that the patient can feel the stimulus. Appreciation of the stimulus is thought to be necessary for potential improvement in sensation (Dannenbaum & Dykes, 1988).

The return of sensation and hand function following hand injury are extremely complex events. Recovery is not just a process of reinnervation but also involves cortical reeducation of the interpretation of altered afferent signals from the periphery (Nishikawa & Smith, 1992). Following nerve repair, there is an inevitable distortion of the profile of neural impulses reaching the sensory cortex because of the misdirection of regrowth of axons. The effect of this misdirection is that a previously well-known stimulus will initiate a different set of neural impulses from that elicited by the same stimulus before the injury. When this altered profile reaches the sensory cortex, the patient may be unable to match it with patterns previously encountered and remembered in the association cortex. The patient is then unable to identify or recognize the stimulus (Fig. 23.1). The purpose of sensory reeducation in these patients is to retrain them to recognize the distorted cortical impression (Dellon & Jabaley, 1982). The goal of sensory reeducation following nerve repair is to help the patient achieve the potential for functional sensory recovery given to him by his surgeon at the time of the nerve repair (Dellon, 1988). Wynn Parry and Salter (1976) believed that "sensory retraining should be a routine part of rehabilitation after suture of the median nerve" (p. 255). They felt that sensory reeducation is not worthwhile following ulnar nerve repair, because patients readily use normal median nerve sensation to compensate for the loss of ulnar sensation.

Techniques

Careful observation of the patient's performance during testing will assist in planning treatment. For instance, the fact that a patient is able to identify that an object is cold and hard even though he cannot identify it, is a significant observation. His sensory retraining might, therefore, begin with differentiation

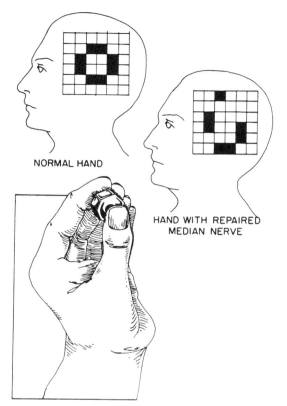

NORMAL HAND

HAND WITH REPAIRED
MEDIAN NERVE

Figure 23.1. "In the normal hand, a stimulus, such as this gripped bolt, elicits a profile of neural impulses which reaches the sensory cortex, and ultimately is perceived, as represented by the checkerboard pattern. After a nerve repair, the same stimulus elicits an altered profile of impulses, which reaches the sensory cortex. The new perception, the altered checkerboard pattern, may be so different from the previous one, that object recognition is at first impossible" (Dellon, 1988, p. 210).

of metal and wood objects (Eggers, 1984). Dellon (1988) emphasized the importance of proper sequencing of the sensory reeducation tasks and instituting them at an appropriate time in recovery. Initiating an exercise before the fiber/receptor system has reunited following nerve repair will cause failure and frustration. Sensory reeducation is provided for the patient who can perceive pinprick, temperature, and touch but who has impaired tactile localization, **two-point discrimination,** and **tactile gnosis** (Callahan, 1990).

Gradation of sensory retraining activities is necessary for the patient to be sufficiently challenged but not frustrated. Gradations can occur along several dimensions. At first, the activity might allow compensation with other senses but will progress to total reliance on tactile sensation. Require a progression of gross to fine discrimination by asking for greater detail as the patient shows progress (Eggers, 1984). Initially, the patient may be asked to tell whether two objects are the same or different. Later, he can identify the object or texture (Callahan, 1990). Progress from objects with

greater differences in size, shape, and texture to those with more subtle differences (Anthony, 1993a; Callahan, 1990; Eggers, 1984). Initially, place the object in the patient's hand. Later, he can search for the named object among others (Eggers, 1984). Increase the number of objects to choose from in a selection or matching task (Callahan, 1990). Progress from three-dimensional objects to two-dimensional objects (Eggers, 1984).

Several general principles apply to sensory reeducation. Each task is done with and without the use of visual feedback for maximal integration of learning. As in sensory testing, the environment needs to be free from distractions to allow optimal patient concentration (Dellon, 1988). Sessions should be brief (10 to 15 min) because of the intense concentration needed for maximal learning (Callahan, 1990). Two to four sessions per day are recommended (Anthony, 1993a; Callahan, 1990; Dellon, 1988; Omer, 1974; Wynn Parry & Salter, 1976); therefore, it is important that the patient be motivated, able to learn the techniques, and able to devote time daily to sensory reeducation (Callahan, 1990). Sensory reeducation needs to be continued for a long time—either until the patient returns to using the hand in work or household tasks or until recovery has reached a plateau (Dellon, 1988). Patients maintain and increase the gains made in sensory reeducation if they continue to use the hand actively for fine activities after discharge from therapy (Callahan, 1990).

Following CVA, there are several detailed programs for motor reeducation. Little information exists about rehabilitation of sensation (Dannenbaum & Dykes, 1988). In the adult hemiplegic, sensory training and motor training are combined in many treatment activities. Eggers (1984) recommended normalization of muscle tone and eliminating abnormal movement patterns first, because abnormal muscle tone interferes with sensory perception. Sensory retraining for the hemiplegic patient requires hundreds of repetitions, and retraining needs to be included in each treatment session for as long as necessary (Eggers, 1984). In the adult hemiplegic patient with severe motor disability, the first stage is incorporating tactile stimuli into activities to enhance motor function. For example, using different textured surfaces during activities requiring weight bearing through the hemiparetic arm can facilitate both motor and sensory function. If deficits in touch sensation exist, apply strong touch stimuli (tapping, rubbing, and brushing) at the beginning of each treatment session; be careful not to increase spasticity (Eggers, 1984).

Activities to increase the amount of tactile input may include (Dannenbaum & Dykes, 1988; Eggers, 1984) the following:

- Applying lotion;
- Rubbing with a terry cloth towel;
- "Drawing" shapes on a piece of pile carpeting;
- Picking up objects that have varied textures between both hands, with fingers interlaced, if necessary, or with hemiparetic hand;
- Making a pattern with sand on the tabletop;
- Kneading dough;
- Washing small garments by hand;
- Making objects from clay;
- Weaving or macramé with sisal twine;
- Stroking of textures across key sensory surfaces;
- Adapting surfaces of utensils held in daily activities to provide greater tactile input;
- Applying electric stimulation.

As motor and sensory function improve, patients may progress to touch localization and sensory discrimination activities, described below for the patient with peripheral nerve involvement.

Dellon (1988) described two phases of sensory reeducation for the patient with injury or insult to the peripheral nerve. The early phase of sensory reeducation is begun when the perception of 30 cycles per second (cps) vibration and moving touch have returned to the area. The goals of this phase are to reeducate in differentiation of moving versus constant touch and to reeducate incorrect localization.

In the early phase, the patient or the therapist uses the eraser end of a pencil to stroke up and down the area being reeducated, while the patient observes what is happening. This is then repeated with his eyes closed while he concentrates on what is happening, stating to himself what he is feeling. He again opens his eyes for reinforcement. When the patient can perceive moving touch, he does a similar reeducation for localization of constant touch by pressing the eraser on one spot, with his eyes open, then closed, and with concentration and verbalization of what he is feeling, followed by visual reinforcement. Callahan (1990) described a similar protocol but recommended that stimuli be applied to one small area of the skin at a time. Callahan recommended this sequence: Start with a purely tactile stimulus, then combine it with visual input, then repeat the tactile stimulus without vision; she believed that this sequence promoted maximal integration of learning. She further suggested that, after the patient can appreciate and localize the eraser stimulus, he progress to smaller and lighter stimuli until he can localize a stimulus that is close to the level of his touch threshold (**Semmes-Weinstein monofilament**).

Late-phase sensory reeducation, as described by Dellon (1988), begins after moving and constant touch can be perceived and localized at the fingertip. The goal is to guide the patient to recovery of **tactile gnosis.** Exercises consist of object identification tasks and are graded by beginning with large objects with greater differences in size, shape, or texture and progressing to smaller objects with more subtle differences. The patient grasps an item, keeping his eyes open, then closes his eyes and concentrates on the perception, then opens his eyes. The patient can be tested periodically to determine the time required to identify correctly each object in his practice set (Fig. 23.2). The patient progresses to objects of similar shape but different texture (pieces of leather, felt, sandpaper, and plastic) and then to small objects differing in size and shape but not in texture (safety pin and paper clip).

Additional sensory discrimination activities have been recommended (Callahan, 1990; Dannenbaum & Dykes, 1988; Eggers, 1984; Vinograd, Taylor, & Grossman, 1962; Wynn Parry & Salter, 1976) and include the following:

- Identify geometric shapes made from Velcro strips on a piece of cardboard;
- Recognize shapes and sizes of different wood blocks;
- Recognize weight using sandbags and cotton bags;
- Sort a group of textures into rough and smooth or sort a group of objects into round versus square;
- Count the number of marbles in a box (place other objects in the box with the marbles to increase difficulty);
- Identify shapes cut out of cardboard;
- Select named object from a group of objects;
- Determine which of two objects is heavier;
- Locate objects hidden in a bowl of sand, unpopped popcorn, rice, Styrofoam, etc.;

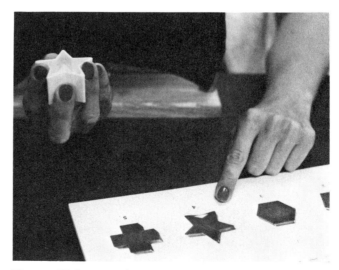

Figure 23.2. Late-phase sensory reeducation following peripheral nerve injury includes identification of various objects by touch.

- Fit wood shapes into a puzzle;
- Assemble wood letters into words or a message;
- Identify whether two pieces of sandpaper or fabric are the same or different (attach sandpaper to both ends of a wood dowel so that the patient can independently work on this task);
- Identify number or geometric shape traced by the therapist on the patient's skin;
- Trace the path of a raised design maze formed by colored epoxy on cardboard;
- Complete self-care and work tasks that require manipulation of objects without vision.

These activities should be attempted without vision, then visual feedback should be provided.

Rehabilitation techniques for impaired **proprioception** and **kinesthesia** are not common and written information about treatment techniques is scarce. Smith and Brunolli (1989) described a program to improve shoulder **kinesthesia** following glenohumeral joint dislocation that included matching various joint positions while using a shoulder wheel apparatus as well as exercises of balancing in a quadruped position with the affected limb on a freely moving platform to facilitate reflexive motor coordination.

Callahan (1990) recommended several methods of documentation of progress in sensory reeducation. Map the improvements in touch localization using the recording chart in Figure 8.6. Use a single dot to indicate a correctly perceived stimulus. For an incorrectly perceived stimulus, draw an arrow from the point of stimulus application to the point at which it was perceived. Record the number of correct responses and the time to complete sensory tasks. Reassess sensation periodically using evaluation methods that are sensitive enough to show change. Record the patient's improvement in functioning in activities of daily living.

Effectiveness of Sensory Reeducation

Table 23.1 shows a classification of the levels of sensory recovery. These levels are frequently used to report research results of the effectiveness of sensory reeducation. Although the number of studies and the number of cases in each study are limited, success has been documented following sensory reeducation (Dannenbaum & Dykes, 1988; Dellon & Jabaley, 1982; Omer, 1974; Szeles, 1992; Vinograd et al., 1962). Dellon and Jabaley (1982) reviewed two other studies as well as their own results following sensory reeducation and recorded achievement of S4 sensation in 50 to 54% of median nerve injuries, 25 to 80% of ulnar nerve injuries, and 64 to 82% of digital nerve injuries. These results are substantial improvements over accepted values for nerve repairs in patients who did not receive sensory reeducation. Dellon (1988) reported

Table 23.1. Classification of Sensory Recovery

Sensory Grade	Recovery of Sensibility
S0	Absent sensation
S1	Recovery of deep pain sensibility
S1+	Recovery of superficial pain sensibility
S2	Recovery of pain and some touch sensibility
S2+	Recovery of pain and some touch sensibility but with overresponse
S3	Recovery of pain and touch sensibility with disappearance of overresponse; static two-point discrimination greater than 15 mm
S3+	Recovery of touch localization; static two-point discrimination 7–15 mm
S4	Complete recovery; static two-point discrimination 2–6 mm

that his program of early-phase reeducation results in virtually 100% correction of false localization. Furthermore, he is almost always successful in achieving moving and constant touch perception in the fingertips of those patients who can perceive vibration (256 cps, tuning fork) at the fingertip. Good improvements in the time and accuracy of recognition of textures and objects as well as improved tactile localization were shown by 23 patients with median nerve lesions following 3 months of retraining (Wynn Parry & Salter, 1976). Omer (1974) found that patients could learn to recognize objects over a period of several months of retraining with the objects but could not generalize this learning to recognize new objects.

The success of sensory reeducation following CVA is less clear. Yekutiel and Guttman (1993) did a study of sensory retraining in stroke patients after the period of spontaneous recovery. Following 18 sessions of retraining activities, the 20 subjects demonstrated significant improvement in touch localization, **two-point discrimination,** stereognosis, and elbow **proprioception** compared with a control group. In studies attempting to link improvements in sensory discrimination with function, one found increased hand usage for functional activities (Dannenbaum & Dykes, 1988), while another found no improvement in spontaneous hand usage (Vinograd et al., 1962). Jongbloed, Stacey, and Brighton (1989) found no significant differences in self-care, mobility, or specific sensory integration test scores among two groups of patients, one of which received functional therapy, including compensation and adaptation, and the other of which received sensorimotor integrative approach, including specific sensory stimulation techniques. Limitations to sensory relearning following CVA seem to be related to the extent and specific region involved. For instance, loss of the function of the entire somatosensory cortex will prevent relearning of tactile discrimination. Some neurons must remain intact within an area for relearning to occur (Dannenbaum & Dykes, 1988).

DESENSITIZATION

Hypersensitivity is a state in which stimuli that do not cause pain in normal tissues do cause pain in the affected region. Hypersensitivity is a poorly studied problem, even though it is fairly common following a number of injuries, including frostbite, burns, nerve trauma, and traumatic crushing forces. Patients with hypersensitivity will typically hold the affected part in a protective manner (Hardy, Moran, & Merritt, 1982). Hypersensitivity can lead to disability through nonuse of the involved body part (Robinson & McPhee, 1986).

Desensitization is based on the belief that progressive stimulation will allow progressive tolerance. The concept of desensitization is of unknown origin. Civil War sailors were known to tap on amputation stumps with silver spoons to improve tolerance of artificial limbs made of wood (Hardy et al., 1982). Through desensitization, the patient learns to filter out unpleasant sensations to permit accurate perception of sensory input (Anthony, 1993b).

Treatment Techniques

Initially, a patient may need to compensate for hypersensitivity by wearing a light splint, lambs wool cuff, or elastomer pad over the sensitive area (Anthony, 1993b). The patient will need to be weaned gradually from the protective device as improvement occurs.

Several hierarchies of progressively irritating sensory stimuli have been published (Anthony, 1993b; Barber, 1990; Hardy et al., 1982; Robinson & McPhee, 1986). One typical program (Hardy et al., 1982) includes five levels. Patients advance to the next level once they demonstrate tolerance of a given level without signs of irritation. Level 1 includes vibration administered via a tuning fork, paraffin, and massage. Level 2 includes vibration administered via a battery-operated massager (Fig. 23.3), **friction massage,** and constant touch pressure administered with a pencil eraser. Level 3 includes the use of an electric vibrator and identification of textures. In level 4, the use of the electric vibrator continues and the patient also works on object identification. Level 5 consists of work and daily activities. Work simulation is believed to be extremely important to ensure that the patient is using the painful site. Activities must be tailored to the patient's interest and occupation.

Table 23.2 shows the hierarchy of textures and vibration used at the Downey Hand Center. Each patient arranges the dowel textures and immersion textures (Fig. 23.4) in the order that he perceives as least to most irritating. He then selects the dowel texture,

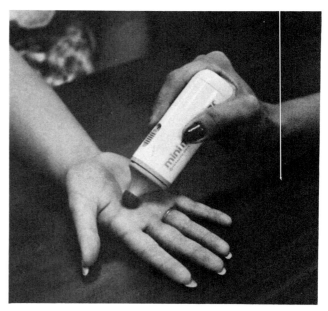

Figure 23.3. The small head on this battery-powered vibrator is useful for desensitization of specific areas of the hand.

Table 23.2. Hierarchy of Texture and Vibration Used in Desensitization

Level	Dowel textures	Immersion textures	Vibration
1	Moleskin	Cotton	83 cps near area
2	Felt	Terry cloth pieces	83 cps near area, 23 cps near area
3	Quickstick[a]	Dry rice	83 cps near area, 23 cps intermittent contact
4	Velvet	Popcorn	83 cps intermittent contact, 23 cps intermittent contact
5	Semirough cloth	Pinto beans	83 cps intermittent contact, 23 cps continuous contact
6	Velcro loop	Macaroni	83 cps continuous contact, 53 cps intermittent contact
7	Hard T-foam	Plastic wire insulation pieces	100 cps intermittent contact, 53 cps intermittent contact
8	Burlap	Small BB's or buckshot	100 cps intermittent contact, 53 cps continuous contact
9	Rug back	Large BB's or buckshot	100 cps continuous contact, 53 cps continuous contact
10	Velcro hook	Plastic squares	No problem with vibration

[a]A closed cell, firm splint padding material.

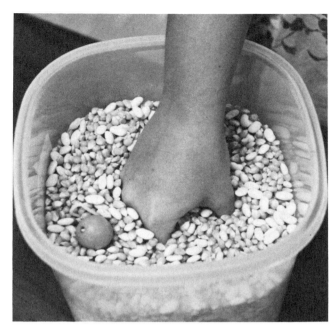

Figure 23.4. Immersion of the hand into a container filled with popcorn kernels and pinto beans for desensitization. Patients can use tactile sensation to locate other objects hidden in the immersion particles.

immersion texture, and vibration level that can be tolerated for 10 min, three to four times daily (Barber, 1990). The patient's initial hierarchy and progress are recorded on the *Downey Hand Center Hand Sensitivity Test* form (Yerxa et al., 1983).

Other activities thought to decrease hypersensitivity include continuous pressure via an Isotoner glove or weight-bearing pressure, massage, transcutaneous electrical stimulation, fluidotherapy, typing, washing hair, macramé, leather link belts, or other activities that encourage use of the hypersensitive part (Anthony, 1993b; Barber, 1990; Waylett-Rendall, 1988). Kenshalo (1986) advocated the use of a **vibrometer** for desensitization, because the amplitude can be increased more gradually than commercially available vibrators.

The success of desensitization has been documented in a case study (Robinson & McPhee, 1986) in which the patient showed marked improvement following 8 weeks of treatment. The patient was seen in the clinic for a total of five sessions, which consisted primarily of reevaluation and revision of the program that the patient completed independently at home. Good success was achieved as measured by the static **two-point discrimination** testing and the use of the involved finger in home, work, and leisure activities. Hardy et al. (1982) reported on the effect of desensitization in 16 patients following nerve and crush injuries. **Two-point discrimination** improved an average of 19.3 mm for 9 of the patients; 13 of the patients were

discharged to their previous occupations. Barber (1990) reported that almost all patients advance at least one level in the hierarchy of the *Downey Hand Center Hand Sensitivity Test* on at least one modality after 2 to 3 weeks of desensitization. A total of 60% to 75% of the patients were able to tolerate all 10 dowel textures within an average of 7 weeks of treatment. Motivation and psychological status do seem to affect the success of desensitization (Barber, 1990).

Compensation for Loss of Sensation

Wood (1969) stated that when hands are used in activities without protective sensory feedback, there is a high frequency of burns, cuts, lacerations, and bruises. Damage or injury to an insensitive limb is the result not of weakness in denervated tissue but instead of external forces that are normally avoided by people who are able to feel the warning pain. Pain is, therefore, considered the most valuable sensation that humans have (Brand, 1979). The goal of treatment for the patient with total sensory loss is to avoid injury. Treatment consists of education for the patient and/or the caregiver in precautions necessary to prevent injury.

Brand (1979) described five mechanisms of damage to insensitive limbs. The first is continuous, low pressure, which causes necrosis from a lack of blood supply. The severity of damage depends on the relationship between the amount of pressure and the time over which it is applied: 1 pound of pressure per square inch will block capillary blood flow and could cause a pressure sore (decubitus ulcer) in 10 hr and 3 pounds of pressure per square inch will cause a pressure ulcer after several hours. Skin areas over bony prominences are particularly prone to pressure ulcers because the cutaneous tissue is trapped between the unyielding bone and the external pressure. This means that frequent position changes are necessary for patients with absent sensation, such as those with spinal cord injuries.

The second mechanism of damage is concentrated high pressure, causing cutting or crushing by mechanical violence. More than 600 pounds per square inch of pressure and shear stress are needed to tear human skin. Pressure equal to 200 pounds per square inch is painful for people with normal sensation. Damage due to concentrated high force occurs from sudden, unexpected accidents and when a force is applied over an area that is too small for the force to be adequately distributed. Compensatory techniques include larger handles on suitcases, drawers and cupboards and large key holders. High pressure can result from splint straps that are too narrow and splints that are too tight; therefore, careful splint construction is needed to prevent injury.

The third mechanism of skin damage is excessive heat or cold, leading to burning or frostbite. The patient's awareness of potential heat or cold sources and how to protect himself from contact with them is important. Oven mitts or quality pot holders are necessary when cooking. Use utensils with wood or plastic handles rather than metal ones. In cold weather, gloves or mittens are necessary protection for insensitive hands.

The fourth mechanism of injury is repetitive mechanical stress of a moderate degree, causing inflammation and **autolysis.** This is the mechanism that can cause cumulative trauma disorders such as tendinitis and tenosynovitis, if the tendons and tendon sheaths are subject to mechanical stress and thus traumatized. Skin trauma can also result from repetitious mechanical force. The amount of damage depends on the relationship between the amount of pressure and the number of repetitions that the pressure is applied. These pressures are so moderate that they are not even uncomfortable for people with normal sensation. For example, the pressure on the foot at the beginning of a hike does not cause any notice. After a few miles, a person may begin to notice soreness in the feet and will rest, change the stride, or limp a little. This changes the distribution of forces. A person without normal sensation who does not become alerted to repeated stress on a given area will not alter his movement pattern, and forces will continue to be applied to the same areas. With numerous repetitions of pressure, the skin will become inflamed and, if repetitive pressure is unrelieved, necrotic. To prevent damage, lower the pressure or the number of repetitions. Inspect the skin for signs of inflammation and give reddened skin areas total relief from pressure. Methods to lower the pressure include using soft shoe insoles, losing weight, wearing gloves, and using enlarged or padded handles on tools. Decrease repetitions by walking shorter distances, resting, using a variety of tools, or alternating hands.

The final mechanism of damage is pressure on infected tissue that results in the spread of infection. Patients with absent sensation often do not give infected tissue a chance to rest, hindering the healing process. Continued use of an infected, insensitive limb will interrupt the body's self-healing mechanisms. Patients without sensation must be instructed to rest completely the infected body part, because pain perception is not present to prevent overuse. Splinting, bedrest, or other means of total immobilization may be necessary.

Other techniques of compensating for absent sensation include reliance on other senses, e.g., vision may be used to prevent contact with sharp objects. Using a body part with intact sensation to test water temperature before immersion of any body part without

sensation is recommended. Auditory cues may also be helpful in preventing injury (Eggers, 1984).

Specific recommendations also include the following:

- Using an insulated coffee cup and using extreme care when smoking (Wood, 1969);
- Avoiding exposure to extreme temperature;
- Becoming aware of using only as much force as necessary in grasping objects and avoiding small handles that concentrate forces on a small area of skin;
- Applying lotion or oil daily for good skin hydration (Callahan, 1990);
- Applying a splint to active but insensate injured areas (because these areas lack the "natural" splint of pain) (Wood, 1969) or splinting to prevent injury in patients who cannot recognize dangerous situations or cannot remember to avoid them.

For the patient with spinal cord injury or for other patients in whom there may be large areas of the body without sensation, special care and instruction are needed to prevent skin breakdown. A variety of wheelchair cushions are available to assist in distributing pressure during sitting. These include cushions filled with air, water, gel, and foam or combinations of these materials. No single cushion is effective for all patients; therefore, careful evaluation is needed. Electronic systems to evaluate pressure have made this evaluation more objective (Garber, 1985).

Garber (1985) used a Texas Interface Pressure Evaluator (TK Applied Technology, Stafford, TX) to compare seven different types of wheelchair cushions. She found that the Roho (air-filled) cushion produced the greatest pressure reduction in the majority of patients; however, each of the other six cushions evaluated was optimal in at least a few of the patients who were referred for a wheelchair cushion evaluation following pressure sores.

Sprigle, Faisant, and Chung (1990) conducted a study comparing custom-contoured cushions with the patient's usual wheelchair cushion. Computer technology allows for individual cutting of a foam cushion to match the patient's contours and pressure patterns. The study results suggested that a custom-contoured cushion distributed pressures more evenly than the cushions regularly used by the subjects. Patients tended to display a positive reaction to the custom-contoured cushions and, in general, displayed improved posture and balance. Precautions include the need to monitor closely skin areas during initial use. Occasionally, modifications are required to correct posture or to improve the pressure profile. Patients are required always to sit in the same location on this cushion for optimal pressure distribution.

While prescription of a wheelchair cushion is important, it needs to be accompanied by proper skin care and position changes to prevent problems (Peterson & Adkins, 1982). The patient should change his body position frequently throughout the day. His skin needs to be visually inspected daily. A reddened area indicates a site of potential breakdown, and extreme care needs to be taken to relieve pressure totally from this area until the color returns to normal. If the time for the skin to recover its normal color exceeds 20 min, it is absolutely essential to discover the cause of the skin irritation and correct it. Modification of orthotics, equipment, schedule, position, and/or procedure is necessary.

SUMMARY

Callahan (1990) stated that "it appears that the motivated client can learn to compensate for sensory deficits and, in a structured program that makes use of learning principles, can improve specific sensory skills that contribute to function" (p. 613).

STUDY QUESTIONS

1. What is the rationale for sensory reeducation following peripheral nerve injury and cerebral vascular accident?
2. Give several examples of gradations in sensory reeducation activities.
3. Describe the goals of early- and late-phase sensory reeducation following peripheral nerve injury.
4. Describe the rationale for using desensitization techniques.
5. List the five mechanisms of injury to insensate skin.
6. What strategies to prevent injury can be taught to a patient with absent sensation?
7. Explain what should be done if a patient develops an area of skin redness.

REFERENCES

American Occupational Therapy Association. (1989). Uniform terminology for occupational therapy—Second edition. *American Journal of Occupational Therapy, 43,* 808–815.

Anthony, M. (1993a). Sensory reeducation. In G. Clark, E. Shaw Wilgis, B. Aiello, D. Eckhaus, & L. Eddington (Eds.), *Hand rehabilitation* (pp. 81–87). New York: Churchill Livingstone.

Anthony, M. (1993b). Desensitization. In G. Clark, E. Shaw Wilgis, B. Aiello, D. Eckhaus, & L. Eddington (Eds.), *Hand rehabilitation* (pp. 73–79). New York: Churchill Livingstone.

Barber, L. (1990). Desensitization of the traumatized hand. In J. Hunter, L. Schneider, E. Mackin, & A. Callahan (Eds.), *Rehabilitation of the hand* (3rd ed., pp. 721–730). St. Louis: C. V. Mosby.

Brand, P. (1979). Management of the insensitive limb. *Physical Therapy, 59,* 8–12.

Callahan, A. (1990). Methods of compensation and reeducation for sensory dysfunction. In J. Hunter, L. Schneider, E. Mackin, &

A. Callahan (Eds.), *Rehabilitation of the hand* (3rd ed., pp. 611–621). St. Louis: C. V. Mosby.

Dannenbaum, R., & Dykes, R. (1988). Sensory loss in the hand after sensory stroke: Therapeutic rationale. *Archives of Physical Medicine and Rehabilitation, 69,* 833–839.

Dellon, A. (1988). *Evaluation of sensibility and re-education of sensation in the hand.* Baltimore: John D. Lucas.

Dellon, A. (1990). The sensational contributions of Erik Moberg. *Journal of Hand Surgery (Edinburgh), 15B,* 14–23.

Dellon, A., & Jabaley, M. (1982). Reeducation of sensation in the hand following nerve suture. *Clinical Orthopedics, 163,* 75–79.

Dorland's illustrated medical dictionary. (1988). (26th ed.). Philadelphia: W. B. Saunders.

Dykes, R. (1984). Central consequences of peripheral nerve injuries. *Annals of Plastic Surgery, 13,* 412–422.

Eggers, O. (1984). *Occupational therapy in the treatment of adult hemiplegia.* Rockville, MD: Aspen Systems.

Garber, S. (1985). Wheelchair cushions for spinal cord injured individuals. *American Journal of Occupational Therapy, 39,* 722–725.

Hardy, M., Moran, C., & Merritt, W. (1982). Desensitization of the traumatized hand. *Virginia Medical Journal, 109,* 134–137.

Johansson, R., & Westling, G. (1984). Role of glabrous skin receptors and sensorimotor memory in automatic control of precision grip when lifting rougher or more slippery objects. *Experimental Brain Research, 56,* 550–564.

Jongbloed, L., Stacey, S., & Brighton, C. (1989). Stroke rehabilitation: Sensorimotor integrative treatment versus functional treatment. *American Journal of Occupational Therapy, 43,* 391–397.

Kenshalo, D. (1986). Somesthetic sensitivity in young and elderly humans. *Journal of Gerontology, 41,* 732–742.

Nishikawa, H., & Smith, P. (1992). The recovery of function after cross-finger flaps for fingertip injury. *Journal of Hand Surgery (Edinburgh), 17B,* 102–107.

Omer, G. (1974). Sensation and sensibility in the upper extremity. *Clinical Orthopedics and Related Research, 104,* 30–36.

Peterson, M., & Adkins, H. (1982). Measurement and redistribution of excessive pressures during wheelchair sitting. *Physical Therapy, 62,* 990–994.

Robinson, S., & McPhee, S. (1986). Case report: Treating the patient with digital hypersensitivity. *American Journal of Occupational Therapy, 40,* 285–287.

Smith, R., & Brunolli, J. (1989). Shoulder kinesthesia after anterior glenohumeral joint dislocation. *Physical Therapy, 69,* 106–112.

Sprigle, S., Faisant, R., & Chung, K. (1990). Clinical evaluation of custom-contoured cushions for the spinal cord injured. *Archives of Physical Medicine and Rehabilitation, 71,* 655–658.

Szeles, D. (1992). Sensory rehabilitation after peripheral nerve injury. *Journal of Hand Therapy, 5,* 237–238.

Vinograd, A., Taylor, E., & Grossman, S. (1962). Sensory retraining of the hemiplegic hand. *American Journal of Occupational Therapy, 16,* 246–250.

Waylett-Rendall, J. (1988). Sensibility evaluation and rehabilitation. *Orthopedic Clinics of North America, 19,* 43–56.

Wood, H. (1969). Prevention of deformity in the insensitive hand: The role of the therapist. *American Journal of Occupational Therapy, 23,* 488–489.

Wynn Parry, C., & Salter, M. (1976). Sensory reeducation after median nerve lesions. *The Hand, 8,* 250–257.

Yekutiel, M., & Guttman, E. (1993). A controlled trial of the retraining of the sensory function of the hand in stroke patients. *Journal of Neurology, Neurosurgery, and Psychiatry, 56,* 241–244.

Yerxa, E., Barber, L., Diaz, O., Black, W., & Azen, S. (1983). Development of a hand sensitivity test for the hypersensitive hand. *American Journal of Occupational Therapy, 37,* 176–181.

Remediating Motor Control and Performance Through Traditional Therapeutic Approaches

Four programs of treatment for patients with motor control problems caused by brain damage were developed in the mid-1950s and early 1960s based on neurophysiological and developmental research of the time as well as careful observation of the responses made by patients when being handled, positioned, touched, or moved in various ways. These traditional therapeutic approaches are

1. Rood Approach
2. Neurodevelopmental (Bobath) Treatment
3. Movement Therapy of Brunnstrom
4. Proprioceptive Neuromuscular Facilitation (PNF) Approach of Kabat and Voss

This chapter consists of an introduction and four subchapters, one for each of the four approaches. Each approach is described as it is presented in the literature. Primary sources of information have been supplemented by the writings of others when necessary.

INTRODUCTION

The approaches discussed in this chapter share the idea of the importance of sensation to the control of movement and the need for repetition for learning, but they differ on other points. The differences have to do with whether conscious attention should be directed toward the movement itself (Brunnstrom and PNF) or only toward the goal of the movement (Rood and Bobath), whether spinal and brainstem reflexes should (Brunnstrom) or should not (Bobath) be used to elicit movement when the patient cannot otherwise move, and whether redevelopment of motor control should be sought in an ontogenetic sequence (PNF and Rood) or in a proximodistal sequence (Bobath and Brunnstrom). None of the approaches addresses methods of developing skilled movement. All emphasize the develop-

ment of basic movement and postures, with the assumption that when movement is "normalized" then skilled movement would occur automatically. These approaches are aimed at reorganizing or permanently changing the central nervous system.

More contemporary neurophysiological and movement science research and clinical observation have called into question some of the assumptions of these approaches (Horvak, 1991). For example, one assumption is that sensory input controls motor output (peripheral motor control theory). Information, gathered from stimulus-response (reflex) research that was conducted on anesthetized, decorticalized animals provided the support for this. This assumption was applied in neurorehabilitation by applying sensory stimulation to elicit motor responses (Marteniuk et al., 1987).

Another assumption is that control of movement is hierarchical, that the higher motor centers control mid-level centers that, in turn, control lower centers (central motor control theory). This hierarchical model was applied in neurorehabilitation by assessing at which level of control the patient moved. The hierarchical model guided the developmental aspect of treatment also. Therapists sought to "integrate" lower-level spinal and brainstem reflexes by eliciting higher-level righting and equilibrium reactions. And they progressed their patients through developmental "motor milestones."

Modern technology has allowed the study of brain function in awake, functioning animals and people. It has been seen that, given a goal, many areas of a person's brain begins to be activated and that this activation precedes movement and sensory feedback from movement (Chollet et al., 1991). Muscles begin contracting before movement starts. Different muscles contract to different levels under various circumstances to achieve the same goal (Trombly & Cole, 1979). Kinematic analysis of normal babies found that their

GLOSSARY

Associated reaction—These are involuntary movements or patterned, reflexive increases in muscle tone and limb position on the hemiplegic side. These reactions occur in situations that are stressful. They are common when yawning; and may occur when other parts of the body are resisted during movement, when the patient exerts effort or when the patient fears loss of balance.

Bilateral asymmetrical—Refers to paired limbs (e.g., arms) moving in different patterns at the same time, e.g., both moving toward one side of the body.

Bilateral symmetrical—Refers to paired limbs (e.g., arms) moving in the same pattern at the same time.

Bridging—A supine treatment activity used to train weight bearing on the hemiplegic foot and to activate hip extensors and abdominal muscles. To bridge, the patient lies supine with the knees flexed and feet on the surface. The patient lifts the hips off the surface, keeping the feet, shoulders, and head against the surface. Used functionally to assist in positioning the bedpan and to move up or sideways in bed.

Contralateral—Refers to the opposite side. For example, after a stroke, the person experiences weakness in the limbs contralateral to the location of the lesion in the brain. A right cerebrovascular accident results in left hemiparesis.

Controlled sensory input—The concept that the neural component of tone can be affected by the number and electrical sign of impulses that impinge on interneurons or motor neurons. Sensory stimuli are applied in a specific manner to increase or reduce the electrical charge on these neurons, making them more or less likely to fire when they receive additional, goal-specific, stimulation from supraspinal centers.

D1 extension—Refers to the final position of shoulder extension, abduction, and internal rotation; elbow extension; and pronation so that the hand passes the hip on the same side of the body. The wrist, fingers, and thumb extend and fingers and thumb abduct.

D1 flexion—Refers to the final position of shoulder flexion, adduction, and external rotation; elbow flexion; and supination so that the hand passes close to the ear on the opposite side of the head. Wrist, fingers, and thumb flex and fingers and thumb adduct.

D2 extension—Refers to the final position of shoulder extension, adduction, and internal rotation; elbow extension; and pronation so that the hand moves past the opposite hip. Wrist flexes; fingers flex and adduct; and thumb opposes.

D2 flexion—Refers to the final position of shoulder flexion, abduction, and external rotation; elbow flexion; and supination so that the hand comes close to the ear on the same side of the head. Wrist extends and fingers and thumb extend and abduct.

Extensor synergy—For the upper extremity: scapular protraction, shoulder horizontal adduction and internal rotation, elbow extension, and forearm pronation. For the lower extremity: hip extension, adduction, and internal rotation; knee extension, plantar flexion and inversion of the ankle; and plantar flexion of the toes.

Facilitate (facilitation); facilitation techniques—To make easier: the state of readying neurons to depolarize and propagate an impulse or to make contraction of a muscle or a reflex response more likely to occur. Manual treatment techniques and hand placements are used to increase muscle tone to produce more nearly normal movement responses in the hemiplegic patient.

Flaccidity—A state of lacking tone; the limb feels limp and falls into place when not supported.

Flexor synergy—For the upper extremity: scapular elevation and retraction, shoulder abduction and external rotation, elbow flexion, and forearm supination. For the lower extremity: hip flexion, abduction, and external rotation; knee flexion; ankle dorsiflexion and inversion; and dorsiflexion of the toes.

Handling—The manner in which the NDT/Bobath therapist uses her hands to stop the patient's abnormal tone and movement and activate normal movement patterns.

Hemiparetic—Weakness of one half of the body, usually following stroke.

Inhibit (inhibition); inhibition techniques—To make more difficult: the state of hyperpolarization of neural cell membrane, decreasing the likelihood of propagating an impulse, or to make contraction of a muscle or a reflex response less likely to occur. Manual treatment techniques and movement patterns are used to decrease spasticity and stop abnormal movement patterns.

Ipsilateral—Refers to the same side. For example, the ipsilateral arm and leg, i.e., the arm and leg on the same side of the body.

Key points of control—Hand placements on the hemiplegic trunk and limbs that are used to change muscle tone and influence the quality of movement. Proximal key points control the trunk and pelvic and scapular girdles, while distal points control the arm and hand or leg and foot.

Muscle tapping—The skin over a muscle is tapped vigorously to provide intermittent mechanical stretch to the muscle to increase the contraction through recruitment of more motor units.

Neutral warmth—The warmth provided by body heat trapped by a wrap of cotton flannel blanket, down quilt, etc., which relaxes the muscle, or inhibits general muscle tension.

Normalization of tone—Process of changing excess tone (hypertonia) or insufficient tone (hypotonia) to a state of "normal" tone needed for normal motor responses.

Ontogenetic—Following the sequence of normal development.

GLOSSARY, *(continued)*

Placing response—The normal adaptation of muscles to passive movement, which allows the body to follow movements and maintain a position when moved there. Muscles with normal tone and motor control will actively assist with passive movements and will briefly maintain a position when placed.

Postural control—The automatic system that functions to maintain posture and balance and forms the basis for functional performance by positioning the trunk to support extremity movement. This system includes righting and equilibrium reactions as well as postural sets used to prepare for movement and adjust to ongoing movement.

Practice—Repetition with the intent to improve.

Reflex inhibiting postures—Positions that inhibit spasticity by passively elongating spastic muscles. This concept of passive positioning was modified by Bobath and Bobath to include the use of movement to inhibit abnormal tone. They called the specific movements used to inhibit tone reflex inhibiting movement patterns.

Reliability—A characteristic of a measuring instrument that indicates the degree to which the test measures consistently from time to time (intrarater reliability or test-retest reliability) or from therapist to therapist (interrater reliability).

Scapula mobilization—A treatment technique used to preserve or restore normal mobility in the scapulothoracic joint, allowing the hemiplegic arm to be moved through its full arc of movement without shoulder pain and to inhibit flexor spasticity in the arm. It can be performed in supine, side lying, and sitting.

Scooter board—A rectangular, flat board with wheels at each corner. It is used to ride on to evoke the pivot prone posture. It should be too short to support the hips and shoulders, thereby requiring the patient to lift these body parts to get a ride (see Fig. 24A.3).

Slow stroking—The flat of the hands are alternately passed slowly and rhythmically down the center of the neck and back, resulting in a generalized relaxation (inhibition of muscle tension).

Spasticity—A state of excess tone and hyperactive response to stretch. If moderately to severely spastic, the limb feels tight and is difficult to move into position.

Stimulation techniques—Specific techniques that use tactile and proprioceptive input to muscles and joints to produce an active muscle response in flaccid limbs.

Tendon tapping—The skin over a tendon is tapped vigorously, which provides a mechanical stretch to the muscle and increases the number of motor units recruited.

Validity—A characteristic of a measuring instrument that means that the test in fact measures what it is supposed to measure.

Vibration—Stimulation using an electrical personal vibrator, which is applied against the skin over the muscle(s) or the tendons of the muscle(s) needing facilitation. The action of the vibrator provides a rapidly repeated mechanical stretch to the muscle, which increases the number of motor units recruited. This is the tonic vibratory reflex (TVR). The response lasts as long as the vibrator is applied.

---

movements represent elegant attempts to solve the motor problem of accessing a particular goal (von Hofsten, 1984). Their movement shows no evidence of obligatory motor responses. Reflexes detected by Sherrington and other early neurophysiologists in decorticalized specimens may simply reflect the basic wiring of the brainstem and spinal cord that can be employed in myriad ways to accomplish the goal. It is the goal of movement and the biomechanical constraints on the person and his or her environment at the moment that appears to organize the sensorimotor responses. This organization is not hierarchical but heterarchical, i.e., distributed around the various parts of the brain, each responsible for its little piece of the whole action (Chollet et al., 1991).

The other major belief of the traditional approaches is that people who have experienced normal movement but who have "regressed" because of brain damage should "recapitulate ontogeny," i.e., start to redevelop control at the earliest motor milestone of normal infant development that they are now unable to accomplish. However, patients with motor dysfunction do not regress to babylike movement. Patients do not move in the nice fluid movements that babies do when they are trying to obtain their goal. Stroke patients, on the contrary, have described attempts to move as "extraordinarily effortful" and as "heavy" (Brodal, 1973), and their movements demonstrate stereotyped qualities—a loss of the many sources of control at higher levels that gives lightness and fractionation to normal movement. Furthermore, newer developmental research has discovered that the universality of the motor milestones does not even exist in normal babies. Rather, development is much more flexible and individual (Touwen, 1978). Some children learn to walk very well without first learning to creep. This implies, e.g., that creeping is not a prerequisite to walking (Van Sant, 1991). Finally, some of the developmental motor tasks are not only socially inappropriate for adults but probably also neurologically inappropriate for them, because they had already attained mature movement skills before brain trauma.

On the other hand, modern motor developmental research has demonstrated newer explanations for so-called developmental phenomena. For example, Thelen and Fisher (1982) discovered an alternate, biomechanical explanation for the "U-shaped phenomenon" of motor development in which the automatic, reflexive movements of newborns (e.g., the stepping reflex) was believed to go through a period of decline and absence before the onset of the "mature" movements of the older child (e.g., walking) as was proposed by McGraw (1945). The decrease seems to be the result of the added weight of the child who has inadequate strength, and if the weight is supported, stepping is evident. Thelen and Whitley-Cooke (1987) have shown that practice of primitive stepping in infants results in earlier independent locomotion. This finding might actually support Brunnstrom's idea of starting stroke patients' motor relearning by using the primitive stereotyped movements they exhibit. The developmental concept should not be totally disregarded. Van Sant (1991) pointed out the usefulness of intratask developmental sequences as opposed to the intertask developmental tasks represented by the motor milestones. An example of intratask developmental sequences are those associated with development of eye-hand coordination or grasp and release.

These newer observations and theories, in effect, invalidate specific procedures used in the traditional approaches presented in this chapter, especially because there are few to no outcome studies supporting the clinical effectiveness of these approaches. There are aspects of these traditional approaches that have been supported and some that have not been improved on, and so we may want to hold on to these aspects. All approaches included procedures to enable the patient to learn to move voluntarily. While newer motor learning research has specified the parameters for teaching and learning in greater detail, that research has not yet been extended to patients with central nervous system dysfunction. The skilled therapists who developed these approaches presented solutions to a problem that current human movement scientists have not yet encountered: how to teach voluntary, "willed" movement to people who can move only in involuntary, stereotypical patterns. The methods these therapists used to teach patients to gain volitional control over their movements need to be reexamined and tested.

Still another aspect of these approaches needs to be preserved: the attention paid to subtle patient responses that indicated his inability to cope with overwhelming stress. When the challenge exceeds the patient's ability to cope, these approaches advocate reducing the task or environmental demands. "The therapist controls the environment, allowing the patient to be a successful problem solver, thereby maintaining or enhancing his motor control and dignity" (Minor, 1991, p. 139).

ˏ   # 24A   ROOD APPROACH

Catherine A. Trombly

OBJECTIVES

After studying this chapter, the learner will be able to:
1. Discuss the major premise and principles of Rood's approach.
2. Understand the process of evaluation used by practitioners of the Rood approach.
3. List the three components of treatment and understand how they are applied.
4. Discuss the developmental sequences included in this approach.
5. Suggest functional activities suitable for adults to encourage **practice** of motor control in developmental sequences.

HISTORY

Rood was both an occupational therapist and a physical therapist. One of her major contributions was the example she set for using research. She kept abreast of research developments of the time. She attempted to bridge between what she learned from basic neurophysiological research and the treatment of brain-injured patients. She invented ways to apply the independent variables that were used in animal studies to people, with the expectation that the results would be the same. She persisted in developing a wonderfully integrated treatment approach.

Rood's treatment was originally designed for cerebral palsy, but she believed it was applicable to any patient with motor control problems (Rood, 1976). As noted in the introduction to this chapter, the peripheral motor control theory has been supplanted. Because some of Rood's assumptions were based on this theory and because no clinician has reported the effectiveness of treatment based on those assumptions, some of Rood's approach is considered invalid. Nonetheless, as anyone who watched her treat patients could attest, she got results. However, those results may have been the result of her responsiveness to patients and her ability to present them with what is now called the "just right challenge" rather than the physiological stimuli and handling she was applying. Without clinical research, it is impossible to know the reasons for Rood's success.

Rood's approach includes three components: (1) controlled sensory stimulation, (2) the use of developmental sequences, and (3) the use of activity to demand a purposeful response. All were part of each treatment

(Ayres, 1974; Curran, 1960). Rood shared her ideas with others through clinical and classroom teaching but published very little. Some of the ideas reported here are based on interpretations of her method by therapists who studied and trained with her.

PRINCIPLES

Rood's basic premise was that

motor patterns are developed from fundamental reflex patterns present at birth which are utilized and gradually modified through sensory stimuli until the highest control is gained on the conscious cortical level. It seemed to me then, that if it were possible to apply the proper sensory stimuli to the appropriate sensory receptor as it is utilized in normal sequential development, it might be possible to elicit motor responses reflexly and by following neurophysiological principles, establish proper motor engrams (Rood, 1954, p. 444).

The four principles of Rood's theory are (Ayres, 1974; Curran, 1960; Stockmeyer, 1967) discussed below.

1. The **normalization of tone** and evocation of desired muscular responses are accomplished through the use of certain, appropriately applied, sensory stimuli. Correct sensory input is necessary for the development of correct motor responses. **Controlled sensory input** is used to evoke muscular responses reflexively, the earliest developmental step in gaining motor control (Rood, 1954, 1962).

2. Sensorimotor control is developmentally based, and therefore, therapy must start at the patient's current level of development and progress sequentially to higher levels of control (Rood, 1962; Minor, 1991). Rood identified several developmental sequences, which are illustrated in Table 24A.1.

3. Movement is purposeful (Ayres, 1963, 1974; Rood, 1962). Rood used purposeful activity to demand a response from the patient to elicit subcortically (unconsciously) the desired movement pattern. The responses of agonists, antagonists, and synergists were believed to be reflexively (automatically) programmed according to a purpose or plan. The cortex does not direct each muscle individually. When the cortex commands "pick up the glass," for example, all the subcortical centers involved in picking up the glass cause **facilitation** or **inhibition** of required muscles to allow the accomplishment of the goal in a coordinated manner. The patient's attention is drawn to the goal, or

Table 24A.1. Integration of Ontogenetic Motor Patterns with Levels of Motor Control [a]

Level I: Mobility		Level II: Stability		Level III: Mobility on Stability		Level IV: Skill	
Skeletal	Vital	Skeletal	Vital	Skeletal	Vital	Skeletal	Vital
1. Supine withdrawal	1. Inspiration	4. Pivot prone (held)	5. Phonation [b]	6. Neck cocontraction (orient head in space)	4. Swallow fluids	9. Prone on elbows (head is doing skilled movement and one arm is free for skilled use; belly crawling)	5. Phonation
2. Roll over	2. Expiration	5. Neck cocontraction	3. Sucking	8. Prone on elbows, (shift from side to side, push backward and pull forward, unilateral weight bearing)	6. Chewing		8. Speech
3. Pivot prone (assume the position)		7. Prone-on-elbows		11. Quadruped (rocking, shifting, unilateral weight bearing)	7. Swallow solids	12. Quadruped (one arm free for skilled use; creeping, trunk rotation and reciprocal movement, crossed diagonal)	
		10. Quadruped		14. Standing (weight shift, unilateral weight bearing)		15. Standing and walking	
		13. Standing					

[a] The steps are numbered sequentially, but they blend together, i.e., one step is not completely mastered before the next begins at the most basic level.
[b] Although out of sequence, phonation is facilitated in the pivot prone position.

purpose, not the movement per se. The sensation that occurs as a result of the movements involved in the activity helps the patient learn the movements.

4. Repetition (**practice**) of sensorimotor responses is necessary for motor learning (Ayres, 1974; Rood, 1956). Activities are used not only to elicit purposeful responses but also to motivate repetition.

EVALUATION

Rood evaluated the patient to determine what the distribution of muscle tone was and to determine what level of motor control, according to her developmental sequences, the patient had achieved. Evaluation and treatment planning involve the following points.

1. Identification of the patient's developmental level. In Table 24A.1 the steps are numbered sequentially for the skeletal and vital function sequences and the motor control sequence, indicating the order used for evaluation and treatment planning. The point at which the patient is easily able to do the task represents his highest level of development. Treatment starts at the point at which the patient has to struggle a little.

2. The plan includes what the activity should be and how the patient should be progressed to the next level of the sequence, using a variation of the same activity or a different one. Treatment is planned so that as the patient is perfecting a lower-level skill, he begins to learn the next (higher-level) skill. The therapist's determination of whether it would be necessary to assist the patient into the desired pattern or if a purposeful

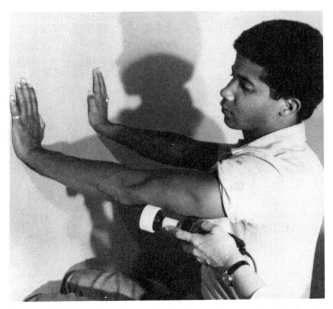

Figure 24A.1. An electrical vibrator being applied to the triceps of a patient in the quadruped posture to facilitate elbow extension.

activity that demanded the movement and/or posture could be used to obtain the desired outcome on a subconscious basis is part of the plan. Even if placed, the patient is immediately presented with an activity that demands the desired sustained posture or repeated movement.

3. Identification of which of the patient's muscles need to be facilitated to effect the pattern desired. Because **facilitation** involves use of particular stimuli to obtain the desired response (tonic or phasic), the plan includes identification of these stimuli and the order of their application. If the patient is spastic, the therapist would have to plan to use **inhibition techniques** to normalize the tone first.

TREATMENT

Controlled Sensory Input

Rood invented tools and methods to administer sensory input, based on the studies of the effects of stimuli on animals and her own clinical practice. She used cutaneous (tactile), thermal, olfactory, gustatory, auditory, visual, and proprioceptive (stretch, resistance) stimuli to **facilitate** or **inhibit** motor responses. The mechanisms of how these stimuli worked were explained according to the peripheral motor control theory of the 1940s and 1950s. Because that theory has been supplanted by newer knowledge, and because there is little research concerning the effects of any of these stimuli on normal subjects or patients, they will not be described in detail here.

The **facilitation technique** of fast brushing has been researched. Fast brushing is described as brushing the hairs or the skin over a muscle with a soft camel hair paintbrush that has been substituted for the stirrer of a hand-held battery-powered cocktail mixer to produce a high-frequency, high-intensity stimulus (Harris, 1969; Huss, n.d.; Rood, 1962; Stockmeyer, 1967). Rood hypothesized that the effect of fast brushing is nonspecific (i.e., not confined to one muscle), has a latency of 30 sec, and does not reach its maximum potency until 30 to 40 min after stimulation, because of processing by the reticular activating system. In controlled studies of normal and poststroke individuals, however, it was demonstrated that although fast brushing produced a significant immediate facilitatory effect, the postapplication effect lasted only 30 to 45 sec (Mason, 1985; Matyas & Spicer, 1980; Spicer & Matyas, 1980) and was not functionally significant. Moreover, the facilitatory effect was seen only in the lower extremity, not in the upper extremity, of normal subjects.

Rider (1971) also examined fast brushing, among other stimuli. She found a statistically significant (P

= .01) increase in the strength of both triceps of eight children with bilateral upper extremity flexor **spasticity** compared with eight children who had normal upper extremities, following a 2-week period of treatment consisting of brushing, stroking, rubbing, icing, and squeezing of the triceps of one limb. She reported a significant mean decrease in strength of both elbow extensors of those children, from both groups, who had been facilitated on the nonpreferred arm following a 2-week period of no **facilitation.**

Stretch, in the form of muscle or **tendon tapping,** is used successfully in the clinic to evoke a stronger response in a muscle that is contracting without added stretch (see Fig. 24C.4). **Vibration,** delivered by an electric personal vibrator (Fig. 24A.1), is a form of stretch. Its effects are apparent even in classroom demonstrations using normal students. It evokes a tonic holding contraction and adds to the strength of contraction of an already weakly contracting muscle. Stretch to the intrinsic muscles of the hand or foot, another **facilitation technique,** is used to **facilitate** cocontraction of the proximal stabilizer muscles (Ayres, 1974; Stockmeyer, 1967). This technique requires the patient to grasp a handle forcefully. It is hypothesized that the best response is gained from use of a cone-shaped handle (with the widest part of the cone at the ulnar border of the hand) or a spherical handle, both of which increase intermetacarpal stretch. If activities that use such handles can be combined with weight-bearing positions, the proximal stabilizers are believed to be further facilitated through the demand placed on them for cocontraction. For example, to develop shoulder cocontraction, a patient can lean on his elbow in a modified prone-on-elbows position while using an electric drill to drill holes in a vertically placed project. Zimny (1979) studied whether scapulohumeral muscles of normal adults showed increased cocontraction in the prone-on-elbows position in combination with resisted grasp. The electromyographic results revealed only a low level of response from these muscles under this condition. It has not yet been tested on patients. Clinical observation suggests resisted grasp is an effective technique to obtain scapulohumeral contraction in some cases.

Prolonged manual stretch is used to **inhibit** spastic muscles so that the patient may move more easily (Carey, 1990). The limb is held so that the muscles are steadily kept at their greatest length for 1 or 2 min until a "letting go" is felt as the muscles adjust to the longer length. It may be that this procedure rebiases the spindles to a longer length and makes them less sensitive to stretch during movement. It certainly also mechanically lengthens the muscles, changing their viscoelastic configuration.

Developmental Sequences of Motor Control and Use of Purposeful Activities

Rood identified several sequences that she used interrelatedly but that will be presented separately here for clarity. One sequence was already mentioned in the list of the principles of the Rood method. To reiterate, a muscular response is first evoked reflexively using sensory stimulation, then responses so obtained are used in developmental patterns, and then the patient uses the response purposefully to gain control over it.

A second sequence that Rood identified was use of muscles in particular patterns according to their classification (Goff, 1972; Rood, 1962). Muscles were classified as light-work or heavy-work muscles based on their anatomical design. Light-work muscles lie superficially, laterally, or distally and have a tendinous origin and insertion. They are multiarthrodial, they are under more voluntary control, and they do phasic work. Rood identified the light-work, or mobilizing, muscles as primarily the flexors and adductors, but multiarthrodial finger and wrist extensors also are included in this category. These muscles are termed *physiological flexors* even though their action is extension of the finger, thumb, or wrist joints. Heavy-work muscles are deep, lie close to the joint, and are uniarthrodial. In the body, they are located proximally and medially. Heavy-work muscles are tonic stability muscles capable of prolonged, sustained contraction. These are primarily the trunk musculature and proximal limb extensors and abductors but also include such muscles as the interossei of the hands and feet. Rood believed that if the normal first response of a muscle was a stabilizing contraction, it should first be facilitated to contract in this manner and not in a mobilizing pattern. However, there is no convenient listing of what the original **ontogenetic** function of each muscle was to guide this aspect of treatment. Therapists are guided by Rood's definitions of heavy-work and light-work muscles in planning treatment.

Another sequence reflects the development of muscle responses. In this sequence, flexion precedes extension, adduction precedes abduction, ulnar patterns develop before radial ones, and rotation develops last (Huss, n.d.).

Another sequence that Rood identified has to do with development of motor control. There are four phases.

1. Movement first appears as phasic, reciprocal shortening and lengthening contractions of muscles that cause movement that subserves a protective function. Muscles contract to cause movement through full range, which, according to Sherringtonian physiology, produces reciprocal **inhibition** of the antagonists (Ayres,

1974; Rood, 1962). Stockmeyer (1967) termed this the mobility phase. The movement of an infant waving his or her extremities back and forth when shown a desired object typifies phasic movement.

2. Tonic, holding contractions are next to develop and are the basis for maintaining proximal posture to allow exploration of the environment and development of skill by the distal segments of the head and limbs. Stability is obtained through cocontraction, i.e., the muscles around the joint contract simultaneously (Ayres, 1974; Stockmeyer, 1967). Development of proximal stability should precede work on developing skilled movement (Rood, 1956). However, this assumption appears not to be true. Research has shown that the proximal and distal motor systems are controlled separately (Freund & Hummelsheim, 1984; Lawrence & Kuyphers, 1965) and, while correlated, follow a separate developmental sequence (Case-Smith, Fisher, & Bauer, 1989; Wilson & Trombly, 1984).

3. Proximal muscles contract to do heavy work superimposed on distal cocontraction (Ayres, 1974; Rood, 1962). "Mobility superimposed on stability" is Stockmeyer's (1967) way of designating this level of motor control in which the distal segment is fixed and the proximal segment moves. This phase is used to develop controlled mobility of the proximal joints. An example of this kind of motion occurs when an infant learns to assume the quadruped position but has not yet learned to move in that position: He or she rocks back and forth with the knees and hands planted firmly on the floor.

4. Skill is the highest level. At this level of motor control, the proximal segment is stabilized and the distal segment moves (Ayres, 1974; Rood, 1962). Examples of this level include walking, crawling, and reaching as well as activities that require coordinated use of the hands.

SKELETAL FUNCTIONS SEQUENCE

These four levels of motor control are developed as the patient is paced through the skeletal functions sequence (**ontogenetic** motor patterns) that are pictured in Figure 24A.2 (Rood, 1962; Stockmeyer, 1967). The eight functional patterns will be described, then the interrelationship between these patterns and the levels of motor control may be studied, using Table 24A.1.

1. Flexor withdrawal supine (Minor, 1991), also called supine flexion, is a position of total flexion toward the vertebral level of T_{10}. The upper extremities cross the chest, and the dorsum of the extended hands touch the face. The lower extremities flex and abduct. This posture demands heavy work of the trunk and proximal parts of the extremities but allows light work

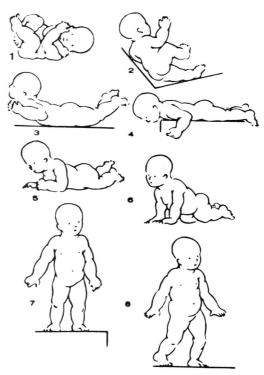

Figure 24A.2. Skeletal functions sequence according to Rood. **1.** Flexor withdrawal supine. **2.** Roll over. **3.** Pivot prone. **4.** Neck cocontraction. **5.** Prone on elbows. **6.** Quadruped. **7.** Standing. **8.** Walking.

of the distal parts of the limbs. It is used to obtain flexor/adductor responses when the patient has no movement or is dominated by extensor responses. It is also used to develop trunk and proximal limb stability or to develop reciprocal phasic movement through normal range. It is thought to integrate the tonic labyrinthine reflex (TLR) by requiring the voluntary contraction of the flexors in spite of reflex **facilitation** of the extensors.

To elicit the flexor withdrawal supine motor pattern, Rood used the following method. First, the low back and the dermatomes of C_{1-4} were fast brushed. Second, small wedge pillows were placed under the head and the pelvis to stretch the short extensors of the back and to put the neck flexors and abdominals in a shortened position. The shortened position allowed the spindles to rebias. Rebiasing the spindles to a short position was believed to make them more sensitive to stretch, and therefore, the muscles were more apt to contract if the patient reverted to a trunk extended position as a result of the influences of the TLR. Finally, after the heavy-work response of the trunk was obtained, a light-work response of the limbs would be elicited by stroking (tactile) or icing (thermal) the sole or palm and immediately demanding a light-work flexion/adduction pattern of the limbs through an activity. The force of the activity is directed toward flexion/adduction, even though reciprocal movement in the opposite direction would be involved. Some examples are tetherball, squeezing a toy accordion, using a cylindrical balloon blower, playing table tennis (forehand shot), and stirring batter in a counterclockwise direction using the right arm or in reverse direction using the left.

According to Rood, this motor pattern also helped develop bowel and bladder function, eye convergence, and respiratory patterns.

If the TLR extensor response in supine was too strong to permit flexor movement, Rood recommended starting treatment with the patient in a side-lying position.

2. Roll over is a movement in which the arm and leg on the same side flex as the trunk rotates. This pattern is used for patients who are dominated by the primitive tonic reflexes or need mobilization of the extremities or activation of lateral trunk musculature. Attempts at rolling over integrate the asymmetrical tonic neck reflex (ATNR), because the top-most limbs—in this case the skull side limbs—flex and adduct proximally and tend to extend at the elbow and knee, which is opposite to the typical ATNR skull-side response. Activity examples are rolling over to reach an attractive or needed object and turning to look at something enticing. To elicit the response on a subconscious level, move the object the person is looking at around to the side, thereby causing the patient's head to turn to maintain visual contact; the body will automatically follow the head, if the righting reactions are developing.

3. Pivot prone, also called prone extension, is a position in which the patient lies prone and extends upper trunk and head; abducts, extends, and externally rotates his shoulders; and extends his hips and knees off the surface so that he rests on the pivot point at approximately the level of T_{10} (Figs. 24A.2 and 24A.3). Assumption of the position is a phasic, reciprocal movement. Holding the position involves a shortened, held, resisted contraction (SHRC) of the extensor/abductor muscles. An SHRC used in combination with the pivot prone position is thought to be a important preparation for weight-bearing postures. Gravity exerts a constant resistive force against holding the position, which causes the central nervous system (CNS) to reprogram more and more motor units. It is reasoned that immediately following an SHRC in prone extension, the spindles of the extensor/abductor muscles are biased short and are, therefore, responsive to small increments of stretch. If the patient moves into a prone-on-elbows or quadruped position, the shoulder and hip extensor/abductor muscles are stretched relative to

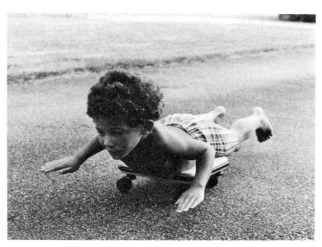

Figure 24A.3. Scooter board being used on an incline and eliciting the pivot prone position automatically.

their new shortened range and are facilitated to contract. When this position can be maintained, it indicates that the symmetrical tonic neck reflex (STNR) and TLR are integrated and the labyrinthine righting reactions are developing.

The procedures to achieve the whole pattern will be described, although for an adult who has trunk control this is modified to a partial pattern. The patient is placed prone on a firm, padded surface large enough to support the trunk only, e.g., on a low stool, bolster, or **scooter board** (Fig. 24A.3). The area over the deep back extensors is fast-brushed, taking care to avoid the L_{1-2} and S_{2-3} areas (believed to cause bladder voiding or retention respectively). The skin over the posterior deltoids, latissimus dorsi, trapezii, proximal hamstrings, and glutei is also fast brushed. Simultaneously with the activity that demands the pivot prone posture, **vibration** is applied to the deep back and neck extensors and other extensor muscles involved in the pattern, starting at the midline. The pivot prone position is held for gradually increasing periods of time up to at least 1 to 2 min. Activities are presented to demand and resist the response. Activity suggestions are doing leather lacing or macramé, using a sling shot, stirring batter in a clockwise direction with the right arm or in the opposite direction with the left (unilateral pattern), riding prone on a **scooter board** (Fig. 24A.3), playing with a "button-on-string" toy, rowing, and tearing apart strips of cloth for rag rugs (bilateral pattern). Note that the force of the activity is in the direction of extension and abduction, although other movements are also involved in the activity.

4. Neck cocontraction is the pattern used to develop head control and is first activated in the prone position. In the prone position, the labyrinth righting reaction stimulates alignment of the head so that the

eyes are parallel and the nose is perpendicular to the surface. Before putting the patient in a prone position, it is necessary to activate the flexors if they are not already active. Rood believed that the short neck flexors could be activated by fast brushing the dermatomal distribution of C2. Next, the long neck flexors, the sternocleidomastoids, are stimulated. The patient is then placed prone and given an activity that prompts him to raise his head against gravity. Sucking a resistive liquid through a straw or playing games in which a small object is picked up by sucking it onto the end of the straw are also activities that result in reflexive cocontraction of the neck muscles. As the patient attempts to maintain neck extension, the upper trapezius is facilitated to maintain the extension by fast brushing and repetitive **muscle tapping.** When the contraction lets go, the head bobs into flexion and the neck and trunk extensors are stretched, thereby facilitated to contract. Neck extension is again sought.

5. Prone on elbows is a pattern of vertical trunk extension, which is thought to **inhibit** the STNR. When the shoulders are brought into forward flexion from a pivot prone posture, so that the patient can bear weight on his elbows, the extensor/abductor muscles of the proximal upper extremity are stretched and facilitated to cocontract with the flexors and adductors in the prone-on-elbows position. A normal infant can be observed assuming the pivot prone position just before going into a prone-on-elbows position, as if to "prime" his or her system.

A procedure to achieve the prone-on-elbows pattern is as follows. The back and neck extensors are fast brushed, as are the glenohumeral extensors and abductors. The patient is asked to assume the pivot prone position or given an activity that demands the pivot prone position. Resistance, for greater **facilitation** in the pivot prone position, may be added manually by pushing the thighs and upper trunk toward the supporting surface. Then the patient is placed in or given an activity to do that demands the prone-on-elbows position. One suggestion is for the person to lie on the floor to watch television; the television set is placed so that neck and upper trunk extension are required for him to look at it. **Vibration** can be applied to the extensor/abductor muscles of the glenohumeral joint as needed to gain cocontraction. An activity that demands resisted grasp can be introduced to obtain reinforcement of shoulder cocontraction. Other activities include playing board games or doing crafts while prone lying. These activities begin to combine the static bilateral position with unilateral positioning and reaching. Unilateral weight bearing is more advanced than bilateral weight bearing. The activities could progress to involve some crawling, which is a higher-level response (see Table 24A.1).

Treatment of adults is more likely to involve a modified prone-on-elbows position (Stockmeyer, 1967), in which the seated patient leans with his elbow on the table or lap tray. Activities are easy to devise for this modified posture and usually involve use of the less-affected limb for the skilled aspect of the activity while the more-affected limb holds down the object being worked on.

6. The all-fours pattern, also called quadruped, occurs after the neck, upper extremities, and upper trunk have developed stability. This position helps the trunk and lower extremities develop cocontraction. At first, the quadruped position is static; later the person is able to shift weight backward and forward, from side to side, and diagonally and then is able to lift one or two of the points of support, i.e., one arm and one leg. Finally, these activities develop into crawling.

A suggested procedure to develop the all-fours pattern is as follows. The back and neck extensors are fast brushed as are the glenohumeral and hip extensors and abductors and the elbow extensors. The patient assumes and holds the pivot prone position while resistance is added. Then the patient is placed into or given an activity to do that demands the all-fours position or a modified version of it. Activity examples include holding a sling shot prepared to shoot (unilateral pattern while upright) (Stockmeyer, 1967), weaving on a large loom adapted to resist elbow extension (while upright), holding wood in place while sawing it with the other hand, painting a large mural on the floor, and playing with a toy truck. While the activity is ongoing, muscle **tendon tapping** and/or **vibration** are applied to the muscles listed above as needed to maintain the posture.

7. Standing is first done as a static bilateral posture, then progresses to shifting weight and to a unilateral posture. Activity suggestions include doing craft activities, playing board or card games, making puzzles while standing at a high table, writing on a wall blackboard, and painting on an easel. Throwing and catching balls, balloons, and bean bags help develop balance while standing.

8. Walking is the skill level of standing. It consists of stance, push off, pick up (swing through), and heel strike. Ambulation training is the responsibility of the physical therapist.

VITAL FUNCTIONS SEQUENCE

The vital functions sequence is related to the skeletal functions sequence (Table 24A.1) (Huss, 1971; Minor, 1991). Both sequences are handled concurrently in treatment, if appropriate. The vital functions developmental sequence leads to speech. Therefore, the occupational therapist, who facilitates this sequence with the goal of treating dysphagia, collaborates with the speech-language pathologist (SLP) to achieve mutual goals. The sequence is as follows.

1. *Inspiration*, which is effected reflexively at birth.

2. *Expiration*, which depends on the depth of inspiration. The depth of inspiration depends on patterns of head and trunk stability set in the flexor withdrawal supine pattern: cocontraction of the deep neck flexors and extensors and cocontraction of the low back musculature with the rectus abdominus (Rood, 1962). The depth of inspiration can be increased by applying ice to the border of the ribs, which stimulates diaphragmatic contraction (Rood, 1976). Crying, sneezing, and coughing are all expiration-type phenomena that occur naturally or can be elicited reflexively (sneezing). Asking an adult patient to increase voluntarily the force of coughing is also used to improve expiratory function.

3. *Sucking*. According to Rood (1962), resisted sucking facilitates neck cocontraction, which in turn facilitates sucking. If pressure is applied to the tip of the tongue, then sucking will ensue after five to seven repetitions of applications of the pressure (Rood, 1976).

4. *Swallowing liquids*. Rood (1956) suggested that swallowing can be facilitated by cutaneous stimulation of the mucous membranes of the palate, tongue, and uvula using a long, cotton-tipped applicator stick. Rood believed that the orbicularis oris was the key to swallowing because she thought that it activated, by direct stretch, the buccinators and superior constrictor of the pharynx (Rood, 1962); therefore, in therapy the orbicularis oris muscle is facilitated by tapping and brushing. Care is taken that the chin is not brushed or stroked because this will cause the patient to be unable to keep his mouth closed to swallow, resulting in drooling. A swipe with an ice cube applied from the sternal notch to the Adam's apple will cause a person to swallow reflexively.

5. *Phonation*, defined as babbling, is controlled expiration as opposed to the reflexive expiration of sneezing, coughing, and crying.

6. *Chewing and swallowing solids.*

7. *Speech*, defined as production of recognizable words.

To illustrate treatment planning using Rood's sequences, this example may be helpful. The evaluation of a hypothetical poststroke patient indicated that he had some voluntary elbow flexion but his shoulder began to abduct simultaneously when he flexed his elbow. He was able to grasp, but unable to release objects. He was able to roll over in bed and rotate his trunk while sitting. In sorting these data out, the therapist noted that the elbow flexors, considered light-work muscles, were contracting in that capacity but the shoulder abductors, heavy-work muscles, should

have been contracting in a tonic pattern first, not in the phasic pattern that they were. She reasoned that if they were active in a stabilizing pattern, they would be prevented from reflexively contracting phasically during elbow flexion. Knowing the developmental sequence, the therapist knew that because flexion developed at the elbow, extension would be the next movement to be sought at that joint. The therapist also knew that prone extension would be the next pattern in the functional sequence to work for, because roll over is already within the patient's repertoire. Therefore, treatment of this patient would begin with controlled sensory stimulation of the extensors/abductors of the shoulder and scapula and with an activity to demand a static pivot prone response at least unilaterally of the affected side. It would proceed to a prone-on-elbows or quadruped position to develop elbow extension as the patient was able to progress.

Huss (n.d.; 1971) suggested some treatment planning guidelines:

1. Hypotonia ("floppy baby syndrome," upper motor neuron **flaccidity**) is treated by overall general stimulation, especially swinging, rolling, spinning in all planes for labyrinth stimulation, and specific exteroceptive and proprioceptive stimulation for specific muscle stimulation. Activities are used to elicit specific motor patterns in sequence.

2. Hypertonia (**spasticity,** which may be seen, e.g., in spastic cerebral palsy, cerebrovascular accident, and multiple sclerosis patients) is treated using **neutral warmth** for relaxation. Exteroceptive and proprioceptive stimulation of the antagonists of the spastic muscles are done. Activity is used in developmental sequence to reinforce normal movement.

3. Hypertonia (rigidity such as seen in Parkinson's disease) is treated using **neutral warmth** for relaxation. Reciprocal movement patterns are stimulated and reinforced using activity.

4. Hyperkinesis (uncontrolled movement such as seen in athetosis, chorea, and ataxia) is treated by **slow stroking** for relaxation. Maintained holding patterns are stimulated at first and then mobility on stability patterns that involve keeping the distal segment stabilized while the proximal segment moves are used. When control of midrange movement is developed in the proximal joints throughout the functional sequence, the patient is progressed to skill level.

EFFECTIVENESS

There are no studies of the effectiveness of the entire approach. Parts of it have been researched. As cited above, Mason (1985), Matyas and Spicer (1980), Spice and Matyas (1980), and Rider (1971) tested fast brushing and determined it was facilitating as predicted, but that it did not have the lasting effects expected by Rood. Carey (1980) verified that prolonged manual stretching results in inhibition of spastic muscles. VanSant (1988, 1991b) observed that the developmental motor sequence was not followed invariably by developing children nor adhered to by adults when rising from supine, as expected.

STUDY QUESTIONS

1. What is the premise on which Rood based her treatment approach?
2. What are the four principles of Rood's theory?
3. What are the three components that are included in each treatment?
4. What is the sequence of muscle activation, according to Rood?
5. What are the four phases of development of motor control used in this approach?
6. What are the eight skeletal function patterns of Rood?
7. Why is pivot prone considered a key developmental step?
8. How are patients evaluated using the Rood approach?
9. How is therapy carried out using the Rood approach?
10. What is the sequence leading to the development of speech?
11. Think of activities, appropriate for adults, that can be used for each of the skeletal functions.

24B   Neurodevelopmental (Bobath) Treatment

Kathryn Levit

OBJECTIVES

The information in this chapter will help the reader to:
1. Identify how the neurodevelopmental treatment/Bobath approach defines the major problems of the adult stroke patient.
2. Describe the important principles of neurodevelopmental/Bobath treatment for the stroke patient.
3. Discuss the role of normal muscle tone and **postural control** in the production of normal movement.
4. Understand the use of neurodevelopmental/Bobath techniques in occupational therapy for the adult stroke patient.
5. List the neurophysiological assumptions that Bobath and Bobath used to support their treatment and explain why these theories are being used to criticize the approach.

HISTORY

K. Bobath and B. Bobath, British neurologist and physiotherapist, respectively, developed methods for the evaluation and treatment of cerebral palsy and adult hemiplegia. Their treatment approach is known as both the Bobath approach and neurodevelopmental treatment (NDT). This chapter provides an introduction to NDT/Bobath theory and treatment as they apply to the adult with hemiplegia from stroke or other neurological condition. A complete description of the treatment approach and its techniques of treatment can be found in Bobath (1990).

Bobath and Bobath began to develop their treatment approach in the 1940s. B. Bobath, trained in Germany as a gymnast and remedial movement specialist, came to England to avoid persecution and began to work with neurologic patients. When working with an adult hemiplegic patient, she noted the stiffness of the patient's arm and leg and his inability to plan and execute normal movement patterns. In her treatment sessions, B. Bobath tried to help this patient and others like him regain normal patterns of coordination in his affected limbs. Through trial and error, she devised techniques to influence the abnormal tone of stroke patients and to retrain more normal patterns of movement in their hemiplegic side. Her method of remediation of movement for the adult stroke patient was not based on the developmental sequence, but on her analysis of the movement components important for use in life tasks.

As the treatment evolved, K. Bobath, a neurologist, reviewed the available neurophysiologic research to provide a scientific explanation for B. Bobath's treatment. Although the clinical techniques were developed first, Bobath and Bobath presented a scientific rationale for their approach based on the theories that were current in the 1940s. The first article describing the approach was published in 1948. Over the next 42 years, at least 70 additional publications were produced. The third edition of B. Bobath's (1990) book was published months before her death.

In their approach, Bobath and Bobath rejected the traditional therapy concept of compensatory training because it neglected the potential of the hemiplegic side for normal function. They also believed that techniques such as passive stretching and exercising individual muscles were of little value to the stroke patient, because these movements did not address the problems of abnormal tone and abnormal coordination. Similarly, they disagreed with the techniques of Knott and Brunnstrom because they reinforced abnormal reflex activity and increased **spasticity** in the hemiplegic side. Bobath and Bobath stressed that potential for more normal movement patterns and improved functional use of the hemiplegic side was present in all stroke patients and that this should be the goal of treatment. Their treatment techniques were designed to decrease the influence of **spasticity** and abnormal coordination and improve control of the involved trunk, arm and leg.

PRINCIPLES

The NDT/Bobath approach is directed toward the goal of retraining normal, functional patterns of movement in the adult stroke patient. To retrain movement in the stroke patient, the therapist must change, or "normalize," the abnormal tone and eliminate unwanted muscle activity. When muscle tone and patterns of muscle contraction are normalized, the therapist introduces and trains normal movement patterns in the trunk and extremities. The training of normal movement patterns includes the activation of postural responses that must be available on an automatic level for function. It also includes reeducation of muscles in the hemiplegic arm and leg for weight-bearing and non–

weight-bearing functions. Muscle reeducation is done both at the level of a single muscle group, i.e., wrist extensors, and at the level of synergistic muscle groups, i.e., wrist extensors with shoulder and elbow flexors and finger grasp to bring a toothbrush to the mouth. Bobath and Bobath believed that permanent reduction in **spasticity** cannot be achieved unless the patient is able actively to move his involved side in normal patterns of coordination (Bobath, 1990). Full potential has not been reached until the patient can use the normal movements in the performance of functional activities.

The following principles of treatment apply to all NDT/Bobath treatment activities:

1. Treatment should avoid movements and activities that increase muscle tone or produce abnormal responses in the involved side.
2. Treatment should be directed toward the development of normal patterns of posture and movement; movement patterns selected are not based on the developmental sequence but on patterns important for function.
3. The hemiplegic side should be incorporated into all treatment activities to reestablish symmetry and increase functional use.
4. Treatment should produce a change in the quality of movement and functional performance of the involved side.

EVALUATION AND TREATMENT PLANNING

Problems in the Adult Stroke Patient

According to Bobath and Bobath, strokes and other types of adult brain damage result in abnormal patterns of posture and movement. These abnormal patterns must be eliminated through treatment because they prevent the patient from regaining normal function on his involved side. The writings of B. Bobath identify four components to the motor disturbance in adult hemiplegia. These problems and their relationship to normal movement are discussed below.

ABNORMAL TONE

Abnormal tone is present in almost all patients with central nervous system (CNS) dysfunction and interferes with the production of normal movement patterns. Muscle tone may be defined as the amount of tension in the muscle. Bobath and Bobath quoted Sherrington (1913) to support their view that normal tone is necessary for the production of normal movement. To be considered normal, muscle tone must be high enough to allow movement against the pull of

gravity but low enough to prevent resistance and allow normal speed and timing of movement (Bobath, 1990). Muscle tone or tension fluctuates in everyone, depending on the situation one is in and the demands of the task. However, in most situations muscle tone matches the demands of the task being performed. During passive movements, bodies with normal tone actively assist and follow movements. If passive movement is arrested and the therapist's hands removed, the body segment will not fall but will remain briefly in the position in which it was placed. Bobath and Bobath called this the **placing response.**

In the adult stroke patient, muscle tone may be higher or lower than normal, both at rest and during movement. In the acute stage, **flaccidity** or low tone is generally present in the affected trunk and limbs. Flaccid limbs feel heavy or floppy and relaxed; they provide no resistance or assistance to passive motion. **Placing responses** are not present. Active motion is difficult because flaccid muscles are weak and cannot easily contract with enough force to lift the weight of the limb against the pull of gravity.

After a stroke, hypertonicity or **spasticity** develops in the muscles of the arm, leg, and trunk on the affected side. **Spasticity** produces stiff limbs that assume abnormal postures. Spastic muscles resist lengthening during passive motion but may assist passive movements that require the spastic muscles to shorten. Similarly, **placing responses** may be possible in patterns of muscle shortening. In the patient with **spasticity,** increased muscle tension may not be evenly distributed throughout the body. Hemiplegic patients frequently have hypertonic arms with hypotonic trunk muscles and may show tightly flexed elbows with flaccid wrists and fingers. When the spastic patient attempts actively to move his arm or leg, the movements are slow and inefficient and limited to mass patterns of flexion and extension.

In the stroke patient, muscle tone fluctuates according to the situation and demands of the task. The hemiplegic side may appear to have low tone at rest but may assume spastic positions during difficult activities. For example, when the stroke patient walks, the hemiplegic arm assumes an abnormal, flexed posture. The hemiplegic leg often stiffens severely during the transition from sit to stand, so that the patient is unable to bend it to take a step. Bobath and Bobath called these nonfunctional and involuntary changes in limb position and muscle tone **associated reactions.** Synergistic posturing of the limbs may vary from position to position. It may also occur when the patient yawns or sneezes and as painful spasms during sleep. Because the flexor posturing of the arm and extensor posturing of the leg are involuntary, the patient cannot change the position of his arm and leg in response to verbal commands such as "Straighten your elbow." **Associated reactions** appear to be linked to the loss of **postural control,** described below, and begin to disappear when balance has improved.

LOSS OF POSTURAL CONTROL

The stroke patient has lost control of the system of postural adjustments that forms "the necessary background for normal movement and for functional skills" (Bobath, 1990, p. 6). Postural reactions can be thought of as the basis for control of movement because they allow people to control the position of their bodies against gravity. Normal postural reactions include the righting reactions that help maintain the correct orientation of the head to trunk and trunk to limbs and equilibrium reactions that help people maintain or regain their balance and keep their body mass over their base of support. These reactions depend on control of the muscles of the trunk and pelvic and scapular girdles in many positions relative to the pull of gravity and on the ability to shift and bear weight on the limbs in many positions.

Postural reactions also include the changes in tone and adjustments in posture that precede and accompany functional movements. For example, in the task of standing up from a chair, people automatically place their feet underneath themselves and move the trunk forward from the back of the chair before standing. Similarly, humans automatically shift their weight over the right hip when reaching to the side with the right arm. During normal movement, postural adaptations and reactions occur automatically and are not under conscious cortical control. Bobath and Bobath use the term **postural control** to describe automatic activation of muscles to maintain control of the body for posture and movement.

In the patient with hemiplegia, the postural system is disrupted by loss of motor control of the hemiplegic trunk and extremities as well as damage to balance centers in the CNS. The patient cannot move the trunk and extremities on one side of his body. Because of poor motor control, he develops asymmetrical posture in his trunk, shoulder girdle, and lower extremity. He is unable to activate trunk muscles to maintain a stable position in sitting or standing and cannot perform functional trunk movements and weight shifts necessary to position the limbs for function or to regain his balance. He cannot move his arm to use it for function or balance or shift his weight onto his hemiplegic hip or foot. Loss of **postural control** forces the patient to rely on his sound side during task performance and to use canes and adaptive equipment to substitute for his poor balance. Because the patient cannot voluntarily

or automatically perform trunk movements and weight shifts in all directions, his functional movements will be limited to the number of postural sets in which he has control.

ABNORMAL COORDINATION

The patient with CNS damage has abnormal patterns of motor coordination, resulting in inefficient, nonfunctional extremity movements. During normal movement of the arm and leg, coordination between agonist, synergist, and antagonist produces smooth, effortless, and efficient patterns of movement. Proximal muscle groups are used to provide appropriate stabilization for distal function. Limb muscles are activated in sequences to position correctly the hand or foot for the desired function. Reciprocal inhibition between agonist and antagonist muscle groups ensures smooth control of limb movements by coordinating muscle firing so that only those muscle groups that produce the correct movement are active at one time. Limb movements are automatically accompanied by postural responses in the trunk to allow full ranges of limb control and production of power. During normal movement, the sequences of muscle activity used to reach for something with the arm, to tie shoes, and to walk are not produced with conscious attention. Once acquired, the plans for these movements are probably stored in the CNS.

In the stroke patient, the timing, sequencing, and coordination of muscle activation are disturbed. This loss of muscle control results in the abnormal patterns of limb movement and coordination typical of CNS patients. In some stroke patients, coordination is abnormal because only some muscles have returned in the arm and leg, while other muscles that should function as synergists are too weak to contribute to movement. A common example of this is found in the hemiplegic arm. The patient may have the ability to flex his shoulder and extend his elbow but be unable to position the hand for grasp because he does not have motor control of the wrist extensors and forearm supinators. In other cases, muscles are activated inappropriately or at the wrong time, producing abnormal limb patterns. In these patients, strong contraction of the scapula elevators and humeral abductors may be used to attempt to reach the arm forward. In a third group of patients, problems of cocontraction may occur. Both agonist and antagonistic muscle groups contract during cocontraction, producing rigid limbs incapable of selective movement. In most stroke patients, conscious attention and effort are necessary to produce any movement of the hemiplegic side. The patient must consciously direct his hemiplegic leg to take a step during ambulation or ask his shoulder muscles to contract to reach for an object.

ABNORMAL FUNCTIONAL PERFORMANCE

The stroke patient has lost the ability to integrate the two sides of his body to perform functional tasks in normal ways. According to Bobath and Bobath, normal movement requires (1) normal muscle tone, (2) normal postural responses, and (3) normal patterns of muscle activation and coordination. Normal task performance is based on sequences of normal movement that integrate movements on both sides of the body. In many functional movements and tasks, the two sides of the body perform the same movements, either at the same time or in alternative sequences. Walking is an example of a movement in which the two sides of the body perform the same movements in alternate sequences; lifting and carrying a laundry basket demonstrates a task in which the two upper extremities do the same movements at the same time. Other tasks such as swinging a golf club or operating a clutch require the two sides of the body to do different movements at the same time. Very few movements or tasks are performed completely with only one arm or hand, and those tasks require postural adjustments on the other side of the body.

With the onset of hemiplegia, the stroke patient loses the ability to coordinate both sides of his body in functional patterns. This affects his ability to perform gross motor movements such as rolling in bed, standing up, and walking. It also interferes with his performance of functional tasks necessary for independence in self-care and vocational or recreation activities. Even though one side of the body is unaffected by the stroke, the patient is unable to use his "good" side normally, because normal movement patterns require interaction and coordination between the two sides of the body. The patient may learn to use one-handed techniques to compensate for the loss of control on the other side, but there will be many tasks that he cannot perform unless he regains some use of his hemiplegic side. Because compensatory techniques tend to increase the patient's orientation toward his uninvolved side, they may increase both postural asymmetry and neglect of the involved side. Even when the patient has some ability to move his involved arm and leg, he often has difficulty using these movements efficiently in task performance.

Common problems in the stroke patients can be summarized as follows:

1. Problems associated with CNS damage includes abnormal tone, abnormal patterns of extremity movement, and atypical posture.
2. Problems associated with deficits in control of posture and movement include poor trunk control, decreased balance and protective responses, and poor weight bearing on the hemiplegic hip.
3. Loss of specific motor abilities and task-specific behaviors such as rolling, sitting up, walking, dressing, or bathing independently.

Although the problems listed in categories 1 and 2 may influence motor and task performance, elimination of these symptoms may not automatically result in improved independence in task performance. In other words, changing the tone in a tightly flexed, spastic upper extremity so that the elbow joint can be fully extended may not result in a patient who is actively able to extend his elbow or put his arm in a sleeve during dressing. Similarly, training active elbow extension does not guarantee that the patient will be able to use the movement to put his arm into a shirt sleeve.

Assessment

The NDT/Bobath method of assessment has three basic goals:

1. To determine the presence and distribution of abnormal tone and abnormal movement patterns that are interfering with the production of normal movement;
2. To identify deficits in normal motor responses, including both automatic postural responses and volitional movement patterns in the trunk and limbs;
3. To analyze the patient's ability to perform functional movement patterns, including gross motor tasks and specific self-care, vocational, and recreational activities.

To gather this information, the therapist uses observation of the patient, direct **handling** of the patient's trunk and limbs, and patient interview to help identify problem areas. For a complete list of motor tasks to assess see Bobath (1990).

Handling techniques are used to help the therapist assess the patient's automatic responses to being moved. By using her hands to direct and **facilitate** movement, the therapist can determine the movements and positions that produce tonal changes and the movement patterns in which the patient is able to assist. The therapist will select the positions and activities for assessment according to the patient's general level of functioning and the areas in which he expresses most interest and concern. For the patient who is not yet ambulatory, it is important for both physical and occupational therapists to assess functioning in standing as well as sitting. The physical therapist will use this information to prepare for gait training, whereas the occupational therapist will be concerned with functional performance of self-care and home-making tasks in standing.

Treatment Goals

NDT/Bobath treatment is directed toward achieving functional goals. Normal movement patterns are facilitated with **handling** techniques, then practiced until the patient can perform them independently in a variety of situations and positions. The movements that are emphasized during treatment are those that are necessary for the development of further independence in task performance. For example, helping the acute stroke patient regain control of trunk movements in sitting will allow the patient to balance himself safely on the edge of the bed while putting on his clothes. Thus during the initial treatment sessions, the therapist's **handling** may emphasize trunk movements in sitting to reestablish the postural basis for task performance before dressing. Because lack of trunk control will interfere with arm function as well, the therapist may begin to **facilitate** arm movements in the supine position until the patient has regained adequate sitting balance to combine trunk and arm treatment in sitting. The occupational therapists should try to combine the **facilitation** of trunk and upper extremity movements with the performance of functional tasks as soon as some control of movement has been established. The therapist helps the acute stroke patient **practice** trunk movements during activities of daily living (ADL) and assists him with upper extremity weight bearing during meal time. In this way, the development of motor control can be immediately incorporated into a normal functional task.

In her writings and courses for therapists, B. Bobath stressed the importance of retraining the following functional tasks in patterns incorporating the involved side:

1. Bed mobility tasks such as rolling, moving from supine to sitting by coming over the involved side and using the involved arm for support, and **bridging;**
2. Weight shift in sitting and standing with controlled shifting over the involved leg;
3. Sit-to-stand and transfers toward the involved side without pushing up with the uninvolved arm;
4. Control of the hemiplegic arm in weight-bearing and functional non–weight-bearing patterns;
5. Gait training and balance activities to increase control of the involved leg and decrease use of canes and braces;
6. Activities of daily living and vocational and recreational activities using the involved arm and avoiding patterns that will increase **spasticity.**

Ideally, these tasks are introduced in the acute stage so that the patient learns to incorporate his involved side into all movements and does not develop compensations that ignore the involved side. However, the patient who does not receive NDT/Bobath treatment in the acute stage may still benefit from this treatment later in the rehabilitation process. For this patient, the therapist will improve function by decreasing reliance on the uninvolved side and on adaptive equipment and by increasing use of the involved arm and leg in tasks that are being performed in an abnormal or compensatory manner. For example, the therapist can increase independence in the patient who puts his pants on lying down by increasing control of the trunk and lower extremities so that he can put his legs in the pants while sitting and pull them up and fasten them safely while standing.

NDT/Bobath treatment has three general goals for the adult stroke patient:

1. To decrease the observable symptoms of upper motor neuron lesion such as hypertonicity, asymmetrical posture, and synergistic movements, using techniques of **inhibition;**
2. To increase the normal patterns of coordinated movement in the involved side and between the two sides of the body, using **facilitation techniques;**
3. To improve functional use of the involved side and decrease compensation and use of adaptive equipment.

ACUTE HEMIPLEGIA

During the initial days or weeks after the stroke, treatment goals for all members of the health care team should be directed toward increasing function on the hemiplegic side and preventing the development of **spasticity** and **associated reactions.** The acute stroke patient exhibits severe loss of **postural control** in the trunk and flaccid paralysis of the hemiplegic arm and leg (Fig. 24B.1). The patient has poor sitting balance and cannot perform functional activities in sitting. Bed mobility tasks and transfers require assistance, as the patient avoids weight bearing on his affected leg and does not spontaneously incorporate his affected arm into any movement patterns or activities. Because of the loss of muscle control of the shoulder, the hemiplegic shoulder frequently subluxes inferiorly.

All members of the health care team will approach these same problems with activities specific to their professional expertise. For the occupational therapist, acute care treatment is directed toward:

1. Regaining balance in patterns important for function in sitting;
2. Incorporating the hemiplegic arm into bed mobility and transfers;

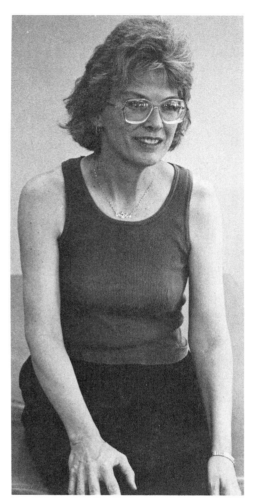

Figure 24B.1. Flaccid hemiplegia with shoulder subluxation on the left side.

3. Developing strategies for self-care activities that involve the affected arm;
4. Maintaining alignment and mobility in the upper extremity;
5. Retraining movement.

HEMIPLEGIA WITH SPASTICITY

Spasticity or hypertonicity develops gradually over a period of weeks or months after the stroke. Although some stroke patients never develop **spasticity,** remaining flaccid on their hemiplegic side or exhibiting motor return without apparent tonal increases, the majority of patients will show signs of hypertonicity in some muscle groups of their involved side. The signs of **spasticity** begin to arise in conjunction with the patient's efforts to become more independent in self-care activities and with the beginning of ambulation. Initially, spastic posturing of the limbs occurs when the patient stands, transfers, and uses

excessive effort to perform self-care activities one handed but is not evident when he is in bed or relaxed in the wheelchair. The first muscles affected are the scapular elevators, flexors of the elbow and fingers, plantar flexors, and extensors of the knee. Gradually, the abnormal posturing of the arm and leg persists for longer periods of the day. At this time, the spastic muscles resist passive stretch and may demonstrate other signs of upper motor neuron syndrome.

The patient at this stage of treatment has more control of his trunk and limbs than in the acute, flaccid stage. Trunk control has improved enough to allow the patient to sit and stand without loss of balance and to walk with a brace and cane. However, the position of the trunk is asymmetrical, with less weight taken on the hemiplegic pelvis and foot, lateral flexion or rotation backward on the hemiplegic ribcage, and flexor **spasticity** in the hemiplegic arm (Fig. 24B.2). Often, the hemiplegic arm has muscle return that allows the pa-

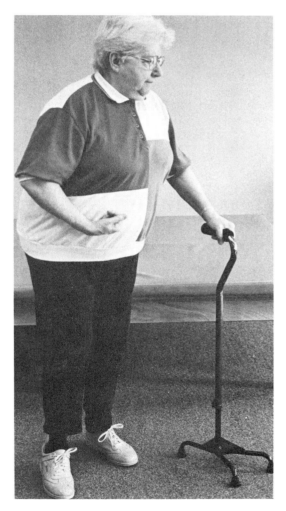

Figure 24B.2. Spastic hemiplegia with flexor spasticity in the hemiplegic arm.

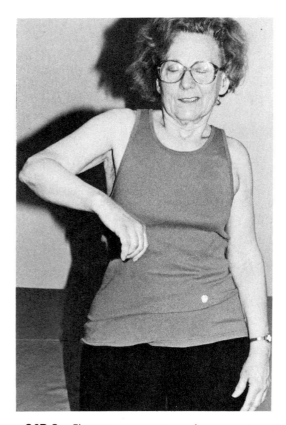

Figure 24B.3. Flexor synergy pattern of movement.

tient to move the arm actively for the first time. However, the patient moves with abnormal coordination and excessive effort in patterns of mass flexion (Fig. 24B.3). The patient cannot isolate individual muscles to perform functional normal movements, nor can he easily stop the muscles from contracting to put his arm back down by his side. Tightness in the muscles connecting the scapula to the trunk and the scapula to the humerus limits the mobility of the scapula and blocks normal scapulohumeral rhythm needed for arm elevation.

During this stage of treatment, the occupational therapist uses NDT/Bobath techniques to **inhibit** the flexor posturing of the arm and to **facilitate** or reeducate normal patterns of upper extremity movement. Upper extremity **spasticity** is inhibited through **scapula mobilization** and upper extremity weight bearing. The therapist also uses NDT/Bobath techniques to train normal patterns of movement in the hemiplegic arm. Weight-bearing activities of the arm are often easiest for the patient to learn, because he does not have to control the weight of the arm as when lifting it for reach. Upper extremity weight bearing activates muscles in the trunk and arm through movements of the body over the arm. The patient should be taught to take weight on his forearm with the arm forward on a table as well

as on the hand with the arm extended by the side of the body. When control of weight bearing has developed, the patient can use his affected arm to help support his body weight during functional activities and transitional movements such as side lying to sitting (Fig. 24B.4). He can also use weight bearing through the hand to help stabilize objects such as paper for writing.

Training of arm movements may begin in supine, in which control of the trunk is not necessary. Sitting treatment is introduced as soon as the patient can sit without support, because he will need to use the arm in an upright position for most functions. Shoulder movements with elbow extension are introduced first, and flexion and extension movements of the elbow are added as shoulder control increases. When the patient can move his arm independently in some patterns, he is encouraged to **practice** using these movements in task performance. For example, the patient who can lift his arm with elbow extension could **practice** using this movement to put his arm in his sleeve, to use a sponge to clean the kitchen counter, or to reach forward to shake hands.

At this stage of treatment, the patient also should learn to grasp objects with a cylindrical palmar grasp, as when holding a cane or hairbrush, and with a flat open hand, as when holding a bowl or a package between two hands. Bilateral grasp activities allow the

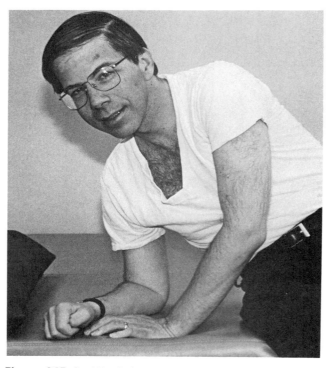

Figure 24B.4. Weight bearing on the hemiplegic arm in moving from side lying to sitting.

patient to **practice** moving independently using the uninvolved side to provide sensory information to the hemiplegic side about how to move (Fig. 24B.5). Grasp activities should be included in treatment only when the wrist and forearm are positioned appropriately, so that the patient learns to contract his finger flexors with wrist extension. As the patient develops control of grasp, he should **practice** carrying objects.

THE HIGHER-LEVEL PATIENT

Many patients with hemiplegia do not progress beyond the problems associated with **spasticity** and do not develop the upper extremity control described earlier. However, some patients never demonstrate **spasticity** in their involved side and other patients respond to treatment techniques designed to **inhibit spasticity** and increase the motor control of their arm and leg. These patients can walk well and do not show marked asymmetries of posture, because they have relatively good control of weight bearing on the hemiplegic leg and minimal flexor posturing of the arm. These patients are able to move their hemiplegic arms with isolated control of the shoulder and elbow and to grasp a variety of objects in their hand when the objects are placed there. They have more problems opening the hand to initiate grasp, extending the fingers with wrist extension for active release of grasp, and controlling humeral and forearm rotation for accurate hand placement. When using their arms functionally, these patients complain of the excessive concentration necessary to produce the desired movement and the slowness and uncoordinated quality of the arm movement. Pro-

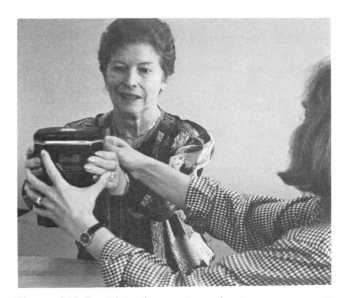

Figure 24B.5. Bilateral grasp to reeducate arm movements and increase arm function.

tective extension and automatic balance reactions in the arm are usually absent or delayed.

Occupational therapy goals for these patients are directed to improving the speed and automaticity of arm movements, introducing variability into hand grasp patterns, and improving control of finger extensors necessary for controlled release of grasp. Hand movements can be practiced in isolation to reeducate specific finger movements or in combination with movements of the forearm and wrist to perfect hand placement. Finger movements and grasp patterns should also be practiced in a variety of arm and body positions and in tasks requiring repetitive grasp and release. For the patient whose finger dexterity and speed have improved, the occupational therapist should introduce tasks that require manipulation of objects and bilateral coordination. At this stage of treatment, the patient should replace one-handed techniques and compensatory task performance with use of the two hands as much as possible. In this way, full potential of the involved arm for function will be realized and any remaining reluctance of the patient to use his arm overcome.

TREATMENT

Handling

Bobath and Bobath called their techniques of treatment **inhibition** and **facilitation** and the implementation of these techniques, **handling.** The term **handling** refers to the way that the therapist uses her hands on the patient's body to change the quality of his movement patterns. **Handling** is used to establish normal alignment, to reduce or eliminate abnormal tone and movement, to reeducate muscles in normal patterns in the trunk and limbs, and to produce an active movement pattern in the stroke patient. Through the experience of being moved by the therapist, the patient relearns the feeling of normal movement, and uses this as a sensory base for his attempts to move independently. Bobath and Bobath believed that the sensory experience of normal movement is the basis for learning new movement patterns and assists the patient in suppressing unwanted abnormal patterns.

During **handling,** the therapist's hands are placed on the patient's body in selected positions. The term **key points of control** describes areas of the body that make it easier to control the quality of the patient's movement pattern. The shoulder, pelvis, and spine/ribcage are key points to control proximal alignment and movement patterns, and the hand and foot are distal key points that are combined with proximal contact to control extremity movement. The therapist selects her hand placement according to the patient's problems and the movement patterns she wishes to reeducate. Proximal hand placements allow the therapist to control the position and movement of the trunk and pelvic and scapular girdles and are generally used with an acute or flaccid patient. As the therapist feels the patient actively assisting in trunk movements and balance, hand placement may move more distally, giving the patient independent control of the trunk or girdles. A combination of shoulder or axillary control with control of the hand is used for training movement in the upper extremity.

Handling is done slowly, to give the patient time to understand what movements are being performed and to organize his response. The therapist is looking for a change in the quality of the patient's muscle tone or active assistance from him, indicating normal muscle activity. Strong and firm hand pressure is used to lengthen spastic muscles and to stop abnormal patterns of coordination. Light pressure is used to guide the patient in a normal movement pattern, to teach the feeling of normal movement, and to elicit an active response from the patient. When the patient is able actively to assist with the movements, the therapist decreases her control and uses repetition and **practice** to let learning occur. In all parts of the NDT/Bobath approach, the patient should be an active and motivated participant.

The patient's hemiplegic side is incorporated into all treatment activities. This may be either by direct **handling** by the therapist, or through bilateral activities in which the patient supports movements of his involved arm or leg with his uninvolved arm. When treating the patient, the therapist positions herself on the hemiplegic side or directly in front of the patient so that his attention and visual regard are directed toward what is happening during the treatment. Because many hemiplegic patients are fearful of falling and do not have accurate processing of sensory information from the hemiplegic side, the therapist uses verbal descriptions and simple commands to tell the patient what she is doing and what his expected and actual responses are. While it is possible to use **handling** with aphasic patients to produce movement without verbal interaction, verbal communication between therapist and patient should be used with **handling** to give the patient feedback on his performance as well as to establish a successful working relationship.

Inhibition techniques are manual techniques and hand placements used to decrease or eliminate **spasticity.** In the early stages of their treatment, Bobath and Bobath used passive positioning to lengthen spastic muscles. They called these positions **reflex inhibiting postures.** Although these patterns were important because they demonstrated to a skeptical neurologic community that **spasticity** could be changed, Bobath and Bobath soon concluded that such patterns did not necessarily improve the patient's ability to function or change the quality of his movements (Bobath, 1990). As the treatment evolved, use of static postures was eliminated and more dynamic **handling** was devised to simultaneously reduce **spasticity** and prepare for movement. The term *reflex-inhibiting movement patterns* describes the active movements that both **inhibit** abnormal tone and encourage or facilitate active movement responses. For the stroke patient, NDT/Bobath **inhibition techniques** are used to:

1. Correct alignment, lengthen shortened muscles, and decrease abnormal tone in specific muscles;
2. Stop unwanted movement patterns from occurring;
3. Teach the patient methods of decreasing the abnormal posturing of his limbs.

Inhibition techniques are not used in patients who do not have **spasticity** or **associated reactions.**

Common techniques of **inhibition** include trunk rotation, weight bearing, and techniques to lengthen muscles and realign joints. Rotational movements of the spine are used to decrease **spasticity** in the trunk, and scapular and pelvic girdles. Weight bearing is used to decrease **spasticity** in the arm and leg, because movements of the trunk over the fixed extremities lengthen tight muscles between the trunk and limbs. In the arm and leg, the pull of spastic muscles is **inhibited** by returning the affected body parts to normal alignment and slowly lengthening the tight muscles in a proximal to distal sequence. **Scapula mobilization** is an example of an upper extremity **inhibition technique** used to reposition the scapula and lengthen the tight muscles around the shoulder girdle.

Facilitation techniques are those patterns of **handling** that help the patient move more normally. The term is taken from the verb, **facilitate,** which means to make easier. Facilitation **handling** techniques are designed to:

1. Teach the sensation of normal movement by moving the limbs in space with proper patterns of initiation and sequencing;
2. Stimulate muscles directly to contract isometrically, eccentrically, and isotonically,;
3. Hold alignment and provide postural stability while the patient **practices** movement;
4. Reeducate normal movement patterns;
5. Teach the patient ways to incorporate the involved side into transitional movements and functional activities.

These techniques are used with both spastic and flaccid hemiplegia.

Facilitation, through guided movement, teaches

the patient the sensation of movement, to allow the patient the opportunity to move with the therapist before moving independently. In the initial stages of treatment, the therapist establishes normal alignment and guides the patient's body and limbs in normal patterns of movement. The patient is encouraged to assist with the movement when he can. As the patient begins to assist, the therapist first lightens, then eliminates a portion of her control so that the patient has opportunities within each treatment session to move independently. Many patients do not know that they can move their arms or bodies in the desired patterns until the **handling** of the therapist makes it possible for them to find the correct muscles. The active assistive quality of **facilitation** also helps to decrease the excessive effort that many hemiplegic patients use to initiate active movement of their involved side.

In cases of flaccid hemiplegia, **facilitation techniques** may be combined with stronger stimulation to increase muscle tone and produce active muscle contraction. For these patients, Bobath and Bobath developed **stimulation techniques,** which use tactile and proprioceptive input to increase the intensity and duration of muscle contraction. NDT/Bobath **stimulation techniques** are applied directly to muscle or via joint approximation to stimulate muscle contraction around the joint. These techniques are performed with the body in normal alignment and directed toward areas of the body that are critical for a normal movement pattern. For example, **stimulation techniques** could be used to increase muscle contraction around the shoulder of a flaccid arm. After carefully aligning the scapula and glenohumeral joint, **stimulation techniques** (tapping over muscle bellies) would be applied to the deltoid and scapular muscles as the patient attempted to bear weight on the glenohumeral joint. **Stimulation techniques** must be used carefully to avoid producing an abnormal response in the muscles being stimulated. Once muscle contraction is established, the therapist returns to guided movement to use the muscle contraction in a movement pattern.

Compensatory Training

Stroke causes long-standing muscle weakness and loss of trunk control, which interfere with the normal use of the involved arm and leg. While many stroke patients eventually regain good use of their hemiplegic side, they must begin the process of becoming independent in life tasks long before they have sufficient use of their arm and leg to perform these tasks normally. For this reason, compensatory training is necessary. In the NDT/Bobath framework, compensatory training is directed toward (1) incorporating the involved arm into task performance and (2) teaching patterns of compensation that do not encourage the development of **spasticity** and **associated reactions.**

Much of the Bobath compensatory training uses symmetrical, bilateral upper extremity patterns to maintain alignment of the upper trunk and shoulder girdle and prevent the arm from being neglected or abnormally positioned. The patient may be taught to clasp his hemiplegic hand with his other hand and maintain the arm in a position of extension during rolling, transfers, and other gross motor activities. The hemiplegic arm can also be placed in a position of weight bearing during task performance in sitting and standing. These concepts will be presented in more detail below.

RETRAINING TRUNK MOVEMENTS

The acute stroke patient is unable to maintain his balance in sitting and cannot perform functional activities such as bathing and dressing in sitting, because he has lost control of the automatic postural patterns that make performance of these activities possible. To help the patient improve task performance in sitting, the occupational therapist must retrain patterns of trunk movement. This training is done first with the therapist assisting the patient in performing the trunk movements. Trunk movements are easiest to reeducate when the patient is seated on a treatment mat or firm chair.

The therapist stands in front of the patient and places both of the patient's hands against her own hips to keep the patient's upper body symmetrical and to protect his hemiplegic shoulder joint. Trunk movements in anterior-posterior, lateral, and rotational directions are then practiced, with the therapist controlling the direction and range of the movements. Movement forward toward the floor and sideways toward the plinth should be practiced as well as movements in upright sitting, because these movements prepare the patient to control body movements in the direction of the pull of gravity (Fig. 24B.6). As muscle control improves and the patient begins to assist in the weight shifts, the patient can **practice** the movements while supporting his hemiplegic hand with his good hand without the assistance of the therapist.

The occupational therapist will make the movements functional for the patient in two ways: (1) combining the weight shifts with reaching tasks and (2) helping the patient incorporate the appropriate movements with the performance of an actual task such as dressing or bathing. The hemiplegic arm is easily positioned for upper extremity dressing by having the patient put his hemiplegic hand in the sleeve, then lean forward toward the floor to assist elbow extension

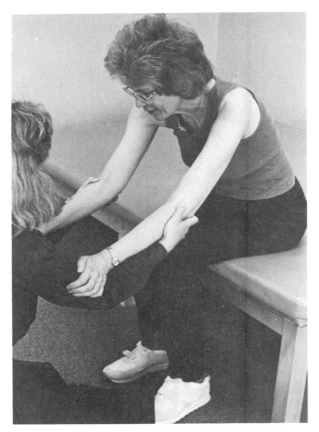

Figure 24B.6. Retraining trunk movements with the hemiplegic arm supported on the therapist's body.

and shoulder flexion, making it easier to pull the sleeve up over the arm.

INCORPORATING THE HEMIPLEGIC ARM

It is important that the hemiplegic arm be incorporated into the early training of gross motor activities such as rolling, coming to sitting, and coming to standing and transfers. Including the arm in training these activities helps decrease neglect of the arm; protects it from injury; and by maintaining good alignment of the shoulder girdle and trunk, prepares the arm for normal participation in the tasks being trained. Bobath and Bobath developed the technique of clasped hands to give the hemiplegic patient a consistent way to hold and move his hemiplegic arm. In the original technique, the patient was taught to interlace the fingers of his hemiplegic hand with his good hand, keeping palms together and thumbs facing up (Fig. 24B.7). The clasped hand grip helps the patient maintain his forearm in mid-position and his wrist in extension, thus preparing the arm for patterns of reach and preventing the wrist flexion that is common in hemiplegic arms. Because many patients have difficulty with the task of interlacing their fingers or cannot maintain the palmar

contact necessary for wrist extension, it is helpful to teach a variation of the technique. For the modification, the patient places the ulnar border of his hemiplegic hand and wrist in the palm of his other hand, with the uninvolved thumb in the palmar arch and the fingers clasping the dorsum of the hand, wrist and ulna. In this way, wrist extension and forearm rotation are easily maintained and the weight of the lower arm and hand are well supported (Fig. 24B.8). Once the hands are clasped, the arms are brought forward with a straight elbow until the desired range of shoulder flexion has been obtained. The patient can use this grip for self-ranging activities in supine and sitting as well as in rolling and transfers.

Bed Mobility

Rolling to both sides is trained by starting in supine with both knees bent and feet on the bed. The patient is directed to locate his hemiplegic arm in the bed and clasp it, using one of the grips described above. Using his uninvolved arm, he extends his elbows and lifts his hands toward the ceiling until the shoulders are flexed to approximately 90°. The patient is then helped to turn his head and shoulders to the involved side, so that the rolling begins with the upper body. Rolling is completed by turning the knees and pelvis to the same side until the side-lying position is achieved. Rolling from side lying to supine is easiest if the pelvis

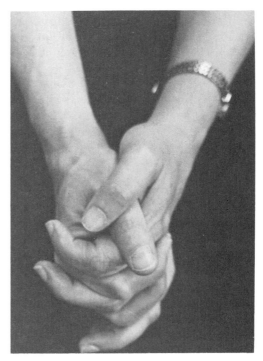

Figure 24B.7. Clasped hands. The patient lifts his hemiplegic arm by interlacing his fingers and holding the palms together.

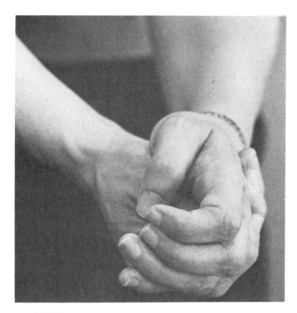

Figure 24B.8. Variation of clasped hands. The patient supports the ulnar border of his hemiplegic hand in the opposite palm.

and knees rotate first, followed by the arms and upper body. The movements can then be practiced toward the uninvolved side (Fig. 24B.9). Lying on the involved side should not be painful using this technique, because the forward reach of the arm that precedes rolling puts the hemiplegic shoulder in a good position. Reaching the clasped hands forward and up can also be used in combination with **bridging** for use of the bedpan and in moving up or sideways on the bed. By reaching the arms forward with elbow extension, flexor **spasticity** of the elbow is inhibited during these activities.

Transfers

For the acute stroke patient, the task of transferring is frightening because he lacks good control of the hemiplegic side. To incorporate the arm into early transfer training, the therapist faces the patient. She supports the patient's arm on her waist and has him place his other arm on her opposite hip (Fig. 24B.10). This grip allows the therapist to support the weight of the patient's arm, to keep his trunk symmetrical, and to **facilitate** the correct forward weight shift while he maintains spinal extension to produce a good stand. As the patient learns to control trunk extension and shift forward over both hips to use both legs to stand, the patient can advance to practicing with the clasped hands grip to control his own arm (Fig. 24B.11). By teaching the patient to stand and transfer without push-

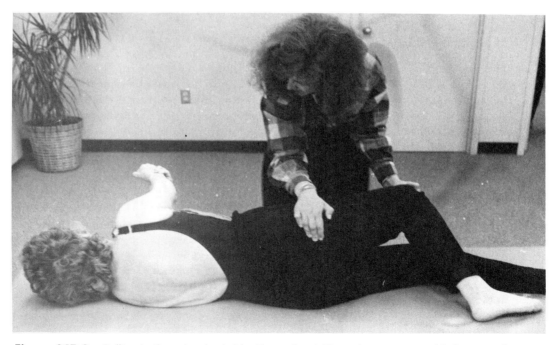

Figure 24B.9. Rolling to the uninvolved side. The patient initiates the movement with the arms, then uses the hemiplegic leg to assist with rotation of the lower body.

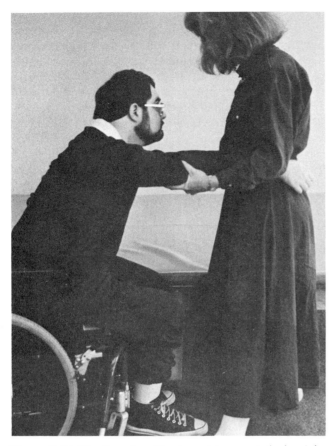

Figure 24B.10. Transfers. The therapist supports the hemiplegic arm against her body and assists the patient in an anterior weight shift with trunk extension to prepare for the stand.

ing with his uninvolved arm, the therapist helps prevent the development of asymmetrical patterns of movement and introduces normal control of the trunk, pelvis and lower extremity. The patient is taught to transfer to both sides, so that he is able to function well in a variety of room arrangements.

TREATMENT OF THE HEMIPLEGIC ARM

Scapula Mobilization

The techniques of **scapula mobilization** are used with the acute hemiplegic patient to maintain scapula/humeral alignment and mobility, to maintain muscle length around the shoulder and elbow, to minimize the development of **spasticity,** and to prevent shoulder pain. They are also used with the patient with upper extremity **spasticity** to restore mobility and alignment to the shoulder girdle and systematically to lengthen tight muscles in the arm. **Scapula mobilization** is done primarily in supine but can also be done in sitting and in side lying on the uninvolved side.

To mobilize the scapula in supine, the therapist sits on the bed on the patient's hemiplegic side, facing

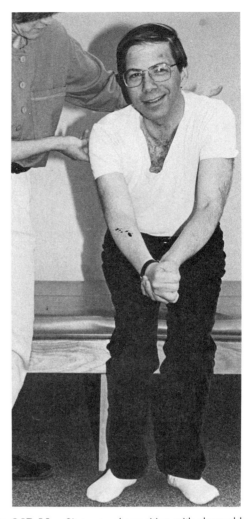

Figure 24B.11. Sit-to-stand transition with clasped hands.

his head. She places her outside hand on the top of the shoulder and her inside hand on the humerus, externally rotating the shoulder joint to neutral. The patient's lower arm is cradled against her body. Then, using both hands together, the therapist moves the scapula up and down into elevation and depression, and forward and back into abduction/adduction (Fig. 24B.12). If the scapula moves freely in these planes with the arm by the side of the body, the patient's arm may be brought forward into 30 to 60° of flexion with external rotation at the shoulder and elbow extension. As the therapist moves the arm into flexion, she must also move her own body position. The scapula movements are then repeated. If no resistance is met, the arm is again brought into a greater degree of flexion, but as the shoulder position approaches 90° of flexion, the therapist moves her hand from the top of the shoulder to position it on the vertebral border of the scapula so that she may assist the scapula to upwardly

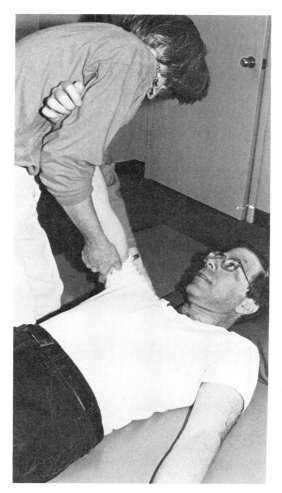

Figure 24B.12. Mobilization of the scapula in supine to maintain or restore normal scapula/humeral rhythm.

rotate. When the patient has no pain and the scapula is rotating, the arm may be brought over the head into full shoulder flexion and out into full abduction to maintain passive range of motion and muscle length. For shoulder movements above 60° of flexion, the humerus must be externally rotated to prevent jamming the head against the acromium process and impinging the supraspinatus tendon. If pain occurs, the arm must be lowered, the humerus externally rotated, and scapular movements repeated in the lowered position.

Place and Hold

Place and hold activities are introduced following mobilization of the scapula when there is no **spasticity**, the arm can be moved passively without pain, and scapulohumeral rhythm is intact. In supine, the arm is brought into 90° or more shoulder flexion as described above. The therapist then moves her hand from the patient's shoulder to take his hemiplegic hand with her hand. Using her two hands together, she guides the arm into abduction and adduction or slight flexion and extension, asking the patient to assist her movements. As she feels the patient assist, she asks him to try to hold his arm in the position it is in, maintaining her own support of the arm but lightening her assistance. The patient may also be guided through elbow flexion to the top of his head and back into extension. As the patient's control of his arm increases, the therapist will be able to let go of her contact with the arm while the patient "places and holds" it in position. With **practice,** the patient will learn to control the arm through a larger range of shoulder and elbow movements as well as forearm rotation and wrist and finger movements.

Arm Movements in Sitting

In sitting, subluxation of the glenohumeral joint must be corrected before the hemiplegic arm can be passively moved or treated. Subluxation or separation of the humerus from the acromium joint of the scapula occurs when the scapula downwardly rotates on the ribcage, changing the angulation of the slope of the glenoid fossa and allowing the humerus to slip out of the joint (Fig. 24B.13). Scapular downward rotation is common in acute hemiplegia, because the muscles

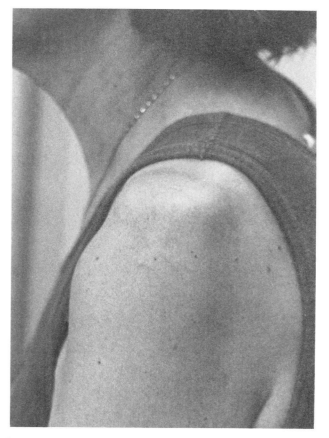

Figure 24B.13. Inferior subluxation of the shoulder.

connecting the scapula to the trunk are flaccid and cannot maintain the weight of the arm against the pull of gravity. Abnormal trunk postures, especially excessive flexion of the upper spine or lateral flexion of the spine with the concavity to the hemiplegic side, encourage malpositioning of the scapula. Inferior subluxation is accompanied by internal rotation of the humerus (Ryerson & Levit, 1991).

To reseat the humeral head into the fossa, the therapist supports the joint from underneath in the axilla, trying first to correct trunk position and upwardly rotate the scapula. She must then use her other hand to lift the humerus up into the fossa and externally rotate it to neutral (Fig. 24B.14).

When the glenohumeral joint has been repositioned, the therapist may progress to reeducation of arm movements. The therapist sits next to the patient on the mat, facing the patient's hemiplegic side. She uses her back hand to support the hemiplegic shoulder and uses her front hand to take the patient's hemiplegic hand as if she were shaking hands with him (Fig. 24B.15). She then uses both her hands to guide the patient's arm into shoulder flexion and abduction, and elbow flexion and extension. Guided arm movements can be practiced using an object target to prepare for reach. They can also be practiced with the patient holding an object in the hemiplegic hand. As motor control of the arm improves, the therapist removes one or both of her hands, allowing the patient to perform part of the movement independently.

Forearm Weight Bearing in Sitting

Forearm weight bearing in sitting can be used to maintain scapular alignment and mobility and to activate muscles of the trunk and arm. Weight bearing on the arm is also one of the earliest ways to incorporate the flaccid upper extremity into functional activities. Forearm weight bearing requires less trunk and arm

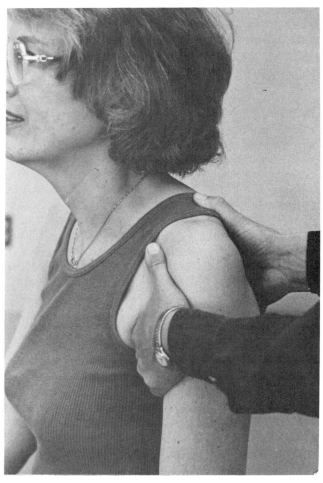

Figure 24B.14.   Reduction of shoulder subluxation by correcting scapular rotation and lifting the humerus up into the glenoid fossa.

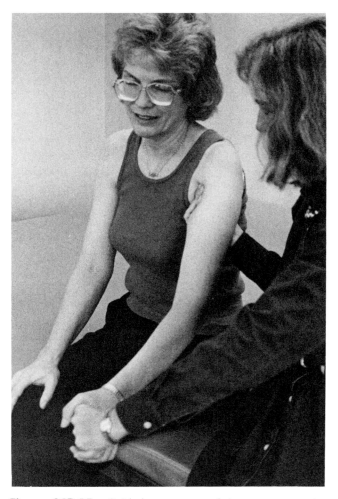

Figure 24B.15.   Guided movements of the upper extremity. The therapist maintains alignment of the shoulder joint while reeducating arm movements.

control than weight bearing on an extended arm and is usually the first weight-bearing task introduced in treatment.

To teach forearm weight bearing, the patient is seated with both forearms resting on a table in front of him, hands in line with the shoulder joint. The therapist may hold the patient's hand on the table if the arm is very floppy or support the glenohumeral joint at the axilla if it is badly subluxed (Fig. 24B.16). The therapist then guides the patient in sitting weight shifts, especially anterior weight shifts to the table (which will develop trunk extension and increase the weight on the hemiplegic arm) and lateral weight shifts to both sides (which will assist in increasing the weight on the hemiplegic hip and activating the muscles of the hemiplegic trunk). As the patient moves his trunk around his arms, the scapula position on the ribcage is changed and muscle length is maintained. The therapist may initially **facilitate** the correct trunk movements, using the spine and ribcage to guide the correct pattern. When the patient is able to move his trunk independently, the therapist can change control to the scapula to **facilitate** the correct shoulder movements. Trunk movements and forearm weight bearing can be used during morning grooming activities with the patient's arm positioned on the sink. They are also easy to combine with eating and other functional tabletop activities (Fig. 24B.17). Having the patient reach with his uninvolved arm while weight bearing on the hemiplegic arm increases the control demands of both the trunk and the arm.

EFFECTIVENESS

As was mentioned earlier, the Bobath techniques were developed through patient treatment, with the goal of improving the control of movement of the hemiplegic side. K. Bobath formulated a scientific explanation for the effectiveness of B. Bobath's clinical techniques based on the scientific research on brain function that was available in the 1940s. Bobath and Bobath believed that the physical impairments associated with stroke (i.e., **spasticity** and disorders of posture and movement) were the result of loss of cortical inhibition and that their treatment, by normalizing sensory feedback from the periphery, helped reorganize motor output from the CNS (Bobath, 1990). Both assumptions were based on a hierarchical model of CNS organization and control of movement that has since been modified (Gordon, 1987). NDT/Bobath treatment has been challenged in the therapy literature because of its outdated scientific theory (Ostrosky, 1990). However, NDT/Bobath continues to be widely used in the clinic, and its techniques could be effective even if the science that was originally used to explain them is no longer current.

Few studies exist that examine the effectiveness

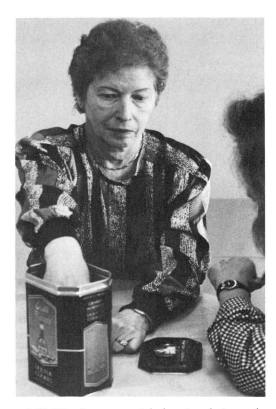

Figure 24B.17. Forearm weight bearing during task performance. The patient uses the hemiplegic arm to support body weight while using the uninvolved arm for skill.

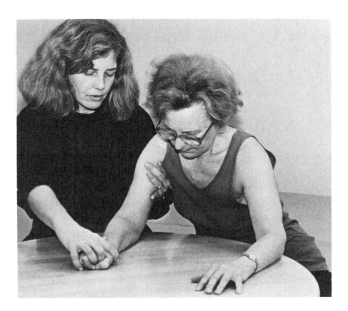

Figure 24B.16. Retraining forearm weight bearing.

of the NDT/Bobath approach with adult stroke patients. A computerized search of all peer-reviewed articles appearing between 1980 and 1990 performed by the Neuro-Developmental Treatment Association (NDTA) research committee identified 41 articles, of which 3 were directly concerned with adult hemiplegia (Royeen & DeGangi, 1992). The remainder were related to NDT/Bobath with cerebral palsy and/or other pediatric diagnoses. The majority of publications do not clearly demonstrate the effectiveness of NDT over other traditional physical and occupational therapy interventions. A major problem contributing to this failure may be the lack of measures sensitive to small changes in movement control, postural responses, and muscle tone.

The studies that related to the treatment of adult hemiplegia did support the effectiveness of NDT/Bobath techniques as well as other treatment approaches in stroke rehabilitation. A study by Basmajian et al. (1987) examined the relative effectiveness of an NDT-based intervention program and a program of cognitive and behavioral training on upper extremity function in 29 stroke patients. The study was well controlled, and the data were subjected to multiple statistical procedures. The authors found that both therapies were effective with stroke patients, but they could identify no significant differences in outcome between the two approaches. These results are similar to those reported by Dickstein et al. (1986) and Logigian et al. (1983).

None of these studies used a control group, and therefore, the possibility of spontaneous recovery causing the observed changes cannot be ruled out. Additional studies on NDT with adult hemiplegia are currently being funded by the NDTA.

STUDY QUESTIONS

1. According to Bobath and Bobath, what are the major problems of the stroke patient?
2. Define the following terms: handling, facilitation, and inhibition. How are these concepts used to treat the problems of adult hemiplegia?
3. What do Bobath and Bobath mean by postural control? What reactions form the parts of this system?
4. What are the scientific theories that Bobath and Bobath used to explain their approach?
5. What is the overall goal of NDT with adult hemiplegia?
6. Why is it important that the occupational therapist help the patient reestablish postural control?
7. How does abnormal tone affect the hemiplegic arm? List several NDT/Bobath techniques that help decrease flexor spasticity in the arm.
8. Why do Bobath and Bobath use bilateral activities and clasped hands with the stroke patient?
9. List several ways that the occupational therapist can incorporate the flaccid arm into gross motor and ADL training.

24C MOVEMENT THERAPY OF BRUNNSTROM

Catherine A. Trombly

Objectives _____

After studying this chapter, the learner will be able to:
1. Understand the premises that underlie Movement Therapy for stroke patients.
2. List the four aspects of movement control that are assessed in the Brunnstrom approach and discuss the methods of evaluating them.
3. Discuss the six stages of recovery for the upper extremity and hand and three stages of recovery for the wrist.
4. Understand the treatment principles of this approach.
5. Understand the treatment procedures to **facilitate** movement control in the trunk and upper extremity of **hemiparetic** patients using this approach.
6. Suggest functional activities suitable to encourage the **practice** of movement control at various stages of recovery.

HISTORY

Brunnstrom, a physical therapist, was particularly concerned with the problems of patients following stroke. Her approach to their treatment has given therapists insight into the behaviors of a master clinician. In developing Movement Therapy, Brunnstrom experimented by applying, in a trial-and-error fashion, procedures that she derived from motor control literature or from observations of patients. She paid careful attention to the patient's motor and verbal reactions to each procedure, interpreted those reactions in light of her knowledge of motor control and development, and adjusted the procedure accordingly. Successful procedures were replicated patient to patient.

The principles of Movement Therapy and the evaluation and treatment procedures presented here are summarized and adapted from Brunnstrom (1970), which describes her approach in detail.

PRINCIPLES

The assumptions that underlie the Movement Therapy approach are as follows.

1. In normal motor development, spinal cord and brainstem reflexes become modified and their components rearranged into purposeful movement through the influence of higher centers. Because reflexes and whole-limb movement patterns are normal stages of development and because stroke appears to result in "development in reverse," reflexes and primitive movement patterns should be used to **facilitate** the recovery of voluntary movement poststroke. Brunnstrom (1956) believed that no reasonable training method should be left untried and stated, "It may well be that a subcortical motion synergy which can be elicited on a reflex basis may serve as a wedge by means of which a limited amount of willed movement may be learned" (p. 225).

2. Proprioceptive and exteroceptive stimuli can be used to evoke desired motion or tonal changes.

3. Recovery of voluntary movement poststroke proceeds in sequence from mass, stereotyped flexor or extensor movement patterns to movements that combine features of the two patterns, and finally to discrete movements of each joint at will. The stereotyped movement patterns are called limb synergies. *Synergy*, in this sense, refers to patterned movements of the entire limb in response to a stimulus or to voluntary effort.

4. Newly produced, correct motions must be practiced to be learned.

5. **Practice** within the context of daily activities enhances the learning process.

The principles of Movement Therapy are listed below.

1. Treatment progresses developmentally, from reflex to voluntary to functional.
2. When no motion exists, movement is facilitated using reflexes, **associated reactions,** proprioceptive **facilitation,** and/or exteroceptive **facilitation** to develop muscle tension in preparation for voluntary movement.
   a. Reflex responses and **associated reactions** elicited in this way combine with the patient's voluntary effort to move, which produces semi-voluntary movement; this allows the patient to experience the sensory feedback associated with movement and the satisfaction of having moved, to some degree, voluntarily.
   b. Proprioceptive and exteroceptive stimuli assist in eliciting movement. Resistance (a proprioceptive stimulus) promotes a spread of impulses to other muscles to produce a patterned response (**associated reaction**), whereas tactile stimulation (exteroceptive) facilitates only the muscles related to the stimulated area.
3. When voluntary effort produces, or contributes to, a response, the patient is asked to hold (isometric) the contraction. If successful, he is asked for an

eccentric (controlled lengthening) contraction and finally a concentric (shortening) contraction.

4. When even only partial movement is possible, reversal of movement from flexion to extension is stressed within each treatment session.

5. **Facilitation** is reduced or dropped out as quickly as the patient shows evidence of volitional control. **Facilitation** procedures are dropped out in order of their stimulus-response binding. Reflexes, in which the response is stereotypically bound to a certain stimulus, are the most primitive and are dropped out of treatment first. Responses to exteroceptive stimulation are least stereotyped, and therefore, tactile stimulation is eliminated last. No primitive reflexes, including **associated reactions,** are used beyond stage 3.

6. Emphasis is placed on willed movement to overcome the linkages between parts of the synergies; willed movement means that the patient is trying to accomplish it. It helps if the person is asked to do a familiar movement, such as reaching for a soft drink can.

7. Correct movement, once elicited, is repeated to learn it; **practice** should include functional activities to increase the willed aspect and to relate the sensations to goal-directed movement.

EVALUATION

Evaluation in the Brunnstrom approach includes determination of the following:

1. The patient's sensory status;
2. The level of recovery of voluntary motor control;
3. The effect of tonic reflexes on the patient's movement;
4. The effect of **associated reactions** on the patient's movement.

Sensation

The sensory evaluation precedes the motor evaluation. The patient's ability to recognize movements of the affected arm and to localize touch in the hand, without looking, are especially noted, because they are associated with better eventual recovery of voluntary movement of the arm and hand, respectively (see Chapter 8 for evaluation procedures). Results of the sensory evaluation guide choice of **facilitation** modalities that the therapist may use to **facilitate** movement or alert the therapist to encourage the patient to substitute visual feedback for lost movement or position senses.

Level of Recovery of Voluntary Movement

Table 24C.1 lists the six stages of recovery of the proximal upper extremity and hand and the three stages of recovery of the wrist that Brunnstrom (1970) identified. Although stroke patients, on average, proceed through these stages, a particular patient may stop at any stage. To date, there are no reliable ways to predict which patients will recover voluntary movement and which will not.

To evaluate stage of recovery, the patient is made physically and psychologically comfortable. The sequential aspects of the motor evaluation (Table 24C.2) are used to determine the patient's level of motor control; no movements beyond the patient's capabilities are demanded. No **facilitation** is used during the evaluation. Each motion is demonstrated to the patient, and he does it with his unaffected extremity before he attempts it with his affected one, so the therapist can be certain that the person understands the request. Instructions should be given in functional terms. For example, to test the **flexor synergy** of the upper extremity, say "Touch behind your ear" and for the extension synergy, "Reach out to touch your [opposite] knee" (Brunnstrom, 1966). The patient's ability to do the requested movement is recorded according to the percentage of range of motion that he completed. For example, when asked for a **flexor synergy** response, if the patient is able to bring the hand only as far as his mouth rather than to his ear, the therapist may observe that he has complete elbow flexion (100%), about 45° of shoulder abduction (50%), supination to midrange (50%), and minimal external rotation (25%). When the patient's response is incomplete, as in this example, it may be necessary to observe the patient's repeated attempts to determine the specific weak areas of the synergy or movement pattern and to decide on the rating. A Polaroid photograph, taken in a standardized way, would provide clear documentation of the patient's abilities before and after a treatment program.

A patient is reported to be in the stage at which he is able to accomplish all motions specified for that stage. Because progress is gradual, there will be instances when the patient is in transition between stages. If he has completed one stage but is just beginning to be able to do the motions of the next stage, many therapists would record his level as "2 going on 3" or "3 going on 4," etc. The upper and lower extremities as well as the hand may all be in different stages of recovery at a given time.

Brunnstrom's evaluation is valid in that it reflects observations made by Twitchell (1951) of the recovery process of 118 patients who had suffered strokes, onset of which ranged from 5 days to 5 years before observation as well as her own observations of 100 patients (Brunnstrom, 1970). A modified, better-defined version of the Brunnstrom and Fugl-Meyer evaluation was used to evaluate recovery of the lower limb of 23 poststroke patients (Clarke et al., 1983). The stage

Table 24C.1.   Recovery Stages of the Upper Extremity

Stage: Arm	Stage: Hand
1. Flaccidity—no voluntary movement	1. Flaccidity
2. Synergies developing—flexion usually develops before extension (may be a weak associated reaction or voluntary contraction with or without joint motion); spasticity developing	2. Little or no active finger flexion
	3. Mass grasp or hook grasp
3. Beginning voluntary movement, but only in synergy; increased spasticity, which may become marked	No voluntary finger extension or release
	4. Lateral prehension with release by thumb movement
4. Some movements deviating from synergy:	Semivoluntary finger extension (small range of motion)
a. Hand behind body;	5. Palmar prehension
b. Arm to forward-horizontal position;	Cylindrical and spherical grasp (awkward)
c. Pronation-supination with elbow flexed to 90°; spasticity decreasing.	Voluntary mass finger extension (variable range of motion)
5. Independence from the basic synergies:	6. All types of prehension (improved skill)
a. Arm to side-horizontal position;	Voluntary finger extension (full range of motion)
b. Arm forward and overhead;	Individual finger movements
c. Pronation-supination with elbow full extended; spasticity waning	
6. Isolated joint movements freely performed with near normal coordination; spasticity minimal	

Table 24C.2.   Hemiplegia—Classification and Progress Record: Upper Limb

Name _____ Age _____ Date of onset _____ Side affected _____

Date   Stage
_____   1. No movement initiated or elicited; flaccidity.
_____   2. Synergies or components may be elicited; spasticity developing. Note extent of response:

Flexor synergy _____

_____

Extensor synergy _____

_____

_____   3. Synergies or components initiated voluntarily; spasticity marked.

Flexor synergy   Percent Active Joint Range

_____   Scapular elevation   _____

_____   Scapular retraction   _____

_____   Shoulder abduction   _____

_____   Shoulder external rotation   _____

_____   Elbow flexion   _____

_____   Forearm supination   _____

Extensor synergy   Percent Active Joint Range

_____   Scapular protraction   _____

_____   Shoulder adduction and internal rotation (pectoralis major)   _____

_____   Elbow extension   _____

_____   Forearm pronation   _____

Table 24C.2.   Continued

_____	4. Movements deviating from basic synergies; spasticity decreasing.	Percent Range of Motion
_____	a. Hand behind back	_____
_____	b. Raise arm to 90° forward flexion	_____
_____	c. Pronation-supination, elbow at 90° flexion	_____
	5. Relative independence of basic synergies; spasticity waning.	Percent Range of Motion
_____	a. Raise arm to 90° abduction	_____
_____	b. Raise arm forward and overhead	_____
_____	c. Pronation-supination, elbow extended	_____
_____	6. Movement coordinated and near normal; spasticity minimal.	

Wrist (describe motion)
_____ 4. Wrist stabilization for grasp
_____   a. Elbow extended _____
_____   b. Elbow flexed _____
_____ 5. Wrist flexion and extension, fist closed
_____   a. Elbow extended _____
_____   b. Elbow flexed _____
_____ 6. Wrist circumduction (stabilize forearm) _____

Digits
_____ 1. Flaccidity; no voluntary movement

_____ 2. Little or no active finger flexion

_____ 3. Mass grasp or hook grasp

_____ 4. a. Lateral prehension; release by thumb movement
_____   b. Semivoluntary mass extension—small range of motion

_____ 5. a. Palmar prehension
_____   b. Voluntary mass extension—variable range of motion
_____   c. Spherical grasp (awkward)
_____   d. Cylindrical grasp (awkward)

_____ 6. a. All types of grasp with improved skill
_____   b. Voluntary finger extension—full range of motion
_____   c. Individual finger movements (do dexterity tests)

of recovery was strongly correlated to key aspects of gait ($r = 0.60$ to 0.88), which supports its **validity.** No data exist concerning the **reliability** of Brunnstrom's version of the evaluation, but the **reliability** can be assumed to be low, because the rating scales are not operationally defined. To improve **reliability,** Fugl-Meyer et al. (1975) operationally defined 50 details of joint motion of the limbs, across the six levels of recovery. The *Fugl-Meyer Motor Test* uses an ordinal level scoring system in which each detail is rated 0 (cannot be performed), 1 (can be partly performed), or 2 (can be performed faultlessly). Total scores range from 0 (**flaccidity**) to 100 (normal motor function). Intrarater and interrater **reliability** of the upper extremity subtest (33 items) were determined to be strong ($r = 0.99$) and significant (Duncan, Propst, & Nelson, 1983).

Because recovery proceeds sequentially, once the stage of recovery is identified, the short-term goal becomes the next step in the recovery sequence.

Tonic Reflexes

Tonic reflexes are assessed to determine whether they can be used in early treatment to initiate movement when none exists. The primitive reflexes that may be present include the symmetrical and asymmetrical tonic neck reflexes, tonic labyrinthine reflexes, and tonic lumbar reflexes. With the exception of the tonic lumbar reflexes, the evaluation of these reflexes was described in Chapter 7.

The tonic lumbar reflex is elicited by helping the patient rotate his upper trunk in relation to his pelvis. If the reflex is active, flexor tone increases in the upper extremity and extensor tone in the lower extremity on the side toward which the trunk is turned. Simultaneously, extensor tone increases in the upper extremity and flexor tone in the lower extremity on the side opposite to the direction of rotation. A change in tone is gauged by comparing the amount of resistance to passive stretch under the test condition to a neutral (unrotated) condition.

Associated Reactions

Associated reactions are involuntary movements or patterned, reflexive increases of tone in those muscles that would be expected to contract to cause the movement. **Associated reactions** are seen in the involved extremities of stroke patients when other parts of the body are resisted during movement or an effort to move is exerted. **Associated reactions** are evaluated to determine which could be used to **facilitate** movement when no voluntary movement exists. They are more easily elicited when **spasticity** is present. **Associated reactions** seen in stroke patients and how to evoke them are as follows:

1. **Flexor synergy** in the involved upper extremity is elicited by applying resistance to shoulder elevation or elbow flexion of the noninvolved upper extremity.
2. **Extensor synergy** in the involved upper extremity is elicited by applying resistance to horizontal adduction of the noninvolved upper extremity, which is equivalent to Raimiste's phenomenon.
3. Raimiste's phenomena are **associated reactions** of hip abduction or adduction. Resistance to hip abduction or adduction of the noninvolved extremity evokes the same motion of the involved extremity.
4. Resistance to flexion of the noninvolved leg causes extension of the involved extremity, and resistance to extension of the noninvolved side causes flexion of the involved extremity.
5. Resisted grasp by the noninvolved hand causes a grasp reaction in the involved hand.
6. Flexor movement or tone may be elicited in the involved arm when the patient attempts to flex the leg or when leg flexion is resisted. This reaction is called homolateral synkinesis.

Basic Limb Synergies

Limb synergies may be elicited as **associated reactions** or may occur as early stages of voluntary control when **spasticity** is present. When the patient initiates a movement of one joint, all muscles that are linked in synergy with that movement automatically contract, causing a stereotyped movement pattern.

In the upper extremity, the **flexor synergy** is composed of scapular retraction and/or elevation, shoulder abduction and external rotation, elbow flexion, and forearm supination. Position of the wrist and fingers is variable. Elbow flexion is the strongest component

of the **flexor synergy** and the first motion to appear (or to be facilitated). Shoulder abduction and external rotation are weak components. Shoulder hyperextension may be seen when abduction and external rotation are weak, although it is not considered part of the **flexor synergy** (LaVigne, 1974).

The **extensor synergy** of the upper extremity is composed of scapular protraction, shoulder horizontal adduction and internal rotation, elbow extension, forearm pronation, and variable wrist and finger motion, although wrist extension and finger flexion may be seen. The pectoralis major is the strongest component of the extension synergy; consequently, shoulder horizontal adduction and internal rotation are the first motions to appear (or to be facilitated). Pronation is the next strongest component. Elbow extension is a weak component.

The upper extremity **flexor synergy** usually develops before the **extensor synergy.** When both synergies are developing and **spasticity** is marked, the strongest components of the flexion and extension synergies sometimes combine to produce the typical upper extremity posture in hemiplegia: The arm is adducted and internally rotated with the elbow flexed, forearm pronated, and the wrist and fingers flexed.

The lower extremity **flexor synergy** is composed of hip flexion, abduction, and external rotation; knee flexion; dorsiflexion and inversion of the ankle; and dorsiflexion of the toes. In this synergy, hip flexion is the strongest component, whereas hip abduction and external rotation are weak components.

The lower extremity **extensor synergy** is composed of hip extension, adduction, and internal rotation; knee extension, plantar flexion and inversion of the ankle, and plantar flexion of the toes. Hip adduction, knee extension, and plantar flexion of the ankle with inversion are all strong components. Weak components of this synergy are hip extension, hip internal rotation, and plantar flexion of the toes. Note that ankle inversion occurs in both lower extremity synergies.

The lower extremity **extensor synergy** is dominant in a standing position, because of the strength of this synergy combined with the influences of the positive supporting reaction and stretch forces against the sole of the foot that elicit plantar flexion.

TREATMENT

The focus of treatment is the recapitulation of normal movement developmentally from its reflexive base to voluntary control of individual motions that can be used functionally.

Rehabilitating Trunk Control

Some patients with hemiplegia may have poor trunk control and may require training to enable them to bend over to retrieve an object from the floor or to dress their lower extremities. To elicit balance responses, the patient is gently pushed in forward, backward, and side-to-side directions. At first, emphasis is given to promoting contraction of trunk muscles on the noninvolved side by pushing the patient off balance toward the involved side while guarding in case of poor response. Then, once it is determined that the person has that skill, recovery from a push toward the noninvolved side is sought. The patient is pushed only to the point at which he is able to hold the position and then regain upright posture and is guarded throughout. Training then progresses to promote trunk flexion, extension, and rotation.

Practice in forward flexion of the trunk is assisted. The patient crosses his arms with the noninvolved hand under the involved elbow and the noninvolved forearm supporting the involved forearm. The therapist, sitting facing the patient, supports the patient under the elbows and assists in trunk flexion forward, avoiding any pull on the shoulders. Some pain-free shoulder flexion is accomplished during this forward movement. The patient is concentrating on trunk control, and shoulder movement occurs without conscious awareness. Return from trunk flexion is performed actively by the patient. Then, while sitting without back support and with the involved arm supported as described above, the patient is pushed backward and encouraged to regain upright posture actively. Forward flexion in oblique directions is then done not only to promote regaining balance but also to incorporate more scapular motion with the shoulder flexion already achieved.

Trunk rotation is then practiced with the patient supporting his involved arm and the therapist guiding trunk motion. Trunk rotation can be combined with head movements in the opposite direction of the trunk rotation, so that the tonic neck and tonic lumbar reflexes can be utilized as one way to begin to elicit the shoulder components of the upper extremity synergies. The arms and trunk move in one direction while the head turns in the opposite direction. Head and trunk movements are combined with increasing ranges of movement of the shoulder, enabling pain-free shoulder and scapular abduction and adduction to be accomplished during trunk rotation.

Retraining Proximal Upper Extremity Control

STAGES 1 TO 3

The goal of treatment is to promote voluntary control of the synergies and to encourage their use in purposeful activities. In these stages, all movements occur in synergy patterns but with increasing voluntary initiation and control of these patterns.

To move the patient from stage 1 (**flaccidity**) to stage 2 (beginning synergy), the basic limb synergies are elicited at a reflex level, using as many reflexes, **associated reactions,** and **facilitation** procedures as are necessary to elicit a response. The effects of these procedures combine to produce a stronger response. The patient tries to move (willed movement) as these **facilitation** techniques are used.

The **flexor synergy** is the first to develop. Within that synergy, the strongest component, elbow flexion, is the first motion to be elicited. Once elbow flexion is seen, the therapist turns concentration from elbow flexion to the proximal components of the synergy with the goal of enabling the patient to "capture the synergy," i.e., bring it under voluntary control (stage 3). Efforts to achieve voluntary control of the **flexor synergy** begin with scapular elevation. Lateral flexion of the neck toward the involved side can be used to initiate scapular elevation because the upper trapezius does both motions although it may have "forgotten" how to elevate the scapula. With the patient's arm supported on a table in shoulder abduction with elbow flexion, resistance is given simultaneously to the head and shoulder while the patient is asked to "hold" the head and not let it be moved away from the shoulder. When the trapezius is felt to respond, both the patient's effort and the therapist's resistance emphasize shoulder elevation when lateral flexion of the neck is repeated. Once elevation begins, active contraction may be promoted by an **associated reaction.** For example, as the patient attempts bilateral scapular elevation, resistance is given to the noninvolved scapula. If the involved scapula elevates as a result of an **associated reaction,** resistance is then added on the involved side as the patient is asked to "hold."

Unilateral scapular elevation of the involved arm is attempted next and may be achieved as a result of the previous procedures. If the patient is unable to accomplish the motion, the therapist supports the patient's arm and assists the patient to elevate the scapula. Percussion or stroking over the upper trapezius will **facilitate** muscle contraction. The patient is then told to hold, "Don't let me push your shoulder down." After repeated holding with some resistance added, the patient does an eccentric contraction—lets the shoulder down slowly. Then a concentric, or shortening, contraction is attempted when the person is told, "Now pull your shoulder up toward your ear." Active scapular elevation evokes other flexor components and tends to **inhibit** the pectoralis major. The patient repeats scapular elevation and relaxation as the therapist gently abducts the shoulder in increasing increments. because many patients with hemiplegia experience shoulder

pain and/or have shoulder subluxation, the shoulder is given special care, and the correct scapulohumeral orientation is maintained. Once shoulder elevation and some active abduction have been achieved, external rotation and forearm supination are then included in the movement. Reversal of movements into the opposite direction are done from the start and this begins to develop some components of the **extensor synergy.**

The **extensor synergy** tends to follow the **flexor synergy** and may need to be assisted in its initiation. Contraction of the pectoralis major, a strong component of the **extensor synergy,** can be elicited by the **associated reaction** in which the therapist supports the patient's arms in a position between horizontal abduction and adduction, instructs the patient to bring his arms together, and resists the noninvolved arm just proximal to the elbow. As contraction occurs bilaterally the patient is instructed, "Don't let me pull your arms apart." Then he attempts to bring his arms together voluntarily.

Because of the predominance of excess tone in the elbow flexors and relative weakness of elbow extensors, elbow extension is usually more difficult to obtain but can be assisted by the following methods. Bilateral "rowing" is the procedure used to initiate elbow extension. In the rowing procedure, movements toward extension combined with pronation are resisted (Fig. 24C.1) and movements into flexion combined with supination are guided (Fig. 24C.2). Rowing is done with the therapist and patient seated facing each other; the therapist's arms are crossed so that she and the patient grasp right hand to right hand and left hand to left hand. First, elbow extension is elicited as an **associated reaction** by resisting the noninvolved arm as it moves into extension and assisting the involved

arm into extension toward the noninvolved knee. Once the affected limb is felt to contract, resistance is offered bilaterally.

"Hold after positioning" is used to reinforce voluntary effort. When the patient's arm is positioned in extension synergy with the elbow in nearly full extension, he is asked to "hold" against resistance. To **facilitate** the extensors, quick stretches are applied to the involved arm by lightly pushing back toward elbow flexion.

When the **extensor synergy** is seen to come under active control, it is further developed through use of bilateral weight bearing. The patient leans forward onto his extended arms supported by a low stool placed in front of him (Fig. 24C.3). The patient uses the noninvolved hand to position the involved hand on a sandbag, pillow, or towel placed on the stool. Vigorous stroking of the skin over the triceps or tapping is done as the patient attempts to bear his weight on both outstretched arms (Fig. 24C.4). Once he is successful, weight is shifted so that the noninvolved extremity attempts to support the weight of the upper trunk. Again tapping and tactile stimulation may be useful. Unilateral weight bearing can be used functionally to hold objects while they are being worked on by the other hand, e.g., holding a piece of wood while sawing, hammering, or painting it; holding a package steady while opening it, addressing it, or fastening it; supporting body weight while polishing or washing large surfaces such as a table or floor.

To encourage active elbow extension, once the triceps is activated via rowing and weight bearing, unilateral resistance is offered to the patient's attempts to move into an extension pattern. Resistance gives

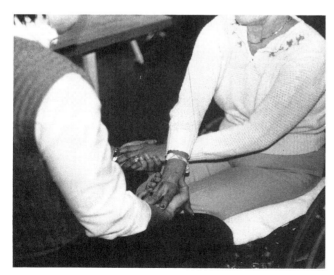

Figure 24C.1. Rowing to encourage elbow extension: resistance to elbow extension combined with pronation.

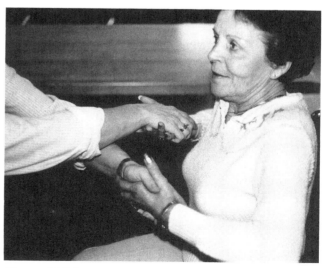

Figure 24C.2. Rowing to encourage elbow extension: guided reversal of motion into elbow flexion and supination. Note the support given to the wrists.

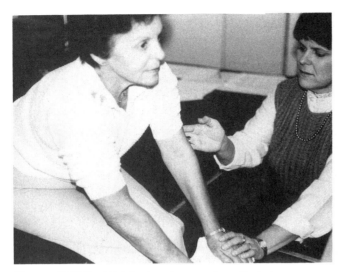

Figure 24C.3. Weight bearing on the affected upper extremity.

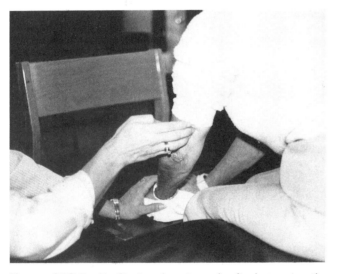

Figure 24C.4. Facilitating the triceps by firmly tapping the tendon and muscle belly.

direction to his effort and facilitates a stronger contraction. Other means that may be used to **facilitate** extension movement include use of supine position (tonic labyrinthine reflex); having the patient watch his extremity, which requires head turning and pulls in the asymmetrical tonic neck reflex; working with the forearm pronated, which is a strong component of the **extensor synergy;** and rotating the trunk toward the noninvolved side to **facilitate** extension of the involved arm via the tonic lumbar reflex.

As the synergies come under voluntary control, they should be used in functional activities. The **extensor synergy** can be used to stabilize an object to be worked on by the other side, to push the arm into the

sleeve of garments, to smooth out a sheet on the bed, or to sponge off the kitchen counter. The **flexor synergy** can be used functionally to assist in carrying items (such as a coat, handbag, or briefcase), feeding oneself, or putting on glasses. Bilateral pushing and pulling activities reinforce both synergies. Sanding, weaving, ironing, and polishing are activities that use the flexor and **extensor synergies** alternately and repeatedly.

STAGES 4 TO 6

To promote movement deviating from synergy, motions that begin to combine components of synergies in small increments are encouraged as a transition from stage 3 to stage 4. For example, as the patient begins to extend his arm consistently in response to the unilateral resistance given by the therapist, the therapist guides the direction of movement toward shoulder abduction in conjunction with elbow extension. This breaks up the synergistic relationship of shoulder adduction to elbow extension. The therapist requests the patient to push his hand into her hand as she directs the movement away from the patient's midline. When the triceps and pectoralis major are disassociated, the synergies no longer dominate.

In stages 4 and 5 the goal of treatment is to condition the synergies, i.e., to promote voluntary movement that combines components of the two synergies into increasingly varied combinations of movements that deviate from synergy. Proprioceptive and exteroceptive stimuli are still used in this phase of training, but tonic reflexes and **associated reactions,** appropriate in the earlier stages when reflex behavior was desirable, are no longer used. Willed movement with isolated control of muscle groups is the desired goal.

The first out-of-synergy motion of stage 4 is hand behind the body, which combines relative shoulder abduction **(flexor synergy)** with elbow extension and forearm pronation **(extensor synergy).** This motion requires that the strongest components of each synergy be subdued. To assist in getting the hand behind the body, a swinging motion of the arm combined with trunk rotation is helpful; if balance is good, this can be done more easily when standing. As the hand reaches the back of the patient, he strokes the dorsum of the hand against the body to complete the sensory awareness of the movement. Stroking the dorsum of the hand on the back is thought to give direction to the attempted voluntary movement. If the patient is unable to do the full motion actively, the therapist passively moves the patient's arm into final position and strokes the dorsum of the patient's hand against his sacrum. The patient, while attempting to do the movement himself, is then assisted into and out of the pattern, which gradually becomes voluntary with **practice. Practice,** using functional tasks as much as possible, continues until the motion can be freely accomplished. Examples of functional tasks, with the patient standing, include putting a belt on, sorting objects by moving certain objects from the table and dropping them into a bucket placed immediately behind the involved foot, swimming using the crawl stroke, and tucking a shirt into trousers.

The second out-of-synergy motion is shoulder flexion to a forward-horizontal position with the elbow extended. If the patient is unable actively to flex the shoulder forward, even with the therapist providing local **facilitation** and guidance of movement, then the arm is brought passively into position. While tapping over the anterior and middle deltoid muscles, the therapist asks the patient to hold the position. If hold after positioning is accomplished, active motion in small increments is then sought starting with lowering of the arm followed by active shoulder flexion. This continues until the full forward flexion motion can be done. Stroking and rubbing of the triceps are used to assist in keeping the elbow straight as the arm is raised. Raising the arm to forward-horizontal is involved in any vertically mounted game such as tic-tac-toe or checkers (using Velcro tabs to secure the pieces). Sponge painting is repetitive and essentially nonresistive and can be mounted vertically on an easel to **practice** the same motion.

The third motion sought in stage 4 is pronation and supination with the elbow flexed to 90°. Supination would not be expected to be a problem unless the pronators retained some *spasticity*. The problem would be to combine pronation of the **extensor synergy** with elbow flexion of the **flexor synergy.** Initially, pronation can be resisted with the elbow extended, and gradually the elbow can be brought into flexion as the resistance to pronation is repeated. An activity to consider when resistance to pronation is still necessary is block printing. It can be positioned to resist pronation with gradual changes in the amount of elbow flexion. Resistance to supination or pronation depends on the direction in which the major force is exerted. When resistance is no longer required and the patient can supinate and pronate with the elbow near the trunk, this motion has been achieved. **Practice** should involve activities that require turning objects such as a knob, a screwdriver, or a dial to reinforce it. Woodworking projects involving sanding of curved edges or assembly with screws can be used. Some games like Skittles are knob operated and require rotary motions, as do card games that require turning the cards over. Wall checkers can be adapted by the use of threaded dowels that must be turned to remove and replace them for each move on the checkerboard. Once the patient is confi-

dent of these stage 4 movements and his performance is fairly consistent, he is ready to enter stage 5 training.

Movement in stage 5 involves active attempts by the patient to move in patterns increasingly away from synergy. Excess effort is avoided, however, so that the limbs will not revert back to stereotyped movements. The attempts are bolstered by use of quick stretch and tactile stimulation. Each new motion is incorporated into functional activities.

The first motion sought in stage 5 is arm raised to side-horizontal, which combines full shoulder abduction with elbow extension. When this can be accomplished, disassociation of components of the synergies has occurred. When the muscles are still under the influence of the synergies, the arm will drift toward horizontal adduction when the elbow is extended or the elbow will flex when the shoulder is abducted. **Practice** with functional tasks assists learning. Activities to encourage side-horizontal movement can employ placement of project or game pieces or materials on a high table to the side of the patient. The table can be gradually moved to require more and more horizontal abduction and elbow extension. The patient would use the materials on a project to be done in front of him. Other activities might include weaving on a floor loom, table tennis, and driving golf balls.

The second motion of stage 5 is arm overhead. To achieve it, the scapula must upwardly rotate. The serratus anterior must be specifically retrained to do this. If the scapula is bound by spastic retractors, passive mobilization may need to be done before seeking an active response. Passive mobilization of the scapula is done by grasping the vertebral border and rotating it as the arm is passively moved into an overhead position. Once mobilized, the serratus is activated in its alternate duty of scapula protraction by placing the arm in the forward-horizontal position and asking, and assisting, the patient to reach forward. It is helpful to rehearse this motion with the patient using the noninvolved extremity. Quick stretches are applied by pushing backward into scapular retraction and the patient is asked to hold. Once activated, a holding contraction of the serratus is sought. These procedures continue, moving the arm in increments toward the arm overhead position. Once the movement has been achieved, **practice** with functional activities reinforces it. Sanding on an inclined plane is an example of an activity requiring a forward push with an increasing range of movement in scapular protraction and rotation and shoulder flexion; doing it bilaterally will allow the stronger, noninvolved arm to help the weaker one. Table tennis would still be useful, so would shooting baskets. Washing or painting a wall would require repeated reversal of movement up overhead and down.

The third motion sought in stage 5 is supination

and pronation (external and internal rotation) with the elbow extended. The best way to achieve this control is by using both hands in activities of interest to the patient that involve supination and pronation in various arm positions. One activity that can be used is grasping a large ball with the arms outstretched and then rotating it so the affected arm is on top (pronated) and the unaffected arm is on the bottom (supinated) and vice versa. The patient can then graduate to handling a basketball. To improve supination, the elbow is at first kept close to the trunk and gradually extended. Brunnstrom had no special treatment recommendations to assist in developing disassociation of supination and elbow flexion.

Patients who recover comparatively rapidly after a stroke may spontaneously achieve stage 6; however, many hemiplegic patients do not achieve full recovery. Twitchell (1951) stated that patients who reached stages 3 and 4 within 10 days after stroke recovered completely; this has never been verified in the literature. In Twitchell's sample, patients who failed to respond to proprioceptive **facilitation** did not recover willed movement at all. He observed, and it is generally accepted, that the longer the duration of the flaccid stage, the less likely was recovery.

Retraining Hand and Wrist Control

Training techniques for return of function in the hand are presented separately because the hand may be at a different stage of recovery than the arm. If the patient is unable to initiate active finger flexion (hand stage 1) or mass grasp (hand stage 2), the traction response in which stretch of the scapular adductors produces reflex finger flexion or an **associated reaction** to resisted grasp by the nonaffected hand may be used in combination with voluntary effort.

In hemiplegia, wrist flexion usually accompanies grasp initially so stability of the wrist in extension must be developed. It is easier for the patient to stabilize the wrist in extension when the elbow is extended; therefore, training starts with the elbow extended and the wrist supported by the therapist. The wrist extensor muscles are facilitated, and the therapist directs the patient to do a forceful grasp by commanding, "Squeeze." The grasp promotes normal synergistic contraction of the wrist extensors. This is repeated until the wrist extensors are felt to respond, allowing the therapist to remove support from the wrist with the command, "Hold." Tapping on the wrist extensor muscles facilitates holding. Once wrist extension and grasp are possible with the elbow extended, the process of positioning, percussion, and hold is repeated in increasing amounts of elbow flexion. Emphasis in this stage of training is on wrist stability, although wrist

flexion and extension and circumduction may then be practiced.

To move from hand stage 3 (flexion) to hand stage 4 (semivoluntary mass extension) **spasticity** of the finger flexors must be relaxed using a series of manipulations. The therapist reflexively releases the patient's grasp by holding the thumb into extension and abduction. Still holding the thumb, the therapist slowly and rhythmically supinates and pronates the forearm. Cutaneous stimulation is given over the dorsum of the wrist and hand while the forearm is supinated. These manipulations continue until a release of flexor tension is seen by some relaxation of the flexed position. If relaxation is incomplete, further manipulations are done. With the forearm still supinated, rapid repeated stretch stimuli are applied to the dorsum of the fingers by rolling them toward the palm with a rapid stroking motion to stretch finger extensors (Fig. 24C.5). When flexor tension is relaxed, the forearm is pronated and the arm elevated above horizontal (Souque's phenomenon). Stroking over the dorsum of the fingers and forearm continues as extension is attempted, but effort exerted should be minimal to avoid a buildup of tension.

Imitation synkinesis, in which the normal side performs a motion that is difficult to achieve on the involved side, may be observed when the patient attempts finger extension. After the fingers can be voluntarily extended with the arm raised, the arm is gradually lowered. If there is an increase of flexor tension reflected by decreased range in extension, it is necessary to repeat the above manipulations to **inhibit** flexion and **facilitate** extension. Reaching and picking up large, lightweight objects and releasing them, such as

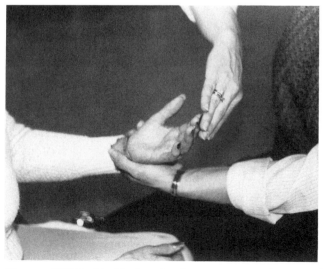

Figure 24C.5. Facilitating the finger extensors by use of quick, light stretch delivered by tapping the dorsal surface of the fingers slightly into flexion.

is required for stacking cones or paper cups, is one example of an activity to **practice** finger extension. The larger the object, the greater the extension required. The other extensor type activities are those that require the hand to be used flat, such as smoothing out a garment while ironing or a sheet while making the bed.

The second motion sought at hand stage 4 is lateral prehension and release. The patient attempts to move the thumb away from the index finger to gain release of lateral prehension while the therapist percusses or strokes over the abductor pollicis longus tendon to **facilitate** this motion. Once the patient has some active release, functional use of lateral prehension is then encouraged. Activities include holding a book while reading, dealing cards, and using a key.

Once the patient is able voluntarily to extend the fingers to release objects, advanced prehensile patterns (hand stage 5) are encouraged through activities. Musical instruments (tambourine, drum, claves, cymbal, tomtom, etc.) provide motivating opportunities for gross use of various hand patterns (Cofrancesco, 1985). As the patient progresses, activities are chosen to reinforce particular prehensions at more precise levels. Holding a pencil or paintbrush encourages palmar prehension. Spherical grasp is used to pick up or hold round objects such as a mayonnaise jar lid or an orange, and cylindrical grasp is used when holding the handles of tools.

Individual finger movements (hand stage 6) may be regained in rare instances. The patient should be given a home program of activities to encourage more and more individual finger use and to increase speed and accuracy of hand movements, but he should also be cautioned about expecting 100% recovery.

Gait patterns, principles used in preparation for walking, and ambulation training are also described by Brunnstrom. These principles and procedures fall under the primary responsibility of the physical therapist.

EFFECTIVENESS

The relative efficacy of Brunnstrom's Movement Therapy and Bobath's neurodevelopment treatment was studied on seven selected poststroke patients (Wagenaar et al., 1990). Each subject was randomly assigned to one treatment for 5 weeks and then to the other for 5 more weeks; this was repeated using a *B-C-B-C*

design. Functional recovery of activities of daily living (ADL), upper limb function, and walking ability were assessed weekly. The treatment program included occupational therapy, physical therapy, and nursing and all members of the treatment team adhered strictly to the written protocol for each treatment that had been developed from primary sources. The only significantly different outcome was greater improvement of gait speed by one patient under the Brunnstrom condition compared with the Bobath condition. This could have reflected the specific training of gait speed in the Brunnstrom method. The lack of difference detected in other subjects and for other assessments could have been the result of alternating short periods of each treatment for each subject, i.e., no subject received a full treatment program that followed one method and these methods have opposite views concerning the use of **associated reactions.** However, the recovery graphs for each patient showed steady recovery, indicating that both methods were probably beneficial. This cannot be stated with finality, however, as no control condition (i.e., no treatment given) was used because of ethical reasons. Patients may have improved spontaneously.

STUDY QUESTIONS

1. What is a synergy?
2. What is an associated reaction and how is it elicited?
3. Describe the flexor synergy of the upper extremity and state which component(s) is strongest.
4. Describe the extensor synergy of the upper extremity and state which component(s) is strongest.
5. List in order the six recovery stages of the proximal upper extremity.
6. List in order the six stages of hand recovery.
7. Name the treatment principles of the Brunnstrom approach.
8. How is the flexor synergy initiated in the upper extremity when the patient is flaccid?
9. How is elbow extension developed?
10. Describe therapeutic activities appropriate for a patient in stage 4 of the recovery of the upper limb.
11. How is finger extension developed?
12. Describe what activities of daily living a patient can be expected to do if he is in stage 5 of upper limb recovery and stage 4 of hand recovery.

24D PROPRIOCEPTIVE NEUROMUSCULAR FACILITATION (PNF) APPROACH

Beverly J. Myers

OBJECTIVES

After studying this chapter. the learner will be able to:
1. Understand the philosophical, neurophysiological, and developmental principles on which PNF is based.
2. List the five aspects of evaluation used in this approach.
3. Discuss the diagonal limb patterns and the combined movements of the upper and lower extremities.
4. Understand the six steps to assist a patient into a total developmental pattern.
5. Apply the diagonal limb patterns and total patterns to functional activities.

The proprioceptive neuromuscular facilitation (PNF) approach embodies broad concepts of human motion derived from normal development. As such, PNF has value to occupational therapists in evaluating and enhancing motor performance. PNF has been defined as "a method of promoting or hastening the response of the neuromuscular mechanism through stimulation of the proprioceptors" (Voss, Ionta, & Myers, 1985, p. xvii). Various techniques are superimposed on patterns of movement and posture with attention to the sensory stimulation from manual contacts, visual cues, and verbal commands to bring as many favorable influences as possible to bear on the patient.

Applying PNF to the treatment of patients in occupational therapy requires that the therapist understands the concepts, learns the motor skills, and then incorporates the approach into activities that meet the individual patient's needs. This introduction presents the principles of PNF and some examples of application to occupational therapy. To learn the motor skills, the patterns and techniques must be performed under the supervision of a knowledgeable instructor. Learning by practicing with other students develops the feeling of how normal balanced antagonistic muscle groups respond in different developmental positions. Then learning may proceed to application and repeated use with patients.

HISTORY

Kabat, a neurophysiologist and physician, developed the method of proprioceptive neuromuscular facil-itation at the Kabat-Kaiser Institute in 1946 to 1951. Sherrington's physiology and philosophy provided the foundation for many of the techniques. Some of the other experimenters who influenced the PNF approach were Gellhorn, a neurophysiologist who studied proprioception and cortically induced movement; Gesell, who studied the development of motor behavior and patterned movement; McGraw, who studied the development of behavior as it relates to the maturation of neural structures; Hellebrandt, who studied combinations of movements and mass movements, finding that one can circumvent fatigue or speed recovery by changing the combination used; and Pavlov, who studied the mechanisms of learning and formation of habit patterns.

The diagonal patterns, PNFs unique feature, were the last aspect to be identified. Specific combinations of motion were carefully analyzed in 1951. Kabat found that when topographically aligned groups of muscles were stretched, they produced a movement in a diagonal direction. Observation of functional movement and sport skills revealed the same spiral and diagonal characteristics.

Kabat began his work in the early 1940s by treating patients with cerebral palsy and multiple sclerosis. However, by the early 1950s PNF had been applied to the treatment of patients with all diagnoses, from those with central nervous system (CNS) deficits to orthopedic conditions, arthritis, and peripheral nerve injuries.

In 1956, Knott and Voss, two physical therapists who worked with Kabat, wrote the first edition of the PNF textbook, which has been revised (Voss et al., 1985) and translated into seven different languages. Occupational therapists used PNF as evidenced by the related articles published during the 1950s (Ayres, 1955a, 1955b, 1955c; Carroll, 1950; Cooke, 1958; Kabat & Rosenberg, 1950; Voss, 1959; Whitaker, 1950).

No courses or workshops were offered for occupational therapists until 1974, when Voss taught the first PNF course for occupational therapists at Northwestern University in collaboration with the curriculum in occupational therapy at the University of Illinois. Continuing education in the form of 1- and 2-week courses and 1-day workshops continues to be offered for occupational therapists.

PRINCIPLES

In developing the PNF method, Kabat relied on authorities in the fields of neurophysiology, motor learning, and motor behavior. The basic principles of PNF encompass the developmental concepts as drawn from these fields (Voss, 1967). The 11 principles are discussed below.

1. All human beings have potentials that are not fully developed (Voss, 1967). This first principle is a statement of philosophy. It provides the base for an attitude toward treating patients. The patient's abilities and potentials become the means to reduce his inabilities. When the patient's progress declines, the idea that the patient has reached a plateau is the last factor to be acknowledged. The cause may not be the result of the patient's natural limitations, but rather because of lack of experience and skills of the therapist, lack of coordination with the rehabilitation team and the patient's family, lack of time for appropriate treatment, or lack of funds. PNF does not disregard the fact that some persons may reach a limit beyond which no further learning may occur. However, the emphasis is on bringing as many favorable influences to bear as possible on developing a patient's potential. Consider the common reaction of a man watching a tennis game for the first time. "Oh, I could never do that," he might exclaim. But after a few lessons, that same man may have channeled his potential and abilities to perform a skill that he previously thought was impossible. This philosophy, inherent in the PNF approach, is compatible with that of occupational therapy, in which emphasis is placed on ability rather than disability.

This philosophy also underlies the approach of PNF in using the patient's stronger movement patterns to strengthen the weaker motions. Thus an indirect approach results. In treatment, when the superior region is intact, as in a person with paraplegia, the movements of the head, neck, upper trunk, and upper limbs are used to **facilitate** and reinforce movements in the weaker lower extremities. When the patient has one involved upper extremity, as in the person with a frozen shoulder, the motions of the intact upper extremity and inferior region are emphasized in bilateral combinations and total patterns to reduce the pain and increase movement in the affected arm.

2. Normal motor development proceeds in a cervicocaudal and proximodistal direction (Voss, 1967). In treatment, this direction is heeded, and attention is given first to the development of motion in the head and neck, then in the trunk, and last in the extremities. For example, with the patient who is comatose, treatment would not begin by quietly performing range of motion on the hand but rather by first directing sensory stimuli to the head, as in greeting and talking to the patient, touching his face or head while talking, or providing other tactile input to the facial region. Positioning the patient in a total pattern, such as side lying, would follow and would stimulate rotation of head, neck, and trunk. Then, if indicated, passive range of motion of the extremities could be administered.

As the head and neck lead the rest of the body in embryonic differentiation and reflex development (Hooker, 1977), so too the position of the head and neck influences the movement of the body's total pattern throughout life. For example, in standing when the head is quickly rotated to one side, the body weight shifts to that side. In treatment, this principle is applied when facilitating weight bearing. When a patient rises to stand from a wheelchair or bed, if weight is not equally distributed, asking the patient to look toward the inefficient side may promote a shift of weight toward that side. Likewise, when working on developing stability of the affected side of the patient who has hemiplegia, positioning the activity on the hemiplegic side will increase a weight shift toward the involved leg or arm, thus facilitating weight bearing on that side.

The development of movement and stability in the limbs proceeds in a proximodistal direction. In therapy, developing the function of the head, neck, and trunk precedes developing the function of the extremities, and that of the shoulder girdle before developing the fine motor skills of the hand. However, coordinated movement proceeds in a distal to proximal direction. When reaching for the telephone on a desk, the shoulder and elbow do not lead the movement, rather the hand opens and reaches to grasp the phone. The rest of the arm supports and follows the movement of the hand.

3. Early motor behavior is dominated by reflex activity. Mature motor behavior is reinforced or supported by postural reflex mechanisms (Voss, 1967). In other words, the reflexes present in the newborn do not disappear completely but become integrated into the child's nervous system as he or she matures. For example, the asymmetric tonic neck reflex (ATNR) supports rolling, the symmetric tonic neck reflex (STNR) supports the assumption of the hands-and-knees posture, and the body-on-body righting reflex supports the assumption of side sitting from prone. In the adult, reflexes are available when needed to support movement. Evidence of this exists frequently in sports and when the body performs under stressful conditions. For example, head and neck extension in the STNR reinforces extension of the arms in pushing a heavy object, such as a bed or box.

Recognizing reflex responses in humans requires good observation skills, as the reflex response may not be complete. Tonus changes and partial movements are common. Hellebrandt, Schade, and Carns (1962) studied the effect of the tonic neck reflex in the normal adult. An adaptation of one of their experiments can be easily performed with a partner. One person assumes a hands-and-knees position and the other person tests the triceps strength unilaterally four times. The first time, the person on hands and knees dorsiflexes the head and maintains this position. The tester waits 15 sec, allowing for the latency of the tonus change, and then resists the triceps by attempting to passively flex the elbow. This procedure is repeated with the head ventroflexed, rotated away from the arm, and rotated toward the arm being tested. One would expect stronger responses when elbow extension is supported by the STNR (head dorsiflexed) and by the ATNR (head rotated toward the resisted arm). In treatment, application occurs when a patient with weakness on one side has difficulty assuming a hands-and-knees posture. Directing the patient to turn his head toward the weaker side will elicit the support of the ATNR to reinforce elbow extension.

4. The growth of motor behavior has cyclic trends as evidenced by shifts between flexor and extensor dominance (Voss, 1967). For example, in the development of the sitting posture, the first cycle is flexion. The newborn child, positioned in sitting with assistance or with support of arms, remains sitting in a flexor-dominant posture. The next cycle is one of extension. Sitting is assumed independently, but usually with extension from prone to hands and knees and then with rotation to side sitting and long sitting. Finally, the cycle shifts to flexion again as the child learns to assume sitting symmetrically from supine.

Interaction between movements of flexion and extension is necessary for functional movement. In the action of rising to stand, one begins by flexing the superior region forward to shift weight onto the feet. Extension of the body follows as the upright position is attained. The normal child facilitates this interaction by rocking alternately from flexion to extension in various postures (McGraw, 1945). Gesell (1977) described this process as reciprocal interweaving in which relationships of opposed functions are established. These reciprocal relationships provide the basis for development of stability and balance of postures.

In treatment, the therapist applies this principle in observing the patient's movements. If flexor tone dominates, then extensor-dominant activities and methods of assumption will be selected. Likewise, if extensor tone is dominant, activities stimulating flexor dominance will be chosen. Care should be taken when stimulating flexion responses, as flexor reflexes are more primitive than extensor reflexes and may become dominant, creating an imbalance. Emphasis of treat-

ment is rarely limited to one dominance, as an interaction between balanced antagonistic movements is sought.

5. Goal-directed activity is made up of reversing movements (Voss, 1967). Early motor behavior occurs in random fashion through full range of motion. The spontaneous limb movements of the newborn usually fluctuate from extremes of flexion to extension. Yet the movements are rhythmic and reversing, qualities that continue throughout life. The act of eating is reversing movement of the arm and jaw. Reversal of a total pattern is commonly found in removing a can of soda from the refrigerator. Initially, the action includes walking forward to open the door and reaching forward to grasp the can. Reversal of direction follows to remove the can from the shelf and walk backward to close the door. If a patient cannot reverse directions, his functional ability will be limited. The rhythmic reversing of direction then becomes a goal of treatment, as reversing movements help to reestablish the balance and interaction between antagonists.

6. Normal movement and posture depend on "synergism" and a balanced interaction of antagonists (Voss, 1967). This principle encompasses the previous three and states the main goal in the PNF approach: to develop a balance of antagonists. A continual adjustment in reflex activity, dominance, and reversing or antagonistic movements is required for the constant changes of movement and posture that occur in functional activity. For example, getting dressed demands interaction in all of these areas. Without a balance of antagonists, the quality of performance decreases, becoming more deliberate and losing its smooth and rhythmical characteristics. Thus in treatment, prevention and correction of imbalances between antagonists are objectives (Voss, 1967).

7. Developing motor behavior is expressed in an orderly sequence of total patterns of movement and posture (Gesell, 1947; McGraw, 1945). The concept of recapitulating the developmental sequence is followed in treatment. The developmental sequence is considered a universal experience, common to all normal human beings. Thus if a person, such as a child with cerebral palsy, has not experienced these total patterns, he has need to do so. With the patient who has developed normally and then becomes disabled, this sequence of developmental positions will have meaning to him (Voss, 1967). In occupational therapy, the developmental sequence has direct application, because functional activities can be performed in a variety of postures. Thus the patient experiences not only total patterns that **facilitate** the use of, and integration of, postural reflexes but reduced frustration. For example, his ability to dress is built through the total patterns of rolling, lower trunk rotation, **bridging,** and assumption

to sitting, rather than through **practice** of inadequate or unstable sitting and standing positions.

The developmental sequence also includes the "combined movements" of the extremities as they interact with the head, neck, and trunk in total patterns (Table 24D.1). The upper or lower extremity movements occur in an orderly sequence (Gesell, 1947; McGraw, 1945). First to appear are **bilateral symmetrical** patterns, then **bilateral asymmetrical** and bilateral reciprocal patterns, and last unilateral patterns. When the upper and lower extremities move together, they begin in an **ipsilateral** pattern, then progress to alternating reciprocal, where **contralateral** extremities move in the same direction one at a time, while opposite **contralateral** extremities move in the opposite direction one at a time. For example, an infant beginning to creep uses an **ipsilateral** pattern. Later, the child uses an alternating reciprocal pattern, moving one extremity at a time. As coordination and rate of movement increase, the child progresses to the most advanced combination, diagonal reciprocal. This combination is similar to alternating reciprocal with only one difference: **contralateral** extremities move in the same direction at the same time, while the other **contralateral** extremities move in the opposite direction at the same time, as in normal creeping or walking. In occupational therapy, these combined movements may

be used to assess a patient's level of performance or to design a treatment activity for stimulation of a response in the total pattern. For example, standing in a **bilateral symmetrical** combination will **facilitate** head, neck, and trunk flexion and extension. Swinging a bat or racquet in a **bilateral asymmetrical** combination will **facilitate** head, neck, and trunk rotation. On the other hand, performing a reciprocal combination, such as throwing a ball or reaching for an item on a high shelf, promotes stability of head, neck, and trunk.

Direction of movement also develops in an orderly sequence. Gesell (1954) observed that a child follows a significant pattern in developing the ability to use a crayon. The strokes move from scrawl, to vertical, to horizontal, to circular, and then to oblique or diagonal. Comparable sequences of direction have been demonstrated in visual behavior, eye-hand coordination, vocalization, percept-concept formation, and postural behavior. Thus the diagonal direction or pattern of movement is a combination of the previous three movements and is the most advanced. Voss (1967), citing Gesell, pointed out that in PNF, total patterns of movement are performed in a diagonal direction, as well as in forward, backward, sideways, and circular directions. A person who has suffered a cerebrovascular accident (CVA) may be able to creep forward and backward. However, difficulty may occur when chang-

Table 24D.1. Combined Movements of Upper and Lower Extremities

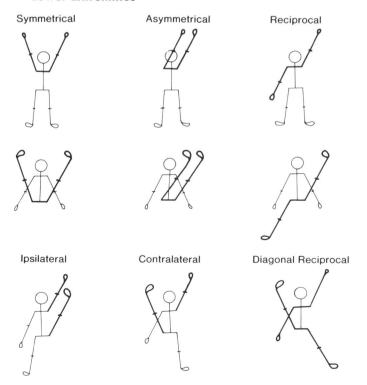

ing direction in circular and diagonal creeping. Thus **facilitation** of circular and diagonal patterns of creeping can be goals of treatment.

8. Normal motor development has an orderly sequence but lacks a step-by-step quality; overlapping occurs (Voss, 1967). In treatment, a patient does not remain in sitting until perfection of balance is achieved before attempting to stand. The order of the developmental sequence aids the therapist in finding a posture or a place to begin when treating the patient. A posture in which the patient is stable and can move successfully becomes a place to begin. The developmental sequence provides a direction in which to progress. However, because the overlapping quality occurs, the patient may benefit from working on activities in postures above and below his level of ability.

Performing activities in developmental postures will enhance a person's adaptive response to the task or movement. However, the activity must be graded in keeping with the physical demands on the patient. If the physical demands are high, the activity must be simple. If the physical demands are low, the activity may be more complex. For example, a patient with brain damage may need to develop balance in kneeling and standing and improve his writing skills. In treatment, activities in kneeling may include simple gross motor activities, such as playing tic-tac-toe on the blackboard or sanding on an inclined board. However, when the patient **practices** writing, a fine motor activity, a more stable posture such as sitting is required. Besides kneeling and sitting, the patient may engage in standing activities, walking to and from each activity, and gait training in physical therapy. Thus overlapping of postures occurs in treatment during an individual therapy session or throughout the day.

9. Improvement of motor ability depends on motor learning (Voss, 1967). The concepts of motor learning that PNF applies to therapeutic exercise are similar to those used by occupational therapists in functional activity training. These concepts will be reviewed briefly with specific emphasis on the PNF approach.

Motor learning extends from the conditioning of responses to the learning of complex voluntary motor acts (Buchwald, 1965). Harlow and Harlow (1962) classified the conditioning of responses as the simplest form of learning. Proprioceptive feedback as received from receptors in the muscles, tendons, joints, and labyrinths plays a significant role in simple conditioned responses (Buchwald, 1965). In addition, stress promotes maturation (Levine, 1960). Levine studied infant rats and their responses to the stresses of handling and electric shock. The rats who received either form of stress developed into normal active adults. Those rats that were not subjected to stress defecated and urinated more frequently and did not explore their environment.

Thus motor learning is facilitated by appropriate stress coupled with sensory and environmental stimulation.

As maturation occurs, more complex acts may be learned. The sequence begins with conditioned responses progressing to an ability to discriminate between objects, to an ability to transfer learning from one problem to another, and then to the ability to solve complex problems requiring concept formation. Learning complex tasks can be facilitated by the use of "stepwise procedures," as demonstrated by Harlow and Harlow (1962). In PNF, the therapist helps the patient learn many complex motor acts, such as transfers and other self-care skills. By selecting and providing appropriate sensory cues and through the use of **facilitation techniques,** the demands of a task or parts of the task that the patient is unable to perform independently may be made more appropriate. PNF emphasizes the stepwise procedures of a task, yet allows the patient to complete the whole task. Thus, by training with repetition, the conditioning of responses occurs and leads to the achievement of the whole task.

Sensory cues include visual, auditory, and tactile stimuli. Vision and hearing give direction to movement (Voss, 1972). Vision may lead movement or follow the movement. For example, in lifting an object up to a shelf, the person will look to the shelf first, then lift the object. Thus, if a patient is not engaging the movement with his eyes, he has a need to do so. Following the movement visually will enhance the motor performance.

Verbal commands increase sensory stimulation and may **facilitate** movement. Tone of voice may influence the quality of the muscle response. A loud, sharp command will yield a quick response and recruit more motor units. A soft, low command will produce a slower response. In the presence of pain, soft commands are always used to avoid stimulating jerky movements and further increasing the pain (Voss, 1967).

Verbal mediation occurs when the patient speaks aloud to direct his movements (Loomis & Boersma, 1982). For example, a patient who has difficulty preparing the wheelchair for a transfer may say, "I am going to lock the brakes, put my feet on the floor, and move the footrests away." Expressing the movement verbally as the task is performed enhances the organization, memory, and execution of the task.

Tactile cues in PNF are mainly provided by the therapist's manual contacts, which **facilitate** movement or promote relaxation. Also, stretch and resistance may be applied by opposing the patient's effort and yet becoming part of his effort (Voss, 1967). Additional tactile stimulation may be provided by adjuncts to treatment, such as **vibration** and cold.

Thus motor learning is enhanced by tracking sensory cues. One may track a visual stimulus, the sound of a voice, or a touch. Tactual tracking is more efficient (Smith, 1967). In cybernetics research, movement with visual tracking was discovered to be less accurate than movement with tactual feedback. In treatment, an application of tracking may occur when a patient reaches for an object but is unable to complete the range of movement. A light touch on the back of the patient's hand, guiding him toward the object, may be the only cue he needs to achieve the goal. Another example may occur when a patient with unilateral weakness in the upper limb attempts to wipe the table with a sponge. The performance may quickly deteriorate with the patient complaining of fatigue. With a light touch on the back of the patient's hand from the therapist hand or with self-touch from the patient's uninvolved hand, the patient's movement becomes less deliberate, endurance improves, and the task is completed. In summary, the application of motor learning concepts in PNF becomes one of combining as many favorable influences as possible to achieve the desired response.

10. Frequency of stimulation and repetition of activity are used for the promotion and retention of motor learning and for the development of strength and endurance (Voss, 1967). Patients, as well as any child or adult learning a new skill, require frequent stimulation and opportunity to **practice** in order for the task being learned to be retained. Motor learning has occurred when the movement is repeated enough to become integrated into the body's repertoire of movements and can be used automatically. In treatment, repetition cannot be overemphasized. Activity has an inherent advantage over exercise because during activity repetition occurs naturally.

11. Goal-directed activities, coupled with **facilitation techniques,** are used to hasten learning of total patterns of walking and of self-care activities (Voss, 1967). **Facilitation techniques** or exercise alone are not as meaningful as when they are coupled with an activity. Activity that directs attention away from the motor aspects of the task and toward a purposeful goal enhances neurological integration (Ayres, 1962). Likewise, purposeful activity alone is not enough. It is necessary but not always sufficient to meet the patient's needs. Therapists need to relate the **facilitation techniques** to activity (Ayres, 1962).

EVALUATION

Assessment becomes an ongoing process in the PNF approach. Following the initial evaluation, a treatment plan is established, using selected procedures and techniques. Modifications in the plan occur as the needs of the patient change or as the therapist observes a change in the patient's performance. As PNF encompasses concepts that may be applied to many diagnoses, the evaluation is general in nature. Forms for evaluation, analysis, and planning treatment programs in physical therapy were developed by Voss (1967, 1969). Descriptions of the evaluation process have been presented in detail in the literature (Voss, 1972; Voss et al., 1985). The evaluation reflects the developmental sequence, proceeding in a proximal to distal direction. A brief summary of the evaluation process is presented here.

1. Vital and related functions of the body, respiration, swallowing, voice production, and facial and tongue motions are evaluated and impairments, weakness, or asymmetry is noted.
2. Movements in response to visual, auditory, and tactile stimuli are elicited to determine which sensory cues may be used to reinforce movement and posture.
3. Head and neck patterns, the key to upper trunk patterns, are observed during the performance of developmental and functional activities. The following are noted:
   a. Dominance of tone (flexor or extensor);
   b. Alignment (midline or asymmetrical);
   c. Stability versus mobility (balanced or deficient in one or both areas).
4. Combinations of diagonal patterns of the extremities are next in the evaluation sequence. The patient is asked to perform **bilateral symmetrical, bilateral asymmetrical,** and bilateral reciprocal combinations. The following areas are assessed:
   a. Influence of head, neck, and trunk postures;
   b. Range of motion, remembering that rotation is not complete in any pattern;
   c. Quality of movement, such as smoothness and rhythm;
   d. Normal timing, with the distal component leading in coordinated movement.
5. Developmental postures are observed by asking the patient to assume and maintain positions in the developmental sequence. These total patterns are assessed to determine how muscle groups function in relation to each other in a given pattern. Previous evaluation centered on individual segments and functions. During observations of total patterns a central problem or imbalance may be identified. For example, is more stability or mobility needed? Is there a dominance rather than a balance of flexor or extensor tone? And does the patient have difficulty shifting from one dominance to another?
6. Functional activities, as performed in self-care tasks and transfers, are observed to determine any discrepancies between the patient's ability to perform individual and total patterns and his ability to com-

bine these movements in performance of a functional task.

TREATMENT

Diagonal Patterns

For every major part of the body—the head, neck, trunk, and extremities—two pairs of diagonal patterns of movement exist. Each pair of antagonistic patterns consists of three motion components. Flexion or extension is always present as the major component. These flexion and extension components are combined with rotation (external or internal) and with abduction or adduction. For example, in diagonal one (D1) flexion of the upper extremity, flexion combines with adduction and external rotation. In diagonal two (D2) flexion, flexion combines with abduction and external rotation. These diagonal patterns were described by Voss et al. (1985), according to shoulder motion components, the original designation by Kabat. The briefer designations of diagonal one and diagonal two were introduced by Voss (1967). In development, the diagonal patterns appear in the functional movements of rolling and prone locomotion. Diagonal one is derived from rolling and diagonal two from crawling on the belly.

Five factors support the use of diagonal patterns in treatment.

1. The patterns agree with the spiral and diagonal characteristics of normal functional movement; most muscles, by virtue of their attachments and alignment of their fibers, support this movement.
2. Scientists who have studied integrative function of the brain support the concept that voluntary movement consists of mass movement patterns rather than individual muscle action; Jackson (1931) was one of the first to stimulate specific areas of the motor cortex and to discover that mass movement patterns were produced.
3. Gesell (1954) noted that diagonal movement occurs last in the normal development of direction and is the most advanced motion; thus diagonal movements are combinations of the three pairs of antagonistic motions of flexion or extension, abduction or adduction, and external or internal rotation.
4. All diagonal patterns cross the midline, thereby facilitating interaction between two sides of the body, which is important to perceptual-motor-sensory integrative functioning.
5. The diagonal patterns always incorporate a rotation component; because rotation is one of the last movements to develop, it is usually the first to be lost following an injury or with aging (Voss, 1967).

Use of diagonal patterns in therapy reinforces the component of rotation, necessary to the performance of functional tasks. Placing an activity in a diagonal direction will elicit a diagonal pattern and the desired rotation. Range of motion may also be performed in diagonal patterns. Rotation is incorporated with each limb motion. This method is more efficient than the traditional range of motion performed in anatomical planes. Figures 24D.1 through 24D.30 are arranged to show the two extremes of the bilateral patterns along with a treatment application of the particular pattern.

Bilateral symmetrical patterns occur when paired extremities perform like movements at the same time. These combining movements are the first to develop; therefore, they are often the easiest to learn. Also, as they influence head, neck, and trunk flexion and extension, they play an important role in facilitating a reciprocal relationship between flexor and extensor dominance. **Bilateral symmetrical** patterns of the upper extremities (Figs. 24D.1 and 24D.2, and 24D.7 and 24D.8) are commonly observed in the daily activities of riding a bicycle, putting a roast in the oven, and removing a pullover shirt overhead. **Bilateral symmetrical** patterns of the lower extremities (Figs. 24D.25 and 24D.26, 24D.28 and 24D.29) are seen in the postures of standing and sitting. **Bilateral asymmetrical** patterns occur when paired extremities perform movements toward one side at the same time. The limbs may move together free from contact as in **bilateral asymmetrical** flexion to the right, with the right arm in **D2 flexion** and the left in **D1 flexion** (Fig. 24D.3). The combining movement may also be performed with the arms in contact, as in the patterns of chopping (Figs. 24D.4 and 24D.5) and lifting (Figs. 24D.10 and 24D.11). **Bilateral asymmetrical** patterns influence the head, neck, and trunk movements in patterns of flexion with rotation or extension with rotation. When the arms perform in contact, the range of trunk flexion and extension with rotation increases. Swinging a baseball bat is an example of a **bilateral asymmetric** pattern in the upper extremities. The same combination in the lower extremities is found in the side-sitting position.

Bilateral reciprocal patterns occur when paired extremities perform movements in opposite directions at the same time. For example, in reciprocal movements of diagonal one, one arm begins in **D1 extension,** the other arm in **D1 flexion** (Fig. 24D.13). As one arm moves toward **D1 flexion,** the other arm moves toward **D1 extension** (Fig. 24D.14). Less flexion and extension of head, neck, and trunk are present in reciprocal motions than in other combined patterns. Rotation of head, neck, and trunk may occur, but the range is incomplete. When antagonistic patterns of both diagonals are performed at the same time, as

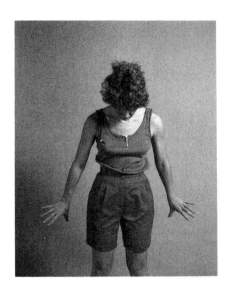

Figure 24D.1. Bilateral symmetrical D1 extension, shortened range; bilateral symmetrical D1 flexion, lengthened range. Shoulders extend, abduct, and internally rotate; elbows extend (as the intermediate joint, the elbow may flex or extend), forearms pronate; wrists extend toward the ulnar side; fingers extend and abduct; and thumbs extend and abduct.

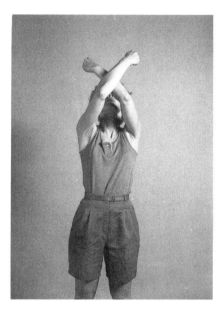

Figure 24D.2. Bilateral symmetrical D1 flexion, shortened range; bilateral symmetrical D1 extension, lengthened range. Shoulders flex, adduct, and externally rotate; elbows flex (as the intermediate joint, the elbow may flex or extend), forearms supinate; wrists flex toward radial side; fingers flex and adduct; and thumbs flex and adduct.

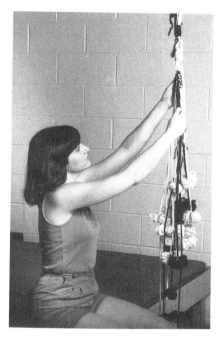

Figure 24D.3. Bilateral asymmetrical flexion to the left to work on a macramé project. Left arm is in D2 flexion, and right arm is in D1 flexion.

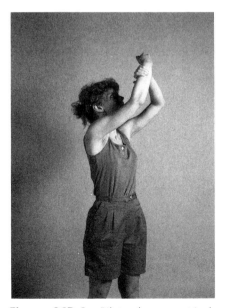

Figure 24D.4. Bilateral asymmetrical pattern with limbs in contact, as in chopping. A chop to the right begins with the right arm in D1 flexion and the left hand grasping the dorsum of the right wrist.

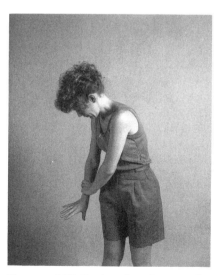

Figure 24D.5. In chopping to the right, the right arm moves in D1 extension, with the left arm assisting in D2 extension.

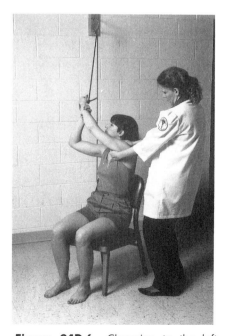

Figure 24D.6. Chopping to the left with pulleys. The left arm will move into D1 extension, and the right arm will assist in D2 extension. Note the rotation of head, neck, and trunk. The therapist resists scapular movement.

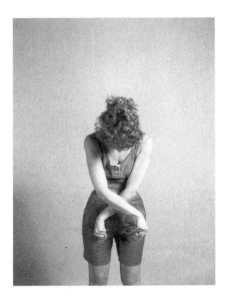

Figure 24D.7. Bilateral symmetrical D2 extension, shortened range; bilateral symmetrical D2 flexion, lengthened range. Shoulders extend, adduct, and internally rotate; elbows flex (as the intermediate joint, the elbow may flex or extend); forearms pronate; wrists flex toward ulnar side; fingers flex and adduct; and thumbs are in opposition.

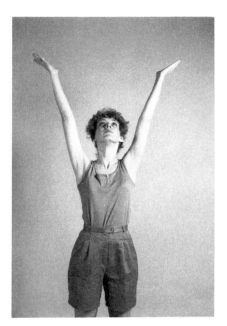

Figure 24D.8. Bilateral symmetrical D2 flexion, shortened range; bilateral symmetrical D2 extension, lengthened range. Shoulders flex, abduct, externally rotate; elbows extend (as the intermediate joint, the elbow may flex or extend); forearms supinate; wrists extend toward radial side; fingers extend and abduct; thumbs extend and adduct.

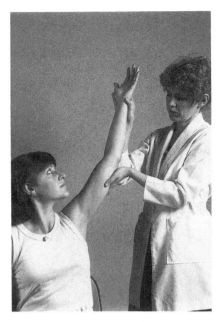

Figure 24D.9. Range of motion in D2 flexion. The therapist's manual contacts are on the extensor surface to facilitate wrist and elbow extension in the D2 flexion pattern. Contacts will switch to flexor surfaces as the patient reverses the pattern in D2 extension.

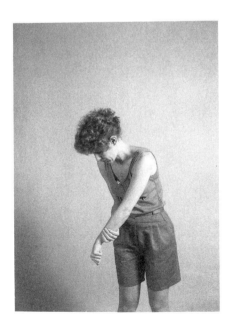

Figure 24D.10. Bilateral symmetrical pattern with limbs in contact, as in lifting. A lift to the left begins with the left arm in D2 extension and the right hand grasping the volar surface of the left wrist.

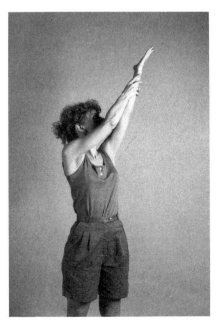

Figure 24D.11. In lifting to the left, the left arm moves in D2 flexion, with the right arm assisting in D1 flexion.

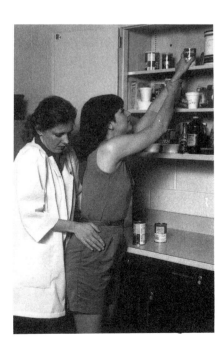

Figure 24D.12. Lifting to the left to place groceries on the shelf. The therapist approximates at the pelvis.

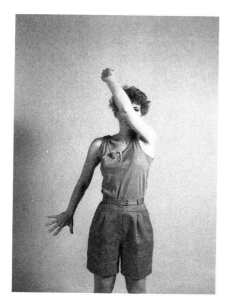

Figure 24D.13. Bilateral reciprocal D1, lengthened range. The left arm begins in D1 flexion, and the right arm begins in D1 extension.

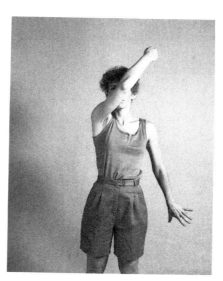

Figure 24D.14. Bilateral reciprocal D1, shortened range. The left arm moves in D1 extension, and the right arm moves in D1 extension.

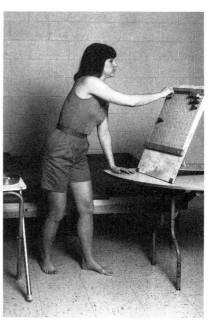

Figure 24D.15. Bilateral reciprocal D1 in a palmar prehension activity. Note the simultaneous static and dynamic position, with the left arm weight bearing (static) in D1 extension and the right arm moving (dynamic) in D1 flexion.

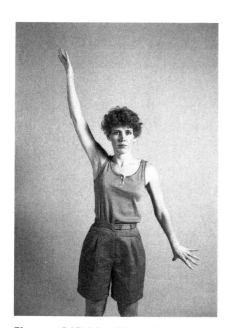

Figure 24D.16. Bilateral reciprocal combined diagonals, lengthened range. The right arm begins in D2 flexion, and the left arm begins in D1 extension.

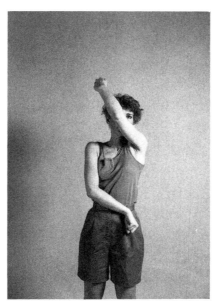

Figure 24D.17. Bilateral reciprocal combined diagonals, shortened range. The right arm moves in D2 extension, and the left arm moves in D1 flexion. The head and neck may rotate, diagonally flex and extend, or remain in midline.

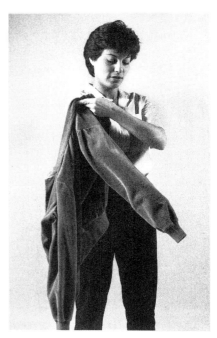

Figure 24D.18. Bilateral reciprocal combined diagonals in donning a jacket. The right arm moves through the sleeve in D2 extension, and the left arm pulls the jacket over the right arm in D1 flexion.

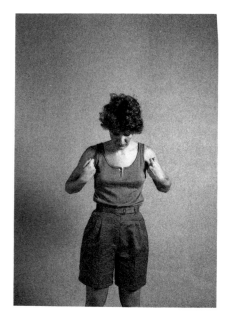

Figure 24D.19. Bilateral symmetrical D1 ulnar thrust, lengthened range. Shoulders extend, abduct, and internally rotate; elbows flex; forearms supinate; wrists flex toward radial side; fingers flex and adduct; and thumbs flex and adduct.

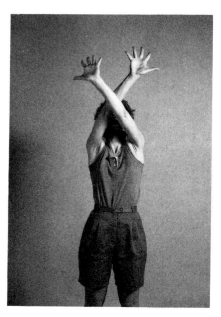

Figure 24D.20. Bilateral symmetrical D1 ulnar thrust, shortened range. Shoulders flex, adduct, and externally rotate; elbows extend; forearms pronate; wrists extend toward ulnar side; fingers extend and abduct; and thumbs extend and abduct.

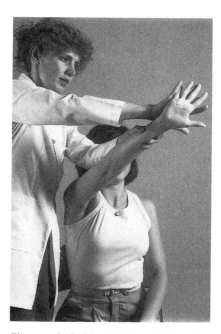

Figure 24D.21. Unilateral D1 ulnar thrust to the left. The therapist resists wrist extension, using the technique of repeated contractions.

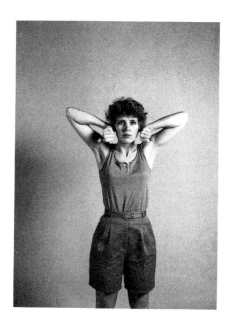

Figure 24D.22. Bilateral symmetrical D2 radial thrust, lengthened range. Shoulders flex, abduct, and externally rotate; elbows flex; forearms pronate; wrists flex toward ulnar side; fingers flex and adduct; and thumbs are in opposition.

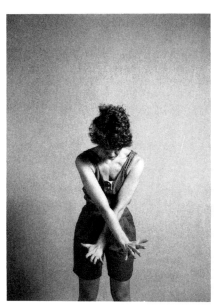

Figure 24D.23. Bilateral symmetrical D2 radial thrust, shortened range. Shoulders extend, adduct, and internally rotate; elbows extend; forearms supinate; wrists extend toward radial side; fingers extend and abduct; and thumbs extend and abduct.

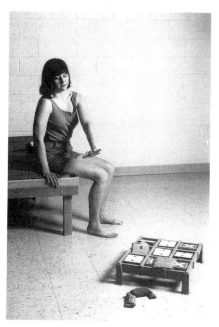

Figure 24D.24. Unilateral D2 radial thrust to the right in a bean bag toss. Thrusting facilitates hand opening with elbow extension.

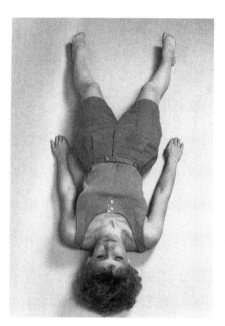

Figure 24D.25. Bilateral symmetrical D1 extension, shortened range; bilateral symmetrical D1 flexion, lengthened range. Hips extend, abduct, and internally rotate; knees extend (as the intermediate joint, the knee may flex or extend), ankles and feet plantar flex and evert; and toes flex and adduct.

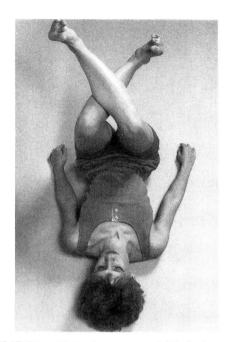

Figure 24D.26. Bilateral symmetrical D1 flexion, shortened range; bilateral symmetrical D1 extension, lengthened range. Hips flex, adduct, and externally rotate; knees flex (as the intermediate joint, the knee may flex or extend), ankles and feet dorsiflex and invert; and toes extend and abduct.

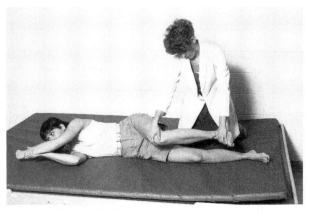

Figure 24D.27. D1 flexion of the lower extremity in rolling. The therapist resists the lower extremity pattern as the patient reverses the chop with the upper extremities. Note the extension and rotation of head, neck, and trunk. Patients with hemiplegia may use this pattern when rolling from supine to prone.

in a reciprocal combination in combined diagonals with one arm in **D1 extension** and the other arm in **D2 flexion,** the movement of the head, neck, and trunk continues to decrease. The position of the head remains in midline. The reciprocal patterns have a stabilizing influence on head, neck, and trunk because one extremity flexes while the other extends, producing stability in the trunk. Examples of reciprocal movements are walking, running, and swimming the crawl stroke. They are also seen in activities that place an increased demand for equilibrium reactions on the body, such as in reaching for an item on a high shelf or performing a lay-up shot during a basketball game.

Unilateral patterns in developing motor behavior emerge from the bilateral patterns. The motions of the unilateral diagonal patterns are the same as those described for **bilateral symmetrical** patterns (Figs. 24D.1 and 24D.2, and 24D.7 and 24D.8). In skilled tasks, the two diagonals may interact or one may dominate. Diagonal one in the upper extremities is observed in the basic activities of feeding and washing the face, right side with left hand. Diagonal two is seen in the self-care activities of zipping a front-opening zipper and winding a watch. Diagonal one in the lower extremities is observed in pushing one foot through a pant leg and in crossing one leg to don a sock. Diagonal two is seen in hurdling and in swimming the breast stroke.

Diagonals change and interact as the hand crosses

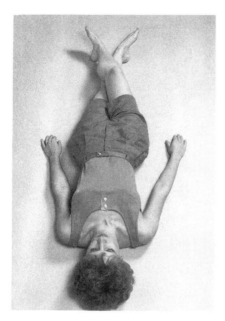

Figure 24D.28. Bilateral symmetrical D2 extension, shortened range; bilateral symmetrical D2 flexion, lengthened range. Hips extend, adduct, and externally rotate; knees extend (as the intermediate joint, the knee may flex or extend); ankles and feet plantar flex and invert; and toes flex and adduct.

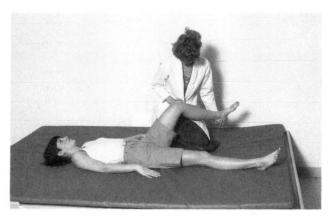

Figure 24D.30. D2 flexion of the lower extremity. The therapist performs rhythmic rotation to relax spastic hip muscles before lower extremity dressing.

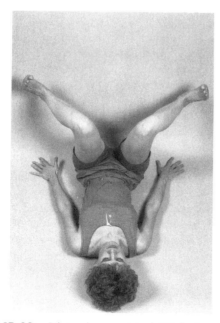

Figure 24D.29. Bilateral symmetrical D2 flexion, shortened range; bilateral symmetrical D2 extension, lengthened range. Hips flex, abduct, and internally rotate; knees flex (as the intermediate joint, the knee may flex or extend); ankle and feet dorsiflex and evert; and toes extend and abduct.

the midline of the face and body. They also interact when the pattern crosses the horizontal plane that transverses at the shoulders. An example occurs when waving good-bye. The right arm begins in extension on the same side of the body in **D1 extension.** When the arm raises above the shoulder to wave good-bye on the same side, it moves into **D2 flexion** with elbows flexed. Another example of the two diagonals interacting occurs in washing the face (Table 24D.2). When the right hand contacts the left face, it is moving into **D1 flexion.** When the right hand washes the right side of the face, it is moving toward **D2 flexion** with elbow flexion.

In all of the above bilateral and unilateral patterns, the intermediate joints, the elbow and the knee, may flex or extend. While the intermediate joints may change, the motions of the proximal and distal joints are consistent with each other. In the upper extremity, the consistency between the proximal and distal joints changes in a variation of the diagonal pattern called thrusting (Figs. 24D.19 and 24D.20, and 24D.22 and 24D.23).

The two pairs of upper extremity thrusting patterns are the ulnar thrust, D1, and the radial thrust, D2. In diagonal one flexion, external rotation is consistent with supination. In the D1 ulnar thrust, the shoulder remains the same, but the forearm is counterrotated in pronation, and the hand opens to the ulnar side. In diagonal two extension, internal rotation is consistent

Table 24D.2. Activity for Analysis: Primitive Washing of Face and Neck[a]

Hand(s)	Side(s) of Face	Diagonal and Sequence[b]	Combined Diagonal[c]
R	L, then R	D1, then D2	
L and R	Both sides	D1, then D2	BS
L contacts R wrist	L, then R	L, D2, then D1 R, D1, then D2	BA, chop and lift
R contacts L wrist	R, then L	L, D1, then D2 R, D2, then D1	BA, chop and lift

[a]Primitive, i.e., using the hands and running water, without a washcloth.
[b]Diagonals change and interact as the hand crosses the midline of the face, nose, or mouth.
[c]BS, both hands use bilateral symmetry, same diagonal. BA, one hand uses one diagonal as other hand uses the second, or other, diagonal. Hands placed in contact as for chopping and lifting permits one hand to guide, or track, the other. This bilateral asymmetrical combination of diagonal patterns may be useful with, e.g., hemiplegic patients.

with pronation. In the D2 radial thrust, the shoulder remains the same, but the forearm is counterrotated in supination, and the hand opens to the radial side. All bilateral combinations can be performed with the thrusting patterns. In the lower extremities, mass extension of hip and knee is a powerful thrusting movement. Thrusting patterns represent primitive patterns of protection, defense, reach, and grasp. The movement of thrusting occurs more forcefully than motions in other diagonal patterns. In treatment, thrusting is a good pattern in which to retrain elbow extension with wrist extension.

The diagonal patterns provide occupational therapists with a framework from which to assess and train functional movements. If a patient performs an incomplete hand-to-mouth pattern, the **D1 flexion** pattern is weak. Thus treatment activities to **facilitate** a stronger **D1 flexion** pattern are designed, e.g., pulleys in chopping pattern (Fig. 24D.6), grasp and release activity in reciprocal D1 using simultaneous static-dynamic positions (Fig. 24D.18), and resisting the D1 pattern using the techniques of slow reversal-hold and repeated contractions.

Total Patterns

PNF has been described as a developmental approach by Knott and Voss. In the course of normal motor development, total patterns of movement precede individual patterns (Hooker, 1952). Each total pattern requires interaction of component patterns of the head, neck, and trunk with those of the extremities. When movement in a forward or backward direction is combined with movement in a lateral direction, the diagonal patterns of **facilitation** become evident. In treatment, performance of total patterns is used to develop the ability to perform diagonal patterns. In PNF, the **facilitation techniques** are superimposed on total patterns

of movement and posture. The total pattern provides the base for all other movement.

The sequence and procedures for assisting patients into the developmental postures were developed by Voss in 1971. In this sequence of total patterns, the therapist elicits reflex support to assist the more severely involved patient. With reflex support, the assumption of postures may be achieved with minimal effort on the part of the therapist and patient (Voss, 1973). One procedure, assisting a patient from prone to prone on elbows, will be described in detail with application to activities.

PRONE ON ELBOWS

The prone-on-elbows posture may be used in daily living to watch television or read on the floor. In active assumption, prone on elbows is a symmetrical movement that is extensor dominant. The tonic labyrinthine prone reflex must be overcome, while the optical and labyrinthine righting reflexes support the assumption. The pattern begins with head, neck, and upper trunk extension followed by adduction of shoulders with forearms pronated and wrist and fingers extended.

To assist a patient from prone to prone on elbows (Fig. 24D.31), the preparatory maneuvers include placing the lower extremities in symmetrical extension and placing the head in a symmetrical position or turned to one side for comfort. Head, turned to one side, will be more difficult for the therapist to control as the shoulder toward which the head is turned will be elevated, with the other depressed against the mat. The upper extremities are placed in symmetrical **D2 flexion** with elbows flexed, fingers pointing to the nose.

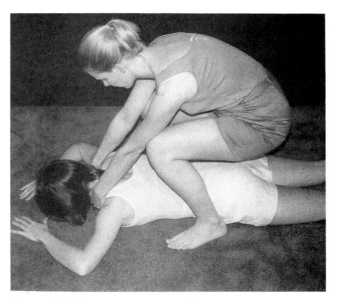

Figure 24D.31. The position of the patient and the therapist for assisting a patient from prone to prone on elbows.

The therapist positions herself astride the patient if the patient is on the mat, or to one side if he is on a bed or plinth. The therapist's hips and knees should be flexed.

Manual contacts, with the hands in a mitt-like position and fingers and thumbs relaxed, apply stretch and assistance or resistance. The hands, placed over the pectoral region with fingers pointing toward the umbilicus, stimulate a muscle response in the shoulder adductors that lends stability to the posture (Fig. 24D.32). Hands should be placed medially to allow the patient's arms to assume a vertical position.

Auditory commands are "When I say three, look up. One, two, three, look up!" Simultaneously with the word *up*, the therapist leans backward, so that the patient's superior region is elevated with forearms falling into place.

In application to activity, prone on elbows provides a good position in which to work for control of head and neck extension with weight bearing to **facilitate** stability in the scapulohumeral joint. Also, any patients who need to spend time prone for healing or prevention of decubitus ulcer or to maintain muscle tone will need to be able to assume and maintain this posture to perform self-care activities. Various activities may be performed, depending on the patient's ability.

In level one, practicing assumption, rocking, raising and lowering the head, and depressing the scapula may be all that the patient can perform. In level two, the patient is able to maintain an adequate posture for

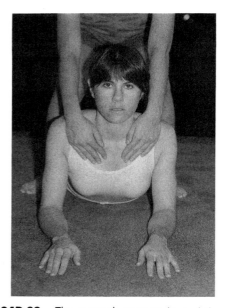

Figure 24D.32. The manual contacts in assisting a patient from prone to prone on elbows. The therapist's hands are placed over the pectoral region with fingers pointing toward the umbilicus.

longer periods of time. Straw or mouth stick activities may be used. Rood demonstrated that sucking and swallowing **facilitate** cocontraction of neck muscles and reinforce head and neck extension (Stockmeyer, 1967). Control of the tongue may be enhanced in this primitive posture.

In level three, the patient will begin to perform manual activities with the elbows immobile and bearing weight. The activity will be confined to a small area as with a drawing or a tile project. Eating finger foods is another facilitatory activity. The tongue receives a stretch stimulus in this position. With **flaccidity** or marked weakness, food may drop out of the mouth unless lip closure is maintained and the tongue is functional. The tongue and lips do not work as hard in the sitting posture. If a patient can perform for short periods in prone, his performance in sitting may improve faster.

In level four, the patient is able to decrease the support needed to maintain the posture and lift one extremity from the surface, as in playing a table game, typing one-handed, or combing one's hair. A brief list of other sequences for assisting patients into developmental postures follows.

SUPINE TO SIDE LYING

Reflex support: ATNR
Preparatory maneuvers: Position uppermost leg and arms in **D1 flexion.**
Position of therapist: On side toward which patient will move.
Manual contacts: Scapula and pelvis.
Commands: "Look here!" Patient is assisted to side lying.
Application to occupational therapy: Patients who must attend therapy on a cart may be positioned in side lying. Also side lying, a very stable posture, may be the place to begin treatment for the severely involved patient.
Examples of activities: Use of a skateboard, stabilizing or rolling a ball, macramé, grasping and releasing objects in diagonal patterns, sliding the hand on the wall in various directions, and writing on the wall.

SIDE LYING TO SIDE SITTING

Reflex support: Body on body righting.
Preparatory maneuvers: Position legs in asymmetric flexion, and arms in asymmetric flexion at shoulder level.
Position of therapist: Behind patient's hips.
Manual contacts: Shoulder girdle.
Commands: "On the count of three, look back at me. One, two, three, look at me!" Patient is assisted to side sitting.

Application to occupational therapy: Side sitting is useful for increasing trunk rotation, facilitating equilibrium reactions, and movement of the free arm, while the supporting arm is stable with compression of joint surfaces and cocontraction of antagonistic muscle groups.

Examples of activities: Table buffer exercises, stacking cones (reaching behind body to pick them up), turning pages of newspaper or magazine, playing chess, watching television, eating a snack, and rug punching (with the frame stabilized in a vise. Response of supporting arm may be enhanced by **vibration** of elbow extensors.

Variation: The patient may move from side lying to leaning on one elbow before progressing to side sitting. Side lying on elbow is often used by patients with paraplegia or quadriplegia during eating and hygiene activities performed on a cart or in a bed.

SUPINE TO LONG SITTING

Reflex support: Labyrinthine righting, optical righting.
Preparatory maneuvers: Place legs in symmetrical extension and abduction.
Position of therapist: Astride patient at knees.
Manual contacts: Dorsum of wrists.
Commands: "On the count of three, look at your feet and sit up. One, two, three, look at your feet!" Patient is assisted to long sitting.
  Alternate sequence: Side sitting to long sitting.
  Preparatory maneuvers: Assist to side sitting.
  Position of therapist: Behind patient.
  Manual contacts: Shoulder girdle, one anteriorly, the other posteriorly.
  Commands: Tell patient to look in direction of turn and reach over for support with moving arm. Assist patient to rotate, distributing weight on both hips.
Application to occupational therapy: Long-sitting improves sitting balance and provides stability for dressing lower extremities in bed. It is easily applied to a variety of one-handed or two-handed activities.
Examples of activities: One-handed: stack cones in a diagonal pattern, play checkers, throw bean bags, hit ball with stick, sanding project positioned on incline board, painting. Two-handed: pull putty, throw and catch ball, roll ball around body, macramé, leather stamping, throw and mold clay, mix ingredients in a bowl, prepare vegetables. For variation, a small lap board with legs can be placed over the patient's legs to provide a solid working surface and expand the type of activities that can be done in this position.

PRONE TO HANDS AND KNEES

Reflex support: STNR (head midline), or ATNR (head rotated).

Preparatory maneuvers: Position inferior region so that hips are flexed and thighs are vertical to floor.
Position of therapist: Astride patient holding hips securely between the therapist's knees.
Manual contacts: Pectoral region.
Commands: "On the count of three, look up. One, two, three, look up!" Patient is assisted to hands and knees.
Application to occupational therapy: The hands and knees posture promotes or enhances balance and stability in hips and shoulders.
Examples of activities: Initially, activity may include use of rhythmic stabilization following or preceding rocking in different directions—forward, backward, sideways, and diagonally to left and right. Simultaneous static-dynamic activity, i.e., stacking cones, sanding, hammering, placing tiles in trivet, and figure-of-eight board may follow as appropriate. Functional activities usually performed in this posture may be used, such as washing and waxing floor, cleaning under bed, picking up item on floor, cleaning low shelves or oven, or working in garden.

KNEELING

Reflex support: Labyrinthine and optical righting, and equilibrium reactions.
Procedure: Varies depending on method of assumption, i.e., from heel sitting, hands and knees, or side sitting.
Application to occupational therapy: Kneeling provides opportunity to develop upper extremity function for free standing as well as hip extension and hip extension with knee flexion necessary for gait.
Examples of activities: Activities will vary according to the patient's ability. Begin with both hands in contact with a supporting surface, as in rocking in various directions. Follow with a surface contact activity, such as sanding or dusting. Later, with both arms free, catching and throwing a ball, writing on a blackboard, or cooking may be tried. Kneeling is the only position other than sitting and standing in which both arms can be used free of the supporting surface.

HANDS AND KNEES TO PLANTIGRADE

Reflex support: Labyrinthine and optical righting and equilibrium reactions.
Preparatory maneuvers: Assist to hands-knees posture.
Position of therapist: Behind patient.
Manual contacts: Pelvis.
Commands: "Straighten your knees" or "Bring one foot forward and place it flat on the floor, then the other."
Application to occupational therapy: Plantigrade posture has minimal application to occupational therapy. However, a modified plantigrade posture with feet

flat on the floor and hands or elbows resting on a supporting surface is easily used in many occupational therapy activities.

Examples of activities: Washing dishes, wiping table, making bed, painting, grasping and releasing objects, playing cards with card holder, throwing bean bags in a game of "toss-a-cross," getting out of bathtub.

Assisting the patient into various postures helps him to experience functional movements with normal environmental and sensory stimulation to the total body. For example, the patient in the wheelchair, with lower limbs supported on footrests, is essentially suspended above the ground in a flexed posture. The sensory cues provided by gravity, body in contact with the ground, will be limited. If activities must be performed in a wheelchair, placing feet on the floor will **facilitate** a better response from the total pattern.

Selected Techniques

Facilitation and **inhibition techniques** include a battery of procedures that may be used singly or in combination, according to the abilities and needs of the patient. All techniques are superimposed on patterns of movement and posture (Voss, 1967).

Sherrington described three principles of neurophysiology from which Kabat (1961) developed many of the PNF techniques. Irradiation, the **facilitation** of one voluntary motion by another, is not haphazard but spreads in a specific pattern of muscle groups. The stimulus for irradiation is generated by tension in contracting muscles and related structures. In treatment, resistance coupled with stretch, as in repeated contractions, may elicit irradiation for the purpose of using the motions of the stronger muscle groups to **facilitate** the weaker motions of a pattern. Successive induction is also a process of facilitating one voluntary motion by another. However, the stronger antagonist facilitates the weaker agonist, as in resisted reversals of antagonists. In treatment, when techniques of slow reversal and slow reversal-hold are used, a contraction of the stronger muscle groups is elicited first to **facilitate** more effectively the weaker muscle groups. If a muscle imbalance is present, this procedure carries the risk of increasing the imbalance. Reciprocal innervation is a process of inhibiting reflexes by voluntary motion. At the time that the agonist is facilitated or contracted against resistance, the antagonist lengthens and provides control as the agonist contracts so that smooth movement is achieved. In treatment a slow reversal-hold-relax technique may be used to relax spastic or tight muscle groups. Relaxation of spastic antagonists can also be achieved by **facilitation** of the

agonist through patterns of irradiation, stretch, and supporting reflexes (Kabat, 1961).

Techniques of positioning, manual contacts, and verbal commands may be used to promote a mobility or a stability response. Because these all have been discussed previously in this chapter, other techniques will be described.

Stretch may be used as a stimulus to initiate movement or to initiate voluntary motion within the pattern and to increase strength and timing of a weak response. When applied as a stimulus, stretch is the positioning of a body part in the extreme lengthened range of a pattern to the point of tension. All motion components are stretched, especially rotation, as it is the rotary component that elongates the muscle fibers in a given pattern. The stretch reflex can be superimposed on a pattern in two ways. (1) After the position for stretch stimulus has been achieved, the body part is quickly and smoothly taken past the point of tension, just before the initiation of movement by the patient. (2) In repeated contractions, stretch stimulates isotonic contractions through increased range or strength of a pattern. Repeated stretch, followed by assisted or voluntary motion, can be an effective technique for patients with little or no voluntary control. For example, repeated stretch of the D2 bilateral reciprocal pattern in the C6 quadriplegic patient may stimulate the pectoral muscles. The increased adductor tonus contributes to functional use of hands at and across the midline, which is important in dressing and feeding.

Traction, separating joint surfaces, stimulates joint receptors to promote movement. Traction is maintained throughout the active range of motion (Voss et al., 1985). Approximation also stimulates joint receptors by compressing joint surfaces. In treatment, approximation promotes stability and postural responses. Application in treatment occurs before demanding a voluntary contraction of muscle groups by the patient. In sitting, with arms extended and bearing weight, pressure may be applied in a downward direction over the shoulders. The pressure occurs in the form of a sustained push or as repeated pushes. The expected result is increased extensor tone in the arm and trunk, which promotes strength and endurance for activity in the posture. Approximation repeated quickly may be contraindicated for the patient with pain and with ataxia as seen in multiple sclerosis (Voss et al., 1985).

Maximal resistance is probably the most misunderstood PNF technique. It does not refer to the maximal effort of the therapist, but rather to the maximal resistance that the patient can receive and still move smoothly through the full range of the pattern or maintain an isometric contraction. Manual contacts must be specifically applied over the agonists to **facilitate** a maximal response. For some patients, maximal resistance may be only a light touch, as resistance is graded to elicit the patient's maximal response. In treatment, maximal resistance is provided by the therapist on motions before and during activity or by equipment, such as pulleys and weighted tools (Voss et al., 1985).

Two techniques directed to the agonist are repeated contractions and rhythmic initiation. Repeated contractions are used to increase range and endurance in weaker components of a pattern through a technique of emphasis. For example, if a patient is unable to reach his mouth for eating, he would be instructed to hold, with an isometric contraction of all components at the point at which the active motion decreases in power. Then the patient is asked repeatedly to "pull again" toward his mouth, shifting from isometric to isotonic contractions. Rhythmic initiation is used to improve the ability to initiate movement. This technique involves passive rhythmic motion, followed by active motion. Resistance may be gradually imposed as the patient's response increases. For example, a patient may lack the ability to initiate reaching for a glass on the table, because of rigidity from Parkinson's disease or severe *spasticity*. The therapist would ask the patient to relax and say, "Let me move you." Then the therapist moves the part through the available range until relaxation is felt. The patient is directed to begin moving actively in the direction of the agonistic pattern with the command, "Now help me move you." As the patient's response increases, resistance may be added to reinforce the movement. The patient is then asked to move actively by himself and complete the task (Voss et al., 1985).

The reversal of antagonists techniques, based on the principle of successive induction, include slow reversal, slow reversal-hold, and rhythmic stabilization. These reversal techniques are primarily used for strengthening or gaining range of motion. Either isotonic, isometric, or a combination of both types of contractions may be used. Slow reversal is an alternating isotonic contraction of antagonists. The procedure begins by asking the patient to perform the weaker agonist pattern. In this example, **D2 flexion** will be the agonist. Manual contacts with maximal resistance are applied to determine the patient's response. The patient then performs the antagonistic pattern **D2 extension** against maximal resistance. The agonistic pattern is now repeated, with an increase in power or range of motion expected because of the law of successive induction. Resistance must be graded to **facilitate** a strong contraction of the antagonist followed by maximal range of motion in the weaker agonist. Activities performed with the assist of a pulley automatically use the slow reversal technique. The pulley assists the

gravity-resisted agonist and then resists the antagonistic movement. Slow reversal-hold proceeds in the same manner; however, an isometric contraction follows the completion of the isotonic contraction. Directions for a slow reversal-hold in the second diagonal would be "Push your arm up and out toward me, and hold. Now, pull your arm down and across, and hold (Voss et al., 1985).

Rhythmic stabilization is the simultaneous isometric contraction of antagonists, which results in co-contraction if the isometric contraction is not broken. This technique promotes stability by eliciting a more balanced response between antagonistic muscle groups. Relaxation is often achieved following the stabilization. As repeated isometric contractions are performed, circulation may increase. Also, the patient may hold his breath. Thus only three or four repetitions are used.

This technique has numerous applications in therapy to provide increased stability and endurance for performance of a task. Rhythmic stabilization cannot be incorporated into an activity, because it is an isometric exercise. However, it is used before an activity to enhance performance, during activity as the performance weakens, and after activity to prevent and correct imbalances built up during the activity. This technique is contraindicated for patients with cardiac problems who are advised not to perform isometric contractions by their physician. Also rhythmic stabilization may be impossible for some patients, such as those with ataxia, who are unable to perform isometric contractions. These patients may be taught to stabilize by using the technique of slow reversal-hold through decrements of range until no motion occurs (Voss et al., 1985).

Relaxation techniques include passive rotation, slow reversal-hold relax, contract-relax, and hold-relax. Rhythmic rotation coupled with range of motion is an effective technique used before dressing or splinting a limb in which the muscles are shortened or spastic (Fig. 24D.27). Place manual contacts on the intermediate and distal joints and perform range of motion. When restriction occurs, repeat rotation of all components of the pattern at the point of limitation, moving slowly and gently. As relaxation is felt, movement may continue through a larger range.

The procedures for the remaining three relaxation techniques follow the same sequence. Because only the stronger pattern of motion is resisted, a danger of creating further imbalances exists. These techniques rely on the principle of reciprocal **inhibition** and can be effective when used appropriately. Contract-relax includes an isotonic contraction of the antagonist, relaxation, then passive movement of the agonistic pattern by the therapist. Hold-relax includes an isometric contraction of the antagonist, relaxation, then active movement of the agonist by the patient. Slow reversal-hold-relax includes isotonic contraction followed by an isometric contraction of the antagonist, relaxation, then active movement of the agonist (Voss et al., 1985). If the patient has the ability to move the agonist, slow reversal-hold-relax is used.

Application to Occupational Therapy

PNF can be used in occupational therapy to (1) evaluate motion, (2) **facilitate** motor function, (3) prepare and position a patient for an activity, and (4) enhance the performance of an activity. The evaluation process was presented earlier in the chapter; this section focuses on the application of PNF in five selected problems of patient care. Then one sample treatment procedure will be explained.

The first problem is commonly seen in patients with C_5 tetraplegia. During the initial recovery, the upper extremities have poor muscle strength. The motion of raising the hand to the mouth and the repetition of that movement to complete a meal are problems that limit independence in self-feeding. Often, mobile arm supports are required to assist the arm against gravity. To **facilitate** feeding without support, the arm must be strengthened. Diagonal one is known as the feeding pattern because the necessary motions of shoulder flexion, elbow flexion, and supination are present in the **D1 flexion** pattern. Therefore, to strengthen these movements, the D1 pattern is resisted with manual contacts on the wrist and shoulder. The techniques of stretch in the lengthened range of **D1 flexion**, slow reversal-hold, and repeated contractions can be used.

The second problem is often found in a person with right hemiplegia from a CVA. **Spasticity** is present with beginning isolated movement in the hand. Grasp and release occur, but coordination of the intrinsic hand muscles is poor. For example, this patient is unable to coordinate palmar abduction of thumb with finger extension to remove the right hand from a drinking glass. Therefore, frequent spilling occurs when the glass is returned to the table. The diagonal pattern is the optimal pattern for the abductor pollicis brevis and the extensor digitorum. The **D1 extension** pattern is resisted using techniques of slow reversal-hold, repeated contractions, and rhythmic stabilization with manual contacts on the thumb and finger. The shortened range of **D1 extension** is emphasized for two reasons: (1) the patient can initiate abduction of the thumb in the lengthened range but has difficulty maintaining the contraction in the shortened range and (2) the patient has **spasticity** in the flexor muscles. By working in the shortened range of **D1 extension,** the influence of the spastic flexors is minimized. In one patient, four repetitions of extension facilitated voluntary release of the glass with coordinated thumb abduction and finger extension.

A third problem is frequently seen in patients with multiple sclerosis who exhibit ataxia. Fine motor tasks such as eating, writing, and applying makeup become difficult because of the incoordination. Several PNF concepts and techniques can be applied. The first priority is to select a stable posture in which the patient can perform the activity. In sitting, the arms are positioned close to the body with elbows and forearms resting on a lapboard or table. Other stable postures include side lying, prone on elbows, and kneeling with both hands in contact with an elevated surface (such as a bench or chair). Rhythmic stabilization, with manual contacts on shoulders or shoulders and pelvis, is used to reinforce the patient's ability to maintain the posture. Then the movements of rocking in different directions are resisted with slow reversal-hold and repeated contractions to build strength and control.

After these preparatory techniques, the patient is ready to perform an activity, such as writing or use of makeup. Self-touching or simultaneous static-dynamic positioning (Hellebrandt et al., 1956) may enhance control. For example, the patient may hold the wrist of the dominant hand while eating (self-touching) or bear weight on one arm (static arm) while writing with the other arm (dynamic arm). Another technique, move and stop, can **facilitate** control in middle range. For example, as the patient raises her arm to apply makeup, stopping at midrange enables her to gain control of the movements in the remainder of the range. Sometimes more than one stop during the range of motion is needed.

A fourth problem, found in a variety of neurological disorders, is difficulty with oral motor function such as sucking, chewing, and swallowing. The patient with dysarthria from a stroke (CVA) has problems of poor tongue control, drooling, inadequate lip closure, and may pocket food between teeth and cheek. Application of the techniques: stretch, slow reversal, slow reversal-hold and repeated contractions can **facilitate** a stronger response in the affected muscles before eating. Voss et al. (1985) provided an illustrated presentation of specific techniques.

A fifth problem occurs in patients with limited shoulder motion caused by joint disease, such as arthritis. Reaching overhead to dress or comb one's hair becomes difficult and often unsuccessful. Both diagonals are used in combing hair. The combing arm demonstrates **D2 flexion** when the shoulder abducts to reach the back of the head. **D1 flexion** occurs as the shoulder adducts to comb the front and opposite side of the head. Bilateral patterns for combing are common as one hand combs and the other adjusts and smoothes the hair. In treatment, bilateral combinations of the upper extremities can be resisted with slow reversals, slow reversal-hold-relax, rhythmic stabilization, and repeated contractions to gain range of motion and strength.

The patient can be taught to apply the techniques of stretch and reversing movement. For example, instead of struggling to move the arm in a partial range from lap level to the head, the motion is reversed. The patient extends the arm in the antagonistic pattern (**D1 extension**). Then stretch is applied by pushing the arms back and down toward the floor. Immediately the hands reach toward the head in **D1 flexion**. The patient can use **bilateral symmetrical** or **asymmetrical** combinations to seek reinforcement from the trunk and a more normal interaction of body segments.

Sequences of PNF treatment procedures vary according to the diagnosis and the individual patient's needs. The sample treatment sequences in this section provide guidelines for application of PNF. Adaptations may be required for the specific patient's age, medical status, and level of ability.

The first sequence outlines treatment activities for a patient with a shoulder-hand syndrome caused by trauma (Table 24D.3). The main goals of treatment include (1) reduction of pain and edema, (2) increase range of motion, (3) restore a balance between antagonistic movements, and (4) increase strength and endurance for functional activity. Steps 1 through 8 (Table 24D.3) are examples of the indirect approach. The therapist does not directly touch the affected hand or arm, because of the severe pain. However, the patient experiences a variety of movement patterns that **facilitate** control and range of movement. Proprioceptive stimulation is applied through weight-bearing activities and resistance to unaffected extremity and trunk.

With success in the preceding steps, the patient is ready for a more direct approach. The affected hand, wrist, elbow, and shoulder are resisted directly in pattern. Stronger components of the pattern are used to reinforce weaker motions. Initiation of motion is emphasized in the lengthened range, while strengthening is resisted toward the shortened range of the pattern. The performance of functional and work-related

Table 24D.3. Sample Sequence of Treatment for the Patient with Shoulder-Hand Syndrome

Preparatory Procedures and Techniques[a]	Patient Position	Manual Contacts
1. Breathing techniques	Sitting	Sternum and dorsal spine
2. Rhythmic stabilization	Sitting	Shoulders
3. Proprioceptive disturbance of balance with resisted recovery	Sitting	Shoulders

Activities	Patterns	Patient Position	Technique	Manual Contacts
4. Grasp and release	Chopping or lifting	Sitting or rolling	Resist unaffected arm Resist scapula of unaffected side, then affected side	Shoulders and wrist Scapula
5. Weight bearing	Bilateral symmetrical D1, D2	Modified plantigrade[b] Hands and knees Sitting with elbows extended Sitting, leaning forward on flexed elbows	Rhythmic stabilization	Shoulders or shoulders and pelvis
6. Rocking	Bilateral symmetrical Bilateral asymmetrical D1, D2	Same as #5	Stretch, resistance Slow reversal Slow reversal-hold Repeated contractions	Shoulders, pelvis, or shoulders and pelvis
7. Surface contact, i.e., washing table, sanding, figure-of-eight	D1, D2	Same as #5	Light touch or self-touch	Back of hand and wrist
8. Free active movement[c]	D1, D2	Modified plantigrade Sitting	Simultaneous static and dynamic	

[a]Breathing techniques and rhythmic stabilization are also used during treatment when the patient fatigues or the motor response deteriorates.
[b]If the patient is unable to bear weight with the wrist fully extended, a pushup block or soft bean bag may be used under the hand to decrease the degree of wrist extension.
[c]Examples of activities are grasp-and-release tasks or games, writing with the marker (built up as necessary), and a one-handed craft such as rug punch. Activities can be placed on an elevated surface to increase shoulder range of motion and reduce edema in the hand.

activities follows. Specific movement problems are analyzed and facilitated as necessary.

A home program would include the following activities:

1. Self-range of motion using the chopping and lifting patterns;
2. Active range of motion, incorporating the distal component of forearm rotation with opening and closing of the hand;
3. Grasp and release activities that involve reaching diagonally in a developmental pattern;
4. Use of door pulleys for chopping and lifting patterns;
5. Functional activities in which the patient incorporates the facilitated pattern into his daily routine.

For example, after bathing, the patient may dry the shower wall with a towel using D1 and D2 patterns. Before morning hygiene, the patient may rock in modified plantigrade position while weight bearing at the sink. Then the patient could reach to grasp the toothpaste and comb from the bathroom shelf in a D1 pattern.

EFFECTIVENESS

Research to support the effectiveness of the PNF treatment approach is limited. The majority of the research reported in the last 15 years analyzed the response of able-bodied subjects to selected techniques by recording electromyographic (EMG) activity. Studies that support the principles and techniques are summarized briefly.

Holt et al. (1968) tested the isometric strength of elbow flexion using EMG and dynamometer readings. Six subjects participated, three able-bodied and three with cerebral palsy. Four muscle contractions were measured with (1) the head in anatomic position, (2) the head turned right, (3) the head turned left, and (4) a prior contraction of the antagonists. The results indicated that the reversal of antagonists was superior to the other independent variables in facilitating strength.

Tanigawa (1972) compared the effects of the PNF hold-relax procedure and passive mobilization on tight hamstring muscles. He used a mathematical method to measure the angle of passive straight leg raising on 30 able-bodied male subjects. The results showed that subjects receiving the PNF hold-relax procedure increased their range of passive straight leg raising to a higher degree and at a faster rate than the subjects receiving passive mobilization.

Markos (1979) compared the effects of the PNF procedures of contract-relax on active hip flexion in 30 able-bodied female subjects. The range of motion increased significantly more in subjects in the contract-relax group, both in the exercised and in the unexercised lower extremities. The author presented application of each technique to treatment, suggesting that contract-relax applied ipsilaterally may prevent disuse atrophy in specific muscles of the **contralateral** lower extremity.

Sullivan and Portney (1980) monitored four shoulder muscles on 29 able-bodied subjects to confirm that each muscle tested would exhibit maximal EMG activity in an optimal diagonal pattern. The anterior deltoid demonstrated maximal activity in the **D1 flexion** pattern; the middle deltoid, in the **D2 flexion** pattern; the posterior deltoid, in the **D1 extension** pattern; and the sternal portion of the pectoralis major, in the **D2 extension** pattern. The authors also reported that performing the patterns with elbows straight, flexing, and extending changed the amount of shoulder muscle activity. This study is of practical value to occupational therapists in that it confirmed the optimum diagonal patterns for four specific shoulder muscles. This may aid the therapist in selecting a place to initiate a treatment program given a particular shoulder limitation.

Pink (1981) measured EMG activity in three muscles of the nonexercised upper extremity. The results from 10 able-bodied female subjects indicated that the following muscles do become active in the nonexercised limb. The sternal portion of the pectoralis major produced similar EMG activity during **D1 flexion** and extension of the **contralateral** limb. The infraspinatus was more active during **D1 flexion,** while the latissimus dorsi was more active during **D1 extension.** The author stated that these results could be used in treatment programs for patients who are unable to exercise one of their upper extremities.

In 1960 Mead reported on a 6-year evaluation of PNF techniques. The author compared an experience using traditional therapeutic exercise to treat patients with poliomyelitis from 1948 to 1953 in a university physical medicine clinic to an experience using PNF to treat patients with varied diagnoses from 1954 to 1960 at the California Rehabilitation Center in Vallejo. Although a controlled study with statistical analysis was not done, the author found that the PNF approach was more effective than the traditional approach. Mead described the therapy program at Vallejo and concluded that PNF techniques have application to all diagnoses.

Nelson et al. (1986) examined the effects of PNF and weight training on muscular strength and performance in 30 healthy college women. Subjects were tested for changes in knee and elbow extension strength, throwing distance, and vertical jump following an 8-week training program. Results indicated the PNF-trained group had greater increases in all of these areas than the weight-trained and control groups. Nelson et al. (1986) suggested this may be attributed to PNF's "incorporation of the theories of irradiation, spatiotemporal summation and stretch reflex" (p. 253). They also concluded that "PNF might be superior to weight-training for athletic training programs and injury rehabilitation" (p. 253).

Some studies have questioned the principles and procedures of PNF. Arsenault (1974) reviewed the literature and reported that success in using PNF techniques to treat neurological disorders was not universally true. Thus he questioned the acceptance of using mass patterns of movement based on the lack of scientific support. Arsenault reviewed several studies on quadriceps function with conflicting results on the effects of PNF irradiation patterns. Toe, ankle, and hip movements made no difference in the augmentation of quadriceps activity. Therefore, further research must be done to confirm the use of the PNF irradiation patterns.

Arsenault and Chapman (1974) studied the effects of movement patterns used to promote quadriceps activity in seven able-bodied subjects over an 8-week period. No consistent response was found. In general, the **D1 flexion** pattern of the lower extremity increased the activity of the rectus femoris but not the vastus medialis. The **D2 flexion** pattern produced a decrease of rectus femoris activity. The findings confirmed **D1 flexion** as the optimal pattern for the medial portion of the rectus femoris and disputed **D2 flexion** as the optimal pattern for the lateral portion of the rectus femoris. Either a proximal or distal resistance provided the **ipsilateral** overflow to the quadriceps. However, it is not clear whether precise PNF manual contacts and procedures were employed.

Synder and Forward (1972) compared the sequential EMG activity in selected muscles of the lower limb during flexion and extension of the knee. A total of 10 able-bodied female subjects performed active range of motion in the sagittal and diagonal planes of movement. An electrogoniometer was used to monitor the degree of knee flexion. The findings showed that selected muscles were more active in the sagittal plane than in the diagonal plane. Also, the authors observed the interaction of antagonists during fast and slow movements and following transiently induced pain in the semisquat position. They concluded that the assumption of increased activity in a diagonal plane of movement appears unjustified.

Surburg (1979) studied the effects of maximal resistance with PNF patterns on reaction, movement, and response times. A total of 50 able-bodied subjects participated for 6 weeks in one of three training programs: weight training, PNF patterning without resistance, and PNF patterning with maximal resistance.

Analysis revealed no significant differences among the training groups.

In summary, scientific studies of the effectiveness of the PNF approach are limited to only one aspect of the approach. Research on the effect of total patterns and combining movements with functional application still needs to be done.

Acknowledgments——The author thanks Dorothy E. Voss, associate professor emeritus of rehabilitation medicine at Northwestern University Medical School, for her assistance and support in developing and reviewing the subchapter as it appeared in the third edition of this textbook. Also, the author is grateful to Mary Herbin, Kathy Knutson, and Cindy Shanker for their time and technical skill in posing for the illustrations and to Laura M. Kearny for her contribution to updating the review of research, introduction to total patterns, and study questions.

STUDY QUESTIONS

1. Discuss 4 of the 11 principles of PNF.
2. From which developmental activities are diagonals one and two derived?
3. What is the advantage of giving passive range of motion in the diagonal patterns?
4. Distinguish the difference between bilateral symmetrical, bilateral asymmetrical, bilateral reciprocal, and unilateral patterns. Give an example of functional activities in which each of these patterns may be observed.
5. Given a patient with a shoulder-hand syndrome, select a therapeutic activity and PNF patterns and techniques that could facilitate more range of motion.
6. Discuss three of the five factors that support the use of diagonal patterns in treatment.
7. Which PNF technique provides increased stability and endurance for performance of a task through a simultaneous isometric contraction of antagonists?
8. List a contraindication for the use of stretch, traction, or approximation during patient treatment.
9. Discuss the importance of the therapist's positioning, appropriate manual contacts, and verbal commands when assisting a patient to a developmental posture.
10. What bilateral asymmetrical pattern could a hemiplegic patient use to put his flaccid arm through the sleeve of a shirt?
11. In a child with cerebral palsy who exhibits a spastic right upper extremity, drooling, and poor sitting balance, which problem would you address first during treatment? What relaxation technique would you use to decrease spasticity in the arm?
12. What is the effect on head, neck, and trunk during bilateral symmetrical D1 extension? Bilateral D2 extension? Which pattern elicits the greatest amount of flexion?

REFERENCES

Arsenault, A. B. (1974). Techniques of muscle re-education: Analysis of studies on the effect of techniques of patterning and neuromuscular facilitation. *Physiotherapy Canada, 26*(4), 190–194.

Arsenault, A. B., & Chapman, A. E. (1974). An electromyographic investigation of the individual recruitment of the quadriceps muscles during isometric contraction of the knee extensors in different patterns of movement. *Physiotherapy Canada, 26*(5), 253–261.

Ayres, A. J. (1955a). Proprioceptive facilitation elicited through the upper extremities. Part I. Background. *American Journal of Occupational Therapy, 9*(1), 1–9.

Ayres, A. J. (1955b). Proprioceptive facilitation elicited through the upper extremities. Part II. Application. *American Journal of Occupational Therapy, 9*(2), 57–62.

Ayres, A. J. (1955c). Proprioceptive facilitation elicited through the upper extremities. Part III. Specific application. *American Journal of Occupational Therapy, 9*(3), 121–126.

Ayres, A. J. (1962). Integration of information. In C. Sattely (Ed.), *Approaches to the treatment of patients with neuromuscular dysfunction* (Study Course VI, 3rd International Congress WFOT, pp. 49–57). Dubuque, IA: W. C. Brown.

Ayres, A. J. (1963). Occupational therapy directed toward neuromuscular integration. In H. S. Willard & C. S. Spackman (Eds.), *Occupational therapy* (3rd ed., pp. 358–459). Philadelphia: J. B. Lippincott.

Ayres, A. J. (1974). Integration of information. In A. Henderson, L. Llorens, E. Gilfoyle, C. Meyers, & S. Prevel (Eds.), *The development of sensory integrative theory and practice: A collection of the works of A. Jean Ayers* (pp. 63–82). Dubuque, IA: Kendall-Hunt.

Basmajian, J. V., Gowland, C. A., Finlayson, A. J., Hall, A. L., Swanson, L. R., Stratford, M. S., Trotter, J. E., & Brandstater, M. E. (1987). Stroke treatment: Comparison of integrated behavioral-physical therapy vs traditional physical therapy programs. *Archives of Physical Medicine and Rehabilitation, 68*, 267–272.

Bobath, B. (1948). A new treatment of lesions of the upper motor neurone. *British Journal of Physical Medicine, 2*(1), 26–29.

Bobath, B. (1990). *Adult hemiplegia: Evaluation and treatment* (3rd ed.). London: William Heinemann Medical Books.

Brodal, A. (1973). Self-observations and neuro-anatomical considerations after a stroke. *Brain, 96*, 675–694.

Brunnstrom, S. (1956). Associated reactions of the upper extremity in adult patients with hemiplegia. *Physical Therapy Review, 36*, 225–236.

Brunnstrom, S. (1966). Motor testing procedures in hemiplegia. *Journal of the American Physical Therapy Association, 46*(4), 357–375.

Brunnstrom, S. (1970). *Movement therapy in hemiplegia.* New York: Harper & Row.

Buchwald, J. S. (1965). Basic mechanisms of motor learning. *Journal of the American Physical Therapy Association, 45*, 314–331.

Carey, J. R. (1990). Manual stretch: Effect on finger movement control and force control in stroke subjects with spastic extrinsic finger flexor muscles. *Archives of Physical Medicine and Rehabilitation, 71*(10), 888–894.

Carroll, J. (1950). The utilization of reinforcement techniques in the program for the hemiplegic. *American Journal of Occupational Therapy, 4*(5), 211–213, 239.

Case-Smith, J., Fisher, A. G., & Bauer, D. (1989). An analysis of the relationship between proximal and distal motor control. *American Journal of Occupational Therapy, 43*, 657–662.

Chollet, F., DiPiero, V., Wise, R. J. S., Brooks, D. J., Dolan, R. J., & Frackowiak, R. S. J. (1991). The functional recovery of motor recovery after stroke in humans: A study with positron emission tomography. *Annals of Neurology, 29*, 63–71.

Clarke, B., Gowland, C., Brandstater, M., & DeBruin, H. (1983). A re-evaluation of the Brunnstrom assessment of motor recovery of the lower limb. *Physiotherapy Canada, 35*(4), 207–211.

Cofrancesco, E. M. (1985). The effect of music therapy on hand grasp strength and functional task performance in stroke patients. *Journal of Music Therapy, 22*(3), 129–145.

Cooke, D. M. (1958) The effects of resistance on multiple sclerosis patients with intention tremor. *American Journal of Occupational Therapy, 12*(2), 89–94.

Curran, P. (1960). A study toward a theory of neuromuscular education through occupational therapy. *American Journal of Occupational Therapy, 14*, 80–87.

Dickstein, R., Hocherman, S., Pillar, T., & Shaham, R. (1986). Stroke rehabilitation: Three exercise therapy approaches. *Physical Therapy, 66*(8), 1233–1238.

Duncan, P. W., Propst, M., & Nelson, S. G. (1983). Reliability of the Fugl-Meyer Assessment of sensorimotor recovery following cerebrovascular accident. *Physical Therapy, 63*(10), 1606–1610.

Freund, H.-J. & Hummelsheim, H. (1984). Premotor cortex in man: Evidence for innervation of proximal limb muscles. *Experimental Brain Research, 53*, 479–482.

Fugl-Meyer, A. R., Jääsko, L., Leyman, I., Olsson, S., & Steglind, S. (1975). The post-stroke hemiplegic patient. I. A method for evaluation of physical performance. *Scandinavian Journal of Rehabilitation Medicine, 7*, 13–31.

Gesell, A. (1954). Behavior patterns of fetal infant and child. *Genetics, 33*, 114–123.

Gesell, A. (1977). Reciprocal interweaving in neuromotor development. In O. Payton, S. Hirt, & R. A. Newton (Eds.), *Scientific bases for neurophysiologic approaches to therapeutic exercise: An anthology* (pp. 105–114) Philadelphia: F. A. Davis.

Goff, B. (1972). The application of recent advances in neurophysiology to Miss M. Rood's concept of neuromuscular facilitation. *Physiotherapy, 58*, 409–415.

Gordon, J. (1987). Assumptions underlying physical therapy intervention: Theoretical and historical perspectives. In J. H. Carr & R. B. Shepherd (Eds.), *Movement science: Foundations for physical therapy in rehabilitation* (pp. 1–30). London: William Heinemann Medical Books.

Harlow, H. F., & Harlow, M. K. (1962). Principles of primate learning: Lessons from animal behavior. *Little Club Clinics in Developmental Medicine* (No. 7). London: William Heinemann Medical Books.

Harris, F. (1969). Control of gamma efferents through the reticular activating system. *American Journal of Occupational Therapy, 23*, 403–408.

Hellebrandt, F. A., Houtz, S. J., Hockman, D. E., & Partridge, M. (1956). Physiological effects of simultaneous static and dynamic exercise. *American Journal of Physical Medicine, 35*, 106–117.

Hellebrandt, F. A., Schade, M., & Carns, M. L. (1962). Methods of evoking the tonic neck reflexes in normal human subjects. *American Journal of Physical Medicine, 41*, 90–139.

Holt, L. E., Kaplan, H. M., Okita, T. Y., & Hoshiko, M. (1968). The influence of antagonistic contraction and head position on the responses of agonistic muscles. *Archives of Physical Medicine and Rehabilitation, 50*(5), 279–291.

Hooker, D. (1952). *The prenatal origin of behavior.* Lawrence: University of Kansas Press.

Hooker, D. (1977). Evidence of prenatal function of the central nervous system in man. In O. Payton, S. Hirt, & R. A. Newton (Eds.), *Scientific bases for neurophysiological approaches to therapeutic exercise: An anthology* (pp. 51–61). Philadelphia: F. A. Davis.

Horak, F. B. (1991). Assumptions underlying motor control for neurologic rehabilitation. In M. Lister (Ed.), *Contemporary management of motor control problems: Proceedings of the II STEP Conference* (pp. 11–27). Alexandria, VA: Foundation for Physical Therapy.

Huss, J. (n.d.). An introduction to treatment techniques developed by Margaret Rood. In S. Perlmutter (Ed.), *Neuroanatomy and neurophysiology underlying current treatment techniques for sensorimotor dysfunction* (pp. 89–94). University of Illinois, Division of Services for Crippled Children.

Huss, J. (1971). Sensorimotor treatment approaches. In H. S. Willard & C. S. Spackman (Eds.), *Occupational therapy* (4th ed., pp. 373–400). Philadelphia: J. B. Lippincott.

Jackson, J. H. (1931). *Selected writings* (Vol. 1). London: Hodder & Staughton.

Kabat, H. (1961). Proprioceptive facilitation in therapeutic exercise. In S. Licht (Ed.), *Therapeutic exercise* (2nd ed., pp. 327–343). New Haven, CT: Elizabeth Licht.

Kabat, H., & Rosenberg, D. (1950). Concepts and techniques of occupational therapy neuromuscular disorders. *American Journal of Occupational Therapy, 4*(1), 6–11, 79.

LaVigne, J. M. (1974). Hemiplegia sensorimotor assessment form. *Physical Therapy, 54*(2), 128–134.

Lawrence, D. G., & Kuyphers, H. G. J. M. (1965). Pyramdial and nonpyramidal pathways in monkeys: Anatomical and functional correlations. *Science, 148*, 973–975.

Levine, S. (1960). Stimulation in infancy. *Scientific American, 202*(5), 80–86.

Logigian, M. K., Samuals, M. A., Falcolner, J., & Zaager, R. (1983). Clinical exercise trial for stroke patients. *Archives of Physical Medicine and Rehabilitation, 64*, 364–367.

Loomis, J. E., & Boersma, F. J. (1982). Training right brain-damaged patients in a wheelchair task: Case studies using verbal mediation. *Canadian Journal of Physiotherapy, 34*, 204–208.

Markos, P. D. (1979). Ipsilateral and contralateral effects of proprioceptive neuromuscular facilitation techniques on hip motion and electromyographic activity. *Physical Therapy, 59*(11), 1366–1373.

Marteniuk, R.G., MacKenzie, C. L., Jeannerod, M., Athenes, S., & Dugas, C. (1987). Constraints on human arm movement trajectories. *Canadian Journal of Psychology, 41*(3), 365–378.

Mason, C. R. (1985). One method for assessing the effectiveness of fast brushing. *Physical Therapy, 65*(8), 1197–1202.

Matyas, T. A., & Spicer, S. D. (1980). Facilitation of the tonic vibration reflex (TVR) by cutaneous stimulation in hemiplegics. *American Journal of Physical Medicine, 59*(6), 280–287.

McGraw, M. (1945). *Neuromuscular maturation of the human infant.* New York: Hafner.

Mead, S. (1960). A six-year evaluation of proprioceptive neuromuscular facilitation technics. *American Journal of Physical Medicine, 39*, 373–376.

Minor, M. A. D. (1991). Merging neurophysiologic approaches with contemporary theories. IV. Proprioceptive neuromuscular facilitation and the approach of Rood. In M. Lister (Ed.), *Contemporary management of motor control problems: Proceedings of the II STEP Conference* (pp. 137–139). Alexandria, VA: Foundation for Physical Therapy.

Myers, B. J. (1981). *Assisting to posture and application in occupational therapy activities.* Videotape. Chicago: Rehabilitation Institute of Chicago.

Nelson, A. G., Chambers, R. S., McGown, C. M., & Penrose, K. W. (1986). Proprioceptive neuromuscular facilitation versus weight training for enhancement of muscular strength and athletic performance. *Journal of Orthopedic and Sports Physical Therapy, 7*(5), 250–253.

Ostrosky, K. (1990). Facilitation vs. motor control. *Clinical Management, 10*(3), 34–40.

Pink, M. (1981). Contralateral effects of upper extremity proprioceptive neuromuscular facilitation patterns. *Physical Therapy, 61*(8), 1158–1162.

Rider, B. (1971). Effects of neuromuscular facilitation on crosstransfer. *American Journal of Occupational Therapy, 25*, 84–89.

Rood, M. S. (1954). Neurophysiological reactions as a basis for physical therapy. *Physical Therapy Review, 34*, 444–449.

Rood, M. S. (1956). Neurophysiological mechanisms utilized in the treatment of neuromuscular dysfunction. *American Journal of Occupational Therapy, 10*, 220–225.

Rood, M. S. (1962). The use of sensory receptors to activate, facilitate, and inhibit motor response, autonomic and somatic, in developmental sequence. In C. Sattely (Ed.), *Approaches to the treatment of patients with neuromuscular dysfunction* (Study Course VI, 3rd International Congress WFOT, pp. 26–37). Dubuque, IA: W. C. Brown.

Rood, M. S. (1976, July 9–11). *The Treatment of Neuromuscular Dysfunction: Rood Approach.* Lecture given in Boston.

Royeen, C., & DeGangi, G. (1992). *Annotated bibliography of NDT peer-reviewed literature 1980–1990, inclusive.* Chicago: Neuro-Developmental Treatment Association.

Ryerson, S., & Levit, K. (1991). The shoulder in hemiplegia. In R. Donatelli (Ed.), *Physical therapy of the shoulder* (2nd ed., pp. 117–149). New York: Churchill Livingstone.

Sherrington, C. S. (1913). Reflex inhibition as a factor in the coordination of movements and postures. *Quarterly Journal of Experimental Physiology, 6*, 251–310.

Smith, K. U. (1967). Cybernetic foundations for rehabilitation. *American Journal of Physical Medicine, 46*(1), 379–467.

Snyder, J. L., & Forward, E. M. (1972). Comparison of knee flexion and extension in the diagonal and sagittal planes. *Physical Therapy, 52*(12), 1255–1263.

Spicer, S. D., & Matyas, T. A. (1980). Facilitation of the tonic vibration reflex (TVR) by cutaneous stimulation. *American Journal of Physical Medicine, 59*(5), 223–231

Stockmeyer, S. (1967). An interpretation of the approach of Rood to the treatment of neuromuscular dysfunction. *American Journal of Physical Medicine, 46*(1), 900–956.

Sullivan, P. E., & Portney, L. G. (1980). Electromyographic activity of shoulder muscles during unilateral upper extremity proprioceptive neuromuscular facilitation patterns. *Physical Therapy, 60*(3), 283–288.

Surburg, P. R. (1979). Interactive effects of resistance and facilitation patterning upon reaction and response times. *Physical Therapy, 59*(13), 1513–1517.

Tanigawa, M. C. (1972). Comparison of the hold-relax procedure and passive mobilization on increasing muscle length. *Physical Therapy, 52*(7), 725–735.

Thelen, E., & Fisher, D. M. (1982). Newborn stepping: An explanation for a "disappearing" reflex. *Developmental Psychology, 18*, 760–775.

Thelen, E., & Whitley-Cooke, D. (1987). Relationship between newborn stepping and later walking: A new interpretation. *Developmental Medicine and Child Neurology, 29*, 380–393.

Touwen, B. C. L. (1978). Variability and stereotypy in normal and deviant development. In J. Apley (Ed.), *Care of the handicapped child* (Clinics in Developmental Medicine, No. 67, pp. 99–110). Philadelphia: J. B. Lippincott.

Trombly, C. A., & Cole, J. M. (1979). Electromyographic study of four hand muscles during selected activities. *American Journal of Occupational Therapy, 33*(7), 440–449.

Twitchell, T. (1951). The restoration of motor function following hemiplegia in man. *Brain, 74*, 443–480.

VanSant, A. (1988). Rising from a supine position to erect stance:

Description of adult movement and a developmental hypothesis. *Physical Therapy, 68,* 185–192.

VanSant, A. (1991a). Should the normal motor developmental sequence be used as a theoretical model to progress adult patients? In M. Lister (Ed.), *Contemporary management of motor control problems: Proceedings of the II STEP Conference* (pp. 95–97). Alexandria, VA: Foundation for Physical Therapy.

VanSant, A. (1991b). Life span motor development. In. M. J. Lister (Ed.), *Contemporary management of motor control problems: Proceedings of the II STEP Conference* (pp. 77–83). Alexandria, VA: Foundation for Physical Therapy.

von Hofsten, C. (1984). Developmental changes in the organization of prereaching movements. *Developmental Psychology, 20,* 378–388.

Voss, D. E. (1959). PNF: Application of patterns and techniques in occupational therapy. *American Journal of Occupational Therapy, 8*(4), 191–194.

Voss, D. E. (1967). Proprioceptive neuromuscular facilitation. *American Journal of Physical Medicine, 46*(1), 838–898.

Voss, D. E. (1969). *Evaluation forms: Introduction and sections 1–3.* Unpublished teaching materials. Northwestern University Medical School, Program in Physical Therapy.

Voss, D. E. (1972). Proprioceptive neuromuscular facilitation: The PNF method. In P. Pearson & C. Williams (Eds.), *Physical therapy services in the developmental disabilities* (pp. 223–282). Springfield, IL: Charles C. Thomas.

Voss, D. E. (1973). *Assistance in the assumption of total patterns of posture, PNF approach.* Videotape. Chicago: Northwestern Medical School, Program in Physical Therapy.

Voss, D. E., Ionta, M. K., & Myers, B. J. (1985). *Proprioceptive neuromuscular facilitation: Patterns and techniques* (3rd ed.). New York: Harper & Row.

Wagenaar, R. C., Meijer, O. G., van Wieringen, P. C. W., Kuik, D. J., Hazenberg, G. J., Lindeboom, J., Wichers, F., & Rijswijk, H. (1990). The functional recovery of stroke: A comparison between neuro-developmental treatment and the Brunnstrom method. *Scandinavian Journal of Rehabilitation Medicine, 22,* 1–8.

Whitaker, E. W. (1950). A suggested treatment in occupational therapy for patients with multiple sclerosis. *American Journal of Occupational Therapy, 4*(6), 247–251.

Wilson, B. N., & Trombly, C. A. (1984). Proximal and distal function in children with and without sensory integrative dysfunction: An E.M.G. study. *Canadian Journal of Occupational Therapy, 51*(1), 11–17.

Zimny, N. (1979). *Effect of position and sensory stimulation on scapular muscles.* Unpublished master's thesis, Boston University.

SUPPLEMENTARY RESOURCES

Suggested Readings

Boakes, M. (1990). Vibrotactile stimulation. *British Journal of Occupational Therapy, 53*(6), 220–224.

Brunnstrom, S. (1961). Motor behavior of adult hemiplegic patients. *American Journal of Occupational Therapy, 25*(1), 6–12.

Davies, P. (1985). *Steps to follow.* Berlin: Springer-Verlag.

Davis, J. Z. (1990). The Bobath approach to the treatment of adult hemiplegia. In L. W. Pedretti & B. Zoltan (Eds.), *Occupational therapy: Practice skills for physical dysfunction* (pp. 351–362). St. Louis: C. V. Mosby.

Delaney, F. Y. (1983). The geriatric patient with central nervous system dysfunction. *Occupational & Physical Therapy in Geriatrics, 2*(3), 5–25.

Eggers, O. (1984). *Occupational therapy in the treatment of adult hemiplegia.* Rockville, MD: Aspen Systems.

Harris, F. A. (1978). Facilitation techniques in therapeutic exercise. In J. V. Basmajian (Ed.), *Therapeutic exercise* (3rd ed., pp. 93–137). Baltimore: Williams & Wilkins.

Hughes, E. (1972). Bobath and Brunnstrom: comparison of two methods of treatment of a left hemiplegia. *Physiotherapy Canada, 24*(5), 262–266.

Kukulka, C. G., Fellows, W. A., Oehlertz, J. E., & Vanderwilt, S. G. (1985). Effect of tendon pressure on alpha motoneuron excitability. *Physical Therapy, 65*(5), 595–600.

Perry, C. E. (1967). Principles and techniques of the Brunnstrom approach to the treatment of hemiplegia. *American Journal of Physical Medicine, 46*(1), 789–812.

Safranek, M. G., Koshland, G. F., & Raymond, G. (1982). Effect of auditory rhythm on muscle activity. *Physical Therapy, 62*(2), 161–168.

Schleichkorn, J. (1992). *The Bobaths.* Tucson, AZ: Therapy Skill Builders.

Wolff, P. H., Gunnoe, C. E., & Cohen, C. (1983). Associated movements as a measure of developmental age. *Developmental Medicine & Child Neurology, 25,* 417–429.

Resources

Neuro-Developmental Treatment Association, Inc. This organization sponsors continuing education courses for therapists interested in learning hands-on treatment for cerebral palsy or adult hemiplegia; courses are offered to graduate therapists at the introductory, basic, and advanced levels and usually incorporate practicum sessions as well as lectures. (P.O. Box 70, Oak Park, IL 60303)

25
Remediating Motor Behavior Through Contemporary Approaches

Newer research on the characteristics of normal human movement, motor skill acquisition in children and adults, robotics, and the mechanisms of motor control have led to new thinking by therapists concerning their approach to the remediation of motor control and performance. Computerized instrumentation allows more sophisticated analysis of movement. Robotics engineers are pushing to learn the mechanisms of skilled movement control. Cognitive and ecological psychologists as well as systems theorists are also contributing heavily to this rethinking. Motor learning problems faced by therapists concerning carryover of a motor skill from one environment to another or generalization of the skill to similar but different conditions have been addressed, for normal subjects, by the human movement scientists. The importance of biomechanical and environmental constraints on the patient's ability to move are also being reconsidered and included in these newer approaches. The procedures used by those who train skilled movement performers (e.g., athletes and dancers) are intriguing to consider for patients.

This chapter consists of two subchapters. The first describes a system of therapy developed by two physical therapists who were influenced by Bobath's neurodevelopmental treatment (NDT) as well as the human movement science literature. The second approach is a synthesis of current knowledge about human movement and occupational therapy theory. The two subchapters are

1. Carr and Shepherd's Motor Relearning Programme for Individuals with Stroke;
2. Contemporary Task-oriented Approach.

The two approaches have similarities. Both are influenced by contemporary skill acquisition and motor development theories. Both emphasize motor performance using functional tasks. Both consider factors other than central nervous system (CNS) damage that may be affecting performance. Both include remediation of performance components and modification of the environment to improve task performance. They stress practice that fits the nature of the task. Both approaches reject assumptions of the reflex-hierarchical model of motor control and of the traditional developmental theories. The two approaches, however, differ in their emphasis. The *Motor Relearning Programme* draws heavily from cognitive motor learning theory, while the contemporary task-oriented approach is strongly influenced by systems theory and ecological psychology. Further developmental and empirical research is encouraged by developers of both approaches.

GLOSSARY

Attractors—Preferred but not obligatory pattern of behavior that emerges from the interaction of a unique person with a particular task and environment.

Blocked practice—Practice that consists of drills and requires many repetitions of the same task in the same way (Schmidt, 1991b).

Closed-loop system—A system of motor control in which accurate performance is based on feedback and the recognition and correction of errors.

Closed task—A task in which there are stable environmental conditions and consistency from one trial to the next.

Collective variables—The fewest number of variables or dimensions that describe a unit of behavior quantitatively.

Compensatory strategies—Motor patterns or fixations that develop in response to obstacles to normal movement to enable an individual to achieve short-term success in movement or balance.

Continuous tasks—Repetitive tasks without a clear beginning or end.

Control parameters—Variables that shift behavior from one preferred pattern to another, do not control the change but act as agents for reorganization of behavior, and must be scalar quantities.

Discrete tasks—Tasks involving movements with a recognizable beginning and end.

Gravitational torque—The net impact that gravity will exert on a body segment as a result of the combined effect of the body segment's weight, its center of gravity, and its angular position.

Kinematics—The area of biomechanics that describes movements in terms of direction, speed, and position of body segments.

Kinetics—The area of biomechanics concerned with the forces producing motion or maintaining equilibrium

Manual guidance—Hands-on, physical cuing by the therapist to facilitate movement by providing a proprioceptive model of task requirements or to constrain movements that are unnecessary for task performance.

Model of the action—A general plan of the most efficient strategy for performing a given functional movement.

Motor learning—The development of general strategies for solving movement problems in a variety of contexts.

Open-loop system—A system of control that does not require use of peripheral feedback; instructions for action are prepared in advance and communicated to various motor centers ahead of the action (feedforward). The instructions are carried out without modification from feedback.

Open task—A task in which there are some features of the environment that are in motion or unstable, and there is variability from one trial to the next.

Part learning—Practice of a task in separate steps.

Phase shift—Transition, often nonlinear, from one preferred qualitative coordinated pattern to another preferred qualitative pattern.

Postural adjustments—Automatic, anticipatory, and ongoing muscle activation that enables an individual to maintain balance against gravity, optimal alignment between body parts, and optimal orientation of the head, trunk, and limbs in relation to the environment.

Random practice—Practice of tasks that vary randomly within the session (Schmidt, 1991b).

Regulatory conditions—Features of the environment that directly influence which movement patterns will be successful in achieving a given goal.

Serial tasks—Tasks involving connected discrete movements.

Whole learning—Practice of a task in its entirety.

25A   CARR AND SHEPHERD'S MOTOR RELEARNING PROGRAMME FOR INDIVIDUALS WITH STROKE

Joyce Shapero Sabari

OBJECTIVES

Reading and studying this section will enable the student to:

1. Identify key concepts and principles from movement science that have influenced the *Motor Relearning Programme*.
2. Describe why the use of task-oriented intervention is compatible with current theories of motor control and **motor learning.**
3. Compare the *Motor Relearning Programme* with the proprioceptive neuromuscular facilitation, Rood, Brunnstrom, and neurodevelopmental treatment approaches.
4. Understand and apply the four-step process used in the *Motor Relearning Programme*.
5. Understand and apply specific evaluation and treatment strategies used in the *Motor Relearning Programme*.

The *Motor Relearning Programme* (MRP) was developed by Australian physical therapists Carr and Shepherd (1983, 1987a) from their clinical experience and extensive review of contemporary movement science theory and research. Carr and Shepherd's approach is particularly relevant to occupational therapists because it emphasizes the relearning of daily activities and it provides a task-oriented strategy for improving motor control.

THEORETICAL FRAMEWORK

Dynamical Systems Model of Motor Control

Contemporary theories in movement science emphasize a distributed control, or dynamical systems, approach rather than a hierarchical model of motor control (Shepherd & Carr, 1991). According to this newer model, responsibilities for motor control are distributed among a number of structures in the central nervous system. Spinal-level structures do not completely depend on higher centers for direct movement commands. Instead, the role of hemispheric structures is to tune and prepare the motor system to respond most efficiently to changing environmental and task demands.

The Brunnstrom (1970; Sawner & LaVigne, 1992), Rood (1954), proprioceptive neuromuscular facilitation (PNF) (Voss, Ionta, & Meyers, 1985), and early neurodevelopmental treatment (NDT) (Bobath, 1978) approaches are based on a hierarchical model of motor control, which predicts that dysfunction in the motor cortex results in a release from inhibition of the more primitive brainstem and spinal networks. Subsequently, the major neuromotor sequelae of stroke are the positive symptoms of spasticity and reflex domination of muscle tone. Treatment focuses on decreasing abnormal reflex activity and primitive movement patterns to facilitate normal movement (Gordon, 1987; Poole, 1991b).

Ecological theories of movement are compatible with distributed control models and emphasize the interaction between the performer and the environment (Saltzman & Kelso, 1987). Motor behaviors emerge as a result of context, or **regulatory conditions** in the environment (Bernstein, 1967; Gentile, 1972, 1987). A successful motor strategy for reaching forward with one arm will vary, depending on several factors: the person's posture (sitting, standing, kneeling) and postural alignment, the shape and stability of the seat or supporting surface, how far away and in what direction the goal object is located, and the presence of any obstacles between the individual and the goal object. Skilled motor performance in any task is the ability to perform in a number of different ways, according to variations in environmental demands (Summers, 1989). Research has shown that simply practicing movements in isolation of a goal or functional task will not lead to skill development (Higgins & Spaeth, 1972; Smyth, 1984). The MRP and its theoretical base lend structure and validation to the long-standing use of purposeful activities in occupational therapy intervention to improve motor control.

POSTURAL ADJUSTMENTS

Evolving views about postural control have strongly influenced Carr and Shepherd's therapeutic approach. Other neuromotor approaches advocate the development of balance in a **closed-loop system.** PNF recommends the rhythmic stabilization technique, which focuses on facilitating alternating contractions of antagonist muscles of the trunk, pelvis, and neck in response to rhythmic alternating resistance by the therapist (Voss, Ionta, & Myers, 1985). Bobath (1978) encouraged therapists to facilitate righting and equilibrium responses by providing manual displacements to a patient's center of gravity. These procedures are based on the theories that (1) postural mechanisms occur in response to a stimulus and (2) stability, or the ability to maintain a static position without falling, is a necessary prerequisite to balance (Carr & Shepherd, 1990).

Balance is now understood to be controlled via an **open-loop system** rather than a **closed-loop system.** **Postural adjustments** (instead of responses) are anticipatory and ongoing. Before the onset of motor activities, widespread changes occur in the muscular organization of persons with intact central nervous systems (Brunia, Haagh, & Scheirs, 1985). These feedforward adjustments occur simultaneously with the plan to move and prepare the person for performing the subsequent task. Well-organized **postural adjustments** prevent major displacements in the center of gravity through a feedforward mode of control.

Postural adjustments are both task and context specific. Early NDT interventions were based on the viewpoint that **postural adjustments** are characterized by specific patterns of muscle activation. However, studies have shown that muscle activation patterns for balance control vary according to (1) the position of the person, (2) the task being performed, (3) the context in which the activity occurs, and (4) the person's perception of which body part is in contact with the more stable base of support (Nashner & McCollum, 1985). Therefore, Carr and Shepherd advocate that **postural adjustments** can be learned only in the context of task performance. Furthermore, balance training in one position, or during performance of one task, is not likely to generalize to improved postural control in other contexts (Shepherd, 1992). Current NDT intervention is compatible with this viewpoint (Bobath, 1990).

COMPENSATORY STRATEGIES

Abnormal motor patterns exhibited by individuals with hemiplegia have typically been attributed to (1) a release of primitive synergies from inhibitory control (Brunnstrom, 1970; Twitchell, 1951), (2) spasticity (Bobath, 1978), and/or (3) a direct result of the brain lesion. Shepherd and Carr (1991) believe these stereotypic movement patterns are **compensatory strategies** that persons with hemiplegia develop as they attempt to move.

Figure 25A.1 illustrates Carr and Shepherd's postulated sequence by which individuals with hemiplegia

develop habitual inefficient movement patterns. It also includes factors that may interfere with smooth, efficient movement and, therefore, lead to the development of **compensatory strategies.**

Carr and Shepherd (1989) are careful to distinguish between function as limited goal attainment via a compensatory strategy and function that is characterized by both efficiency and flexibility of performance. They believe that the continual practice of fundamentally inappropriate **compensatory strategies** is a critical mechanism that limits recovery following brain damage. Therefore, a major goal of intervention is to ensure that compensatory behavior is not learned as a substitute for optimal performance.

One way to prevent the development of compensatory behaviors is to reduce the obstacles to efficient movement (Fig. 25A.1). Ways to do this are discussed below.

Prevention of Abnormal Muscle Shortening

Prevention of abnormal muscle shortening is an important component of the *Motor Relearning Pro-*

ATTEMPT TO MOVE

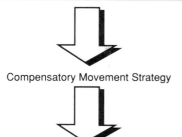

Obstacles to Efficient Movement:

Diminished soft tissue extensibility
Impaired balance
Postural insecurity and resultant fixation patterns
Specific muscle weakness

Compensatory Movement Strategy

Repeated "Practice" of the Compensatory Strategy

Learned Use of the Compensatory Strategy

Figure 25A.1. Development of abnormal movement patterns in individuals with hemiplegia.

gramme. This is achieved by establishing appropriate postural alignment in bed, when sitting, and when standing. In addition, patients are instructed to follow daily routines to maintain muscle length through the practice of a variety of motor tasks. For example, frequent practice of standing up will maintain length and flexibility of the gastrocnemius muscle if feet are sufficiently dorsiflexed at the start of the movement. Activities performed while bearing weight on a paretic hand will prevent shortening of upper extremity flexors, adductors, and internal rotators.

Prevention of Fixation Patterns

When people feel unable to maintain their balance in posturally threatening situations, the natural strategy is to fixate selected body parts and thus decrease the number of motor elements (or degrees of freedom) the central nervous system must control. An example of this strategy is a person's tendency to cocontract all the flexors and extensors of the trunk when attempting to ski or ice skate for the first time (Lemkuhl & Smith, 1985). Individuals with postural adjustment deficits as a result of stroke feel insecure about their ability to maintain balance, even in routine sitting or standing positions. The strategy of fixating one's pelvis on the lumbar spine or the scapula on the thorax has short-term benefits for enhancing the person's sense of postural security. A negative consequence is that these fixation patterns lead to difficulty disassociating the scapula and pelvis from adjacent proximal structures. This lack of sufficient mobility at the limb girdles subsequently limits the normal **kinematics** of upper and lower extremity movement. The MRP seeks to prevent the development of fixation patterns through the early introduction of techniques to enhance balance and postural security.

Prevention of Compensations Caused by Weakness

The MRP encourages therapists to "actively search for and detect small amounts of muscle activity as soon as they occur" (Carr & Shepherd, 1987a, p. 47). Early control of weak muscles is facilitated by finding an optimal length for muscle contraction and by positioning the limb so that gravity assists, rather than resists, the muscle. An example, which is also used in the NDT approach, is to elicit early contraction of the deltoid when the individual lies supine, with the shoulder flexed to 90°. In this position, gravity provides a stabilizing force on the shoulder. Therefore, activation of fewer motor units is required for the individual successfully to hold the arm and move it slightly from this position.

When patients demonstrate compensatory move-ment patterns of the limbs because of weakness in specific muscles, the MRP proposes the following therapeutic interventions.

1. Change the position of task performance to optimize conditions of muscle length and **gravitational torque.**
2. Teach the patient which movements are inefficient compensations, so he will be aware of which strategies he should attempt to avoid.
3. Teach the patient to consciously eliminate muscle activity unnecessary to the movement being attempted.
4. Provide light **manual guidance** to direct a patient's movement pattern as he attempts to perform a task.

In **manual guidance,** therapists should avoid holding a limb too firmly or providing support once sufficient muscle activity has been regained. Such excessive guidance may prevent the patient from activating muscles by removing the need to do so (Carr & Shepherd, 1987a).

ANALYSIS OF NORMAL MOTOR PERFORMANCE OF FUNCTIONAL TASKS

Carr and Shepherd believe that systematic research on how average people perform motor activities can provide a framework for the treatment of motor-disabled people who must relearn what were once habitual, everyday tasks. Such systematic descriptive and biomechanical information about the motor performance of daily activities has been limited, but recently, studies of rolling (Richter, VanSant, & Newton, 1989), rising from bed (VanSant, 1988), reaching (Morasso, 1981), and grasp (Jeannerod, 1984) have appeared in the literature.

These analyses were based on data collected with video cameras, force plate sensors, and electromyographic polygraphs. They provide information about (1) kinematic features of the action, such as angular displacements and body part trajectories, and (2) kinetic features such as muscle activation, ground reaction forces, and muscular and **gravitational torque** values. Carr and Shepherd (1990) contend that information generated from such movement analyses can provide therapists with a **model of the action,** based on what is known of normal performance.

The MRP presents descriptions of normal function for selected activities (Carr & Shepherd, 1987a). Therapists can then compare their detailed observations of a patient's movement during task performance with the description of normal function for that activity. Carr and Shepherd acknowledge that the understanding of normal function may continually change in response to ongoing descriptive and data-based biomechanical research.

Carr and Shepherd also call for descriptive studies of the **kinetics** and **kinematics** of everyday activities performed by subjects with hemiplegia. They think that such data will add insight to therapists' knowledge of underlying control and dyscontrol processes. Most important, such analysis will allow for the systematic development of strategies therapists can use when analyzing patients' task performance. One recent study (Trombly, 1993a) described upper extremity reaching patterns in five individuals with hemiplegia.

The MRP presents descriptions of common problems and compensatory problems associated with the performance of selected tasks by individuals with hemiplegia. These descriptions are currently based on the authors' own clinical experience rather than on the results of empirical research.

MOTOR LEARNING

Current theories about motor skill acquisition emphasize the active, problem-solving aspects of learning (Schmidt, 1988, 1992). Cognitive processes play a critical role in the development of motor behaviors (Marteniuk, 1986). Correspondingly, Carr and Shepherd's (1989) approach views the individual as an active participant whose major goal in rehabilitation is to relearn effective strategies for performing functional movement.

The *Motor Relearning Programme* has a significantly different approach to motor learning from the previous approaches designed to improve motor control.

Nature of Practice

PNF, Rood, Brunnstrom, and early NDT approaches viewed practice as the repetitive performance of one action for the purpose of improving motor skill (Gordon, 1987). It was assumed that practice of an exercise will generalize into improved performance of functional tasks. Unfortunately, empirical research has failed to support this assumption, even with learners who have no motor control deficits (Higgins & Spaeth, 1972). Instead of learning specific movements, participants in the MRP learn general strategies for solving motor problems. Rather than performing exercises without functional goals, patients practice tasks that require mild variations in movement patterns during successive repetitions. Furthermore, limb movements and **postural adjustments** are always learned simultaneously and in the context of task performance.

Neurodevelopmental Sequence of Intervention

Other approaches have assumed that the practice of developmentally earlier actions, such as rolling over and crawling, will aid a person in regaining control over motor activities that develop later in normal in-

fancy (e.g., standing, walking, and reaching). This assumption is based on a hierarchical view of motor control and is not supported by current views of distributed control. Therefore, Carr and Shepherd's (1987a) interventions do not follow a developmental sequence. They believe that rolling over is often given excessive emphasis in rehabilitation. In fact, they prefer to focus on teaching patients to assume sitting and standing positions, which will allow for optimal active engagement with the environment.

Carr and Shepherd also disagree with those who suggest that therapeutic intervention should proceed in a proximal to distal sequence. When working to improve upper limb function, therapists are encouraged to capitalize on small demonstrations of active movement in wrist and finger muscles. Whenever possible, hand function is practiced simultaneously with shoulder girdle control, within the context of functional reaching tasks.

In summary, previous therapeutic interventions for individuals with hemiplegia have focused on the patient as a recipient of facilitation and inhibition techniques provided by the therapist. In the MRP, the patient is an active participant in learning how to move functionally and how to problem solve during attempts at novel tasks. **Postural adjustments** and limb movements are linked together in the learning process. The therapist's role is to guide the individual in this process and to prevent or remove obstacles that may lead to the use of inefficient **compensatory strategies**. Successful task learning has occurred when an individual can perform activities effectively and automatically in a variety of environmental contexts.

INTERVENTION

The MRP provides guidelines for evaluating and improving motor control in seven categories of functional daily activities:

1. Upper limb function;
2. Orofacial function;
3. Sitting up over the side of the bed;
4. Balanced sitting;
5. Standing up and sitting down;
6. Balanced standing;
7. Walking.

Carr and Shepherd do not propose any specific sequence for intervention among these seven functional categories. However, when working to improve skill in a selected function, a four-step sequence is followed (Table 25A.1).

In Step 1, evaluation is administered in the context of task performance. Steps 2 and 3 actually overlap during treatment. Step 2, the practice of specific task components, precedes task practice only when a patient

Table 25A.1.   The Four Steps of the *Motor Relearning Programme*

1. Analysis of task
   Observation
   Comparison
   Analysis
2. Practice of missing components
   Explanation—identification of goal
   Instruction
   Practice plus verbal and visual feedback plus manual
      guidance
3. Practice of task
   Explanation—identification of goal
   Instruction
   Practice plus verbal and visual feedback plus manual
      guidance
   Reevaluation
   Encourage flexibility
4. Transference of training
   Opportunity to practice in context
   Consistency of practice
   Organization of self-monitored practice
   Structured learning environment
   Involvement of relatives and staff

cannot contract or control the required muscles and needs to practice this component before incorporating it into the complex task. Step 4 provides a link between progress in therapy sessions and actual task performance during the individual's daily routines.

Evaluation

Evaluation is a detailed analysis of the patient's performance of tasks within each of the seven categories of daily activities. The MRP provides a description of normal function and a list of essential components for performing each task. These are based on the authors' clinical experience and published normative descriptive studies (Jeannerod, 1984; Morasso, 1981; Richter, VanSant, & Newton, 1989; VanSant, 1988).

The therapist observes the patient as he performs each task and then compares his performance with the normal kinesiology associated with the task. Specifically, the therapist notes

1. Any missing components, such as a lack of anterior pelvic tilt and hip flexion when rising to stand;
2. Incorrect timing of components within a movement pattern, e.g., an inappropriate interplay among extrinsic and intrinsic finger muscles during attempts at grasp;
3. The absence of specific muscle activity;
4. The presence of any excessive or inappropriate muscle activity;
5. Compensatory motor behavior, such as elevation of the entire shoulder girdle on attempts to reach forward.

A major focus of the analysis is to hypothesize the underlying reasons for the individual's development of the **compensatory strategies** he has chosen. Based on what she has just observed, the therapist asks a series of questions to determine which primary and secondary problems will be addressed in treatment. Primary problems are the underlying obstacles to movement, some of which are listed in Figure 25A.1. Secondary problems are the observable movement dysfunctions. Carr and Shepherd (1987a) offered a list of common problems and **compensatory strategies** for each of the functional tasks included in the MRP. However, they acknowledged that each patient will demonstrate unique combinations of motor assets and limitations.

The patient is included as an active participant in the analysis of his performance. This allows the therapist to see how well an individual is able to detect his own movement problems. In addition, this encourages patients to develop insight about their own movement, develop problem-solving skills, and understand the goals of the treatment program.

Although Carr and Shepherd recommend using a qualitative assessment style as a guide to treatment planning, they developed a quantitative scale that is useful for documenting progress and conducting research. The *Motor Assessment Scale* (MAS) (Carr et al., 1985) consists of one item, which measures general tone, and eight motor activity items (supine to side lying, supine to sitting over the side of the bed, balanced sitting, sitting to standing, walking, upper arm function, hand movements, and advanced hand activities). Each motor activity is scored on a 7-point ordinal scale, ranging from 0 to 6. A score of 6 indicates optimal behavior. Clear criteria are provided for score assignment on each item. High interrater ($r > 0.97$), intrarater ($r = 0.98$), and test-retest reliability ($r = 0.98$) have been established (Carr et al., 1985; Loewen & Anderson, 1988; Poole & Whitney, 1988). High concurrent validity has been determined in studies that compared scores on the MAS with scores on the *Fugl-Meyer Assessment* (Poole & Whitney, 1988) and a modified version of the MAS with scores on the *Barthel Index* (Loewen & Anderson, 1988). Content validity of the scoring criteria needs to be determined and seems especially weak for the two items related to hand function.

Treatment

Many treatment principles in the MRP are compatible with basic occupational therapy theory. The key to therapy is to adapt the task or the environment so that the person can achieve successful performance without compensation. Occupational therapy principles of grading and synthesizing activities are consistent with Carr and Shepherd's suggestions for structuring the **regulatory conditions** of a task. Therapists select motor tasks with goals that are clear, relevant, and worthwhile in the eyes of the patient. Appropriate tasks are challenging yet attainable without reliance on **compensatory strategies.** The therapist creatively alters the patient's position and the position of tools and goal objects to match the level of motor demand to each patient's current abilities. In addition, the supporting surfaces on which the patient sits or stands are carefully chosen for each patient's level of postural control. Furthermore, the nature and amount of the therapist's handling, or **manual guidance,** is adapted to the patient's needs (Sabari, 1991). Although Carr and Shepherd focus on improving motor skills, they believe that task-specific training improves the person's sensory perception concurrently with motor performance. Engagement in activity provides individuals with opportunities to select and attend to relevant environmental cues. Cognitive skills are used and developed as the patient is encouraged to analyze his own movements and to make decisions about effective sequences and strategies for task performance (Carr & Shepherd, 1987b).

Treatment is viewed as a teaching-learning process. Learning will proceed most smoothly when the patient has a clear idea of the motor goal as well as which strategies are appropriate or inappropriate for reaching that goal. Carr and Shepherd recommend that therapists routinely ask patients to describe or demonstrate (with the unaffected side, if necessary) the specific movements required to achieve a task. This provides the therapist with a clear understanding of what the patient thinks he is being asked to do. Instructions can then be modified to ensure that the patient and therapist are truly working toward the same goal.

The *Motor Relearning Programme* relies on five strategies for teaching the patient what he needs to learn. Therapists choose the most appropriate combinations of these strategies to suit the needs of individual patients.

1. Verbal instruction is a useful teaching strategy, but only when words are kept to a minimum. The therapist identifies the most important aspect of the movement on which the patient will concentrate during task performance. Verbal instructions presented in terms of an object goal will be easier to follow than abstract directions to move. For example, "Touch the checker" will be more likely to elicit active forward reach than "Reach forward." Of course, verbal instructions are replaced or reinforced by nonverbal communication if the patient is dysphasic.

2. Visual demonstration is generally provided through the therapist's own performance of the task, with a focus on one or two components most important

to the patient's development of control. Carr and Shepherd report success with photographs of a patient's maladaptive alignment during task performance as well as stick figure drawings that indicate the essential task components (Carr & Shepherd, 1987b). These strategies seem particularly effective in teaching tasks that are inherently sequential, such as rising from supine to sitting, standing up, and sitting down.

3. **Manual guidance** helps to clarify the model of action by passively guiding the patient through the path of movement or by physically constraining inappropriate components. During attempts at task-related forward reach, the therapist may provide passive movement to the scapula, with simultaneous cues over the acromium for the patient to limit elevation of the entire shoulder girdle. When a patient attempts to sit down from standing, the therapist's **manual guidance** behind the shoulders reinforces the concept that the individual must move forward at the shoulders to achieve the necessary hip and knee flexion for smooth, controlled descent. **Manual guidance** has similarities to the NDT strategy of handling, but Carr and Shepherd caution that the patient must always be participating actively and even be given some opportunities to make mistakes during practice.

4. Accurate, timely feedback about quality of performance helps the patient learn which strategies to repeat and which strategies to avoid. The therapist reserves positive comments for actual improvements in performance. If effort is rewarded in addition to success, the patient receives confusing feedback about the correctness or incorrectness of the motor strategy he has chosen.

5. Consistency of practice facilitates development of skill in task performance (Johnson, 1984). Because patients learn what they practice, it is important that they do not revert to using compensatory movement strategies during daily activities outside of therapy. Carr and Shepherd emphasize that significant motor improvements will be achieved only if patients practice movement, according to therapist guidelines, throughout each day. Therefore, the therapist structures a practice program for each patient to reinforce activities performed during therapy sessions. Friends and relatives learn effective ways to assist the patient in this program. The therapist provides clear written directions, photographs, drawings, and/or performance checklists to ensure that the additional practice is consistent with the motor strategies promoted during therapy.

Treatment is task specific and based directly on movement analysis of the patient's performance of that task. The therapist continues to reevaluate and analyze the patient's performance throughout each treatment session to make ongoing decisions about intervention. If a patient's performance does not improve, the therapist checks her original analysis of his problems and considers whether or not the training approach should be modified.

Steps 2 and 3 of the *Motor Relearning Programme* (see Table 25A.1) are integrated during treatment. Selected tasks are generally practiced in their entirety, with the aid of the teaching and grading strategies described earlier. The therapist encourages flexibility of performance by requiring small modifications of movements during task repetitions. Occupational therapists' use of naturalistic activities like simple crafts and games ensures variations through the creative placement of tools, materials, and goal objects.

When the patient is unable to perform a task in its entirety successfully, the therapist divides the task into its component parts. For example, the component of moving from weight bearing on the forearm at one's side to weight bearing on an extended elbow may be practiced in preparation for the total activity of rising from supine to sitting. This is similar to the NDT strategy of practicing transitional movements within a larger movement sequence. Occupational therapists use this strategy when engaging patients in sitting tasks that require hip flexion and forward reach as preparation for rising from sit to stand. The component of hip flexion and anterior displacement of the shoulders has been isolated from the larger task of standing up.

Step 4 of the *Motor Relearning Programme* (see Table 25A.1) ensures that the patient applies what he has learned during therapy sessions to motor performance in other environments. Active participation in problem solving during therapy will facilitate the patient's development of similar strategies when he practices on his own. In addition, the therapist provides clear guidelines for incorporating newly learned movement patterns into daily activities. At the end of each session, the therapist teaches the patient and family members or friends how to reinforce the improvements the patient has achieved.

EVALUATION AND TREATMENT OF SELECTED FUNCTIONAL ACTIVITIES

Balanced Sitting

Although Carr and Shepherd do not specifically recommend starting therapy with intervention to improve sitting balance, it is assumed that this function serves as a prerequisite to standing up, sitting down, and upper limb control. Analysis of sitting consists of (1) observation of the patient's alignment in quiet sitting and (2) analysis of his ability to adjust to self-initiated movement of his limbs, trunk, and head as he performs a variety of motor tasks. These tasks may include looking at the ceiling; turning to look behind; reaching forward, sideways, backward, and toward the floor to touch or grasp an object; and lifting his intact foot off the floor. The therapist observes for normal **postural adjustments** of the head, trunk, and limbs. Specific features of these adjustments have been previously described by Bobath (1978, 1990) and Davies (1985, 1990), but Carr and Shepherd emphasize that these adjustments are preparatory, ongoing, and context specific. The therapist notes any extraneous or limited movements and analyzes the reasons for problems or **compensatory strategies.** Common signs of balance impairments include the following:

1. Use of a wide base of support, achieved by placing the feet and/or knees apart;
2. A tendency to hold the breath and maintain a stiff body posture;
3. A strategy of shuffling the feet instead of making adjustments with appropriate body segments;
4. Use of protective support by the upper limb—either by grasping for support or by weight bearing on the hands to increase stability;
5. A tendency to lean forward or backward when the task requires that body weight should be shifting sideways, which indicates impaired control over lateral flexion of the trunk.

Treatment techniques are similar to those used in the NDT approach, with a major difference being that the therapist never passively displaces the patient's center of gravity. The patient practices each of the tasks included in the assessment, while the therapist provides cues and **manual guidance** at selected body segments. The therapist uses her knowledge about normal **postural adjustments** to provide guidance that will teach the patient the appropriate models of action. All displacements are self-initiated and unresisted. The therapist draws the patient's attention toward his affected side, making sure he bears weight on that side when appropriate. Because **postural adjustments** are rarely used in isolation of limb movements, treatment to improve balanced sitting is combined with limb training during the performance of goal-oriented tasks.

Standing Up and Sitting Down

To do functional tasks like wheelchair transfers and use of the tub or toilet, a person must know how to stand up and sit down safely and efficiently. A major problem in task performance is the inability to shift the center of gravity of one's upper body sufficiently forward during the early stages of standing up and the late stages of sitting down. Patients may demonstrate difficulty flexing their hips, protracting the shoulder girdles, or dorsiflexing the ankles to bring the knees forward. Often, patients try to shift weight forward by flexing the head and thorax instead of the hips.

A second problem is the tendency to bear body weight predominantly on the intact lower limb. This is accentuated when patients position their intact foot far posterior to the involved foot. In this position, the posteriorly placed lower limb will automatically support more body weight than the forward foot.

Empirical research (Ada & Westwood, 1992) supports a therapeutic emphasis on the temporal characteristics of task performance. Once individuals have learned the basic angular displacements required for standing up and sitting down, further improvements are related more to changes in movement time and joint angular velocities than to changes in range of motion at the hips and knees.

Based on an assessment of individual performance, the therapist uses the teaching strategies described above to help the patient learn the key components of these tasks. The patient learns that both standing up and sitting down require the same motor strategies, only in an opposite sequence. Isolated practice of key components may precede performance of standing up or sitting down in their entirety.

Balanced Standing

Evaluation and treatment are similar to the interventions for balanced sitting. The therapist observes the patient's alignment in quiet standing and analyzes his ability to adjust to self-initiated movements of his limbs, trunk, and head as he performs a graded variety of motor tasks. In addition to the common signs of balance impairments noted above, the therapist will take note of any tendency (1) to take steps prematurely in an attempt to compensate for insufficient balance and (2) to move proximal, rather than distal, body parts when shifting center of gravity. For example, when reaching forward, the patient will flex his hips instead of dorsiflexing at his ankles, which is normal. When reaching sideways, he will move his trunk, instead of his hips and ankles.

Carr and Shepherd recommend that patients stand early in treatment. Once a person has learned to stand in physical therapy, the occupational therapist can incorporate balanced standing into functional activities. Maintaining one's balance when moving while standing increases awareness of bilaterality, position in space, and positioning of body parts. Furthermore, standing with the affected leg bearing weight in normal alignment may minimize the development of spasticity in the leg (Carr & Shepherd, 1987a).

Upper Limb Function

The therapist assesses and elicits muscle activity at the scapula and shoulder when the patient is supine, until the patient can control his shoulder girdle while sitting without excessive compensatory movements. Common problems of the upper arm include the following:

1. Impaired scapular movement, especially rotation and protraction, and persistent depression of the shoulder girdle;
2. Impaired control over the deltoid muscle, with an inability to sustain positions of shoulder abduction or flexion; patients may compensate when attempting to move by using excessive shoulder girdle elevation and lateral flexion of the trunk;
3. Excessive and unnecessary elbow flexion, shoulder internal rotation, and forearm pronation.

Movement problems in the upper limb are often secondary to shortening of soft tissues, which is caused by habitual posturing, use of the intact arm to move or compensate for the affected arm, and learned nonuse of the affected arm. Therefore, active use of the affected arm in functional patterns is encouraged as early as possible to prevent learned nonuse and shortening of soft tissues. The authors caution that inappropriate passive exercises of the shoulder that do not accommodate the normal kinesiologic relationship between the scapula and humerus can lead to damage of soft tissue, chronic inflammation, and joint stiffness.

Common problems in hand function include the following:

1. Difficulty maintaining wrist extension while attempting grasp;
2. Difficulty extending and flexing the metacarpophalangeal joints while maintaining appropriate flexion of the interphalangeal joints to position the fingers for grasping and releasing objects (an intrinsic muscle activity);
3. Difficulty abducting and opposing the thumb for grasp and release;
4. Tendency to flex the wrist and/or extend the fingers and thumb excessively when attempting to release objects;
5. Tendency to pronate the forearm excessively while grasping objects;
6. Inability to maintain grasp while moving the arm;
7. Difficulty cupping the hand.

Carr and Shepherd (1987a) present specific activity sequences involving grasp, release, and manipulation of common objects. Occupational therapists can expand these sequences to a variety of functional tasks through which patients will improve upper limb function in combination with sitting or standing balance.

EFFECTIVENESS

Recent clinical studies provide support for the efficacy of the MRP. Dean and Mackey (1992) conducted a retrospective, descriptive study of patients who participated in a multidisciplinary program based on Carr and Shepherd's model. Comparison of initial scores and discharge scores on the *Motor Assessment Scale* revealed significant mean differences for all eight items assessed. Furthermore, performance outcomes were higher than outcomes reported in previously published studies of stroke rehabilitation programs (Gowland, 1986; Parker, Wade, & Langton Hewer, 1986). Ada and Westwood's (1992) kinematic analysis of recovery of the ability to stand up following stroke provides construct validation for both the *Motor Assessment Scale* and Carr and Shepherd's theoretical approach to teaching the task of standing up.

Trombly's (1992) study of reaching in subjects with left hemiparesis supports Carr and Shepherd's view that deficits in generating appropriate models of action are the primary problem after stroke, not spasticity or pathological movement synergies. Sietsema et al. (1993) provided empirical support for use of task-oriented intervention to improve motor control in patients with central nervous system dysfunction. Ford-Smith and VanSant's (1993) descriptive study of normal subjects provides support for some aspects of the MRP's strategy for teaching patients to rise from supine. However, their findings indicate that strategies vary widely among individuals and that age may influence which strategy is chosen to perform this task.

Carr and Shepherd's writings have played a role in influencing occupational and physical therapists to integrate contemporary theories of motor control into intervention for individuals with stroke and other central nervous system disorders (Abreu & Schmidt, 1992; Lister, 1991; Poole, 1991b; Sabari, 1991). The NDT approach has been particularly responsive to the recommendations of these authors and others to place increased emphasis on active movement and functional tasks in treatment.

The effectiveness of the MRP depends on the individual therapist's knowledge of biomechanics and motor control and her problem-solving ability. The therapist must be able to recognize and analyze the motor problem, select the most essential missing component, effectively teach the patient the required movement, monitor the patient's response, give meaningful feedback, and create an environment that promotes a drive toward recovery and relearning.

The MRP is still relatively new and has some inconsistencies between its stated theoretical framework and its actual intervention strategies. Carr and Shepherd repeatedly speak about the need for functional, task-oriented intervention. Yet their program to improve balanced sitting and standing calls for patients to move their heads and bodies in various directions without involvement in actual goal-oriented tasks. They state that they do not consider spasticity to be a significant residual problem of stroke, and they offer no recommendations for reducing abnormal tone. Yet they included an evaluation of tone on their *Motor Assessment Scale*. Their proposed sequences for assessing and training hand skills need to be confirmed or challenged through empirical research. Furthermore, the MRP's applicability to patients with severe cognitive deficits needs to be assessed. Occupational therapy's emphasis on the therapeutic use of purposeful activities provides occupational therapists with a unique ability to expand on the ideas presented in the MRP.

Acknowledgments—The author wishes to thank Roberta Carr and Janet Shepherd for their helpful suggestions.

STUDY QUESTIONS

1. How does the MRP differ from the approaches described in Chapter 24? How is it similar?
2. How have movement science theories and research influenced the MRP?
3. How does the MRP attempt to prevent the development of compensatory motor strategies?
4. What is the therapist's role in this approach? What is the patient's role?
5. Which occupational therapy principles are inherent to the MRP?
6. What are the four steps of the MRP?
7. How does the MRP intervene to improve balance in sitting and standing?
8. How does the MRP intervene to improve the ability to stand up and sit down?
9. How does the MRP intervene to improve functional use of the arm and hand?

25B   Contemporary Task-Oriented Approach

Julie Bass Haugen and Virgil Mathiowetz

OBJECTIVES

After studying this chapter, the reader will be able to:
1. Discuss how the assumptions of the contemporary task-oriented approach influence evaluation and treatment.
2. Discuss the ideas from the contemporary perspective that are the basis for the contemporary task-oriented approach.
3. Explain the primary concepts of the systems model and contemporary theories that influence the approach.
4. Describe a general approach to evaluation using the approach.
5. Discuss treatment planning and implementation using the approach.
6. Explain the roles of the client and the therapist in a contemporary task-oriented approach.
7. Contrast traditional and contemporary approaches to evaluation and treatment.

The contemporary task-oriented approach emerges from a systems model of motor control and is influenced by contemporary developmental and **motor learning** (skill acquisition) theories (see Figs. 7.1 and 7.8). Before reading further, review the model, theories, assumptions, and basic evaluation ideas of the contemporary perspective outlined in Chapter 7. This chapter examines specific strategies related to evaluation and treatment.

The interpretation presented here of the contemporary task-oriented approach for occupational therapy is influenced by recent literature. Horak (1991) introduced the term *contemporary task-oriented approach* in an article on motor control and neurologic rehabilitation models. Literature that has provided the basis for assumptions and principles of this approach include Lister (1991); Rothstein (1991); Royeen (1990–1991); Forssberg and Hirschfeld (1992); Kamm, Thelen, and Jensen (1990); Thelen (1989); Thelen and Ulrich (1991); Davis and Burton (1991); and Gentile (1987, 1992).

Many ideas presented as part of a contemporary task-oriented approach are as old as the profession itself. Functional performance, person, and environment are not new ideas in occupational therapy. However, the traditional neurodevelopmental approaches deemphasized some of these ideas. Contemporary motor behavior literature challenges therapists to return

to some of the original assumptions of the profession. It provides a stronger theoretical basis for using purposeful activity as the primary treatment modality. The development of this approach is still in its infancy. At present, therapists frequently rely on the motor behavior, physical therapy, and adapted physical education literature for identification of principles and key concepts. The hypothetical examples presented in this chapter translate these new ideas into treatment principles for occupational therapy. Like the traditional neurodevelopmental approaches, there is very little empirical support for this treatment approach. However, it is an exciting time of transition in approaches to central nervous system (CNS) dysfunction. Occupational therapists look forward to further development of the contemporary task-oriented approach and empirical research that will provide direction for practice.

In Chapter 7, the assumptions of the contemporary task-oriented approach and their implications for evaluation were discussed. From the contemporary perspective, achieving functional goals is the focus of motor behavior; thus therapists should facilitate performance of tasks that are a part of their clients' roles. The contemporary perspective also promotes the use of a holistic view in working with individuals. Multiple personal characteristics and environmental factors are considered as having a potential influence on the way a person performs movements. None of these variables automatically deserves more attention than others. The interaction of all these systems is unique to the individual, and thus the approach adopted must be unique to the performance needs of the individual, i.e., the therapist should take a client-centered approach. To understand these needs, it is important to look at movements in their different contexts and in settings that are or closely resemble the clients' environments. It is also necessary to consider the actual movements used to perform the task as well as the outcome of performance. These assumptions are the basis for the evaluation and treatment principles outlined in this chapter.

Concepts from the contemporary perspective were also introduced in Chapter 7. Many of these terms have origins in other disciplines and thus may be hard to understand initially. However, these terms and their implications for practice are consistent with other ideas in occupational therapy and the contemporary task-oriented approach. **Attractors, phase shifts, control parameters,** and **collective variables** are terms that originated in mathematics and the sciences. They are used to explain the behavior of complex phenomena like weather patterns and water turbulence. Motor behavior scientists have begun to find that these ideas are useful in understanding the complexities of human movements. Other concepts are proposed by **motor learning** theorists, who have introduced new ideas about the classification of tasks and the characteristics of effective feedback and practice. These terms and their implications for evaluation and treatment are discussed under the related assumptions.

CONCEPTS AND PRINCIPLES RELATED TO ASSUMPTIONS

Assumption: Functional Tasks Help Organize Motor Behavior

CONCEPTS

Functional Tasks

A primary reason for moving is to achieve functional goals. Thus it seems natural to focus on functional tasks whenever one is looking at motor behavior. Functional tasks and task (or activity) analyses have always been part of the occupational therapy process. In task analysis, therapists recognize that their clients have different capabilities and that different tasks require different skills. Thus evaluation involves an examination of the task requirements and the personal capabilities to determine if there is a match that permits task performance. If there is not a match, the occupational therapist plans interventions that address the problems of the client or the characteristics of the environment or both. Many approaches to task analysis (e.g., Trombly, 1989; see also Chapters 11 and 17) emphasize personal characteristics or performance component requirements.

Classification schemes of motor behavior may also be useful in a task analysis (Davis & Burton, 1991; Gentile, 1987; Schmidt, 1988). Tasks and the required movements for tasks are discribed as **discrete, serial,** or **continuous** (Schmidt, 1988). Skilled performance in a **continuous task** is generally retained even when there are periods of time when practice is impossible (Crutchfield & Barnes, 1993). For example, most people learn to ride a bike when they are quite young. As an adult, there may be long periods of time when there is no opportunity to practice this skill. However, biking is one of those skills that once you learn it, you easily remember it later after only brief practice. On the other end of the continuum are tasks requiring discrete movements. Many skilled movements used in sports with balls (e.g., hitting, slam-dunking, and pitching) are discrete in that they have a definite beginning and

end. Frequent practice of the movements is required to maintain performance at a high-skill level, i.e., if you do not use it, you lose it. Neither **discrete** nor **continuous tasks** are easily broken into steps.

Gentile (1987) proposed a two-dimensional taxonomy of tasks based on characteristics of the environmental context and the function of the action. The environmental context is analyzed in terms of the features of the environment (i.e., the **regulatory conditions**) and changes in these features from one performance to the next (i.e., intertrial variability). The environment, which includes objects, supporting surfaces, and other people, may be stationary or in motion during a given performance. In addition, there may be variation or consistency in the environmental features from trial to trial. When the **regulatory conditions** are stationary and do not change from one trial to the next, the task is categorized as a **closed task.** Signing your name on a check at a desk could be considered an example of a **closed task,** because the environmental context is generally stable and unchanging. In an **open task,** some features of the environment are in motion and vary from one performance to the next. These tasks are very complex and place many demands on the person, because the performance context is unstable and changes for different trials. Driving a car is an **open task** (Poole, 1991b), because the driver must process the motions of other cars, pedestrians, and the broader performance context (e.g., snow or rain). Furthermore, these features of the environment vary dramatically from one trip to another.

The function of the action is the second dimension in Gentile's (1987) taxonomy. This dimension consists of the person's actions during task performance and includes body orientation and object manipulation. In a given task, body orientation might involve stabilization or transport. Gentile states that this component of action is similar to the different roles of the postural support system. For example, during a word-processing task, the trunk and lower extremities primarily provide stability. In a tennis match, however, the trunk and lower extremities transport or move toward the general location of the ball. Actions are also analyzed in terms of whether the upper extremities are a part of the postural support system or involved in object manipulation. For example, the upper extremities help maintain balance and thus are part of the postural support system when walking on a wet kitchen floor. In this situation, there is no object manipulation. In the task of washing the floor, however, arms and hands are used for object manipulation (e.g., mop or sponge). The complete taxonomy proposed by Gentile (1987) combines the environmental context and the function of the action dimensions and results in 16 possible task categories.

Organization of Motor Behavior

How are movements organized to do a common task? For example, how would you describe the movements used to write your name? One characteristic is that there is a fair amount of consistency in the way a person moves during the task of writing. These preferred movements are usually the best movements for a given situation (e.g., writing on a piece of paper using a pencil at a desk). There may be some variation in the ways people move in this situation, but the movements do not vary a lot. However, there is also some flexibility in the movements, so that if a need arises (e.g., one has a blister on a finger or wants to use a stick to write in the sand) a person can temporarily or permanently change the movements used to complete the task.

The preferred movement patterns that emerge for a given task in a given context are called **attractors.** For most people, these patterns are stable and are the optimal way to achieve the functional goal, because they are efficient and effective (Kamm et al., 1990). An attractor can be illustrated by how a marble moves on different surfaces (Fig. 25B.1). Wells depict the stability of the patterns (Thelen, 1989). The marble on a surface with a shallow well (Fig. 25B.1A) illustrates movement patterns used for everyday tasks, i.e., the movements used for a familiar task (e.g., writing) in its usual context (e.g., on paper, using a pencil, at a desk). These movements tend to be stable or fall in the same well. However, this well is shallow enough so that a person can modify movements or move to a new attractor state if his or her personal characteristics or environment changes.

Now consider the first few times a new sport is tried (e.g., skating or skiing). The movement patterns are unstable and similar to a marble on a flat or bumpy surface—very irregular and unpredictable (Fig. 25B.1B). A tiny perturbation or disturbance of the marble would cause the marble to move and it would be hard to predict where the marble would stop; there is no attractor. It is also possible that the wells are so

deep that it is difficult to perform the task with any flexibility at all (Fig. 25B.1C). In this situation, a large perturbation would be needed to move the marble, and it would rapidly return to the well. Most people with intact CNS have few deep wells; humans adapt their movement patterns to meet the demands of the environment.

EVALUATION AND TREATMENT PRINCIPLES

1. Use functional tasks as the focus in evaluation and treatment. Therapists' ultimate goal in remediation of motor behavior problems is to enable their clients to do the things they want to do now and in the future. Thus, at each evaluation point—from the initial evaluation to recording progress to discharge to follow-up—the determination of the effectiveness of interventions is performance on functional tasks. In addition, the interventions emphasize the practice of real functional tasks. There is renewed interest in functional tasks and goals in applied settings and in basic research. Recently developed evaluations in occupational therapy include measures of functional task performance, e.g., *Assessment of Motor and Process Skills* (AMPS) (Fisher, 1990), the *Occupational Therapy Functional Assessment Compilation Tool* (OT FACT) (Smith, 1990), and *A-One Evaluation* (Arnadottir, 1990). Treatment protocols for motor behavior problems emphasize functional tasks (Burton & Davis, 1992; Carr & Shepherd, 1987a; Carr et al., 1987; Harris, 1991). In basic research, many studies are examining the role of functional goals on motor behavior. Thelen and Fisher (1983) studied kicking behavior in 3-month-old infants. They found that kicking increased when a mobile was tied to the leg by way of a control line. The results of this study and other research support the idea that therapists' evaluations of, and interventions for, motor behavior problems must revolve around functional goals. The functional goals of interest in occupational therapy are broad. Traditional activities of daily living (ADL) and instrumental activities of daily living (IADL) tasks are important. However, the tasks considered must also address functional needs in other self-care, work, and leisure roles.

2. Work on functional tasks that are important in the client's roles. This principle clearly follows the first principle because functional tasks of importance are often unique to the individual. What is important for one person to do may not be important for another. So how do therapists determine the key tasks for a given individual? They should examine a client's occupational roles and the meaning of these roles to the person. Satisfaction with life is not defined by successful completion of a random set of functional tasks

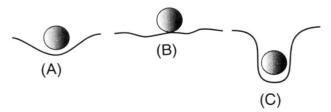

Figure 25B.1. Various attractor states. **A.** Shallow well—stable and flexible attractor state. **B.** No well—no attractor state. **C.** Deep well—stable and inflexible attractor state.

(e.g., changing a diaper and taking out the garbage). Satisfaction or reward comes from the feeling that roles are fulfilled (e.g., parent and homemaker). Roles are described using the general terms of self-maintenance (ADL and IADL), self-advancement (work), or self-enhancement (leisure); specific roles, however, are operationally defined by the client in terms of the tasks and related activities that are of interest or importance (Fisher & Short-DeGraff, 1993; Pollock, 1993; Trombly, 1993b). For example, two clients may view the role of parent differently. One client may identify washing a child's clothing as a key functional task, whereas another client might view playing touch football as more important. These two functional tasks vary greatly in their environments and in the motor behaviors required to achieve the functional goals.

A detailed examination of roles will also help the occupational therapist tap in to the personal motivations of clients for performing particular tasks. When a client attempts to change motor behaviors it usually reflects an internal desire to perform, acquire, or accomplish something (Crutchfield & Barnes, 1993). This motivation may be prompted because the degree of skill in performance is not personally satisfactory (Higgins, 1991) or because of other personal and environmental influences (Lewthwaite, 1990). Selection of tasks that are within the realm of capabilities are goal oriented, have meaning for the client, and motivate him to increase participation and improve functional outcomes in the therapy program (Lewthwaite, 1990).

3. Analyze the functional tasks. After a specific task has been selected for evaluation or treatment, a task analysis is necessary. The outcome of a task analysis will help in designing appropriate **motor learning** experiences and selecting practice and feedback strategies that fit the nature of the task. The task is described in terms of general personal requirements and performance contexts using one or more of the classification systems described above (e.g., Gentile, 1987; Schmidt, 1991b). It is important to recognize, however, that the specific strategies used for task performance may be unique to the person.

4. Evaluate the movements used for particular functional tasks. The motor behavior of clients can also be depicted in terms of three types of patterns or attractor states (Kamm et al., 1990). Clients in the acute stage of recovery often use movement patterns that show little stability. It may appear as if an attractor did not exist (Fig. 25B.1*B*). Every time they do a task they do it in a different way. As a result, task performance is not efficient or effective. The preferred movement patterns are likely in transition.

Other clients seem obligated to perform a task in only one way (Fig. 25B.1*C*). Although a single movement pattern may be effective for performance of a task in one context, the person may be unable to achieve functional goals in the real world because of its ever-changing context, e.g., a client may use a flexor pattern for all tasks that require reaching. This pattern may be effective when the arm is only an assist in some bilateral reaching tasks; however, most reaching tasks require complex and varied motor skills. For these tasks, the client may be unable to adapt movements and so cannot achieve the functional goals. Finally, some clients show good motor recovery after CNS damage. They resume stable, but flexible performance of tasks in their daily lives (Fig. 25B.1*A*).

An analysis of the organization of motor behavior helps therapists estimate stability and flexibility, understand changes, and prevent fixation of movement patterns (Kamm et al., 1990; Scholz, 1990). Scholz (1990) described two strategies for evaluating the stability of movement patterns. The first strategy is to look at fluctuations in one or more quantitative measures of movement patterns during task performance. The second strategy is to determine what happens when an occupational therapist tries to disturb or perturb the movement patterns by changing some critical personal or environmental factors. Therapists can ask, "How big of a change is needed to disturb the patterns?" and "How long does it take for the movement patterns to return to the previous state?" The quantitative measures of movement patterns are **collective variables,** and the critical factors influencing behavior are **control parameters;** these concepts are discussed later in this chapter.

An example of these strategies was described by Scholz (1990). Consider the locomotion of a child with cerebral palsy. The preferred pattern for this child may be a "bunny-hop," and a goal of therapy may be to move toward a reciprocal pattern for locomotion. One quantitative measure of movement patterns might be the relative phase of the hip motions as measured by videography, i.e., are the hip motions in the same phase (e.g., both hips are in flexion) or in opposite phases during locomotion (e.g., one hip is in flexion and the other is in extension)? The therapist analyzes the fluctuations in the relative phase when the child is using the preferred pattern, the bunny hop. Next, she perturbs this pattern by slowing the speed of locomotion or by imposing a physical restraint on one lower extremity. The therapist gains understanding of the child's movement patterns for this task by analyzing how much slowing or restraint is needed to change to a reciprocal pattern and how long it takes to return to a bunny hop after the critical factors are removed. Similar strategies can be devised for other tasks in occupational therapy.

Assumption: Occupational Performance Emerges from the Interaction of Multiple Systems that Represent the Unique Characteristics of the Person and the Performance Context

CONCEPTS

Occupational Performance

Occupational performance was defined by Nelson (1988) as the doing of occupation. Thus occupational performance helps people achieve their functional goals and fulfill their occupational roles.

Emerges from the Interaction of Multiple Systems

Movements are not controlled or prescribed by any one system (Horak, 1991). Multiple systems interact and cooperate to organize the many elements that are hypothetically free to vary in motor behavior. Emergence or self-organization is used to explain how the task of walking has such simplicity and stability even with all the possible combinations of influences by neurons, muscles, bones, and joints (Heriza, 1991). These multiple systems cooperate for a given task in a given context so that efficient and effective movements emerge to achieve a functional goal (Kamm et al., 1990).

Unique Characteristics

Personal characteristics include all those requirements of task performance that can be ascribed to the individual. Occupational performance requires doing, and doing generally involves movement. Movement requires the use of many personal characteristics like strength, postural support, memory, motivation, and attention. There are different ways to classify the various systems that are part of the person. The authors chose to adapt the performance components outlined by the American Occupational Therapy Association (1989). *Sensorimotor, cognition,* and *psychosocial* are identified as the major personal systems (see Fig. 7.8). For each of these systems, there are many subsystems that can also influence performance.

Performance Context

The performance context or environment consists of all the characteristics of the task itself and features of the broader environment. Several options are available for describing and classifying the performance contexts. The classification schemes used by Christiansen (1991) and Barris et al. (1985) have been adapted here to describe the task and broader environment in terms of physical, socioeconomic, and cultural systems.

Interaction of Person and Environment

In a systems model (see Fig. 7.8), there is no inherent ordering of personal and environmental factors in the interaction process. The nature of the interaction is dynamic or changing (Fisher & Short-DeGraff, 1993) and emerges as does occupational performance. The unique characteristics of the person and the unique characteristics of the environment interact in unpredictable ways. Thus in this type of model it is impossible to identify starting and ending points.

EVALUATION AND TREATMENT PRINCIPLES

1. Use personal characteristics, the performance context, and the interaction of person and environment to affect task performance. The therapist begins the occupational therapy process by identifying tasks that are difficult for the person to perform and by describing the preferred movement patterns for these tasks. The therapist then evaluates the personal and environmental systems that support optimal performance and contribute to ineffective performance. (Other chapters in this text are helpful in identifying evaluation and treatment strategies for specific personal characteristics and performance contexts.) The interactions of various systems are also important to consider (see Chapter 7). A qualitative analysis (i.e., observation and description) is used to understand the influence of interactions on task performance.

As therapists become more knowledgeable about the personal characteristics and contexts that are related to specific tasks, they can identify the important systems in more appropriate terms. VanSant (1990, 1991a, 1991b) and others have attempted to identify the systems for tasks requiring righting (e.g., rising from a bed and getting up from a chair or the floor). The results of these studies suggest that the preferred movement patterns used for these tasks are influenced by body dimensions (e.g., ratio of leg length to body length, size of body relative to bed or chair, height, weight, body build, and topography), age, gender, and activity level. Such studies are critical in helping occupational therapists identify the major systems for a task.

2. Consider neural and nonneural factors of the sensorimotor system as possible influences on occupational performance. The sensorimotor system is important in both traditional and contemporary approaches to CNS dysfunction. However, the focus in the traditional approaches is primarily on neural subsystems (e.g., reflex, muscle tone, and postural control). Until recently, it was believed that normalization of muscle tone in the antagonist (e.g., biceps) would allow normal voluntary movement to occur in response to agonist contraction (e.g., triceps) (Bobath, 1978).

Bourbonnais and Vanden Noven (1989) and Nwaobi (1983) reviewed research studies that suggested this is not true and that the effect of nonneural factors on movement (e.g., range of motion, strength, endurance, soft tissue integrity) should also be considered.

Studies show that many subsystems of the sensorimotor system, not just neural subsystems, may have a role in motor behavior after CNS damage. For example, improved functional performance in clients with hemiparesis is associated with increases in muscle strength (Andrews et al., 1981; Bohannon, 1986). Sabari (1991) summarized the sensorimotor factors constraining movement in adults with hemiplegia as the inability to dissociate the scapula from the thorax or the pelvis from the lumbar spine, weakness of specific muscles, inability to counteract gravitational forces, abnormalities in muscle tone, and incorrect timing of components within a movement pattern.

In evaluating and remediating motor behavior problems, therapists need to consider alternative explanations for the movement patterns that are currently used. For example, a client with hemiparesis may use a flexor pattern for reaching or lifting because of muscle weakness. A person without CNS damage uses this pattern, too. Imagine lifting a very heavy object, say a television. Describe the positions of the arms. The arms are pulled in close to the body (i.e., a flexor pattern), because arm strength relative to the weight of the object requires use of a more biomechanically efficient pattern (i.e., a shorter resistance arm). Clients may use this same pattern when lifting something as light as a feather, because arm strength relative to the weight of the feather—and, more important the force of gravity on the arm—requires it (Flynn, personal communication, 1993). Thus biomechanical factors, such as those described by Spaulding (1989) for prehension and those discussed in Chapters 6 and 22 are important to include in treatment approaches for clients with CNS dysfunction.

3. Consider characteristics of the task or broader environment as possible influences on occupational performance. The performance context is just as important as the personal characteristics in evaluation and treatment (Fisher & Short-DeGraff, 1993). Consider the following examples. People with motor impairments can scuba dive without special equipment and do so as well as any other person (Burton & Davis, 1992). On the other hand, walking can be difficult for even a person without physical impairments if the walking is attempted at an altitude of 15,000 ft. What are the factors that influence motor behavior in these two examples? In both cases, the ability or inability to perform a task is context dependent.

There are various ways to characterize the physical context of the task. The environmental dimension in Gentile's (1987) taxonomy provides one way of describing the context. Other task dimensions and examples of possible adaptations have been described (Davis & Burton, 1991; Sabari, 1991; Trombly, 1989). The support surface may be adjusted in terms of the slope and height from ground. The size, shape, and texture of the object used in a task may be varied. Equipment used to act on an object may be modified in terms of length and weight. The accuracy and speed requirements for task performance can be altered. The information required or provided as part of task performance can be changed in terms of timing, precision, and abstractness of the response. These adaptations are similar to the compensatory strategies described in other occupational therapy approaches.

Systems other than the physical context must also be considered. Heriza (1991) and Thelen (1989) emphasized the importance of social influences on motor behavior. They reviewed studies that show that locomotion in infants changes and develops faster when there is social reinforcement for the behaviors. The social and cultural context for performance is also emphasized in several recent approaches to assessment (Dunn, 1993; Spencer, Krefting, & Mattingly, 1993). The role of environmental systems on motor behavior needs to be explored further.

4. Develop and implement treatment plans that are unique to the individual and his environment. Many therapists refer to the art and science of occupational therapy. The art of the contemporary task-oriented approach is the identification of interventions for the unique needs of each client, taking into account his unique personal and environmental systems. Thus treatment planning cannot be prescriptive. There are no cookbook strategies that are correct for every person in every environment. This can seem overwhelming to the student who is trying to process lots of new information. However, these challenges in clinical practice can be the very things that make occupational therapy so exciting and rewarding.

Assumption: After CNS Damage or Other Changes in Personal or Environmental Systems, Clients' Behavioral Changes Reflect Attempts to Compensate to Achieve Functional Goals

CONCEPTS

Change in Systems

All motor behaviors undergo change. A **phase shift,** or change in the preferred movement patterns, occurs because of changes in personal characteristics or the performance context. During a period of change, there is more variation in movement patterns used for a given task. Periods of transition are the optimal times to facilitate change to new movement patterns.

Measuring change is important in occupational therapy. Therapists have developed measures of change related to outcomes, but quantitative measures of change are needed for the process or actual movements used in task performance. For example, it was noted that a change in the movements used for writing may occur as a result of changes in some systems (e.g., a blister or writing utensil). In this situation, a therapist might record the outcome of the writing task the same as before (e.g., independent). However, this measure of the outcome does not depict the real changes in the preferred movement patterns (i.e., change to a different attractor state). The challenge is to identify a measure of the change in how a person moves. These quantitative measures are called **collective variables,** and they describe the complex interaction of multiple systems in simple terms (Heriza, 1991). Examples of **collective variables** identified in basic research are described later in this chapter.

Attempts to Compensate to Achieve Functional Goals

There are several explanations for the different movement patterns seen in individuals with CNS damage. The traditional perspective suggests that CNS damage causes loss of higher-level control and release of lower-level reflexes and abnormal muscle tone, resulting in abnormal patterns of movement (Bobath, 1978) or synergies (Brunnstrom, 1970). The contemporary perspective proposes that the person is simply trying to control all the elements that are now free to vary and use the remaining systems to compensate to achieve functional goals. These patterns may or may not be optimal for a given task in its context given the client's capabilities and limitations.

EVALUATION AND TREATMENT PRINCIPLES

1. Consider whether the motor behaviors are stable or in transition. Changes in motor behavior, or **phase shifts,** observed in clients may be the result of aging, CNS damage, a new environment, and many other factors. When a change is occurring, the motor behaviors seen during task performance are more variable or unstable. It may be hard to identify a preferred movement pattern or an attractor for a task. The marble on the flat or slightly bumpy surface illustrates this period of change.

Part of the evaluation process is to determine if the patterns of behavior are stable or in a period of transition. This information is important, because it helps the therapist identify the optimal times to provide treatment and the strategies that are needed to produce

a change in the preferred movement patterns (Kamm et al., 1990; Scholz, 1990). Data are gathered through analyzing movements used for task performance (**collective variables**) and by constructing an individual developmental profile that provides an historical overview of previous changes in motor behavior (Thelen, 1989). If the movement patterns are stable in a particular performance context, it is difficult to produce a change in the way the task is performed. In this scenario, change in motor behavior is less likely to be observed and the person is apt to return easily to the preferred pattern, even if it is possible temporarily to produce a change. This stability may be characterized as shallow wells or deep wells (Fig. 25B.1, *A* and *C*). For example, neuromotor synergy patterns may represent the stable, obligatory movement patterns of a damaged system. On the other hand, if the motor behavior is in a period of transition, there is increased variability in the movements used to complete a task and increased susceptibility to change or perturbation by the influence of some personal or environmental systems. In addition, movement patterns take longer to return to a somewhat stable state if perturbed (Heriza, 1991). These findings in an evaluation mark a transition period, or **phase shift,** and may be characterized as a marble on a smooth or bumpy surface (Fig. 25.1*B*).

When the movement patterns are unstable or in transition, therapists are more likely to facilitate a change to different patterns—ones, it is hoped, that are more efficient and effective in achieving the task goal. Remediation of motor behavior problems should begin before the movement patterns fall into an obligatory, stereotyped pattern (Kamm et al., 1990). Occupational therapists must also consider the possibility that if the movement patterns for a person have been obligatory or in transition for a long time, the interventions might not effect a change to an optimal attractor state. Perhaps only a trial period of therapy is warranted.

2. Determine whether the motor behaviors seen represent ineffective movement patterns or are optimal given the constraints on the person and environment. After CNS damage, a client may have to learn strategies for task performance given personal limitations. When the client understands the idea of the task, his own personal limitations and capabilities, environmental resources, and a basic solution to the problem, he may begin to practice the task. The inefficient and ineffective movements sometimes seen at this time are consistent with the limited understanding and control one has during the early stages of learning and at the lower levels of skill (Higgins, 1991). Perhaps the client simply needs further practice and time to develop skill. On the other hand, therapists need to identify ineffective movement patterns that are hindering task performance or contributing to future problems in per-

sonal and environmental systems. Mulder (1991) added one more caution regarding the analysis of preferred patterns: The achievement of functional outcomes may be more important to the client and family than the therapist's goal of "normal" movement patterns. Again, a client-centered approach is important.

3. Analyze the functional outcomes and processes used for task performance. One of the challenges in the contemporary task-oriented approach is identification of **collective variables** that can describe in simple terms all the systems that cooperate to produce movements (Heriza, 1991; Thelen, 1991). **Collective variables** are a way of objectively measuring the motor behavior and changes in motor behavior. Identification of **collective variables** that are measurable in clinical practice represents a great challenge for occupational therapists in the next decade. Therapists are beginning to discover ways to measure the outcomes of functional performance. However, sometimes occupational therapy interventions are not intended to result in a substantial change in the outcome. For example, a client may already be independent in bathing. The goal in occupational therapy may be to help him change the movement patterns used for getting out of the tub so that performance is more optimal in terms of efficiency and safety. An inability to document changes in movement efficiency may represent a potential problem related to reimbursement for occupational therapy services.

Evaluation of the process of occupational performance is a description of the preferred pattern of motor behavior for completing a task (i.e., the attractor) and the stability or instability of the pattern. The person performs the same task several times in the same context and then in different contexts. Intervention is not needed if the attractor is relatively efficient and effective for a given task and is stable but also flexible so that it can be modified for different contexts. On the other hand, if there is no attractor (Fig. 25B.1*B*) or if the attractor well is fixed, the therapist may consider treatment to facilitate a transition to a different attractor state.

The results of basic research may help the therapist identify **collective variables.** Disorders of movement have been characterized by slow reaction times, slow movement times, increased variability in performance, movement trajectories with discontinuities, and rate or speed limitations (Campbell, 1991; Corcos, 1991). A possible collective variable that would be easy to use in practice might simply be a measure of time (e.g., time to begin task, task completion time, and time until movement patterns regress to previous pattern after being perturbed). As videographic and movement analysis methods become more accessible in clinical settings, occupational therapists may mea-

sure the relative timing of one motion with respect to another (relative phase), the curvature or straightness of movements (trajectories), the distance and the direction of movement (displacement), and the speed or constancy of speed (velocity, accelerations, and decelerations) (Corcos, 1991; Fetters, 1991; Heriza, 1991; Scholz, 1990). Finally, movement pattern categories are comprehensive descriptors of movement that may be helpful in describing sequences of movements and natural variability in movement patterns for certain tasks. For example, VanSant (1990, 1991a, 1991b) described four unique movement pattern categories used by different age groups for the task of rising from a supine to a standing position.

Assumption: Personal and Environmental Systems are Heterarchically Organized

CONCEPTS

Heterarchical Organization

A heterarchy has no automatic or inherent ordering of the systems in terms of their importance or influence on motor behavior. Thus muscle tone or soft tissue contracture, or any other factor for that matter, is not automatically addressed first in evaluation and treatment for all persons. For each individual, one or more systems will no doubt have a bigger role than others. The challenge is to identify those systems or **control parameters** that are the most important for a given client. **Control parameters** are personal characteristics or environmental factors that constrain movement into specific patterns and can cause a shift from one pattern of behavior to another (Heriza, 1991). These parameters may promote use of optimal or dysfunctional patterns for task performance. **Control parameters** can change and can be graded to cause a **phase shift** (Burton & Davis, 1992).

EVALUATION AND TREATMENT PRINCIPLES

1. Consider all personal and environmental systems as possible positive or negative influences of motor behavior. **Control parameters** may be highly specific (e.g., muscle tone) or general (e.g., attitude), but they cannot be known in advance (Kamm et al., 1990). Thelen (1989) studied treadmill stepping in infants and found that neurological and morphological maturation and the postures of the leg were the major factors influencing the movements used. Velocity is identified as a control parameter in the locomotion patterns used by people and animals (Scholz, 1990). If a horse is forced to increase its speed, changes in movements associated with a walk, trot, and gallop can be observed (Crutchfield & Barnes, 1993). Body dimensions are

identified by VanSant (1990) as factors influencing movement patterns used for righting tasks.

2. Identify the personal and environmental systems that serve as major influences on motor behavior for each individual. Once the therapist describes the preferred movement patterns and their current and past status, she must identify the personal and environmental systems that constrain movement to an ineffective pattern and those that may act as agents of change or elicit optimal movement patterns. Part of the occupational therapy process, then, is systematically to manipulate personal characteristics (e.g., attention and positioning) and environmental context (e.g., size of object and stability of base of support) and observe the effect on occupational performance. This process can help identify one or several **control parameters** that can cause a shift in motor behavior.

It may seem an impossible task to identify only a couple of systems from the multiple systems and subsystems that influence motor performance. However, occupational therapists already do this, using quantitative and qualitative measures. Several hypothetical examples are described below to illustrate these ideas and propose other possible **control parameters** for motor behavior. An analogy might be helpful in understanding why therapists often identify one or two control variables or parameters that influence performance when multiple systems are involved. Some people were discussing the factors that led to a major flood in their town. In a sense, they were considering the role of various systems on the complex behavior of flooding. One person suggested that the critical variable was farming practices upstream. Another person claimed the control parameter was the removal of wetlands in the area. Yet another person argued it was the failure to implement a flood-control plan. Although all of these systems indeed had a role in the behavior of flooding, it was a toddler who revealed the real control parameter for flooding as too much rain.

In the same way, occupational therapists can identify one or several **control parameters** for an individual client. Consider the task of placing items on a shelf above shoulder level. Now imagine, or better yet actually try, placing various items on the shelf. Consider the different movement patterns used to lift an empty paint can and a full paint can to the high shelf. What is the control parameter that explains the change in movement patterns when lifting an empty can versus a full can? It is likely the weight of the can relative to arm strength. What is the control parameter that explains the change in movement patterns when lifting a tennis ball versus a beach ball in the same task (assuming weight is held constant)? In this situation, it is the size of the object relative to hand size. Both of the **control parameters** in these examples are

performer-scaled variables (Davis & Burton, 1991), or parameters that link a characteristic of the person (e.g., strength or hand size) to a characteristic of the task or an object that is used in the task (e.g., weight or size).

Thelen (1989) stated that it is important to consider nonobvious and distantly related factors as possible **control parameters.** She described studies showing that the onset of crawling, a motor skill, is an influential factor in cognitive, affective, and social phase shifts in children. The ability to locomote to different environments then is a control parameter that can cause a dramatic change in the problem-solving, communication, and play behaviors of children.

One last example is used to propose other systems that might serve as **control parameters.** In one long-term care setting, health care professionals were wondering why older men who had suffered a cerebrovascular accident (CVA) in this home were not achieving independence in dressing. One therapist hypothesized it was loss of automatic reactions and postural control. Another therapist claimed the critical factor was motor planning problems. A nurse argued that general loss of strength and endurance explained the performance deficit. Again, all of these systems did indeed influence motor behavior. However, a nursing assistant who had worked at the institution for 20 years revealed that the control parameter for the motor behaviors related to dressing was because of a different culture. That is, most residents in this setting represented a culture that did not place value on independence in self-care for older adults—especially men who had disease-related impairments. In fact, it was an expectation that women in the extended family would come to the residence every day to complete activities of daily living.

There are several purposes in relating these examples. One purpose is to challenge therapists to use more creativity and common sense in the evaluation and treatment process; sometimes, the control parameter may be as simple as "too much rain." Second, for given individuals with given tasks, the **control parameters** may be neural or nonneural sensorimotor components (e.g., soft tissue contracture, muscle weakness, and abnormal muscle tone). Third, occupational therapists sometimes neglect important factors like "a different culture" and look only at performance components that seem directly related to the motor behaviors. The traditional approaches have overemphasized the role of the CNS and the sensorimotor system to the neglect of other equally important personal and environmental systems. The point again is that no system automatically deserves more attention than others until research indicates otherwise.

3. Anticipate that the critical variables influencing motor behavior will change. The **control parameters** of motor behavior change. CNS damage affects

each system differently relative to occupational performance. This idea is illustrated in Figures 25B.2 and 25B.3, which depict hypothetical changes in systems and subsystems over time for a unique person. The y axes represent the degree of impact (positive or negative) the system has on occupational performance, and the x axes represent these changes over time from onset of CNS damage to the rehabilitation stage to postdischarge or home. Some systems are highly affected immediately after CNS damage, while other systems become more important at later times. For example, the physical environment in Figure 25B.2 may become a more critical variable when the person returns home. The home environment may or may not support performance of previous occupational roles and tasks. In current rehabilitation settings, the physical environment is designed for persons with physical disabilities and thus may not be as important because the setting is so unlike the natural environment. Therefore, systems that influence occupational performance at one time may not be the critical systems at other times. Figure 25B.3 shows the effects of neural and nonneural components of muscle tone at different points in time. Based on the authors' clinical experience, neural factors (e.g., spasticity) are important immediately after the onset of CNS damage but have less of an effect on performance later. The influence of nonneural factors (e.g., soft tissue contracture), however, is almost the inverse of the neural systems.

A client's occupational performance at any one time reflects the interaction of all these systems. The **control parameters** at a given point in time may vary

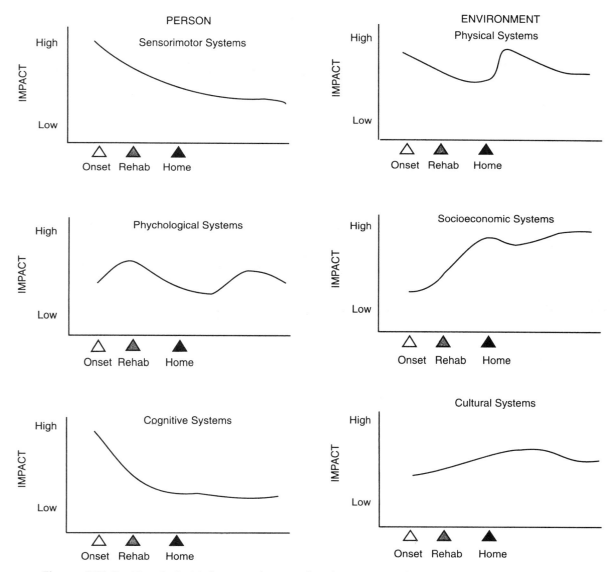

Figure 25B.2. Hypothetical influences of personal and environmental systems on occupational performance for a unique person at different points in time.

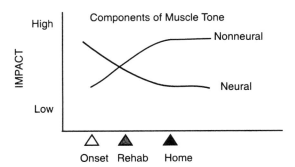

Figure 25B.3. Hypothetical influences of neural and nonneural components of muscle tone on occupational performance at different points in time.

greatly, depending on the characteristics of the unique person and his environment. What is effective for one client may not be effective for the next client with similar CNS dysfunction. In addition, systems that enhance performance at one time may actually interfere with task performance at a later time (Kamm et al., 1990). What is effective early in treatment may not be effective later. Therapists need to identify the major influences on motor behavior at a specific time for a specific person and anticipate future changes in the **control parameters.**

4. Manipulate critical personal or environmental systems to cause change in motor behavior. After a control parameter is identified, the therapist manipulates this personal or environmental characteristic until a shift in motor behavior is observed. Relatively small changes in a critical personal or environmental system may produce large changes in the movement patterns used for a task (Thelen, 1989). For example, putting an infant in water or on a treadmill dramatically affects walking (Thelen, 1989). Use of an orthotic device in a shoe or a splint that provides wrist support may change the movement patterns and thus change the functional ability (Kamm et al., 1990). The goals of occupational therapy are to help individuals to identify and use **control parameters** that support optimal performance and to determine the optimal value for producing the best performance outcome (Burton & Davis, 1992).

Assumption: A Person Needs to Practice and Experiment with Varied Strategies to Find the Optimal Solution for a Motor Problem and Develop Skill in Performance

CONCEPTS

Practice and Experiment with Movement Strategies

Practice is defined as "repeated attempts to produce motor behaviors that are beyond present capabili-

ties" (Schmidt, 1991b, p. 49). The outcome of practice is **motor learning.** The contemporary perspective on **motor learning** proposes that practice should lead to "relatively permanent changes in the capability of responding" (Schmidt, 1991b, p. 51) rather than simply changed performance during the practice session.

The word *experiment* suggests that the person has an active role in the learning process. The client finds solutions to motor problems, using information or feedback from his own sensory system (i.e., intrinsic feedback) and from outside sources (i.e., extrinsic feedback) (Crutchfield & Barnes, 1993). Feedback is information about the success of motor behavior in meeting a functional goal (Schmidt, 1991a, 1991b).

Optimal Solution and Skill

Higgins (1991) proposed a framework for understanding motor skill acquisition based on the contemporary perspective. She suggested that individuals are problem solvers who use their personal characteristics or resources to interact meaningfully and adaptively with their environments. "Problems are goals that arise as a function of an encounter between the individual and the surround [environmental context], occurring under an infinite variety of conditions across a lifespan. Skill is the ability to solve problems with a degree of consistency and economy" (Higgins, 1991, p. 125). Thus skillful individuals use the optimal biomechanical and physiological solution for a motor problem. Different people will reach different levels of skill for a given task.

EVALUATION AND TREATMENT PRINCIPLES

1. Provide practice opportunities that fit the nature of the task. As discussed in the first assumption, there are a number of classification schemes that are used to describe the nature of the task. Research shows that different types of tasks require different types of practice sessions to facilitate learning. One decision made in designing a practice session is whether to have the client practice the task in its entirety (i.e., **whole learning**), in separate steps (i.e., **part learning**), or in some combination of **whole** and **part learning.** **Motor learning** studies by Winstein (1991) and others suggested that the effectiveness of the strategies selected depends on the type of task. Winstein (1991) studied weight shifting as a possible **part learning** task for locomotion in persons with hemiparesis. She found that persons in the treatment group using **part learning** did improve in the symmetry of standing posture but showed no significant improvement over a control group in actual locomotion. Thus **whole learning** rather than **part learning** is recommended for **discrete** and **continuous tasks** (Crutchfield & Barnes,

1993). **Discrete** (e.g., throwing a ball) and **continuous** (e.g., riding a bicycle and walking) **tasks** cannot be easily broken down into steps. Separate practice of the discrete components of a **serial task** is beneficial. Kerr (1982) stated that the complexity of the task should also be taken into consideration. When the task is low in complexity, **whole learning** is recommended. **Part learning** is suggested for more complex tasks.

2. Provide practice opportunities that are appropriate for the client's stage of learning. The stages of learning are discovery (cognitive), mastery (associative), and generalization (autonomous) (Fitts & Posner, 1967; Higgins, 1991). Many clients will be in the discovery stage as they develop an understanding of the task, identify the performance problems, and find a general solution. This stage is characterized by slow performance, clumsiness, and self-imposed rigidity or freezing of body parts to control all the elements (i.e., degrees of freedom) that are normally free to vary in high levels of skill. In this stage, clients attempt to exert control over some parts of the body to learn the influence of changes in their personal systems and relationships to the environment (Higgins, 1991). Later stages of learning help the client refine the solutions identified in the discovery stage and generalize these solutions to other tasks. The behaviors in these stages are more consistent, accurate, faster, and coordinated (see Chapter 13).

3. Provide practice opportunities that result in permanent changes in the capability for responding. Occupational therapists have always incorporated practice into treatment sessions. Recent **motor learning** research suggests that although the idea of practice is still a critical factor in **motor learning,** therapists need to think differently about the structure of practice opportunities and measures of the outcome of practice (i.e., **motor learning**). In this section, the traditional and contemporary perspectives on practice and **motor learning** are contrasted (Poole, 1991a).

The traditional perspective on practice and **motor learning** is used in many therapy and training programs. Practice sessions consist of drills and require clients to perform many repetitions of the same task in the same way (Schmidt, 1991b). This is called **blocked practice.** For example, in the task of dressing, the client is presented a series of steps that must be practiced again and again in the same manner. Learning, or the outcome of these practice experiences, is measured in terms of observable changes in performance seen during practice or immediately after.

The contemporary perspective argues that therapists must rethink the characteristics of practice and the timing of the measures of **motor learning.** Although measurement of learning during the practice session is efficient, the occupational therapist's inten-

tion for the outcome of practice is that clients can perform better once they leave treatment. Research in **motor learning** (Schmidt, 1991b) shows that measures of the outcome of performance during practice is not the same as later performance. If the goal is to improve motor performance on a relatively permanent basis, then therapists need to evaluate the effectiveness of the practice sessions in terms of later performance.

Recent studies have examined the type of practice that is most valuable for changing the capability for later performance. A review of the literature by Schmidt (1991b) suggested that practice of tasks should vary randomly **(random practice),** i.e., therapists should ask clients to try a variety of tasks within one session. For example, a treatment session might involve practice of all tasks in a morning routine (e.g., feeding, dressing, hygiene, and toileting). One thing to remember when adopting a **random practice** approach is that performance during the practice session may actually look worse than performance after **blocked practice.** This is acceptable because the goal is to enhance **motor learning** or the capability for later performance rather than change observable behaviors during a practice session.

Variation of the context within a task is also important in practice (Keshner, 1991; Lee, Swanson, & Hall, 1991; Mulder, 1991; Sabari, 1991; VanSant, 1991a, 1991b). Because the occupational therapist's goals relate to independence in solving motor problems, variation in practice experiences is critical. Varied contexts promote development of preferred movement patterns for specific contexts and flexibility in movement patterns for different contexts (Heriza, 1991). If the client practices only in a narrow context, then a limited number of solutions will be learned. On the other hand, if the client practices the task in many contexts, many solutions are learned and varied performance is possible (Higgins, 1991). Manipulating the context of the task can cause changes in the preferred movement patterns for task performance (Thelen, 1989). Possible task dimensions can be identified for support surfaces, objects, equipment, task demands, and information required (Davis & Burton, 1991). Bernstein (1967) summarized this principle by stating that people need repetition without repetition.

4. Provide practice opportunities in natural environments. If therapists hope that clients develop stable, but flexible, movement patterns for the tasks and contexts in their home and community, then it is important to use natural environments for practice sessions (Burgess, 1989). The rehabilitation unit should simulate the real-life setting, if interventions cannot be provided in the actual situation (Poole, 1991b; Mulder, 1991). Easy Street and other therapeutic modules (Stahl, 1993) provide simulations of community-based environments.

Many rehabilitation units have apartments with furniture commonly found in homes. Other resources within the institution can also serve to simulate community settings (e.g., gift shop, cafeteria, and chapel).

5. Provide feedback that facilitates **motor learning** and encourages experimentation with solutions to motor problems. When therapists recognize that a goal is to have clients rely on intrinsic feedback for task performance in the future, therapists realize that careful planning of the extrinsic feedback during treatment is important. Using intuition and a traditional perspective, therapists assume that frequent, immediate, and consistent feedback is best. Lee et al. (1991), Schmidt (1991b), and Winstein (1991) reviewed their own and other studies that shed light on more appropriate feedback strategies related to the knowledge of results (KR) or the outcome of performance. Studies of people without motor problems suggested that feedback should be less frequent, scheduled randomly or intermittently, faded over time, and given as summary information or when performance is outside a given error range. These feedback strategies resulted in better retention of motor skills over time than control groups who were provided traditional feedback. Of course, it is critical that research on feedback also be conducted on subjects with motor problems, and that therapists carefully analyze the effect of their feedback conditions on individual client performance.

6. Encourage active participation in the learning process and collaborate with the client during evaluation and treatment. Clients should have an active role in the selection of tasks for evaluation and treatment and in solving occupational performance problems. There are several ways to elicit active participation. Teach clients the principles of task analysis (Higgins, 1991). Clients also need to evaluate their own performance in terms of the outcomes of their efforts and the efficiency and effectiveness of the movement patterns used. Thus a goal of therapy is to help clients understand the movement patterns and the performance contexts that contribute to optimal performance for given tasks (Burton & Davis, 1992). The therapist promotes an understanding of personal capabilities and limitations and encourages exploration of the available environmental resources that can be modified (Higgins, 1991). These strategies assist clients in developing skills needed for solving motor problems in their home and community environments.

There is one last idea that should be embraced by occupational therapists. Therapists need to give skilled clients permission to solve their own motor problems and to use movement patterns that are the most functional for them, regardless of how these strategies are perceived by others (Burton & Davis, 1992). When a person becomes skilled in task analysis and

solving motor problems, therapists can celebrate their participation in various tasks and autonomy in learning (Higgins, 1991). This is possible even when clients' solutions are not traditional or identical to the strategies therapists would recommend. For example, Mattson, a wheelchair racer with a C_{6-7} spinal cord lesion, found he could propel faster using a backhand stroke that maximized use of his remaining muscle groups (Burton & Davis, 1992). This technique is unconventional, but Mattson's performance dramatically improved, and soon after many other wheelchair racers were using the same approach. Thus people may use unique movement patterns because they require the least amount of energy and are efficient means of performing the task (Kamm et al., 1990).

EVALUATION OF MOTOR BEHAVIOR PROBLEMS

As stated in Chapter 7, the evaluation process from the contemporary perspective will require use of both qualitative and quantitative measures. Because motor behavior is organized by the functional goals of the clients, therapists need to spend more time getting a picture of the client's and significant others' perspective on past occupational performance and future goals as well as current observable behavior. The therapist also gathers information on the preferred movement patterns for given tasks and their stability, quantitative measures of change in performance, the major influences on motor behavior, and the characteristics of tasks.

Figure 25B.4 presents some guidelines for data collection in evaluation. *The Canadian Occupational Performance Measure* (COPM) (Law et al., 1990) has greatly influenced these guidelines. These guidelines can help therapists gather information on past and current performance, identify goals for the future, and consider occupational roles and tasks as the starting points in the evaluation process.

REMEDIATION OF MOTOR BEHAVIOR PROBLEMS

Summary of Principles

A brief summary of treatment principles is possible (Davis & Burton, 1991; Duncan & Badke, 1987; Montgomery & Connolly, 1991).

1. Collaborate with the client in identifying problematic tasks of interest and importance.
2. Encourage an active learning process by allowing the person to discover and experiment with various movements that can be used to optimally perform a task.

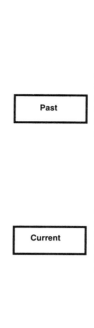

Occupational Roles	Occupational Performance
Past	
• Description of past roles • Importance of roles from perspective of client and others • Past role changes and factors influencing these changes • Roles immediately prior to OT referral • Stabilty and changes in roles immediately prior to OT referral • Tasks that are now a problem and are considered important or necessary for roles	• Preferred movement patterns used to complete past tasks • Flexibility in movement patterns used to complete tasks • Stability or instability of the movement patterns • Personal characteristics required and affected in tasks • Typical performance contexts and variability in contexts • Factors that caused previous changes in performance
Current	
• Current roles • Differences between current and past roles • Factors influencing shift to current roles • Satisfaction of current roles to client and others • Stability of current roles • Tasks associated with each role that can and can't be done satisfactorily	• Tasks that can and can't be satisfactorily performed • Independence in solving motor problems • Stability of preferred movement patterns • Efficiency, effectiveness, and safety of preferred patterns • Personal characteristics affecting performance • Typical performance contexts and variability in contexts • Effects of environmental manipulation on performance • Ability to learn new strategies • Optimal practice and feedback strategies to be used
Future	
• Roles of importance to resume • New roles that might be explored by self and others • Tasks that need to be performed in future roles	• Movement patterns that might be used in future tasks • Difference between current and future movement patterns • Need for a shift to new movement patterns • Possible control parameters that may used to shift behavior

Figure 25B.4. Evaluation guidelines for gathering information on occupational roles and occupational performance along a continuum of time.

3. Analyze the preferred movements for task performance and the outcome.
4. Perturb dysfunctional movement patterns by manipulating a critical personal or environmental factor.
5. Record changes in the preferred movements for task performance and the outcomes.
6. Grade manipulations until movements approximate an efficient and effective pattern.
7. Vary the practice conditions to facilitate learning and flexible task performance.

Treatment Goals

The goals of a therapist who uses a contemporary task-oriented approach are to help the person:

1. Discover the optimal movement patterns for performing a task;
2. Achieve flexibility in task performance by providing practice opportunities with varying contexts;
3. Maximize use of personal characteristics and environmental factors that make efficient and effective task performance possible;
4. Facilitate problem solving by the client so he can identify his own solutions to motor problems in home and community environments.

Roles of the Therapist

Many roles for the therapist are proposed in the literature (Burton & Davis, 1992; Gentile, 1992; Heriza, 1991; Higgins, 1991; Kamm et al., 1990). The therapist collaborates with the client in selecting a variety of tasks for practice. She may modify the task initially so the learner can succeed. The therapist teaches task analysis, structures learning opportunities, provides feedback, and facilitates understanding of unique personal and environmental systems that promote optimal performance. If the client cannot learn using this approach, the therapist will need to use a different approach and provide nongeneralizable solutions that the client can memorize. The therapist may also serve as a coach for the client during the learning process by directing the focus to the functional outcome, suggesting movements to try, recording progress, and assisting with decision making when new challenges arise. The final role is to manipulate the personal and environmental factors and to identify optimal times to effect changes in movement. **Manual guidance** may be used but should allow some elements to vary so that the client can experiment with movement patterns. Assistance provided through handling should also be faded as soon as possible. All of these roles are important in helping the client to become autonomous in solving motor problems.

Treatment Techniques

Most proponents of approaches based on the contemporary perspective use a variety of techniques to facilitate the learning process. Verbal instructions, visual input, positioning or passive movement, and structuring environments will continue to be important in treatment using a contemporary task-oriented approach (Crutchfield & Barnes, 1993).

Recording Progress and Outcomes

There are no clearly defined measures of progress in the contemporary task-oriented approach. However, therapists can ask their clients and themselves a number of questions to determine if the interventions made a difference (see Fig. 25B.4). These and other questions might provide a starting point in evaluating the effectiveness of interventions for an individual.

LIMITATIONS

There are some limitations to the contemporary task-oriented approach. Evaluation and intervention strategies must be developed or refined, and efficacy studies need to be done. It is difficult to simulate natural environments in many clinical settings. However, as therapy clinics are remodeled and new clinics are designed, there is potential to create more natural environments in the hospital setting. In addition, some work and leisure tasks are not easily simulated in clinical settings. The latter two limitations suggest that therapy interventions should ideally occur in clients' home, school, leisure, and work settings. The increased pressure to shorten hospital stays, and the increased development of community-based treatment programs should support this trend. Because this approach requires problem solving of clients, it might appear to be inappropriate in acute settings and for clients with cognitive impairments. However, it is argued that aspects of the contemporary task-oriented approach, e.g., use of natural environments, may be better for clients with cognitive impairments than previous approaches that often used contrived tasks in clinical settings. Implementation of a client-centered approach may not be possible in some acute settings or with clients who adopt a passive role. Another limitation of this approach relates to communication problems when using concepts that originate outside of occupational therapy and the testability of an approach based on such abstract, complex ideas (Horak, 1991).

FUTURE DIRECTIONS

All treatment approaches evolve over time. Through clinical practice and research, the assumptions of this approach will be tested. Some assumptions will be supported and developed further. Other assumptions will not be supported and may need to be dropped or modified. The contemporary task-oriented approach provides occupational therapists with new ideas about the remediation of motor behavior problems. Basic and clinical research is needed. Development of evaluation tools and measures of change is critical. Identification of **control parameters** and **collective variables** will lead to more effective treatment strategies. Empirical testing of this approach with persons having CNS dysfunction is needed to provide support for its use in practice. The authors challenge the reader to join us in this process.

Acknowledgments—Thanks to our families, our colleagues, and our students for the ideas, feedback, and encouragement they have provided us. This chapter is dedicated to Sister Genevieve Cummings (Miriam Joseph).

STUDY QUESTIONS

1. Define and give examples of discrete, serial, and continuous movements.
2. Describe the optimal type of practice to facilitate motor learning for discrete, serial, and continuous movements.
3. Identify the two dimensions and related components of Gentile's taxonomy.
4. Describe the characteristics of the different attractor states in Figure 25B.1 and give examples of these states in clients.
5. What are some strategies for making the evaluation and treatment process more client centered?
6. Give examples of possible systems and subsystems that might influence motor behavior for a given individual.
7. What are optimal and nonoptimal times for producing a change in motor behavior?
8. How is change in motor behavior measured?
9. What are collective variables and why are they important in evaluation and treatment?
10. What are control parameters and how should they be used in evaluation and treatment?
11. What are the characteristics of skilled motor behavior and how can therapists facilitate development of skill in their clients?
12. Describe feedback that facilitates development of skilled motor behavior?
13. Why are natural environments important to use in treatment?

References

Abreu, B., & Schmidt, R. (1992). *The Neuroscience Institute: Motor control, learning, and cognitive rehabilitation*. Workshop sponsored by the American Occupational Therapy Association.

Ada, L., & Westwood, P. (1992). A kinematic analysis of recovery of the ability to stand up following stroke. *Australian Journal of Physiotherapy, 38*, 135–142.

American Occupational Therapy Association. (1989). Uniform terminology for occupational therapy (2nd ed.). *American Journal of Occupational Therapy, 43*, 808–815.

Andrews, K., Brocklehurst, G. C., Richards, B. & Laycock, P. J. (1981). The rate of recovery from stroke and its measurement. *International Rehabilitation Medicine, 31*, 155–161.

Arnadottir, G. (1990). *The brain and behavior: Assessing cortical dysfunction through activities of daily living*. St. Louis: C. V. Mosby.

Barris, R., Kielhofner, G., Levine, R. E., & Neville, A. M. (1985). Occupation as interaction with the environment. In G. Kielhofner (Ed.), *A model of human occupation: Theory and application* (pp. 42-62). Baltimore: Williams & Wilkins.

Bernstein, N. (1967). *The coordination and regulation of movements*. Oxford, UK: Pergamon Press.

Bobath, B. (1978). *Adult hemiplegia: Evaluation and treatment* (2nd ed.). London: William Heinemann Medical Books.

Bobath, B. (1990). *Adult hemiplegia: Evaluation and treatment* (3rd ed.). London: William Heinemann Medical Books.

Bohannon, R. W. (1986). Strength of lower limb related to gait velocity and cadence in stroke patients. *Physiotherapy Canada, 38*, 204–206.

Bourbonnais, D., & Vanden Noven, S. (1989). Weakness in patients with hemiparesis. *American Journal of Occupational Therapy, 43*, 313–319.

Brunia, C. H. M., Haagh, S., & Scheirs, J. G. M. (1985). Waiting to respond: Electrophysiological measurements in man during preparation for a voluntary movement. In H. Heuer, U. Kleinbeck, & K. Schmidt (Eds.), *Motor behavior: Programming, control and acquisition* (pp. 35–78). Berlin: Springer-Verlag.

Brunnstrom, S. (1970). *Movement therapy in hemiplegia*. New York: Harper & Row.

Burgess, M. K. (1989). The issue is—Motor control and the role of occupational therapy: Past, present, and future. *American Journal of Occupational Therapy, 43*, 345–348.

Burton, A. W., & Davis, W. E. (1992). Optimizing the involvement and performance of children with physical impairments in movement activities. *Pediatric Exercise Science, 4*, 236–248.

Campbell, S. K. (1991). Framework for the measurement of neurologic impairment and disability. In M. J. Lister (Ed.), *Contemporary management of motor control problems: Proceedings of the II STEP Conference* (pp. 143–154). Alexandria, VA: Foundation for Physical Therapy.

Carr, J. H. (1992). Compensatory and substitution movements following acute brain lesions: Useful or not? In *Proceedings of the World Confederation for Physical Therapy* (pp. 985–987). London.

Carr, J. H., & Shepherd, R. B. (1983a). *Early care of the stroke patient: A positive approach*. London: William Heinemann Medical Books.

Carr, J. H., & Shepherd, R. B. (1987a). *A Motor Relearning Programme for stroke* (2nd ed.). Rockville, MD: Aspen Systems.

Carr, J. H., & Shepherd, R. B. (1987b). A motor learning model for rehabilitation. In J. H. Carr, R. B. Shepherd, J. Gordon, A. M. Gentile, & J. M. Held (Eds.), *Movement science: Foundations for physical therapy in rehabilitation* (pp. 31–91). Rockville, MD: Aspen Systems.

Carr, J. H., & Shepherd, R. B. (1989). A motor learning model for stroke rehabilitation. *Physiotherapy, 75*, 372–379.

Carr, J. H., & Shepherd, R. B. (1990). A motor learning model for rehabilitation of the movement-disabled. In L. Ada & C. Canning (Eds.), *Key issues in neurological physiotherapy* (pp. 1–24). Kent, UK: Butterworth.

Carr, J. H., Shepherd, R. B., Gordon, J., Gentile, A. M., & Held, J. M. (1987). *Movement science: Foundations for physical therapy in rehabilitation*. Rockville, MD: Aspen Systems.

Carr, J. H., Shepherd, R. B., Nordholm, L., & Lynne, D. (1985). Investigation of a new motor assessment scale for stroke patients. *Physical Therapy, 65*, 175–180.

Christiansen, C. (1991). Occupational therapy: Intervention for life performance. In C. Christiansen & C. Baum (Eds.), *Occupational therapy: Overcoming human performance deficits* (pp. 3–44). Thorofare, NJ: Slack.

Corcos, D. (1991). Strategies underlying the control of disordered movement. *Physical Therapy, 71*, 25–38.

Crutchfield, C. A., & Barnes, M.R. (1993). *Motor control and motor learning in rehabilitation*. Atlanta, GA: Stokesville.

Davies, P. M. (1985). *Steps to follow—A guide to the treatment of adult hemiplegia*. New York: Springer-Verlag.

Davies, P. M. (1990). *Right in the middle: Selective trunk activity in the treatment of adult hemiplegia*. New York: Springer-Verlag.

Davis, W. E., & Burton, A. W. (1991). Ecological task analysis: Translating movement behavior theory into practice. *Adapted Physical Activity Quarterly, 8*, 154–177.

Dean, C., & Mackey, F. (1992). Motor assessment scale scores as a measure of rehabilitation outcome following stroke. *Australian Journal of Physiotherapy, 38*, 31–35.

Duncan, P. W., & Badke, M. B. (1987). *Stroke rehabilitation: The recovery of motor control*. Chicago: Year Book.

Dunn, W. (1993). The issue is—Measurement of function: Actions for the future. *American Journal of Occupational Therapy, 47*, 357–360.

Fetters, L. (1991). Measurement and treatment in cerebral palsy: An argument for a new approach. *Physical Therapy, 71*, 244–247.

Fisher, A. (1990). *Assessment of motor and process skills* (rev. ed. 6.1). Unpublished manuscript. (Available from Colorado State University, Occupational Therapy Department, Fort Collins, CO 80523)

Fisher, A., & Short-DeGraff, M. (1993). Nationally speaking— Improving functional assessment in occupational therapy: Recommendations and philosophy for change. *American Journal of Occupational Therapy, 47*, 199–201.

Fitts, P. M., & Posner, M. I. (1967). *Human performance*. Belmont, CA: Brooks/Cole.

Ford-Smith, C. D., & VanSant, A. F. (1993). Age differences in movement patterns used to rise from a bed in subjects in the third through fifth decades of age. *Physical Therapy, 73*, 300–307.

Forssberg, H., & Hirschfeld, H. (Eds.). (1992). *Movement disorders in children* (Vol. 36). Basel: S. Karger.

Gentile, A. M. (1972). A working model of skill acquisition with application to teaching. *Quest, 17*, 3–23.

Gentile, A. M. (1987). Skill acquisition: Action, movement, and neuromotor processes. In J. H. Carr, R. B. Shepherd, J. Gordon, A. M. Gentile, & J. M. Held (Eds.), *Movement science: Foundations for physical therapy in rehabilitation* (pp. 93–154). Rockville, MD: Aspen Systems.

Gentile, A. M. (1992). The nature of skill acquisition: Therapeutic implications for children with movement disorders. In H. Forssberg & H. Hirschfeld (Eds.), *Movement disorders in children* (pp. 31–40). Basel: S. Karger.

Gordon, J. (1987). Assumptions underlying physical therapy intervention: Theoretical and historical perspectives. In J. H. Carr, R. B. Shepherd, J. Gordon, A. M. Gentile, & J. M. Held (Eds.), *Movement science: Foundations for physical therapy in rehabilitation* (pp. 1–30). Rockville, MD: Aspen Systems.

Gowland, C. (1986). Predicting the outcome of stroke. In M. Banks, (Ed.), *International perspectives in physical therapy 2: Stroke* (pp. 17–47). Edinburgh: Churchill Livingstone.

Harris, S. (1991). Functional abilities in context. In M. J. Lister (Ed.), *Contemporary management of motor control problems: Proceedings of the II STEP Conference* (pp. 253–260). Alexandria, VA: Foundation for Physical Therapy.

Heriza, C. (1991). Motor development: Traditional and contemporary theories. In M. J. Lister (Ed.), *Contemporary management of motor control problems: Proceedings of the II STEP Conference* (pp. 99–126). Alexandria, VA: Foundation for Physical Therapy.

Higgins, J. R., & Spaeth, R. K. (1972). Relationship between consistency of movement and environmental condition. *Quest, 17*, 61–69.

Higgins, S. (1991). Motor skill acquisition. *Physical Therapy, 71*, 123–139.

Horak, F. B. (1991). Assumptions underlying motor control for neurologic rehabilitation. In M. J. Lister (Ed.), *Contemporary management of motor control problems: Proceedings of the II STEP Conference* (pp. 11–27). Alexandria, VA: Foundation for Physical Therapy.

Jeannerod, M. (1984). The timing of natural prehension movements. *Journal of Motor Behavior, 16*, 235–254 .

Johnson, P. (1984). The acquisition of skill. In M. Smyth &, A. Wing (Eds.), *The psychology of human movement* (pp. 215–240). London: Academic Press

Kamm, K., Thelen, E., & Jensen, J. L. (1990). A dynamical systems approach to motor development. *Physical Therapy, 70*, 763–775.

Kerr, R. (1982). *Psychomotor learning.* New York: CBS Publishing.

Keshner, E. (1991). How theoretical framework biases evaluation and treatment. In M. J. Lister (Ed.), (1991). *Contemporary management of motor control problems: Proceedings of the II STEP Conference* (pp. 37–47). Alexandria, VA: Foundation for Physical Therapy.

Law, M., Baptiste, S., McColl, M., Opzoomer, A., Polatajko, H., & Pollock, N. (1990). The Canadian Occupational Performance Measure: An outcome measurement protocol for occupational therapy. *Canadian Journal of Occupational Therapy, 57*, 82–87.

Lee, T., Swanson, L., & Hall, A. (1991). What is repeated in a repetition? Effects of practice conditions on motor skill acquisition. *Physical Therapy, 71*, 150–156.

Lemkuhl, L. D., & Smith, L. K. (1985). *Brunnstrom's clinical kinesiology* (4th ed.). Philadelphia: F. A. Davis.

Lewthwaite, R. (1990). Motivational considerations in physical activity involvement. *Physical Therapy, 70*, 808–819.

Lister, M. J. (Ed.). (1991). *Contemporary management of motor control problems: Proceedings of the II Step Conference.* Alexandria, VA: Foundation for Physical Therapy.

Loewen, S. C., & Anderson, B. A. (1988). Reliability of the Modified Motor Assessment Scale and the Barthel Index. *Physical Therapy, 68*, 1077–1081.

Marteniuk, R. G. (1986). Information processes in movement learning: Capacity and structural interference effects. *Journal of Motor Behavior, 18*, 55–75.

Montgomery, P. C., & Connolly, B. H. (Eds.). (1991). *Motor control and physical therapy: Theoretical framework and practical applications.* Hixson, TN: Chattanooga Group.

Morasso, P. (1981). Spatial control of arm movements. *Experimental Brain Research, 42*, 223–227.

Mulder, T. (1991). A process-oriented model of human motor behavior: Toward a theory-based rehabilitation approach. *Physical Therapy, 71*, 157–164.

Nashner, L. M., & McCollum, G. (1985). The organization of human postural movements: A formal basis and experimental synthesis. *The Behavioral and Brain Sciences, 8*, 135–172.

Nelson, D. L. (1988). Occupation: Form and performance. *American Journal of Occupational Therapy, 42*, 633–641.

Nwaobi, O. M. (1983). Voluntary movement impairment in upper motor neuron lesions: Is spasticity the main cause? *Occupational Therapy Journal of Research, 3*, 131–140.

Parker, V. M., Wade, D. T., & Langton Hewer, R. (1986). Loss of arm function after stroke: Measurement, frequency and recovery. *International Rehabilitation Medicine, 8*, 69–73.

Pollock, N. (1993). Client-centered assessment. *American Journal of Occupational Therapy, 47*, 298–302.

Poole, J. L. (1991a). Application of motor learning principles in occupational therapy. *American Journal of Occupational Therapy, 45*, 531–537.

Poole, J. L. (1991b). Motor control. In C. B. Royeen (Ed.), *AOTA Self-study series: Neuroscience foundations of human performance* (Monograph No. 11, pp. 1–31). Rockville, MD: American Occupational Therapy Association.

Poole, J. L., & Whitney, S. L. (1988). Motor assessment scale for stroke patients: Concurrent validity and interrater reliability. *Archives of Physical Medicine & Rehabilitation, 69*, 195–197.

Richter, R. R., VanSant, A. F., & Newton, R. A. (1989). Description of adult rolling movements and hypothesis of developmental sequences. *Physical Therapy, 69*, 63–71.

Rood, M. S. (1954). Neurophysiological reactions as a basis for physical therapy. *Physical Therapy Review, 34*, 444–449.

Rothstein, J. M. (Ed.). (1991). *Movement science.* Alexandria, VA: American Physical Therapy Association.

Royeen, C. B. (Ed.). (1990–1991). *AOTA self-studies series: Neuroscience foundations of human performance.* Rockville, MD: American Occupational Therapy Association.

Sabari, J. S. (1991). Motor learning concepts applied to activity-based intervention with adults with hemiplegia. *American Journal of Occupational Therapy, 45*, 523–530.

Saltzman, E., & Kelso, J. A. S. (1987). Skilled actions: A task-dynamic approach. *Psychological Review, 94*, 84–106.

Sawnerm J,m & LaVigne, J. (1992). *Brunnstrom's movement theory in hemiplegia.* Philadelphia: J. B. Lippincott.

Schmidt, R. A. (1988). *Motor control and learning: A behavioral emphasis* (2nd ed.). Champaign, IL: Human Kinetics.

Schmidt, R. A. (1991a). *Motor learning and performance: From principles to practice.* Champaign, IL: Human Kinetics.

Schmidt, R. A. (1991b). Motor learning principles for physical therapy. In M. J. Lister (Ed.), *Contemporary management of motor control problems: Proceedings of the II STEP Conference* (pp. 49–63). Alexandria, VA: Foundation for Physical Therapy.

Schmidt, R. A. (1992). *Motor performance and learning: Principles for practitioners.* Champaign, IL: Human Kinetics.

Scholz, J. (1990). Dynamic pattern theory—Some implications for therapeutics. *Physical Therapy, 70*, 827–843.

Shepherd, R. B. (1992). Adaptive motor behaviour in response to perturbations of balance. *Physiotherapy Theory and Practice, 8*, 137–143.

Shepherd, R. B., & Carr, J. H. (1991). An emergent or dynamical systems view of movement dysfunction. *Australian Journal of Physiotherapy, 37*, 4–5.

Sietsema, J. M., Nelson, D. L., Mulder, R. M., Mervau-Scheidel, D., & White, B. E. (1993). The use of a game to promote arm reach in persons with traumatic brain injury. *American Journal of Occupational Therapy, 47*, 19–24.

Smith, R. (1990). *Administration and scoring manual. OT Fact (Occupational Therapy Functional Assessment Compilation Tool)*. Rockville, MD: American Occupational Therapy Association.

Smyth, M. M. (1984). Memory for movements. In M. M. Smyth & A. M. Wing (Eds.), *The psychology of movement* (pp. 83–117). London: Academic Press.

Spaulding, S. (1989). The biomechanics of prehension. *American Journal of Occupational Therapy, 43,* 302–306.

Spencer, J., Krefting, L., & Mattingly, C. (1993). Incorporation of ethnographic methods in occupational therapy assessment. *American Journal of Occupational Therapy, 47,* 303–310.

Stahl, C. (1993). Rehab in the rain or in a rowboat: New environments bring the outdoors indoors. *Advance for Occupational Therapists, 9,* 14–15.

Summers, J. J. (1989). Motor programs. In D. Holding (Ed.), *Human skills* (2nd ed., pp. 49–69). New York: John Wiley & Sons.

Thelen, E. (1989). Self-organization in developmental processes: Can systems approaches work? In M. R. Gunnar & E. Thelen (Eds.), *Systems and development* (pp. 77–117). Hillsdale, NJ: Lawrence Erlbaum.

Thelen, E., & Fisher, D. M. (1983). The organization of spontaneous to instrumental behavior: Kinematic analysis of movement changes during very early learning. *Child Development, 54,* 120–140.

Thelen, E. & Ulrich, B. D. (1991). Hidden skills. *Monographs of the Society for Research in Child Development, 56*(Serial No. 223). Chicago: University of Chicago Press.

Trombly, C. A. (1989). Activity selection and analysis. In C. Trombly (Ed.), *Occupational therapy for physical dysfunction* (3rd ed., pp. 303–310). Baltimore: Williams & Wilkins.

Trombly, C. A. (1992). Deficits of reaching in subjects with left hemiparesis: A pilot study. *American Journal of Occupational Therapy, 46,* 887–897.

Trombly, C. A. (1993a). Observations of improvement of reaching in five subjects with left hemiparesis. *Journal of Neurology, Neurosurgery, & Psychiatry, 56*(1), 40–45.

Trombly, C. (1993b). The issue is—Anticipating the future: Assessment of occupational function. *American Journal of Occupational Therapy, 47,* 253–257.

VanSant, A. (1988). Rising from a supine position to erect stance: Description of adult movement and a developmental hypothesis. *Physical Therapy, 68,* 185–192.

VanSant, A. (1990). Life-span development in functional tasks. *Physical Therapy, 70,* 788–798.

VanSant, A. (1991a). Motor control, motor learning, and motor development. In P. C. Montgomery & B. H. Connolly (Eds.), *Motor control and physical therapy: Theoretical framework and practical applications* (pp. 13–28). Hixson, TN: Chattanooga Group.

VanSant, A. (1991b). Life-span motor development. In M. J. Lister (Ed.), *Contemporary management of motor control problems: Proceedings of the II STEP Conference* (pp. 77–83). Alexandria, VA: Foundation for Physical Therapy.

Voss, D. E., Ionta, M. K., & Myers, B. J. (1985). *Proprioceptive neuromuscular facilitation: Patterns and techniques* (3rd ed.). New York: Harper & Row.

Winstein, C. J. (1991). Knowledge of results and motor learning—Implications for physical therapy. *Physical Therapy, 71,* 140–149.

Remediating Perceptual Impairments

Lee Ann Quintana

Evaluation and treatment of perceptual dysfunction have traditionally been emphasized by occupational therapists working with adults with brain injury (Abreu & Toglia, 1987; Warren, 1993a). Although there is extensive literature on the identification and evaluation of perceptual dysfunction, there is limited information on the effectiveness of treatment. Much of the research on diagnosis and evaluation has been carried out by psychologists and neuropsychologists who have only recently begun to focus on function. Unfortunately, occupational therapists, who see the effects of perceptual dysfunction on a person's daily living skills, have been slow to generate research and, subsequently, support for their treatment.

Remediation of perceptual deficits generally falls under the realm of cognitive rehabilitation, which is provided by occupational therapists, speech and language pathologists, neuropsychologists, and psychologists (Harley et al., 1992). Historically, occupational therapists have emphasized the area of perception, whereas speech and language pathologists and psychologists have emphasized cognition.

This chapter discusses specific treatment for visual foundation skills; body scheme, including right/left

discrimination, body part identification, finger agnosia, and anosognosia; unilateral neglect; spatial relations and position in space, including topographical orientation and figure/ground perception; and apraxia, including limb apraxia, constructional apraxia, and dressing apraxia. Treatment approaches and general treatment principles to consider in the remediation of perceptual and cognitive deficits are discussed in Chapter 27.

REMEDIATION OF SPECIFIC SKILLS

Visual Foundation Skills

Visual foundation skills include acuity, visual fields, and oculomotor function. Following a screening of these skills, patients may then be referred for a rehabilitation optometry evaluation. Gianutsos, Ramsey, and Perlin (1988) found that more than half of patients who were admitted for head injury rehabilitation and who were eligible for cognitive services had visual sensory impairments sufficient enough to warrant further evaluation. The decision to refer included the existence of problems in one or more of the following areas: reduced acuity; visual field loss; oculomotor dysfunction; and impaired binocular function. In addition, characteristics of patients in this study included the ability to transfer to an examining chair, manageable behavior, alertness, and the ability to make a consistent response. Treatments included new glasses to correct refraction errors, different glasses for near and far viewing, prisms, patching or occlusion of one eye, fusion training, and occasionally devices (e.g., hand-held magnifier and enlarged print reading material). Although not formally evaluated, the staff noted changes in function such as increased awareness and mental status.

Farber and Zoltan (1989) suggested that vestibular-based treatment (such as rocking and inversion over a large ball) "would facilitate the organization of visual behavior in individuals who have suffered from head trauma" (p. 14). But they noted that this suggestion

GLOSSARY

Anchoring—Method of providing a visual cue on the side contralateral to brain damage in the presence of unilateral neglect

Cancellation tasks—Tasks that require the patient to draw a line through, or in some way mark, a targeted stimulus on a sheet of paper that has random letters, numbers, or symbols printed on it.

Chaining—Method by which a task is broken down into steps. The patient learns the first step, then the next, and then puts the two together. He then learns the next step and puts them all together, and so on. In backward chaining, the therapist completes the task except for the last step, which the patient does; then the therapist completes all except the last two steps, which the patient does; and so on.

Density—Controlling the amount of stimuli present during a cancellation task. Many letters and numbers close together have a higher density than symbols presented with more space between them. Organized presentation of stimuli (e.g., in rows) is less dense than a random presentation of stimuli.

Fresnel prisms—Prisms (used with a patient with hemianopsia or unilateral neglect) that are applied to a patient's glasses over the affected hemifield, the purpose of which is to shift the peripheral images more toward the central field.

Limb activation—Active motion initiated by the patient.

must be validated through research with head injury patients.

Rossi, Kheyfets, and Reding (1990) found that the use of press-on **Fresnel prisms** improved visual perception in stroke patients with homonymous hemianopsia or unilateral visual neglect. Zihl (1980) found that intensive stimulation of the blind hemifield can decrease the size of the patient's visual field deficit.

Manipulation of the environment may also decrease the effect of the visual deficit (Warren, 1993b). This includes increasing the contrast in the environment and providing increased lighting.

Body Scheme

Body scheme is the awareness of body parts and the position of the body and its parts in relation to themselves and objects in the environment. Related deficits include right/left disorientation, impaired body part identification, finger agnosia, anosognosia, and unilateral neglect.

The goal of treatment of body scheme disorders is to increase the patient's awareness of his body and decrease his disorientation. Treatment starts in a low-stimulation environment. As the patient becomes less disoriented, treatment can be expanded to the clinic. Marmo (1974) suggested a sensory integrative approach to treatment of body scheme disorders that included controlled sensory stimulation and developmental motor patterns administered under conditions of decreased stress to help the patient in reorganizing his body scheme. She recommended beginning with tactile rubdowns, progressing to rolling over, following up with prone-on-elbows posture. There is no documentation of the effectiveness of this treatment approach.

RIGHT/LEFT DISCRIMINATION

Right/left (R/L) discrimination denotes the ability to understand the concepts of right and left. Boone and Landes (1968) observed that they were unable to retrain aphasics in R/L discrimination (no information is given as to what the training included). If the patient is unable to regain automatic knowledge of the difference between right and left, he may have to learn to compensate cognitively (e.g., use the ring on his left hand as a cue for the left side).

Treatment can include activities that stress right and left (e.g., using the words *right* and *left* in directions) or the use of increased cutaneous or proprioceptive input to one extremity (Zoltan, Siev, & Freishtat, 1986). For example, the therapist may have the patient wear a weight cuff on one arm during treatment to provide increased proprioceptive input while calling his attention to that side. It is important to apply the input to the same side consistently. If *right* and *left* only confuse the patient, it would be useful to avoid using these words during treatment (Boone & Landers, 1968; Zoltan et al., 1986).

BODY PART IDENTIFICATION

Body part identification is the ability to identify body parts on self and others. Anderson and Choy (1970) reported a program to increase awareness of body image, space perception, and unilateral neglect. To increase body awareness, they suggested the following activities: the patient verbally identifies parts of the body as they are touched; the therapist names a part followed by the patient rubbing the area; the patient mimics the therapist, who moves her head and limbs in different positions.

FINGER AGNOSIA

Finger agnosia denotes an inability to identify one's own fingers and difficulty naming fingers or being able to indicate which finger has been touched. Fox (1964) found that using pressure and cutaneous stimulation improved finger agnosia in hemiplegic patients.

This treatment consists of rubbing vigorously using a corduroy-covered, padded wood stimulator that is applied to one or more of the following areas: dorsal surface of forearm, hand, and fingers and the ventral surface of fingers. In addition, grasping a rough-surfaced cardboard cone is used to provide pressure to the volar surface of the hand. This stimulation should feel comfortable to the patient to avoid a protective response; therefore, the area of stimulation depends on the patient's response. Rubbing and pressure should be done for a minimum of 2 min each, although they can be alternated (30 sec of rubbing and 30 sec of pressure) (Zoltan et al., 1986).

ANOSOGNOSIA

Anosognosia, which refers to an unawareness of hemiplegia, can range from an unawareness of hemiparesis, to lack of concern, to total denial. Calvanio, Levine, and Petrone (1993) found that patients with persistent anosognosia also presented with severe hemisensory loss, severe left spatial neglect and "at least moderate impairments of intellect and memory" (p. 46). These cognitive deficits, the sensory loss, and the neglect all hinder the patient's insight and his ability to participate in treatment. If the patient denies he has a problem, little can be done to teach him to compensate. As the patient begins to recover and denial lessens, efforts must be made to make the patient aware of his deficit (see Chapter 10 for a discussion of denial).

Unilateral Neglect

Unilateral neglect is referred to by a variety of names, including hemiinattention, hemispatial neglect, and unilateral spatial agnosia. It is manifested by a failure to respond or orient to stimuli presented contralateral to a brain lesion (Heilman, Watson, & Valenstein, 1985). It is observed functionally in the patient who eats the food on only half of his plate, shaves only one side of his face, and walks into objects on the side contralateral to the brain lesion.

The treatment of unilateral neglect can be approached in several ways (Table 26.1). Documentation

Table 26.1. Treatment Approaches for Unilateral Neglect

Scanning training (King, 1993; Robertson et al., 1990; Ross, 1992; Wagenaar et al., 1992; Weinberg et al., 1977)	Tasks presented at tabletop (e.g., paper-and-pencil tasks and computer activities) or in extrapersonal space (e.g., scanning grocery shelf items and chalkboards); tabletop resulted in improvement in academic skills and reading but did not carry over to functional tasks
Table 26.1. Continued	
Increase awareness of neglected side through tactile stimulation	Stroking, brushing, and icing of involved extremity; may be carried out by therapist and/or patient (Anderson & Choy, 1970); the above followed by gross visual perceptual activities requiring orientation toward neglected side (Fox, 1983)
Activation of the right hemisphere (Heilman & Watson, 1978)	Use of perceptual tasks instead of verbal tasks (e.g., use of shapes instead of letters) Monocular patching of eye ipsilateral to brain damage (Butter & Kirsch, 1992) Lateral visual stimulation (Butter & Kirsch, 1992)
Spatiomotor cuing (Halligan, Manning, & Marshall, 1991; Robertson & North, 1992; Robertson, 1991; Robertson et al., 1992)	Use of involved extremity as a motor cue to increase awareness (e.g., movement of left hand while ambulating to decrease neglect and pointing to answers with the left hand rather than the right)
Cognitive compensation	Megacognitive training (Toglia, 1991) Use of videofeedback (Söderback et al., 1992) Teaching patient to cue cognitively the start of a movement or attention to left hemispace (Van Deusen, 1988)
Environmental compensation	Fresnel prisms (Rossi, Kheyfets, & Reding, 1990) Arrangement of living space so that important items are on uninvolved side (to allow patient to benefit from intact visual field) or involved side (to force patient to scan involved field); but bed orientation is not related to rehabilitation outcome (Loverro & Reding, 1988)
Comprehensive programs	Scanning training, somatosensory awareness and size estimation training, and complex visual perceptual training (Gordon et al., 1985) Multicontext approach (Toglia, 1991)

of the effectiveness of these approaches is scarce, and the influence of treatment on a person's functional ability is even more scarce. Visual scanning training is the most common treatment discussed in the literature

(Cooke, 1992). This training includes paper-and-pencil tasks (Carter, Howard, & O'Neil, 1983; Gordon et al., 1985), the use of computer programs (Robertson et al., 1990; Ross, 1992), and tracking a series of lights across a panel (Weinberg et al., 1977). Although the research often provides support for improvement on visual perceptual tests, reading, and academic skills, this type of training does not generalize to gross motor tasks (Wagenaar et al., 1992).

When practicing scanning using **cancellation tasks,** a structured array (symbols arranged in neat, straight rows across the page) should initially be used, because patients with right brain damage (RBD) have difficulty with organized search (Weintraub & Mesulam, 1988). This array could be made increasingly more complex (e.g., requesting two target letters, decreasing the spacing between letters, or decreasing the size of the letters) as the patient progresses (Cooke, 1992). Scanning tasks must be practiced in a variety of settings, because patients can improve on a task without an improvement in neglect. An excellent therapeutic intervention is the use of Toglia's (1991) multicontext treatment approach. An example of levels of transfer for a letter **cancellation task,** consisting of crossing out a specific letter on a page of four rows of random letters, can be seen in Table 26.2.

A recent study evaluated the effect of computer visual scanning training on a functional scanning task (Ross, 1992). It was found that although the subjects' scanning times and accuracy improved, the results did not generalize to the functional grocery-shelf scanning task. It was noted that the inherent limitations of the computer (e.g., two-dimensional, small size of the screen, and decreased visual motor demands on the patient) may hinder generalizability.

In an attempt to compensate for some of these limitations, King (1993) projected a computer visual scanning program onto a large screen (5 feet wide). Although there was significant improvement of scanning from the beginning to the end of treatment, correlation to a functional task was not attempted in this study. It would be interesting to evaluate the effects of this training on the grocery-shelf scanning task (Ross, 1992), because this task more closely resembles the training provided by King.

The literature indicates that the effects of scanning training are specific to the situation. If the goal is to improve the patient's ability to read or scan at tabletop, then tabletop scanning training is appropriate; but if the therapist wants to improve a patient's ability to scan in the community, then practice in the community is needed. Warren (1993b) provided guidelines for selection of treatment activities for patients with deficits in visual attention and visual scanning (Table 26.3).

Another approach to the treatment of unilateral neglect, is to increase activation of the right hemisphere and thereby decrease neglect. Heilman and Watson (1978) found that perceptual stimuli lessen neglect by activating the right hemisphere, whereas verbal stimulation can increase left neglect by increasing arousal asymmetries. Cermak et al. (1991) designed a study to determine if activities that stimulate the right hemisphere decrease neglect and if activities that stimulate the left hemisphere increase neglect. Their results failed to support this hypothesis. Cermak et al. (1991) indicated that facilitation of the targeted hemisphere may not have occurred and in fact "selective activation

Table 26.2. Levels of Transfer for a Letter Cancellation Task

Transfer Distance	Task
Near	Patient is instructed to cross out the number 5 (number cancellation task)
Intermediate	Four horizontal rows of various coins are presented. Patient is instructed to place a marker over all the nickels (tabletop task)
Far	Patient is presented with a spice rack and is asked to pick out all of the jars that need to be refilled (standing and reaching at kitchen cabinets)
Very far	Patient is evaluated on the ability to initiate spontaneously left-to-right scanning in the context of simple, everyday life tasks (reading four lines in a large-print magazine or locating an item in the medicine cabinet or on a shelf)

Table 26.3 Training Guidelines for Visual Attention and Visual Scanning

Train patients to reorganize their scanning strategy	Use of anchoring techniques and scanning devices (Weinberg et al., 1979)
Broaden visual field that patient must scan	Use of activities that require the patient to turn his head or change body positions to complete the task (e.g., scanning items on a kitchen shelf)
Reinforce visual experience with sensorimotor experiences	Use of activities in which the patient is required to manipulate what is seen (e.g., reach for or touch items scanned)
Emphasize conscious attention to detail and careful inspection of objects	Use of matching tasks in which the patient may be encouraged to slow down and double-check his interpretation of what is seen
Practice the skill in context to ensure carryover	Treatment may begin in the clinic, but strategies must be practiced in a variety of real-life situations

of a specific hemisphere may be too complex to manipulate in a clinical setting" (p. 285).

Butter and Kirsch (1992) found that patching the right eye of patients with left neglect decreased the patients' left neglect score. When lateralized visual stimulation was added, the relative benefits were larger. It should be noted that the beneficial effects were present only when the eye patch was on and that the study did not include generalization to functional tasks.

If there are two types of neglect—as has been suggested (Bisiach et al., 1990; Coslett et al., 1990; Tegner & Levander, 1991)—then it is reasonable to expect that each has its own form of treatment. For a patient with primarily a motor or output neglect, encouragement of left hand activation may reduce neglect to a greater extent than visual perceptual cuing. An example might be having the patient move the left hand (whatever movement he is able to do) while performing a scanning task instead of using a visual **anchoring** technique (supplying a visual cue on the impaired side to indicate starting position). Robertson and North (1992) found that left motor activation in left hemispace reduced neglect to a greater extent than did left motor activation in right hemispace, right motor activation in left hemispace, or visual cuing. Robertson (1992) further reported that (1) left lower extremity activation reduced neglect, (2) passive movement of the left extremity had no effect on neglect, (3) bilateral movements produced no effect, and (4) there was no effect if the movement became automatic.

If the patient has more of a perceptual or input neglect, he may benefit from visual cuing such as **anchoring** (Table 26.4) or reminders to look to the left. Training the patient to use the left upper extremity as an anchor during functional activities provides both a perceptual anchor and a means of left **limb activation** (Robertson et al., 1992).

Adaptation of the environment includes such things as arranging the patient's bed so that his uninvolved side is toward the activity in the room and always interacting with the patient on his uninvolved side (Heilman et al., 1985). While this might be a good idea initially, to evaluate the patient and to keep him from harming himself, it does nothing to help the patient overcome his deficit. It is recommended that both the remedial and adaptive approaches be used.

Weinberg et al. (1977) developed a training program for left neglect that included reading, writing, and calculation activities. They used the principles of **anchoring,** pacing (controlling speed), **density** of stimuli (facilitating response by increasing the distance between stimuli), and offering immediate feedback; they found that following training RBD patients improved on tests of academic skill. This program was later expanded to include training to increase sensory

Table 26.4 Anchoring Technique

Sequence of Cuing	Task Demand
1. A vertical anchoring line is used on the left side; the beginning and ending of the line are sequentially numbered	Patient uses the vertical line to find the beginning and the numbers to avoid skipping lines.
Example: 1 2 3 4 ⎢ The law was passed to allow the 1 state to conduct a national FBI 2 criminal records check before 3 certifying teachers. 4	
2. A vertical anchoring line is used on the left side; only the beginning of the line is sequentially numbered	Patient uses the vertical line and numbers on the left; the number cue on the right has been eliminated
Example: 1 2 3 4 ⎢ Family members, followed by co-workers, are the most frequent targets of anger.	
3. A vertical anchoring line is used on the left side	Patient uses only the vertical line to find left side
Example: ⎢ Environmental groups hope to minimize the divisiveness and avoid mistakes made in the Pacific Northwest.	
4. No cues are provided	Patient must read without any cues
Example: The state distributes its lottery proceeds without regard to which communities generate the revenue.	

awareness and spatial organization (Weinberg et al., 1977). The new tasks included practice in identification of locus of touch on the back and estimation of gross size of objects. It was found that combining the two phases of training resulted in even more improvement in reading and math skills than using the initial phase alone. Weinberg et al. (1979) further suggested that these training principles (**anchoring,** pacing, etc.) could be applied to activities of daily living (ADL) tasks. A description of their training program is available (Diller et al., 1980).

A third phase, which was aimed at improving complex visual perception, was added to the training program (Weinberg et al., 1982). These three training modules (scanning, somatosensory awareness and size estimation, and complex visual perception) were combined into one program. Improvements in basic scanning functions and complex visual perceptual skills were found following all three phases, but generalization of skills was not as extensive as that found following just the initial two phases (Gordon et al., 1985). To increase generalization, it was suggested that therapists provide a wider range of stimuli to which patients must use their newly learned compensatory strategies (i.e., always use an anchor on the left when dressing, eating, walking down the hall, etc.).

Spatial Relations and Position in Space

A patient with a deficit in position in space has difficulty with concepts such as over, front, back, and below, whereas a patient with a deficit in spatial relations has difficulty perceiving himself in relation to other objects. Zoltan et al. (1986) suggested various tabletop activities in which the patient is given the opportunity to practice discriminating different orientations in space by copying designs set up by the therapist or from pictures using blocks, pegs, puzzles, or matchsticks. A functional activity such as organizing a closet requires use of the concepts of position in space. This type of activity can be graded from simple to complex. To improve spatial relations, the patient can be asked to navigate through a maze or to follow a path through an obstacle course. If the patient has poor body scheme, he may experience difficulty perceiving himself in relation to other objects. If this is the case, treatment to increase the patient's awareness of his body, such as a sensory integrative approach may be indicated.

TOPOGRAPHICAL ORIENTATION

The patient with a deficit in topographical orientation exhibits difficulty finding his way from one place to another. Zoltan et al. (1986) suggested several methods of treatment, including rote practice and memorization of routes. As a means of compensation, markers can be used to identify a route, and the markers can gradually be removed (Charness, 1986). If the difficulty in topographical orientation is left neglect, spatial relations, and so on, then treatment should be aimed at the more basic visual perceptual skills.

Borst and Peterson (1993) described a program that included both adaptive (practice using a map to find one's way around) and remedial (practice with mazes and parquetry for spatial relations and orientation) approaches to the treatment of topographical orientation deficit. At the end of 4 weeks of treatment, their patient was able to follow three-step directional instructions 75% of the time and was able to find her way around the clinic independently 75% of the time, if she looked at her map first. Generalization to other areas is not known, but recommendations were given to the family regarding use of mazes and map activities.

For patients with intact language skills, the development and use of verbal maps may assist them in getting around. Jarvis and Hamlin (1991) described

nine steps in the development of a verbal map (Table 26.5). The patient is taught how to use maps to different locations, and then he and family members are taught how to create new maps so that this idea can be carried over to new and different situations. Jarvis and Hamlin (1991) noted that if there is a language deficit, use of tactile cues (e.g., a model of the environment) may be needed.

FIGURE/GROUND PERCEPTION

Figure/ground perception is the ability to distinguish the foreground or figure from the background. A deficit in this area can be seen functionally in the patient who is unable to find a white shirt on the bed, the brakes on his wheelchair, or eyeglasses in a cluttered drawer.

Treatment can include remedial activities such as word-search games and scanning activities. Word-search games (finding words embedded in a group of letters) are commonly found in crossword puzzle books.

Table 26.5   Steps in the Development of a Verbal Map

1. Choose a common route that is troublesome for the patient, e.g., from the patient's bedroom to the dining room or occupational therapy area
2. Walk through the route with the patient, identifying the starting point, all choice points such as turns, and the end point or destination
3. At the starting point, all choice points, and the destination, ask the patient to stop, look around, and identify a visible "marker" that he can label (e.g., a phone booth or a fire extinguisher on the wall) and the instructions to be executed at that point (e.g., turn right)
4. Each time the patient is to turn, have him pat the appropriate thigh while verbalizing the instructions; model for him "Turn right," while patting your right thigh
5. Print the "verbal map" as a series of instructions that will direct the patient from one visual marker to the next until the destination is reached; "When you see x, do y," e.g., (a) go to the door of your room and find the phone booth; (b) walk to the phone booth; (c) when you get there, pat your left thigh and turn left; (d) walk to the Exit sign; and so on
6. Walk through the route behind the patient, listening to make sure that the "verbal map" is complete and accurate and that the patient vocalizes the instructions and gives the appropriate motor cues (thigh pats) at each turn correctly
7. Have the patient travel the route regularly, using the "verbal map" as a guide, and evaluate his ability to do this accurately
8. Once the patient is able to do this accurately and efficiently, begin to wean him from the use of the printed "verbal map" and to rely on the memory of it to increase independence of functioning
9. Teach the patient how to reverse the map to get back to the original starting point; some patients may be able to learn this fairly easily, but for others it may be necessary to repeat the first eight steps in the reverse direction—this is important to give a sense of "spatial security"

Scanning activities, such as having the patient find certain objects within pictures taken from magazines or from a random scattering of objects, can be used and graded from easy to difficult as the patient improves. Treatment can include development of compensation techniques, such as keeping the environment as simple and uncluttered as possible, and marking significant objects (e.g., wheelchair brakes) with a bright color (Zoltan et al., 1986).

Functional difficulties (e.g., finding a white wash-cloth on a white sheet) may also be the result of decreased visual acuity and contrast sensitivity. If this is the case, proper referral and environmental modifications to improve acuity are important.

Apraxia

Apraxia is the inability to carry out purposeful movement in the presence of intact sensation, movement, and coordination (Poeck, 1985). Three types of apraxia are addressed here: limb, constructional, and dressing.

LIMB APRAXIA

There are two types of limb apraxia: ideomotor and ideational (see Table 9.4). Although there are volumes of literature on apraxia, little is written on treatment. Treatment recommendations are usually based on neurobiological principles but have not been tested in controlled research to determine outcome (Farber, 1993).

Poeck (1985) stated that there is a strong tendency for spontaneous recovery in apraxia and that treatment is usually not necessary with ideomotor apraxia, because the patient is able to use the limbs spontaneously. The question the therapist needs to ask is, "Does the patient's clumsiness and/or difficulty with gestures interfere with his daily living skills?" If so, then this area should be addressed. In the case of the patient with an ideational apraxia who has difficulty with the use of objects, the need for treatment is more obvious.

Some treatment activities suggested include gross motor activities, involving interpretation and use of tactile, kinesthetic, and proprioceptive stimulation to influence motor patterns; manual contact or guiding of the apraxic extremity through the task; and **chaining** techniques (Farber, 1993). The therapist should keep verbal commands to a minimum and ask the patient to perform activities in the environment in which they would normally be done. Furthermore, the patient can be asked to visualize the movement before attempting to carry it out (Zoltan et al., 1986). The therapist may need to break down the activity into component parts and teach each part separately; then, as each is learned, the parts are integrated into more complex activities.

CONSTRUCTIONAL APRAXIA

Patients with constructional apraxia have difficulty with copying, drawing, and constructing designs in two- and three-dimensions. It has been found that some left brain damaged (LBD) patients benefited from the use of landmarks on a drawing task (Hecaen & Assal, 1970). Performance of LBD patients on a drawing task should be assessed to determine the effect of the use of landmarks on simple designs. If performance improves, the number of landmarks is gradually reduced and treatment progresses to more complicated designs (Zoltan et al., 1986). Both RBD and LBD patients benefited from visual cues on a block design task (Hadano, 1984). Training (Warrington, James, & Kinsbourne, 1966) and provision of a model (Piercy, Hecaen, & Ajuriaguerra, 1960) have also been found to benefit the performance of LBD patients, but not necessarily that of RBD patients.

Treatment for patients having difficulty with block design tasks includes having the patient copy simple block designs, beginning with three blocks and gradually increasing the number of blocks and the complexity of the design. The task can begin with plain wood cubes, proceed to colored cubes (which adds the second dimension of color), and finally to blocks of various sizes and shapes. The patient can be required to transfer a two-dimensional design to three dimensions, as when using blocks to copy a design from a photograph or pattern on paper. Stick designs and peg-board designs can be used in a similar fashion.

Neistadt (1989) developed performance criteria for college educated young adults on a parquetry block assembly task. She suggested that the treatment sequence using parquetry block designs (from least to most difficult) proceed as follows: colored card with full detail, black-and-white card with full detail, colored card with partial detail, and black-and-white card with partial detail.

Neistadt (1992) compared the effects of adaptive training (preparing snacks and beverages) and remedial training (using parquetry blocks) on head-injured patients' performance. She found that those patients who received training with parquetry blocks improved most on the parquetry block test and least on the food preparation task, whereas those who received the functional training, improved more on the food preparation task. The results suggested that learning in adult head-injured males, at least 6 months after injury, is task specific; this supports the use of the functional approach.

DRESSING APRAXIA

Dressing apraxia refers to an inability to dress oneself, and little is written specifically regarding treatment. Treatment generally consists of teaching the patient a pattern of dressing. Cognitive cues—such as using the label to tell front from back or talking himself through the steps of putting on each item of clothing—are used, and the patient eventually learns through practice (Zoltan et al., 1986). Cook, Luschen, and Sikes (1991) described the use of an audiotape and a specific method of stacking (sequencing) clothing to improve dressing in an elderly woman with cognitive and perceptual impairments. If the basis for the dressing apraxia is found to be constructional apraxia, unilateral neglect, or body scheme disturbances, treatment is aimed at ameliorating those deficits.

SUMMARY

This chapter presented treatment strategies for rehabilitation of deficits in visual foundation skills, body scheme (including right/left discrimination, body part identification, finger agnosia, and anosognosia), unilateral neglect, spatial relations and position in space (including topographical orientation and figure/ground discrimination), and apraxia (including limb apraxia, constructional apraxia, and dressing apraxia). The majority of today's research is in the areas of unilateral neglect and apraxia, with emphasis on evaluation rather than treatment. The results of much of the research presented seem to indicate that there is little generalization from one treatment task to another or from more remedial tasks to function. An approach such as that developed by Toglia (1991) seeks to promote generalization of remedial treatment to functional tasks. To provide meaningful treatment of perceptual deficits, occupational therapists must generate relevant research and continue to expand the base of effective treatments that these patients need and deserve.

STUDY QUESTIONS

1. Under what conditions would you refer a patient to a rehabilitation optometrist?
2. What is the goal of treatment for body scheme disorders?
3. List five treatment ideas for body scheme, including both remedial and adaptive.
4. List five guidelines for visual scanning training.
5. List five approaches to treatment of unilateral neglect and an example of an activity for each approach.
6. What is a verbal map and how is it used in the treatment of a patient with a deficit in topographical orientation?
7. List five treatment activities for limb apraxia.
8. What would be the treatment sequence using the following parquetry block design cards: colored

card with full detail, colored card with partial detail, black-and-white card with full detail, black-and-white card with partial detail?
9. Deficits in what areas could be the basis for dressing apraxia?
10. Why is it important for occupational therapists to become involved in research?

REFERENCES

Abreu, B. C., & Toglia, J. P. (1987). Cognitive rehabilitation: A model for occupational therapy. *American Journal of Occupational Therapy, 41*, 439–448.

Anderson, E. K., & Choy, E. (1970). Parietal lobe syndromes in hemiplegia. *American Journal of Occupational Therapy, 24*, 13–18.

Bisiach, E., Geminiani, G., Berti, A., & Rusconi, M. L. (1990). Perceptual and premotor factors of unilateral neglect. *Neurology, 40*, 1278–1281.

Boone, D. R., & Landes, B. A. (1968). Left-right discrimination in hemiplegic patients. *Archives of Physical Medicine & Rehabilitation, 49*, 533–537.

Borst, M. J., & Peterson, C. Q. (1993). Overcoming topographical orientation deficits in an elderly woman with a right cerebrovascular accident. *American Journal of Occupational Therapy, 47*, 551–554.

Butter, C. M., & Kirsch, N. (1992). Combined and separate effects of eye patching and visual stimulation on unilateral neglect following stroke. *Archives of Physical Medicine & Rehabilitation, 73*, 1133–1139.

Calvanio, R., Levine, D., & Petrone, P. (1993). Elements of cognitive rehabilitation after right hemisphere stroke. *Behavioral Neurology, 11*, 25–57.

Carter, L. T., Howard, B. E., & O'Neil, W. A. (1983). Effectiveness of cognitive skill remediation in acute stroke patients. *American Journal of Occupational Therapy, 37*, 320–326.

Cermak, S. A., Trombly, C. A., Hausser, J., & Tiernan, A. M. (1991). Effects of lateralized tasks on unilateral neglect after right cerebrovascular accident. *Occupational Therapy Journal of Research, 11*, 271–291.

Charness, A. (1986). *Stroke/head injury: A guide to functional outcomes in physical therapy management.* Rockville, MD: Aspen Systems.

Cook, E. A., Luschen, L., & Sikes, S. (1991). Dressing training for an elderly woman with cognitive and perceptual impairments. *American Journal of Occupational Therapy, 45*, 652–654.

Cooke, D. (1992). Remediation of unilateral neglect: What do we know? *Australian Occupational Therapy Journal, 39*, 19–25.

Coslett, H. B., Bowers, D., Fitzpatrick, E., Haws, B., & Heilman, K. M. (1990). Directional hypokinesia and hemispatial inattention in neglect. *Brain, 113*, 475–486.

Diller, L., Weinberg, J., Piasetsky, E., Ruckdeschel-Hibbard, M., Egelko, S., Scotzin, M., Couniotakis, J., & Gordon, W. (1980). *Methods for the evaluation and treatment of the visual perceptual difficulties of right brain damaged individuals* (Monograph No. 67). New York: New York University Medical Center.

Farber, S. (1993, March). *OT intervention for individuals with limb apraxia,* paper presented at the AOTA Neuroscience Institute, Baltimore, MD.

Farber, S. D., & Zoltan, B. (1989). Visual-vestibular systems interaction: Therapeutic implications. *Journal of Head Trauma Rehabilitation, 4*(2), 9–16.

Fox, J. (1964). Cutaneous stimulation—Effects on selected tests of perception. *American Journal of Occupational Therapy, 18,* 53–55.

Fox, J. (1983). Unilateral neglect: Evaluation & treatment. *Physical and Occupational Therapy in Geriatrics, 2*(4), 5–15.

Gianutsos, R., Ramsey, G., & Perlin, R. R. (1988). Rehabilitative optometric services for survivors of acquired brain injury. *Archives of Physical Medicine & Rehabilitation, 69,* 573–578.

Gordon, W. A., Hibbard, M. R., Egelko, S., Diller, L., Shaver, M. S., Lieberman, A., & Ragnarsson, K. (1985). Perceptual remediation in patients with right brain damage: A comprehensive program. *Archives of Physical Medicine & Rehabilitation, 66,* 353–359.

Hadano, K. (1984). On block design constructional disability in right and left hemisphere brain-damaged patients. *Cortex, 20,* 391–401.

Halligan, P. W., Manning, L., & Marshall, J. C. (1991). Hemispheric actuation vs spatio-motor cueing in visual neglect: A case study. *Neuropsychologica, 29,* 169–176.

Harley, J. P., Allen, C., Braciszeski, T. L., Cicerone, D. K., Dahlberg, C., Evans, S., Foto, M., Gordon, W. A., Harrington, D., Levin, W., Malec, J. F., Millis, S., Morris, J., Muir, C., Richert, J., Salazar, E., Schiavone, D. A., & Smigielski, J. S. (1992). Guidelines for cognitive rehabilitation. *Neurological Rehabilitation, 2*(3), 62–67.

Hecaen, H., & Assal, G. (1970). A comparison of constructive deficits following right and left hemispheric lesions. *Neuropsychologia, 8,* 289–303.

Heilman, K. M., & Watson, R. T. (1978). Changes in the symptoms of neglect induced by changing task strategy. *Archives of Neurology, 35,* 47–49.

Heilman, K. M., Watson, R. T., & Valenstein, E. (1985). Neglect and related disorders. In K. M. Heilman, & E. Valenstein (Eds.), *Clinical Neuropsychology* (pp. 243–293). New York: Oxford University Press.

Jarvis, P. E., & Hamlin, D. H. (1991). The use of verbal maps to help people with right cerebral hemisphere lesions compensate for perceptual spatial deficits. *Journal of Rehabilitation, 57*(3), 51–53.

King, T. (1993). Treatment of visual inattention using computerized overhead projection. *Journal of Cognitive Rehabilitation, 11*(2), 32–35.

Loverro, J., & Reding, M. (1988). Bed orientation & rehabilitation outcome for patients with stroke hemianopsia or visual neglect. *Journal of Neurologic Rehabilitation, 2,* 147–150.

Marmo, N. A. (1974). A new look at the brain-damaged adult. American *Journal of Occupational Therapy, 28,* 199–206.

Neistadt, M. E. (1989). Normal adult performance on constructional praxis training tasks. *American Journal of Occupational Therapy, 43,* 448–455.

Neistadt, M. E. (1992). Occupational therapy treatments for constructional deficits. *American Journal of Occupational Therapy, 46,* 141–148.

Piercy, M., Hecaen, H., & Ajuriaguerra, J. (1960). Constructional apraxia associated with unilateral cerebral lesions—Left and right sided cases compared. *Brain, 83,* 225–242.

Poeck, K. (1985). Clues to the nature of disruptions to limb praxis. In E. A. Roy (Ed.), *Neuropsychological studies of apraxia and related disorders* (pp. 99–109). Amsterdam: Elsevier Science.

Robertson, I. (1991). Use of left vs right hand in responding to lateralized stimuli in unilateral neglect. *Neurophsychologia, 29,* 1129–1135.

Robertson, I. (1992, October). *Treatment of neglect.* Paper presented at the conference for Evaluation and Treatment of Disorders of Memory, Attention and Visual Neglect, Philadelphia, PA.

Robertson, I. H., Gray, J. M., Pentlan, B., & Waite, L. J. (1990). Microcomputer based rehabilitation for unilateral left visual ne-

glect: A randomized controlled trial. *Archives of Physical Medicine & Rehabilitation, 71,* 663–668.

Robertson, I. H., & North, N. (1992). Spatio-motor cueing in unilateral left neglect: The role of hemispace, hand and motor activation. *Neuropsychologia, 30,* 553–563.

Robertson, I. H., North, N. T., & Geggie, C. (1992). Spatiomotor cueing in unilateral left neglect: Three case studies of its therapeutic effects. *Journal of Neurology, Neurosurgery, and Psychiatry, 55,* 799–805.

Ross, F. L. (1992). The use of computers in occupational therapy for visual scanning training. *American Journal of Occupational Therapy, 46,* 314–322.

Rossi, P. W., Kheyfets, S., & Reding, M. J. (1990). Fresnel prisms improve visual perception in stroke patients with homonymous hemianopsia or unilateral visual neglect. *Neurology, 40,* 1597–1599.

Söderback, I., Begtsson, I., Ginsburg, E., & Eleholm, J. (1992). Videofeedback in occupational therapy: Its effect in patients with neglect syndrom. *Archives of Physical Medicine & Rehabilitation, 73,* 1140–1146.

Tegner, R., & Levander, M. (1991). Through a looking glass. A new technique to demonstrate directional hypokinesia in unilateral neglect. *Brain, 114,* 1943–1951.

Toglia, J. P. (1991). Generalization of treatment: A multicontext approach to cognitive perceptual impairment in adults with brain injury. *American Journal of Occupational Therapy, 45,* 505–516.

Van Deusen, J. (1988). Unilateral neglect: Suggestions for research by occupational therapists. *American Journal of Occupational Therapy, 42,* 441–448.

Wagenaar, R. C., Van Wierignen, P. C. W., Netelenbos, J. B., Meijer, O. G., & Kuik, D. J. (1992). The transfer of scanning training effects in visual inattention after stroke: Five single-case studies. *Disability and Rehabilitation, 14,* 51–60.

Warren, M. (1993a). A hierarchical model for evaluation and treatment of visual perceptual dysfunction in adult acquired brain injury, Part 1. *American Journal of Occupational Therapy, 47,* 42–54.

Warren, M. (1993b). A hierarchical model for evaluation and treatment of visual perceptual dysfunction in adult acquired brain injury, Part 2. *American Journal of Occupational Therapy, 47,* 55–66.

Warrington, E. K., James, M., & Kinsbourne, M. (1966). Drawing disability in relation to laterality of cerebral lesion. *Brain, 89,* 53–82.

Weinberg, J., Diller, L., Gordon, W. A., Gerstman, L. J., Liberman, A., Lakin, P., Hodges, G., & Ezrachi, O. (1977). Visual scanning training effect on reading-related tasks in acquired right brain damage. *Archives of Physical Medicine & Rehabilitation, 58,* 479–486.

Weinberg, J., Diller, L., Gordon, W. A., Gerstman, L. J., Liberman, A., Lakin, P., Hodges, G., & Ezrachi, O. (1979). Training sensory awareness and spatial organization in people with right brain damage. *Archives of Physical Medicine & Rehabilitation, 60,* 491–496.

Weinberg, J., Pcasetsky, E., Diller, L., & Gordon, W. (1982). Treating perceptual organization deficits in nonneglecting RBD stroke patients. *Journal of Clinical Psychology, 4,* 59–75.

Weintaub, S., & Mesulam, M. M. (1988). Visual hemispatial inattention: Stimulus parameters and exploratory strategies. *Journal of Neurology, Neurosurgery and Psychiatry, 51,* 1481–1488.

Zihl, J. (1980). "Blindsight": Improvement of visually guided eye movements by systematic practice in patients with cerebral blindness. *Neuropsychologia, 18,* 71–77.

Zoltan, B., Siev, E., & Freishtat, B. (1986). *The adult stroke patient: A manual for evaluation and treatment of perceptual and cognitive dysfunction.* Thorofare, NJ: Slack.

Remediating Cognitive Impairments

Lee Ann Quintana

OBJECTIVES

After studying this chapter the reader will be able to:
1. Define **cognitive rehabilitation.**
2. Define and discuss two treatment approaches for cognitive impairment.
3. Describe how to choose and modify a treatment task for cognitive impairment.
4. Identify and describe specific treatment for deficits in attention, orientation, memory, and problem solving.
5. Recognize the need for generalization of treatment.

Cognitive rehabilitation (CR) has been defined by the American Academy of Rehabilitation Medicine as "a systematic functionally oriented service of therapeutic cognitive activities based on an assessment and understanding of the person's brain-behavior deficits" (Harley et al., 1992, p. 63). The American Occupational Therapy Association further states that the occupational therapist specifically identifies how cognitive impairment affects the performance of daily living tasks (Poole et al., 1991). The overall goal of occupational therapy is to improve daily living skills. Current literature of other professions includes terms such as functional adaptation (Berrol, 1990), functional dimension (Beh-Yishay & Diller, 1993), real-life tasks (Webb, 1991), ecologically relevant (Lynch, 1992b; Ruff et al., 1989), and functional behavior (Ben-Yishay, Piasetsky, & Rattock, 1987). Generalization of treatment to daily activities has become the focus and goal of CR. Improving test scores is not sufficient, treatment must be generalized to promote improvement in daily life.

CR generally includes the areas of memory, atten-tion, problem solving, and perceptual abilities. It is provided by occupational therapists, speech and language pathologists, neuropsychologists, and psychologists (Harley et al., 1992). CR is not the same as cognitive remediation. CR is a broader term that includes cognitive remediation. Cognitive remediation is a "systematic endeavor aimed at improvement of cognitive functions" (Ben-Yishay & Diller, 1993, p. 206). Cognitive remediation is focused on a specific deficit; CR includes a broader approach to treatment. This chapter examines different treatment approaches, general treatment principles, and specific treatment strategies for remediation of attention, orientation, memory, and problem solving.

TREATMENT APPROACHES

Treatment approaches can generally be put into one of two categories: remedial or adaptive (Table 27.1). **Remedial treatment approaches** attempt to affect specific cognitive functions (e.g., memory). This approach assumes treatment will promote recovery of function of the central nervous system. Remedial approaches have had limited direct impact on functional activity (Ben-Yishay & Diller, 1993). The research literature indicates that while patients show changes in specific cognitive functions they may fail to show improvement in daily living skills (Carter, Howard, & O'Neil, 1983; Gordon et al., 1985; Riddoch & Humphreys, 1983). With the increased interest in functional activities, several studies have reported improvement in daily living skills, but the authors did not provide specific measurements (Benedict & Wechsler, 1992; Ben-Yishay et al., 1987; Ruff et al., 1989). There is a need for research that specifically measures the effects of CR on daily living skills in a standardized manner.

Table 27.1   Treatment Approaches

Adaptive	Remedial
Compensatory, substitutive, functional	Retraining, direct, restorative
Attempts to bypass deficit, emphasis on task rather than underlying skill	Focuses on impaired area
Direct retraining of activities of daily living, use of strategies	Use of tabletop and sensorimotor activities
Environmental adaptation, domain-specific training, compensatory strategies	Sensory integration, neurodevelopmental training, multicontext treatment approach
Less requirement for generalization	Assumes that generalization will occur automatically (but this has not been found to be the case)

The use of computer-assisted cognitive remediation (CACR) has increased. Some see CACR as "inexpensive substitute therapists or as cognitive prostheses" (Ben-Yishay & Diller 1993, p. 204), but research on its effectiveness is lacking. CACR has been criticized for the lack of information regarding generalization and its inflexibility (Gordon, Hibbard, & Kreutzer, 1989). Before using CACR with a patient, the therapist needs to determine the answers to such questions as: How well does the patient follow directions? How does the patient manage the keyboard? How well does the patient manage other input devices? Are there any problems with vision or hearing? How difficult does the patient find the software? (Lynch, 1992a). The therapist must continually evaluate the patient and software, being sure to adapt the software to meet the needs of the patient.

Adaptive treatment approaches attempt to bypass the deficit by teaching the patient strategies or by changing the environment. This approach assumes that one can facilitate substitution of intact behaviors for impaired behaviors (Neistadt, 1990). An example is teaching the patient with left brain damage (LBD) to

use visual imagery to remember a name. The adaptive approaches have met with greater acceptance than remedial approaches, because they are generally geared toward facilitation of activities of daily living (Ben-Yishay & Diller, 1993).

Toglia (1991, 1993) described a treatment model called the **multicontext treatment approach** (Table 27.2). This approach emphasizes **generalization** and the importance of training self-awareness and metacognitive skills. **Generalization** is the ability to transfer what is learned in the treatment situation to everyday activities. For this to happen, strategies and skills are practiced in multiple environments and tasks. The surface characteristics of a task are varied, while the underlying strategy remains the same (Table 27.3).

GENERAL TREATMENT PRINCIPLES

There are several issues that must be considered when selecting a treatment approach. One factor is the patient's level of awareness of his deficits. If the patient is not aware of, or denies, his deficits, it is difficult to get him to participate in treatment. This level of awareness will determine the type of **compensation** a patient is able to use.

Crosson et al. (1989) described three levels of awareness: intellectual, emergent, and anticipatory. Intellectual awareness ranges from an understanding that one is having difficulty with some activities to understanding the implications of one's deficits (e.g., a person with spatial deficits cannot be a graphic artist). Deficits in abstract reasoning and memory may limit a patient's intellectual awareness. Emergent awareness is recognition of a problem when it is happening. If a patient does not have emergent awareness, he will not be able to use compensatory techniques, as he is not aware that a problem exists. In the next level, anticipatory awareness, the patient is able to anticipate when a problem will occur and either to use compensatory strategies or to avoid the situation. Crosson et al. (1989) also described four types of compensatory strategies based on the way their implementation is

Table 27.2 Components of the Multicontext Treatment Approach

Component	Definition	Example
Processing strategies	Situational strategies: those strategies effective in specific tasks and environments	Rehearsal, visual imagery left-to-right scanning, etc.
	Nonsituational strategies: those strategies effective in a wide range of tasks and environments	Planning ahead, prioritizing information before begining task, use of self-monitoring, etc.
Task analysis and establishment of criteria for transfer	Identify series of tasks that decrease in degrees of physical and conceptual similarity to the original task	Task: donning a pullover T-shirt in the therapy area
	Near transfer: only one or two surface characteristics are changed	Donning a pullover sweater (color and texture are changed)
	Intermediate transfer: three to six surface characteristics are changed, tasks share some physical similarities	Donning a button-down silk blouse in the patient's room (type of clothing, color and texture, movement requirements, and environment are changed)
	Far transfer: tasks are conceptually similar; surface characteristics are different or only one surface characteristic is similar	Donning pants or socks (strategy of dressing affected side first remains the same, while almost everything else changes)
	Very far transfer: generalization, spontaneous application of what is learned to everyday functioning	Use of an external aid within everyday activity such as reading a checklist posted on the closet door before dressing
Use of multiple environments	The patient is asked to practice a strategy in multiple situations or environments to facilitate generalization	Left-to-right scanning is practiced on cancellation tasks, and then used to located items in a medicine cabinet or to count books on a shelf, etc.
Relation of new knowledge to previously learned knowledge or skill	Information is learned and retained better when the patient can relate it to previously learned skills or knowledge	Choose treatment tasks with the patient's personality, interests, and experiences in mind; connect each new treatment task with prior tasks and experience
Metacognitive training	Metacognitive skills include task evaluation, prediction of consequences, formulation of goals, plan, self-monitoring performance, self-control, and self-initiation	Self-estimation (e.g., of task difficulty, time required, and amount of cues needed); self-questioning ("How am I doing?"); focus on the process rather than the end product of the task; role reversal (the therapist performs the task and the patient identifies the therapist's errors)

Table 27.3   Analysis of Surface Task and Underlying Task Characteristics

Task	Characteristics	Examples
Surface	Type of stimuli	Objects, shapes, numbers, letters, words, sentences, symbols
	Presentation mode	Three-dimensional, two-dimensional, photographs, drawings, written form, auditory mode, tactile mode
	Variable attributes	Color, texture, size, thickness
	Stimuli arrangement	Scattered, horizontal, rotated, overlapping
	Movement requirements	Body alignment, positioning, active movement pattern
	Environmental context	Physical surroundings, familiarity, number of people
	Rules or directions	Number of steps required
Underlying	Underlying skills	Eye-hand coordination, selective attention, memory, visual discrimination, categorization
	Nonsituational strategies	Planning, self-questioning, pacing speed, checking outcomes, anticipating results
	Situational strategies	Grouping, association, left-to-right scanning, rehearsal, elaboration, visual imagery

triggered (Table 27.4). Therapist and patient alike can become frustrated when the patient does not have sufficient awareness to support the compensatory technique that is being taught.

Webb (1991) described a therapy program to teach compensatory strategies. The patient should be receiving ongoing cognitive remediation in addition to Webb's program. The first stage of Webb's program is evaluation and development of appropriate strategies. Next, structured practice provides training in the target compensatory strategy. Initially, cues are visual symbols that progress to written cues, then to auditory cues, and eventually to self-cuing. Carryover is the final stage, as the patient learns to implement and use strategies in daily activities.

Basic issues such as severity and location of injury, time since injury, prognosis, and age will affect selection of treatment procedures. In the case of traumatic brain injury, the deficits tend to be more general, whereas with a cerebrovascular accident, the deficit will be more specific. Generally, the left hemisphere is dominant for language, and the right hemisphere is dominant for visuospatial tasks. The left hemisphere processes information by breaking it down into details and storing it as verbal symbols on the basis of conceptual similarities. The right hemisphere processes information visually or spatially and on the basis of structural similarities (Lezak, 1976). These deficits have a definite impact on treatment. Patients with LBD have difficulty processing information in the auditory modal-

ity, whereas patients with right brain damage (RBD) have difficulty processing information in the visual modality (Ross & Mesulam, 1979). As a result, LBD patients generally respond better to visual demonstration and RBD patients generally respond better to verbal instructions.

Certain types of training depend on the severity of the injury. Patients who are severely involved are not likely to benefit from or use compensatory strategies (Webb, 1991) or memory retraining (Benedict & Wechsler, 1992).

Almost any activity can be adapted for use in the treatment of a variety of deficits. Things to consider when choosing an activity include the following:

1. The activity must demand a response that involves the impaired skill;
2. The level of difficulty must be variable so that the demand can start within the patient's capabilities and progress to higher levels;
3. Progress should be quantifiable and objective;
4. The patient should receive immediate feedback;
5. The activity should be such that the patient is prevented from making an inordinate number of errors (Golden, 1978).

Activities can be varied in many ways, including speed of presentation, modality of presentation (auditory, visual, or tactile), speed of response required, number of items presented at one time, number of spatial dimensions included (two- and three-dimensional),

Table 27.4 Compensatory Strategies

Type	Definition	Example
Anticipatory compensation	Strategies triggered by anticipating that a problem will occur; most desirable level, as it allows the patient to avoid or minimize problems; requires anticipatory awareness	A patient with memory deficit who anticipates difficulty remembering new information and initiates note taking appropriately
Recognition compensation	Strategies triggered by the patient's recognition that a problem is occuring; strategies are applied only when needed; requires emergent awareness	A patient recognizes nonverbal signals that his conversation is becoming tangential; he then implements appropriate strategies to alter the course of the conversation
Situational compensation	Strategies triggered by specific type of circumstance; these depend on habit not recognition; requires intellectual awareness	A patient with a memory deficit is taught to take notes every time he receives new instructions
External compensation	Compensatory techniques initiated by an outside agent or a modification of a environment; used with patients who have intellectual awareness deficit	The patient uses visual cues such as a sign on the door that reads "Have I turned off the lights?"

level of concreteness of directions, and amount of supplementary information available from other sensory modalities (Diller, 1976). Surface task characteristics noted in Table 27.3 can be varied as well.

Activities are presented that gradually and systematically increase demands on the information-processing system (Abreu & Toglia, 1987). Treatment generally flows from simple to complex, from automatic to requiring effort, and from the ability to respond to the external environment to the ability to respond to and analyze the internal environment. Emphasis in treatment is not on the task but on the process the patient uses. The therapist must keep in mind that an intervention may be successful without "repairing" the underlying deficit (Whyte, 1992). For example, the patient may exhibit improvement on letter cancellation tasks, suggesting that his neglect has improved, but performance during a timed task may still reveal a neglect. This is another reason that the patient must practice the underlying skill in multiple environments.

Aphasia, a language disorder that has been well described and researched, generally occurs following LBD. In recent years a similar disorder of affective language called **aprosodia** has been described following RBD (Diller & Weinberg, 1972; Ruckdeschel-Hibbard, Gordon, & Diller, 1986). Prosody is the coloring, melody, and cadence of speech (Ross & Mesulam, 1979). The aphasic patient may not understand the phrase *I'm happy*, because he does not understand the words. The patient with **aprosodia** may understand only the words and may miss the real meaning if it is spoken in a sad voice. Such a patient's use and appreciation of gestures may be disturbed as well.

After brain damage, different emotional reactions, depending on side of lesion, are generally described. RBD patients frequently deny their deficits, appear indifferent and euphoric. Their reaction is termed an indifference reaction. LBD patients are generally said to show a catastrophic reaction often characterized by depression, agitation, and restlessness (Ross, 1981). These descriptions are being challenged. The label of indifference reaction in RBD patients may be the result of their difficulty with affective language. For the RBD patient, a more accurate assessment of his emotional state would be a verbal report of his feelings rather than a judgment based on nonverbal behavior.

Patients must be shown the relevance of treatment to daily life. The more relevance they see, the more likely they are to become involved in their treatment and use the techniques taught to them. The therapist's goal is to improve the patient's daily living skills, and only by relating treatment to activities of daily living will therapist and patient know they are on the right track.

REMEDIATION OF SPECIFIC SKILLS

Attention

Because the environment has an effect on attention, treatment should begin in a quiet, uncluttered environment. When ability to attend improves, treatment can progress to a more normal environment. Be aware of the patient's emotional status, as this too will affect his ability to attend. If the patient is distracted by internal factors (e.g., worry or preoccupation with personal concerns), it may be necessary to focus on decreasing these first (Sohlberg & Mateer, 1989).

It is sometimes difficult to differentiate between decreased arousal and slowed information processing. If a new task is presented that is more complex or of greater interest to the patient and an increase in information processing is noted, the problem is more likely to be the result of decreased arousal (an interesting, complex task elicits greater arousal). On the other hand, if increased complexity only makes the problem worse, it is probably the result of slow information processing (Whyte, 1992).

The patient who has difficulty attending is usually poorly oriented; his gaze is not focused on the task and he may appear passive and uninvolved. The therapist may have to prepare the patient for the task. This is done by (1) focusing the patient's gaze and attention on the task (i.e., verbally calling his attention to the task and using items that are provocative—bright, colorful, etc.), (2) activating the patient (stating what is to be done and if necessary, physically moving the patient's hand to start the activity), and (3) engaging the patient's interest in the activity (perhaps with a pep talk) (Ben-Yishay & Diller, 1983).

In a study of two patients, contingent token reinforcement (tokens, which could be exchanged for a reward, were given to the patient when he exhibited attention to task behavior) was found to improve attention significantly in one patient, and improve attention, although not significantly, in the other patient (Wood, 1986). In another study of four patients, token reinforcement was linked to training in tasks of auditory and visual attention. A significant improvement in attention to task behavior was exhibited following training, but the improvement in attentional behavior did not translate into improvement of performance on tests of auditory recall memory. Wood (1986) believed this may have been the result of the small sample size,

insufficient training, or the presence of other cognitive deficits.

Computer programs, which offer graphic reinforcement for correct responses, may be beneficial for use with attentional deficits. Sohlberg and Mateer (1989) studied the effects of their *Attention Process Training* program on four brain-injured patients. This training addressed sustained, selective, alternating, and divided attention (see Table 9.8). Improvement was found in all subjects and improvement remained above baseline for 8 months following cessation of treatment. Examples of the treatment are given in Table 27.5.

Table 27.5   Treatment Activities for Attention

Type	Activity
Sustained attention (tasks that require consistent response to either visually or auditorily presented stimuli)	The therapist reads a list of letters; the patient indicates when he hears the letter *b*; then every time he hears a *b* or an *h*; then every time he hears each of those letters come just after the one before it in the alphabet (e.g., *k*, *q*, *g*, **h,** *m*, *l*, *v*, *a*, **b,** etc.)
Selective attention (tasks that incorporate distracting or irrelevant information during task performance)	While performing a task (e.g., math exercises, peg-board designs, etc.) a tape is played that may be distracting to the patient (e.g., conversations, news broadcast, music, etc.); the tape used is determined individually, depending on the patient's interests
Alternating attention (tasks that require flexibility, redirection, and reallocation of attention)	Big-little task: the words *big* and *little* are written in big and little letters; the patient is to read what is written as words or size (e.g., *BIG*, *little*, *LITTLE*, *big* when read as words is "big, little, little, big" but when read as size is "big, little, big, little")
	The patient is given a sheet with numbers on it and is asked to cross out the even numbers; at some point while doing this he is asked to change and cross out the odd numbers
Divided attention (tasks with multiple kinds of information or those that involve simultaneous use of two or more tasks)	The patient is asked to sort cards by suit and specific cards (e.g., those that contain the letter *e*: 1's, 3's, 5's, etc.) must also be turned as they are sorted

Orientation

Following brain injury, patients are frequently disoriented as to person, place, and/or time. Treatment is often compensatory. The patient uses cue cards, calendars, rehearsal, and other such techniques to remember these facts. Patients who are disoriented about self, time, and place are often able to benefit only from external **compensation** or, if they have some intellectual awareness, situational **compensation.** Patient's are often given a memory book; but without sufficient awareness, they are unable to use it without cuing from family and staff around them.

One mode of treatment has been described in which groups meet daily to practice skills related to goals set by the group (Corrigan et al., 1985; Lundgren & Persechino, 1986). One such group defined seven behavioral objectives related to orientation to time, locale, identity of group members and staff, general facts, personal facts, and episodic information. Members of the group were rated daily by one of the group leaders on each of the behavioral objectives. This information was combined over a week and used to reflect the patients' development of dynamic cognitive skills over time rather than the acquisition of individual skills in a serial manner (Corrigan et al., 1985). Although more research is needed to determine the effectiveness of this treatment, this type of daily monitoring of cognitive skills provides a means of justifying further treatment. If the therapist can objectively show that the patient is progressing, it is easier to justify treatment rather than basing continued need for treatment on the subjective description that the patient is "improving."

Memory

Treatment of memory deficits focuses on remediation and/or compensatory interventions. General principles for treatment of memory disorders are given in Table 27.6. Although CACR is frequently used for remediation, the data regarding its efficacy are not optimistic. In a study using computer programs for memory retraining, patients made significant gains from the first to last (12 total) session, but this gain was not maintained when retested 15 days later (Kerner & Acker, 1985). Towle, Edmans, and Lincoln (1988) found that although memory skills improved with CACR, the skill did not generalize to untrained memory tasks. Another study, conducted in an acute medical rehabilitation unit, used a general memory retraining program consisting of visual imagery, verbal mediation, and other techniques. No change was found in memory after 12 sessions, indicating that it may be more appropriate in the acute stage to work on attention/concentration deficits, rather than memory deficits (Fussey & Tyerman, 1985). If the patient's performance improves in a quiet room or if he is interested in the material, then the memory deficit may be secondary to an attentional problem, and therefore, treatment should focus on attention rather than memory.

Sohlberg and Mateer (1989) proposed a three-part model of memory rehabilitation that included attention training, prospective memory process training, and training in the use of a compensatory notebook system. Their preliminary data demonstrated that significant improvement in memory ability was seen following attention training; this type of training is appropriate with patients whose memory deficit is related to atten-

Table 27.6   General Treatment Principles for Memory Disorders

Difficulty with	Treatment Principles
Encoding information (decreased ability to encode stimuli or impaired ability to analyze information)	Simplify the information given; reduce the amount of information given at any one time; make sure the information is understood; link or associate the information; encourage organization and processing (e.g., group it, ask questions about it)
Storing information (may analyze information appropriately but is unable to hold it in storage)	Test, rehearse, practice; use expanding rehearsal (e.g., present information, test immediately, retest after a delay of 1 to 2 sec, retest after a slightly longer delay; try to get three correct responses after an 8-sec delay)
Retrieving information (difficulty with retrieval but can retrieve with cues)	Present information in several different contexts; use first-letter prompts, alphabetical searching, and/or mental retracing

tion. Prospective memory is memory for things that will happen in the future (e.g., appointments, to turn off the oven in an hour, etc.). Sohlberg and Mateer's (1989) program *PROMPT* is used with patients who have a primary deficit in memory, and its overall goal is to increase systematically the amount of time a person is able to remember to carry out specific tasks.

For those patients with more severe impairments, a systematic training procedure was developed for use of a compensatory notebook system (Sohlberg & Mateer, 1989). Using this system, Sohlberg and Mateer were able to train four globally amnesic patients to use the memory notebook. It should be noted that in one case study presented, it required 6 months of intensive training for independent use of the system, but the patient was able to live alone, with only 1 hr of assistance per day, whereas before training, he required 24-hr supervision.

There are various compensatory techniques that can be used with patients who have memory deficits. These include both internal and external aids. Various internal aids are presented in Table 27.7. External memory aids include storage devices (e.g., diaries, notebooks, lists, calculators, and computers), cuing devices (e.g., alarm watches and bell timers), and structured environments that reduce memory load (e.g., labeling and/or color coding of drawers and cupboards) (Glisky & Schacter, 1986). These aids, as well as others that the therapist can develop, should be applied

to the specific functional problems the patient is experiencing.

In determining which strategy to use, it is important to understand the patient's strengths and weaknesses. If the patient has difficulty with writing and reading, he may benefit more from imagery than first-word mnemonics or from the use of pictures in conjunction with words rather than words alone. When using imagery with a patient with RBD, involved images that require verbal mediation may be easier than simple images (Wilson, 1982). More recent studies with visual imagery have found that severely involved patients do not benefit from this technique but that moderately impaired patients can benefit when the image is drawn for them, rather than when the image is self-generated (Wilson, 1987).

It is important that the patient and his family be involved in developing and using these strategies (Milton, 1985). The patient may initially require cuing to use the techniques learned, and the family must know the techniques and how to assist the patient when at home and in the community.

Problem Solving

The literature on remediation of problem solving is fragmented, and treatment effectiveness has not been adequately evaluated (Goldstein & Levine, 1987). If problem solving is broken down into the three stages

Table 27.7 Compensatory Memory Aids

Technique	Description
Rehearsal	Patient repeats out loud or to self the information to be remembered
Visual imagery	Patient consolidates information to be remembered by making a mental picture that includes the information (e.g., to remember the name *Barbara*, the patient pictures a barber holding the letter A)
Semantic elaboration	Patient consolidates information by making up a simple story (e.g., if patient is to remember the words *lawyer, game,* and *hat,* he develops a sentence such as: The lawyer wore a hat to the game)
First letter mnemonics	Patient consolidates information to be remembered by using the first letter of each word to make up a word or phrase to be remembered (e.g., to remember a shopping list of salt, ham, olives, peanut butter, pickles, ice cream, napkins, and grapes, he uses the word *SHOPPING* to help him recall the items)
PSQRTA rehearsal method	Patient (1) previews (skims the material for general content), (2) questions (asks questions about the content), (3) reads (actively reads to answer the questions), (4) states (rehearses or repeats the information read), and (5) tests (tests himself by answering the questions)
Establish motor routines and environmental predictability	Patient develops habits (e.g., if he cannot remember where he puts his watch, he sets up a routine in which he always places the watch in the same place when undressing and learns to associate that place with "Where is my watch?")

of preparation, production, and judgment (Bourne, Dominowski, & Loftus, 1979), it is closely related to executive functions of anticipation, goal selection, planning, initiation, self-regulation, and use of feedback (Sohlberg & Mateer, 1989). Sohlberg and Mateer (1989) reported a treatment program for remediation of executive functions consisting of selection and execution of cognitive plans (e.g., listing steps in an activity, sequencing an activity, errand completion, group planning, and modification of plans), time management (e.g., time estimation and scheduling activity), self-regulation (e.g., increasing awareness of behavior), and **compensation** as needed. The patients that have participated in this program have shown improvement of executive function in daily activities.

Treatment may include exercises such as anagrams, puzzles (Zoltan, Siev, & Freishtat, 1986), analysis of proverbs, categorization exercises, or functional problem-solving tasks (Carberry & Burd, 1985). The patient is given different problems to solve. The therapist observes his manner of doing so and provides him with different strategies, as needed, to complete the tasks. Such strategies might include introducing chaining (or breaking the activity down into its component parts, in which one part triggers the next response, etc.), having the patient do the problem one step at a time, having the patient check for errors, providing the patient with external cues, and having the patient write down the steps to increase his memory of them (Zoltan et al., 1986).

Group treatment is frequently used. As the patient's deficits in higher-level cognitive skills become readily apparent in a functional situation, this type of treatment provides a means of interaction and **generalization** to everyday life. It is a means for the patient to become more aware of his strengths and weaknesses, his social interactions, and the importance of compensatory strategies as well as providing the opportunity to use the skills he has learned. Goals of these groups can vary according to the patient population. Goals of the group may be to provide strategies for problem solving and memory storage (Lundgren & Persechino, 1986; Wilson, 1992), training in attention/concentration and abstract reasoning (Carberry & Burd, 1985), or help with reality orientation (Corrigan et al., 1985).

SUMMARY

The purpose of this chapter was to present a definition of **cognitive rehabilitation;** discuss treatment approaches and general treatment principles; and provide specific treatment strategies for rehabilitation of attention, orientation, memory, and problem solving. It is imperative that occupational therapists be constantly mindful of the importance of generalization and the need for systematic research on the influence of cognitive rehabilitation on daily living skills.

STUDY QUESTIONS

1. Define cognitive rehabilitation. How is it different from cognitive remediation?
2. Compare and contrast remedial and adaptive treatment approaches.
3. Describe the five components of Toglia's multicontext treatment approach.
4. Why is it important to know a patient's level of awareness?
5. What task characteristics can be manipulated when developing a treatment task for a specific patient?
6. List five different ways to vary the surface task characteristics of a cognitive remediation task that uses a set of blocks.
7. Define and describe aprosodia.
8. List five treatment activities that can be used for a patient with a deficit in attention.
9. Define compensation and list specific internal and external compensatory strategies for patients with a memory deficit.
10. Define and discuss the need for generalization of treatment.

REFERENCES

Abreu, B. C., & Toglia, J. P. (1987). Cognitive rehabilitation: A model for occupational therapy. *American Journal of Occupational Therapy, 41,* 439–448.
Ben-Yishay, Y., & Diller, L. (1983). Cognitive remediation. In M. Rosenthal, E. R. Griffith, M. R. Bond, & J. D. Miller (Eds.), *Rehabilitation of the head injured adult* (pp. 367–380). Philadelphia: F. A. Davis.
Ben-Yishay, Y., & Diller, L. (1993). Cognitive remediation in traumatic brain injury: Update and issues. *Archives of Physical Medicine & Rehabilitation, 74,* 204–213.
Ben-Yishay, Y., Piasetsky, E. B., & Rattock, J. (1987). A systematic method for ameliorating disorders in basic attention. In M. J. Meier, A. L. Benton, & L. Diller (Eds.), *Neuropsychological rehabilitation* (pp. 165–181). New York: Churchill Livingston.
Benedict, R. H. B., & Wechsler, F. S. (1992). Evaluation of memory retraining in patients with traumatic brain injury: Two single-case experimental designs. *Journal of Head Trauma Rehabilitation, 7*(4), 84–93.
Berrol, S. (1990). Issues in cognitive rehabilitation. *Archives of Neurology, 47,* 219–220.
Bourne, L. E., Dominowski, R. L., & Loftus, E. F. (1979). *Cognitive processes.* Englewood Cliffs, NJ: Prentice-Hall.
Carberry, H., & Burd, B. (1985). The use of psychological theory and content as a media in the cognitive and social training of head injured patients. *Cognitive Rehabilitation, 3*(4), 8–10.
Carter, L. T., Howard, B. E., & O'Neil, W. A. (1983). Effectiveness of cognitive skill remediation in acute stroke patients. *American Journal of Occupational Therapy, 37,* 320–326.
Corrigan, J. D., Arnett, J. A., Houck, L. J., & Jackson, R. D. (1985). Reality orientation for brain injured patients: Group

treatment and monitoring of recovery. *Archives of Physical Medicine & Rehabilitation, 66,* 626–630.

Crosson, B., Barco, P. P., Velozo, C. A., Bolesta, M. M., Cooper, P. V., Werts, D., & Brobeck, T. C. (1989). Awareness and compensation in postacute head injury rehabilitation. *Journal of Head Trauma Rehabilitation, 4*(3), 46–54.

Diller, L. (1976). A model for cognitive retraining in rehabilitation. *Clinical Psychologist, 29,* 13–17.

Diller, L., & Weinberg, J. (1972). Differential aspects of attention in brain-damaged persons. *Perceptual & Motor Skills, 35,* 71–81.

Fussey, I., & Tyerman, A. D. (1985). An exploration of memory retraining in rehabilitation following closed head injury. *International Journal of Rehabilitation Research, 8,* 465–467.

Glasgow, R. E., Zeiss, R. A., Barrera, M., & Lewisohn, P. M. (1977). Case studies on remediating memory deficits in brain-damaged individuals. *Journal of Clinical Psychology, 33,* 1049–1054.

Glisky, E. L., & Schacter, D. L. (1986). Remediation of organic memory disorders: Current status and future prospects. *Journal of Head Trauma Rehabilitation, 1*(3), 54–63.

Golden, C. J. (1978). *Diagnosis and rehabilitation in clinical neuropsychology.* Springfield, IL: Charles C. Thomas.

Goldstein, F. C., & Levin, H. S. (1987). Disorders of reasoning and problem-solving ability. In M. J. Meier, A. L. Benton, & L. Diller (Eds.), *Neuropsychological rehabilitation* (pp. 327–354). New York: Churchill Livingston.

Gordon, W. A., Hibbard, M. R., Egelko, S., Diller, L., Shaver, M. S., Lieberman, A., & Ragnarsson, K. (1985). Perceptual remediation in patients with right brain damage: A comprehensive program. *Archives of Physical Medicine & Rehabilitation, 66,* 353–359.

Gordon, W. A., Hibbard, M. R., & Kreutzer, J. S. (1989). Cognitive remediation: Issues in research and practice. *Journal of Head Trauma Rehabilitation, 4*(3), 76–84.

Harley, J. P., Allen, C., Braciszeski, T. L., Cicerone, D. K., Dahlberg, C., Evans, S., Foto, M., Gordon, W. A., Harrington, D., Levin, W., Malec, J. F., Millis, S., Morris, J., Muir, C., Richert, J., Salazar, E., Schiavone, D. A., & Smigielski, J. S. (1992). Guidelines for cognitive rehabilitation. *Neurological Rehabilitation, 2*(3), 62–67.

Kerner, M. J., & Acker, M. (1985). Computer delivery of memory re-training with head injured patients. *Cognitive Rehabilitation, 3*(6), 26–31.

Lezak, M. D. (1976). *Neuropsychological assessment.* New York: Oxford University Press.

Lundgren, C. C., & Persechino, E. L. (1986). Cognitive group: A treatment program for head-injured adults. *American Journal of Occupational Therapy, 40,* 397–401.

Lynch, W. J. (1992a). Selecting patients and software for computer-assisted cognitive retraining. Part 2: Key patient variables to consider. *Journal of Head Trauma Rehabilitation, 7*(2), 106–108.

Lynch, W. J. (1992b). Suggestions for the next generation of cognitive rehabilitation software. Part I: Memory software. *Journal of Head Trauma Rehabilitation, 7*(4), 109–111.

Malec, J., & Questad, K. (1983). Rehabilitation of memory after craniocerebral trauma: Case report. *Archives of Physical Medicine & Rehabilitation, 64,* 436–438.

Milton, S. B. (1985). Compensatory memory strategy training: A practical approach for managing persistent memory problems. *Cognitive Rehabilitation, 3*(6), 8–15.

Neistadt, M. E. (1988). Occupational therapy for adults with perceptual deficits. *American Journal of Occupational Therapy, 42,* 434–440.

Neistadt, M. E. (1990). A critical analysis of occupational therapy approaches for perceptual deficits in adults with brain injury. *American Journal of Occupational Therapy, 44,* 299–304.

Poole, J., Dunn, W., Schell, B., Tiernan, K., Barnhart, J. M., Abreu, B., Fine, S. B., Hayes, M., Holtz-Yotz, M., & Toglia, J. (1991). Statement: Occupational therapy services management of persons with cognitive impairments. *American Journal of Occupational Therapy, 45,* 1067–1068.

Riddoch, M. J., & Humphreys, G. W. (1983). The effects of cueing on unilateral neglect. *Neuropsychologia, 21,* 589–599.

Ross, E. D. (1981). The aprosodias. *Neurology, 38,* 561–569.

Ross, E. D., & Mesulam, M.-M. (1979). Dominant language functions of the right hemisphere? *Archives of Neurology, 36,* 144–148.

Ruckdeschel-Hibbard, M., Gordon, W. A., & Diller, L. (1986) Affective disturbances associated with brain damage. In S. Filskov & T. Boll (Eds.), *Handbook of clinical neuropsychology* (pp. 305–337). New York: John Wiley & Sons.

Ruff, R. M., Baser, C. A., Johnston, J. W., Marshall, L. F., Klauber, S. K., Klauber, M. R., & Minteer, M. (1989). Neuropsychological rehabilitation: An experimental study with head-injured patients. *Journal of Head Trauma Rehabilitation, 4*(3), 20–36.

Sohlberg, M. M., & Mateer, C. A. (1989). *Introduction to cognitive rehabilitation.* New York: Gilford Press.

Toglia, J. P. (1991). Generalization of treatment: A multicontext approach to cognitive perceptual impairment in adults with brain injury. *American Journal of Occupational Therapy, 45,* 505–516.

Toglia, J. (1993, March 19, 20). *OT intervention for individuals with constructional apraxia,* paper presented at the AOTA Neurosciences Institute, Baltimore.

Towle, D., Edmans, J. A., & Lincoln, N. B. (1988). Use of computer-presented games with memory-impaired stroke patients. *Clinical Rehabilitation, 2,* 303–307.

Webb, D.-M. (1991). Increasing carryover and independent use of compensatory strategies in brain injured patients. *Cognitive Rehabilitation, 9*(3), 28–35.

Whyte, J. (1992). Neurologic disorders of attention and arousal: Assessment and treatment. *Archives of Physical Medicine & Rehabilitation, 73,* 1094–1103.

Wilson, B. (1982). Success and failure in memory training following a cerebral vascular accident. *Cortex, 18,* 581–594.

Wilson, B. (1987). *Rehabilitation of memory.* New York: Guilford Press.

Wilson, B. (1992, October). *Approaches to memory therapy.* Paper presented at the conference for Evaluation and Treatment of Disorders of Memory, Attention and Visual Neglect, Philadelphia, PA.

Wood, R. L. (1986). Rehabilitation of patients with disorders of attention. *Journal of Head Trauma Rehabilitation, 1*(3), 43–53.

Zoltan, B., Siev, E., & Freishtat, B. (1986). *The adult stroke patient: A manual for evaluation and treatment of perceptual and cognitive dysfunction.* Thorofare, NJ: Slack.

Adjunctive Therapies

Sometimes, for patients to engage in meaningful occupational tasks or to benefit from developmental or learning therapies, some outside instrumentation is needed. Splints or orthoses provide support and function when the patient has lost strength or is at risk for developing potentially limiting postures or cumulative trauma injury. Chapters 28 and 29 describe the various types of orthoses and how to construct splints from thermoplastic materials. Wheelchairs may be necessary for nonambulatory persons; how the particular type and options are chosen and prescribed are described in Chapter 30. Persons with severe motor or sensory impairments have greater access to and engagement in meaningful occupations and recreational opportunities because of electronic technology. Chapter 31 describes these adaptations. Chapter 32 describes biofeedback, which is used to assist people who are relearning how to move correctly. Individuals who are not aware of their muscular or movement responses can use biofeedback to improve performance. Chapter 33 is a primer in the use of physical agent modalities recently accepted by the Representative Assembly as legitimate tools of occupational therapy. The modalities prepare the patient to engage in activity by decreasing pain and swelling or activating muscle not under voluntary control.

Orthoses: Kinds and Purposes

Cheryl A. Linden and Catherine A. Trombly

OBJECTIVES

After reading this chapter, the student will be able to:
1. Define and discuss key concepts and terms.
2. Identify the goals of static and dynamic splinting.
3. Identify precautions relative to the use of slings with various types of injuries.
4. Select an appropriate **splint** or **orthosis** based for a particular diagnosis.
5. Given a picture, identify the **splint** or **orthosis** according to the function of the **splint** and describe the lost or diminished function for which it is used.

Orthotic rehabilitation involves the prescription, design, fabrication, checkout, and training in the use of special devices applied to patients to substitute for lost function. Several rehabilitation professionals bring their special expertise to different aspects of the orthotic rehabilitation process. The physician is responsible for prescribing the device. The certified orthotist is an expert in design and fabrication of all types of permanent orthoses, especially complicated spinal and lower extremity orthoses and upper extremity orthoses used to restore function. The occupational therapist is an expert in the adaptive use of the upper extremities in occupational performance tasks and has taken major responsibility for the checkout and training in the use of permanent orthoses for the upper extremities as well as design and fabrication of thermoplastic **splints.** The physical therapist is an expert in mobility, especially locomotion and gait, and is responsible for the checkout and training in the use of trunk and lower extremity orthoses. The rehabilitation engineer is an expert in technical problem solving involving mechanical and/or electrical solutions to unique problems of particular patients. Occupational therapists and rehabilitation engineers often collaborate to solve problems encountered by patients in performing their tasks of daily life. The

therapist presents the parameters of the problem to the engineer in terms of patient abilities and disabilities and the functional and psychological goals that the device needs to meet or allow. The engineer then proposes technical solutions, and together they apply them to the patient and evaluate the outcome.

An **orthosis** is a device added to a person's body to support, position, or immobilize a part; to correct deformities; to assist weak muscles and restore function; or to modify tone. Orthoses are classified descriptively according to the part they include. For example, a wrist cock-up **splint** is a wrist-hand **orthosis** (WHO) (Long & Schutt, 1986) and a long leg brace is a knee-ankle-foot **orthosis** (KAFO). Within that classification, there may be several types. For example, a wrist cock-up **splint** and a flexor hinge hand **splint** are both WHOs. In this chapter, the traditional names that communicate exactly which **splint** is meant will be used. Orthoses for the hands are often called **splints.**

There are two basic classifications of **splints:** static and dynamic (also known as lively) (Long & Schutt, 1986). Static **splints,** which have no moving parts, prevent motion and are used to rest or rigidly support the splinted part (Cailliet, 1982; Long & Schutt, 1986). Static **splints** are also used to stretch joint contractures progressively or align specified joints after a surgical procedure for optimal healing. Because immobilization causes such unwanted effects as atrophy and stiffness, a static **splint** should never be used longer than physiologically required and should never include joints other than those being treated (Cailliet, 1982). A dynamic **splint** is preferable if it is equally effective. Dynamic **splints** have moving parts to permit, control, or restore movement (Cailliet, 1982; Shafer, 1986). The movement in dynamic **splints** may be intrinsically powered by another body part or electrical stimulation of the patient's muscles (Long & Schutt, 1986). Extrinsic power can be provided by elastic or pulley traction systems (Dovelle, Heeter, & McFaul,

GLOSSARY

Arm sling—Orthosis that supports the proximal upper extremity; may be used to prevent shoulder subluxation or assist weak muscles.

Lapboard—A portable table top that is applied to a wheelchair and provides a working surface.

Mobile arm support—Frictionless arm support that is mounted to a wheelchair, table, or belt around the waist and uses gravity in an inclined plane to assist movement of the arms when shoulder and elbow muscles are weak.

Orthokinetic cuff—Based on Rood's theory, it is a cuff made from an elastic bandage applied over a weak muscle to provide tactile stimulation of that muscle, because the cuff-skin interface moves when the patient's muscles contract.

Orthosis—A device that is added to part of a person's body to support, position, or immobilize that part; to correct deformities; to assist weak muscles and restore function; or to modify tone.

Serial casting—Process of applying casts, of increasingly greater degrees of joint position, every few days, to stretch a limb progressively away from a contracted spastic posture.

Splint—Type of orthosis, usually for the hand, which can be custom made or purchased commercially; referred to as static (no moving parts) or dynamic (moving parts).

Universal hemiplegic sling—A sling that is used to support a nonfunctional shoulder and prevent shoulder subluxation by restricting active motion and keeping the humerus in adduction and internal rotation; commonly used in patients with hemiplegia.

1988; Dovelle, Heeter, & Phillips, 1987) springs, gas-operated devices, and motors (Long & Schutt, 1986), and new systems are continually being researched to enhance function (May & Silfverskiold, 1989).

Orthoses are categorized here by the most common goal for which they are used; however, that goal is not necessarily their only goal. The same **orthosis** may fulfill several functions. For example, a dynamic **splint** that provides prehension function also provides static positioning of the thumb in a functional position. The therapist should clearly have the goal(s) and precautions in mind when selecting a **splint** for a particular patient. The therapist must incorporate functional objectives into the fabrication of the **splint** and, throughout, monitor the functional performance of the patient through activities that provide the patient with practice in the use of the **splint** (Canadian Association of Occupational Therapists [CAOT], 1987). Another important factor to keep in mind is that the patient's acceptance of a **splint** is based on comfort level, the stability (reliability) and the value of the **splint** or **orthosis** to the person (CAOT, 1987), and the cosmesis of the **splint** (Rossi, 1988). The representative sampling of orthoses in this chapter is not meant to be exhaustive; the references provide additional information.

TO SUPPORT OR IMMOBILIZE A PAINFUL JOINT AND TO POSITION TO PREVENT DEFORMITIES OR ENHANCE FUNCTION

When a patient lacks the ability to keep the joint aligned or to hold a part in a functional position, such as with weakness of the extensor pollicis brevis, or has suffered soft tissue injury that may result in deformities

as healing progresses, such as with burns, orthoses to maintain a functional position are needed. During acute episodes of rheumatoid arthritis or other instances when rest of a joint is required to relieve pain or to protect joint integrity, supportive types of **splints** are used.

These types of **splints** are often worn all day, all night, or both, to provide the most benefit. However, in every case, the **splint** is removed several times a day for gentle passive range of motion exercises to maintain the patient's mobility. It is imperative to understand that if these procedures are not followed, further splinting will probably be needed to correct deformities developed through immobility.

Some common examples of these kinds of orthoses are discussed below.

Proximal Supports

The suspension sling is a device that supports the upper extremity with cuffs that fit under the elbow and wrist. These cuffs are suspended from a spring attached overhead. Suspension slings can be used unilaterally or bilaterally. Some are designed for suspension from a rod that attaches to the wheelchair and are thus referred to as an overhead rod and sling (Fig. 28.1); some are mounted on floor stands, such as the Swedish Aid and operate on a system of counterbalanced weights (Fig. 28.2); and others are suspended directly from the ceiling. Regardless of how the sling is suspended, the distance between the point of suspension and the cuffs should be as far as is practical, because the longer the pendulum, the wider the arc of motion and, consequently, the longer the relatively flat section of the arc (Long & Schutt, 1986). Movement is easier for the patient in the flatter area of the arc because the resistance offered by the inclined ends of the arc is eliminated or minimized (Long & Schutt, 1986). Adjust-

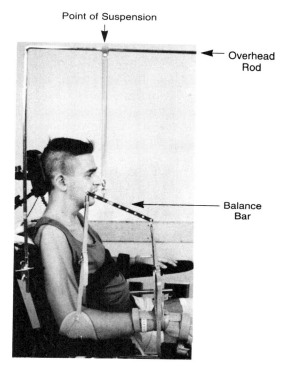

Figure 28.1.   Suspension sling.

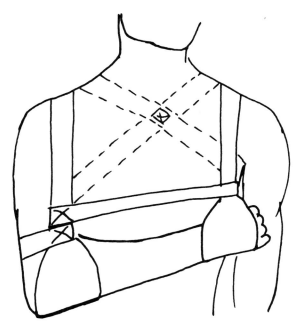

Figure 28.3.   Double trough arm sling to support a flaccid shoulder. Dashed lines indicate placement of the straps on the back.

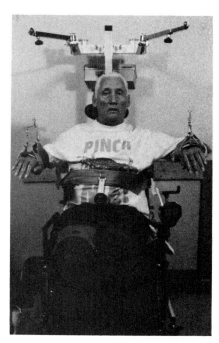

Figure 28.2.   Swedish Aid.

ments can be made to the balance bar to promote more flexion or extension of the elbow, depending on the activity. For example, the bar would be balanced more toward flexion if the patient needed assistance in hand-to-mouth activities. Other adjustments to assist function are described later in this chapter.

Arm slings have been developed to prevent shoulder subluxation in patients with brachial plexus injuries (DeVore, 1970; Kohlmeyer, Weber, & Yarkony, 1990; Robinson, 1986), polymyositis (Neal & Williamson, 1980), hemiplegia (Bobath, 1990), and central cord syndrome injuries (Kohlmeyer et al., 1990). Some slings support and immobilize the whole arm (DeVore, 1970) (Fig. 28.3). These slings, such as the figure-of-eight and the **universal hemiplegic sling** restrict active motion by keeping the humerus in adduction and internal rotation and putting the elbow into flexion (Sullivan & Rogers, 1989). These slings take the weight of the arm off the shoulder, but do not approximate the humeral head back into the glenoid fossa. It was noted in a study by Moodie, Brisbin, and Morgan (1986) that the downside of slings that immobilize is that they also reinforce synergy patterns and fail to provide motor and sensory feedback. Other slings support the shoulder but leave the rest of the arm free for function (Bobath, 1990; Neal & Williamson, 1980; Sullivan & Rogers, 1989) (Fig. 28.4).

There are numerous styles of slings; however, there is no consensus as to which type of sling is best for a particular goal or whether a sling should be used

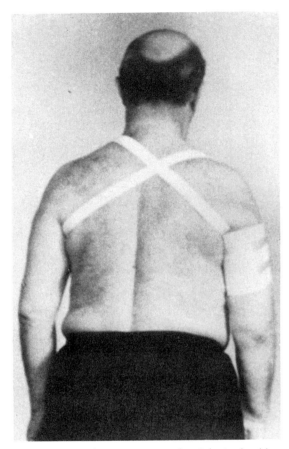

Figure 28.4. Arm sling to support a hemiplegic shoulder.

at all for the subluxed shoulder. A survey of Canadian physical and occupational therapists determined that the most frequently used slings for the hemiplegic shoulder were the cuff type arm sling (76%) and the Bobath axilla roll (62%) (Boyd & Gaylard, 1986). The cuff type arm sling has an elbow cuff attached to the strap that goes across the patient's back, over the unaffected shoulder, and ends in a wrist cuff so that the patient's hand is positioned about waist high (Fig. 28.5). The Bobath axilla roll is described below. One study documented by x-ray that a sling designed to support both the shoulder and forearm during ambulation, but only the shoulder when the patient is seated and using a **lapboard,** does in fact reduce subluxation; patients also reported reduced pain (Rajaram & Holtz, 1985). The sling is complicated and difficult to don, however. Some slings are commercially available, while others are made by occupational therapists. Instructions for the sling pictured in Fig. 28.3, called the double trough arm sling by Boyd and Gaylard (1986), are as follows. Elbow and wrist cuffs are connected by 2-inch webbing that extends from the elbow cuff, up the front of the chest, over the affected shoulder, across

the back, around the unaffected side to the wrist cuff, around the wrist cuff, up the front of the chest, and over the unaffected shoulder, across the back to the elbow cuff under the affected arm. The webbing makes a figure-of-eight on the patient's back. The crossed areas are permanently sewn, as is the webbing to the cuffs. Stabilizing pieces are added behind the elbow and between the elbow and wrist straps in front. Needless to say, the nursing staff and the patient must have careful instruction in applying this sling correctly.

The Bobath axilla roll holds the humerus slightly abducted, which orients the humeral head more directly into the glenoid fossa while supporting the joint (Bobath, 1990). The patient wears the sling when he is ambulating or in his wheelchair. It is constructed by rolling up an 8- to 10-inch-wide piece of soft foam rubber jelly roll fashion to fit under the axilla. The roll is secured in place with a figure-of-eight harness, similar to that used for upper extremity prostheses, made from an ace bandage or webbing. An alternative strapping procedure uses a chest strap that passes through the roll; the chest strap is suspended by two straps over the affected shoulder, one directly attached and the other diagonally attached (Walker, 1983). When using this axilla roll sling, care must be taken that the humerus is not displaced laterally and the radial nerve is not compressed (Bobath, 1990). The addition of a distal support component could help prevent these risks while still encouraging arm swinging during ambulation (Claus & Godfrey, 1985). It must be noted however, that in a study by Moodie, Brisbin, and Morgan (1986) the Bobath axilla roll did not effectively reduce humeral subluxation. Sullivan and

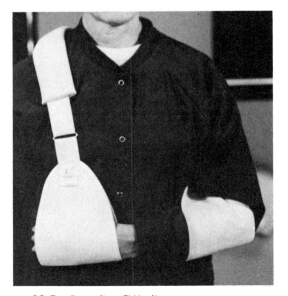

Figure 28.5. Bunnyline CVA sling.

Rogers (1989) suggested a modification to the Bobath sling. Their design added a distal piece that supported the hand so that the thumb was extended and abducted and the wrist was in neutral. This distal piece was attached to the chest strap rather than the shoulder harness to decrease the pull on the glenohumeral joint. The other slight modification was reducing the diameter of the foam roll to reduce lateral displacement of the humeral head.

The use of a humeral cuff suspended by a figure-of-eight harness to support the humerus while allowing use of the extremity was also suggested by Bobath (1990) (Fig. 28.4) and is now commercially available (Smith & Nephew Roylan, Germantown, WI).

For the patient who has a brachial plexus injury, a full flail arm **splint** or an elbow lock **splint** was suggested by Robinson (1986). The full flail arm **splint** is recommended for the patient who has involvement from C_5-T_1 (whole upper limb involvement). It provides stability at both the shoulder and elbow required to place the hand for function. The elbow lock **splint** is used with the patient who has involvement at C_{5-6} only. This **splint** provides stability at the elbow so that the patient may place the hand closer to or away from the body for function. The Kohlmeyer-RIC **orthosis** has also been suggested for brachial plexus injury, in addition to the central cord syndrome (Kohlmeyer et al., 1990). This **orthosis** allows the patient with greater proximal weakness than distal weakness in the upper extremity to participate early in activities of daily living. The **orthosis** is described as follows: It is a figure-of-eight shoulder harness with unilateral or bilateral forearm cuffs made of Orthoplast. These cuffs are connected to the harness by flexible rubber tubing, and the tubing length is adjustable via clamps that are connected to the forearm cuff, which allows for different arm positions. The arm position can be independently changed by the patient, using trunk flexion and by adjusting the degree of arm flexion, using the **orthosis.** This **orthosis** was found to improve arm swing and balance during ambulation, decrease shoulder pain and subluxation, and increase independence in activities of daily living (Kohlmeyer et al., 1990).

In using any sling, the therapist not only must check for size and comfort but also must be sure the sling does not prevent function the patient has and should be using, create new problems for the patient such as edema in the dependent hand, or increase disability by positioning in patterns of spasticity or pulling the head of the humerus out of the glenoid fossa. Patient compliance and acceptance of the sling also need to be considered. Relative ease of donning and doffing the sling is imperative so the limb is not damaged further from an improperly worn sling. A

checklist of 19 desirable and 4 undesirable characteristics of slings has been published to aid in selection of a sling for a particular patient (Smith & Okamoto, 1981). Further research on the effectiveness of slings and orthoses in the management of the flaccid or subluxed shoulder is recommended, and therapists should consider carefully all of their options before prescribing slings for their patients.

Wheelchair arm boards are often preferred to the use of slings for a wheelchair-bound patient, because they allow the humeral head to approximate the glenoid fossa at an angle, its more natural position, and they support the hand so that edema is less likely to occur. The arm board is approximately 10 to 12 cm wide, is padded, and may have straps to hold the arm in place. It attaches over the regular wheelchair armrest. Depending on the design of the arm board, it can be more aesthetically appealing to the patient than a sling. There is none of the difficulty of donning/doffing as is sometimes the case with slings. Arm boards can be removable to allow transfers and performance of activities of daily living. Ideally, the board also supports the wrist and fingers in a functional position. A total of 64% of therapists in one survey (Boyd & Gaylard, 1986) chose arm boards to protect the hemiplegic shoulder, although the sling was preferred while patients were ambulating. There have been no studies of the effectiveness of arm boards to maintain the humerus in a correct anatomical orientation to the scapula at the glenoid fossa. Arm boards and troughs are now commercially available, although the occupational therapist may need to custom make one to suit a particular patient's problem. Various designs have been published (Bobath, 1990; Ferreri & Tumminelli 1974; Goold, 1976; Iveson, Phillips, & Ream, 1972; Salo, 1978).

An alternative to an arm board is the use of a wheelchair **lapboard.** It is generally used when a patient has either decreased trunk control, has visual field deficits, needs a wider variety of positioning possibilities, or needs a surface to work on (Walsh, 1987). It was used by 81% of the therapists responding to a survey about support devices for the hemiplegic shoulder (Boyd & Gaylard, 1986). The **lapboard** provides all the advantages of the arm board plus allows the arm to be positioned forward to pull the scapula forward, a position of choice for hemiplegic patients (Bobath, 1990). In the opinion of some, the **lapboard** seems more natural and less a badge of disability than a sling or arm board. Clear acrylic plastic **lapboards** allow the patient to see his whole body. **Lapboards** do make independent wheelchair propulsion difficult, however. An alternative is a half **lapboard** (similar to those on a school desk) that is positioned on the armrest; it can be rotated up and out of the way during transfers instead of having to be taken off (Walsh, 1987).

Distal Supports: Hand Splints

Volar wrist cock-up **splints** (Fig. 28.6) support the wrist in a position of 20 to 30° of dorsiflexion. The person for whom a wrist cock-up **splint** would be appropriate would generally have use of the fingers, however, this is not always the case. This **splint** can be made of plaster of Paris bandage, thermoplastics, or metal. It is a simple **splint** that extends from the distal palmar crease, over the wrist, to approximately two-thirds the length of the forearm. Small hands do not require such a long **splint** because that amount of leverage offered by the forearm piece is not needed for the light weight of the small hand. The palmar piece is trimmed and rolled to avoid interfering with the thenar eminence and the metacarpophalangeal joints and is molded to the palm to support the arches of the hand. Prefabricated wrist cock-up **splints** can also be purchased; however, because these are not made specifically for a particular patient's hand, it is difficult to get the support of the palmar arches.

Other wrist support **splints** are elasticized cuffs with metal stays to support the wrist. Such a **splint** may be worn while working or engaging in sports. One study (Carlson & Trombly, 1983) found that although immobilization was not complete with this style of **splint,** working speed on hand tasks was subtly slower, a factor to be weighed for the working patient. A similar wrist support **splint** is the economy wrist support (Fig. 28.7). This dorsal **splint** supports the wrist in a neutral position and is used in positioning the tetraplegic hand such as in a C_5-level injury. This **splint** has a palmar cuff in which, e.g., an eating utensil can be inserted for use in self-feeding. The **splint** is readily available and relatively inexpensive; the drawbacks are lack of

ulnar wrist support, which results in an ulnar deviation deformity over time and failure to support the palmar arches adequately.

Wrist **splints** are also used on persons with arthritis. The purposes of such a **splint** are to reduce pain and synovitis by resting the joint, to increase hand function by proper positioning, and to support and protect the joint during activities (Anderson & Maas, 1987; Backman, 1988). Common **splints** used are the elastic or leather gauntlet **splint,** the dorsal or palmar Orthoplast **splint** (Stewart & Maas, 1990), and the spandex wrist **splint** (Backman, 1988). These types of **splints** fit either dorsally or volarly and hold the wrist in a neutral position, providing external support to the wrist during activities. These **splints** all have assets and drawbacks, so it is imperative that the therapist be aware of the activities the patient wants or needs to accomplish so that the most appropriate **splint** can be prescribed. The modification of wrist **splints** to incorporate a type of wrist ulnar deviation block has also been suggested for use with arthritic patients (Johnson et al., 1992; Sofer, Pagnotta, & Bitensky, 1987); however, there are no significant data to support the claim that these types of **splints** actually prevent ulnar deviation.

A resting-pan **splint** (Figs. 28.8 and 28.9) is chosen for patients who need to have the wrist, fingers, and thumb supported in functional position. A resting **splint** may be of volar or dorsal design, depending

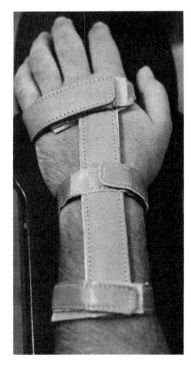

Figure 28.7. Economy wrist support.

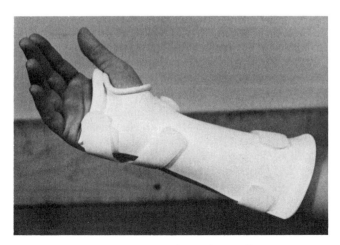

Figure 28.6. Thermoplastic volar cock-up splint.

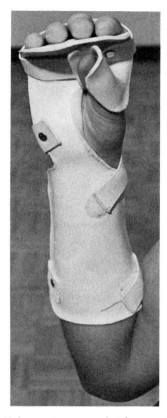

Figure 28.8. Volar resting-pan splint from underneath.

because the joint stress is too great. An alternative for arthritic patients who require both wrist and finger support would be a volar resting **splint** with ulnar support; this type of **splint** was found to decrease pain and increase grip strength (after removal of the **splint**) in the arthritic hand (Johnson et al., 1992).

Long and short opponens **splints** (Figs. 28.10 to 28.14) are designed to support the thumb in an abducted and opposed position. The long opponens hand **splint** also supports the wrist and has been used effectively for positioning the tetraplegic hand and/or resting the hand following trauma, deQuervain's syndrome, or thumb tendon repair (LMB Hand Rehab Products, San

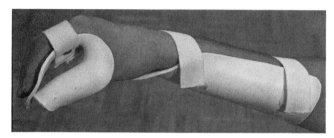

Figure 28.9. Volar resting-pan splint from the side.

on patient needs and preferences. The commercially available **splints** may be adjusted somewhat, such as reforming the palmar arch or trimming the **splint.** It saves time to have a stock of these **splints** already made for use with average-size persons, especially in the case of burn patients for whom time is of the essence and because a **splint** cannot be formed directly on the newly burned skin.

A variation of the resting pan has been devised to **splint** the burned hand after primary excision and early skin grafting (Fishwick & Tobin, 1978; Tenney & Lisak, 1986). The **splint** is made before surgery. A large circular piece of **splint** material is added to the finger part of the **splint** to act as an outrigger. Dress hooks are cemented to the fingernails of the patient; rubber bands are attached to them and stretched to the perimeter of the circular piece. This setup holds the fingers abducted and partially flexed at the metacarpophalangeal (MP) joints and extended at the proximal interphalangeal (PIP) and distal interphalangeal (DIP) joints.

Another variation is to **splint** the hand in an intrinsic plus position, in which the PIP joints are extended fully to promote increased flexion of the MP joints. This would be used for a spinal cord–injured patient but would be detrimental to the arthritic hand,

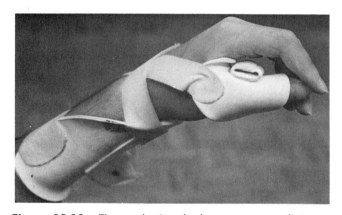

Figure 28.10. Thermoplastic volar long opponens splint.

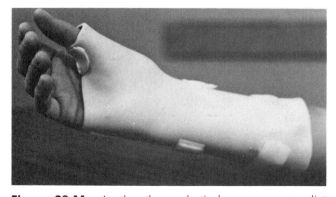

Figure 28.11. Another thermoplastic long opponens splint, sometimes referred to as a thumb spica splint.

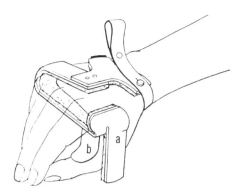

Figure 28.12. Schematic of short opponens splint. **a,** Opponens bar. **b,** C-bar.

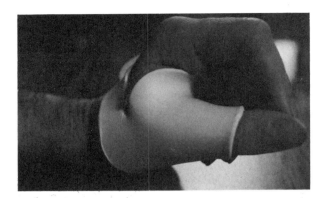

Figure 28.13. Short opponens splint made from Orthoplast.

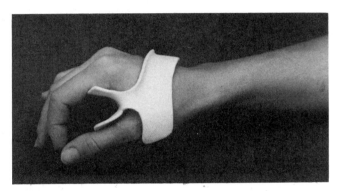

Figure 28.14. Another short opponens splint made from Orthoplast.

Luis Obispo, CA; Tenney & Lisak, 1986). The **splint** can be made so that the support bar is located volarly, dorsally, or radially (Hunter et al., 1990). For example, a volar long opponens **splint** (Fig. 28.11) immobilizes the wrist and the carpometacarpal and metacarpophalangeal joints of the thumb. This **splint** positions the thumb in opposition for light prehension activities (Hunter et al., 1990). Both the long and short opponens **splints** can be modified by adding a platform to support nonfunctioning fingers and provide a functional position of the hand and wrist. By protecting the functional position, especially in C_6 spinal cord–injured patients, there is a greater likelihood that a palmar or three-jaw chuck prehension pattern can be accomplished through wrist extension when the **splint** is removed. Whereas the long opponens **splint** is used when the wrist is flaccid, the short opponens is used when there is a motorically functional wrist (Krajnik & Bridle, 1992).

The thumb carpometacarpal (CMC) stabilization **splint** (Melvin, 1982; Parks, Barrett, & Voss, 1983) is a short, static **splint** that slips over the first metacarpal to relieve thumb pain and increase hand function. The thumb CMC stabilization **splint** restricts motion of the thumb CMC and MP joints but allows motion of the IP joint and wrist. It is indicated for patients

with degenerative joint disease who experience pain during activities.

Thumb metacarpophalangeal (MCP) stabilization **splint** (Moore & Braverman, 1990) is a short static **splint** used for instability of the radial collateral ligament of the MCP joint. The thumb MCP stabilization **splint** immobilizes the MCP joint while allowing functional CMC and IP motion during activity. It is indicated for patients who have tenderness and swelling at the MCP joint. The **splint** can also be used after removal of a thumb spica **splint** worn postoperatively.

The finger deviation support **splint** (Fig. 28.15), a static variation of the Rancho finger deviation dynamic **splint,** is used to support the MP joints of rheumatoid arthritic patients in semiextension and neutral alignment during hand use (LMB Hand Rehab Products, San Luis Obispo, CA) to counteract the normal tendency for the MP joints to sublux and deviate ulnarly during grasp, which is believed to stress the already disease-weakened ligaments.

Finger stabilizer **splint** (Fig. 28.16) refers to a variety of **splints** designed to stabilize one or more joints of a finger in flexion or extension. These **splints** are easily constructed from thermoplastic materials and are also commercially available in a variety of materials; including silver and gold.

Wrist-hand **splints** are a conservative treatment for mild cases of carpal tunnel syndrome, considering the other options, i.e., surgery, steroid injections, and other medications (Kruger et al., 1991). Carpal tunnel syndrome results from compression of the median nerve within the carpal tunnel space. This causes pain, numbness, stiffness and tingling, which can exacerbate at night or through repetitive activity involving maximum wrist flexion, especially in combination with pinch or grasp (Dolhanty, 1986; Jackson & Clifford, 1989). The hand is splinted with the wrist in neutral or in a few degrees of flexion to minimize compression in the carpal tunnel space. Ideally, the **splint** should be worn during activity. A volar cock-up **splint** (Fig. 28.6)

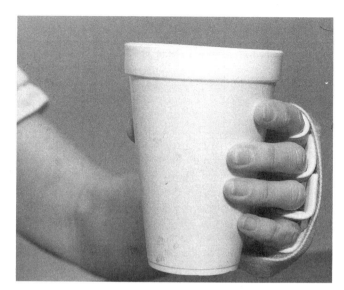

Figure 28.15. Wire-Foam proximal phalangeal splint (ulnar deviation splint) for the arthritic patient.

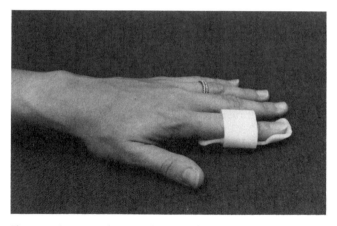

Figure 28.16. A finger stabilizer splint. This splint immobilizes the proximal interphalangeal and distal interphalangeal joints.

can be used. A semiflexible support **splint** has been suggested for those people who do not require a rigid **splint** but need to restrict extremes of motion (Henshaw, Satren, & Wrightsman, 1989). In a study by Dolhanty (1986), patients wearing **splints** for carpal tunnel syndrome noted that the intensity of numbness, pain, and tingling decreased significantly.

TO CORRECT DEFORMITIES

Static and dynamic orthoses are used to provide prolonged stretch, to correct contractures, or to provide prolonged pressure to reduce scarring. Orthoses to stretch out contractures are adjusted to provide stretch of the tissue to the point at which the patient indicates discomfort rather than at the point of maximal stretch, which would result in intolerable pain if prolonged. As

in manual stretching, gentle pressure over a long time is preferred to rapid, forceful stretching. Adjustments to static **splints** are required as the tissue adjusts to each new position. An adjustable **orthosis** is better than refabricating one for each new position.

Wearing time of the **orthosis** is gradually increased as the patient is able to tolerate the device. The importance of wearing the **splint** for the designated time must be emphasized to the patient. After wearing tolerance has increased to several hours, it might be preferable for the patient to wear the device at night when he is asleep, freeing the part for active use during the day. If sleep is interrupted because of discomfort from the **splint,** the force is too great (Long & Schutt, 1986).

Splints designed to correct or prevent scarring secondary to burns must provide firm, even pressure over the entire surface. These **splints** are worn constantly, except for the brief period needed for hygiene, to prevent contractures and deformities (Pratt & Allen, 1989).

The following orthoses were selected to illustrate the principles involved in increasing range of motion or preventing scarring. Others types are available, and the therapist may need to design one to suit a particular patient's unique problem.

Proximal Correction

Neck extension **splint** (Fig. 41.2), also called the conformer neck **splint,** is used for patients whose neck has been burned; it holds the neck extended and prevents the fusion of the chin to the chest during the healing process (Larson, 1973; "Making the Least of Burn Scars," 1972). It can also be used to reduce the thickness of scar tissue through the constant, uniform pressure offered against the developing scar tissue.

The transparent face mask has been used successfully to prevent hypertrophic scarring of facial tissue after deep, partial, or full-thickness thermal injury. The mask is made of cellulose acetate butyrate (Uvex), a clear, high-temperature plastic. Directions for making the negative and positive molds and the mask are published (Rivers, Strate, & Salem, 1979).

The shoulder abduction **splint,** also called an airplane **splint** (Fig. 28.17), is designed to maintain or increase range of motion in shoulder abduction and can be fabricated to place the shoulder in internal or external rotation as well as any degree of abduction. A similar **splint,** simply called a shoulder elevation **splint,** is less expensive and can be fabricated by the therapist (McClure & Flowere, 1992). The **splint** consists of a waist resting pad and forearm trough made of thermoplastic material; an adjustable aluminum rod connects the two pieces, and a belt attached to the waist piece holds the **splint** in place. The angle of

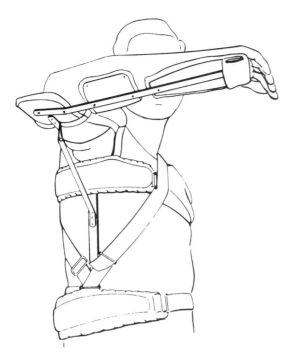

Figure 28.17. Shoulder abduction or airplane splint.

the arm in relationship to the body should closely approximate the plane of the scapula (30 to 40° anterior to the frontal plane). The shoulder should rest near its available end range of pure glenohumeral abduction (120°), although this **splint** can hold the arm up to 150° of elevation (McClure & Flowere, 1992).

Elbow flexion contractures can be corrected by use of a turnbuckle **splint** (Fig. 28.18), a Dynasplint (Dynasplint Systems, Inc., Baltimore, MD), or **serial casting** (discussed below). The turnbuckle **splint** uses a turnbuckle on the lateral aspect of a hinged elbow brace to exert force toward extension. A turnbuckle is a piece of hardware that can be adjusted in fine gradations to hold rigidly two points at a given distance from each other. The turnbuckle **splint** was used successfully to stretch contractures in 12 of 15 patients (80%) on whom it was researched (Green & McCoy, 1979). The average increase in range of motion was 43°; the average reduction of deformity was 37°. The Dynasplint is a precisely adjustable **splint** composed of two stainless-steel struts, which are placed laterally and medially; upper arm and forearm cuffs; and compression-coil springs, which are located at the axis of elbow motion and can be adjusted with a screwdriver (Hepburn & Crivelli, 1984).

Elbow extension contractures are rare. To increase range toward elbow flexion, a **splint** can be made that incorporates upper arm and forearm cuffs with springs or elastic traction for continual stretch. Alternatively, turnbuckles or Klenzak or Lehrman frac-

ture brace joints (Collins et al., 1985) can be used to provide the adjustable traction. The **splint** would be similar to that shown in Figure 28.18, but the direction of force would be reversed. This would also be true in **serial casting.**

The drop-out **splint** is used to immobilize the elbow to prevent elbow flexion of greater than 45° in the case of ulnar nerve entrapment (Harper, 1990). Before the use of this **splint,** patients used to be placed in long arm **splints,** but acceptance was not good. The drop-out **splint,** which allows elbow extension, forearm rotation and wrist motion for function, has been found to be more acceptable (Harper, 1990).

The dynamic pronation-supination **splint** (Fig. 28.19) is designed to increase forearm pronation or supination (Smith & Nephew Roylan Inc., Germantown, WI). The tubing controls the forces and direction of sustained stretch. The components of the **splint** are commercially available; alternatively, the therapist can fabricate the wrist and elbow supports and purchase the metal housing and tubing kit. An example of someone who may use this **splint** is the C_5 tetraplegic who may be developing a supination contracture as a

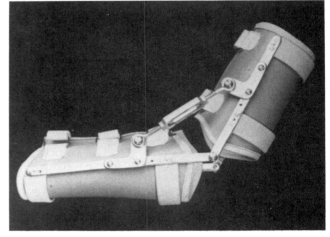

Figure 28.18. Turnbuckle splint for elbow flexion contractures.

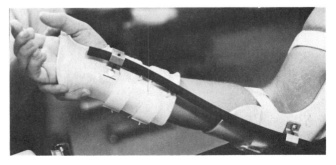

Figure 28.19. Preformed dynamic pronation-supination splint.

result of lack of innervation to pronators. This **splint** would be applied to increase forearm pronation. Complete directions for fabrication and application of this **splint** are available from the manufacturer.

Distal Correction

Volar cock-up **splints** (Fig. 28.6) can be used to provide a gentle force toward wrist hyperextension to stretch the wrist flexors while permitting active finger flexion. If the wrist contracture is secondary to spasticity, however, the resting-pan type **splints** (Fig. 28.9), or similarly styled **splints,** must be used to exert traction not only on the wrist flexors but also the extrinsic finger flexors.

The metacarpophalangeal flexion **splint** with outrigger (Fig. 28.20) can be easily constructed using thermoplastics (Tenney & Lisak, 1986). Finger loops are placed over the proximal phalanges and attach via rubber bands to a volar outrigger to force the MP joints into flexion. For the angle of pull of the rubber bands to be perpendicular, the outrigger must extend the correct distance from the surface of the **splint** and be changed as the patient improves. If the patient can actively maintain wrist extension, a "knuckle bender" type **splint** (Fig. 28.21) can be used to provide the force toward MP flexion. This type of **splint** is commercially available from several manufacturers. All fingers are forced into the same degree of flexion, whereas the MP flexion **splint** with outrigger can be used when some of the fingers need a force different from what others need. The reverse knuckle bender forces the MP joints into extension.

The glove flexion mitt is a **splint** used to force the fingers into flexion (Malick, 1974). It has sometimes been used as exercise equipment to resist finger extension. The **splint** is made from a cotton gardener's glove. Rubber bands are attached from the fingertips to a button secured at the wrist. Directions for construction of an adaptation of the mitt for a patient whose impairment is limited to less than all fingers has been published (Heurich & Polansky, 1978).

The interphalangeal extension **splint** with lumbrical bar (Anderson, 1965) prohibits MP joint hyperextension (Fig. 28.22), and a dorsal outrigger provides attachment for finger loops and rubber bands set at an angle of 90°, which exert a rotary force to pull the interphalangeal joints into extension. A craning traction **splint** (CTS) has been suggested as an alternative to this **splint** (Chesher, Schwartz, & Kleinert, 1988).

The finger knuckle bender (Bunnell, 1956) is a commercially available **splint** that works on the same principle as the knuckle bender for MP joints, except that this one forces flexion of one PIP joint only. Reverse finger knuckle benders (Fig. 28.23) are also available for extension of the PIP joints.

The fingernail **splint** uses dress hooks that are cemented to the dorsal surfaces of the fingernails. Rubber bands extend from these hooks to an outrigger to pull all joints of the fingers into flexion or extension (Von Prince, Cureri, & Pruitt, 1970). The length and location of the outrigger controls the direction and extent of pull. This type of **splint** may be used for burn patients and others for whom skin contact is contraindicated.

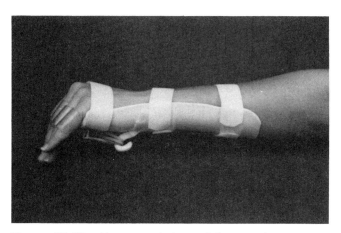

Figure 28.20. Metacarpophalangeal flexion splint with outrigger.

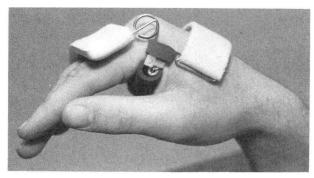

Figure 28.21. Wire-Foam knuckle bender.

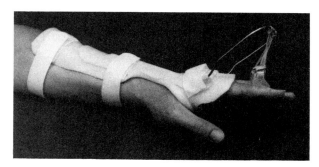

Figure 28.22. Interphalangeal extension splint with lumbrical bar.

The spring safety pin **splint** (Bunnell, 1956), or spring coil finger extension assist (also called the Capener or Wynn-Parry **splint**), is commercially available (e.g., LMB Hand Rehab Products, San Luis Obispo, CA) and uses spring steel wires to stretch out a PIP joint flexion contracture and/or to assist the joint into extension, while permitting active finger flexion (Fig. 28.24). To correct a flexion contracture of both PIP and DIP joints, a spring coil long finger extension assist **splint** or a belly gutter **splint** (Wu, 1991) can be used. To stretch a PIP joint extension contracture or to assist flexion, a spring coil finger flexion assist can be used (LMB Hand Rehab Products, San Luis Obispo, CA). For DIP or PIP joints, finger flexion spring **splints** (Fig. 28.25) and finger extension spring **splints** (Fig. 28.26) are available. It should be noted,

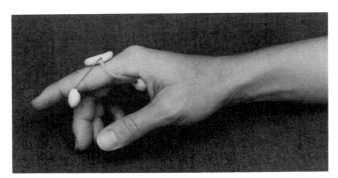

Figure 28.23.   Reverse finger knuckle bender.

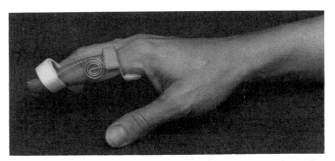

Figure 28.24.   Spring safety pin splint (see text for other names for this splint).

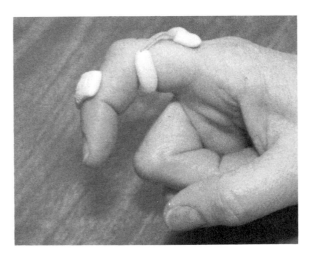

Figure 28.25.   Finger flexion spring splint.

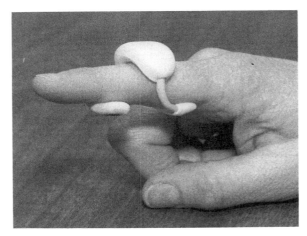

Figure 28.26.   Finger extension spring splint.

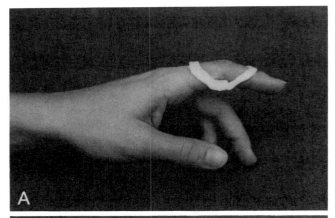

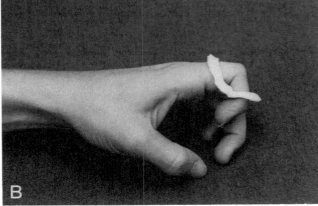

Figure 28.27.   Finger splint for swan neck deformity. **A,** Prevents hyperextension of proximal interphalangeal joint. **B,** Allows flexion.

however, that these types of **splints** must be carefully monitored, because they may produce too much torque to the joints, resulting in further injury and deformity (Fess, 1988).

Static PIP extension block **splints,** designed by Hollis (Fess, Gettle, & Strickland, 1981), are easily constructed from bits of thermoplastic splinting material to prevent or correct swan neck deformity, because the **splint** will prevent PIP hyperextension (Fig. 28.27). In a study by McPhee (1987), patients adapted to the **splint** because of its small size; this type of **splint** does not impede hand function. Extension block **splints** can also be purchased commercially. When used on the PIP and DIP joints (Fig. 28.28), the commercially available **splint** provides lateral stability and joint protection during activity.

Static PIP flexion block **splints** (Fig. 28.29) are easily constructed out of thermoplastic material. These **splints** prevent boutonniere deformity, which is a rupture of the central extensor tendon over the PIP joint (Hunter et al., 1990). A position of PIP flexion and DIP extension results. The finger is splinted with PIP extension, leaving the DIP joint free for flexion exercises.

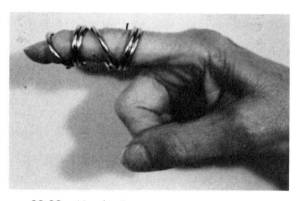

Figure 28.28. Murphy rings.

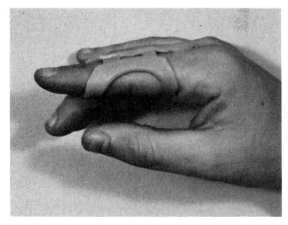

Figure 28.29. Thermoplastic PIP flexion block splint.

A foot-drop **splint** is used when a person with a neurologic or orthopedic condition is confined to bed and lacks the ability to keep his feet dorsiflexed (Seligman & Burack, 1989). This **splint** prevents development of plantar flexion contractures that are detrimental to future ambulation. Foot-drop **splints** are made to hold the foot perpendicular to the leg, as if the patient were standing upright. Adjustable **splints** made of aluminum, with and without foam lining, are commercially available (Fig. 28.30).

ORTHOSES TO RESTORE FUNCTION

Orthoses that assist weak muscles or substitute for absent motor power may enable functional activities to be performed more easily by the patient.

Distal Function: Hand Splints

The following dynamic **splints** have been selected to illustrate orthoses used to assist weakness and increase strength. Assistance may be given to a motion by use of rubber bands that are adjusted to complete the motion after the patient has moved as far as he can. Assistance can also be provided by use of springs or coiled wire. The weak muscle is strengthened by actively moving the part as far as it can before the assisting mechanism completes the motion. The therapist needs to realize that opposing muscles may be strengthened at the same time, because they are required to work against the elastic, wires, or springs. Corrective **splints,** described earlier, may be used alternatively to assist weak muscles. For example, a spring safety pin **splint,** described above to correct a PIP flexion contracture, could be used to assist weak extensor movement.

A long opponens hand **splint** with action wrist and dorsiflexion assist (Fig. 28.31) is a dorsal **splint** that supports the thumb and assists the weak wrist

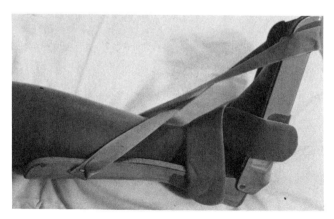

Figure 28.30. Southpaw flex splint, an adjustable ankle dorsiflexion splint.

extensors via the rubber band that extends from the proximal band of the **splint** to the hand piece.

The wrist-hand **orthosis** with metacarpophalangeal extension assist (Fig. 28.32) is used for radial nerve injuries, commonly referred to as wrist-drop, or following tendon transfers (Colditz, 1987). The **splint** supports the wrist in extension and the thumb in abduction and extension; it assists weak MP extension while allowing finger flexion. The MP extension assist is a dorsal outrigger from which cuffs are suspended via rubber bands to support the fingers individually. The pull of the rubber bands must be perpendicular to the proximal phalanx so the full benefit is applied to moving the finger around the axis of the joint and not to traction or compression of the joint. The tension of the rubber bands is adjusted to complete the extension motion while allowing the patient actively to extend and flex to his limits. This orthotic design may also be used to increase range of motion of the fingers when there is a

flexor contracture by increasing the tension of the rubber bands to stretch the fingers into extension. Lucas (1988) designed an alternative one-piece design **splint** that uses a roll of **splint** material as the pulley.

For the metacarpophalangeal stop or lumbrical bar (Fig. 28.33), the bar is attached to a hand **splint** dorsally and exerts a force over the proximal phalanges to hold the MP joints into slight flexion (Tenney & Lisak, 1986). The force of the extensor digitorum is thereby transferred to the interphalangeal joints. For these reasons, this bar prevents the development of claw hand deformity (intrinsic-minus hand) that is the result of absent interossei and lumbricales. The bar can be constructed to exert the force against all or selected fingers. It may be used in conjunction with DIP extension outriggers and/or thumb abduction-extension assist.

The MP extension assist with thumb abduction and extension assist (Fig. 28.34) is used for a low radial nerve injury (i.e., one in which the patient still has control of wrist extension). It allows active grasp of objects and assists release.

Permanent Functional Orthoses

Residual weakness of the upper extremity that results in an inability to move the limb effectively to orient the hand to objects or an inability to pinch or grasp an object can be partially compensated for by the use of permanent orthoses. For a permanent **orthosis** to be useful to the patient, he must accept it, value it, and incorporate it into his body image. A prime prerequisite to acceptance is that the device allow the patient to do something he wants to do that he cannot do without the **orthosis** (Long & Schutt, 1986; Nichols et al., 1978; Yasuda, Bowman, & Hsu, 1986). Other

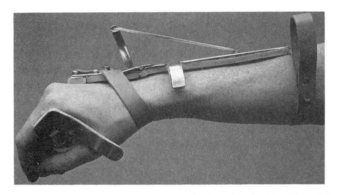

Figure 28.31. Long opponens wrist-hand orthosis with wrist extension assist.

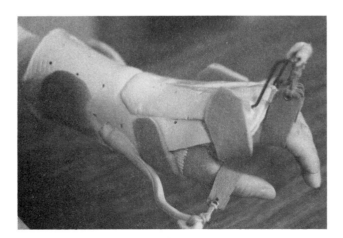

Figure 28.32. Wrist-hand orthosis with metacarpophalangeal stop or lumbrical bar.

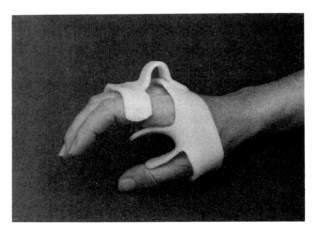

Figure 28.33. Lumbrical bar attached to short opponens splint.

factors that influence the acceptance are mechanical reliability, cosmesis, ease of application and control, and thorough training to the point of automatic control.

The principles of orthotic training are borrowed from the field of prosthetics and include checkout of the fit and mechanical aspects of the **orthosis;** instruction in the names of the parts; care of the **orthosis** and how to put it on and remove it; controls training; and use training. Intensive practice under various conditions is an essential aspect of the training.

FLEXOR HINGE HAND SPLINTS

Palmar prehension, or three-jaw chuck prehension, is provided by flexor hinge hand **splints** by these three factors: (1) the thumb is posted into a position of abduction and partial opposition; (2) the MP and interphalangeal joints of the thumb are posted into extension; and (3) the index and middle fingers are splinted into a semiflexed position so that when the mechanical joint at the MP joint flexes, the pads of the fingers meet the pad of the thumb (Fig. 28.35). If the wrist is included in the **splint,** it is usually held in about 15° of dorsiflexion.

The power for the pinching motion of the fingers is supplied by power from the person's remaining musculature, which is mechanically harnessed. If that is not possible, an external power source, such as a motor, carbon dioxide artificial muscle, or electric stimulation, is used.

Finger-driven Flexor Hinge Hand Splint

For the patient who has active flexion of the ring and/or little fingers, prehension is powered by these fingers. Prehension is accomplished by the force obtained when the patient presses down on a rod that extends from the middle and index fingers to under the ring and little fingers. When the patient wants to pinch, he flexes the ulnar fingers, and the bar transfers this power to the radial fingers. If the patient lacks active extension, a spring can be added to pull the fingers away from the thumb. This **splint** may be a hand **splint** only or may also incorporate the wrist, to which it would give static support.

Checkout involves inspection of the **splint** both on and off the patient for proper construction and fit. The criteria of fit outlined in Chapter 29 apply to these hand **splints.** In addition, the mechanism must operate smoothly and allow pinch of thin flat objects as well as large objects. The joint of the **splint** must exactly coincide with the axis of the patient's second MP joint. Straps and fastenings must facilitate independent application and removal.

The patient will probably be able to apply and remove his own hand **splint** and should practice this until he is able to do so in less than 1 min. Speed is important because the **splint** impedes some tasks, such as propelling a wheelchair; and unless it can be quickly put on and off as needed, it will be discarded as just one more hindrance (Nichols et al., 1978).

Controls training teaches the patient to pick up, move, and release objects of different sizes, textures, weights, and crushability. Firm objects of about 1 inch (2.5 cm) in circumference and with semirough texture are easiest to handle. As the patient's skill increases, objects are graded in size, smoothness, flatness, and fragility. Marshmallows, paper cups, fresh jelly donuts, playing cards, coins, pencils, and metal or glass objects are all challenges. For a person with a posted thumb

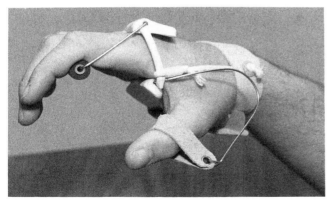

Figure 28.34. Wire-Foam metacarpophalangeal extension spring with thumb abduction extension assist.

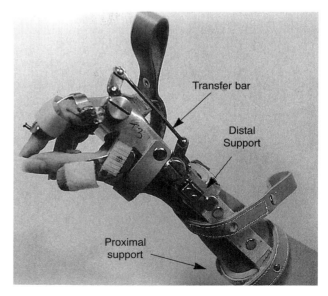

Figure 28.35. Wrist-driven flexor hinge hand splint.

to pick up flat objects, the objects must be pushed so that they partially overhang the table or must be placed on a soft surface, such as a sheet of foam rubber, to allow the thumb to get under the object. Tip prehension, which the **splint** does not provide, is normally used to pick up these types of things. The absence of active wrist motion in a **splint** requires that the patient compensatorily abduct and internally rotate at the shoulder to pick something up. If the patient has proprioceptive feedback along with the fine control of the extrinsic hand muscles, controls training will be rapidly accomplished.

Use training involves a systematic trial of occupational performance tasks to discover which require the **splint,** how these tasks may best be accomplished, and if metal or glass objects need to be coated or covered to provide friction. If slipping of objects is a frequent problem it is preferable to have the patient wear a large-size secretary's rubber finger cover over the thumb post to provide friction. The maximal weight of any object that can be lifted will depend both on the strength of pinch and the strength of the proximal extremity. A pinch meter that records in ounces (grams) is used to measure amount of pinch possible when using a prehension **splint.**

Wrist-driven Flexor Hinge Hand Splint (Tenodesis)

In a wrist-driven flexor hinge hand **splint,** the thumb is posted and the radial fingers are splinted as described above. In addition to the joint located at the patient's second MP joint to allow finger flexion, there is also a joint located at the exact axis of the wrist on the radial side to allow wrist movement. The proximal and distal supports can be fabricated in an under-over position (Fig. 28.35) or in an over-over position, where both the proximal and distal supports are on the dorsal

side of the forearm (Fig. 28.36). The C_6 tetraplegic patient who has active wrist extension can pinch using this **splint,** because the power of wrist extension is transferred to prehension through a power transfer bar. This **splint** augments the natural tenodesis grasp the patient has and enlarges his scope of abilities. In a properly adjusted **splint,** the wrist:pinch strength ratio is 2:1. A more cost-effective **orthosis** is the RIC tenodesis **orthosis** (Fig. 28.37), which is quickly fabricated for use in early tenodesis training (Hill, 1986).

Using the tenodesis **splint,** the patient must abduct and internally rotate his shoulder to approach an object on a table properly. Ratchet-type mechanisms are available that lock the **splint** into position to relieve the patient of the necessity of maintaining active wrist extension during holding (McKenzie, 1973). The ratchet mechanism is released by pressure. Some C_5 tetraplegic patients who cannot actively use a wrist-driven flexor hinge hand **splint** because they lack active wrist extension use a ratchet **splint** in preference to an externally powered **splint** (McKenzie, 1973). They passively engage the mechanism by pushing their wrist into extension against their body, wheelchair, or a table. The mechanism remains locked in that position until the release push button is depressed (Fig. 28.38).

The checkout procedure for a wrist-driven flexor hinge hand **splint** is the same as described above for the finger-driven flexor hinge hand **splint,** with the addition of checking the exactness of the location of the wrist joint axis. The strength of pinch is also measured, because the length of the transfer bar can be changed by the orthotist to increase the strength of pinch if this is necessary (Stenehjem, Swenson, & Sprague, 1983). The patient must learn to put on and remove this hand **splint** rapidly for the same reasons as stated for the finger-driven flexor hinge hand **splint.**

Controls and use training are also the same as described above, although patients using this type of **splint** will require more practice, because the patient

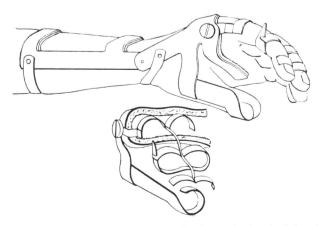

Figure 28.36. Flexor hinge hand splint with detail of thumb post and finger piece.

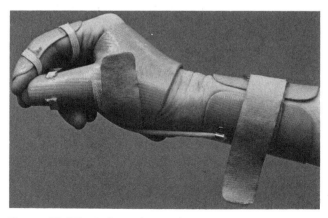

Figure 28.37. RIC tenodesis orthosis.

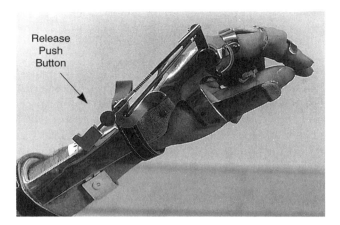

Figure 28.38. Ratchet orthosis.

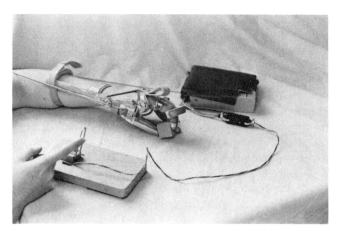

Figure 28.39. Demonstration of microswitch control of externally powered (motor) flexor hinge hand splint. A fingertip's pressure is sufficient to activate the switch, which would be mounted where the patient could voluntarily control it.

who uses this **splint** usually lacks sensory feedback from the fingers. Also, the patient must learn how to orient the **splint** to approach objects of different shapes and must practice until this becomes automatic.

Externally Powered Flexor Hinge Hand Splint

For the externally powered flexor hinge hand **splint,** the **splint** is the same as that used for the wrist-driven flexor hinge hand **splint** with these exceptions: The wrist joint is fixed at about 15 to 20° of dorsiflexion, there is no transfer bar, a short bar extends from the finger piece to allow distal attachment of the external power mechanism, and a spring provides motion of the radial fingers in one direction, usually extension. Because the power source is located outside the patient's body, the learning process for the patient is complicated by the need to learn to control switches, valves, or other transducers to operate the power source. Power to drive hand **splints** can be obtained from any of the following methods.

1. *A small rotary motor that runs forward, backward, and holds when stopped.* One end of a cable is attached to the motor and the other end of the cable is attached to the bar that extends from the finger piece of the **splint** (Fig. 28.39). As the cable is pulled in by the motor, the fingers are flexed and pinch against the thumb. As the cable is reeled out, the spring pulls the fingers into extension. The patient can control the extent of the opening by turning the motor on and off more or less quickly. Some motors are proportional and operate fast or slow, depending on the force the patient exerts on the control switch. The control switch itself can be mounted wherever the patient can access it, using whatever available musculature he has for operation.

2. *Electrical stimulation of one of a patient's muscles over which he has no control* (Long & Masciarelli,

1963). When the electrical stimulation is on, the muscle contracts, and when the stimulation ceases the muscle relaxes. The opposite motion, usually flexion, is accomplished by a spring. Originally, this type of **splint** seemed to have limited value for tetraplegics, because the stimulated muscle rapidly fatigued. This fatigue phenomenon occurred when the finger extensor muscles were repetitively stimulated with enough voltage to overcome the strong pull of the spring that is needed for the pinch used in daily tasks (3 to 4 pounds) and these muscles lost their ability to continue to contract. Stimulating the flexor muscles instead of the extensor was not a satisfactory solution; fatigue developed because of the prolonged tetany needed for maintained holding. This problem seems to have been overcome by using a program of electrically induced exercise to hypertrophy the muscles and by using a sequential stimulation technique. Contractions that are strong, fatigue-resistant and smooth and have controllable strength have been produced (Peckham & Mortimer, 1977).

3. *An artificial muscle made of a tubular, helically woven nylon sleeve covering a leakproof rubber bladder* (Fig. 28.40). When gas (carbon dioxide) is allowed to flow into the bladder it enlarges as a balloon would; however, the constraint of the helical weave of the sleeve causes the ends of the "muscle" to move closer together as the circumference increases. When the gas is released, the "muscle" gets thin and long again. A Chinese finger trap operates on the same principle. The end of the muscle is attached to the finger piece and causes the fingers to flex when it is distended, while a spring causes extension when the tension in the muscle is reduced.

The control transducer of the externally powered

splint is operated by a part of the patient's body over which he has voluntary control, where he has normal sensation, and which does not activate the transducer accidentally during habitual motions. For a C_4 tetraplegic this means upper trapezius-, tongue-, or chin-operated controls. If shoulder elevation is to be used, the opposite shoulder is usually chosen to reduce the likelihood of associated unintentional activation. The C_5 tetraplegic may use upper trapezius, deltoids, or biceps of the opposite extremity. Spotty muscle weakness such as occurs in polio may preserve control sites in the lower extremities if none exist in the upper body.

The motor can be controlled by microswitches that require about 1 ounce of pressure to activate (Fig. 28.39). These microswitches may be mounted over the patient's shoulder so he can elevate or retract the shoulder to touch and activate them (Fig. 28.41), near his face so his tongue can press them, in a joystick arrangement that can be controlled by the chin pushing on the stick, in a figure-of-eight harness configuration so that scapular protraction activates it (Long & Schutt, 1986), or in any other position where the patient can exert voluntary pressure. The microswitches must be mounted so that the patient can activate two switches—

forward and reverse—for each motor. The motor also can be controlled by myoelectric signals that when amplified can electronically switch the motor (Silverstein, French, & Siebens, 1974; Trombly, Prentke, & Long, 1967). The electrical activity of the voluntarily contracting control muscle is picked up using surface electrodes. Forward and reverse directions of the motor are achieved by using a low-amplitude signal to switch forward and a high-amplitude signal to switch backward or vice versa instead of using two muscles. A protocol for determination of suitable controller muscles has been published (Rudin et al., 1987). Voice activation of the motor is a possible, but as yet unreliable, method of control, because extraneous noise also activates the motor.

In electrical stimulation **splints,** the flow of electrical stimulation can be controlled by myoelectric signals, by a potentiometer (an electrical component that increases or decreases the resistance to the flow of electricity as the armature is moved), or by a switch. The switch or potentiometer can be arranged so it can be controlled by shoulder elevation or any other movement the patient can control.

The artificial muscle (also known as the McKibben muscle after the physicist who invented it) is controlled by a three-position valve: When the stem of the valve is pushed all the way in, the gas flows to activate the muscle; when released, the valve holds the gas in place, and the fingers remain in whatever position they were (Fig. 28.42). When the stem of the valve is pushed halfway in, the gas is allowed to escape, which deflates the muscle. The gas can be allowed to escape in short, quick spurts, thus opening the fingers a little at a time; this is called feathering the valve.

Checkout of externally powered hand **splints** involves all that was discussed for the flexor hinge hand

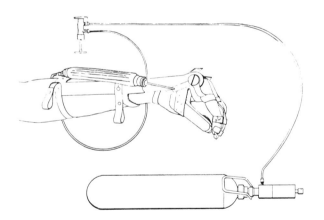

Figure 28.40. Artificial muscle–driven flexor hinge hand splint.

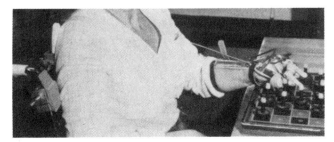

Figure 28.41. Microswitch activation of motor-driven flexor hinge hand splint via retraction of the opposite shoulder.

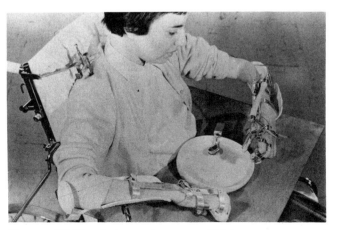

Figure 28.42. Patient using an artificial muscle–powered flexor hinge hand splint on the left hand with control valve mounted over right shoulder, activated by scapular elevation.

splints. In addition, the reliability of the control mechanism must be carefully checked: The signal used to close the **splint** must always close the **splint** and always work with the same amount of pressure of the control site. If the cable is too short or the spring too forceful, pinching thin objects (paper) will be prevented and the cable or spring will need adjustment. Adjustments would need to be made also if large (2-inch) items could not be grasped. A stop can be incorporated into this **splint** to prevent excessive pressure on the fingertips in the closed position; however, it should still allow the patient to hold paper or playing cards.

Rarely will a patient who needs this type of **splint** be able to put it on and off by himself. However, he should be able to instruct another clearly and should receive supervised practice in giving this instruction. He must also instruct others in the care and recharging of the power unit. Battery-powered **splints** (motor and electrical stimulation) can be charged overnight using the charger that comes with the unit. The CO_2 gas bottle refill may need to be obtained from the orthotist; fire station supply houses have CO_2 and often are willing to fill the empty bottle using the proper adapter obtained from the orthotist. A full 12-inch bottle of CO_2 lasts about 3 weeks if the **splint** is opened and closed once every 5 min, 8 hours per day. This amount of use is rare, because the **splint** is opened and closed once to grasp something that is then usually held; no gas is used during the holding phase.

CARE AND TRAINING

All hand **splints** should be treated like fine jewelry: washed, polished, and stored where they cannot be bent or misaligned. An out-of-kilter hand **splint** can cause decubitus ulcers and can exert undesired forces on the joints.

Controls training must be thoroughly completed before use training is attempted, to decrease the inevitable frustration. Controls training begins with observation of the effect of the control motion on the hand **splint** (Trombly, 1966, 1968). The hand **splint** may be on the patient's hand, but if it cannot be seen easily, the **splint** is best mounted some other place so the patient can watch it while simultaneously feeling his controlling movement. Electronic feedback devices are helpful adjuncts to training (Seeger, Caudrey, & McAllister, 1985). Once the effect of the control motion is learned, the patient begins the same practice of picking up, moving, and releasing various objects as described above. A good test of the patient's ability to automatically control the **splint** is to have him pick up, on signal, a cube that has been placed on a premarked spot and to release it into a small box placed 6 to 8 inches away. The time in tenths of

seconds is recorded. This is repeated 20 or so times during each training session. The mean and the standard deviation are computed (Table 29.1). A low standard deviation indicates consistency of operation, a sign of skill. Tasks attempted during use training will be limited by the patient's disability. Adaptations beyond the **orthosis** will probably be necessary to accomplish these, and the reader is referred to Chapter 39 for specifics.

Proximal Function

The suspension sling (Fig. 28.1) can be adjusted to assist certain movements of the upper extremities. Remember that whenever a motion is assisted, its opposite is resisted. For example, the patient must have relatively strong shoulder horizontal abductor muscles if the suspension sling is adjusted to assist weak shoulder horizontal adductors. Motions that can be assisted using an overhead suspension sling are shoulder horizontal abduction and adduction, shoulder external and internal rotation, shoulder abduction, and elbow flexion and extension. Adjustments to assist weak muscles in shoulder motions are made to parts of the suspension sling as follows.

Motion Assisted by Suspension Sling	Adjustment
Horizontal abduction	The overhead rod is rotated laterally, i.e., the top part of the rod is turned out away from the patient, which carries the suspended arm out toward horizontal abduction
Horizontal adduction	The overhead rod is rotated medially, i.e., the top part of the rod is turned in toward the patient; the suspended arm is thereby carried in toward horizontal adduction.
Abduction	The distance between the spring and the overhead rod is shortened to pull the arm into abduction.

Some adjustments are made by moving the position of the cuffs on the balance bar.

Motion Assisted by Suspension Sling	Adjustment
External rotation	The cuffs are moved back on the bar to shift the weight toward the elbow
Internal rotation	The cuffs are moved forward on the balance bar to shift the weight toward the hand

Adjustments for elbow motions are as follows:

Motion Assisted by Suspension Sling	Adjustment
Flexion	The point of suspension is moved backward on the overhead rod, which puts the hand back toward the patient's face
Extension	The point of suspension is moved forward on the overhead rod, which puts the hand out away from the patient's face

Each adjustment is made in as small an increment as is necessary to assist the patient's motion. Similar adjustments can be made when using the Swedish Aid (Fig. 28.2).

Mobile Arm Supports

The term **mobile arm supports** (MAS), once inclusive of suspension **arm slings** and feeders, now refers only to feeders. Their former name was ball-bearing forearm orthoses (BFO), and are also referred to as ball-bearing feeders or ball-bearing feeder orthoses. MAS are frictionless arm supports that are usually mounted on a wheelchair but also may extend from a waist belt for ambulatory patients or attach to a table by a clamp mechanism (Fig. 28.43). They use the principle of the inclined plane in which gravity causes movement when something is inclined away from horizontal. They assist weak shoulder and elbow muscles to place the hand in space as needed. Adjustments are made individually to tailor the assistance of the MAS for each person's disability.

The neutral setup and adjustments for a Rancho Los Amigos type **mobile arm support** are described here. The Georgia Warm Springs feeder (Fig. 28.44) is very similar to the Rancho one (Fig. 28.45), with

two exceptions: the proximal ball-bearing wheelchair bracket assembly and the rocker arm assembly. The bracket of the Georgia Warm Springs feeder is adjustable and the rocker arm assembly is offset, which allows unimpeded vertical motions. The Michigan feeder (Fig. 28.46) allows more precise adjustment of the position of the proximal ball-bearing and the rocker assembly. The Michigan rocker assembly allows adjustment in the Z coordinate of movement (up and down), which allows the therapist to match the axis of the motion of the forearm trough to the exact axis of the bulk of the forearm, thereby enabling a weaker patient to use the feeder effectively.

The principles of setup and balancing described below apply generally to all designs of **mobile arm supports,** although the exact methods of adjusting the pieces are slightly different. Neutral setup of the MAS is sufficient for the patient who has generalized, balanced weakness throughout the upper extremity. Modi-

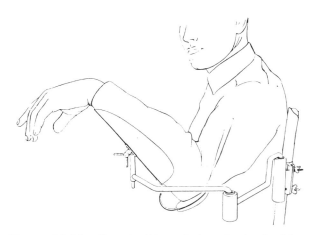

Figure 28.44. Georgia Warm Springs feeder (mobile arm support).

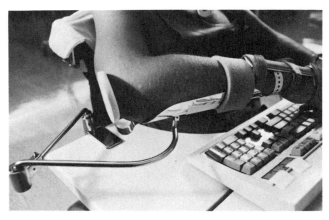

Figure 28.43. Mobile arm support temporarily clamped to a table.

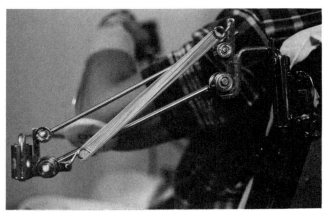

Figure 28.45. Rancho mobile arm support with optional elevating arm.

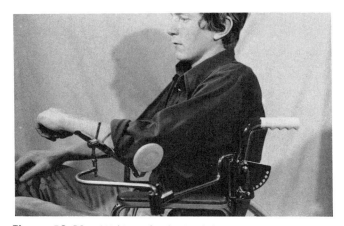

Figure 28.46. Michigan feeder (mobile arm support).

fications of this neutral setup must be made for patients with other patterns of weakness. Many therapists prefer to adjust the MAS initially into neutral position before proceeding to make modifications in the balance as required by the patient's particular pattern of weakness. A properly balanced MAS will hold the forearm in a position of 45° from the horizontal and the upper arm in approximately 45° of combined shoulder abduction and flexion, without any effort on the patient's part.

For MAS to be fitted to the patient, he ought to be able to sit for 1 hour. The Rancho assembly requires that the patient sit upright, whereas the Georgia Warm Springs or Michigan types allow 5 to 10° of recline of the wheelchair back. The patient must have good lateral trunk stability, which may be provided by corsets, seat adaptations, braces, or restraints, if he does not have it actively. MAS cannot be used in bed or when the patient is semireclined in his wheelchair. He can use suspension slings in these positions, however.

The patient must have some source of power to operate the MAS, although some external power can be added for very weak patients. If the patient is too weak to operate a MAS, the alternative is use of environmental control units (Long & Schutt, 1986; Warren & Enders, 1986). Passive range of motion (PROM) must be within normal limits to obtain the most benefit from the MAS. Limited range of motion combined with very limited strength precludes the use of feeders in most cases (Yasuda et al., 1986). Incoordination and poor head or trunk control are contraindications for the use of MAS.

If the patient wears a hand **splint,** this is put on before beginning to balance the feeders. MAS are applied bilaterally, one at a time. All screws, nuts, etc. must be secured to prevent slipping of the MAS while the patient is attempting to use it, even during fitting.

Parts, Functions, and Adjustments of Mobile Arm Supports

Ball-bearing Feeder Bracket Assembly

The bracket is the piece that attaches to the wheelchair upright (Fig. 28.47). The ball-bearing assembly is the piece that fits into the bracket and holds the proximal ball-bearing rings. There are right and left assemblies; the bevel for the screw head indicates the back of the bracket. It may be necessary to put tape on the wheelchair upright before applying the bracket to prevent the bracket from slipping down the smooth wheelchair upright under the weight of the patient's arm.

This assembly determines the height of the feeder in relation to the patient's body. The neutral position is set at a height equal to midhumerus. Raise the assembly to enable the patient to get his hand to his mouth or for the elbow dial of the trough to clear the **lapboard.** Lower the bracket if the patient's shoulders are pushed into elevation. The height of the patient's seat cushion affects this setting. This assembly holds the proximal swivel arm. To prevent pushing the bottom ball-bearing ring out, be sure that the proximal arm is pushed all the way down so that the first 90° angle of the proximal arm rests against the top of the assembly. This assembly also determines the horizontal motion at the shoulder. Neutral is when the ball bearing is

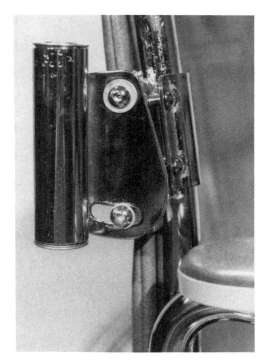

Figure 28.47. Ball-bearing feeder bracket assembly (Rancho type).

perpendicular to the floor so that the proximal arm, when inserted, falls neither forward nor backward. Move the bracket out (posteriorly around the wheelchair upright) to assist horizontal abduction; move it in (anteriorly around the upright) to assist horizontal adduction.

Proximal Swivel Arm

The proximal swivel arm permits humeral motion (Fig. 28.48). The distal ball bearing is located at the end of the proximal swivel arm to hold the distal swivel arm. The distal ball bearing may be angled down to assist elbow extension or upward to assist elbow flexion. The patient's permanent feeders will be angled by the orthotist; there is an adjustable proximal arm available for trial purposes (Figs. 28.43 and 28.49). The proximal arms are interchangeable, unless adapted, in which case the right and left ones must be marked.

Elevating Proximal Arm

The elevating proximal arm (Fig. 28.45) is a component that may be selected in lieu of the standard proximal arm. This component is used to assist a weak $(F-)$ deltoid. Strong rubber bands assist the weak deltoid muscle to abduct and flex the shoulder, thus allowing the hand to be brought toward the head. Rubber bands can be added or subtracted to increase or decrease the assistance.

Distal Swivel Arm

The distal swivel arm (Figs. 28.43 and 28.50) corresponds to the forearm; it permits elbow motion in the horizontal plane. It supports the rocker arm assembly and feeder trough. Right and left distal swivel arms

differ; to distinguish them, hold the solid end in your hand, the arm should angle in toward you in both cases (R or L). The hollow post at the distal end of the arm may need to be cut lower if the patient is having trouble inwardly rotating. The curvature of the distal arm occasionally may need to be different from standard for a particular patient to allow the elbow dial of the trough to clear the distal arm during vertical motion. The orthotist will do this. Be sure the patient is using a proper motion pattern before you take the problem to the orthotist. The length of the distal arm, like the proximal arm, is standard; however, an unusually small or large patient may need special length arms. When fitted correctly, the distal ball bearing would be located directly opposite the patient's elbow.

Post

The post (Fig. 28.51) provides added height at the distal end of the distal arm for specific activities. This part must be added by another person whenever it is needed; therefore, an effort should be made to balance the feeders without using this. If one must be used permanently, the orthotist can make the permanent post of the distal arm higher to alleviate the need for this piece.

Horizontal Stop

The horizontal stop (Figs. 28.45 and 28.52) limits horizontal motion to within the patient's controllable limits. The horizontal stop can also be used to transfer motion from the shoulder to the elbow by applying it at the proximal ball bearing to prevent horizontal abduction; this will result in elbow extension when the patient attempts horizontal abduction. If the patient lacks shoulder power, it can be used to transfer power

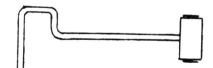

Figure 28.48. Proximal swivel arm.

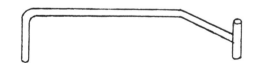

Figure 28.50. Distal swivel arm (left).

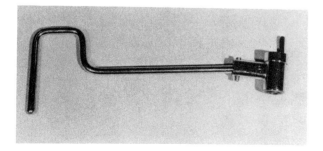

Figure 28.49. Adjustable type proximal swivel arm.

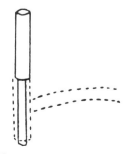

Figure 28.51. The post.

proximally by applying it at the distal ball bearing. The horizontal stop is usually applied to the ball bearing on the outside to limit horizontal abduction or extension rather than inside to limit adduction or flexion. Neutral setup is no stop used.

Rocker Arm Assemblies

Five rocker arm assemblies are described here. Any one of these may be used on any MAS setup.

1. The Rancho type (Figs. 28.43 and 28.53) permits vertical motion of the feeder trough. It swivels to produce added horizontal motion at the elbow. Right and left are indistinguishable. The trough is attached to this part, which is inserted into the distal end of the distal swivel arm.

2. The Georgia Warm Springs type (Fig. 28.54) provides an offset that permits the elbow dial of the trough to clear the distal arm. The functions listed for the Rancho type are also offered. The right and left differ; when inserted into the distal arm, the assembly should angle toward the patient.

3. The Michigan type (Figs. 28.46 and 28.55) allows, in addition to the features of the Rancho and Georgia Warm Springs types, adjustment in the Z axis (vertical), thus allowing the pivot point to be located directly opposite the center of mass of the forearm. A weak patient is more easily able to use this type.

4. The modular adjustment mechanism (Fig. 28.56) improves on the Rancho type assembly by alleviating the need for unscrewing the assembly when making proximal and distal adjustments on the trough (Drew & Stern, 1979).

5. The supinator assist (Fig. 28.57) is a special rocker arm assembly that provides mechanical supination: humeral external rotation during flexion and reciprocal pronation (internal rotation) during extension. The amount of supination-pronation can be controlled by limiting the length of the wire loop. The supinator assist can be mounted in lieu of a Rancho or offset

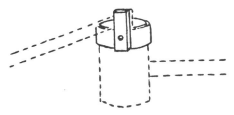

Figure 28.52. The horizontal stop.

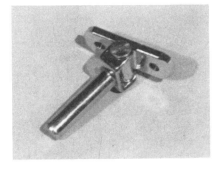

Figure 28.53. Rancho type rocker arm assembly.

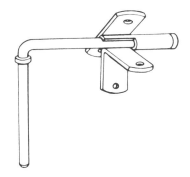

Figure 28.54. Georgia Warm Springs type offset rocker arm assembly.

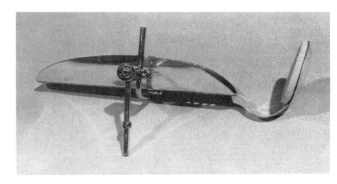

Figure 28.55. Michigan type rocker arm assembly attached to trough.

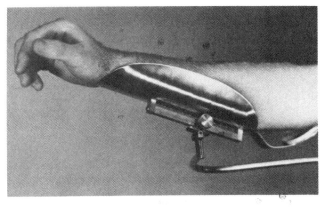

Figure 28.56. Modular adjustment mechanism attached to Rancho type rocker arm assembly. In this photograph the trough is too long for the person (see text).

rocker assembly. Right and left differ; the wire loop is on the side toward the patient.

Vertical Stop

The vertical stop (Fig. 28.58) is attached to the offset rocker assembly to limit vertical motion. It keeps the motion within the controllable limits of the patient. It may be used to limit both up and down motions or only one or the other by adjusting the screws. The neutral setup is with no stop.

Troughs

The trough supports the forearm. Two types are described.

1. In the trough with elbow dial (Figs. 28.43 and 28.59), the length of the trough is 2 inches less than the distance from the olecranon to the head of the ulna so that motion at the wrist is not be impeded. The distal lip is flared so it does not limit circulation in the patient's hand. It is possible to adjust the location of the trough on the rocker assembly to assist either internal rotation (hand heavy—move the trough forward on the rocker assembly) or external rotation (elbow heavy—move the trough backward on the rocker assembly). For neutral setting, set the trough on the rocker assembly so that the forearm rests at an angle of 45° in relation to the **lapboard.** The elbow dial can be bent forward or backward to provide fine adjustment to assist internal or external rotation. The dial offers good, stable elbow support, although it restricts some elbow extension in the process. However, this does not limit function significantly. To accommodate right and left arms, the dials are angled in slightly toward the patient.

2. The flying saucer feeder trough (Fig. 28.60) supports the forearm. It is used in cases in which the patient has active elbow flexion and external rotation of the humerus and does not need the vertical motion. This part supplants the distal arm, the trough, and the rocker arm assembly.

Once the MAS is assembled, always mark the location of pieces in relation to one another before making changes during the balancing so that it is easy to return to the previous position, which may prove to be the better adjustment after all. When the MAS is finally balanced, erase all extraneous marks and remark all final positions, in case the MAS are knocked out of adjustment and need to be rebalanced. Be sure all screws are tight.

Movement Patterns and Equipment Adjustments to Achieve Motion in Mobile Arm Supports

It is preferable to instruct the patient in movement patterns to achieve certain motions in the neutrally adjusted **mobile arm supports.** However, as is fre-

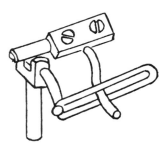

Figure 28.57. Supinator assist.

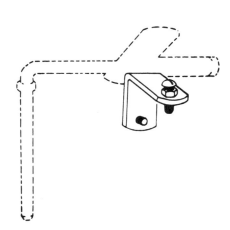

Figure 28.58. Vertical stop.

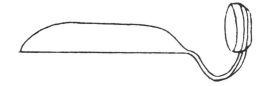

Figure 28.59. Forearm trough with elbow dial.

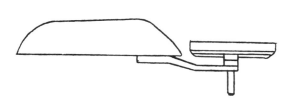

Figure 28.60. Flying saucer forearm trough for feeder. This replaces the distal arm, the trough, and the rocker arm assembly.

quently the case, the patient may be too weak to be able to do these motions. In that case the equipment can be adjusted to assist the motions that are weakest. It is not advisable to require the patient to practice the motions a long time before making the equipment adjustments, because he will become discouraged and may reject the **orthosis.** The movement patterns and the equipment adjustments are not listed here in any order of preference. One motion, or one adjustment, may be all that is necessary; or for greater effect, a combination of two or more motions, two or more adjustments, or a combination of a motion plus an adjustment may be necessary for the extremely weak patient. Use only the movement patterns and adjustments that are completely safe for the patient, use the least energy, most nearly approximate normal or acceptable movement, and are most effective. The process of discovery of the correct combination is one of trial and error. The patient should not be allowed to become fatigued in the process, however, because fatigue invalidates the adjustments. The movement patterns listed below are adapted from a manual once available from Georgia Warm Springs Rehabilitation Center. The instructions should be worded to suit the level of patient understanding.

DESIRED MOTION: HAND TO MOUTH

Instructions for movement patterns
1. Depress your shoulder while adducting your humerus.
2. Externally rotate your shoulder.
3. Shift your body weight toward the side that the MAS you want to move is on [only if the patient has enough strength to regain balance].
4. Straighten up or lean back in the chair.
5. Rotate your trunk toward the side that the MAS that you want to move is on.
6. Turn your head toward the MAS that you want to move.
7. Press the elbow dial against a friction pad placed on the **lapboard** near the waist by depressing your scapula. This may cause enough supination to aim the eating utensil toward your mouth.

Equipment adjustment
1. Move the rocker assembly forward on trough [make it elbow heavy].
2. Turn the ball-bearing bracket assembly toward the patient.
3. Adjust the proximal swivel arm up.
4. Position the anterior vertical stop to decrease internal rotation.
5. Raise the ball-bearing bracket assembly on the wheelchair upright.
6. Adapt the utensil's length or angle.

7. Raise the trough by use of a post.
8. Lower the posterior vertical stop under the trough to permit additional shoulder external rotation.

DESIRED MOTION: HAND TO TABLE

Instructions for movement patterns
1. Elevate and internally rotate your shoulder to lower the hand.
2. Roll the shoulder forward, which encourages horizontal adduction with shoulder flexion, internal rotation, and elbow extension.
3. Shift your body weight to the side opposite from the MAS that you want to move [if the patient has enough strength to regain balance].
4. Rotate your trunk toward the side opposite from the MAS that you want to move.
5. Tilt or turn your head away from the MAS that you want to move.

Equipment adjustment
1. Move the rocker assembly farther back on the trough [make it hand heavy].
2. Turn the ball-bearing bracket assembly backward, away from the patient.
3. Adjust the proximal swivel arm down.
4. Position the anterior vertical stop under the trough to allow more elbow extension (internal rotation).
5. Lower the ball-bearing feeder bracket assembly on the wheelchair upright.
6. Lower the trough by removing the post or cutting down the distal channel into which the rocker arm assembly fits.

DESIRED MOTION: HORIZONTAL ABDUCTION

Instructions for movement patterns
1. Shift your body weight toward the side that the **orthosis** you want to move is on.
2. Rotate your trunk toward the side that the **orthosis** you want to move is on.
3. Turn your head briskly toward the **orthosis.**

Equipment adjustment
1. Rotate the ball-bearing bracket assembly on the wheelchair upright backward, away from the individual.
2. Shorten the proximal swivel arm.

DESIRED MOTION: HORIZONTAL ADDUCTION

Instructions for movement pattern
1. Shift your body weight away from the side that the **orthosis** you want to move is on.
2. Rotate your body away from the side that the **orthosis** you want to move is on.

3. Turn your head briskly away from the **orthosis.**

Equipment adjustment

1. Rotate the ball-bearing bracket assembly on the wheelchair upright forward, toward the patient.
2. Lengthen the proximal swivel arm.

CHECKOUT AND TRAINING FOR MOBILE ARM SUPPORTS

The patient will not be able to put on his MAS independently but must instruct others in their proper application. Patients can remove the MAS by lifting their arms slightly, allowing the MAS to move away. The MAS, except for the ball-bearing bracket assembly, is removed when the wheelchair is stored. Care must be taken that the bracket assembly does not get knocked out of alignment when the chair is put into the car or when the patient is wheeled through doorways, because this will change the entire balance of the MAS.

Checkout may be done using Table 28.1. Controls training involves teaching the patient the effects that his trunk, head, and proximal movements will have on the movement of the MAS. The patient learns to control first one feeder, then the other. Both are usually worn for balance, but if the patient is tall and has lateral instability he may be more stable if his nontraining arm is out of the feeder and resting on the **lapboard.**

Controls training begins with having the patient move the MAS as far as he can horizontally from side to side and then from front to back. If the patient needs practice to do these motions effortlessly, then activities such as drawing with felt-tipped pens, turning large magazine pages, playing board games, etc. provide motivation. Next, vertical motions are learned, first out to the side, which is easiest, then in front of the face, and then at any point within horizontal range. Games that require picking up playing pieces and movement in space are motivating to the patient.

Use training is not initiated before the patient has excellent control of the feeders and his hand **splint,** if he has one. Use training activities include feeding, grooming, use of telephone, typewriter, calculators, computers and other electronic devices, page turning, games, possibly writing and drawing, and powered wheelchair mobility skills using a hand drive control.

ORTHOSES TO MODIFY TONE

Through splinting, therapists have implemented the principle of prolonged stretch to reduce spasticity. According to that principle, when a muscle is held in an elongated position, the muscle spindles will be rebiased to a longer length, making them less likely to become activated by small movements. Other treatment principles incorporated into some splinting designs for the spastic patient include neutral warmth or grasp of

Table 28.1. **Checkout Sheet for Mobile Arm Supports**

Patient's Name _____ Type Feeder (R)___

Date Fitted _____ (L)___

I. Patient's position in wheelchair

Yes	No	Is patient able to sit up straight?
Yes	No	Are hips well back in chair?
Yes	No	Is spine in good vertical alignment?
Yes	No	Does patient have lateral trunk stability?
Yes	No	Is chair seat adequate for comfort and stability?
Yes	No	If patient wears hand splints, are they on?
Yes	No	Does patient meet requirements for passive ROM and coordination?

II. Mechanical checkout

Yes	No	Are all screws tight?
Yes	No	Is bracket tight on wheelchair?
Yes	No	Are all joints freely movable?
Yes	No	Is proximal arm all the way down into the bracket?
Yes	No	Is bracket at proper height so shoulders are not forced into elevation?
Yes	No	Does elbow dial clear lapboard when trough is in up position?
Yes	No	Is patient's hand (in up position) as close to mouth as possible?
Yes	No	Can patient obtain maximal active reach?
Yes	No	Is feeder trough short enough to allow wrist flexion or to prevent pressure on blood vessels?
Yes	No	Are trough edges rolled so that they do not contact forearm?
Yes	No	Is elbow secure and comfortable in elbow support?
Yes	No	In vertical motion, does the dial clear the distal arm?

III. Control checkout

Yes	No	Can patient control motion of proximal arm from either extreme?
Yes	No	Can patient control motion of distal arm from either extreme?
Yes	No	Can patient control vertical motion from either extreme?
Yes	No	Have stops been applied to limit range within controllable limits if necessary?

a hard cone to inhibit spasticity (Rood), positioning opposite to patterns of spasticity to inhibit or prevent development of spasticity (Bobath), tactile stimulation of antagonists to facilitate them and reciprocally inhibit the spastic muscles (Rood), and quick stretch to facilitate hypotonic muscles.

Splinting of the spastic hand is controversial. Some therapists choose volar **splints;** others choose dorsal **splints,** fearing the effects of sensory stimulation of the flexor surface and hoping to use the sensory stimulation of the dorsal surface to facilitate extension. In a study of 10 hemiplegic patients, Kaplan (1962) reported increased free range of motion (decreased spasticity) at the wrist and fingers following splinting of the affected arm into maximal extension. The wrist was hyperextended to approximately 90° and the fingers and thumb to 0°. The fingers were adducted. This dorsal **splint,** with textured lining for sensory stimulation, was worn at least 8 hr per day as tolerated by the patient. Another study of 3 hemiparetic subjects found that none of three volar **splints** (resting pan, finger spreader, and hard cone) immediately reduced electromyographic (EMG) activity of flexor muscles of hemiparetic patients (Mathiowetz, Bolding, & Trombly, 1983). The resting-pan **splint** actually produced higher EMG activity than no **splint.**

In a study of 10 subjects with hypertonic wrist flexors, half of whom were assigned to use of a volar resting pan with finger separators and half to a spasticity-reduction **splint** with dorsal forearm piece, static splinting reduced the viscoelastic components of hypertonicity (McPherson et al., 1982), but no measure of the neural component was made. No significant differences were found between the two **splint** styles. Age was found to be an intervening variable: Subjects 35 years old and younger showed a greater change than those 65 years old and older. This study points out that some of the controversy about splinting may reflect differential effects of splinting on the two components of spasticity. Successful reduction of the viscoelastic component without change in the neural component has been reported (Booth, Doyle, & Montgomery, 1983).

Inhibitory splinting can be considered a neurorehabilitation treatment when aimed at the neural component of spasticity. Like other such treatments, it is successful for some and may provide a low-cost, noninvasive treatment method for decreasing upper extremity tone (Langlois, Pederson, & Mackinnon, 1991) but may not be successful with others. Another aspect to consider is carryover of results. One study found immediate reduction in hypertonus of the upper extremity up to 2 hr after removal of **splints** (Rose & Shah, 1987), but the long-term effects of splinting requires further study. Continued research on the effectiveness of splinting for spasticity reduction and the key patient variables that contribute to that effectiveness is needed. Therapists must not assume effectiveness but must carefully monitor the outcome with each patient.

A spastic patient, or potentially spastic patient, if splinted at all, must have a **splint** that incorporates both the wrist and the fingers because, e.g., the effect of splinting one part of the spastic hand in extension is to cause flexion contractures of the unsplinted part.

Splint designs for the hemiplegic hand include the dorsal or volar resting pans (Fig. 28.9), the finger abduction **splint** (Figs. 28.61 and 28.62), the orthokinetic **splint,** and others (Scherling & Johnson, 1989).

The spasticity reduction **splint** (Fig. 28.61) is a variation of the resting-pan **splint** (Snook, 1979). The **splint** is molded to provide 30° of wrist hyperextension; 45° of MP flexion; and full interphalangeal extension, finger abduction, and thumb extension and abduction. This position duplicates a reflex-inhibiting pattern of Bobath. No data on the effectiveness of this **splint** in reducing spasticity have been published.

The finger abduction **splint** for the spastic hand (Fig. 28.62) also uses Bobath's reflex-inhibiting pattern theory. Originally, the **splint** was constructed of a block of foam with holes punched through the foam to allow insertion of the fingers and thumb in an abducted position (Bobath, 1990). A more permanent **splint** has been designed for the same purpose, using low-temperature splinting materials (Doubilet & Polkow,

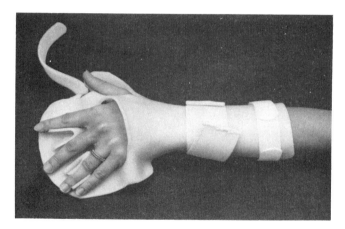

Figure 28.61.   Spasticity reduction splint.

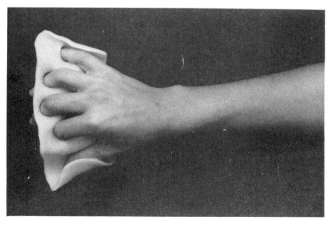

Figure 28.62.   Finger abduction splint for the spastic hand.

1977); a more recent modification prevents MP ulnar drift (Woodson, 1988).

The orthokinetic **splint** for the spastic hemiplegic hand was developed by Huss and used ideas from Rood as its theoretical base: a firm surface in the palm of the hand to inhibit the extrinsic flexor muscles and tactile stimulation of the extensor surface of the forearm to facilitate extensor tone. The hand and forearm pieces are made of low-temperature plastics. The hand piece is shaped into a cone; the larger end of the cone is ulnar directed. The forearm shell extends two-thirds of the length of the forearm from approximately 3 cm from the wrist crease. The cone is attached to the forearm piece by two side supports that are bent to follow the contour of the hand laterally. The side supports are attached loosely, using rivets, so that the wrist is free to move. The forearm piece is secured to the patient using an elastic bandage for straps (Kiel, 1974) to simulate the benefits of an **orthokinetic cuff.** No data on the effectiveness have been published.

The inflatable **splint** is a double plastic cuff long enough to envelop the part to be splinted. It was originally designed as an emergency immobilizer **splint** for the limbs, but has been adopted for use with spastic patients. It is blown up like a balloon and provides deep-pressure therapy (Johnstone, 1983) and warmth. The **splint** is worn for 15 to 20 min before movement therapy begins (Johnstone, 1975). The patient may continue to wear it in conjunction with simulated weight-bearing exercise to position the intermediate joints of the arm correctly and to provide sensory stimulation to reduce spastic tone during exercise (Johnstone, 1983). There is debate as to the long-term effects of inflatable **splints** (Poole et al., 1990).

Serial casting of spastic limbs is developing as a treatment choice for brain-injured (Booth et al., 1983), stroke (Brennan, 1959; King, 1982), and tetraplegic (Cruickshank & O'Neill, 1990) patients. The casts are replaced as the limb is stretched more and more away from the contracted spastic posture with each cast change, so that greater free ROM is obtained over time. There is some evidence that prolonged immobilization of the limb (3 months with removal for washing and free movement twice daily) in a position of full stretch will decrease the spasticity, increase the range of free movement, and increase the tone of the antagonists (except in cases of wrist and finger extensors) (Brennan, 1959). Pain and skin damage may occur during prolonged immobilization unless the device is well constructed and the condition of the limb is frequently monitored (Brennan, 1959). Another study in which immobilization was followed by night casting in a half-shell cast for a total of 16 days showed benefits to one patient with severe elbow flexor spasticity (King,

1982). In this study, a plaster cast was preferred to plastic **splints.**

Two types of casts are described here. A dropout cast is used when a supination contracture is not present and the elbow is minus no more than 35 to 40° of extension. This type of cast focuses on gaining elbow extension before trying to manage supination (Hill, 1986). The cast is most effective when the patient can be up most of the day so the arm can "drop out" with gravity assisting. A patient may be casted two to three times in a drop-out cast before enough elbow extension is gained to begin casting in a long arm cast (Hill, 1986).

The long arm cast is used when there is less than a 35 to 40° elbow contracture and a supination contracture or tightness is occurring. There may be from three to five casts used, gradually extending and pronating the elbow. Casting is discontinued when full range of motion (ROM) has been gained, functional ROM is gained, or no increase in ROM is seen after two casts (Hill, 1986). A final long arm cast made from

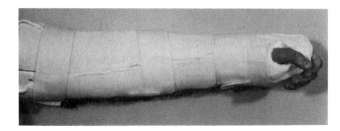

Figure 28.63. Bivalved long arm fiberglass cast.

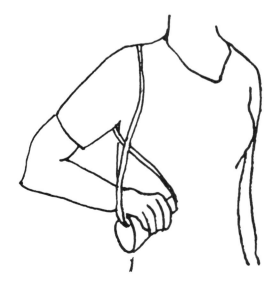

Figure 28.64. Dynamic sling to facilitate hypotonic elbow extensor muscles of a hemiparetic patient.

fiberglass and then bivalved (Fig. 28.63) may then be used temporarily as a night-positioning **splint.**

A dynamic sling, designed by Winsinky, has been used to facilitate the elbow extensors via stretch and resistance offered by a surgical tubing strap as the patient walks. It also is believed to inhibit finger flexion, and possibly the whole flexor pattern, by use of the cone held in the hand. To construct this sling, the plastic cone is placed on a length of rubber tubing or strapping long enough to loop over the patient's shoulder while the patient holds the cone and has the elbow flexed to 90° or less. A knot is made in the tubing and pushed inside the cone out of view. The large end of the cone is worn to the ulnar side, and the tubing crosses under the axilla if the sling is applied correctly (Fig. 28.64). It may be necessary to fasten the tubing onto the shoulder and to strap the hand onto the cone (Farber & Huss, 1974).

Acknowledgments—We would like to thank Annette Russell Farmer and Eleanor Marshall for their feedback, Joyce Bryant for the new photography, Lisa Link for her literature search, and Julie Pope for bibliographic assistance.

STUDY QUESTIONS

1. What is the role of the occupational therapist in orthotic rehabilitation?
2. Define orthosis.
3. Name the goals for which splinting may be used.
4. Discuss the pros and cons of slings that immobilize the arm and slings that leave the arm free for function relative to the shoulder of a hemiplegic patient.
5. Discuss why a static splint might be chosen and the precautions related to such splints.
6. Describe two dynamic splints and the purposes for which they are used.
7. Select an orthosis to decrease an elbow contracture, discuss the reasons for your choice, and state the principle(s) that it implements.
8. Discuss two types of finger or hand orthoses that assist in restoring function while stabilizing a joint.
9. When would you choose a wrist-driven flexor hinge hand splint? A RIC wrist orthosis?
10. Select the correct styles of all parts of a mobile arm support for a weak patient with particular weakness of the internal rotators and absent triceps. State how each part will be adjusted for this patient.
11. Describe a treatment session to improve a patient's hand-to-mouth and hand-to-table control of a MAS.
12. What are the pros and cons of various orthoses designed to modify tone?

REFERENCES

Anderson, K., & Maas, F. (1987). Immediate effect of working splints on grip strength of arthritic patients. *Australian Occupational Therapy Journal, 34*(1), 26–31.

Anderson, M. (1965). *Upper extremity orthotics.* Springfield, IL: Charles C. Thomas.

Backman, C. (1988). Spandex wrist splint: An alternative for the client with arthritis. *Canadian Journal of Occupational Therapists, 55*(2), 89–91.

Bobath, B. (1990). *Adult hemiplegia: Evaluation and treatment* (3rd ed.). London: William Heinemann Medical Books.

Booth, B. J., Doyle, M., & Montgomery, J. (1983). Serial casting for the management of spasticity in the head-injured adult. *Physical Therapy, 63*(12), 1960–1966.

Boyd, E., & Gaylard, A. (1986). Shoulder supports with stroke patients: A Canadian survey. *Canadian Journal of Occupational Therapy, 53*(2), 61–67.

Brennan, J. B. (1959). Response to stretch of hypertonic muscle groups in hemiplegia. *British Medical Journal, 1*(5136), 1504–1507.

Bunnell, S. (1956). *Surgery of the hand* (3rd ed.). Philadelphia: J. B. Lippincott.

Cailliet, R. (1982). *Hand pain and impairment* (3rd ed.). Philadelphia: F. A. Davis.

Canadian Association of Occupational Therapists (1987). *Position paper on the use of orthoses in occupational therapy.* Toronto, Ont.: CAOT Publications del l'ACE.

Carlson, J. D., & Trombly, C. A. (1983). The effect of wrist immobilization on performance of the Jebsen Hand Function Test. *American Journal of Occupational Therapy, 37*(3), 167–175.

Chesher, S., Schwartz, K., & Kleinert, H. (1988). A new early-mobilization splint for proximal interphalangeal joint replacements. *Journal of Hand Therapy, 2*(4), 200–203.

Claus, B. S., & Godfrey, K. J. (1985). Brief or new: A distal support sling for the hemiplegic patient. *American Journal of Occupational Therapy, 39*(8), 536–537.

Colditz, J. (1987). Splinting for radial nerve palsy. *Journal of Hand Therapy, 1,* 18–23.

Collins, K., Oswald, P., Burger, G., & Nolden, J. (1985). Customized adjustable orthoses: Their use in spasticity. *Archives of Physical Medicine & Rehabilitation, 66*(6), 397–398.

Cruickshank, D., & O'Neill, D. (1990). Upper extremity inhibitive casting in a boy with spastic quadriplegia. *American Journal of Occupational Therapy, 44*(6), 552–555.

DeVore, G. L. (1970). A sling to prevent a subluxed shoulder. *American Journal of Occupational Therapy, 24*(5), 580–581.

Dolhanty, D. (1986). Effectiveness of splinting for carpal tunnel syndrome. *Canadian Journal of Occupational Therapy, 53*(5), 275–280.

Doubilet, L., & Polkow, L. S. (1977). Theory and design of a finger abduction splint for the spastic hand. *American Journal of Occupational Therapy, 31*(5), 320–322.

Dovelle, S., Heeter, P. K., & McFaul, T. V. (1988). A dynamic finger flexion loop. *American Journal of Occupational Therapy, 42*(8), 535–537.

Dovelle, S., Heeter, P. K., & Phillips, P. D. (1987). A dynamic traction splint for the management of extrinsic tendon tightness. *American Journal of Occupational Therapy, 41*(2), 123–125.

Drew, W. E., & Stern, P. H. (1979). Modular adjustment mechanism for the balanced forearm orthosis. *Archives of Physical Medicine & Rehabilitation, 60*(2), 81.

Farber, S. D., & Huss, A. J. (1974). *Sensorimotor evaluation and treatment methods for allied health personnel* (2nd ed.). Indianapolis: Indiana University Foundation.

Ferreri, J., & Tumminelli, J. (1974). A swivel cock-up splint-type arm trough. *American Journal of Occupational Therapy, 28*(6), 359.

Fess, E. (1988). Force magnitude of commercial spring-coil and spring-wire splints designed to extend the proximal interphalangeal joint. *Journal of Hand Therapy, 1,* 86–90.

Fess, E. E., Gettle, K. S., & Strickland, J. W. (1981). *Hand splinting: Principles and methods.* St. Louis: C. V. Mosby.

Fishwick, G. M., & Tobin, D. G. (1978). Splinting the burned hand with primary excision and early grafting. *American Journal of Occupational Therapy, 32*(3), 182–183.

Goold, N. J. (1976). A versatile wheelchair armrest attachment. *American Journal of Occupational Therapy, 30*(8), 502–504.

Green, D. P., & McCoy, H. (1979). Turnbuckle orthotic correction of elbow-flexion contractures after acute injuries. *Journal of Bone & Joint Surgery, 61A*(7), 1092–1095.

Harper, B. (1990). The drop-out splint: An alternative to the conservative management of ulnar nerve entrapment at the elbow. *Journal of Hand Therapy, 3*(4), 199–201.

Henshaw, J., Satren, J., & Wrightsman, J. (1989). The semi-flexible support: An alternative for the hand-injured worker. *Journal of Hand Therapy, 2*(1), 35–40.

Hepburn, G. R., & Crivelli, K. J. (1984). Use of elbow Dynasplint for reduction of elbow flexion contractures: A case study. *Journal of Orthopaedic and Sports Physical Therapy, 5*(5), 269–274.

Heurich, M., & Polansky, S. (1978). An adaptation of the glove flexion mitt. *American Journal of Occupational Therapy, 32*(2), 110-111.

Hill, J. (1986). *Spinal cord injury: A guide to functional outcomes in occupational therapy.* Gaithersburg, MD: Aspen Systems.

Hunter, J., Schneider, L., Mackin, E., & Callahan, A. (1990). *Rehabilitation of the hand: Surgery and therapy* (3rd ed.). St. Louis: C. V. Mosby.

Iveson, E., Phillips, M., & Ream, W. D. (1972). A removable arm trough for wheelchair patients. *American Journal of Occupational Therapy, 26*(5), 269.

Jackson, D., & Clifford, J. (1989). Electrodiagnosis of mildcarpal tunnel syndrome. *Archives of Physical Medicine & Rehabilitation, 70,* 199–204.

Johnson, M., Sandkvist, G., Eberhardt, K., Liang, B., & Herrlin, K. (1992). The usefulness of nocturnal resting splints in the treatment of ulnar deviation of the rheumatoid hand. *Clinical Rheumatology, 11*(1), 72–75.

Johnstone, M. (1975). Inflatable splint for the hemiplegic arm. *Physiotherapy, 61*(12), 377.

Johnstone, M. (1983). *Restoration of motor function in the stroke patient* (2nd ed.). London: Churchill Livingstone.

Kaplan, N. (1962). Effect of splinting on reflex inhibition and sensorimotor stimulation in treatment of spasticity. *Archives of Physical Medicine & Rehabilitation, 43*(11), 565–569.

Kiel, J. L. (1974). Making the dynamic orthokinetic wrist splint for flexor spasticity in hand and wrist. In S. D. Farber & A. J. Huss (Eds.), *Sensorimotor evaluation and treatment procedures for allied health personnel* (2nd ed., pp. 82–88). Indianapolis: Indiana University Foundation.

King, T. I. (1982). Plaster splinting as a means of reducing elbow flexor spasticity: A case study. *American Journal of Occupational Therapy, 36*(10), 671–673.

Kohlmeyer, K., Weber, C., & Yarkony, G. (1990). A new orthosis for central cord syndrome and brachial plexus injuries. *Archives of Physical Medicine & Rehabilitation, 71,* 1006–1009.

Krajnik, S., & Bridle, J. (1992). Hand splinting in quadriplegia: Current practice. *American Journal of Occupational Therapy, 46*(2), 149–156.

Kruger, V., Kraft, G., Deitz, J., Ameis, A., & Polissar, L. (1991). Carpal tunnel syndrome: Objective measures and splint use. *Archives of Physical Medicine & Rehabilitation, 72,* 517–520.

Langlois, S., Pederson, L., & Mackinnon, J. (1991). The effects of splinting on the spastic hemiplegic hand: Report of a feasibility study. *Canadian Journal of Occupational Therapy, 58*(1), 17–25.

Larson, D. (1973). *The prevention and correction of burn scarcontracture and hypertrophy.* Galveston: University of Texas Medical Branch, Shriner's Burn Institute.

Long, C., & Masciarelli, V. (1963). An electrophysiological splint for the hand. *Archives of Physical Medicine & Rehabilitation, 44*(9), 499–503.

Long, C., & Schutt, A. (1986). Upper limb orthotics. In J. B. Redford (Ed.), *Orthotics etcetera* (3rd ed., pp. 198–270). Baltimore: Williams & Wilkins.

Lucas, B. (1988). Roll splints: An option in low-profile dynamic splinting. *American Journal of Occupational Therapy, 42*(1), 49–52.

Making the least of burn scars. (1972). *Emergency Medicine, 4,* 24–25.

Malick, M. H. (1974). *Manual on dynamic hand splinting with thermoplastic materials.* New York: ABC.

Mathiowetz, V., Bolding, D. J., & Trombly, C. A. (1983). Immediate effects of positioning devices on the normal and spastic hand measured by electromyography. *American Journal of Occupational Therapy, 37*(4), 247–254.

May, E., & Silfverskiold, K. (1989). A new power source in dynamic splinting: Experimental studies. *Journal of Hand Therapy, 2*(3), 164–168.

McClure, P., & Flowere, K. (1992). Treatment of limited shoulder motion using an elevation splint. *Physical Therapy, 72*(1), 57–62.

McKenzie, M. (1973). The ratchet hand splint. *American Journal of Occupational Therapy, 27*(8), 477–479.

McPhee, S. (1987). Extension block splinting for the proximal interphalangeal joint. *American Journal of Occupational Therapy, 41*(6), 389–390.

McPherson, J. J., Kreimeyer, D., Aalderks, M., & Gallagher, T. (1982). A comparison of dorsal and volar resting hand splints in the reduction of hypertonus. *American Journal of Occupational Therapy, 36*(10), 664–670.

Melvin, J. L. (1982). *Rheumatic disease: Occupational therapy and rehabilitation* (2nd ed.). Philadelphia: F. A. Davis.

Moodie, N. B., Brisbin, J., & Morgan, A. M. (1986). Subluxation of the glenohumeral joint in hemiplegia: Evaluation of supportive devices. *Physiotherapy Canada, 38*(3), 151–157.

Moore, J., & Braverman, S. (1990). Splinting for radial instability of the thumb MCP joint. *Journal of Hand Therapy, 3*(4), 202–204.

Neal, M. R., & Williamson, J. (1980). Collar sling for bilateral shoulder subluxation. *American Journal of Occupational Therapy, 34*(6), 400–401.

Nichols, P. J. R., Peach, S. L., Haworth, R. J., & Ennis, J. (1978). The value of flexor hinge hand splints. *Prosthetics and Orthotics International, 2*(2), 86–94.

Parks, B. J., Barrett, K. P., & Voss, K. (1983). The use of Hexcelite in splinting the thumb. *American Journal of Occupational Therapy, 37*(4), 266–267.

Peckham, P. H., & Mortimer, J. T. (1977). Restoration of hand function in the quadriplegic through electrical stimulation. In F. T. Hambrecht and J. B. Reswick (Eds.), *Functional electrical stimulation* (pp. 83–95). New York: Marcel Dekker.

Poole, J., Whitney, S., Hangeland, N., & Baker, C. (1990). The effectiveness of inflatable pressure splints on motor function in stroke patients. *Occupational Therapy Journal of Research, 10*(6), 361–367.

Pratt, P., & Allen, A. (1989). *Occupational therapy for children* (2nd ed). St. Louis: C. V. Mosby.

Rajaram, V., & Holtz, M. (1985). Shoulder forearm support for the subluxed shoulder. *Archives of Physical Medicine & Rehabilitation, 66*(3), 191–192.

Rivers, E. A., Strate, R. G., & Salem, L. D. (1979). The transparent face mask. *American Journal of Occupational Therapy, 33*(2), 108–113.

Robinson, C. (1986). Brachial plexus lesions. Part 2: Functional splintage. *British Journal of Occupational Therapy, 49*, 331–334.

Rose, V., & Shah, S. (1987). A comparative study on the immediate effects of hand orthoses on reduction of hypertonus. *Australian Occupational Therapy Journal, 34*(2), 59–64.

Rossi, J. (1988). Concepts and current trends in hand splinting. *Occupational Therapy in Health Care, 4*(3–4), 53–68.

Rudin, N. J., Gilmore, L. D., Roy, S. H., & DeLuca, C. J. (1987). New motor control assessment techniques for evaluating individuals with severe handicaps: A case study. *Journal of Rehabilitation Research and Development, 24*(3), 57–74.

Salo, R. E. (1978). A hammock wheelchair armrest. *American Journal of Occupational Therapy, 32*(8), 525.

Scherling, E., & Johnson, H. (1989). A tone-reducing wrist-hand orthosis. *American Journal of Occupational Therapy, 43*(9), 609–611.

Seeger, B. R., Caudrey, D. J., & McAllister, G. M. (1985). Skill evaluator and trainer for electrically operated devices: An evaluation of the SET. *Archives of Physical Medicine & Rehabilitation, 66*(6), 387–390.

Seligman, D., & Burack, E. (1989). A customized ankle foot positioning support. *Canadian Journal of Occupational Therapy, 56*(2), 80–82.

Shafer, A. A. (1986). *Common problems, useful solutions in hand rehabilitation*. Dedham, MA: AliMed.

Silverstein, F., French J., & Siebens, A. (1974). A myoelectric hand splint. *American Journal of Occupational Therapy, 28*(2), 99–101.

Smith, R. O., & Okamoto, G. A. (1981). Checklist for the prescription of slings for the hemiplegic patient. *American Journal of Occupational Therapy, 35*(2), 91–95.

Snook, J. H. (1979). Spasticity reduction splint. *American Journal of Occupational Therapy, 33*(10), 648–651.

Sofer, S., Pagnotta, A., & Bitensky, N. (1987). Ulnar deviation adaptation for the wrist cock-up splint. *Canadian Journal of Occupational Therapy, 54*(2), 81–84.

Stenehjem, J., Swenson, J., & Sprague, C. (1983). Wrist driven flexor hinge orthosis: Linkage design improvements. *Archives of Physical Medicine & Rehabilitation, 64*(11), 566–568.

Stewart, D., & Maas, F. (1990). Splint suitability: A comparison of four wrist splints for arthritics. *Australian Occupational Therapy Journal, 37*(1), 15–24.

Sullivan, B., & Rogers, S. (1989). Modified Bobath sling with distal support. *American Journal of Occupational Therapy, 43*(1), 47–49.

Tenney, C. G., & Lisak, J. M. (1986). *Atlas of hand splinting*. Boston: Little, Brown.

Trombly, C. (1966). Principles of operant conditioning related to orthotic training of quadriplegic patients. *American Journal of Occupational Therapy, 20*(5), 217–220.

Trombly, C. (1968). Myoelectric control of orthotic devices for the severely paralyzed. *American Journal of Occupational Therapy, 22*(5), 385–389.

Trombly, C., Prentke, E., & Long, C. (1967). Myoelectrically controlled electric torque motor for the flexor hinge hand splint. *Orthopedic & Prosthetic Appliance Journal, 21*, 39–43.

Von Prince, K., Cureri, W., & Pruitt, B. (1970). Application of fingernail hooks in splinting burned hands. *American Journal of Occupational Therapy, 24*(8), 556–559.

Walker, J. (1983). Modified strapping of roll sling. *American Journal of Occupational Therapy, 37*(2), 110–111.

Walsh, M. (1987). Half-lapboard for hemiplegic patients. *American Journal of Occupational Therapy, 41*(8), 533–535.

Warren, C. G., & Enders, A. (1986). Introduction to systems and devices for the disabled. In J. B. Redford (Ed.), *Orthotics etcetera* (3rd ed., pp. 708–738). Baltimore: Williams & Wilkins.

Woodson, A. M. (1988). Proposal for splinting the adult hemiplegic hand to promote function. *Occupational Therapy in Health Care, 4*(3–4), 85–95.

Wu, S. (1991). A belly gutter splint for proximal interphalangeal joint flexion contracture. *American Journal of Occupational Therapy, 45*(9), 839–843.

Yasuda, Y. L., Bowman, K., & Hsu, J. D. (1986). Mobile arm supports: Criteria for successful use in muscle disease patients. *Archives of Physical Medicine & Rehabilitation, 67*(4), 253–256.

SUGGESTED READINGS

American Occupational Therapy Association. (1986). *Adaptive equipment rehabilitation technology*. Information packet. Rockville, MD: author.

Bielawski, T., & Lehman, J. (1986). Brief or new: A gauntlet work splint. *American Journal of Occupational Therapy, 40*(3), 199–201.

Bowen, M., & Germanos, L. (1988). Orthotic management of the flaccid upper limb in hemiplegia: Two case studies. *Australian Occupational Therapy Journal, 35*(3), 130–138.

Casey, C., & Kratz, E. (1988). Soft splinting with Neoprene: The thumb abduction supinator splint. *American Journal of Occupational Therapy, 42*(6), 395–398.

Fairleigh, A., & Hacking, S. (1988). Post-operative metacarpophalangeal arthroplasty dynamic splint for patients with rheumatoid arthritis. *Canadian Journal of Occupational Therapy, 55*(3), 141–146.

Gajiwala, K., Sams, S., Pandya, N., & Wagh, A. (1991). A new dynamic lumbrical simulating splint for claw hand deformity. *Plastic and Reconstructive Surgery, 87*(1), 170–173.

Garber, S. L., & Gregorio, T. L. (1990). Upper extremity assistive devices: Assessment of use by spinal cord-injured patients with quadriplegia. *American Journal of Occupational Therapy, 44*(2), 126–131.

Goodman, G., & Bazyk, S. (1991). The effects of a short thumb opponens splint on hand function in cerebral palsy: A single-subject study. *American Journal of Occupational Therapy, 45*(8), 726–731.

Langlois, S., MacKinnon, J., & Pederson, L. (1989). Hand splints and cerebral spasticity: A review of the literature. *Canadian Journal of Occupational Therapy, 56*(3), 113–119.

Roberson, L., Breger, D., Buford, W., & Freeman, M. J. (1988). Analysis of the physical properties of SCOMAS springs and their potential use in dynamic splinting. *Journal of Hand Therapy, 1*, 110–114.

Saldana, M., Choban, S., Westerbeck, P., & Schacherer, T. (1991). Results of acute zone III extensor tendon injuries treated with dynamic extension splinting. *Journal of Hand Surgery, 16A*(6), 1145–1150.

Silver Ring Splint Company. (1994). *Catalogue*. Charlottesville, VA: author.

Steadman, A., & Netscher, D. (1990). A detachable thumb spica combined with an outrigger brace simplifies postoperative management of the rheumatoid hand. *Journal of Hand Therapy, 3*(4), 205–208.

29
Construction of Hand Splints

Colleen T. Lowe

OBJECTIVES _____

After studying this chapter, the reader will be able to:
1. Discuss the anatomical principles important to splint making.
2. Discuss the mechanical principles important to splint making.
3. Understand an approach for selecting and designing the appropriate splint.
4. Understand the process of pattern making.
5. List the capabilities and limitations of the more commonly used materials.

The goal of splinting is to maintain the structures of the wrist and hand in balance to preserve prehension and functional ability (Fess & Philips, 1987; Kiel, 1983; Malick, 1985; Tenney & Lisak, 1986). The use of orthotics in the treatment of upper extremity dysfunction is not a contemporary concept. In *Bunnell's Surgery of the Hand* (Boyes, 1970). there are references to splints and pictures of splints used in the 1500s, which were constructed from wood, metal, and leather. Over time the materials used have evolved but the mechanical principles of construction are still similar.

Splints are introduced into the treatment of hand injuries or dysfunction to maintain or improve a patient's functional ability. Low-temperature thermoplastic splints are most often considered temporary. If a splint is needed permanently to assist function (e.g., to provide prehension for a tetraplegic patient), then a splint would be machined from metals by a certified orthotist. Anderson (1974) graphically illustrated the process. The fabrication and fitting of permanent orthoses require advanced postgraduate training. If a therapist is to have this duty, then further training is recommended. Occupational therapists sometimes make the prototypes for these splints out of low-temperature thermoplastics.

The occupational therapist is the most appropriate

health care provider to determine when a splint is indicated, when it should be modified, and how it should be designed. Splints are applied at different stages of tissue healing. The purposes of splints are threefold:

1. To protect or support joints and soft tissue to encourage healing or to reduce inflammation;
2. To assist or to substitute for absent or weak muscles as seen in patients with peripheral nerve injuries;
3. to correct an existing deformity, such as a web space contracture.

The classification of splints is complicated by a number of variables including materials, biomechanics, and anatomical considerations. For this chapter, splints will be classified as static or dynamic. A **static splint** is a rigid orthosis used for the prevention of movement of a joint or for the fixation of a displaced part. A **dynamic splint** is an orthosis that achieves its effect by movement and force. "It is a form of manipulation" (Brand, 1990, p. 1095).

SELECTING THE SPLINT DESIGN

Much of the complexity surrounding splinting can be eliminated with a thorough understanding of upper extremity anatomy and kinesiology, good clinical observation skills during the hand evaluation and activity analysis, and an understanding of the capabilities and limitations of splinting. To decide whether a hand splint is needed and what type is indicated, the therapist examines the patient's hand (see Chapter 38) to determine the causes for the imbalances. What is the effect of pain and swelling on the hand? What prevents the hand from normal grip and prehension? What is required to place the hand and wrist in a functional position?

The functional position of the hand—that which places the muscles, tendons, and ligaments at resting length and in good anatomical alignment—is 15 to 30°

GLOSSARY

Dynamic splint—An orthosis that achieves its effect by applying movement and force to the body part.
Metacarpophalangeal descent—The length of the metacarpals decrease from the radial to ulnar border, which is noted in the obliquity of the metacarpal heads when the hand is fisted.

Outrigger—A projecting support attached to a splint from which finger loops are suspended.
Stabilizing block—An extension on a splint that limits the motion of the joint proximal to the joint to which dynamic traction is applied.
Static splint—A rigid orthosis used for the prevention of movement of a joint or for the fixation of a displaced part.

of wrist dorsiflexion and neutral to slight ulnar deviation, 75° of metacarpophalangeal (MCP) joint flexion and 10° of interphalangeal joint flexion of the fingers, palmar abduction, and 30° rotation of the carpometacarpal joint and extension of the metacarpophalangeal and interphalangeal joints of the thumb (Fess & Philips, 1987; Malick, 1985). At rest, the uninjured hand assumes this position due to the balance of biomechanical forces related to the distinctive shape of the joints and the viscoelastic properties of the ligaments, tendons, skin, and innervated muscles (Brand & Hollister, 1993). Changes in form of any of those structures may result in a hand problem that might require a hand splint. As previously stated, the ideal goal of hand splinting is to preserve normal hand function.

The traditional position of function is not always the most appropriate position for improved function. The aforementioned functional position is appropriate for patients with a flaccid hand or a hand with inflammation or an exacerbation of arthritis. At times, however (e.g., following dorsal hand burns or metacarpal fractures), more metacarpophalangeal flexion is indicated. This position is referred to as the position of safety. In the position of safety, the wrist is immobilized in 20 to 30° of dorsiflexion and neutral to slight ulnar deviation, there is 90° of metacarpophalangeal flexion and 0° of extension at the interphalangeal joints, and the thumb is positioned in palmar abduction and 30° rotation of the carpometacarpal joint (Malick, 1985). In the presence of a radial nerve injury, when the wrist and metacarpophalangeal joints are unable to actively extend, then the best position for function would be with the wrist positioned in neutral to 5° of dorsiflexion and the metacarpophalangeal joints of all digits in 0° extension. The radial nerve injury highlights the relationship that exists between the position of the wrist and the position and operation of the digits as a result of the tenodesis effect. The tenodesis action relates to the passive extension of the joints of the digits when the wrist is flexed and its converse, i.e., passive flexion of the digits when the wrist is extended. This is an important anatomical principle to remember when determining if the splint should be forearm based and immobilize the wrist or hand based and not immobilize the wrist.

To determine what splint design is indicated to achieve a good functional outcome, the therapist must do a careful and thorough assessment of the patient's hand to delineate the patient's limitations. The assessment will reveal where the assistive or corrective forces need to be applied to place the hand in a good anatomical position to facilitate return of function.

Anatomical Principles

Knowledge of anatomy is basic to good splint construction. Anatomical considerations important to splint design are discussed below (Fess & Philips, 1987, Kiel, 1983, Malick, 1985).

1. Maintain the three arches of the hand: (1) the proximal carpal arch, (2) the distal transverse metacarpal arch, and (3) the longitudinal arch. The proximal carpal arch is made up of the eight carpal bones, which are divided into two rows of four, and the annular ligaments. The distal transverse arch consists of the relatively immobile second and third metacarpals around which the mobile thumb metacarpal and ulnar fourth and fifth metacarpals rotate (Boyes, 1970; Brand & Hollister, 1993; Fess & Philips, 1987). If viewed in the transverse plane, the metacarpal heads of the normal, fisted hand define an oblique line that descends from high to low from the radial to ulnar side. The splint accommodates this obliquity by being higher on the radial side than the ulnar side. The longitudinal arch includes the carpus, metacarpals, and phalanges. The metacarpophalangeal joints are the apex of this arch. The longitudinal arch allows approximately 280° of total active flexion of each finger (Fess & Philips, 1987).

2. Maintain the normal axis of motion.

3. Permit balanced function of unaffected muscles. Do not splint a joint that is not injured.

4. Permit contact of palmar surface of palm and digits with the environment to allow greater sensory discrimination.

Mechanical Principles

The fitting and fabrication of splints require the application of external forces to the upper extremity. An understanding of a few basic mechanical principles is essential to effective splint design. The mechanical principles inherent in splinting are as follows (Colditz, 1983; Fess & Philips, 1987; Malick, 1974; Pearson, 1990):

1. *Area of Force Application.* The area of force application is the relationship between the total force exerted and the area over which that force is applied. Stated differently, increasing the area of the force application will minimize the pressure forces on the skin; or the smaller the area of force application, the greater the force. To prevent pressure sores and skin breakdown, especially over bony areas and at those areas proximal to the application of dynamic tension, the force should be distributed over as large an area possible. This principle is considered when determining the width of the forearm trough, palmar bars, the dorsal and volar **stabilizing blocks** for dynamic traction, and the width of the straps and finger loops. Rolling the edges of the splints and applying dynamic traction over a greater distance also relates to the principle of force application.

2. *Mechanical Advantage.* The principle of mechanical advantage relates to a class I lever system in which three points of pressure are applied in parallel (Fess & Philips, 1987). It refers to the relationship between the length of the force arm and that of the resistance arm of the lever system. A volar splint is an example of a class I lever system in which the axis is located at the wrist joint, the weight of the hand is the resistance, and the weight of the forearm is the force. Remembering from kinesiology that $F \times FA = R \times RA$, or $F = (RA \times R)/FA$, it can be deduced that if the resistance and resistance arm (palmar support) remain constant, the force exerted on the forearm skin can be reduced by increasing the length of the force arm (forearm trough).

Clinically, these two principles, which relate to forces applied in parallel, explain why a forearm-based splint that is long (two-thirds of the length of the forearm) and wide (from the midaxis medially and laterally) is more comfortable and more durable than a short, narrow one (Fess & Philips, 1987).

3. *Perpendicular Traction Application.* The third principle, to apply dynamic traction perpendicularly, relates to **outrigger** design and placement. Inherently, force has both rotational and translational components. The rotational component provides motion that brings the part in a circular arc around the joint axis. The translational, or linear, component compresses or distracts the joint surfaces. If the force to correct passive joint motion is applied perpendicularly, i.e., at 90° to the axis of rotation, then the force is entirely rotational. As the angle of application moves away from the perpendicular, the translational component increases. If the force is applied at greater than 90°, it tends to

compress the joint surfaces, whereas at angles less than 90°, it tends to distract the joint surfaces. Oblique forces, forces to the right or left of the perpendicular, are not wanted in splint design or application. Clinically, this means that the therapist must continually monitor the angle of pull in a **dynamic splint** to maintain a 90° angle of pull, which is the most effective angle of corrective force for improving limited passive range of motion (Colditz, 1983; Fess & Philips, 1987). Corrective force application is not a state of static symmetry; it is a process of constant adjustment. As the patient shows an improvement in range of motion, the angle of pull (dynamic traction) needs to be readjusted to maintain the correct angle of force application at all times.

4. *The Application of Torque at the Joint.* The torque of rotational force at the joint is equal to the product of the force and the length of the moment arm on which it acts. The longer the moment arm, the greater the torque for a given force. This applies clinically when considering that the amount of torque acting on the MCP joint is influenced by the distance between the joint axis and the finger cuff. Optimal torque is applied just distal to the joint being mobilized, which results in a glide between the adjoining joint surfaces instead of a tilt (Fess & Philips, 1987). The exact placement of finger cuffs and proximal stabilizers to provide a counterbalancing force, if necessary, depends on the relative degree of passive mobility of the proximal and distal joints. If the proximal joint has normal range of motion, a stabilizer or block will be necessary to direct the pull to the restricted joint. If all joints are limited, e.g., unable to flex through full range of motion, then the traction can be applied distally to achieve composite flexion.

It is important to consider the patient's age, ability to accept responsibility, level of independence, occupational demands, and the distance the patient lives from his therapist before selecting a splint design (Fess & Philips, 1987; Tenney & Lisak, 1986). All of these considerations have an influence on the design of a splint. For example, if the patient requires assistance to apply a splint or lives far from the clinic and cannot come to the therapist for frequent splint adjustments then a simpler design would be constructed.

FITTING THE PATTERN

A well-designed pattern usually leads to a well-fitting splint with relative ease. Problems associated with splint construction occur when therapists try to make the leap from the splint prescription to splint fabrication without assessing the patient or making a good pattern. For each splint, a paper pattern should be fitted to the patient. It is rare for standard patterns to fit perfectly. There are two stages to the fitting process: gross adaptation of the pattern to the patient's hand and the final fitting.

Gross adaptation, or drawing, of the pattern is done directly from the involved hand or the nonaffected hand. The patient's hand is placed flat onto a piece of paper and an outline of the patient's hand and forearm is traced. The locations of the patient's joints are indicated on this drawing. Important markings, to aid in drawing the pattern once the patient's hand has been removed, are made between the thumb and index finger; between the middle and ring fingers; the radial and ulnar border of the wrist; the distal palmar crease, radially and ulnarly; the interphalangeal joint of the thumb; and two-thirds the length of the forearm (Fig. 29.1).

After the hand and forearm have been traced and the markings indicated, the outline of the splint pattern is drawn over the drawing of the hand, connecting the landmarks of the hand as indicated in Figure 29.2. This is a two-dimensional process, and the thickness of the splinting material to be used must be allowed for in the paper pattern; any part that curves around must be longer by twice the thickness of the material.

Final fitting is done by cutting the pattern out of paper toweling and placing it onto the patient's hand (Fig. 29.3*A*). An alternative method is to draw the pattern on a paper towel that is placed over the entire surface of the hand and arm that the splint is to cover. The pattern is drawn freehand to fit the contour of the hand, which is beneath the paper towel. If the therapist finds it difficult to draw the contour of the splint freehand, she may use the too small or too large patterns available in the literature cited at the end of this chapter and change the size by adding to or trimming away the pattern until it fits without altering the basic shape of the pattern.

Final adjustment of the pattern is done by carefully checking the fit at every point with the hand stationary and when the fingers and wrist are gently moved if movement is meant to take place. Extra material is trimmed away and/or marks are made to

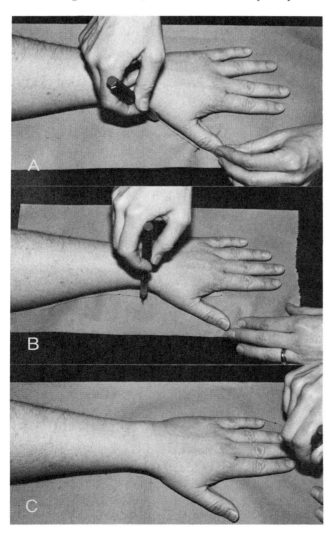

Figure 29.1. Important points of fit are marked onto the paper pattern. **A.** Volar long opponens splint. **B.** Volar wrist cock-up splint. **C.** Volar resting hand splint.

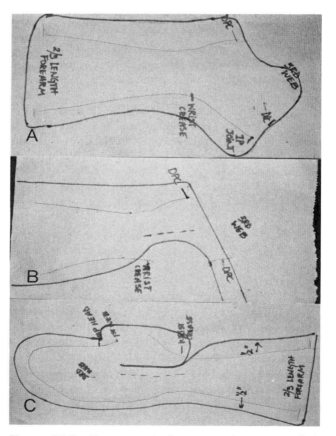

Figure 29.2. The pattern is drawn onto the paper to fit the tracing of the patient's hand. **A.** Volar long opponens splint. **B.** Volar wrist cock-up splint. **C.** Volar resting hand splint.

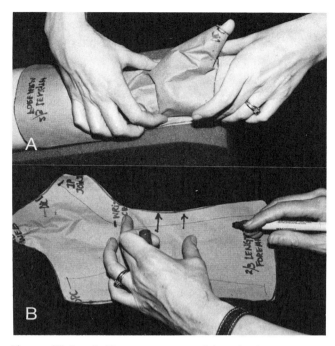

Figure 29.3.   A. The paper pattern of the volar long opponens splint is fitted to the patient's hand. **B.** Arrows are placed on the pattern to indicate where the pattern needs to be wider when traced onto the thermoplastic material.

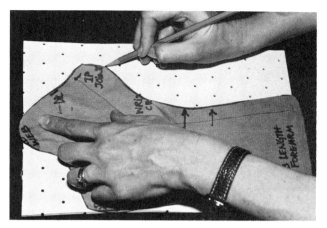

Figure 29.4.   The pattern is transferred to the material (here, Multiform plastic).

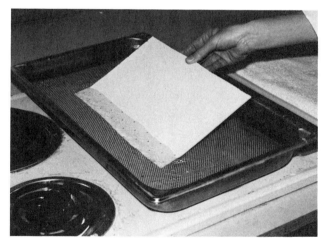

Figure 29.5.   Multiform plastic is warmed in 140 to 160°F water before it is cut.

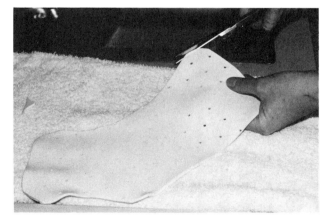

Figure 29.6.   The splint is cut out. The plastic material must be kept horizontal while being cut to avoid stretching the material.

indicate where the pattern needs to be extended when it is transferred to the splinting material (Fig. 29.3*B*). Attention to detail in the fitting of the pattern makes fabrication of the splint easier. The three patterns shown in Figure 29.2—volar long opponens, volar wrist cock-up, and volar resting hand splints—are the roots of all the other variations of splints. It is essential to know how to construct these splints well, as they are the most commonly requested splints. The splint-making procedures described below detail the construction of a volar long opponens splint (Figs. 29.4 to 29.14).

Recommended Criteria of Fit of a Hand Splint

Because of the need to apply correct forces and to make the splint comfortable and safe, certain recommendations for fitting hand splints have evolved (Brand, 1990; Brand & Hollister, 1993, Pearson, 1990; Tenney & Lisck, 1986). They are noted below.

1. To prevent pressure points and/or friction, splints should be molded well, following the contours of the hand and forearm closely.

2. The longitudinal and transverse arches should be maintained in the splint to preserve the ability to grasp various-shaped objects. The splint should have a molded palmar support to maintain the distal transverse arch. The obliquity of the **metacarpophalangeal de-**

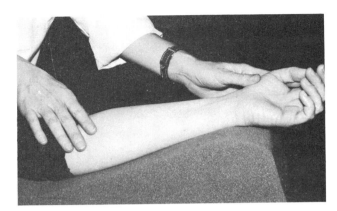

Figure 29.7. When using a plastic-based material, position the patient's forearm, wrist, and hand in the gravity-assist position before applying the splint to aid the molding process and to prevent finger indentations.

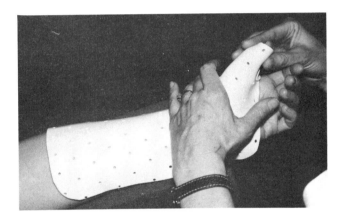

Figure 29.8. The splint is fitted to conform to the contours of the forearm, thumb, and distal palmar arch.

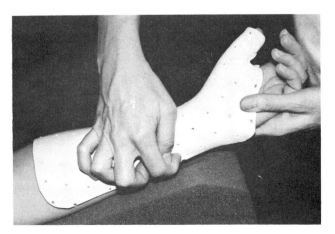

Figure 29.9. The splint is marked where it is too high on the lateral borders of the forearm. The forearm trough should align midaxially to enable the straps to secure the splint to the arm. If the edges of the forearm trough are too high, the straps just lie across the dorsum of the arm and do not secure the splint, allowing it to slip distally.

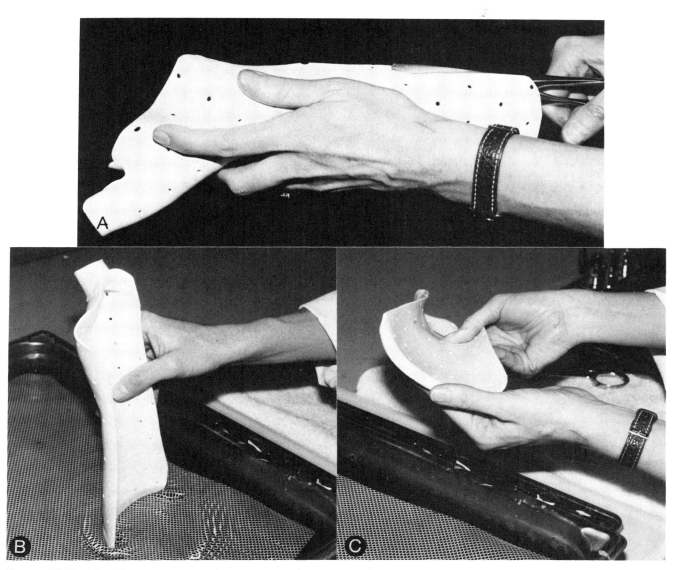

Figure 29.10.   A. Adjustments are made as necessary by snipping off any excess material. **B and C.** The edges are rolled to displace pressure.

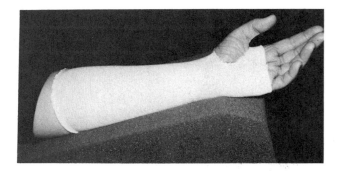

Figure 29.11. A stockinette sleeve is applied before the final fitting to protect the skin from irritation secondary to sweating and/or from a reaction to the plastic.

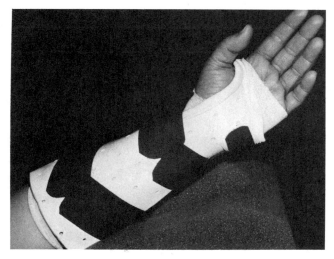

Figure 29.14. Final fitting for volar wrist cock-up splint.

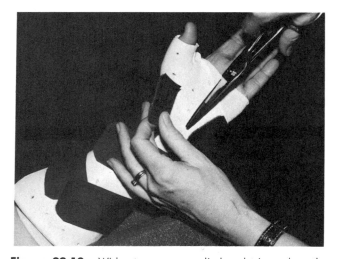

Figure 29.12. Wide straps are applied and trimmed on the volar long opponens splint

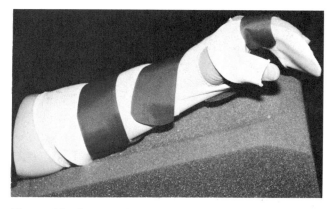

Figure 29.13. Final fitting for volar resting hand splint.

scent should be checked to see if it is present with the splint on. To ensure this obliquity, the splint will be higher on the radial side than the ulnar side so as not to block full flexion of the metacarpophalangeal joint of the fourth and fifth digits.

3. Except in special circumstances, volar hand splints must allow 90° of metacarpophalangeal flexion and, therefore, should not extend beyond the distal palmar crease. The distal palmar crease also guides the correct oblique angle the splint should incorporate to allow for the decreased length of the metacarpals from the radial to ulnar fingers (Fess & Philips, 1987; Malick, 1985).

4. The fingers should be in the appropriate functional position to maintain function. Usually this is 60 to 75° flexion at the metacarpophalangeal joint and 0 to 10° of flexion at the interphalangeal joints.

5. The thumb should be in a functional position. Palmar abduction and 30° rotation at the carpometacarpal joint and 0° extension at the metacarpophalangeal and interphalangeal joints provide a gentle stretch to the first web space.

6. The wrist should be in a neutral position or in 15 to 30° of dorsiflexion, depending on the patient's diagnosis and the purpose of the splint.

7. A forearm-based splint should extend two-thirds the length of the forearm for proper leverage and to decrease the pressure at the distal and proximal edges.

8. A splint should not restrict the motion of any uninvolved joints. Hence a hand-based splint should extend from the most distal wrist crease.

9. Finger and thumb pieces should be long enough to give adequate support but not so long as to

interfere with prehension, if allowed, or cause pressure on opposing fingers.

10. The splint should not cross the thenar eminence crease and restrict motion.

11. The width of the forearm trough should extend from the lateral to medial midline of the forearm for better splint stability and comfort.

12. Bony prominences should be free from pressure either by not covering them or by molding the splint to include space over them. Well-molded splints are critical over the dorsum of the hand; especially over the metacarpophalangeal heads. If padding is to be used, it should be placed onto the splint material before it is molded to the hand to ensure a good fit and no translation of pressure to a different area of the hand or forearm.

13. The straps should be wide to distribute the pressure; tight and narrow circumferential parts must be avoided.

14. **Outriggers** should be positioned so that the rotational force is applied perpendicularly to the axis of motion (Brand & Hollister, 1993; Colditz, 1983; Malick, 1974).

15. The dynamic traction force exerted by spring wire, springs, or elastics should be not so strong as to distort the joint or cause pressure breakdown on the skin. Brand and Hollister (1993) recommended 200 to 250 g of force for up to 8 hr at a time.

16. Splints that have joints must fit so that the axis of splint motion aligns with the axis of anatomical joint motion.

17. There should be no evidence of excessive pressure after 1 hr of splint wearing, i.e., reddened skin areas that continue beyond 20 min after removal.

These criteria of fit are used also during the checkout process, described later in this chapter.

SELECTION OF MATERIALS

The quest for new and improved materials has continued into the field of splinting. Materials for splinting have evolved from the plaster of Paris bandage to a variety of low-temperature thermoplastics (Breger-Lee & Buford, 1991; 1992). Influences on choice of splinting materials include patient pathology and the resultant needs, the demand for greater efficiency in patient care, and technological advances. A representative sampling of the available thermoplastics are discussed; the advantages and disadvantages of each can be judged by the reader on the basis of the properties of each and the methods required to work with each. This is not a comprehensive list of available materials; the reader is referred to Breger-Lee and Buford (1992) for greater detail and to rehabilitation supply catalogs and conference displays for the latest materials.

High-Temperature Thermoplastics

TYPES OF MATERIALS

High-temperature thermoplastics were once the primary type of orthotic material available. While today they are used less frequently by therapists, it is still important to understand how these materials are used. Many preformed splints are made of high-temperature thermoplastics that can be modified and adapted with a heat gun in much less time than is required for custom fabrication.

High-temperature thermoplastics are available in sheets of varying thicknesses and are either hard and rigid or soft and pliable. Examples of hard/rigid thermoplastics are Royalite, Kydex, and Plexiglas. Examples of soft/pliable thermoplastics are Plastizote, AliPlast, Nickelplast, and Evazote.

HEATING PROCEDURES

Royalite, Kydex, and Plexiglas require heat between 300 and 350°F to become pliable. Plastizote, AliPlast, Nickelplast, and Evazote require less heat; from 225 to as much as 350°F. While both types of materials can be heated in a conventional oven, this is not recommended, because oven heat is not evenly distributed. Small convection air ovens are inexpensive, readily available, and safer to use for orthotic fabrication. The shape of preformed splints made of these materials can be adapted with a heat gun. For example, preformed functional position splints are typically fabricated in 30° of wrist extension. To use a high-temperature preformed splint with a patient who needs the wrist in neutral, carefully heat the wrist area of the splint by slowly moving a heat gun back and forth over the area. Allow approximately 6 inches between the splint and the heat source. In 60 sec or less, the spot-heated area will become pliable so that the wrist angle can be adjusted.

Fabrication of a hand splint with any rigid high-temperature material first requires construction of a positive plaster mold of the hand to be splinted. The soft materials when heated at a lower temperature range (225 to 250°F) can be applied directly to the patient over an appropriate thermal barrier such as several layers of cotton stockinette.

APPLICATIONS

Rigid thermoplastic materials are most often used to fabricate splints for patients who have significant spasticity or when a splint is likely to be used for many months or years. The soft thermoplastic materials are often used in contact sports applications, in splinting long-term care patients, and for protective splinting for patients with chronic arthritis.

Low-Temperature Thermoplastics

MATERIAL CLASSIFICATION ACCORDING TO BASE

Low-temperature materials are now the principal type of material used in orthotic fabrication. As a group, they are easy to use, they heat quickly in 160°F water, and they can be safely applied directly to the patient without a thermal barrier. Because there are so many low-temperature materials available, it is helpful to understand that all materials of this type can be classified according to their base. Once the base is known, behavior of a particular material can be anticipated.

Materials with a Transpolyisoprene Base

The first low-temperature material available for orthotic fabrication was called Prenyl. Its first application was custom foot orthotics. This transpolyisoprene-based (or rubber-based) material was unique at the time. Within a few years it was replaced by a second, more rigid transpolyisoprene-based material from Johnson & Johnson called Orthoplast. This brand name has become as familiar as other brand name products such as Kleenex and Xerox. Rubber-based materials are made by blending varying amounts of "filler" with transpolyisoprene (TPI) pellets, which is then formed into sheets of varying thickness ($^1/_8$ or $^1/_{16}$ inch) over large rollers. Today there are many rubber or rubber-like materials available, yet it is not uncommon for a therapist to receive a prescription for an "Orthoplast splint." Materials with a transpolyisoprene (or isoprene) based material share similar working characteristics, described below. Examples of low-temperature materials manufactured in the United States having a TPI or rubber-like base are Orthoplast, Ezeform, Synergy, Multiform Isoprene, NCM Spectrum, and ContourEase (Table 29.1).

Materials with a Polycaprolactone Base

Several years after Orthoplast became available, the husband of an occupational therapist observed her making a splint for an elderly patient. He noticed that considerable force was required to get the TPI-based material to take the desired shape. His company manufactured products from a material with a polycaprolactone (PCL) base, and he wondered if that material could be used in orthotic fabrication. He developed a material known as Polyform which was the first material available in the United States with a PCL (or plastic) base. There is a significant difference between TPI- and PCL-based materials. With a PCL base, it is possible to obtain significant anatomical detail without the manipulation or force required to form a rubber-based material like Orthoplast. Examples of materials manufactured in the United States with a PCL or plastic

Table 29.1.   Principal U.S. Sources of Low-Temperature Splinting Materials

Brand Name	Base Type	Manufacturer, Principal Source
Orthoplast	TPI (rubber)	Johnson & Johnson (New Brunswick, NJ)
Orthoplast II	PCL (plastic)	Johnson & Johnson (New Brunswick, NJ)
Polyform	PCL (plastic)	Smith & Nephew/Rolyan (Germantown, WI)
Polyflex	TPI/PCL blend	Smith & Nephew/Rolyan (Germantown, WI)
Ezeform	Rubber-like	Smith & Nephew/Rolyan (Germantown, WI)
Synergy	Rubber-like	Smith & Nephew/Rolyan (Germantown, WI)
Aquaplast	Clear (no fillers)	Smith & Nephew/Rolyan (Germantown, WI)
Multiform plastic	PCL (plastic)	AliMed, Inc. (Dedham, MA)
Multiform isoprene	TPI (rubber)	AliMed, Inc. (Dedham, MA)
Multiform clear	Clear (no fillers)	AliMed, Inc. (Dedham, MA)
NCM Clinic	PCL (plastic)	North Coast Medical, Inc. (San Jose, CA)
NCM Preferred	TPI/PCL blend	North Coast Medical, Inc. (San Jose, CA)
Orfit	Clear (no fillers)	North Coast Medical, Inc. (San Jose, CA)
ContourForm	PCL (plastic)	Sammons, Inc. (Brookfield, IL)
ContourEase	TPI (rubber)	Sammons, Inc. (Brookfield, IL)
ContourBlend	TPI/PCL blend	Sammons, Inc. (Brookfield, IL)

base are Polyform, Multiform plastic, Orthoplast II, NCM Clinic, and ContourForm.

TPI/PCL Blended Materials

By blending TPI and PCL with sheet fillers, a third group of materials was created and are referred to as blended, or plastic/rubber combinations. As might be expected, these materials heat in the same way as all the other low-temperature materials but behave slightly differently. They are not as quick to conform as a plastic (TCL) based material yet they are more conforming than materials made of rubber (TPI) alone. Examples of blended materials are Polyflex II and NCM Preferred.

Low-Temperature Materials That Turn Clear

A fourth category of materials is unique in its ability to turn totally clear when heated. These materials are formed without fillers and the sheets are manufactured by pouring formulated liquid plastic into sheet molds. The first material of this type available in the United States was called Aquaplast. Initially, it was primarily marketed for use in x-ray and in burn treatment applications, because with this material it was possible to determine that total contact had been made with the body part to which it was applied. Today Aquaplast is available in several grades, in multiple thicknesses, and with a variety of surface perforation configurations. It is also available in several colors under the brand name Watercolors. These colored materials do not turn clear. In addition to Aquaplast, materials that turn clear are also available under the brand names Orfit and Multiform Clear (see Table 29.1).

FABRICATION CHARACTERISTICS BY MATERIAL BASE

To fabricate effectively with any material, the first step is one that most people forget. To be successful, read the instruction sheet each manufacturer packs with the material. While there are more similarities than differences among materials with the same base, the therapist will get the best performance if she reads the "fine-tuning" instructions the manufacturers provide. For example, some plastic-based materials heat more quickly than others and any plastic-based material when overheated becomes more difficult to control. Be sure to read and retain the instruction sheets.

Fabrication Characteristics of Rubber-Based Materials

Because rubber-based materials tend to retain heat longer than plastic-based materials it is particularly important not to overheat them. Use the temperature recommended by the manufacturer, and have a thermometer available to check the water. Rubber-

based materials do not become more pliable with increased heating time. In fact, prolonged heating has been associated with shrinkage and is thought to be a possible cause of rubber-based splints breaking under stress. Rubber-based materials will adhere to themselves when hot, but the bond will probably not hold when the splint is cool. If the therapist intends to attach **outriggers** or add other components to a rubber-based splint, she must be sure to apply a bonding solvent as recommended by the manufacturer.

Rubber-based materials require more pressure and more manipulation than do plastic-based materials. It is necessary to press and manipulate to achieve good contact with areas such as the palmar arch and the thenar web space.

The strength of a splint is more a function of the contoured surfaces than any other factor. For a functional position splint to support a spastic wrist, the ulnar edge must be brought up higher than the ulnar styloid. The therapist can achieve this and avoid pressure on the ulnar styloid by padding the skin with a self-adhesive foam disc during the fabrication process. Rubber-based materials are not influenced by gravity, making them easier to use for large constructions (leg splints, shoulder orthoses with trunk supports, jackets, and fracture bracing) than plastic-based materials. A rubber-based material is easier to reform than a plastic-based material, because when reheated, it will approximate its original shape more readily so long as bonds or overlapped areas have not been used.

Fabrication Characteristics of Plastic-Based Materials

Plastic-based materials are exceptionally sensitive to overheating. To be successful, the therapist must be fully organized and prepared to complete the fabrication process before she puts the material into the hot water bath. The patient must be correctly positioned, and all tools she intends to use must be available. If an **outrigger** is going to be applied, it should be lined up; the bonding solvent should be open and ready to use.

Plastic-based materials, as a group have a working temperature of 140 to approximately 165°F. At less than 140°, the material will not soften enough to be malleable and at over 165° these materials will become overly pliable. The effects of gravity on an overheated plastic-based material can significantly reduce success by stretching the material beyond its ability to recover. If the water temperature is at the high end of the recommended range, the material will take less time to heat. None of the plastic-based materials should ever be heated for more than 60 to 80 sec unless the heat is at the lowest setting. Many materials will be ready to use in 30 to 45 sec! It is preferable to heat plastic-based materials in a horizontal heating pan as opposed to using a Hydrocollator in which material can be heated only in the vertical position.

Plastic-based materials are either self-bonding or nonbonding, depending on whether the manufacturer has treated the surface or not. Most nonbonding materials have a silicone derivative sprayed on their surfaces. Bonding solvents can be used to remove this coating. The edges of nonbonding materials self-bond easily because the cut edges no longer have a coating. Self-bonding materials will hold aggressively when overlapped, and the bond will be permanent. This is helpful when applying **outriggers,** but for the inexperienced therapist, self-bonding materials can be difficult to work with. If you have a plastic-based material that is self-bonding, one easy way to render it nonbonding is to add a few drops of liquid detergent to the hot water bath. Alternatively, the application of hand lotion or liquid soap to the surface will have the same effect.

Fabricating with Materials That Turn Clear or with Blended Materials

The therapist will be successful using either materials that turn clear or blended materials if she treats them as if they had a plastic base. Other considerations for these materials are described in the instruction sheets provided by each manufacturer.

GENERAL FABRICATING CONSIDERATIONS

Here are some general instructions that apply to all low-temperature materials regardless of their base.

Marking the Pattern

The best device for marking a pattern on any splinting material is a scratch awl. It is possible to use a ballpoint pen, but if one is used it will be necessary to cut inside the marked line, because it will not be possible to remove the pen marks later. A pencil marks well but the line is faint.

Cutting the Pattern

After the pattern has been marked, preheat the material for 10 to 20 sec and remove. The preheated material can be cut with scissors without undue effort or stress. It is important to cut with long strokes of the scissors rather than short nips, because long strokes ensure smooth edges. Place the material into the deepest part of the scissors and pull the blades together with one motion. Once the pattern has been cut, reheat the material for the amount of time recommended by the manufacturer.

Heating the Material

Splint pan netting should be in the bottom of the heating pan no matter what material is used. Because most heating pans are coiled on the base of the pan, without splint pan netting, the material will sit directly on the heating element. When heating low-temperature splinting material, be sure to follow the manufacturer's instructions. Err on the side of heating the material too little, never too much. If using a frying pan, be sure to move the material as it heats and to turn it at least once during the process. Have a spatula handy for this purpose.

Edge Finishing

If the therapist was careful in cutting the material, the edges will require very little extra finishing. If the edges are not as smooth as needed, wait until the splint is fully cooled, then dip the edge into the hot water for 20 sec. Run a finger along the warmed edge to smooth out any irregularities.

Adding Straps

Self-stick Velcro hook and loop tape is the most frequently used material for anchoring straps. To ensure good adhesion, warm the backing of the Velcro with a heat gun for a few seconds before placing it on the splint. Straps can be made of Velcro, or for extra patient comfort, select a padded material such as Beta Pile II or Velfoam. Straps may be added to self-bonding materials by cutting a narrow strip of the splinting material 1.5 times longer than the width of the strap and heating the splint near the edges of the strap and through holes cut in the strap. The little strip of splint material is heated and bonded to either side of the strap and to the splint below the holes (Fig. 29.15).

Reinforcing Stress Points

Aluminum wire may be sandwiched between two layers of splinting materials when extra strength is

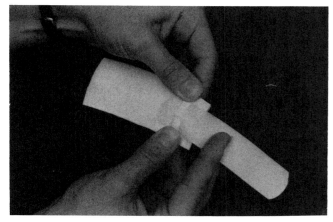

Figure 29.15. Demonstration of self-bonding method of applying straps to thermoplastic, using a scrap piece of the same thermoplastic.

required. Form the splint first and allow it to cool. Heat another piece of the same material in hot water and embed the wire into the warmed material. Apply bonding solvent to both the splint and the reinforcing piece. Spot heat the area of the splint to which the reinforcement will be applied, using a heat gun. Bring the two surfaces into contact and hold firmly for 15 sec or so.

Adding Outriggers

The process for adding **outriggers** is the same as for reinforcing stress points (Figs. 29.16 to 29.19). Be sure that the area on the splint base that will hold the **outrigger** and the material that will cover it have been heated properly. Apply bonding solvent (even with self-bonding materials) to both surfaces to ensure a permanent bond. Follow the directions from the manufacturer for best results.

CHECKOUT OF THE SPLINT

It is the responsibility of the occupational therapist to check out the fit of any upper extremity orthosis or any splint that she has made. The checkout is the process of examining the fit, function, and effectiveness of the orthosis. The checkout is done before establishing a wearing schedule and before either controls or use training. Periodic recheck of the orthosis may be necessary for those patients who wear the orthosis on a permanent or long-term basis.

The checkout considers the following points:

1. Does the orthosis actually accomplish the purpose for which it was intended? If not, it must be remade or redesigned.
2. Are the insides, edges, rivets, etc. padded and/or smooth to prevent skin abrasions? If not, they must be smoothed or padded. Many manufacturers of orthotic materials also manufacture self-adhesive

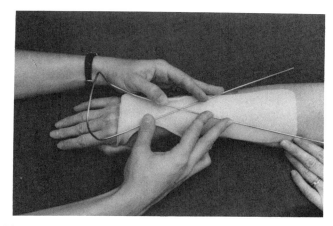

Figure 29.17.   After it has been shaped, the outrigger's length is measured.

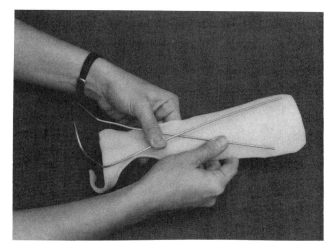

Figure 29.18.   After it has been cut, the outrigger's fit is rechecked.

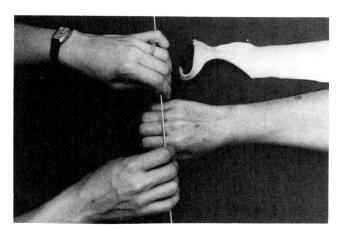

Figure 29.16.   The width of the outrigger is measured.

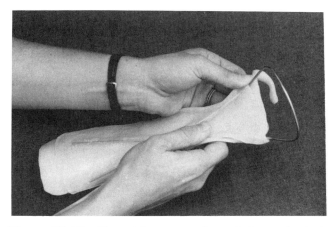

Figure 29.19.   The reinforcement piece of thermoplastic is added to hold the outrigger in place.

padding material, which can be cut with scissors and applied to the splint before molding. The size of the splint must allow for the extra room needed for adding padding.

3. Are there red areas on the patient's skin, indicating pressure, which remain for 20 min after the splint has been removed following wear for 30 min? If so, pressure must be relieved by spot heating the thermoplastic splint and pushing the material out away from the patient. Do not add padding; this increases the pressure.

4. Does the splint conform to the recommended criteria of good fit stated previously? If not, it must be corrected by cutting, reshaping, or even remaking.

Table 29.2 is an example of a form that may be used for orthotic checkout.

ESTABLISHING THE WEARING SCHEDULE

A patient adjusts to his new splint over time by following a wearing schedule that designates the amount of time the splint is to be worn and the amount of time the splint should remain off. The wearing schedule for a splint designed to correct deformity will start with a very brief wearing period, whereas a supportive splint may be indicated all of the time. When the splint is off, the patient will exercise the part or do his hygiene or other tasks permitted by the physician.

The wearing period is gradually increased to the full amount of time prescribed. The time is increased as the discomfort subsides or as the patient learns to

Table 29.2.   Checkout for Hand Splints

		General Considerations
Yes	No	Is the splint on the patient correctly?
Yes	No	Does this splint needlessly immobilize a joint?
Yes	No	If the splint, or parts of it, immobilizes a joint, is the splint removed periodically and the joints moved through passive range of motion?
Yes	No	Does this splint actually accomplish the function for which it was intended?
Yes	No	Does this splint cover the least amount of skin area to permit tactile sensation, but also provide good distribution of force over sufficiently large areas?
Yes	No	After wearing the splint for 30 min does the patient have reddened areas?
Yes	No	Do these disappear within 15 to 20 minutes?
Yes	No	Is the splint cosmetically acceptable to the patient?
		Traction Splints
Yes	No	If elastics are used, do they pull perpendicularly to the part as they should?
Yes	No	Is the tension in the elastics exactly right (just enough to provide a small force beyond that needed to pull the part to the limit of range of motion)?
Yes	No	If this is a static traction splint, is the force just enough to push slightly beyond the limit of range of motion?
Yes	No	Is the traction force distributed over as large an area as possible?
Yes	No	Is the force adjusted periodically to keep up with the changes in the patient's limits of range of motion?
Yes	No	Has a wearing schedule been established?
Yes	No	Does the splint prevent the patient from doing any functional activity he can otherwise do? What? _____ Why? _____
		Function Splints
		Can the patient pick up correctly:
Yes	No	Squashable things (paper cup, marshmallow, cotton, etc.)
Yes	No	Glass or metal objects
Yes	No	Thin things (cards, paper, checkers)
Yes	No	Small things (pencil, dice)
Yes	No	Eating utensils
Yes	No	Large things (beer can, cup, razor)
		What is the prehension force without the splint? _____ With the splint? _____
		As an indication of the patient's level of learning to control an externally powered orthosis, evaluate the variability of performance over trials by calculating the standard deviation. Measure the time (in 0.1 sec) to do a repetitive task 10 to 20 times, such as pick up a 1-inch cube on command and release it into a small box. Be sure the cube and box are located in the exact same spots each time and that the patient starts from the same position each time. Graphing each day's standard deviation will allow the patient to track his progress and the therapist to know when learning is leveling off.

tolerate the sensation of a device attached to him. A reasonable tolerance to a splint that is meant to be used at night is developed during the day so that the patient's sleep will not be repeatedly interrupted by discomfort or the handling of the splint by the nurse as it is removed and reapplied.

The wearing schedule may be established by the physician who ordered the orthosis or by the therapist who made or checked it out. Preferably, it is determined by these two professionals in collaboration.

DEVELOPING COMPLIANCE

Splinting complements therapy. It is not meant to be the only therapeutic tool for the treatment of hand dysfunction. Splint use is sometimes resisted by the patient who perceives the splint to be an inconvenience, functionally limiting, and interfering with occupational performance. Patient compliance with splint use improves when the splint's purpose and goal have been explained to the patient, when it fits comfortably, when it can be applied independently and when it meets the needs of the patient and allows him to continue with his life's occupations. The key to success of the splinting regimen is patient education, including the wearing schedule.

Acknowledgments—I would like to acknowledge Alice Shafer for her invaluable assistance in defining and delineating the current available thermoplastic materials used for the fabrication of splints and their unique methods of management.

STUDY QUESTIONS

1. What is the goal of hand splinting?
2. What is the functional position for a flaccid hand and wrist?
3. Explain the mechanical principles that support the clinical observation that long, wide splints cause fewer secondary problems than do short, narrow ones.
4. Why are outriggers mounted so the line of pull is perpendicular to the part?
5. What should a therapist do before making a splint pattern?
6. How would you know if a splint was exerting too much pressure on a patient's skin?
7. What points are considered during checkout of a splint?

8. Which of the splinting materials described here would you choose to make a thumb carpometacarpal stabilization splint for a 50-year-old female gardener with degenerative joint disease? On what factors is your choice based?

REFERENCES

Anderson, M. (1974). *Upper extremity orthotics* (3rd ed.). Springfield, IL: Charles C. Thomas.

Boyes, J. H. (Ed.). (1970). *Bunnell's surgery of the hand* (5th ed.). Philadelphia: J. B. Lippincott.

Brand, P. (1990). The forces of dynamic splinting: Ten questions before applying a dynamic splint to the hand. In J. Hunter, L. Schneider, E. Mackin, & A. Callahan (Eds.), *Rehabilitation of the hand* (3rd ed., pp. 1095–1100). St. Louis: C. V. Mosby.

Brand, P., & Hollister, A. (1993). *Clinical mechanics of the hand* (2nd ed.). St. Louis: C. V. Mosby.

Breger-Lee, D. E., & Buford, W. E. Jr. (1991). Update in splinting materials and methods. *Hand Clinics*, 7(3), 569–585.

Breger-Lee, D. E., & Buford, W. E. Jr. (1992). Properties of thermoplastic splinting materials. *Journal of Hand Therapy*, 5(4), 202–211.

Colditz, J. C. (1983). Low profile dynamic splinting of the injured hand. *American Journal of Occupational Therapy*, 37(3), 182–188.

Fess, E. W., & Philips, C. A. (1987). Hand splinting: Principles and methods (2nd ed.). St. Louis: C. V. Mosby.

Kiel, J. (1983). *Basic hand splinting: A pattern-designing approach*. Boston: Little, Brown & Co.

Malick, M. H. (1974). *Manual on dynamic hand splinting with thermoplastic materials. Low temperature materials and techniques*. Pittsburgh: Harmarville Rehabilitation Centers.

Malick, M. H. (1985). *Manual on static hand splinting. New materials and techniques* (Vol. 1, 5th ed.). Pittsburgh: Aren.

Pearson, S. O. (1990). Dynamic splinting. In J. Hunter, L. Schneider, E. Mackin, & A. Callahan (Eds.), *Rehabilitation of the hand* (3rd ed., pp. 452–456). St. Louis: C. V. Mosby.

Tenney, C. G., & Lisak, J. M. (1986). *Atlas of hand splinting*. Boston: Little, Brown & Co.

SUPPLEMENTARY READINGS

Mildenberger, L. A., Amadio, P. C., & An, K. N. (1986). Dynamic splinting: A systemic approach to the selection of elastic traction. *Archives of Physical Medicine & Rehabilitation*, 67(4), 241–244.

Roberts, S. L., & Falkenburg, S. A. (1992). *Biomechanics: Problem solving for functional activity*. St. Louis: C. V. Mosby.

Schultz-Johnson, K. (1992). Splinting—A problem solving approach. In B. G. Stanley & S. M. Tribuzi (Eds.), *Concepts in hand rehabilitation* (pp. 238–271). Philadelphia: F. A. Davis.

Ziegler, E. (1986). A problem-solving approach to orthotic design. *AOTA Physical Disabilities Special Interest Newsletter*, 9(2), 4–5.

Wheelchair Selection Process

Jean Deitz and Brian Dudgeon

"For man, mobility is a fundamental part of living. Being able to move about, to explore, under one's volitional control is a keystone of independence."—Warren, 1990

OBJECTIVES

After completing this chapter, the reader will be able to:

1. Describe the factors that should be considered in the wheelchair selection process and explain how they interrelate.
2. Describe the three basic types of wheelchairs and why each would be selected.
3. Demonstrate knowledge of the components common to many wheelchairs and describe why each merits consideration in the wheelchair selection process.
4. Demonstrate an understanding of the measurements that are typically taken to determine wheelchair and related seating system sizes for a particular individual.
5. Demonstrate an awareness of the role and responsibilities of the occupational therapist in the wheelchair selection process.
6. Demonstrate an understanding of how the occupational therapist can facilitate the client's participation in the wheelchair selection process.

The wheelchair selection process involves the client, the interdisciplinary team, and the equipment supplier or vendor. Family members, primary care providers, and others from the client's home, work, and leisure environments also can contribute important information useful in choosing an appropriate wheelchair system.

The selection process has a functional orientation and includes the consideration of multiple factors: (1) the client's needs and goals; (2) the client's home, work, recreational, and other community environments; (3) the client's physical and mental status and antici-

pated course of the disease or disability; (4) financial and community resources; (5) appearance and social acceptability issues related to both the client and to others in the client's environment; and (6) the ability of the wheelchair system to interface with other assistive technology used by the client. Throughout this process, attention should be focused on task as well as role specific uses of the wheelchair system. Essential issues include changing needs of the client and family, training needs for wheelchair use and maintenance, and anticipated advances in technology. Unfortunately, although a large range of wheelchair options are available, funding and community-based resources for monitoring and servicing sometimes limit choices.

Some individuals use wheelchairs only occasionally to meet brief transportation needs, while others use them continuously to meet the majority of day-to-day positioning and mobility demands. Especially in the latter case, the events that require the use of a wheelchair may be dramatic. For some individuals the stress or confusion represented by acquiring a wheelchair system can hinder their contribution to the assessment of needs and selection of a system. Others will view the acquisition of a wheelchair as a positive move toward greater independence and freedom. In either case, the perceived needs of the client are central to the overall process of wheelchair selection, prescription, and training, with the wheelchair viewed not just as a means for mobility but as a highly personal device that should be chosen with care and precision (Phillips & Nicosia, 1990).

To contribute to the wheelchair selection process, the occupational therapist must have a thorough grasp of the potential user's medical needs and personal profile, including environment, daily routines, and

GLOSSARY

Angle in space—The angle (in degrees) of the seat back in relation to the true vertical when the seat and back are rotated counterclockwise as a unit. This angle is typically a 5 to 10° backward tilt.
Prone—Lying horizontal with the face downward.
Proximity sensing systems—Systems that remotely sense the position of a body part (e.g., head) and use that position to control the wheelchair without physical contact between the part of the body used for control and the switch.
Scanning—A control option that presents choices one at a time (grouped or singly) until the desired choice

is offered for the user to select by switch activation.
Seat-back angle—The angle (in degrees) of the seat surface relative to the back surface. This angle is typically between 90 and 100°.
Sip and puff—A system typically involving a dual-action switch, in which one action is controlled by the user sipping on a tube held in the mouth and the second action is controlled by puffing on the same tube. (In wheelchair operation the chair functions can be controlled by patterns of switch closures.)
Third-party payer—An individual (other than the person receiving the services) or an organization (i.e., insurance company) that pays for services.

goals. In addition, the therapist should have a current understanding of wheelchair types, control mechanisms, and features and accessories; should be skilled in wheelchair size determination; and should be able to apply principles of seating and positioning. Though this information is presented as components, within the clinical reasoning process, all of these factors interrelate in comprehensive planning for functional mobility.

ASSESSMENT OF THE INDIVIDUAL

The assessment process typically evolves around concerns for both sitting posture and mobility needs. The therapist can best assist in the seating and wheelchair selection process by understanding the client's medical and personal profiles (Behrman, 1990). The medical profile includes the individual's medical history and physical assessment. The physical assessment should focus on neuromuscular status (e.g., muscle tone, postural control, reflexes, and coordination), musculoskeletal status (e.g., range of motion, deformity, and strength), sensory status (e.g., anesthetic skin and skin integrity), and physiologic status (e.g., temperature regulation and respiration). The therapist should be aware of the client's diagnosis and prognosis, considering whether the medical condition is temporary, stable, or progressive. Such factors influence choices related to rental or purchase as well as overall costs, complexity of options, and needs for adjustment. For example, if a condition is temporary, a chair may be selected with greater concern for cost factors. Thus a low-cost or rental chair might be considered. In contrast, if a client's condition is chronic and stable, necessitating full-time use of a wheelchair, then durability and individualization to meet needs are priorities. If a condition is progressive (e.g., amyotrophic lateral sclerosis), then a chair with a range of adjustment options to accommodate changes would be chosen.

The client's personal profile that should be considered in the wheelchair selection process includes

factors such as the individual's age, developmental status, living environment, educational and work history and plans, recreational pursuits, and other assistive technology needed or used. In examining these factors, a functional perspective is warranted, with special attention focused on the fit and operation of the chair within both private and public environments. Specifically, the therapist should consider factors such as floor surfaces, outdoor terrain, doorways, hall spaces, restroom dimensions, workspace design, transportability, and parking areas. If a client has used a wheelchair before, it is important for the therapist to determine the individual's assessment of the pros and cons of the client's current wheelchair system. Therapists should recognize that public accessibility is based, in part, on engineering concepts in which the typical wheelchair user sits at a 19-inch height and propels a manual wheelchair that is 32 inches wide and 48 inches long (Allan & Moffett, 1992). Many people are served well by environmental designs that accommodate this type of user, but other users continue to be constrained by the environment and need individualized guidance about making appropriate accommodations.

WHEELCHAIR TYPES

Once the therapist has a comprehensive understanding of the client's medical and personal profile, it is important for her to understand the types and uses of wheelchair systems. Wheelchairs can be divided into three general categories: (1) attendant-propelled chairs, (2) manual chairs, and (3) power mobility devices (Hobson, 1990).

Attendant-propelled Chairs

Attendant-propelled chairs are designed to be pushed by another individual because of the user's brief or chronic inability to propel or operate manual and power wheelchair systems in a functional or safe manner. Attendant-propelled chairs may be full size (e.g., those used in nursing homes) or may be smaller and created for use in limited spaces (e.g., folding stroller types). Such chairs may be used briefly, such as for transport in the community, or may be used for extended periods, thus requiring careful attention to postural needs and functional activities. Attendant-propelled chairs are also employed as a substitute for power mobility when the individual's typical mobility system is being repaired or when space constraints, such as in airline aisles, preclude power mobility use. When assisting a client in selecting an attendant-propelled chair, it is necessary to consider not only the fit and comfort of the chair for the person who will be seated in the chair but also the fit and comfort of the chair for the person most likely to be pushing it (Kettle, Rowley, & Chamberlain, 1992). Besides chairs specifically designed to be attendant propelled, many manual wheelchairs (described below) can also serve as attendant-propelled devices.

Manual Chairs

The manual wheelchair is typically selected if the person is able to propel the wheelchair independently (Fig. 30.1). These chairs have a variety of frame types, with differing weights and transport features. In general, manual wheelchairs have rigid frames or folding frames, the latter of which are either free or fixed. Quick-release wheels also may be used. These characteristics allow relative ease in transporting the wheelchair in automobiles. The most conventional manual wheelchair frame has large rear wheels, used to propel the chair, with smaller caster wheels in the front. Wheelchairs of this design are highly maneuverable and easy to propel, and they allow greater freedom for tilting, which is necessary when ascending or descending curbs. Standard designs weigh ≥ 50 lb without specialized seating systems. In recent years, sturdy but lighter weight metals and designs have been adapted from sport wheelchairs, resulting in lightweight and

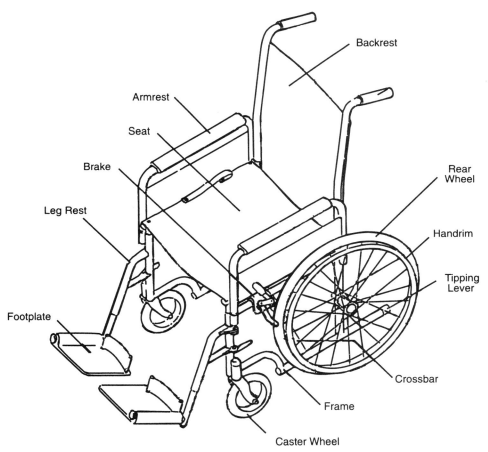

Figure 30.1. Conventional wheelchair.

ultra-lightweight wheelchairs ranging from about 40 to ≤25 lb. These lighter weight chairs are now often used by active wheelchair users on a full-time basis. Many newer designs allow adjustable wheel positions and seat heights, making it possible to optimize biomechanical efficiency for the user (Masse, Lamontagne, & O'Riain, 1992). Along with reduced weight, these changes can enhance propulsion and ease transport (Brubaker, 1990; Parziale, 1991).

Other types of manual wheelchair designs include the amputee frame for the person with loss of, or severely reduced, weight of the lower limbs. In this design, the rear axle is offset farther behind the seat back. This concentrates a person's weight farther in front of the rear axle, thus reducing the risk of the chair tipping over backward. Another type of manual wheelchair is the indoor frame. It has large front wheels, used for propulsion, with smaller casters in back. While it rolls easily over door sills and rug edges, curbs are difficult to traverse and transfers may be more awkward.

Manual wheelchairs are characterized by propelling and braking using the upper limbs. Typically, handrims are attached to the outside of the large wheels. Optimally, the user is seated so that with elbows extended to about 120°, each hand rests at the 12 o'clock position of each handrim (Brubaker, 1990). Maneuvering generally occurs between the 11 and 2 o'clock positions on each side. Circular steel tube handrims are typical. However, for users who have difficulty with grip, handrims can be covered with vinyl coating, knobs or other projections can be added to the rims so that grip is not required, and/or gloves or mitts can be worn to improve traction. The latter have the additional benefit of protecting the hands. Handrims vary in size. Smaller handrims, often used on racing chairs, result in a slower and more difficult start, but provide for a faster top speed that is sustainable with less effort (Ragnarsson, 1990). A common means of maneuvering the wheelchair by persons with hemiplegia is to use the appropriate handrim as well as the leg and foot to steer and provide additional propulsion or braking. This requires removal of the footrest and may require dropping the seat height or using smaller-diameter wheels to optimize foot contact with the floor. For the user who plans to propel the wheelchair using only one arm, a chair can be ordered with both hand rims on one side so that each wheel can be controlled independently or together. Learning to maneuver two handrims on the same side can be difficult. Another alternative for unilateral control involves single lever drives. Typically, this involves a forward and backward motion to propel the chair and rotation of the lever to turn the chair.

The manual nature of wheelchairs in this category applies to both propulsion and to braking. As an aid to propelling on inclines, hill climbers or grade-aid devices can be used, which restrict the counterclockwise movement of wheels through a friction stop engaged by a lever on each tire. Speed control and braking to a stop simply depend on slowing wheel rotation by use of the arms or legs. Parking brakes restrict wheel turning but are not recommended for slowing or bringing the chair to a stop. These brakes are used on each large wheel and are engaged through a variable length single or dual action lever, depending on reach and force abilities. Such levers impinge on the tire to resist rolling and require periodic tightening after tire wear. Antirotation locks also can be used on casters. Dynamic braking systems that allow continuous braking on hills or when coming to a stop can be obtained with some wheelchairs in Europe, but are not generally available in the United States.

Unconventional mobility devices also should be considered when selecting a manual mobility system for a specific user. Examples of these are row cycles and gurneys. Row cycles are large, low to the ground, three-wheeled cycles that are propelled by a rowing action that activates chain-driven rear wheels (Bergen, Presperin, & Tallman, 1990). Gurneys allow the individual to be positioned in **prone,** and they are propelled by using the upper extremities.

Power Mobility Devices (Motorized Wheelchairs)

Power mobility devices are used by individuals (1) who cannot propel a chair using either the hands or the feet, (2) for whom the energy expenditure required to walk or propel a manual chair is contraindicated, (3) who have musculoskeletal complications such as arthritis in upper limb joints, (4) who are prone to repetitive stress injury, and/or (5) who have neuromuscular dysfunction that may cause associated reactions in the lower extremities when the upper extremities are used for wheelchair propulsion.

There are a number of different types of power mobility devices. Conventional power wheelchairs may resemble the manual frame with large powered rear wheels and casters in front. Power-base wheelchairs are designed so that the wheels are independent of the seating components. Such bases may have front- or rear-wheel drive with small and/or large wheel diameters. For both types of designs, the wheels may be connected to the drive motors through exposed or concealed belts, chains, or gear systems. Both of these types of power wheelchair designs are noted for being sturdy and appropriate for the full-time user in both indoor and outdoor environments. Some conventional styles leave more space beneath the chair for respirators and other equipment than do power-base chairs. Power-base designs generally allow for ease in changing seating dimensions, such as for a growing child.

Several power-base chairs have options that enable the user independently to change seat height or elevate to a standing position. Similarly, some manual wheelchair systems have manual lever systems that allow the user to rise into a near standing position. These allow the person greater flexibility in movement and environmental accessibility than do fixed height designs. Consider the student trying to access books in a library or a person working in a shop using power equipment or needing access to higher-than-standard counters.

The primary disadvantages of conventional power chairs and power-base chairs are that they are large and heavy and may be difficult to transport. Special lifts are required in vans or buses, and the sizes of some chairs necessitate enlarged openings in these vehicles. Alternatively, in some cases, ramps can be used by an attendant to load power wheelchairs into vans or trucks. Most often this is accomplished with the user not seated in the chair.

Lightweight power wheelchairs designed to be taken apart for transport in more conventional vehicles are available. These chairs are usually built on folding frames and have lower powered motors, making hill climbing and use on uneven surfaces less successful. Assistance with taking apart and reassembling the chair is often required. Another option for power mobility is the use of an add-on unit placed on a manual wheelchair to provide power assistance. Such systems can be engaged or unengaged for the option of either manual or power mobility. Because a significant amount of weight is added to the chair and units are not easily taken on and off the frame, this option may be more commonly suggested for trial purposes or as a transition toward regular power wheelchair use.

An increasingly popular type of power wheelchair is the scooter. These are typically three-wheeled, although some four-wheeled designs are available, and may have either rear- or front-wheel drive (National Rehabilitation Hospital, 1991). Most often, these designs are characterized by tiller control, wherein users steer the scooter by rotating the front wheel while using a switch for forward and reverse power. This type of chair is appropriate for the marginal walker and is often used to compensate for a person's inability to comfortably travel distances outside the home (Warren, 1990). These chairs are noted for ease of mounting and dismounting, cosmetic appearance, and in some cases for ease of transportability. Often they are modular and can be loaded in the trunk of a car or the back of a station wagon.

A variety of more novel designs has been devel-oped for power mobility. For example, a chair, referred to as the Access Mobility System, was developed to enable ascent and descent of stairs. This chair rolls on wheels for regular surfaces and has a track system for stairs. It is very heavy with limited maneuverability in small spaces. A contrasting example, is the Hoverround (Hoverround Corp.), which advances and rotates through a single powered wheel. This device has four other wheels that are small and move freely. Low profile footrests and armrests permit easy access to tables. While the small wheels and single motor facilitate maneuverability, these features also limit its use on inclines and uneven surfaces.

Numerous factors that are unique to power wheelchairs require consideration when making a selection. The therapist should determine whether the device will be used primarily indoors or indoors and outdoors. If the device is to be used in both settings, it will need more stability, power, distance capability, and durability. In addition, the therapist should consider the batteries, which at present are the best solution for power. Deep-cycle lead acid batteries, either wet cell or sealed cell types, are generally recommended ("Rechargeable," 1991). Noise factors, braking systems, ride quality, and portability (including ease of assembly and disassembly, if appropriate) also must be determined. If the device can be disassembled, the weight and size of each part should be carefully evaluated for transportability.

Selection of appropriate controls for driving the power mobility device is critical. Power mobility devices are typically driven using one of two types of options: proportional or microswitch control. Most commonly, a proportional joystick is used in which directions and speeds are linked to angle and magnitude of displacement. An alternative is microswitch control activated either with a joystick or a multiple-switch array. Each switch activation engages a single preset speed and direction. Less responsive than proportional control, such switch systems generally require less skilled movements to achieve control, albeit learning to use such controls is not simple. Besides activating a switch using a body part (i.e., hand/arm, chin, foot, head, mouth/lips/tongue), wheelchair switches can be operated using special techniques such as **sip and puff, scanning,** and **proximity sensing systems.** When selecting controls, the therapist should consider the adjustment capabilities of various systems in relationship to the needs to the individual. For example, clients with poor motor control might benefit from programmable electronics so that wheelchair speeds are automatically restricted when turning thus requiring less refined movements on the part of the user.

Modern power wheelchairs and scooters are electronically braked, meaning that drive wheels do not rotate unless under power. Belts or gears are released by levers that allow the chair to roll freely. Parking brakes, like those on manual wheelchairs, typically are provided for additional stability and safety.

COMMON WHEELCHAIR COMPONENTS

Armrests of wheelchairs can be fixed, detachable, or swing away. The latter two styles may allow greater ease in sliding-board and other sideways transfers than fixed armrest. Height adjustment is an option with many detachable styles. Desk-arm styles can be selected that are low in front with a raised padded area for the elbow. The low part allows the wheelchair to be rolled under the edge of a table or desk to enable the person to move closer to these surfaces. Guards can be used on fixed or detachable armrests to keep clothes from coming in contact with wheels. Stable armrests, typically seen in fixed or detachable styles, are often preferred by users who perform wheelchair push-ups for pressure release. Attachment of lap trays may require use of full-length armrests or other specialized hardware.

The front rigging consists of leg rests and footplates. Leg rests may be fixed, swing away, or detachable. The latter two options can be important for transfers. Elevating leg rests are appropriate for users who have limited knee flexion or who need lower extremity elevation because of edema or other medical concerns. They also are typically necessary for comfort when wheelchair recline systems are used. Footplates can be fixed but generally swing up to allow the foot to reach the floor. They come in a variety of sizes and can be equipped with heel loops, ankle straps, and/or other foot harnessing. Footplates that allow for angle adjustment for special needs at the ankle joint can be obtained. To keep the foot from colliding with front wheels, a calf pad, strap, or other block is often attached to leg rests or footplates.

Tires can be either pneumatic (air filled), semipneumatic (airless foam inserts), or solid-core rubber and are mounted on spoke or molded wheels. Air-filled tires require regular maintenance but provide a more cushioned ride and have a shock absorber function that tends to improve comfort and prolong the life of the chair. Semipneumatics provide good cushioning and less maintenance, but tire wear many be more of a problem. Solid-core tires are noted for minimal maintenance. Newly designed nonpneumatic tires approach the light weight and low rolling resistance of high-pressure pneumatic tires (Gordon, Kauzlarick, & Thacker, 1989).

Casters vary in diameter, with smaller ones facilitating maneuverability. Pneumatic and semipneumatic caster tires provide some shock absorption for use outdoors and on rough surfaces. Solid-core caster tires are best for use indoors and on smooth surfaces.

Placement of the rear wheel axles is fixed on most wheelchairs but adjustable on others, especially newer manual lightweight and ultralight styles. Backward placement of the axle tends to increase stability; by contrast, forward placement of the axle decreases stability but increases maneuverability and shortens turning radius. Sometimes rear wheels can be cambered (tilted inward at the top). This orients the handrim for easier propulsion and may slightly widen the wheel base for better stability.

Antitipping extensions can be used on a wheelchair to prevent the chair from tipping backward and/or forward. Typically used on the back, these fixed or adjustable extensions can improve safety during wheelchair mobility training.

Seatbelts, safety vests, and harnesses vary in design and are used for both safety and positioning purposes. These devices should be considered for individuals who require restraint because of poor judgment and for individuals with severe neuromuscular impairments who need control for posture and safety.

Frame color and upholstery color and material options are numerous. Users can personalize their appearance through selections of colors and other styling. Durability, repair, and compatibility of materials with the concerns of temperature regulation, friction, moisture, and skin protection also require careful planning.

Recline and tilt-in-space options enable postural changes for rest and pressure relief. In attendant-propelled wheelchairs a $\leq 30°$ semireclining option or a $\leq 90°$ full-reclining option can be considered. Some systems allow tilt-in-space for reclining, whereby the seat and back assembly pivot together. This feature makes the use of postural seating components less awkward because the angle between the seat and the back remains unchanged. Power recline systems can be used with conventional or power-base designs. Such systems may involve tilt-in-space and/or low-shear back recline, both of which provide pressure relief and rest positioning (Hobson, 1992).

Narrowing devices are available for some folding frame manual chairs to reduce chair width temporarily for fitting through smaller openings. The device mounts on one side of the seat and arm. By turning a crank the chair narrows by starting the folding process.

Wheelchair tie downs are necessary as safety mechanisms to keep chairs stabilized when traveling in vans or buses. Different styles may be required based on wheelchair design. Such devices secure the wheelchair to the base of the vehicle, while the individual is independently secured in the wheelchair seat or in another seating device within the vehicle.

WHEELCHAIR SIZE DETERMINATION AND SEATING AND POSITIONING

Wheelchair Sizing

Modern wheelchairs are engineered as modular systems, assembled to match best the physical dimensions of the user. Measurements of the individual form the basis for determining wheelchair frame size, needs for adjustable ranges in component parts, or need for customization to meet special requirements.

Appropriate size determinations of the wheelchair frame, seat and back, and leg rests and armrests are based on measurements typically taken of the client while in an optimally seated position. If difficult to position, the therapist may position the individual on a mat in supine or side lying and take careful measurements of distances between key landmarks. Then these measurements can be confirmed for accuracy in a seated position. The individual's typical or specialized clothing needs should be considered during measurement. If thoracolumbar bracing or other lower limb orthotics and prosthetics are likely to be used in the wheelchair, they should be worn during wheelchair sizing measurements. Manufacturers of wheelchairs and seating systems have differing standards for measurement and sizing, but typically included are measures of pelvic or hip width; thigh and leg lengths; heights of mid-back, mid-scapula, and shoulder levels; and elbow position (Fig. 30.2).

SEAT WIDTH

To measure for seat width, the widest point across the hips and thighs is determined, and a total of 5 cm (2 inches) are typically added for adequate clearance on each side. Overall wheelchair width may be dictated by the seat width measure. Because narrower wheelchairs are likely to improve ease of handrim propulsion and maneuverability, wheelchairs should be as narrow as possible while allowing for comfort, ease of repositioning, and transfers.

SEAT DEPTH

For seat depth, the greatest lengths of both the left and right sides are taken from the most posterior part of the buttocks, under the thigh, to the popliteal fossa of each knee. About 5 cm (2 inches) are then subtracted from the measure. This allows as much weight bearing through the thigh as possible, without the front edge of the seat pressing into the back of the knee. Right and left leg length discrepancies can be apparent because of hip dislocation, pelvic rotation and obliquity, or other anatomical factors. The shorter side may be used to determine seat depth, or if a

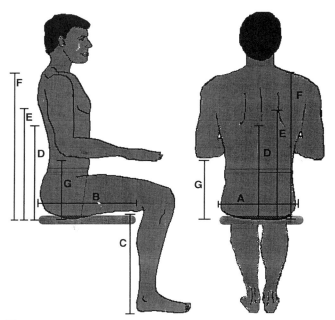

Figure 30.2. Measurements taken for wheelchair sizing: *A,* hip and thigh width, *B,* thigh length; *C,* leg length; *D,* back height to below scapula; *E,* back height to mid-scapula or axilla; *F,* back height to top of shoulder; *G,* elbow and forearm height. For B through G, all measurements are taken on both the left and the right sides.

greater than 1-inch discrepancy is found, the front seat edge may be offset to accommodate the length of each side.

BACK HEIGHT

For back height, three measures are generally taken of the back: from the seat surface upward (1) to the mid-back just under the scapula, (2) to the mid-scapula or axilla, and (3) to the top of the shoulder. Back height is affected by seat cushions, which should be considered in sizing decisions. Height of the back is determined based on the needs for postural stability and freedom of arm movements for propulsion or other functions. For those who exclusively self-propel, a chair back height of 2 to 5 cm (1 to 2 inches) under the tip of the scapula may be preferred. For sporting activities, the optimal back height may be even lower. By contrast, for power wheelchair users, back heights to mid-scapula or to the top of the shoulder may be necessary to allow use of postural supports for the upper trunk and the head. Back width may also need to be measured due to deformity or to determine the space available for lateral trunk supports.

SEAT HEIGHT AND LEG RESTS

For seat height and leg rests, right and left leg lengths are determined with the individual's knees and ankles positioned at about 90°. Measures are taken from under the distal thigh to the heel of the individual's commonly used footwear or shoe. Several centimeters of adjustment are typically available in leg rest lengths to accommodate left and right side discrepancies. Unusual leg length needs may require special ordering. Overall wheelchair seat height is based on positioning of the individual such that footrests have at least 5 cm (2 inches) clearance from the floor. Use of seat cushions impact this decision by raising overall seat height.

ARMREST HEIGHT

For armrest height, a measure is taken—with the shoulder complex in neutral, the arms hanging at the sides, and the elbows flexed to 90°—from under each elbow to the cushioned seating surface. Armrests need to provide forearm support with neutral shoulder position but should not obstruct reach to handrims for propulsion or to brakes for locking.

Wheelchair Seating and Positioning

Effective seating of the individual in the wheelchair has several broad goals, including promoting (1) posture, (2) comfort, (3) physiologic maintenance and tissue protection, (4) sensory readiness, (5) upper limb function, and (6) cosmetic appearance and social acceptance. A process of evaluation and intervention related to positioning includes all team members. This ongoing concern may be coordinated by the occupational therapist who incorporates perceived needs of the individual and family with medical care concerns in making recommendations regarding the selection of a seating system and the type of wheelchair appropriate for the individual. Functional abilities also need careful analysis, because the seating and positioning recommendations should maximize rather than restrict the individual's access to activities in various environments (i.e., home, school, work, and community). Effective use of seating systems may have an impact on the abilities of the user to such an extent that basic decisions about choice of wheelchair will be affected.

Seating strategies and particular techniques are both age and diagnosis specific (Letts, 1991). Generic principles can be identified and include the need to provide the individual with a solid base of support. The sling seat, common to free-folding wheelchair frames, is the seating element most often criticized because it tends to create pelvic instability and malalignment of the thighs (Bergen et al., 1990) and is often the primary component of seating modification (Krasilovsky, 1993). A solid seating base is accomplished by stabilizing the pelvis on a firm surface with pressure distributed throughout the buttocks and throughout the full length of each thigh. Postural control is influenced in part by the firm seat and back surfaces as well as by adjustments to the **seat-back angle** and the **angle in space.** A sitting position with 90° hip, knee, and ankle positions and with the seat fully upright is often preferred. This position distributes weight through the buttocks and thighs, and for some individuals this position inhibits abnormal reflexive responses. A standard wheelchair frame generally has a 95° seat-back angle with a 3 to 5° angle-in-space recline. Adjustments of these angles is usually accomplished through brackets that secure the modular seat and the back components to the frame. The seat and back surfaces can be either planar (flat), precontoured or custom contoured. Planar designs are appropriate only for individuals who need little or no postural support and who can successfully move to reposition themselves for comfort. Contoured designs are used to provide added contact for postural support and distribution of pressure. Customized contouring is often needed by individuals with fixed deformity of the pelvis or spine or who experience discomfort from lack of support at the lumbar spine. Cushioning of the seat and back surfaces may call for use of single materials or combinations of variable density foams, air, fluid, or gels. Surface materials also should be selected considering factors such as heat and moisture, friction, durability, and cosmetic appearance.

A seatbelt is routinely recommended for safety and can serve an important role in stabilizing the pelvis. This anterior support is typically mounted on the wheelchair frame so that it pulls on the pelvis at a 45° angle to the base of the seat back, fitting just under the anterior superior iliac spines. Additional seating supports should be used as needed to improve posture, restrict abnormal movements, and promote head control and voluntary use of the limbs. If sitting balance and posture continue to be problematic, lateral trunk and thigh supports may be suggested. Additional use of anterior supports also may be necessary across the upper trunk, knee, or ankle. Neck and head supports are sometimes recommended for safety, and may involve the use of continuous contact devices to aid posture and head alignment. Upper extremity positioning also may be of concern, in which case, contoured armrests or the wheelchair laptray can be used for effective positioning.

Remembering that sitting is a dynamic rather than a static state, seating devices should allow some element of pressure relief and freedom of movement. The principle of less may mean more can be suggested for applying specialized seating systems. As more seating apparatuses are used, freedom of movement will likely diminish. Therefore, only those components that maximize individuals' abilities to function, correct their positions, and maintain comfort should be suggested.

To justify expenses associated with therapeutic positioning, the experienced therapist can employ clinical observation and literature reviews to justify use of specialized seating. Although improved motor skills (Myhr & von Wendt, 1991; Nwaobi, 1987), comfort and participation (Hulme, Gallacher, et al., 1987), physiologic supports (Nwaobi & Smith, 1986; Stewart, 1991), and functional independence (Hulme, Shaver, et al., 1987; McEwen, 1992; McEwen & Lloyd, 1990; Trefler, Nickey, & Hobson, 1983; Trefler & Taylor, 1991) are widely recognized as benefits, several claims should be viewed cautiously. Specialized seating mostly provides a prosthetic effect, meaning that it works well only when used. Little evidence can be cited that verifies the beneficial use of seating apparatuses to correct or prevent deformity, speed developmental gains or recovery, or reduce the need for additional therapies (Borello-France, Burdett, & Gee, 1988; Mac Neela, 1987).

FINAL DETERMINATION

In making a final determination regarding wheelchair style and size, control systems, and seating components, the team needs a comprehensive and functional view, simultaneously considering the needs, desires, and resources of the user as well as anticipated advances in technology. During this process, costs and related funding issues are of critical concern. More expensive technology and options should not be ordered unless justifiable for increased function, health (e.g., skin protection), user satisfaction, or safety. When more-expensive choices are being considered, it is important to rule out the feasibility of using less-expensive options. For example, before selecting power mobility, it is important to rule out the feasibility of using a manual chair, because the cost of providing and maintaining a powered system is estimated to be approximately three times that required for a manual system (Warren, 1990). In such cases, appropriate justification must be clearly delineated for clients and **third-party payers.**

Also, in the wheelchair selection process, it should not be assumed that the optimal choice involves only one means of mobility. Instead, it should be recognized, that for some, the optimal choice might be the use of multiple means of mobility (York, 1989). For example, an individual might benefit from having a manual chair for traveling short distances such as those required in a home and a power chair for traveling longer distances in the community and at work. Because funding sources may only pay for one of these options, priorities must be established.

The occupational therapist can facilitate the client's participation in the wheelchair selection process in at least three ways. First, the therapist can help the client identify functional needs and planned uses of mobility and seating systems. Second, the therapist has an educational role in helping the client understand various wheelchairs, related options, and seating systems. Third, the therapist should assist the client in prioritizing needs, because it may not be possible to identify a chair and options that will necessarily meet all the recognized needs. This involvement of the client is essential. As Ragnarsson (1990) stated, "Ultimately, the most important factor in the success of a wheelchair prescription is the user's total level of acceptance and satisfaction with his chair as it combines looks, comfort, and function" (p. 8).

CLINICIAN RESPONSIBILITIES

Technology is changing rapidly. Therefore, it is a continual challenge for occupational therapists to remain current. Therapists have a responsibility to keep abreast of new product development and product evaluation research (Phillips & Nicosia, 1990). They need to be able to provide clients with current information on the advantages and disadvantages of various wheelchairs and different components and features. In addition, they must have current knowledge of issues related to availability, serviceability, and performance of various wheelchairs and options (Behrman, 1990). The following are some sources of information about wheelchairs; related options; and manufacturers of mobility systems, controls, and seating systems (addresses are given under "Supplementary Resources," below):

Paraplegia News & Sports 'N Spokes
Accent on Living
Assistive Technology
TeamRehab Report
Exceptional Parent

Therapists also are encouraged to explore wheelchair standards that have been developed by RESNA (an interdisciplinary association for the advancement of rehabilitation and assistive technologies), the International Standards Organization, and the American National Standards Institute. These voluntary standards for wheelchair developers and manufacturers provide guidelines for product specifications based on uniform measurements and testing. Use of these standards facilitates product comparisons. Besides being aware of wheelchair standards, the therapist is also responsible, in combination with the interdisciplinary team, to develop relationships with appropriate vendors of seating and wheelchair systems. The National Association of Medical Equipment Suppliers (Alexandria, VA) can assist in identifying qualified vendors.

The occupational therapist's responsibility to the

individual does not end with selecting a wheelchair and seating system. Because safe and efficient operation of mobility systems are essential, once the chair has been provided a checkout should be conducted and appropriate training of the user and care providers should commence. This should include review of the chair for fit and adjustment, use of the chair indoors and outdoors and on a variety of surfaces (e.g., level, incline, and uneven), transfers (e.g., bed, toilet, and car), transport of the wheelchair (e.g., cars, trucks, vans, and buses), and maintenance of the wheelchair (e.g., cleaning the chair, lubricating moving parts, monitoring tire pressure and wear, adjusting brakes, and caring for batteries). Throughout training, safety issues should be emphasized, because accidents, though infrequent, do occur and in some cases appear to be preventable (Calder & Kirby, 1990). Along with the initial checkout and training, periodic follow-up should be planned to address further safety issues and fit and adjustment, to meet the changing needs of the individual, and to provide the individual with updated information about new options.

Acknowledgments—We would like to thank and acknowledge the following people for critiquing this manuscript and for contributing their knowledge and expertise: Laura Shillam, occupational therapy specialist, Assistive Technology Clinic, University of Washington Hospital and Medical Center, Seattle; Joyce Engel, assistant professor, University of Washington, Seattle; Sharon Greenberg, senior lecturer, University of Washington, Seattle; and Cynthia Dudgeon, community home health therapist, Seattle. In addition, we would like to express our appreciation to Bill Abelson, secretary, Occupational Therapy Division, University of Washington, for his editorial skills.

STUDY QUESTIONS

1. Who should be involved in the wheelchair selection process?
2. What are the three basic types of wheelchairs and why would each be selected?
3. What factors should be taken into consideration in the wheelchair selection process?
4. Describe a situation in which the optimal decision for an individual might involve the selection of more than one mobility device.
5. Compare and contrast conventional power wheelchairs and power-base wheelchairs.
6. Name and describe two types of controls for power mobility devices. Which would be preferable for a person with cerebral palsy and extremely poor upper extremity control? Why?
7. In determining wheelchair and related seating system sizes for a particular individual, what measurements typically are taken?
8. What are the six broad goals of wheelchair seating and positioning?
9. How can an occupational therapist keep abreast of new product development and research related to these products?
10. How can the occupational therapist facilitate the client's participation in the wheelchair selection process?
11. Once the wheelchair and seating system have been selected, what is the role of the occupational therapist?

REFERENCES

Allan, B. L., & Moffett, F. C. (1992). *Accessibility design for all: An illustrated handbook, Washington State regulations* (5th ed.). Olympia: Washington Council/A.I.A.

Behrman, A. L. (1990). Factors in functional assessment. *Journal of Rehabilitation Research and Development: Clinical Supplement, 2,* 17–30.

Bergen, A. F., Presperin, J., & Tallman, T. (1990). *Positioning for function: Wheelchairs and other assistive technologies.* Valhalla, NY: Valhalla Rehabilitation Publications, Ltd.

Borello-France, D. F., Burdett, R. G., & Gee, Z. L. (1988). Modification of sitting posture of patients with hemiplegia using seat boards and backboards. *Physical Therapy, 68*(1), 67–71.

Brubaker, C. (1990). Ergonometric considerations. *Journal of Rehabilitation Research and Development: Clinical Supplement, 2,* 37–48.

Calder, C. J., & Kirby, R. (1990). Fatal wheelchair-related accidents in the United States. *American Journal of Physical Medicine and Rehabilitation, 69*(4), 184–190.

Gordon, J., Kauzlarich, J. J., & Thacker, J. G. (1989). Tests of two new polyurethane foam wheelchair tires. *Journal of Rehabilitation Research and Development, 26*(1), 33–46.

Hobson, D. A. (1990). Seating and mobility for the severely disabled. In R. Smith & J. Leslie Jr. (Eds.), *Rehabilitation Engineering* (pp. 193–252). Boca Raton, FL: CRC Press.

Hobson, D. A. (1992). Comparative effects of posture on pressure and shear at the body-seat interface. *Journal of Rehabilitation Research and Development, 29*(4), 21–31.

Hulme, J. B., Gallacher, K., Walsh, J., Niesen, S., & Waldron, D. (1987). Behavioral and postural changes observed with use of adaptive seating by clients with multiple handicaps. *Physical Therapy, 67,* 1060–1067.

Hulme, J. B., Shaver, J., Acher, S., Mullette, L., & Eggert, C. (1987). Effects of adaptive seating devices on the eating and drinking of children with multiple handicaps. *American Journal of Occupational Therapy, 41*(2), 81–89.

Kettle, M., Rowley, C., & Chamberlain, M. A. (1992). A national survey of wheelchair users. *Clinical Rehabilitation, 6,* 67–73.

Krasilovsky, G. (1993). Seating assessment and management in a nursing home population. *Physical and Occupational Therapy in Geriatrics, 11*(2), 25–38.

Letts, R. M. (1991). *Principles of seating the disabled.* Boca Raton, FL: CRC Press.

Mac Neela, J. C. (1987). An overview of therapeutic positioning for multiply-handicapped persons, including augmentative communication users. *Occupational and Physical Therapy in Pediatrics, 7*(2), 39–60.

Masse, L. C., Lamontagne, M., & O'Riain, M. D. (1992). Biomechanical analysis of wheelchair propulsion for various seating positions. *Journal of Rehabilitation Research and Development, 29*(3), 12–28.

McEwen, I. R. (1992). Assistive positioning as a control parameter of social-communicative interactions between students with profound multiple disabilities and classroom staff. *Physical Therapy, 72*(9), 634–647.

McEwen, I. R., & Lloyd, L. L. (1990). Positioning students with cerebral palsy to use augmentative and alternative communication. *Language, Speech and Hearing Services in Schools, 21,* 15–21.

Myhr, U., & von Wendt, L. (1991). Improvement of functional sitting position for children with cerebral palsy. *Developmental Medicine and Child Neurology, 33*(3), 246–256.

National Rehabilitation Hospital. (1991). *Product comparison and evaluation: Scooters.* Washington, DC: Author, Rehabilitation Engineering Center.

Nwaobi, O. M. (1987). Seating orientations and upper extremity function in children with cerebral palsy. *Physical Therapy, 67*(8), 1209–1212.

Nwaobi, O. M., & Smith, P. D. (1986). Effect of adaptive seating on pulmonary function of children with cerebral palsy. *Developmental Medicine and Child Neurology, 28*(3), 351–354.

Parziale, J. R. (1991). Standard v. lightweight wheelchair propulsion in spinal cord injured patients. *American Journal of Physical Medicine and Rehabilitation, 70*(2), 76–80.

Phillips, L., & Nicosia, A. (1990). An overview . . . with reflections past and present of a consumer. *Journal of Rehabilitation Research and Development: Clinical Supplement, 2,* 1–7.

Ragnarsson, K. T. (1990). Prescription considerations and a comparison of conventional and lightweight wheelchairs. *Journal of Rehabilitation Research and Development: Clinical Supplement, 2,* 8–16.

Rechargeable, deep-cycle, lead-acid batteries for powered wheelchair and scooter users. (1991). *Health Devices, 20*(12), 474–494.

Stewart, C. P. (1991). Physiological considerations in seating. *Prosthetics and Orthotics International, 15*(3), 193–198.

Trefler, E., & Taylor, S. J. (1991). Prescription and positioning: Evaluating the physically disabled individual for wheelchair seating. *Prosthetics and Orthotics International, 15*(3), 217–224.

Trefler, E., Nickey, J., & Hobson, D. A. (1983). Technology in the education of multiply-handicapped children. *American Journal of Occupational Therapy, 37*(6), 381–387.

Warren, C. G. (1990). Powered mobility and its implications. *Journal of Rehabilitation Research and Development: Clinical Supplement, 2,* 74–85.

York, J. (1989). Mobility methods selected for use in home and community environments. *Physical Therapy, 69*(9), 736–747.

SUPPLEMENTARY RESOURCES

Suggested Readings

Herzberg, S. R. (1993). Positioning the nursing home resident: An issue of quality of life. *American Journal Occupational Therapy, 47*(1), 75–77.

Hughes, C. J., Weimar, W. H., Sheth, P. N., & Brubaker, C. E. (1992). Biomechanics of wheelchair propulsion as a function of seat position and user-to-chair interface. *Archives of Physical Medicine and Rehabilitation, 73,* 263–269.

Hulme, J. B., Bain, B., Hardin, M., McKinnon, A., & Waldron, D. (1989). The influence of adaptive seating devices on vocalization. *Journal of Communication Disorders, 22*(2), 137–145.

Kayner, B. (1992). Meeting the seating and mobility needs of the client with traumatic brain injury. *Journal of Head Trauma Rehabilitation, 7,* 81–93.

Mayall, J. (1990). *Positioning in a wheelchair: A guide for professional care givers of the disabled adult.* Thorofare, NJ: Slack.

McLaurin, C. A. (1990). Current directions in wheelchair research.

Journal of Rehabilitation Research and Development: Clinical Supplement, 2, 88–99.

McLaurin, C. A. (1991). Biomechanics and the wheelchair. *Prosthetics and Orthotics International, 15,* 24–37.

McLaurin, C. A., & Axelson, P. (1990). Wheelchair standards: An overview. *Journal of Rehabilitation Research and Development: Clinical Supplement, 2,* 100–103.

Ozer, M. N. (1990). A participatory planning process for wheelchair selection. *Journal of Rehabilitation Research and Development: Clinical Supplement, 2,* 31–36.

Reed, R. L., Yochum, K., & Schloss, M. (1993). Platform motorized wheelchairs in congregate care centers: A survey of usage and safety. *Archives of Physical Medicine & Rehabilitation, 74,* 101–103.

Wilson, A. (1992). *Wheelchairs: A prescription guide* (2nd ed.). New York: Demos.

Zacharkow, D. (1988). *Posture: Sitting, standing, chair design and exercise.* Springfield, IL: Charles C. Thomas.

Sources of Information about Wheelchairs

Accent on Living. (P.O. Box 700, Bloomington, IL 61702)

Assistive Techology. (RESNA, 1700 North Moore Street, Suite 1540, Rosslyn, VA 22209)

Exceptional Parent. (P.O. Box 3000, Department EP, Denville, NJ 07834)

National Association of Medical Equipment Services. (625 Slaters Lane, Suite 200, Alexandria, VA 22314)

Paraplegia News & Sports 'N Spokes. (2111 East Highland Avenue, Suite 180, Phoenix, AZ 85016)

TeamRehab Report. (Miramar Publishing Co., 6133 Bristol Parkway, P.O. Box 3640, Culver City, CA 90231)

Wheelchair Manufacturers

Allied Medical Supply. (P.O. Box 5122, Richmond, VA 23220)

Amigo Mobility International. (6693 Dixie Highway, Bridgeport, MI 48722-0402)

Braun Corporation. (1014 South Monticello, P.O. Box 310, Winamac, IN 46996)

Convaid Products, Inc. (P.O. Box 2458, Rancho Palos Verdes, CA 90274)

DAMACO Inc.. (20542 Plummer Street, Chatsworth, CA 91311)

ENDURO, Wheel Ring Inc.. (199 Forest Street, Manchester, CT 06040)

Everest and Jennings. (1100 Corporate Square, St. Louis, MO 63132)

Falcon Rehabilitation Products. (4404 East Sixtieth Avenue, Commerce City, CO 80022)

Fortress. (P.O. Box 489, Clovis, CA 93613-0489)

Gendron, Inc.. (P.O. Box 197, Archbold, OH 43502)

Hoverround Corporation. (1748 Independence Boulevard, Suite B1, Sarasota, FL 34234)

Invacare Corporation (Action Technology). (Box 4028, Elyria, OH 44036)

Kushall of America. (708 Via Alondra, Camrillo, CA 93012)

LeBac Systems. (8955 South Ridgeline Boulevard, Highlands Ranch, CO 80126)

Mulholland Positioning. (P.O. Box 391, Santa Paula, CA 93060)

Ortho-Kinetics, Inc. (P.O. Box 1647, Waukesha, WI 53187)

Permobile, Inc.. (6-B Gill Street, Woburn, MA 01801)

Quickie Designs, Inc. (2842 Business Park Avenue, Fresno, CA 93727)

XL Manufacturing Co. Inc. (1020 Marauder Street, Suite 102, Chico, CA 95926)

31
High-Technology Adaptations to Overcome Disability

Patricia Weber Dow and Nancy Pearson Rees

OBJECTIVES

After completing this chapter, the student will be able to:

1. Recognize which patients are appropriate for, or could be helped by, assistive technology.
2. Describe general categories and components of a typical assistive technology system.
3. Describe how a client's motor, sensory, and cognitive performance components influence the selection and successful use of assistive technology equipment.
4. Analyze specific products according to their possible function in the assistive technology system as a whole.
5. Demonstrate an understanding of issues affecting assistive technology selection outside of client and device characteristics.
6. Discuss the roles of the occupational therapist as a member of an assistive technology multidisciplinary team.

Like it or not, technological devices have become a part of everyday life for the vast majority of us. A remote control for the television, an alarm system in the car, and a microwave oven are just a few examples of technology in daily use. In part, these products have become possible because of manufacturing developments in the computer industry. This industry began in the space and scientific fields, but as the technology moved from large vacuum tubes to tiny microchips, commercial applications became inevitable. With more companies becoming involved in the industry, the products have become increasingly available and affordable, and of course, the companies have needed to look for new markets for their products.

Coincidentally, the advance of medical technology has allowed more victims of severe diseases and injuries to survive but often only with extensive limitations that affect their ability to function in many, if not all, aspects of their lives. As this population (from premature babies to the elderly) has increased, there has been a growing awareness of needs of these individuals and their right to have equal opportunities. Legislation has been passed to address the needs and rights of people with disabilities in all occupational performance areas (Reed, 1992).

Two pieces of legislation that significantly affected the practice of occupational therapy with this population are the Technology-Related Assistance for Individuals with Disabilities Act (Tech Act) of 1988 and the Americans with Disabilities Act of 1990. These two acts mandated, among other things, that assistive technology be made available to persons with disabilities to enhance their functional capabilities and also that employers provide reasonable accommodation, including electronic aids if necessary. According to the Tech Act of 1988, an assistive technology device is defined as "any item, piece of equipment, or product system, whether acquired commercially off the shelf, modified or customized, that is used to increase, maintain, or improve functional capabilities of individuals with disabilities" (*Congressional Report*, 1988, §3).

Smith (1991) made a distinction between two major roles of technology: assistive or adaptive technology and rehabilitative or educational technology. Examples of technology that are used for rehabilitation or remediation of function include software for cognitive rehabilitation, biofeedback, and electrical stimulation (Smith 1991; see also Chapters 27, 32, and 33). Assistive or adaptive technology, however, consists of products or devices that substitute for an impaired function and allow the individual to perform an activity more independently (Smith, 1991). This chapter does

GLOSSARY

Alternate keyboard—A device consisting of a matrix, keys in different shapes and sizes, or switches that can be attached to the computer and used to input data.

Analog signal—An electrical signal that is a continuous, oscillating, or modulating waveform. The telephone uses the analog signal of soundwaves.

Augmentative and Alternative Communication (AAC) Devices—Electronic devices to supplement a person's ability to communicate. These devices, similar to a keyboard, have pictures, letters, symbols, words, or encoded language systems in squares that are pressed or indicated by the user to communicate with someone else. AAC devices have text-to-speech synthesis; in addition, some have a visual display.

Bulletin boards—A service available on some on-line systems, such as CompuServe. These boards contain information about the system itself, what it is capable of doing, and may also contain databases of software programs or of news and information. People with particular hobbies may communicate with each other on various organized bulletin boards.

Digital signal—An electrical signal that is transmitted as a series of discrete, unmodulated numerals. A computer operates with a binary digital signal: the switch is either on or off (1 or 0).

Environmental control systems (ECSs)—A system or device attached to electronic or electrical equipment (such as appliances, televisions, lights, and telephone) to enable a person with impairment to operate the equipment through a remote-control device, computer, or switch.

Ergonomics—The study and development of general principles that govern the interaction of humans and their working environment. The primary goal of ergonomics is to improve worker performance and safety.

Keyboard emulating interface—A hardware device connected to the computer or a software program installed on the computer that allows input from an alternate device to be accepted as standard keyboard input.

Mouse—A standard device for computer input that moves the cursor on the screen, via a small ball, in the same direction as the device is moved across a surface; a push button on the top indicates selection. It operates with software written for mouse functions and requires good fine and gross motor coordination to operate.

On-line services—Services accessed through the modem, such as electronic mail or databases. Electronic mail (also called e-mail and net-mail) is the exchange of messages with other computer users electronically via the computer. Databases are systems with information that can be searched by computer for pertinent information. For example, Hyper-ABLEDATA is a database for rehabilitation products.

On-screen keyboard—A virtual keyboard provided on the computer monitor by specific software (e.g., ScreenKeys and HandiKEY). The on-screen keyboard can then be used with an alternate access device such as the HeadMaster Plus or Freewheel II Optical Head Pointer.

Optical character recognition—Technology used in scanning to convert the images of typed text into a computer code, i.e., translating the analog signal from the voltage of reflected light to a digital value readable by the computer.

Scanning activation methods—Methods of scanning that require varying degrees of motor and perceptual control from the user. (1) Inverse (momentary) scan—the user presses a switch and scanning continues only until the pressure is released for the choice. (2) Latched (regular) scan—once begun, the device scans automatically until the user activates a switch to stop the scan on his choice. (3) Step scan—the user pushes a switch to advance to each choice and must activate another switch or wait a specified interval on the selection to indicate choice.

Scanning techniques—Variations to increase scanning speed. (1) Block or cluster scan—the user scans preset blocks of the grid and changes to linear scanning when block containing desired selection is reached. (2) Directed scan—the user indicates via a joystick or multiple switches to go up, down, left, or right, and select. (3) Row/column scan—the user scans row by row and, when the row containing his choice is reached, presses a switch to scan each choice (column) in that row, making a selection by another switch activation.

Screen-reading software—Program capable of reading menus, format commands, and punctuation as well as text on the monitor (screen).

Telecommunications Device for the Deaf (TDD)—A device that consists of a small screen or display, a modem, a connection to a phone line, and some means of input (such as a keyboard).

Text-to-speech synthesis—Translation of written communication (text) into speech sounds and messages.

Utilities—the operating system for the computer, the system file, or software.

not discuss technology used for remediation of function but focuses on technology used to assist clients' independence in occupational performance roles.

The traditional focus of occupational therapy has always been increased independence and increased function of the client in all areas of his life. Occupational therapists have historically looked at the entire range of human performance roles and the possibilities for adaptation of the environment or the use of adapted devices in determining how to achieve this increased function. With the explosion of computer and microchip technology, it is only natural for adaptive devices to incorporate technology. As with other adaptive devices, assistive technology (AT), when carefully selected for a specific client, has the capacity to improve substantially that person's quality of life. Therefore, AT is swiftly emerging as one of the modalities used by therapists in the overall treatment of adults with physical (and cognitive) disabilities.

Therapists may encounter clients who already have an AT system but who need to be trained in its use. Some clients may have problems using their AT systems and need a therapist's help to begin the troubleshooting process. Sometimes the occupational therapist has a client whose function may be enhanced by AT. After referring such a client to a specialized technology assessment team, the therapist will work closely with the technology specialists to match their knowledge of the available devices with her specific knowledge of the client's capabilities and limitations. Therefore, whether the therapist was introduced to computers in nursery school or is baffled by the controls of a new VCR, she must have a working knowledge of AT to use it as a therapeutic tool to increase a client's functional independence and enable him to lead a productive life.

This chapter introduces the realm of AT and provides a general framework for understanding its role in physical rehabilitation. Because of the rapid change and development in this area, new products and new technological advances are emerging daily. Thus the information provided here should be used to begin a knowledge base in this area.

DEVICE CHARACTERISTICS

Although it is impossible to be familiar with all assistive devices currently manufactured, the therapist needs to understand certain basic categories and characteristics of assistive devices and systems before evaluating the client. Knowledge of basic parts of an AT system and the potential of these components to be changed or expanded to keep pace with the client's changing situation will enable the therapist to select

components that function together and that also match the client's residual abilities.

The most successful assistive device or AT system is not always the most elaborate one; it is whatever combination of devices or aids that easily, reliably, and quickly accomplishes the intended function(s). Such a system typically strikes a balance between low technology and high technology (Musselwhite, 1993). *Low technology* refers to devices with less complexity and few moving parts, such as glasses, hearing aids, and reaching sticks. *High technology* refers to devices with greater complexity such as computer systems, **environmental control systems (ECSs), and augmentative and alternative communication (AAC) devices** (Smith, 1991). An example of a system with combined elements used by a person with a spinal cord injury (SCI) would be the use of a mouthstick (low-tech device) to access a computer keyboard and the use of a software program on the computer (high-tech device) to change the layout of the keyboard letters for easier, more efficient access and to provide **mouse** keys to enhance the user's ability to access software features.

Another way to substitute for the intended or desired function does not precisely qualify as either low or high technology but does involve more complicated aids such as electric feeders, electric bed controls, and electric page turners. These devices are unifunctional, usually contributing to only one occupational performance area.

The high technology with which an occupational therapist is typically involved includes electronic devices such as computers, AAC devices, powered wheelchairs, and/or ECSs.

High-tech Systems: Typical Features

Any high-tech electronic device requires some means of activation (input) to produce some result (output). Between the input and the output, the device or system processes or manipulates the information to produce the result. Thus such an electronic system typically requires an input device as well as an output device connected to the processing component.

Increasingly, the AT devices or systems substituting for a client's function in the areas of work, communication, or control of the daily environment involve a computer as the processing component. Personal computers are more familiar than an ECS, and because they incorporate almost all the elements of other AT systems, the computer will be used as an example to illustrate input, interfaces, processing, and output before discussing the full potential for modification of these components for accessibility.

Parts of a Computer

The parts of a computer will be presented somewhat out of the order of input, processing, output described above so that the discussion can correlate with the terminology used by vendors of computers and so that the computer system components can be fully explicated.

HARDWARE

The hardware of a computer is the physical components of the system. These components are discussed below.

Central Processing Unit

The central processing unit (CPU) is the control parts of the computer that, following instructions (a program), make the computer parts work together and perform arithmetic and logical operations.

Memory and Storage

Read-only memory (ROM) is permanently contained within the computer and is not erased or changed when the computer is turned on or off. It cannot be written on or changed by the user. ROM chips typically contain basic instructions to guide the operation of the CPU components and to "boot up" the computer, i.e., get it ready to run the software (White, 1993). Random access memory (RAM) is temporary storage and is also referred to as read/write memory; its contents change. Information (data and files) from the disc containing the software program must be loaded on the RAM chips for the data to be accessed and manipulated quickly. The RAM chips are the "desk" on which the computer spreads its files, writes its papers, and does its work according to the instructions of the software program chosen by the user. Because RAM depends on electricity going through the machine, it is not permanent and is lost when the computer is turned off. Secondary, or long-term memory is possible on diskettes (or floppy discs), an external hard-disc drive, or a hard drive inside the computer itself. To save the changes made to the data on the desk, the user must transfer the changed file to such long-term memory. Compact disc read-only memory (CD-ROM) discs are increasingly available. These discs contain audio, visual, and text files that are retrieved by a special disc drive using a laser beam. Because the files on these discs cannot be changed by the user, they are primarily used for storage of large databases, encyclopedias, and other references materials.

Peripherals

Peripherals are input devices (such as a keyboard or **mouse**) that enter information into (i.e., to access) the computer and output devices (such as a monitor or a printer) that display the product to the client or others. Some peripherals, such as a modem, both send information (output) and receive information (input).

The modem (short for modulator/demodulator) is a peripheral that allows one computer to exchange information with another over telephone lines (Whipp & Freeman, 1993). Modems require communications software to interface user's computer with the other computer. The modem converts the telephone's **analog signal** into the computer's **digital signal**. Modems can also have built-in fax capabilities and allow access to **on-line services** and **bulletin boards.**

SOFTWARE

Software is a computer program. Such programs are a set of instructions to be executed by a computer. The hardware components and the software programs must be compatible, i.e., they must be designed to work together. The computer must also have enough RAM to operate the software. There are two categories of software.

Operating Software

Operating software is an internal set of programmed running instructions that execute the programs from the application software via the hardware of the computer. The operating software also details things such as how to send data to the printer and how to operate the disc drives. When the computer is turned on and booted up, the operating system must be loaded onto RAM chips so that the machine can perform its function.

Application Software

Application software is a set of programmed instructions that accomplish or do something specific, e.g., type a paper using word processing, do spreadsheets or math calculations, create databases (like a filing system that allows the user to sort through the information in any number of ways), play games, and run programs with musical output.

The operating system used by the computer surrenders the computer functions to the application software used. However, this application software must interface with the operating system. Once the application software use has stopped, control returns to the operating system.

INTERFACES OR ADAPTERS

Interfaces, or adapters, connect the peripherals to the computer, permit new capabilities to be added to the originally purchased computer system, and expand the RAM available on the computer. There are three basic types of interfaces.

Specialized Circuit Boards or Cards

Specialized circuit boards or cards are inserted into an expansion slot on the main circuit board (the motherboard) inside the computer. Circuit cards can be added to allow the computer to operate a new disc drive such as a CD-ROM drive, change the display on the monitor, or provide voice output.

Software Programs

Software programs provide new capabilities or give instructions for using the newly added peripherals or specialized circuit boards for a modem, CD-ROM drive, etc.

Cables

Cables connect a peripheral to the computer via an external port (serial or parallel) in the computer. The computer's serial port (also called a communications port) is typically used for a **mouse,** modem, or joystick. Only one bit of datum at a time can be sent or received over the serial port. The computer's parallel port can send or receive several bits of data at one time. The parallel ports typically are used for printers, connections with another computer, hard drives, or components that produce speech.

High-tech Systems: Possible Modifications

There are several ways to intervene with electronic devices to allow access for a person with a disability. Changes can be made anywhere along the chain of input, processing, to output. Modifications can be made to:

1. The way in which the user actually interacts with the device to produce the input;
2. The actual input device itself;
3. The type of connection between the device and the processing unit (electronic or wireless interface or connection);
4. The way that the processing itself is done;
5. The interface between the processing and the output device;
6. The actual output device itself.

The parts of the system changed depend on the diagnosis of each client, which performance components are lost or impaired, and for what function(s) the assistive technology is expected to substitute. Depending on the client's roles and expectations and on the results of the assessment (see below), a therapist may need to change several parts of the system or adapt only one for access by that client.

INPUT MODIFICATIONS

Method of User Interaction with Input Device

The manner in which the user interacts with the device can vary in two ways: the type of input from the user and the selection method. The type of input used can involve physical contact (i.e., pressure, movement, or contact from the hand or other body part) or no physical contact (i.e., sound, eye movement, light activation, magnetic attraction, or proximity/capacitance). The three major selection methods include direct selection, scanning, and encoding.

Direct Selection

In direct selection, one choice is selected from among available choices. The most common examples of this are selection of keys on a typewriter or keyboard using both hands and the use of a **mouse.** For users who do not have fine motor control of one or both hands, direct selection may also be made by one finger, mouthstick, headstick, or a pointer using ultrasound or infrared reflection.

Scanning

Scanning involves a cursor moving sequentially through the choices; the user indicates when the desired selection is reached. A scanning display may be configured in a grid, with scanning done linearly (scanning left to right and top to bottom through the selections until the choice is reached) or configured in a circle, with scanning done in a rotary fashion. Other variations of linear **scanning techniques** are row/column, block or cluster, and directed scanning (Fig. 31.1).

Scanning is activated by a switch and, therefore, is the access mode considered for clients with motor control insufficient for direct selection. **Scanning activation methods** include latched, step, or inverse scanning. Feedback provided to the user during scanning can be visual or auditory. Visual feedback consists of a light scanning past the choices. Auditory feedback can state the location or contents of a cell, the icon name, or a customized scan prompt.

Encoding

Encoding involves letters, words, or phrases that are represented by a code. Encoding can also be done with icons (symbols or pictures). The icons selected by the user take on sightly different meanings, depending on the other icons chosen with them. MINSPEAK (Prentke Romich Co., Wooster, OH) is a semantic compaction (encoding) system using icons with multiple meanings to represent concepts. For example, selection of an eye and a cup will prompt the voice synthesized

Direct Selection

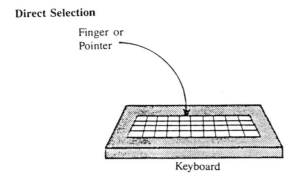

Input	Output
Press S	S

Directed Scanning

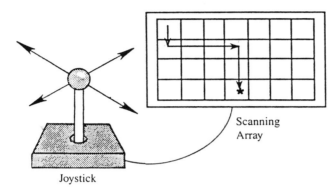

Input	Output
Move Joystick: Down Right Right Right Down	S

Scanning (Row-Column)

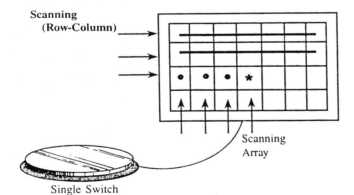

Input	Output
Press Switch Wait Wait Press Switch Wait Wait Wait Press Switch	S

Figure 31.1. Selection techniques.

message: "I am thirsty" (Banajee, 1993). Another form of encoding is used in computer software programs. Abbreviation expansion is one example of such a program that prints whole words or phrases when the user indicates the preselected abbreviation. A different method of encoding uses one or more switches to input Morse code.

Direct selection is 5 to 10 times faster than scanning and, therefore, is the method of choice. Scanning requires less motor skill than direct selection but is cognitively more difficult. Encoding is faster than scanning, but slower than direct selection. However, encoding requires a higher level of cognition than direct selection, as the user must remember the nonvisible code.

Modifications of Actual Input Devices

A variety of devices can provide input to electronic products by either direct selection or **scanning techniques.** Each input device has particular characteristics that can be matched with the client's abilities and functional needs.

Devices Used with Direct Selection and Physical Contact

Keyboard and modifications. A number of products have been developed that modify access to the standard keyboard or modify the keyboard itself and allow the user with gross or fine motor impairment or incoordination to continue to use direct selection to access it. Such products can be low-tech devices or high-tech adaptations.

Examples of low-tech adaptations for the hand of a client include use of a universal cuff with the eraser end of a pencil to key in, a mitten with the hand sewn down and one hole for a finger to assist with finger isolation, and splints to stabilize or position a finger for typing. Mouthsticks and headsticks are low-tech adaptations that allow access to the keyboard by those clients who are unable to use their arms and legs but who have good head control, e.g., individuals with spastic cerebral palsy, amyotrophic lateral sclerosis, or tetraplegia. These devices are rubber-tipped sticks that are positioned on a headset (Fig. 31.2) or on a mouthpiece that is held between the teeth. They function like a finger to select a choice as the client leans his head forward to the keyboard. Problems noted with mouthsticks include fatigue, jaw/tooth pain, and actual strain on the teeth. Mouthsticks require good head control and have been found by users to be faster than some high-tech alternate input methods (Lau & O'Leary, 1993).

Low-tech adaptations for the keyboard itself are key guards, key latches, overlays, and key-top changes. A key guard (Fig. 31.3), usually made of firm plastic to fit over the keys with holes over each key, helps the patient target one key at a time, without accidentally pressing multiple keys. This improves typing accuracy for clients with motor control problems or clients learning to use a mouthstick. Key guards with decreased number of holes reduce the number of key options available for clients who are cognitively impaired.

Key latches attach to the side of the keyboard or to rockers built into a key guard and are available to press two or more keys simultaneously (e.g., to do control functions that involve more than one key such as the ctrl, alt, and delete keys on an IBM-compatible system). This would allow the computer to be operated by one hand, a mouthstick, or head pointer. This feature is available in some software programs or as a hardware modification to the computer.

Larger letters or color-coded letters can be glued on the keyboard keys themselves. Braille dot pads for each key can be added, or the texture of the keys can be changed for those clients with low vision.

Keyboards typically attach to the computer (or to the interface) with a thin cable. Thus they can be easily positioned for access by a user in a bed or wheelchair.

High-tech adaptations for the keyboard itself can include keyboard redefinition: software or hardware programs that change the keyboard letter arrangement to one that is more suitable to the client's needs and patterns of use. The standard keyboard is called QWERTY, which refers to the letters on the top left row of keys. The DVORAK system was designed for more efficient and ergonomic keyboard input; keys are located according to comparative finger strengths and use frequency (Fig. 31.4). Approximately 75% of the typing is done on one line. Such an arrangement may be helpful to someone not already familiar with the QWERTY keyboard, someone who does not need to use a QWERTY keyboard elsewhere, or someone with decreased finger strength. However, if the client was an experienced typist before disability, it may be diffi-

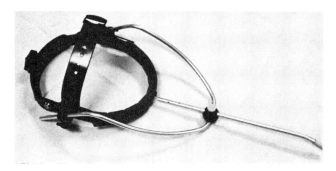

Figure 31.2. Headstick.

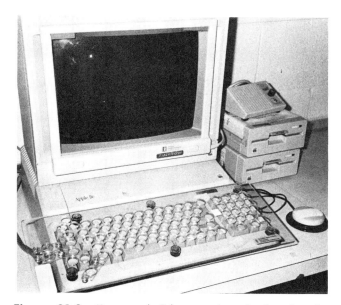

Figure 31.3. Key guard, Echo speech synthesizer (on disc drives), and TouchWindow (attached to computer monitor).

cult and time-consuming to unlearn the QWERTY keyboard and learn the new configuration.

Alternate keyboards. An **alternate keyboard** may be necessary. An **alternate keyboard** used with a computer is considered "transparent" to the computer if its input can be translated into a form indistinguishable from that of an ordinary keyboard. The advantage of transparency is that the adapted device can operate any standard software written for keyboard input to that computer. This avoids the expense of software written only for that one input device, which might be limited in application and availability. The **alternate keyboard** may not be able to control or operate software written for a keyboard and a **mouse,** however. It is important to ascertain what software the client will be using and whether the chosen input method will be totally transparent. Compatibility and transparency between components also become issues as more features are added to the basic computer system to improve access (Russell, 1993).

Keyboard size, shape, and surface may be changed to enable users to input with direct selection by hand, foot, mouthstick, or optical pointer. Enlarged keys (e.g., Key Largo, Don Johnston Developmental Equipment, Inc., Wauconda, IL; PC King, TASH Inc., Ajax, Ont., Canada) assist the client with poor targeting skills and poor fine motor coordination (Fig. 31.4). Miniature keyboards (Fig. 31.4) allow clients with

restricted range of motion or decreased endurance for arm and hand movements to access the computer; they do require greater fine motor control to target the smaller keys. Other keyboards are being designed with different configurations; some are hinged in the middle so that the client's hands access the keys in a thumbs-up position. A touch-sensitive or membrane keyboard requires less pressure for key activation and provides access for those users who cannot exert enough pressure to depress keys. Certain keyboards currently available allow the user to define the size and location of the key press areas (e.g., Concept Keyboard, Sammons, Inc., Brookfield, IL; IntelliKeys, IntelliTools, Richmond, CA). Another **alternate keyboard** is Ke:nx On Board (Don Johnston Developmental Equipment, Inc.), which allows portable use with the Macintosh PowerBook (Fig. 31.5).

Membrane keyboards can be used with key guards and/or overlays. Overlays are typically made of laminated paper or thin plastic and are used to delineate visually the target area for direct selection or make the letters meaningful to the client by including pictures representing the function of that key (Figs. 31.5 and 31.6). Overlays can be used as a training tool or permanently. Software programs such as the Overlay Manager for the Concept Keyboard, the IntelliKeys Overlay Maker, and Ke:nx Create can be customized to meet a specific client's motor or communication needs.

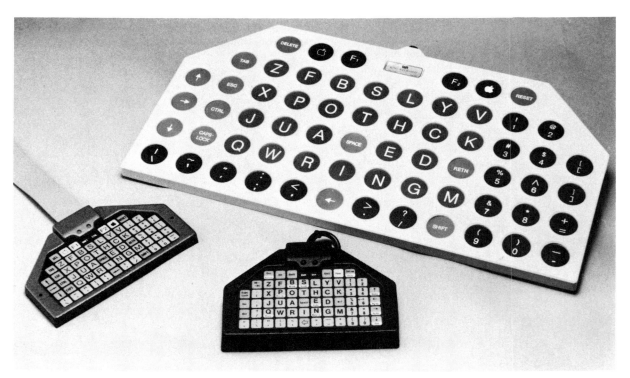

Figure 31.4. TASH Mini Keyboard with ribbon cable (for Apple and Macintosh), PC King keyboard, and PC Mini keyboard (for IBM compatibles).

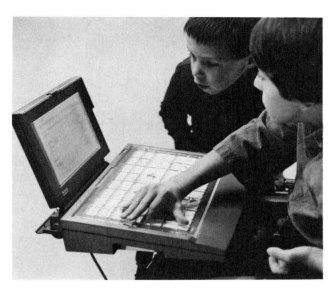

Figure 31.5. Ke:nx On Board placed over the Macintosh PowerBook. The child is using a key guard and overlay to customize access.

Mouse and trackball. Other forms of input using direct selection with physical contact are the **mouse** and the trackball. The trackball is an upside-down **mouse,** with the exposed ball being moved by the user to obtain the **mouse** movements. This device may be useful for a client with limited arm range of motion but some controlled finger motion. Cursor accuracy is difficult to achieve. The Trackerball (Penny & Giles, Santa Monica, CA) consists of a trackball with various switches to substitute for the drag and click motions necessary with a standard **mouse.** Unwanted movement on the vertical or horizontal planes can also be inhibited in this device.

There are alternate input devices to substitute for, or emulate, the **mouse** functions of pointing at and selecting icons or text on the computer screen. **Mouse** emulators take the form of multiple switches, touch screens, or software programs with **on-screen keyboards,** such as ScreenDoors (Madenta Communications, Edmonton, Alta., Canada) and WiViK2 (Prentke Romich Co.) with scanning (Fig. 31.7). Software programs can be used with any pointing device (headstick; **mouse;** trackball; HeadMaster Plus, Prentke Romich Co.) with a click (or switch closure) to indicate the user's selection or allowing "dwell" on the choice instead of a click to make the selection (DButton for Windows, Pointer Systems, Inc., Burlington, VT). Recently developed, the Tongue Touch keypad (New Abilities System, Mountain View, CA) can be used as a **mouse** emulator to control a computer. This keypad fits into the roof of a user's mouth like a retainer. The user's pressure on selected keys on the keypad, with tongue elevation, sends radio frequency signals to a

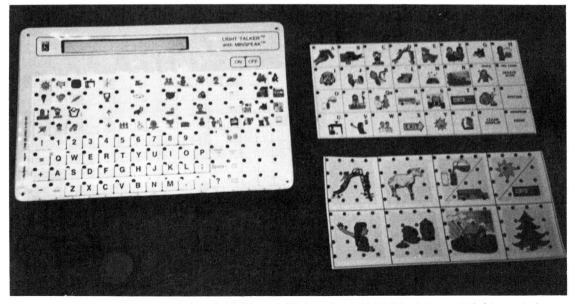

Figure 31.6. LightTalker showing overlays for 8, 32, and 128 locations with TASH minicup switch for row/column scan.

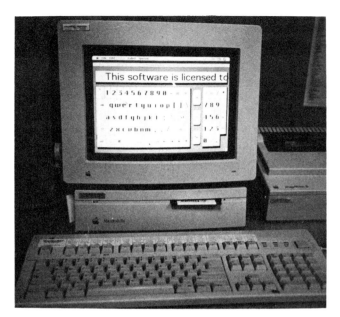

Figure 31.7. Macintosh computer (CPU and monitor) with on-screen keyboard in QWERTY format (ScreenDoors software) with standard keyboard.

controller device that then relays infrared signals to the computer, fitted with appropriate software.

Increasingly, computers are relying on graphical user interface (GUI) operating environments, i.e., a **mouse,** a pointing device, or **mouse** keys are used to select from the available menus or icons (e.g., Windows, Microsoft Corp., Redmond, WA). The GUI system is inaccessible to users with visual impairment (Rizer, 1992). For them, software is now available (outSPOKEN, Berkeley Systems, Inc., Berkeley, CA) to make the Macintosh completely accessible, by replacing visual icons with spoken words and software is being developed to access a Windows format by providing auditory tracking of information (WinVision, Artic Technologies, Troy, MI).

Nontransparent alternate input. Alternate sources of input, which have been nontransparent in the past, include touch screens on the computer monitor (Fig. 31.3) and other tactually accessed devices, such as the PowerPad (Dunamis, Inc., Suwanee, GA), and certain graphics pads such as the KoalaPad+ (Koala Technologies, San Jose, CA). Input occurs from directly touching the choice on the touch screens or by drawing on the pressure-sensitive graphics pads. Whatever is drawn on the pad is displayed on the computer screen. The touch screens are particularly helpful for clients with impaired cognition, because there is no separation between the input device and the choice. Most of these devices can run only software specifically written for them. For example, the TouchWindow (Edmark Corp., Redmond, WA) is com-

patible with all Macintosh software and many programs for the Apple II but only some IBM and IBM-compatible computer software (Fig. 31.3). Programs to create customized applications for these types of input are now becoming available, e.g., Tool Kit 4 (Dunamis, Inc.) and Talking TouchWindow (Edmark). Sometimes this software allows for designation of special key press areas on the pad surface to be used with overlays to increase the target area. Touch screens are usually attached over the existing computer monitor and graphics/input pads are typically connected to the computer via the game port or serial port in the back of the computer. The TouchWindow can also be put on the table surface for clients unable to reach up to the screen.

Devices for Direct Selection with no Physical Contact

If a person is unable to use physical contact to select choices directly from a keyboard, other input methods, such as eye gaze, light activation, and sound, can still be used. Eyegaze vests (vests with Velcro on which can be stuck a limited number of pictures) and E-Tran frames (clear plastic panels with choices placed around the perimeter) are low-tech eye gaze systems. The therapist, wearing the eyegaze vest, sits opposite the client or sits on the other side of the E-Tran frame. The user selects his choice by looking at the picture and the therapist notes the direction of the gaze. The high-tech method of eyegaze involves a camera under the Eyegaze Control monitor, which shines infrared light into the user's eye to illuminate the pupil and provide a reflection off the cornea (Eyegaze Computer, LC Technologies, Inc., Fairfax, VA). Coordinates of the difference between the corneal reflection and certain measurements of the illuminated pupil are compared with the coordinates of a calibration program run before the client uses the program. These coordinates are translated into eye direction by the computer. Selection is made by a timed dwell of eye gaze. The Eyegaze computer can be used to run an ECS and provide speech output.

The Eyegaze system is expensive, requires relatively good head control and good control of at least one eye, and is hampered by an environment with extra sources of infrared signals such as sunlight or incandescent lamps (Cleveland & Doyle, 1993). Currently, the system is unable to do word processing. Only seven lines of text can be viewed on the monitor or printed at one time, and no storage of text is available (Lahoud, 1994). If word processing is necessary, this computer must either be equipped with additional hardware and software and interfaced with a second monitor or must be connected to a second computer, thus becoming the second computer's alternate input.

Light pointers, which simply direct a beam of light toward a selection, such as the LightBeam Lightweight (Ability Research, Inc., Minnetonka, MN), are available as well as more complicated high-tech models that use a laser light pointer with a board containing light sensors (Scan-It-All, Innocomp, Warrensville Heights, OH). The Infrared Pointing System (Prentke Romich Co.) uses infrared signals to provide direct access to the Liberator. Other pointer systems are available: FreeWheel II Optical Head Pointer (Pointer Systems, Inc.) and HeadMaster Plus with Remote Adaptor (Prentke Romich Co.).

Sound waves (ultrasound or voice transmission) provide an alternate input to achieve direct selection. HeadMaster Plus (Fig. 31.8) moves a cursor on the screen. The ultrasonic transmitting unit positioned on top of the monitor sends signals to the user's headset that contains sensors to measure the relative strength of the ultrasound signal to determine changes in the user's head position. This information is then sent by cable to the computer's **mouse** port to change the cursor position on screen. Selection is typically indicated by a single pneumatic switch attached to the headset.

Other devices use voice as an alternate input. Some of these voice recognition systems require "training" of the system by the user, who uses a microphone to speak several repetitions of the word or phrase to program voice patterns. When the user inputs voice commands, they are compared with the stored voice patterns and the keystrokes equivalent to that command are implemented. The speaker needs to have consistent speech patterns or the system has difficulty recognizing the speech input and translating it to words. Other systems require no training; instead word models for commonly used terms and statistical language models are implemented to recognize accurately the client's speech and language patterns. Kurzweil VOICE (Kurzweil Applied Intelligence, Inc., Waltham, MA) and DragonDictate (Dragon Systems, Inc., Newton, MA) are two examples of this type of system (Fig. 31.9). These systems have the ability to update the models according to user patterns, thus becoming quickly personalized. These systems do not require the same consistency of voice patterns and breath control as do the systems that need to be trained. This breath control is sometimes difficult for the most common user of this system, i.e., a high tetraplegic.

Optical scanners do not really permit direct selection per se by the user but enable those with visual impairment, dyslexia, or motor impairment to access printed material. Scanners (e.g., DeskScan-3000, Chinon America, Inc., Torrance, CA) equipped with **optical character recognition** (OCR) software (such as OsCaR, TeleSensory, Mountain View, CA, and CALERA WordScan for Windows, Talktronics, Inc., Lake Forest, CA) encode printed material into machine-readable material. The text can then be projected to a computer monitor where, in addition to being viewed and magnified if necessary, it can be manipulated as a standard computer file, using a keyboard. The text can also be sent to a speech synthesizer (Fig. 31.3), a printer, or a refreshable braille display (Fig. 31.10).

Devices Used with Scanning or Encoding

If the client is unable to use direct selection to access a computer or other AT device, then switch access is considered. Various switches are available that are activated by physical contact or other methods

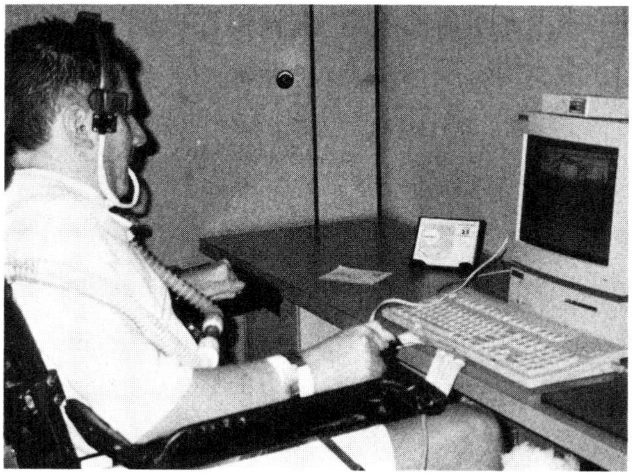

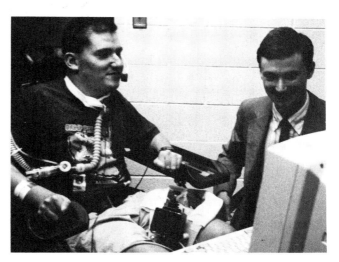

Figure 31.8. Buck using the HeadMaster Plus and a sip and puff switch for computer input.

Figure 31.9. Buck trying out the DragonDictate voice recognition system. Note that the chin-mounted joystick was removed for trials.

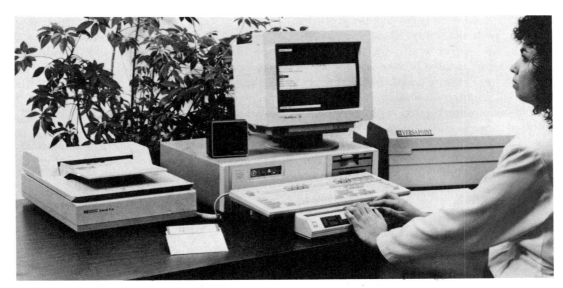

Figure 31.10. Flatbed OsCaR scanner, Vert speech synthesizer (on CPU), the Navigator (a refreshable braille display, positioned underneath computer keyboard), and the VersaPoint braille embosser (printer).

(Table 31.1). Switches can be connected via an interface to the internal input/output (I/O) port of the computer with a ribbon cable (Fig. 31.4) or to the joystick port on the back of the computer with a standard cable. When switches are used for access, software programs need to have instructions for accommodating switch input. Such programs are available from Don Johnston Developmental Equipment Inc., Laureate Learning Systems (Winooski, VT), and Marblesoft (Blaine, MN), among others.

Switches activated by physical contact include those operated pneumatically (e.g., sip and puff; Fig. 31.8), those requiring contact but no pressure or some slight movement, and those requiring pressure of some degree (Table 31.1). Certain characteristics of switches that require physical contact need to be understood when trying to match a client with an input type (Goossens' & Crain, 1992). The size of the switch (i.e., the target area it presents) must be considered in terms of the client's coordination, cognitive-perceptual status, and visual status. The shape of the switch (button, pad, lever, plate, or flexible tube) must be correlated with the client's control site and the physical comfort of the switch positioning. The weight of the switch itself is a factor when mounting the switch for access by the client. The client must be able to generate and sustain the pressure necessary to activate the switch (Table 31.1). The amount of travel in the switch (i.e., how far it must be moved before being activated) must be carefully matched with the client's motor abilities. The durability of the switch is a factor if client makes many uncontrolled or forceful movements or is going to be accessing the switch continuously, or if the switch will be moved frequently. The delay between the switch

activation and the device operation must also be considered. The type of feedback provided by the switch must be matched with the client's needs and impairments. Some switches click when activated, some provide visual feedback, and some provide proprioceptive feedback of the end of the switch's movement. And, finally, the aesthetics of the switch, the cost, and the availability must be considered and matched with the client's needs, expectations, and resources. Depending on the client's gross motor coordination and access needs, a single switch, dual switch, or multiple switches will be selected.

Modifications to the Connection or Interface Between Input and Processing Devices

There can be an actual physical connection between the input device and the processing device or the method of activation of the target device can be wireless or remote (via sound or infrared signals). Cables connecting the input device to the other system components may limit the user's mobility and may also necessitate setup by another person, thus inhibiting the user's spontaneous use of the system. Remote activation, on the other hand, fosters independence by the user.

The AT system can also be modified by placing an interface along this path from the input device to the processing component. This component can be a separate box-like device, a software program, and/or a circuit card. The interface accepts the nonstandardized (adapted) signal sent by the input device, changes it to a signal understood by the processing device, and transmits that input, thus making accessibility possible.

Table 31.1. Common Switch Types

Category and Specific Switches	Company	Primary Activation Site	Activation Pressure or Range
No Physical Contact			
Eye movement/gaze			
IST switch (infrared, sound, touch)	Words+	Eyes	
Light sensitive			
Light activated	Ability Research	Head	
Photo eye (beam interruption)	Creative Switch	Body part or object	0–6 inches
Infrared reflex	Adaptive Switch Labs	Hand	0.5–3 inches from sensor
Blink	VME Technologies	Eye blink	
Sound			
IST	Words+	Slight vocalization, breath	
Voice activated	Toys for Special Children	Mouth (microphone)	
Magnetic			
Magnetic finger	Luminaud	Finger magnet sleeve and small external switch nearby	0.38-inch movement
Nearness			
Proximity	Adaptive Switch Lab	Head, hand	0–0.5 inches from sensor
Capacitive sensor	Adaptive Switch Lab	Head, arm, hand	0–0.25 inches from sensor
Physical Contact			
Pneumatic			
Sip and puff	Zygo	Mouth	0.02 psi
Air cushion	Creative Switch; Prentke Romich	Hand, body part	2 ounces
Contact/no pressure or slight movement			
P-switch or sensor	Prentke Romich; Don Johnston	Eyebrow, forehead, fingers	
Mercury or tilt	TASH; Creative Switch	Head	
Pressure			
Light touch	Don Johnston; Dunamis	Hand, arm, head	0.75 ounces
Tongue	DU-IT; Prentke Romich	Tongue	0.75–3 ounces
Pillow	TASH	Cheek	0.5–7 ounces
Leaf	TASH; Zygo	Head	0.5 ounce
Wobble	Prentke Romich	Arm, hand	1–3 ounces
Plate	Zygo; TASH	Hand, feet	2–7 ounces
Tread	TASH	Feet	5–25 ounces
Rocker	Don Johnston; TASH; Prentke Romich	Arm, hand	2–8 ounces
Grasp	TASH	Hand	6–11 ounces
Joystick	Prentke Romich; Zygo	Hand, chin	7–11 ounces
Penta	TASH	Thumb	4–5 ounces
Mat	Creative Switch	Wheelchair	6 pounds

Alternate input devices (such as switches or **alternate keyboards**), whether accessed by direct selection, scanning, or encoding, traditionally have had to be connected to the computer via a **keyboard emulating interface** (KEI), or a switch interface, which renders this alternate input transparent to the computer.

KEIs can either be software, hardware, or a com-

bination of both. The type of KEI used depends on the type of adaptive input and the computer used. A few examples of KEIs follow.

1. The Adaptive Firmware Card (AFC) (Don Johnston Developmental Equipment, Inc.) is a combination circuit card and external component that plugs into an expansion slot in Apple II computers, permits

various input methods (switch, direct selection, encoding), and has the potential for voice output and **mouse** emulation (Fig. 31.11).

2. Ke:nx (Don Johnston Developmental Equipment, Inc.) is a combination of an external interface system and customizing software for the Macintosh computer that allows access via switch, encoding, **mouse,** touch, or AACs (Fig. 31.5); it plugs into the Apple Desk Bus (ADB) port; and customized overlays can be created.

3. PC A.I.D. (Designing Aids for Disabled Adults, Toronto, Ont., Canada) is an external device used with IBM and compatibles that allows keyboard redefinition and input via keyboard or switch(es).

4. T-Tam (Prentke Romich Co.) is an external interface component used with an Apple II GS, a Macintosh, or IBM-compatible computer that allows for access by a **mouse, alternate keyboard,** or an AAC; when used with the T-Tam, Mouse Interface and Keyboard Emulation (MIKE; Prentke Romich Co.), a software program, interfaces the Liberator (Prentke Romich Co.) and a Macintosh.

5. HandiCODE (Microsystems Software, Inc., Framingham, MA) is a software program for IBM and compatibles that permits input by Morse code through the keyboard or one, two, or three switches; these switches connect via a cable interface to the serial, parallel, or game port of the computer.

6. RevolvingDoors (Madenta Communications, Inc., Edmonton, Alta., Canada) is a software program that allows single switch access to a Macintosh computer; a switch input device must be used (e.g., SwitchBack, Madenta Communications, Inc.); the program contains an **on-screen keyboard** with three rows that can be scanned (one of these rows contains the alphabet, another has word prediction, and the third has common symbols and function keys); and it provides **mouse** emulation.

The need for a KEI is diminishing rapidly. More recent products, e.g., IntelliKeys (IntelliTools Co.) and PC Mini (TASH Inc.) are being manufactured with interface capabilities, avoiding the need for an external KEI to operate standard computer software. Such alternate input devices are built to plug directly into the standard keyboard port.

PROCESSING DEVICE MODIFICATIONS

The processing device can be a computer, a stand-alone component (such as an AAC device), or a control box (for an ECS or a powered wheelchair). These can be adapted to improve access for a person with a disability. Knowledge of computer systems, possible modifications, and software programs is essential when designing a workable, adapted computer system that meets the client's needs.

The three most common personal computer (PC) systems used today are Apple, Macintosh, and IBM (or IBM compatibles). Historically, these three computers have functioned with different operating systems, and thus products designed for IBM are not compatible with Apple or Macintosh and so on. Now "conversion bridges" are available that can translate information produced on one type of computer to that of another. Originally, IBM computers were designed to function primarily in a business setting and Apple computers were targeted for the personal computer market. Thus software for the Apple computer was developed for educational settings and was easily used in rehabilitation facilities, whereas IBM software was predominantly business oriented and had little applicability to rehabilitation. That is rapidly changing, however; software for both Macintosh and IBM computers suitable for children, rehabilitation, and adapted access is being developed. Both IBM and Apple Computer have worked to increase the accessibility of their products and have technical departments for answering specific questions.

One feature that becomes important in computer adaptation is the memory capacity of the computer. Memory is measured in kilobytes (Kb = 1000 bytes) or megabytes (Mb = 1,000,000 b). Computer memory may be expanded by the purchase of additional circuit

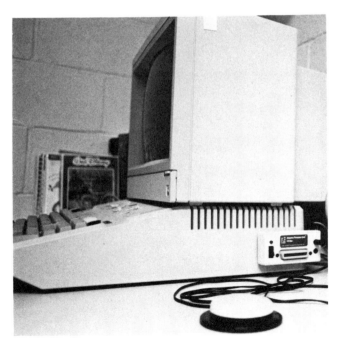

Figure 31.11. Apple IIe with Adaptive Firmware Card I/O box, with Jelly Bean switch connected. Circuit card of AFC is in place inside the CPU.

cards. Such expansion may be necessary because each additional component or software program requires a specific amount of memory to run. Product literature for each component under consideration must be carefully examined.

Software packages are available that will modify standard processing of the input to allow easier access. These software packages can be separate programs within the **utilities** in the operating system (such as Access Pack for Windows, Microsoft Corp., and HandiWARE, Microsystems Software, Inc.) or they can be standard parts of a word processing program (AccessDos, IBM, Boca Raton, FL, and WiViK2, Prentke Romich Co.). Some common methods for adaptive processing are listed below.

1. Macros are single keystrokes that are programmed with whole phrases or messages, i.e., preset little programs are called up by a single keystroke or combination of keystrokes.
2. With abbreviation expansion, the number of key strokes required is decreased by allowing the user to store frequently used words, phrases or paragraphs and retrieve them by an abbreviation only.
3. For word prediction, the computer provides a list of frequently used words based on the beginning letter sequence entered. If the desired word is on the list, the user selects it and further keystrokes are not needed; next-word prediction (based on words already entered) is also available.
4. With auto repeat defeat, the repeat rate of the keys can be adjusted or removed altogether (so that keys will not repeat if the person cannot quickly lift off the key).
5. Keyboard delay means that keystrokes not held down for a certain period of time are disregarded, thus avoiding input of keys contacted indirectly and eliminating time spent correcting unintentional input.
6. The control of typical **mouse** features is done from the keyboard's numeric pad rather than from the **mouse** itself.
7. Toggle keys can be modified by auditory feedback to notify the user with visual impairment when a toggle key (such as the capital lock) is on or off.
8. HyperCard and Linkway are software systems developed for the Macintosh and IBM, respectively, that allow control of arrangement, storage, and access to information using "buttons" to link the cards to other information; authoring systems, using HyperCard stacking, are available that allow a nonprogrammer to create customized software (e.g., the Gateway Authoring System, Don Johnston Developmental Equipment, Inc., combined with a Macin-

tosh Switch Interface, allows switch users to create their own stories).

Other Access Issues

Disc guides are low-tech pieces of equipment designed to assist clients who have motor coordination difficulties with insertion of the disc into the disc drive or computer monitor. The guides typically provide a channel or surface on which the disc can be aligned with the internal or external disc drive.

A multioutlet power strip on the front of the computer allows all hardware components (the computer, monitor, printer, and peripherals) to be plugged in and turned on and off from the front (instead of the typical location in the back of the computer) by turning the power strip's switch on and off. This improves accessibility for clients who have difficulty bending forward and reaching around to the back of the computer. To further improve accessibility for clients using a switch to access a computer, a switch jack can be added to a power strip to turn all components on and off.

OUTPUT MODIFICATIONS
Modification to the Output Interface and Connections

Interfaces, or connections, to the output device are similar to those of input device interfaces. They consist of cables, sound, infrared signals, and radio frequencies. Software programs and circuit boards may also be needed to allow the computer to use a particular output device (such as a speech synthesizer) to translate the computer text file into signals understood by a braille printer, or to read aloud the screen contents to allow a person with visual impairment to access certain computer files or commands.

Modifications of Actual Output Devices

The traditional output from electronic devices is auditory or visual. These can be modified for accessibility or tactile output can be produced.

Auditory

Auditory output can be in the form of synthesized or digitized speech. Digitized speech is actual recorded human voices, whereas synthesized speech (**text-to-speech**) is generated from stored speech sounds and pronunciation rules. Some AAC devices, such as Talking Screen (Words +, Inc., Palmdale, CA) are able to provide both digitized and synthesized speech.

An auditory output device commonly used is a speech synthesizer. Speech synthesizers can be either an external component (Fig. 31.3)—Echo II (Street Electronics Corp, Carpinteria, CA) and DECtalk (Digital Equipment Corp., Merrimack, NH)—or the synthesizer can be built into the computer itself and use the computer's own speakers—MacinTalk Pro (Apple Computer, Cupertino, CA).

For visually impaired clients, speech synthesis can be combined with **screen reading software,** such as MasterTouch ScreenReading Software (HumanWare, Loomis, CA), Write:OutLoud (Don Johnston Developmental Equipment, Inc.), and IBM Screen Reader/2. This software allows the user to navigate the screen via a standard keyboard or special keypad and find the specific commands, icons, text line, or paragraph desired. Instant or delayed speech output of selected text sequences is available (WinVision, Artic Technologies). These programs are helpful not only for persons with visual impairment but also for those with a learning disability or cognitive impairment.

Visual

The most common forms of visual output are the monitor screen itself and the hard copy from the printer. Attaching a magnifying lens in front of the monitor to enlarge the text; changing the foreground or background contrast and colors; using a color or monochrome monitor, a large closed-circuit television or larger monitor, or screen-magnification software to enlarge the print; and changing the fonts to something more legible on screen are options to make the text on the monitor more accessible to people with low vision. Screen-magnification software is available for GUI-based programs and graphics programs as well as for standard software programs: inLARGE (Berkeley Systems) and MAGic Deluxe (Microsystems Software Inc.). Software programs that produce a visual beep instead of an auditory beep to indicate completion of some function or some error message (See Beep, Microsystems Soft-

ware, Inc.) can be important for computer users with hearing impairments. Some printers' hardware can be modified or software programs can be added to allow output with enlarged letters or braille (Braille-Talk, G W Micro, Loomis, CA).

Tactile

Tactile output (i.e., braille) can be produced in a temporary or permanent form. The computer user with visual impairment can use a refreshable braille display device containing tiny filaments that are electronically pushed up to form braille characters corresponding to the screen information being scanned at that moment. Software is now available to translate off-the-shelf software programs into refreshable braille display (Navigator, TeleSensory) (Fig. 31.10). Translation of braille keyboard input to standard text and vice versa for manipulation on the monitor or for printed output can be accomplished by software programs such as MegaDots (Raised Dot Computing Inc., Madison, WI) or by a braille keyboard (embosser) connected to a computer equipped with special software (Mountbatten Brailler, HumanWare). Software used in conjunction with a speech synthesizer is available to allow braille input with speech synthesis output (Braille 'n Speak, Blazie Engineering, Forest Hill, MD) or both braille embossing output and speech output (Hot Dots, Raised Dot Computing, Inc.)

Augmentative and Alternative Communication Devices

AAC devices, or speech output devices, can be simple or extremely complex language systems. A low-tech version of a communication device is a picture board by which the user points to indicate choice (direct selection). A simple version of an electronic communication device is the IntroTalker (Prentke Romich Co.) (Fig. 31.12). AAC devices can be accessed

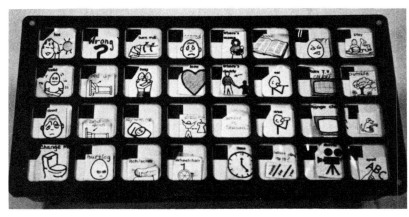

Figure 31.12.   Point and Scan IntroTalker showing 32 locations.

by direct selection or scanning with a switch. Overlays are typically used with an AAC to reduce the target area, e.g., to decrease the selection areas from 128 to only 32, thus providing larger areas with larger pictures (Fig. 31.6).

Increasingly, however, AAC devices are becoming more elaborate with parts similar to those of a computer, as described above. These AAC devices typically consist of a hardware device with varying capacities of open versus programmable memory; ports for connections to peripherals such as a printer, speech synthesizer, and/or a computer; and device-specific language application software. AAC devices vary in the intelligibility of speech synthesis, the speed of conversation, and the organization of available memory for vocabulary. Some AAC devices (such as the Dac, acs Technologies, Coraopolis, PA; and the Liberator, Prentke Romich, Wooster, OH) have several levels or pages (Fig. 31.13). If the user is able to understand and remember the various levels, the amount of vocabulary and phrases contained in the device can be maximized. Other devices (such as the DynaVox (Sentient Systems Technology, Pittsburgh, PA) have dynamic display of various categories, i.e., the display is changed electronically when the client indicates (Fig. 31.14). This avoids manual change of overlay displays and provides additional capacity for language.

Environmental Control Units or Systems

With the advances in technology in recent years, it has become increasingly possible for clients with disabilities to operate single devices or various electrical devices that were not previously accessible and thus control much of their environment. This remote operation of electrical equipment, accomplished by simple devices or complex systems, is known as an **environmental control system.** The term environmental control unit (ECU) was once used when such a control base operated only a few devices at most. If more devices needed to be controlled, separate ECU bases were necessary. Now with the integration of wheelchair controls and the interface with computers, environmental control is really a system.

Control over the environment is crucial so the client with a disability can avoid the passivity and learned helplessness that results from dependence on someone else for all activities of daily living (ADL) function and for initiation of any social interaction (Abramson, Seligmann, & Teasdale, 1978; Symington et al., 1986; Weisz, 1979). The independence gained, e.g., by a person with C_{4-5} tetraplegia, might allow a decrease in the amount of paid attendant care that was needed (Bach, Zeelenberg, & Winter, 1990), but more

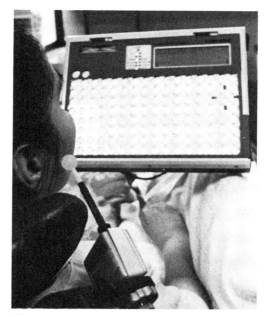

Figure 31.13. Client using the Liberator with a wobble switch to control scan functions and select.

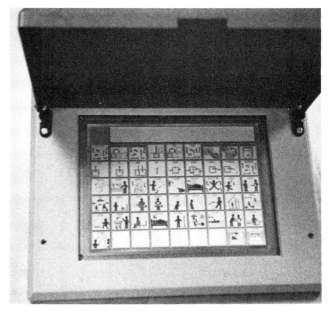

Figure 31.14. DynaVox, an icon-based communication system with dynamic display of overlays.

important, it gives the client a sense of control over his own life (Gross, 1992; Mann, 1989). ECSs can affect occupational performance in many ways, such as offering safety (burglar alarms, sensing systems, lights turning on automatically for a bedridden person, and intercom units), providing leisure activities (television, stereo, and computer games), assisting household functions (operate lights, fan, power doors, and an electric bed), and allowing a person with a disability to return to school or become a participating member of the work force (operate telephones, modems, computers, and fax machines).

An ECS can range from simple (single control of a few devices affecting only one area of occupational performance) to more complex high-tech systems. This variation depends on the client's needs and functional abilities. Low-tech examples of a simple ECS are a reacher to switch off lights, a remote control with larger buttons for the television, lamps operated by touch instead of a switch, and alarm clocks or phones that signal with vibration or lights to alert a client with hearing impairment. For a person in a nursing home, simple switch devices (such as the HECS-1, Prentke Romich Co.) are available that control the bed, phone, television, and lights.

Another example of a moderately simple ECS that is activity specific is a **telecommunications device for the deaf (TDD).** This device translates auditory information from the phone to written information for people with hearing impairment (and vice versa). Newer technology permits the TDD to be operated through a computer system, allowing communication to other people (nonhearing impaired) via touch-tone phones or other TDDs.

Complicated ECSs operate through an ECS base or through a computer to control the necessary devices. Examples of ECSs controlling all the functions in a house include the SmartHouse (Zygo Industries, Inc., Portland, OR) and The Future Home (VME Technologies, Inc., Baltimore, MD) (Stahl, 1993).

BASIC PARTS OF THE ECS

As described above for the computer, high-tech electronic devices used in an ECS typically require some form of input or activation sent to the processing unit that results in some form of output. It was stated above that modifications to allow access could occur anywhere along this continuum of method to achieve input, input device, interface, processing, interface, and output. When thinking about an ECS, the terminology changes slightly, but the concept remains the same. An ECS basically consists of the following (Haataja & Saarnio, 1990):

1. An input method (direct selection or scanning via single, dual, or multiple switches);
2. A control or signaling device (the transmitter) to change input into a sendable form such as infrared pulses, ultrasound, voice, radio frequencies, and electrical signals;
3. A receiving device to receive the input signals;
4. A target device or device (peripherals such as appliances, computer, and phone) that responds to the signals relayed by the receiving device;
5. The connection or interface between the signaling devices and the target device(s) and/or receiving unit, which can be electrical or wireless (remote) and may be a switch, computer, AAC device, ECS base, or integrated controller from a wheelchair;
6. The output or feedback mechanism (visual, auditory, etc.) to inform the user of the results and actions

If the client in Figure 31.15 is using the switch to turn on a lamp, his method to achieve input is scanning, the signaling device is the ECS base unit and the X-10 control unit, the receiving device is the X-10 module plugged into the wall, the target device is the lamp, and the connection is the radio frequency signal between the X-10 control unit and the lamp module and the electrical connection between the module and the lamp.

SPECIFIC TYPES OF ACTIVATION

Infrared

Devices in common use activated by infrared (IR) signals are televisions, CD players, and radios. Digital signals representing control codes or commands for the specific device are converted into IR pulses that are transmitted, received, and converted into **digital signals** again to activate the desired command (e.g., to change the television channel). The control device (e.g., the acs Controller, acs Technologies, Inc.) must be within the line of sight of the transmitter (i.e., it cannot be blocked by furniture or walls) unless used with a Powermid (X-10 USA Inc., Northvale, NJ), to convert IR to radio frequency. Trainable remotes are increasingly used to learn the control schemes of and, therefore operate, several target devices.

Radio Frequency

Some common devices that can be operated by radio frequency (RF) waves include lamps, electric beds and doors, and small appliances such as coffee machines. X-10 modules (X-10 USA, Inc.), the receiving devices for this type of transmission, plug into wall electrical outlets and are designed for a specific appliance (lamp, fan, etc.) that is then plugged into the module. Transmission of an RF specific to that module's control code is sent to switch the appliance on or off. An electrician should assist with system setup. The advantages of RF are portability, no line of sight requirement, and the use of existing wiring. Disadvantages include inadvertent device operation because of overcrowded frequencies and the need to be

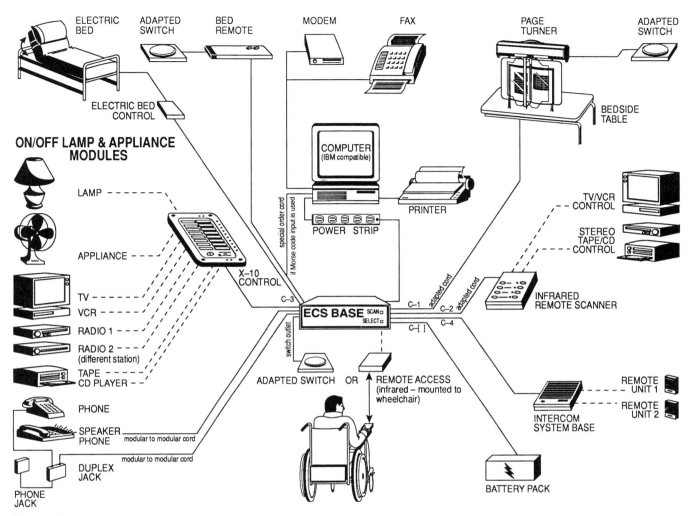

Figure 31.15. A schematic of an environmental control system, demonstrating common devices controlled and methods of activation. Only four control outlets are available on certain ECS bases. C-1, the cord from the first outlet; C-[ ], indicates that a choice must be made if other options are desired.

within about 50 feet of the target device for most RF systems (Bischof, 1986). Some RF systems can be operated up to a maximum of 200 feet away (Church & Glennen, 1992), but this depends on the specific characteristics of the transmitter, its antenna orientation, and the radio frequency being used (Jerome, 1994).

Ultrasound

Systems using ultrasound (US) waves to activate a control command for an appliance operate similarly to the RF method, incorporating color-coded modules with the appliance plugged into them (Ultra 4, TASH Inc.). Advantages of this system include no line of sight operation and no inappropriate operation of devices in another room. A major disadvantage is that only

appliances in the same room as the transmitter can be controlled.

Electrical Wiring

Control of devices (such as air-conditioners, washers, and computers) through household AC wiring requires a transmitter for IR signals or RF that may be interfaced with a computer, a base receiver plugged into the wiring to signal the appropriate appliance, appliance modules plugged into outlets, and the target appliances plugged into the modules. A few examples of ECS bases include DEUCE (DU-IT Control Systems Group, Inc., Shreve, OH), Control 1 (Prentke Romich Co.), and CHEC2 (Bloorview Children's Hospital, Willowdale, Ont., Canada). Advantages of this type of activation are that no expensive rewiring needs to be done and the user needs only a single portable control unit. The system can be comprehensive if careful grouping of devices is done.

Voice

Activation by voice requires a microphone on a headset worn by the client or mounted on the wheelchair or table. Such a system (e.g., Simplicity Series 6, Quartet Technology, Tyngsboro, MA, and Hal-B, Voice Connexion, Irvine, CA) typically gives both auditory feedback (an actual reply from the computer: "Dialing the number") and visual with lights indicating the selected operations.

Multiple Types of Activation

Some ECSs are able to operate multiple devices in the environment, including telephones, appliances, and infrared-controlled devices. Some that interface with a computer (e.g., PROXi, Madenta Communications) can in fact control up to 256 target devices, with access possible via voice, keyboard, or single switch.

ACCESS TO AND CONFIGURATION OF THE ECS SELECTED

An ECS can be operated by direct selection or by switches. Access through switches may require scanning first through a menu of the devices controlled and then through a menu of the functions of the particular selected device. For example, if the user chooses to turn on the television, the selection menu would then branch to choices about channels, volume levels, and so on (e.g. LIASON, DU-IT Control Systems Group, Inc.). The ECS type of activation will be chosen on the basis of the devices most frequently accessed by the client and by the client's cognitive, motor, and sensory status (which determines the type of feedback necessary from the ECS device).

The client's physical access to the ECS must also be considered. Some systems have a portable transmitter, a stationary transmitter, or both. In the latter case, the client could operate the stationary console from the bed and the portable one from the wheelchair to control various devices in each room.

Figure 31.15 shows various possibilities of an ECS. Each ECS will, of course, be configured to the client's needs and abilities. Clients may require only simple X-10 control of devices, may add in control of infrared devices, or may want additional options such as security systems or door opening capabilities. The ECS shown in Figure 31.15 demonstrates the computer system operated through the ECS base. This setup would be necessary if the computer was unable to run multitask environments. A computer with a multitask environment allows the user to access ECS features (e.g., dim lights, answer the phone, turn the television

down, etc.) without stopping his computer application (e.g., word processing or sending a transmission via modem). With an ECS base, the user can similarly operate the computer and control the environment simultaneously.

ECS CONTROL INTEGRATED WITH POWERED WHEELCHAIR CONTROL

As a result of technological advances, it is now possible to control one or more AT devices from the controls of a powered wheelchair. Known as an integrated controller, this system has advantages and disadvantages. Integrated control is typically recommended when the client has only one access site with reliable, voluntary movement, when each necessary piece of AT can be best accessed by the same input device, or when the client prefers such integration to decrease his need for assisted donning or positioning of the other switches(es) and access devices (Guerette, Caves, & Gross, 1992). However, the controller can only operate one AT device at a time, i.e., the wheelchair user cannot operate his computer or AAC device simultaneously with the wheelchair. Also, if the controller malfunctions, control of all AT devices is lost.

Integrated control may be not recommended if the client needed to access AT devices from positions other than his wheelchair, had cognitive and/or perceptual impairment that did not permit learning integrated control operation, or had greatly diminished speed and/or accuracy of AT use with a single input device (e.g., he may have the necessary control to access a computer with a switch, but may control his wheelchair more efficiently with a joystick) (Guerette et al., 1992).

ROBOTICS

At present, robotic systems available provide a specialized type of environmental control, although companies are beginning to focus on development of robots to perform everyday functions (Bach et al., 1990, Marlewski-Probert, 1993). Robotics are not universally used because of cost and limited applicability (Hammel, 1993). The present cost of the systems can really only be justified in workstations, where a person is able to be a productive job holder solely because of the robotics aid (Taylor, Cupo, & Sheredos, 1993). Currently available robotics products such as the Desktop Vocational Assistant Robot (DeVAR; Independence Works, Inc., Stanford, CA) function from a fixed location to pick up and move objects on a surface, handle files, answer phones, and perform other office tasks. The Robotics Work Station Attendant (Regenesis Development Corp., North Vancouver, B.C., Canada) is a robotics device for office tasks that is controlled by voice input, scanning or encoding, or keyboard.

INDICATIONS FOR ASSISTIVE TECHNOLOGY USE

Assistive technology as a modality could potentially be used with clients of all ages and with just about any diagnosis. How, then, do you make decisions about whether the use of technology is appropriate for a given client? Begin by asking the following questions.

1. What occupational performance areas (i.e., what ADL tasks, vocational and educational activities, and leisure activities) are affected? For instance, does the client need assistance in the areas of mobility, verbal or written communication, and/or environmental control? This will help to determine the configuration of the technical devices that may be of use to the client.

2. Are these impairments likely to be temporary? For impairments that may be temporary, a complex technological solution is unnecessary. A better use of personal and financial resources would be to provide low-tech adaptations to improve function while working toward remediation of the impairment(s) through typical therapeutic modalities. However, if a client's safety, self-esteem, or sense of well-being is threatened by his impairments and a technological device is available that could significantly impact these areas, then the therapist would strongly consider use of such a device in the overall care plan of the client. A C_{1-2} SCI client in the acute phase after injury, unable to speak because he has a tracheostomy, would be unable to use a standard hospital call button. A switch activated by eyebrow movements attached to a call signal and communication device could significantly impact his emotional recovery by giving him control over at least one aspect of function.

3. If a client's status is considered permanent, or not likely to improve significantly, even with maximum rehabilitation, then AT that can increase functional independence is strongly indicated. At this point, the client would be referred to AT specialists for further evaluation of specific impairment in motor, sensory, cognitive, or other functional areas. The rehabilitation team members, if not specialists themselves, would be expected to work closely with the AT team to provide specific details of client performance, needs, and limitations that would affect technology use.

ASSESSMENT FOR TECHNOLOGY USE

As technology has evolved and shared knowledge has increased, the evaluation process has become more refined and systematic evaluation formats have begun to be published (Bain, 1989; Bristow, Pickering, & Fristoe, 1993; Petty & Teal, 1991; Williams et al., 1993). While personnel of each facility may differ slightly in the process by which they evaluate clients for technology access, certain key factors seem to be common across all settings. Assistive technology evaluations are a collaborative process carried out by a multidisciplinary team of professionals, each of whom brings a slightly different set of skills, information, and point of view to the assessment. The team may consist of any or all of the following: the client (consumer), the family and caregivers, occupational therapists, physical therapists, speech language pathologists, audiologists, rehabilitation engineers, educators, physicians, vocational rehabilitators, and psychologists. The exact makeup of the team is decided by several factors, including the specific needs of the client, the range of expertise of the individual team members, the purpose of the technology, and the specific environment in which the technology will be used (Rizer, Ourand, & Rein, 1991).

Occupational therapists on the assessment team serve as interface specialists (Hammel, 1993; Hussey, 1993; Johnson, 1993). In this context, the term *interface* refers to the connection between the client; the environment, including the tools (electronic or nonelectronic) used to manipulate that environment; and the community in which the client functions on a daily basis. The occupational therapist works with the client and the team to determine if assistive technology could improve the client's ability to interface with his world. The occupational therapist's perspective is unique because she looks holistically at the entire range of human performance when determining ways to integrate low- and high-technology into the client's daily routine so that function and quality of life are maximized. Specifically, the therapist is responsible for:

1. Analyzing occupational performance roles in the areas of daily life tasks, vocation and education, and leisure;
2. Contributing to assessment of positioning and seating to promote functional motor control needed to use the device(s);
3. Assessing sensorimotor function related to technology access (including evaluation of fine motor and/or visual-motor and perceptual motor skills for accurately targeting and activating computer keys, AAC devices, and/or switches) and perhaps evaluating the ability of the client to use effectively sensory feedback from the equipment once activated;
4. Determining optimum placement of technology components in relation to the client and to the environment in which they will be used so that function is maximized;
5. Recommending and/or fabricating any orthotics or low-tech adaptive equipment necessary to access technology components and/or devising alternate methods for performing desired activities, which may or may not involve technology use;

6. Training in the use of the equipment or interface technology;
7. Evaluating the effectiveness of the AT solutions to increase occupational performance.

The sequence of steps of the assessment process is presented graphically in Figure 31.16. The typical progression of AT assessments is circular or cyclical (Galvin & Barnicle, 1993). Information gathered at each step of the assessment process determines what is to be done at the next step. After the nine steps of the assessment process are described, a case study that follows this process is presented.

Step 1: Assessment of Client Needs

INFORMATION GATHERING

If the referral to the AT team is from an outside source and members of the team are not familiar with the client, the assessment process is begun by compiling and reviewing available background information on the client. This will help determine if the referral was appropriate and if the client is a potential AT user. Specific types of information needed include the following.

1. What is the client's specific diagnosis or disability area and what is the potential for changes?
2. What are the client and family needs and expectations for assistive technology? What are the current and possible future life roles or occupational perfor-

mance areas of the client? Which performance areas are a priority for the client? What is his motivation to be independent in this area? Do family and caregiver goals match client goals? What are the desired or necessary functional performance activities in the areas of work, play, and self-care?

3. What specific problems is the client having with performance of the targeted activity? Are component skills impaired and, therefore, hindering performance in these areas? Is there technology available that will perform or assist with performance of these activities? Could a low-tech solution be as effective?
4. In what environments will the technology be needed?
5. What prior exposure has the client had to technology and what was his reaction? Does he use technology as part of his routine now and how is this working?

Having as much of this information as possible beforehand allows the team to prepare for assessment by assembling potential systems or pieces of technology, assigning relevant team members, and selecting appropriate application software and/or language systems. By reviewing this information, the team can also identify areas in which more specific information is needed. For example, the client may be looking for computer adaptations to be used at work. The team would need to have information about the specifics of the employment site, e.g., types of computer system(s) in use, space availability, and software requirements. The team may decide to include the employer as a

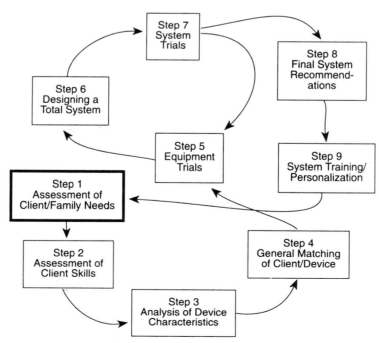

Figure 31.16. Steps in the assessment process for assistive technology.

team member and/or do a job analysis as part of the assessment.

GOAL SETTING

Once background information is gathered, the team is ready to determine the goals of the assessment process. Open communication and team dialogue are used to define desired outcomes and/or establish realistic goals for technology use. Goals will need to be prioritized so that options can be considered methodically and decisions can be made effectively. After clear goals are established, the client's skills are systematically assessed. Throughout, the team must not only consider what the client is capable of now but also make predictions as to future capabilities.

Step 2: Assessment of Client Skills

POSTURAL CONTROL

Occupational and physical therapy evaluation of postural control and of seating and positioning equipment needs is often the first step in evaluation of motor functioning for technology access. The purposes of this portion of the assessment are discussed below.

1. It is important to determine what positioning is possible given the patient's medical needs, orthopedic considerations, etc. Ideally the more upright, the better for technology access. This allows more normal placement of components on the tabletop, and equipment is within the visual field of the user. Upright is the normal position of function for occupational performance. However, many clients have preferred positioning, and/or cannot tolerate being upright for long periods of time. They may not be able to function efficiently in the upright position because of poor trunk or head control.

2. The therapist should determine which positions allow the patient maximum control over voluntary movements and, therefore, maximum control over the technology. Kangas (1992) noted that the 90-90-90 posture (hip-knee-ankle position) that has been the accepted optimal position for client seating is in fact a posture human beings assume only when waiting (i.e., for a lecture to begin). She further observed that the posture we assume when getting ready to do something is to lean forward, bring our hands forward and usually shift our feet behind our knees. Her point was that humans are dynamic beings and use multiple positions for function. She maintained that therapists must sacrifice strict therapeutic positioning if a different position increases function. In light of this, the therapist on the assessment team must carefully analyze various positions and positioning equipment to determine movement patterns that are functional but have the lowest potential for developing deformity. In general,

a stable base of support proximally improves mobility distally. However, some clients are oversupported and movement is restricted. The occupational therapist must observe the client in a functional context to make accurate judgments about optimal positions both for the client and the device. A particular client may use different positions for different functions.

3. It is important to determine what type of equipment is needed to provide these optimum positions, the team may decide to provide or refer the client for provision of seating services before continuation of evaluation for technology access if current positioning does not permit functional access. It is important that any positioning equipment prescribed be integrated with other devices used by the client, such as ventilators, orthotics, and mobile arm supports. Mobility equipment, particularly wheelchairs, may be part of the total AT system recommended for a client. Therefore, it is essential that the seating team work closely with the AT team to coordinate recommendations.

MOTOR CONTROL

Once the client is positioned appropriately, the therapist evaluates the client's ability to control voluntary movements consistently and reliably to determine possible methods of physical access to the technology. The therapist notes purposeful movements during observation of the client in a functional activity and considers the following factors.

Body Site Selection

At this point in the evaluation process, the occupational therapist probably will have one or more possible control sites in mind. A control site must be one over which the client has voluntary control, i.e., not activated by reflexive or by habitual movements (e.g., laughing and talking). The most commonly accepted hierarchy of desirable control sites is hands, head (including eyes, chin, lips, and tongue), other parts of the upper extremities, and finally the lower extremities. The hands are generally preferred over other sites, because they are typically used to manipulate or operate equipment. The therapist determines if one or both hands are able to be used. If both hands are used, bilateral coordination and the ability to isolate one or more fingers are assessed. If the hands are not functional, other sites are considered. The head is considered as a control site most often after the hands because of the importance of visual monitoring. For the user who inputs without being able to see the input device, kinesthesia and touch localization are crucial. The body site with the greatest degree of fine control offers the greatest chance for successful direct selection of characters from a display (Wright, 1992). If a client has only gross control of a movement, it is more likely that he will have to use a switch to scan and select characters and messages.

Range of Motion

The range of motion (ROM) possible at each site, together with the degree of control as assessed above, will determine possible input devices and methods. If a client is able to move through a large range and has fine motor control, then he probably can use standard input methods such as a **mouse** or keyboard. If he can move through large ranges but with poorly controlled movements, then larger targets are necessary, such as expanded keyboards or switch arrays. If he has diminished range but fine control, then a **mouse,** trackball, or mini-keyboard may be appropriate. If decreased range with decreased control are noted, then a switch may be the only possible input device.

Speed and Reaction Time

How fast can the client respond motorically to auditory or visual stimuli from the device? This information is important in determining device and software parameters that need to be adjusted to accommodate a client's abilities. For example, if a person requires 3 to 5 sec to hit the switch after hearing or seeing the target letter or message, the scan speed of the device must be programmed to allow that minimum reaction time.

Recovery Time

Can the movement be reversed or released quickly? Some input devices require only a momentary activation to perform their intended function. Sustained pressure on a standard computer key, for example, results in multiple inputs of that key character. This effect can be eliminated through the use of software and hardware options discussed earlier. Similarly, sustained switch closure is undesirable when using step scanning, as the switch must be hit repeatedly to move through the scan sequence.

Accuracy

As noted previously, the ROM and degree of control of a particular body site help to determine possible input devices and methods. Unless these parameters are easily ascertained by informal observation, the occupational therapist will need specifically to determine the client's ability to activate accurately targets of varying size and distance from the starting point. This information will be necessary to establish optimum placement of switch(es) and/or configuration of **alternate keyboards** or communication devices. To assess and record these performance variables ob-

jectively, Petty (1991) used a grid to measure, mark, and record a client's ROM at selected body sites. This same grid format could be used to determine targeting ability by measuring client ability to hit single targets on successively smaller grids. Accidental activations of adjacent targets could indicate the need for low-tech equipment such as key guards and pointing aids.

Force and Endurance Factors

How much force or pressure can be generated once a target is reached? Can a position or movement be sustained or repeated sufficiently to accomplish the desired task? This information helps in the selection of an input device that matches client strength and endurance.

SENSORY STATUS

General information about a client's visual and auditory status would typically be included in referral or preassessment documentation. Having test scores or standardized measures does not always help to determine functional use of technology. The team needs to test specific client abilities.

Auditory

Can the client adequately hear the auditory feedback given by the device so he can respond efficiently? If partially deaf, the client may require sound augmentation through hearing aids, external speakers, etc. If auditory discrimination or processing is a problem, he may require better quality speech synthesis. If his hearing impairment is great, he may require products that provide visual or vibratory feedback.

Visual

There are three aspects of vision that are important to evaluate when assessing a client's ability to use technology. Visual acuity affects the type of visual output required by the client as well as placement of that output in regard to distance from the client. Large print texts, enlarged key labels, screen magnification (all or parts of the display) may be sufficient for mild visual impairment. Visual discrimination, figure/ground perception, and visual neglect affect choice of icon size, format (line drawings versus colored icons), and arrangement (spacing or location on screen). The contrast of the visual materials used must be considered. Antiglare screens or varied background colors on the monitor may be necessary. For the client with figure/ground discrimination difficulties, the visual format of the software on-screen display must be as uncluttered as possible. A flat screen monitor instead of a curved monitor may make a difference. Tracking, peripheral vision, and oculomotor control affect placement of materials for viewing by the client. Horizontal and vertical placement and the ability to shift focus from hands to screen, text to screen, etc. must be considered. The angle of the viewing materials may affect the client's visual performance. This becomes particularly important when the client is not 90° upright or when he wears bifocals. If functional vision is sufficiently limited, devices designed for use by blind persons (discussed above) are indicated.

COGNITION AND COMMUNICATION

Cognition and communication would primarily be assessed by speech language pathologists and/or psychologists and educators. The speech language pathologist typically assesses the status of speech production, receptive and expressive language skills, syntactic and pragmatic use of language, and general cognitive abilities relating to use of representational language systems. While an in-depth cognitive assessment is not usually done at the time of the technology assessment, having this information available, preferably beforehand, can help determine appropriate software complexity and the ability to use input methods with a higher cognitive load, such as encoding. In addition, planning for academic and vocational potential is essential so the therapists can recommend a flexible system with adequate growth capabilities. The occupational therapist may have input here in regard to the client's memory (visual and auditory), ability to follow directions, attention span, sequencing abilities, and optimum learning style.

PSYCHOSOCIAL FACTORS

While psychosocial factors may not be formally assessed, they are extremely important in client acceptance and successful use of technology and must be considered by the evaluation team. Passive clients with a history of difficulty initiating interactions, seeking support, asserting rights, or taking responsibility for self-management may not be effective technology users. However, the team must consider whether a client has learned helplessness from oversupportive caregivers, lack of opportunities to participate and build skills in this area, or ineffective interactions secondary to inadequate equipment (Weisz, 1979).

Therefore, the team must consider the client's motivation to use technology and to be independent. Will he be able to take responsibility for upkeep of the equipment, seeking necessary maintenance and repairs and/or technical help when needed? Does he have concerns about "looking different" or an aversion to technology or gadgetry? Patience and frustration tolerance play a large role in the user's ability to interact successfully with technology (Johnson, 1993).

Step 3: Analysis of Device Characteristics

At this point the team reviews its knowledge of specific devices and their features to determine which will match the ascertained client skills and meet the stated needs for function. The team already has knowledge of basic features and has been considering and selecting possibilities throughout the needs and skills assessment part of the evaluation. But now the team more directly begins the process of considering device specifics by consulting product literature, comprehensive AT resources (e.g., Berliss et al., 1991–1992; *Closing the Gap Annual Resource Directory*, 1993), vendors, or other professionals or consumers who may have had experience with the products under consideration.

Step 4: General Matching of Client and Device Characteristics

After the client's skills are carefully assessed and general device characteristics are considered, the team will propose general system features that appear necessary for the client, including probable input method (direct selection versus scanning), possible input devices (expanded or regular keyboard, pneumatic or chin switch), possible control sites (head or hand), and necessary processing modifications and output characteristics (Varga & Swengel, 1993). The possibilities for specific system components are carefully discussed by the team (with client as equal participant) to determine client preferences and to weigh advantages and disadvantages of the proposed system(s). They may select one or several possible system components to take to equipment trials. This next step may not be necessary if the client's skills are easily defined and matched or if the client is already using a system and just wants modifications or upgrades. However, for those with multiple impairments or complex issues affecting performance, equipment trials provide additional information for final system design.

Step 5: Equipment Trials

During equipment trials, the team evaluates the match of selected system components to the client's skills and abilities. Using the specific devices and equipment under consideration, the team collects data to determine objectively and systematically the optimum system components. For example, the team might feel certain that a client will not be able to use direct selection with efficiency but may want to give the client the opportunity to try various direct selection methods at various control sites before definitely ruling this out.

Ideally during equipment trials, the client's specific skills or abilities would be assessed using the exact piece(s) of equipment or device(s) that would be finally prescribed. However, depending on what had to be assessed, the therapist could use a device that closely matched the desired device in the key aspects to be considered (e.g., an older version of a communication device that has the same locations, sizes, and pressure requirements as the newer model). If such equipment substitution was made, the occupational therapist must use her training in activity analysis to ensure that the actual technology and client performance variables under consideration were still accurately matched.

If devices with the specific features the team thinks the client may need are not available at its facility, then the team must explore resources for making that equipment available for client trials. Programs that loan equipment on a temporary basis are established in some areas. Other options are to contact the manufacturer or the local representative to see if demonstration equipment or loaners are available. The team must be sure to make equipment fit the client's needs rather than making the user fit the equipment that the team may have available or with which the team has had prior experience.

If the client's skills are improving or show the potential to improve with training or practice, the team might decide to recommend a period of training before selecting the final piece of equipment or system. Or the team may decide to recommend an intervention that would give the client some immediate independence but continue to train him simultaneously for increased control, if that increase in control would give him greater efficiency or independence. For example, if the client could potentially use a direct selection input method rather than scanning, this would greatly increase his speed and efficiency and should be a goal pursued in therapy.

When working with a client to improve motor control for input, the therapist should use graded activities that do not require the client to learn system software simultaneously. For example, computer games that require a timed motor response but little problem solving are a motivating way to train motor control. Task analysis skills are essential in the training process to identify activities that target the specific skills the therapist wishes to train (Musselwhite, Goossens', & Elder, 1991). It is also important to remember that motor learning requires a significant amount of practice. If the client is to be using a particular input setup, the client should practice with that identical setup in as many activities and environments as possible. If the client has primitive reflex activity or increased muscle tone, training should begin in a quiet nondistractible environment to reduce the effects of excitement on motor performance. However, training

should move as quickly as possible to the types of environments in which the client will be expected to perform (Petty & Teal, 1991).

Step 6: Designing a Total System

Now the team is ready to put together a specific system with all the components that have been selected to match client performance variables. The team will be able to identify certain key features that are necessary in the client's final system. The most important aspect of a system is that it truly increases the user's functional performance in the area desired. For example, if the client is using a communication device or method that is so slow that his impatient peers leave before he's finished, the device is not increasing his functional communication.

The team must consider the amount of setup required in relation to caregiver skills as well as practicality, the speed with which the technology (or the user) performs the intended function, and the flexibility of the system to change with the client's changing needs. These factors greatly affect the client's acceptance of the system and the extent to which the technology will be integrated into the client's daily activities (Galvin & Barnicle, 1993).

Device characteristics must be considered in the context of the environments in which the system will be used. Physical factors, such as lighting or noise levels, can greatly affect the way a device functions for the user (Cleveland & Doyle, 1993). If the device will be used in multiple occupational performance areas, the entire system must be easily transported with the client. Power availability for the system from the wheelchair battery or other sources must be considered. Weather resistance may be important to consider if the device will be used outdoors. Durability of system components must be considered. The amount of use expected in different environments should be determined. If heavy use is expected at work or in school but only minimal use is anticipated at home, the major components of the system could remain in the heavy-use environment and smaller components (or low-tech equivalents) might be used adequately at home.

If the client is using his system at work, the compatibility of the processing system and application programs with those already in use is important. The team must determine the type of application programs the client will need to operate as part of his job, the peripherals needed, and the ability of fellow workers to use the system. In making the work environment accessible for the client, it should not be made inaccessible for another worker. The team must also consider whether the client's system will be networked or will be an independent workstation. The ability to network enables some clients with disabilities to be employed but work in the environment in which they are able (e.g., at home, from bed, in a small area office).

Systems designed for vocational applications must also include work space design. Considerations here include the availability of work surface area required for the device and the proximity of any electrical outlets necessary for power. Safety issues must be considered carefully. The arrangement of cords and cables connecting components of the system must be considered for the safety of the user as well as those who share the same environment. Most AT equipment is electrical and, therefore, poses hazards to the client and others if not properly setup and maintained. It may be necessary for the occupational therapist or the team to consult rehabilitation engineers or physical plant personnel if major modifications to the work space or electrical system will be necessary.

The physical layout or placement of system components is also important at home, at school, or even on the wheelchair, if that is the client's usual work space (Lewis, 1993). There must be adequate access for the user (i.e., enough room for a wheelchair to maneuver up to the computer), all necessary input devices must be within easy reach, and output devices must be adequately placed. If other activities need to be carried out in the same space, system components should be easily removable or swing away. If a device is mounted on the wheelchair, the client must still be able to fit through doorways.

The field of **ergonomics** is increasingly being applied to designing offices and work spaces for the able-bodied population as well as for the disabled worker. Adaptations to increase comfort and productivity and decrease strain injuries are in common use in many offices. These include wrist rests, adjustable-height furniture, and document holders. The therapist and the assessment team should not fail to consider these low-tech adaptations when designing a total system for the client.

The way in which system components are mounted or held in place is extremely important when designing an AT system. A wide variety of mounting systems are available—both commercially and through therapist ingenuity. The most important consideration is the safety of the user and the stability of the mounting system.

Finally, consideration of the past reliability of a particular device and its manufacturer's service record is crucial. Warranty information, the expense of potential repairs, and the availability of local maintenance and repair services should also be judged when selecting system components. Whenever possible, a manual backup system for crucial functions should be recommended for when the AT system is in the shop (Johnson, 1993).

Technological interventions, as all adaptations, should be as reliable and as simple as possible while still meeting client needs. The most successful system will integrate low-and high-tech components, consist of the fewest components, and make the fewest changes in the standard configuration.

Step 7: System Trials

The team has now defined and designed a specific system that will be recommended for the client. Client trials with the specific system recommended should be completed before pursuing funding and ordering the equipment (Cottier, 1993). Ideally, this would take place in the environment(s) in which the system will be used. The client and training team may discover unexpected obstacles not predicted or planned for when designing the system—the inevitable system glitches that occur with all high-tech systems. For example, while product literature may have advertised transparency or compatibility between components, the actual performance of the system may be less than expected. Hardware or software modifications, such as additional memory, may be necessary to run all applications simultaneously. System trials help the client discover firsthand how the recommended system works for him. This will help to keep client and family expectations realistic. On the other hand, the team may need to encourage the client who was expecting miracles and help him understand that training is necessary to develop proficiency with any system.

Step 8: Recommend Final System

Once trials are completed and the team is reasonably sure the system will achieve the client's goals, the team documents the evaluation results and recommends the final system. At this point, the issue of funding must be considered. The occupational therapist is responsible for justifying AT equipment through documentation of how this equipment will increase the user's functional independence in ADLs, work, and leisure activities. This documentation, along with a letter from the physician stating that the system is a medical necessity, is submitted to traditional funding sources such as Medicare, Medicaid, vocational rehabilitation agencies, and private insurance companies. If these sources are pursued and adequate funding is not forthcoming, then it may be necessary to seek creative funding (Leubben et al., 1993).

Step 9: System Training and Personalization

Once the system is in place, the client usually will require some level of training with system operation. The amount of training required depends on the complexity of the system, the client's prior exposure to the technological components to be used, and the specific level of client skill when technology is provided.

Especially for the new technology user, it is important to begin training with successful experiences. Once the user becomes familiar with his new system, he will begin to identify features of his system he wishes to modify, add, or delete to improve speed or efficiency of task accomplishment. Specific vocabulary, macros, keyboard or communication device configuration, etc. will be created to personalize the system for its user.

It is also essential to train the client's family and any caregivers who will be working with the client. Identifying and training support personnel, including other therapists, teachers, and coworkers helps minimize system dysfunction. These support people may be required to set up the device, adjust switch positions, add paper, etc. Someone also must be responsible for taking care of daily maintenance of the equipment, such as charging batteries.

It must be stressed that assessment and training of clients and caregivers for appropriate AT use are ongoing processes. Consistent follow-up by the team is necessary to ensure continued use of the AT system and assist with necessary modifications (Cottier, 1993; Galvin & Barnicle, 1993).

CASE STUDY

Buck, a 20-year-old male with an incomplete spinal cord injury at C$_{1-2}$, was injured in a bicycle accident at age 19 (Fig. 31.17).

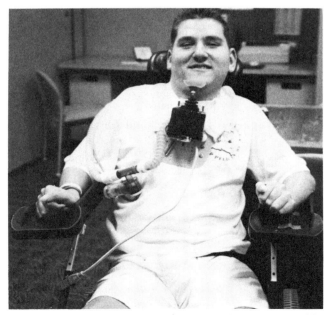

Figure 31.17. Buck demonstrating control components of his powered wheelchair.

He was referred to the AT assessment team for recommendations on any technology that would decrease his need for a full-time attendant.

Step 1: Assessment of Client Needs

INFORMATION GATHERING

Buck's injury was incomplete, so slight improvement in muscle function or in his ability to use functional return may occur, but major functional changes were not anticipated. At the time of the evaluation, Buck was living at home. He had completed high school before injury and was now ready to continue his education to prepare for entry into the work force. Buck also wanted to move to an apartment and reduce his dependence on his family and his attendant. In addition, he expressed a desire to have more social interaction with his peers.

Buck's parents had been caring for him at home but were concerned about their ability to do so as they aged. They were also interested in having him develop skills that would provide him with financial security.

In keeping with these stated goals, the team gathered the following information about specific problems in occupational performance areas. Buck was ventilator dependent and, therefore, needed someone within calling range at all times in case of an emergency. He was able to communicate verbally, with speech quality and intelligibility varying secondary to muscle spasms, breath control, and general endurance. Buck had no means of written communication and no means of accessing a standard computer keyboard without adaptations. He completely depended on others for all ADLs and control of devices in his environment, such as television, lights, air-conditioning, and telephone.

During his rehabilitation, Buck had used various low- and high-tech devices. A LightTalker (Prentke Romich Co.) with a light pointer was initially used for improved oral communication, but Buck adamantly did not wish to rely on an AAC device for communication. He found it easier, faster, and more personal to mouth words, even when he had to repeat. A headpointer for access to a computer keyboard, equipped with a key guard, was tried briefly to play computer games and do limited word processing. Buck fatigued rapidly with this method and was uncomfortable with the head mount. At the time of the AT assessment, Buck had a power wheelchair with a chin joystick for maneuvering and a simple pressure switch on his left arm trough to allow him to change the modes (tilt, on/off) independently (Fig. 31.17). Buck demonstrated no difficulty using this means of control to maneuver his wheelchair skillfully and safely.

GOAL SETTING

Goals for Buck were set and prioritized as follows:
1. Education or vocational program;
2. Environmental control;
3. Leisure activities.

Education or enrollment in a program leading to development of marketable job skills was the top priority identified by both Buck and his parents. Enrollment in such a program would also qualify him for vocational rehabilitation funding to assist with purchase of recommended technology. Computer access would be a major factor in allowing Buck to participate successfully in this type of program. Environmental control and a more independent living situation were identified as the second priority. As much as Buck desired to move out of his parents' house, he recognized that he needed to develop a means of financial support, because he would always need some assistance with self-care and ADLs. His family also could not afford an ECS without outside financial aid.

Step 2: Assessment of Client Skills

POSTURAL CONTROL

Buck demonstrated excellent head control limited by decreased endurance. He exhibited no trunk control. Buck was already adequately positioned in his wheelchair with a headrest, trunk supports, and adjustable armrests. His positioning allowed him fully to use the movements available to him.

MOTOR CONTROL

Buck had no functional hand movement on either side. He was able to control a single switch with his left upper extremity using slight supination but exhibited no other reliable movement in his upper extremities, except for shoulder elevation and scapular retraction. He was already using head movements to control his wheelchair. He had full control of head, neck, and oral motor musculature.

SENSORY STATUS

Buck had normal visual acuity, perceptual skills and auditory function. He demonstrated only slight, inconsistent sensory return in his upper extremities.

COGNITION AND COMMUNICATION

Buck was evaluated by a psychologist and assessed to be of normal intelligence. The team's speech pathologist found Buck's speech had only fair intelligibility to the unfamiliar listener because of limited breath control.

PSYCHOSOCIAL FACTORS

Buck was quite assertive and verbal about his needs during the goal-setting process and appeared to have realistic expectations for possible technological devices. Therefore, the team felt confident he would be a successful technology user.

Step 3: Analysis of Device Characteristics

The team at this point began researching computer access methods more specifically to address the first prioritized goal. Identification of a viable input method would not only apply to the computer system recommended but could also be used to access an ECS through the computer.

Step 4: General Matching of Client and Device Characteristics

At this time, the team felt certain that Buck would be able to use direct selection to access a computer system, because he had already mastered proportional control of his wheelchair using good fine motor control of his head and neck. Possible input devices and control sites under consideration included a head-pointing system such as the HeadMaster Plus with an **on-screen keyboard** or a voice-recognition system such as DragonDictate or Kurzweil VOICE. Processing modifications to speed up keyboarding were also considered (e.g., HandiWORD, Microsoft Systems, Inc.).

The team, Buck, and his family discussed the advantages and disadvantages of the specific input methods being considered. Buck was very excited about the possibility of a voice-recognition system, as it would eliminate the need for initial setup by the attendant. He also was interested in the more normal appearance of speaking into a microphone. The team expressed concerns about Buck's ability to maintain speech production for the extended periods of time necessary for completion of assignments. They were also concerned with the ability of the voice-recognition system to recognize accurately Buck's speech patterns as they changed with his level of fatigue and his ability to provide breath support.

Step 5: Equipment Trials

Buck first tried the HeadMaster Plus, because this device was available in the facility and was less expensive than a voice-recognition system (Fig. 31.8). Buck quickly mastered the use of the pointing device to access the **on-screen keyboard,** because of his previous experience with the light pointer. Software was then tried to speed up Buck's rate of input. Despite the use of such software, Buck expressed disappointment at the slowness of the input. The headset also slipped, requiring frequent repositioning, and felt uncomfortable to him.

Subsequently, the local vendor for DragonDictate was contacted to demonstrate this system and assist the team in assessment of this possible input method for Buck (Fig. 31.9). Following readjustment of the system to accommodate Buck's inconsistent voice quality, Buck was successfully able to use this method for input, producing recognizable voice patterns for more than 1 hr. Buck clearly expressed a preference for this method of input and was able to generate text with greater speed than with the HeadMaster Plus.

Step 6: Designing a Total System

The team now had enough information to recommend the following equipment to enhance Buck's independence in the educational setting as well as contain future expansion capabilities for environmental control and vocational applications.

1. A portable full-sized computer with the body of the computer located behind the wheelchair and the screen mounted in front on a power swing-away screen mount. Systems such as Synergy PC (Synergy, East Walpole, MA) or the Access-1 computer (WorkLink Innovations, Walnut Creek, CA) are specially designed in this fashion to avoid having the entire computer on the laptray. A portable computer system was considered essential as Buck would be moving between several environments in the educational setting (classroom, library, and home). The motorized screen mount would allow Buck to move the computer screen down when traveling to his next class, interacting with peers in a more informal setting between classes, or when he needed to be transferred from his chair.

2. A DragonDictate voice-recognition system with the microphone mounted on the wheelchair. This system was selected because Buck clearly preferred this method and it provided faster, more efficient data entry, especially for long assignments.

3. A flatbed scanner with OCR software (Fig. 31.10) to be used at home to input text pages into the computer for independent manipulation by Buck. The actual scanning (handling) of the documents would be done by another person.

4. A printer for home, with printer cables for the school's printer so that Buck could produce in-class assignments or take exams independently.

FUTURE EXPANSION CAPABILITIES

The following software and hardware could eventually be added to Buck's system.

1. A computer-controlled ECS (such as Synergy Integrated Remote, Synergy) or a switch-controlled ECS (such as Relax, TASH Inc.) if a more portable method of environmental control was desired; both types could be controlled from the wheelchair or in bed (if the wheelchair was near the bed);

2. A speaker phone with switch access for independent communication, recreation, and future work contacts;

3. Computer games software for recreational pursuits;

4. A computer card (such as LinkCard, Synergy) to network with other computers and expand Buck's employability.

Step 7: System Trials

To begin system trials, a local distributor for the Synergy PC was contacted, and he agreed to bring a demonstration model to the evaluation center with the DragonDictate system installed. Buck wanted to try using a swing-away microphone, and this was temporarily mounted for trial purposes. Buck was successfully able to use the microphone mounted on the wheelchair for input to the portable PC with the voice recognition system installed. The team's seating specialists and rehabilitation engineers measured the PC components and decided on the optimal mounting on Buck's wheelchair to prevent interference with the ventilator equipment and wheelchair tilt mechanisms and to distribute the weight of the components safely on the wheelchair base. Specifications for final mounting of the microphone and computer screen were determined.

Step 8: Recommend Final System

The team's recommendations were documented, with careful justification of each component. At this point, Buck's case worker assisted with funding applications to Medicaid and vocational rehabilitation.

Step 9: System Training and Personalization

Buck returned to the team when all system components were delivered. At this time, mounting and setup of the components on the wheelchair were completed. Buck was accompanied by his father and his personal care attendant. The local vendors for the Synergy PC and DragonDictate were present to train Buck and his caregivers in the basic operation and care of these components. The seating specialists on the team explained how computer components interfaced with the wheelchair system. Product literature, warranties, and specific contact personnel for service/maintenance were provided to Buck and his father. Buck and his father, in turn, identified specific caregivers who would take responsibility for each part of the system maintenance and for communication with the AT team.

Buck returned to the team several months later with a request for an alternate system for input. He was having difficulty in the classroom with noise interference and with using voice input while trying to listen to the lecture. The team recommended a backup system consisting of software for an **on-screen keyboard,** a Switch-Mouse (Synergy) to allow his chin joystick to function as a **mouse,** and a switch mounted in his wheelchair headrest to perform the select function of the **mouse.** Buck was still living at home, adjusting to his computer system and the school routine. He promised to contact the team when he was ready to move into an apartment and needed ECS capabilities.

FUTURE TRENDS

The ability to operate increasingly sophisticated technological devices to perform everyday activities has become a survival skill in today's world and is a necessary component of human occupation (Hammel & Smith, 1993). Predicted future developments in this field read like a science fiction novel but are rapidly proceeding through the research and development stages to marketing. One such trend is known as virtual reality (VR) technology.

Virtual reality is a term describing any optical or sensory simulation of something real, to the point of confounding the senses into accepting that simulation. Virtual reality technology combines high-speed computers with sensors capable of measuring motion, heat, and spatial relationships. Data received from the sensors are used by the computer to create virtual worlds in which the user experiences sensations that he or she perceives as real (Reingold, 1991). The applications of VR technology for the disabled population seem unlimited. Architects are using computer simulations to provide clients with a walk through of a newly designed building to check for architectural barriers before the plans are finalized (Trimble, Morris, & Crandall, 1992).

As exciting as these trends are, at the time of this writing appropriate technology services are reaching only a handful of disabled individuals because of the lack of trained personnel to provide AT services (Hammel & Smith, 1993) as well as a general lack of understanding on the part of agencies responsible for funding as to the necessity of technology for the disabled community (Leubben et al., 1993).

As students of human performance, occupational therapists have unique qualifications to use technology as a modality with clients with disabilities. Recognition of the need for technology training for occupation therapists has prompted the American Occupational Therapy Association to create its Technology Special Interest Section and charge the section with defining core competencies for therapists in this area (Hammel & Smith, 1993). Other organizations have also begun to develop advanced training programs and certification programs for technology specialists.

In the future, clients will be assessed for technology needs from the moment of entry or admission to the health care system as a patient. The entire process of evaluation and matchup of client and technology will be more thorough and will proceed faster, because of increased acceptance of and familiarity with technology on the part of clients and their families, increased knowledge and experience on the part of therapists, and the rapid improvement and evolution of the whole field of technological products.

Acknowledgments—The authors would like to thank the following people: Geralyn Provenzano for her support and encouragement, Diane Ostdiek for her technical advice and generosity in sharing information, Dawn Russell at Synergy, and the numerous people at various other companies who willingly shared their expertise.

STUDY QUESTIONS

1. Discuss the role of the occupational therapist on the AT team.
2. List the parts of a computer system, classify these parts as software or hardware, and explain the difference between software and hardware.
3. Describe characteristics of the patient who would be the most appropriate for each of the three selection methods (direct selection, scanning, and encoding).
4. Discuss the difference between an alternate keyboard and an on-screen keyboard.

5. List seven characteristics considered in selection of an appropriate switch for a client.

6. Discuss all the ways a computer system could be made more accessible for a client with moderate visual impairment. How would these modifications need to be further changed to accommodate someone with no vision?

7. List the basic parts of an ECS and describe two different types of activation for such a system.

8. Explain the specific role of the client and the family in each step of the assessment process.

9. ROM and voluntary control are typically assessed for almost all adult patients referred for occupational therapy. Explain what additional information the AT team needs in these areas to assist their selection of the most appropriate AT system.

10. Design an AT system for a 23-year-old client, who suffered a traumatic brain injury as the result of a motor vehicle accident. She has gross control of her arms, but very little fine motor control in her hands and fingers. She is unable to press buttons or point effectively. She has good control of her knees and feet when sitting, but is nonambulatory. She has some cognitive impairment in short-term memory, e.g., she has difficulty recalling information after a 5-min delay. She has no functional speech. She would like to attend the local college and live in an apartment with a good friend.

REFERENCES

Abramson, L. Y., Seligmann, M. E. P., & Teasdale, J. D. (1978). Learned helplessness in humans: Critique and reformation. *Journal of Abnormal Psychology, 87,* 49–74.

Americans with Disabilities Act of 1990, 42 U.S.C. §12101.

Bach, J. R., Zeelenberg, A. P., & Winter, C. (1990). Wheelchair-mounted robot manipulators. *American Journal of Physical Medicine and Rehabilitation, 69*(2), 55–59.

Bain, B. K. (1989). Assessment of clients for technological assistive devices. In American Occupational Therapy Association (Ed.), *Technology review '89: Perspectives on occupational therapy practice* (pp. 55–59). Rockville, MD: AOTA.

Banajee, M. (1993, November). Personal communication.

Berliss, J. R., Borden, P. A., Ford, K., & Vanderheiden, G. C. (Eds.). (1991–1992). *Trace resource book: Assistive technologies for communication, control, & computer access.* Madison, WI: Trace Research/Development Center.

Bischof, J. (1986). Technical aids. In J. P. Hill (Ed.), *Spinal cord injury: A guide to functional outcomes in occupational therapy* (pp. 205–223). Rockville, MD: Aspen Systems.

Bristow, D. C., Pickering, G. L., & Fristoe, M. W. (1993, March). *SAAT: Systematic assessment in assistive technology evaluation form.* Paper presented the Northridge Conference on Technology and Persons with Disabilities, California State University, Los Angeles.

Church, G., & Glennen, S. (1992). *The handbook of assistive technology.* San Diego: Singular Publishing Group.

Cleveland, N. R., & Doyle, P. (1993). The Eyegaze computer system: How does it work? Who can use it? *Closing the Gap Newsletter, 12*(1), 15–17.

Closing the Gap annual resource directory of hardware, software, producers, organizations. (1993). Henderson, MN: Closing the Gap.

Congressional report on PL 100-407. (1988). The Technology-Related Assistance for Individuals with Disabilities Act. Washington, DC: U.S. Government Printing Office.

Cottier, C. A. (1993, March). *How good is our first guess?* Paper presented at the Northridge Conference on Technology and Persons with Disabilities, California State University, Los Angeles.

Galvin, J., & Barnicle, K. (1993). *How to evaluate and select appropriate assistive devices.* Paper presented at the Northridge Conference on Technology and Persons with Disabilities, California State University, Los Angeles.

Goossens', C., & Crain, S. S. (1992). *Utilizing switch interfaces with children who are severely physically challenged.* Austin, TX: Pro-Ed.

Gross, K. (1992). Controlling the environment. *TeamRehab Report, 3*(6), 14–16.

Guerette, P., Caves, K., & Gross, K. (1992). One switch does it all. *TeamRehab Report, 3*(2), 26–29.

Haataja, S., & Saarnio, I. (1990). An evaluation procedure for environmental control systems. In *Proceedings of the 13th Annual RESNA Conference* (pp. 25–26). Arlington: VA: RESNA Press.

Hammel, J. (1993). Notes on the making of an interface specialist. *AOTA Technology Special Interest Newsletter, 3*(1), 3–4.

Hammel, J. M., & Smith, R. O. (1993). The development of technology competencies and training guidelines for O.T. 's. *American Journal of Occupational Therapy, 47*(11), 970–979.

Hussey, S. (1993). A framework for interface specialists. *AOTA Technology Special Interest Newsletter, 3*(1), 2–3.

Jerome, J. (1994, February). Personal communication.

Johnson, A. (1993). Interface technology: Low tech as a stepping stone to high tech. *AOTA Technology Special Interest Newsletter, 3*(1), 1–2.

Kangas, K. (1992, October). *The myth of the optimal position, and other mysteries revealed.* Paper presented at the 10th Annual International Conference on Microcomputer Technology in Special Education and Rehabilitation, Minneapolis, MN.

Lahoud, J. (1994, February). Personal communication.

Lau, C., & O'Leary, S. (1993). Comparison of computer interface devices for persons with severe physical disabilities. *American Journal of Occupational Therapy, 47,* 1022–1030.

Leubben, A. J., Harpe, S. B., Collins, R. A., Alvey, T. C., Buedel, J. K., Edwards, M. M., Foders, R. M., Sawyer-Gaslin, S., Herrington, M., Kitchell, S. L., Oxley, R. J., & Woodsmall, M. M. (1993). Funding questions. *AOTA Technology Special Interest Newsletter, 3*(2), 1–4.

Lewis, D. O. (1993). Work station wheelchair. *Mainstream, 18*(2), 31, 38–41.

Mann, W. C. (1989). Use of environmental control devices by nursing home patients. *Journal of Rehabilitation, Research, and Development, 25*(Suppl.), 1–8.

Marlewski-Probert, B. (1993). Robot helpers for the disabled community—Wave of the future. *Closing the Gap Newsletter, 12*(1), 12.

Musselwhite, C. (1993). *Merging technology and whole language: Reading activities project for older students (RAPS).* Paper presented at the Northridge Conference on Technology and Persons with Disabilities, California State University, Los Angeles.

Musselwhite, C., Goossens', C., & Elder, P. (1991, June). *Learn to play, play to learn: Clinical strategies for children who are severely physically challenged.* Paper presented at a conference at the United Cerebral Palsy Center, Birmingham, AL.

Petty, L. (1991). *Physical functional assessment.* Willowdale, Ont., Canada: Bloorview Children's Hospital.

Petty, L., & Teal, C. (1991, October). *The client who can't access:*

Assessing and training the hard-to-fit client for switch access. Paper presented at the 9th Annual International Conference on Microcomputer Technology in Special Education and Rehabilitation, Minneapolis, MN.

Reed, K. L. (1992). History of federal legislation for persons with disabilities. *American Journal of Occupational Therapy, 46,* 397–408.

Reingold, H. (1991). *Virtual reality.* New York: Summit.

Rizer, H. (1992). Alternative mouse control devices: Advantages for persons with physical disabilities. *AOTA Technology Special Interest Newsletter, 2*(3), 2–3.

Rizer, H., Ourand, P., & Rein, J. (1991, October). *Evaluation of computer input methods for persons with physical disabilities.* Paper presented at the 9th Annual International Conference on Microcomputer Technology in Special Education and Rehabilitation, Minneapolis, MN.

Russell, D. (1993, June). Personal communication.

Smith, R. O. (1991). Technological approaches to performance enhancement. In C. Christiansen & C. Baum (Eds.), *Occupational therapy: Overcoming human performance deficits* (pp. 746–786). Thorofare, NJ: Slack.

Stahl, C. (1993). In environmental control, it's the simple things that count. *ADVANCE for Occupational Therapists, 9*(29), 9.

Symington, D. C., Lywood, D. W., Lawson, J. S., & Maclean, J. (1986). Environmental control systems in chronic care hospitals and nursing homes. *Archives of Physical Medicine & Rehabilitation, 67,* 322–325.

Taylor, B., Cupo, M. E., & Sheredos, S. J. (1993). Workstation robotics: A pilot study of a desktop vocational assistant robot. *American Journal of Occupational Therapy, 47,* 1009–1013.

Trimble, J., Morris, T., & Crandall, R. (1992). Virtual reality: Designing accessible environments. *TeamRehab Report, 3*(8), 32–36

Varga, T. E., & Swengel, K. E. (1993, March). *Feature match: An essential component of the assessment process.* Paper presented at the Northridge Conference on Technology and Persons with Disabilities, California State University, Los Angeles.

Weisz, J. R. (1979). Perceived control and learned helplessness among mentally retarded and nonretarded children: A developmental analysis. *Developmental Psychology, 15,* 311–319.

Whipp, D., & Freeman, T. (1993). *The modem manual.* Dunbar: West Virginia Research and Training Center.

White, R. (1993). *How computers work.* Emeryville, CA: Ziff-Davis.

Williams, W. B., Stemach, G., Wolfe, S., & Stanger, C. (1993, March). *Lifespace access profile: Assistive technology assessment and planning for individuals with severe or multiple disabilities.* Paper presented at the Northridge Conference on Technology and Persons with Disabilities, California State University, Los Angeles.

Wright, C. (1992). Access to technology: The multidisciplinary team approach. *AOTA Technology Special Interest Newsletter, 2*(1), 1–2.

Supplementary Resources

Ability Research, Inc. (P.O. Box 1721, Minnetonka, MN 55345; 612-939-0121)

AbleNet. (1081 Tenth Avenue SE, Minneapolis, MN 55414; 612-379-0956; 800-322-0956)

acs Technologies, Inc. (1400 Lee Drive, Coraopolis, PA 15108; 800-227-2922)

Adaptive Switch Laboratories. (1181 Brittmoore Road, Suite 500, Houston, TX 77043; 713-827-7766; 800-626-8698)

Apple Computer, Inc. (Worldwide Disability Solutions Group, MS 2SE, 20525 Mariani Avenue, Cupertino, CA 95014; 408-974-7910; 800-776-2333)

Artic Technologies International, Inc. (55 Park Street, Troy, MI 48083; 313-588-7370)

Berkeley Systems, Inc. (2095 Rose Street, Berkeley, CA 94709; 510-540-5535)

Blazie Engineering. (105 East Jarrettsville Road, Forest Hill, MD 21050; 410-893-9333)

Bloorview Children's Hospital. (Communication & Assistive Technology, 25 Buchan Court, Willowdale, Ont., Canada M2J 459; 416-494-2222)

Chinon America, Inc. (660 Maple Avenue, Torrance, CA 90503; 213-533-0274; 800-441-0222)

Creative Switch Industries. (P.O. Box 5256, Des Moines, IA 50306; 515-287-5748; 800-257-4358)

Designing Aids for Disabled Adults (DADA). (249 Concord Avenue #2, Toronto, Ont., Canada ONM6H 2P4)

Digital Equipment Corporation. (Continental Boulevard, Merrimack, NH 03054; 603-884-8990)

Don Johnston Developmental Equipment, Inc. (1000 North Rand Road, Building 115, P.O. Box 639, Wauconda, IL 60084-0639; 708-526-2682; 800-999-4660)

Dragon Systems, Inc. (320 Nevada Street, Newton, MA 02160; 617-965-5200; 800-825-5897)

DU-IT Control Systems Group, Inc. (8765 Township Road #513, Shreve, OH 44676; 216-567-2906)

Dunamis Inc. (3620 Highway 317, Suwanee, GA 30174; 404-932-0485; 800-828-2443)

Edmark Corp. (P.O. Box 3218, Redmond, WA 98073; 206-556-8400; 800-362-2890)

G W Micro. (310 Racquet Drive, Fort Wayne, IN 46825; 219-483-3625)

Hear Our Voices. A support group. (55-301 Hanover Circle S, Birmingham, AL 35205; 205-930-9025)

HumanWare, Inc. (6245 King Road, Loomis, CA 95650; 916-652-7253; 800-722-3393)

IBM Corp. (Special Needs Systems, 1000 Northwest 51st Street, Boca Raton, FL 33432; 800-426-4832)

Independence Works, Inc. (831 Esplanada Way, Stanford, CA 94305)

Innocomp. (26210 Emery Road, Suite 302, Warrensville Heights, OH 44128; 216-464-3636; 800-382-8622)

IntelliTools (Formerly Unicorn Engineering). (5221 Central Avenue, Suite 205, Richmond, CA 94804; 510-528-0670; 800-899-6687)

International Society for Augmentative and Alternative Communication (ASAAC). (P.O. Box 1762, Staion R, Toronto, Ont. M4G 4A3 Canada

J. A. Preston Corp. (P.O. Box 89, Jackson, MI 49204; 800-631-7277)

Koala Technologies Corp. (70 North 2nd Street, San Jose, CA 95113; 408-287-6311)

Kurzweil Applied Intelligence, Inc. (411 Waverly Oaks Road, Waltham, MA 02154; 617-893-5151)

Laureate Learning Systems, Inc. (110 East Spring Street, Winooski, VT 05404; 800-562-6801)

LC Technologies, Inc. (9455 Silver King Court, Fairfax, VA 22031; 703-385-7133; 800-733-5284)

Luminaud, Inc. (8688 Tyler Boulevard, Mentor, OH 44060; 216-255-9082)

Madenta Communications Inc. (9411 A 20th Avenue, Edmonton, Alta., Canada T6N 1E5; 403-450-8926; 800-661-8406)

Marblesoft. (12301 Central Avenue NE, Suite 205, Blaine, MN 55434; 612-755-1402)

Microsoft Corp. (One Microsoft Way, Redmond, WA 98052; 206-882-8080; 800-426-9400)

Microsystems Software, Inc. (600 Worcester Road, Framingham, MA 01701; 508-879-9000; 800-828-2600)

New Abilities System. (1940 Colony Street, #2, Mountain View, CA 94043)

Penny & Giles Computer Products. (1640 Fifth Street, Suite 224, Santa Monica, CA 90401; 310-393-1497)

Pointer Systems, Inc. (One Mill Street, Burlington, VT 05401; 802-658-3260; 800-537-1562)

Prentke Romich Co. (1022 Heyl Road, Wooster, OH 44691; 800-262-1984)

Quartet Technology, Inc. (52 Davis Road, Tyngsboro, MA 01879; 508-692-9313)

Raised Dot Computing. (408 South Baldwin Street, Madison, WI 53703; 608-257-9595; 800-347-9594)

Regenesis Development Corp. (1046 Deep Cove Road, North Vancouver, B.C., Canada V7G-1S3; 604-929-2414)

Rehabilitation Engineering Society of North America (RESNA). (1700 North Moore Street, Suite 1540, Arlington, VA 22209-1903; 703-524-6686)

Sammons, Inc. (P.O. Box 32, Brookfield, IL 60513; 708-325-1700; 800-323-5547)

Sentient Systems Technology, Inc. (2100 Wharton Street, Suite 630, Pittsburgh, PA 15203; 412-682-0144; 800-344-1778)

Street Electronics Corp. (6420 Via Real, Carpinteria, CA 93013; 805-684-4593)

Synergy. (68 Hale Road, East Walpole, MA 02032; 508-668-7424)

Talktronics, Inc. (27341 Eastridge Drive, Lake Forest, CA 92630; 714-768-4220; 800-421-7668)

TASH Inc. (Unit #1, 91 Station Street, Ajax, Ont. L1S 3H2 Canada; 905-686-4129)

TeleSensory. (455 North Bernardo Avenue, P.O. Box 7455, Mountain View, CA 94039; 415-960-0920; 800-227-8418)

Toys for Special Children, Inc. (385 Warburton Avenue, Hastings-on-Hudson, NY 10706; 800-832-8697)

Trace Research/Development Center. (Room S-151, Waisman Center, 1500 Highland Avenue, Madison, WI 53705; 608-262-6966)

VME Technologies, Inc. (5202 Westland Boulevard, Baltimore, MD 21227; 410-455-6397)

Voice Connexion. (17835 Skypark Circle, Suite C, Irvine, CA 92714; 714-261-2366)

Words+, Inc. (43700 17th Street W, Suite 202, Lancaster, CA 93584; 800-869-8521)

WorkLink Innovations. (2328 Tice Valley Boulevard, Walnut Creek, CA 94595; 510-937-9347)

X-10, USA Inc. (185 LeGrand Avenue, Northvale, NJ 07647; 201-784-9700)

Zygo Industries, Inc. (P.O. Box 1008, Portland, OR 97207; 503-684-6006; 800-234-6006)

32
Biofeedback

Catherine A. Trombly and Jeannette Tries

OBJECTIVES _____

After studying this chapter, the reader will be able to:
1. Define biofeedback.
2. Understand the uses of electrogoniometric and electromyographic biofeedback.
3. Organize treatment sessions using biofeedback to recruit or inhibit muscle activity.

Feedback is necessary for motor learning (Mulder & Hulstyn, 1984). To illustrate the role of feedback, Miller (1978) used the analogy of a basketball player acquiring the skill of making foul shots. The player receives visual feedback regarding the result of each shot, compares that information with proprioceptive and kinesthetic stimuli, and corrects subsequent throws as a result of this informational reinforcement. Motor performance is refined as the external consequence, or feedback of knowledge of results of a response, is paired with internal kinesthetic cues associated with that response. As a result, the person learns to discriminate the specific kinesthetic stimuli linked to the more desired response. In other words, better, more efficient motor responses are learned if they are differentially reinforced through neurophysiological feedback systems. Without immediate and accurate feedback, the skill cannot be developed easily and motivation to continue at the task will diminish. When trying to learn muscle control in a limb that does not move or does not move predictably, the individual is like a blindfolded basketball player in need of augmented feedback.

Biofeedback, a coined term meaning "biological feedback," refers to the process of using instrumentation to feed back to the patient sensory information not usually in conscious awareness or unavailable secondary to injury or disease. By receiving and processing such information, the person can learn to control the monitored function because he knows the effects of his efforts.

The use of biofeedback by occupational therapists is a natural extension of their use of feedback to motivate and inform the patient about his success and progress. Biofeedback may be used as an adjunct to therapy to remediate motor impairments through occupation or may be used as an enabling therapy at a time when the person is unable to engage in occupation. If the patient is paralyzed and cannot move, biofeedback becomes the therapeutic modality of choice to inform the patient that his efforts are having an effect (DeWeerdt & Harrison, 1986; Mulder & Hulstyn, 1984). Because he cannot move, he cannot gain knowledge of results by observing his own movements, and so, without feedback, neither the patient nor therapist can know whether the adopted strategy is useful in reorganizing the motor system. Likewise, if the patient is spastic and trying to learn to relax muscle contraction, electromyographic (EMG) biofeedback gives him information concerning the effectiveness of his strategies and rewards his efforts. For patients who can move, but not with controlled speed and accuracy, kinesthetic (electrogoniometric) biofeedback allows the patient to learn correct movement patterns. Figure 32.1 shows the use of biofeedback instrumentation to detect abnormal synergistic muscle recruitment before treatment planning.

This chapter focuses on electrogoniometric and EMG biofeedback. Electrogoniometric biofeedback informs the patient of joint position or small increments of movement he may not notice and makes him aware of the speed and smoothness of his movement (Fig. 32.2). EMG biofeedback is used to make the patient aware of the state of contraction of his muscles.

BIOFEEDBACK INSTRUMENTATION

All biofeedback instruments have three major components: the transducer, the processing unit, and the output display. The transducer is what detects the change in the parameter being measured. Different

GLOSSARY

AC signal—AC is the acronym for alternating current. The polarity of the signal reverses periodically, and its magnitude changes over time. EMG is an AC signal.

Artifact—An electrical signal that originates from a source other than what is being monitored. The artifact is included in the feedback signal and presents the patient with erroneous information. It cannot be discerned by the patient or the therapist, and therefore, great care must be taken to prevent the likelihood of artifact becoming part of the feedback signal.

DC signal—DC is the acronym for direct current. The polarity and magnitude of the signal stay the same over time until turned off or modified by changing resistance in the circuit. The electrogoniometer changes the resistance in a DC circuit.

Electrode-electrolyte interface—The junction between the electrolyte (gel) and the metal electrode. An ionic exchange occurs there and if unstable can contaminate the EMG feedback signal with artifact.

Operant conditioning—A theory developed by B. F. Skinner to modify behavior by rewarding (reinforcing) desired behavior and ignoring or punishing undesired behavior. One of the techniques, shaping, rewards behavior that approximates the desired response and once the person or animal responds correctly, the reward is given only for improved performance. Measuring the rate of correct responses is one way to document effectiveness (Ince & Leon, 1987).

Resistor—An electronic component, or equivalent, that hinders the flow of electricity. The outer layer of dead skin acts as a resistor.

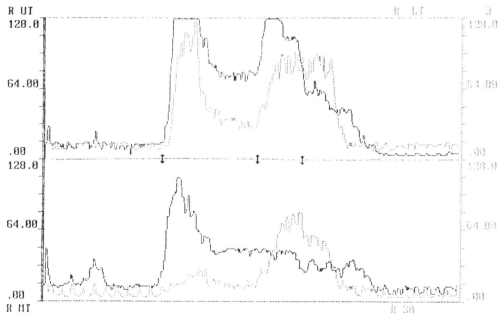

Figure 32.1. EMG measures taken over 36 sec during humeral abduction from the right scapular muscles of a 57-year-old woman with right hemiplegia, 1 year after cerebrovascular accident (CVA). This patient complained of pain with humeral abduction and forward flexion and exhibited subtle incoordination in the affected extremity despite full AROM. Recruitment levels of specific muscles are displayed in the upper trace by (1) the dark line—right upper trapezius (*R UT*) and (2) the light line—right lower trapezius (*R LT*). Recruitment levels are displayed in the lower trace by (3) the dark line—middle trapezius (*R MT*) and (4) the light line—right serratus anterior (*R SA*). The left event marker (*double-pointed arrow*) indicates the beginning of the movement into humeral abduction to 90°, the middle event marker denotes movement from 90° abduction through 180°, and the right event marker shows the beginning of adduction from the fully abducted position. The EMG analysis demonstrates that this patient recruited the upper trapezius with far greater intensity relative to the lower trapezius. It can be seen that at the beginning of the movement, the upper and middle trapezius precede the lower trapezius recruitment by about 2 sec and the serratus anterior is poorly recruited before the humerus reaches 90° abduction. When the humerus is stabilized at 90° abduction (just left of the middle event marker) a considerable decay is seen in lower trapezius recruitment. As the humerus is elevated through 180°, the SA appropriately increased its recruitment but the lower trapezius recruitment was attenuated relative to upper trapezius. This pattern is pathokinetic because the lower trapezius should be the primary scapular rotator in abduction, especially as the humerus elevates above 90°. With this analysis, the therapist can develop a treatment plan to strengthen and encourage the recruitment of the lower trapezius and serratus anterior muscles and limit the overactivity of the upper trapezius.

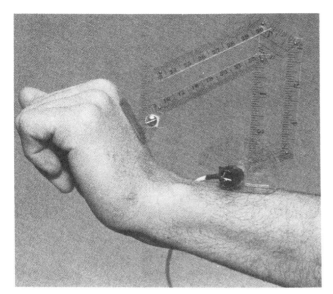

Figure 32.2. Electrogoniometer for biofeedback.

transducers are used to pick up different types of signals. In general, there are two types of signals monitored for biofeedback purposes. One type is the actual electrical signal produced by physiological processes in the body, e.g., muscle fiber depolarization. The transducers to pick up this biological signal are electrodes, i.e., small pieces of metal that convert ionic bioelectric current to electronic current (DeWeerdt & Harrison, 1986; Reiner & Rogoff, 1980). The electrodes are taped to the patient's skin over the muscle to detect the tiny electrical signals that skeletal muscle generates during contraction.

The other type of signal used for biofeedback purposes is the result of a mechanical or chemical change of the transducer secondary to the change in the body. The electrogoniometric transducer, the potentiometer, is a type of variable **resistor** that changes resistance when rotated. One arm of the potentiometer is connected to the movable arm of the goniometer and the other, to the stationary arm. When the positions of the arms of the goniometer change in relation to each other, the potentiometer changes the amount of resistance it offers to the flow of electricity in the circuit. The electrical signal that is spoken of in this case comes from a battery or other voltage source outside of the patient.

The processing unit contains electrical circuits that amplify (enlarge), rectify (make all positive polarity), filter (smooth), and integrate (collect, store, or sum) the signal in preparation for its display (Cohen, 1983). Different processing systems are required for EMG biofeedback, which is an **AC signal,** and electrogoniometric biofeedback, which is a **DC signal.**

Preferably, the output of the feedback display changes instantaneously in proportion to the effort to give the patient immediate information about his response. The biofeedback signal can be thought of as a switch to turn a display device on or off. The type of display can take many forms. One type is a computer monitor on which the signal can be plotted over time. Another type of display is sound broadcast over a speaker. Other types of displays include buzzers of various types, lights, or meters. One particularly motivating type of display for children or adolescents to reward maintained response is the use of a switching unit that turns some electrical appliance on and keeps it running as long as the desired level of signal indicates maintained effort. The switching unit can be reversed to keep the equipment running as long as no unwanted signal is detected, e.g., in the case of control of spasticity or maintained upright posture. Any type of appliance can be attached to the switching unit: radio, television, electronic toys, tape player, etc. The selection of type of display is usually limited in any occupational therapy department, but there is always a choice between audio or visual displays. Some patients may know which type of feedback would be most helpful to them; others may need to discover it by trial and error. If the patient is confused by one, another can be tried.

Biofeedback instruments have either a detector that requires the signal to reach a certain level or threshold before the display is activated or a goal line on the computer display. This allows shaping of the patient's response by requiring improvement to obtain the reward of the display. According to **operant conditioning** methodology, a response that in any way approximates the final performance is rewarded at first, then, as that is learned, only a better response is rewarded, and so on until the final level of performance is achieved.

There may be times when two channels of information are of interest. If the display devices are meters, lights, or lines on a monitor, visual monitoring of both channels simultaneously is too difficult. Monitoring of one visual display (agonist) and one auditory display (antagonist) is one way of accomplishing dual monitoring. Another way to monitor dual outputs is to use a unit that links the outputs so that only when both conditions are correct will the display reward the effort. Examples of when this type of monitoring is desirable are contraction of agonist and relaxation of antagonist, contraction of two synergistic muscles, and contraction of the anterior deltoid to raise the arm while straightening the elbow (monitored using an electrogoniometer) by stroke patients.

PATIENT SELECTION

The patient must be able to understand the relationship between his effort and the feedback. Characteristics reported to be associated with success include some voluntary movement at the start of treatment and less spasticity (Wolf & Binder-Macleod, 1983). Variables that do not seem to affect success include age, sex, side affected by stroke, type of injury (peripheral or central nervous system), amount of previous rehabilitation or duration of injury, and number of biofeedback treatments (Greenberg & Fowler, 1980; Middaugh & Miller, 1980; Wolf, Baker, & Kelly, 1979, 1980). Proprioceptive loss, however, has been found to greatly impair functional success (Wolf et al., 1979).

ELECTROGONIOMETRIC BIOFEEDBACK

Electrogoniometric biofeedback is more useful than EMG when increased range of motion is the goal (Brown, DeBacher, & Basmajian, 1979). EMG biofeedback is not relevant to improve goal-directed actions, because the same goal can be achieved using different muscles (Mulder, Hulstyn, & Van Der Meer, 1986; Scholz, 1990). EMG output does not linearly relate to force generated or joint angle; therefore, EMG is more helpful for learning specific muscle contraction or relaxation but not for learning goal-directed action (Harris, 1980). Electrogoniometric biofeedback provides easily codable information and relates the person's effort in a straightforward way to movement. Therefore, kinesthetic biofeedback should result in greater success than has been reported for EMG biofeedback (Newell & Walter, 1981; Schmidt & Young, 1991; Young & Schmidt, 1992).

The electrogoniometer is a goniometer that measures joint angle electronically. It is fastened over the bones adjacent to the joint so that the axis of the potentiometer is aligned with the axis of joint motion, similar to a manual goniometer used to measure range of motion (ROM) (Fig. 6.56). A parallel linkage electrogoniometer (Figs. 32.2 and 6.56) needs to be aligned so that the hinge in the linkages is located directly above the joint when the joint is in neutral position. The signal that is processed is a DC voltage signal, the amplitude of which varies, depending on the position of the arms of the goniometer.

Training to Modify Movement

The procedures found useful in training persons using electrogoniometric biofeedback are the following (Brown et al., 1979):

1. Baseline measurements of the patient's active range of motion (AROM) and passive range of motion (PROM) are measured using a standard goniometer and recorded.

2. The dysfunctional joint, or a key joint if many are dysfunctional, is selected, and the electrogonio-

meter is carefully positioned over it as described above.

3. If the goal is to increase range of movement, the target angle or threshold should be set so that the patient is required to move a certain, achievable range. Facilitation techniques may be useful to initiate motion. The target angle is changed in small increments so that the goal is always achieved at each session.

If the goal is to improve speed and control of movement, instrumentation that will allow repeated traces to be visible on the monitor at once is used. The therapist moves the person's arm, with the electrogoniometer in place, at a certain speed and to particular limits of motion. This puts the first trace on the screen. The patient then attempts to trace over this pattern by duplicating the previous movement. At first the reversals of movement are slow. As this is learned, the speed is increased and the range made less regular, requiring more planning to initiate the reversal.

4. The session should last no more than 10 to 15 min, as tolerated, with the person working at his own pace and with ample rest periods. Later sessions can increase in duration and frequency, as tolerated.

5. As the patient improves, the feedback can be used in combination with therapeutic activities to maintain motivation.

ELECTROMYOGRAPHIC BIOFEEDBACK

Each motor unit is composed of many muscle fibers that depolarize more or less simultaneously when the neuron belonging to that unit activates them. When a muscle fiber depolarizes, a small electrical charge or voltage is generated. If many motor units depolarize at the same time, their signals are combined, and the amplitude of the resultant signal increases as the number of muscle fibers depolarizing increases. When no contraction of extrafusal muscle is occurring (when the muscle is at rest), no signal is generated.

Instruments

For biofeedback to be effective for learning, the signal must be valid, i.e., must actually represent the monitored change. The signal of one large motor unit has an amplitude of 0 at rest and approximately 250 μV at contraction. Many motor units firing simultaneously result in voltages of 1000 μV or higher (Basmajian & De Luca, 1985). Because the biological signal is so small, and ambient, non-EMG electrical signals produced by house current are so large, **artifact** can be processed. This would give the patient false information. Therefore, the amplifier of the processing unit needs to be not only sensitive enough to detect and amplify the tiny signal but also discriminative enough to process only the EMG signal. Such an amplifier is called a differential amplifier, i.e., one that processes that part of the signal that is different from the ambient signals held in common among the electrodes.

When monitoring one muscle, three electrodes are used: two are placed on the skin over the muscle. They pick up not only the muscle signal but also the ambient signals that the antenna-like body has captured from the atmosphere. The other electrode (common or ground) can be located anywhere on the body, preferably over a bony prominence or on the earlobe, where no muscle is actively contracting. That single electrode also picks up the ambient signals but not the muscle signals. The differential amplifier then processes that part of the signal that is different among the three electrodes—the muscle signal (Basmajian & De Luca, 1985; Reiner & Rogoff, 1980). If the electrodes are different in size or composition or the resistances are different because of incomplete skin preparation or a dirty electrode, then instead of the differential amplifier receiving a common level of ambient noise signal from each electrode, it receives different levels from each. Therefore, the interference is not all canceled out. What happens then is that this **artifact** become part of the signal and gives false information to the patient.

High impedance (resistance) of the electrode-skin combination in relation to the input impedance of the amplifier results in attenuated EMG signals and **artifact** (Cohen, 1983). The input impedance of the amplifier is specified by the manufacturer. It should be high (>100 times the expected electrode impedance) (Bergveld, 1980). The therapist has some control over the electrode-skin resistance through proper care of electrodes and skin preparation (discussed below).

Biofeedback instrumentation adjustments are gain (amplification factor) and filtering (frequency). The amplification is specified in terms of microvolt ranges and can be set more sensitively to amplify signals as weak as 10 μV or set less sensitively for larger signals. Frequency refers to the harmonics of the waveform. If you were to visualize the output of one motor unit, it would have a characteristic shape that is composed of many frequencies of waveforms. Figure 32.3 schematically illustrates this concept. Near the baseline are low-frequency waves and near the peak are high-frequency waves. The waves represent electrical energy. To present the shape of that motor unit, waveforms of various frequencies are represented, and their electrical values summate (Reiner & Rogoff, 1980; Yack, 1984). A frequency range of 10 Hz to 1 kHz will give a good representation of the EMG signal for biofeedback purposes. The high and low filters can be set separately or in tandem (bandwidth). Figure 32.4 illustrates the effect of use of a 20- to 200-Hz bandwidth filter. Frequencies <200 but >20 Hz are passed, but those above or below those frequencies are not. Whenever some frequencies are filtered out, the resultant electri-

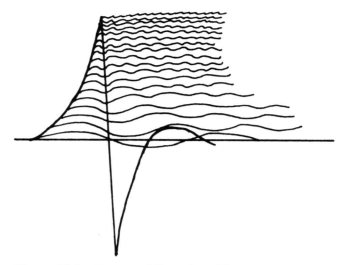

Figure 32.3. Conceptual illustration of frequency.

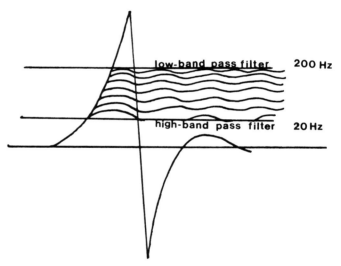

Figure 32.4. Conceptual illustration of the effects of filters. A low-band pass filter allows low-frequency waves to pass but blocks high-frequency waves. A high-band pass filter acts in the opposite direction. Taken together, they form a band pass filter that allows a certain bandwidth of frequencies to be processed.

cal signal is less than it would be if not filtered (Cohen, 1983). However, if not filtered, the signal fed to the patient would be contaminated with low-frequency **artifact** (movement **artifact**) and/or high-frequency **artifact** (internal processor noise). In many systems the low end of the frequency band is set higher than 60 Hz to filter out 60-Hz (house current) **artifact.** Because the filters have an effect on the amplitude of the signal, the setting of the filter switch should be the same for each visit so that the output signal will reflect the patient's effort, not the difference in settings.

ELECTRODE SELECTION

Two electrodes are used to transmit the signal of each muscle being monitored. Surface electrodes are small metal discs. Any type of metal may be used. However, because the electrical conductivity differs among metals, both electrodes should be of the same material. If they are not, then the signal is contaminated by differences in ionic interchange between the gel and the different metals. Most surface electrodes used today are the silver–silver chloride type. The chloride provides a stable ionic transmission between the electrode and the electrolyte (gel) (DeWeerdt & Harrison, 1986).

The size of electrodes affects validity of the signal, because the pickup area is circumferential around the electrode configuration on the skin and conical in depth (Fig. 32.5). Small electrodes allow more specific monitoring than large ones and should absolutely be used to monitor muscles of the hand or the closely packed muscles of the forearm. Even then, the signal may contain output from surrounding muscles.

ELECTRODE PLACEMENT

The muscle to be trained is carefully palpated to determine its margins so that the electrodes can be located over the belly of the muscle. Palpation, not simply a chart of electrode placement sites, should be used to locate the electrodes. The electrodes are aligned parallel to the muscle's line of pull.

The spacing of the electrodes affects the size and specificity of the signal. Closely placed electrodes pick up signals more superficially and from a more circumscribed area than do widely spaced electrodes (Fig. 32.6). During early sessions to reeducate a weak muscle, the electrodes are spaced apart but still within the margins of the muscle belly to pick up whatever signals may be generated by the muscle and its synergists and to give the patient positive reinforcement. On the other hand, to relax spasticity, close spacing will reduce the pickup area, making it more specific, and consequently increase the likelihood of early success.

ELECTRODE APPLICATION

The electrical signal generated by ionic exchange during depolarization of muscle fibers moves away from the muscle, through the saline of the tissues, and toward the surface of the body (as well as deeper into the body). The body is a volume conductor, i.e., electrical signals are conducted throughout its volume as opposed to a wire, which conducts electricity along its length. At the surface, the skin has a dead, horny layer that is in effect a **resistor.** This layer needs to be removed or its resistance reduced to allow valid

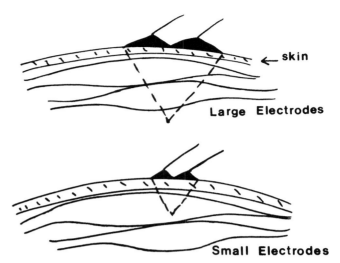

Figure 32.5. Schematic denoting the pickup area of different size electrodes.

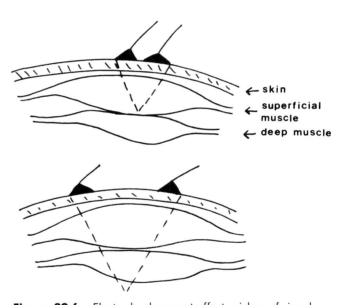

Figure 32.6. Electrode placement affects pickup of signals.

conduction of the signal via electrodes. One way to reduce the resistance is to rub the skin with rough material (gauze pad) and then rub a little electrode gel into the skin. The electrode gel is also put into the cup of the electrode housing. When the electrode is placed over the skin where the gel was rubbed in, the electrical signal continues its journey from body saline to gel to electrode and up the wires to the amplifier. Disposable electrodes, some pregelled, are available; therapists should follow the manufacturer's directions for application. The following process applies to cup-type, commercially available electrodes.

1. If the patient is hairy, the hair is shaved off the electrode sites.

2. The skin is rubbed with gauze and alcohol to remove body oil and the layer of dead skin cells. When the site is reddened, it is ready. Do not cause an abrasion. Some gel is rubbed into the skin where each electrode will be placed. The gel cannot be allowed to communicate between the sites because it will short-circuit (stop) the signal.

3. The electrode is prepared by peeling the double-sided adhesive electrode collar off the backing. The collar is placed exactly around the bottom of the plastic rim of the electrode. The cup of the electrode is filled with electrolyte and leveled off. The remaining gel is inspected for bubbles and, if found, these are broken. Bubbles cause **artifact** due to the disturbance of the **electrode-electrolyte interface.** The electrode with its leveled amount of gel is attached to the skin after removing the protective ring from the collar. The periphery of the electrode is pressed into place.

4. It is useful to tape the leads (wires) to the skin to prevent them from swinging, which causes **artifact,** and the electrodes from being accidentally removed.

Training for EMG Biofeedback

Although there is no universally correct method of training, some procedures for training persons using electromyographic biofeedback are the following.

1. The frequency filter range is set, e.g., 100 to 500 Hz.

2. Range of activity of the monitored muscle is determined and the amplification factor (gain) is set, e.g., 100 to 1000 μV.

3. The threshold goal is set so that the patient must make an effort to reach the goal and gain feedback. If the muscle is being reeducated, the baseline level is low, and because the goal is to produce greater output, the threshold is set a small increment greater than baseline. If the muscle is being inhibited, the baseline is high, and because the goal is to decrease output, the threshold is set a small amount below baseline. Baseline refers to the level of muscle activity present before feedback is offered.

4. The patient is oriented to the apparatus and procedure. A trial using the unaffected limb allows the patient to understand the treatment and begin to determine strategies for achieving the goal with the impaired limb.

5. For brief (10- to 15-min) treatment periods, the patient follows a treatment protocol appropriate for the goal.

GOAL: REEDUCATION OF MUSCLE CONTRACTION

The techniques discussed here are appropriate for reeducating weak (O or T) or flaccid muscles. To start, the electrodes are large and are spaced apart but within the muscle's borders. As the patient improves, the electrode spacing and size are reduced (Kelly, Baker, & Wolf, 1979). The patient is encouraged to contract the muscle and facilitation techniques may be used. As the patient achieves success, the threshold goal is raised. The performance is shaped by increasing the threshold as success occurs at each previous level. When success consistently occurs at the maximum threshold level for that patient, the patient is gradually weaned from EMG feedback. Weaning is done by preventing the patient from receiving the feedback while the therapist continues to monitor the output. If his performance deteriorates, then feedback is allowed so that he can regain control. Once control is regained, feedback is removed again. The weaning process continues until the patient is successful during functional activities without the feedback.

GOAL: REDUCTION OF SPASTICITY

For reduction of spasticity, the atmosphere should be relaxing, and the therapist should use a soothing voice. The electrodes are small and closely spaced. The best position for achieving relaxation of the target muscle is determined. The goal threshold is set slightly below baseline level. The patient is encouraged to relax. Relaxation methods such as imagery and contract/relax (see Chapter 24D) are used to aid the process (Brown & Nahai, 1983; DeBacher, 1983).

The patient seeks to maintain the relaxation for as long as possible. Then he tries to keep the muscle relaxed despite contraction of contralateral muscles, arousal, or mental effort (counting backward for example). When relaxation can be achieved in various positions under these conditions, relaxation during unresisted contraction of the antagonist is aimed for (Fig. 32.7). Once the patient is consistently successful, he is weaned from the instrument.

GOAL: RECOVERY OF SHOULDER CONTROL POSTSTROKE

Even minimal upper extremity function depends on the complex interaction of many muscles acting on many joints from the scapula to the fingers, with most joints having more than one degree of freedom (Phillips, 1986). Upper limb function demands the complex interaction of force couples to provide rotation and stabilization (Schenkman & DeCartaya, 1987). A force couple is a pair of equal and opposite forces acting on either side of the fulcrum (axis) of a lever, e.g., the action of two hands placed opposite each other when turning the steering wheel of a car (Wells, 1955).

The upper extremity after stroke is often characterized by hypertonicity of some muscle groups and

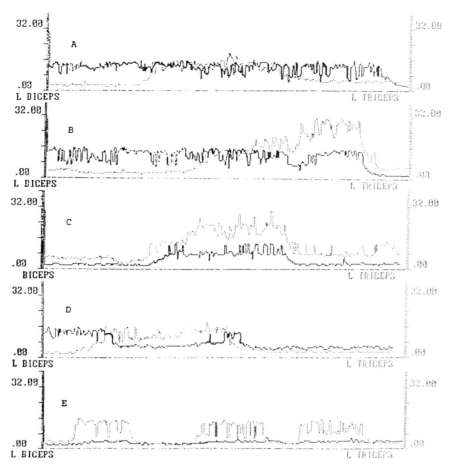

Figure 32.7. Five EMG tracings over reinforcement trials within a single session structured to improve isolated recruitment of triceps and inhibit a hypertonic biceps in a 38-year-old female with left hemiplegia. The dark line represents biceps activity, and the light line represents triceps activity. Tracing A shows elevated biceps activity at rest, which remains elevated while the patient attempts triceps recruitment. Tracing B shows greater triceps recruitment followed by relaxation of both the triceps and biceps. Tracing C shows a reduced biceps baseline, but as the triceps are recruited, there is abnormal cocontraction of the biceps. Tracing D shows reciprocal biceps inhibition with triceps recruitment. Tracing E is taken at the session end, demonstrating that the patient has learned to relax the biceps while producing three isolated triceps contractions without abnormal biceps cocontraction.

weakness of others. Motor control returns unevenly. For example, patients can often elevate the scapula before they can reach forward. The balance of other scapular muscles that normally combine with the upper trapezius to provide the appropriate force couple required to rotate the scapula in preparation for forward reaching is not there. As a result, scapular movement becomes dominated by a disinhibited upper trapezius, leading to habitual and maladaptive scapular elevation, which forms the basis for the abnormal flexor synergy pattern seen poststroke.

For the therapist, it is frustrating when, after working with such an individual to reduce upper trapezius activity with verbal and manual cuing, the patient is observed to precede spontaneous functional movement with scapular elevation. This maladaptive pattern is maintained because (1) upper trapezius activity is reinforced by observable movement, (2) kinesthetic feedback from excessive contraction of the upper trapezius muscle masks feedback from lesser functioning scapular rotators (lower trapezius and serratus anterior), (3) the weaker synergists required for scapular rotation are not directly reinforced by observable movement, and (4) sensory and perceptual deficits associated with stroke disrupt internal feedback processing that form the basis for learning or updating of motor skills. Biofeedback could both reinforce inhibition of the maladaptive upper trapezius contraction and concurrently recruit the less active antagonists.

Restoring Muscle Balance

In the flexor synergy pattern of poststroke patients, the upper trapezius, pectoralis major, and scapular retractors are chronically overused, while other muscles (lower trapezius, serratus anterior, infraspinatus, and anterior deltoid) are relatively inactive. As a result, e.g., the normal force couple between the upper and lower trapezius, which upwardly rotates the scapula to allow full and painless scapulohumeral range of motion, is never reestablished. Moreover, hypertonic responses to stretch and learned muscle substitutions contribute to maintain a nonfunctional extremity. For example, when scapular elevation is part of all movement attempts, a hypertonic biceps is stretched through its attachment to the coracoid process. The resultant spastic response fixes the elbow in flexion and inhibits the triceps.

A seemingly obvious strategy to address this problem would be to inhibit the upper trapezius. This approach has limited success, however, if the upper trapezius is overresponding to compensate for weakness in the other scapular stabilizers and rotators. If one muscle, or even fibers of a muscle, is weak, other muscles attempt to substitute for the weak component as a natural response to achieve the goal (Basmajian, 1980). With upper extremity dysfunction after stroke, scapular protraction, humeral external rotation, and forward flexion of the shoulder are most often weak. As a result, attempts at functional movement will encourage the more reactive muscles to contract in an effort to complete the goal-directed action. However, the resulting movement will be inefficient. Therefore, treatment strategies that simply train inhibition of the overactive and spastic muscles without improving muscle balance are limited, because the overactive muscles will remain so during functional movements in which the focus is on the goal and not the process of balanced muscle recruitment.

Operating scapulohumeral force couples are essential for normal shoulder flexion. The serratus anterior, the levator scapulae, and the upper and lower trapezius constitute force couples that rotate and stabilize the scapula so that the anterior deltoid, as the prime mover, can move the humerus through forward flexion. If the scapular rotators cannot provide the required stability during attempts at forward flexion, the stability function will be shifted to less suited muscles, e.g., the upper trapezius. The movement that results is often shoulder elevation, retraction of the scapula, and trunk flexion. Scapula elevation further facilitates internal rotation of the humerus and elbow flexion. The weak prime mover, the anterior deltoid, is unable to compensate for the mechanical disadvantage produced by the scapular elevation and internal humeral rotation, which locates the insertion of the anterior deltoid medially rather than laterally. The resulting movement is either an absence of any humeral flexion if the anterior deltoid is exceedingly weak or, if the

deltoids have greater recruitment ability, a pull of the humerus into abduction rather than forward flexion.

What follows is a brief discussion of certain EMG feedback strategies that are useful in increasing recruitment of muscles that are often difficult to strengthen with traditional therapy.

Serratus Anterior

The serratus anterior (SA) upwardly rotates the scapula and draws it forward (protraction; abduction). Because of its location and because it is frequently weak after stroke, the serratus is a difficult muscle to palpate accurately to provide verbal feedback to the patient as to its changing recruitment. It is generally necessary to demonstrate proper scapular protraction on the uninvolved side so that the patient can conceptualize the appropriate movement.

Surface electrodes are placed over the fifth and sixth ribs just anterior to the lateral border of the latissimus dorsi (Basmajian & Blumenstein, 1983). Proper trunk alignment is maintained, weight is distributed evenly on both hips, and surrounding scapular muscles (i.e., the upper trapezius and pectoralis major) are relatively relaxed. Then the patient is assisted to achieve SA recruitment. The patient's affected arm is cradled in the therapist's arm and held at 90° forward flexion with the elbow extended and the humerus externally rotated to at least neutral. The therapist's other hand is placed on the patient's scapula, with her thenar eminence and medial surface of the thumb outlining the lateral border of the patient's scapula and her fingers extending obliquely to outline the medial border of the patient's scapula (see Fig. 6.63). The therapist gently glides the scapula into protraction by pulling anteriorly at the scapula's medial border to rotate it around the ribs. This is done several times before any active movement is requested of the patient both to loosen the scapula and to provide a kinesthetic image of the scapula moving around the thorax. The patient is then asked to move the arm forward actively. Once achieved, the humerus is held at greater levels of elevation, and contraction is requested. After the patient can control SA activity in isolation, the therapist asks for active forward flexion and monitors the recruitment of the SA.

Focusing on the action of scapular protraction, even at the beginning of training for forward flexion, seems to promote scapular stabilization and limits the frequently observed tendency to retract and elevate the scapula as movement is initiated. Before advancing to active forward flexion, however, it is generally advisable to integrate recruitment training for humeral external rotation and lower trapezius stabilization as well as inhibition of excessive upper trapezius activity.

Lower Trapezius

As with the serratus anterior, the lower trapezius (LT) is often profoundly weakened after stroke, which disinhibits the upper trapezius (UT) and allows for its unrestricted scapula elevation. To record EMG activity from the LT, the most proximal electrode is placed just medial to the lower one-third of the scapula's medial border with the second electrode placed more medially and obliquely, in line with the LT fibers, 1.5 cm from the first. To reinforce the kinesthetic sense of scapula depression, the therapist sits behind the patient and identifies the inferior scapular angle for the patient with her fingertips. The patient is asked to move the inferior angle down into depression without scapular elevation (here it may be useful to record from the upper trapezius to train its inhibition). Slight resistance at the inferior angle may improve proprioceptive feedback for depression. The patient should be able to increase LT recruitment without any upper trapezius activity. Next, the patient is asked to use EMG feedback to guide LT recruitment without the proprioceptive or tactile stimuli from the therapist, and then perform the movement without visual feedback so that it can be generalized outside the feedback condition. Scapular depression can also be reinforced by having the patient attempt to push downward onto a mat with elbows extended bilaterally and weight bearing through the humerus. EMG monitoring during this activity ensures that, indeed, the LT is being recruited rather than other, less suited muscles.

There are several movements that normally recruit considerable LT activity. For example, humeral abduction requires a greater LT contribution to scapular stabilization than does UT. Several activities can be used during EMG feedback to condition the LT to maintain a sustained contraction during abduction. At first, bring the patient's extended and externally rotated arm into approximately 30° abduction. Ask the patient to depress the scapula using LT recruitment as practiced in isolation. Then ask the patient to produce an isometric contraction to maintain the slightly abducted position while resistance is applied in the direction of horizontal adduction. The patient receives feedback about LT contraction. Care again should be taken to maintain minimal UT recruitment during this procedure. As the patient can perform this contraction, raise the arm into greater abduction range and apply resistance. As with other movements and recruitment exercises described herein, the initial training is introduced while the therapist passively stabilizes the limb in the desired position. As the patient can maintain the position using the appropriate muscles, passive support is gradually removed. Also, the movements described to improve external rotation can be used to strengthen the LT if instrumental feedback is provided for its recruitment simultaneously with feedback for the infraspinatus (see below).

External Rotation

Some degree of external rotation is required to move the arm effectively into any functional position and to allow pain-free humeral elevation. Without activity of the lateral rotators during forward flexion, activity of the deltoid would force the head of the humerus into the glenoid cavity, increasing the probability for soft tissue impingement (Schenkman & DeCartaya, 1987).

The infraspinatus and teres minor are the primary lateral rotators of the humerus. Electrodes for the infraspinatus are placed 1.0 to 1.5 cm apart on the muscle located just below the spine of the scapula in the infraspinatus fossa. The infraspinatus is superficial and accessible lateral to the fibers of the LT and medial to the fibers of the posterior deltoid, approximately level with the fifth thoracic vertebra.

To begin reinforcing external rotation, seat the client so the humerus is in the dependent position and the elbow passively flexed to 90° with the forearm supinated. Stabilize the humerus against the chest wall while passively moving the client's forearm into internal rotation toward the body, placing the external rotators in their lengthened position. While supporting the forearm and stabilizing the elbow, ask the client to rotate the forearm outward. It is essential to control with verbal and instrumental feedback any tendency to abduct or extend the humerus, retract or elevate the scapula, or flex the elbow more than 90°.

A useful image that may aid the patient in visualizing the isolated external rotation movement is that of a clock, where the patient's forearm forms one of the clock's hands and the elbow marks the center of the clock. As the patient's arm moves into internal rotation toward the body, it can be thought to move toward either 9 or 3 o'clock, depending on whether it is the right or left extremity, and as the patient moves into external rotation, the forearm is brought to 12 o'clock. Cuing the patient to fix the elbow in the middle of the imaginary clock also seems to decrease the tendency to abduct the humerus during the rotational movements.

As the patient is moving the humerus in external rotation, apply low-load resistance in the direction of internal rotation to stimulate a sustained contraction. If the patient cannot externally rotate to the 12 o'clock position, provide resistance within the range before active external rotation breaks down. The amount of resistance applied should be sufficient to increase the EMG output but not enough to cause the patient's contraction to decay or generate muscle substitution. The conditioning of tonic contractile ability in the external rotators is essential, because these muscles must maintain the appropriate glenohumeral alignment as the arm is lifted through greater range by the anterior deltoid.

After the patient has displayed the ability to sustain a contraction in the humeral dependent position, advance the training to different levels of humeral elevation. For example, passively abduct the humerus to 90° while maintaining the initial elbow flexion. In this position the imaginary clock can be viewed just off to the side of the patient. As before, ask the patient to move from either the 3 o'clock or the 9 o'clock position into external rotation (12 o'clock) as slight resistance is applied. Alternatively, with the forearm at neutral external rotation, ask the patient to maintain

contraction against resistance. The patient should acquire the ability to perform both isometric and isotonic contractions with increasing resistance loads.

After the scapular and humeral stability functions are addressed, training can proceed to integrate anterior deltoid recruitment with these stabilizing functions, working toward a forward reaching movement. Multichannel EMG allows for the concurrent reinforcement of anterior deltoid synergists (infraspinatus, SA) as well as inhibition of responses that are counterproductive to efficient anterior deltoid recruitment, such as that generated by the UT and pectoralis major. It is often the case that infraspinatus recruitment decays when the patient first attempts concurrently to recruit the AD. Biofeedback at this stage is thus useful, allowing

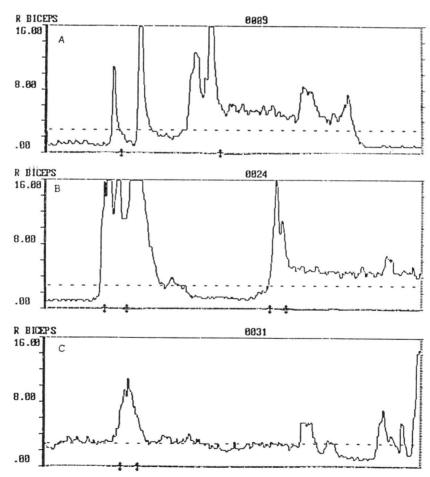

Figure 32.8. EMG measures from the hypertonic biceps of a 7-year-old boy with hemiplegia taken over several biofeedback trials within a single session. The treatment goal was to improve voluntary control of the spastic biceps and improve discrimination for various states of muscle activity. Tracing A shows an attempt to contract the biceps voluntarily followed by a request to relax the muscle as quickly as possible and bring the output below the threshold line. The event marker (*double-pointed arrow*) on the bottom left records the therapist's cue to the patient to contract the biceps, and the event marker on the right records the cue to relax. Note the long latency to recruit the muscle followed by a long latency to achieve relaxation, indicating poor voluntary control. Tracing B demonstrates an improved recruitment latency but a delayed relaxation response. Tracing C shows an improved recruitment and relaxation pattern after approximately 10 feedback-reinforcement trials.

the selected reinforcement of synergistic responses that are requisite to the functional forward reaching pattern and hand-to-mouth pattern.

EFFECTIVENESS

Outcome of electrogoniometric biofeedback is limited (Greenberg & Fowler, 1980; Young & Schmidt, 1992). By far the most commonly reported use of EMG biofeedback for recovery of motor control has been with stroke patients. For individual subjects, the benefits are obvious (Figs. 32.7 and 32.8) However, in one review of 32 papers (which were published during the last 25 years) on the use of EMG biofeedback for stroke patients, the conclusion was equivocal: No solid scientific evidence exists for or against the use of EMG biofeedback with stroke patients (DeWeerdt & Harrison, 1986). A recent metaanalysis of all published randomized controlled trials of EMG biofeedback used to reeducate motor control in poststroke patients came to the same conclusion (Agency for Healthy Care Policy and Research, 1994).

However, Schleenbaker and Mainous (1993) concluded from a metaanalysis that EMG biofeedback increases functional improvement in hemiplegic patients. They defined function as complex neuromuscular activity needed to execute activities of daily living and included, for instance, the ability to trace a circle with the olecranon, gait speed, and pinch strength. Because the results are equivocal and the definitive study has not been done and because new information on motor control (e.g., dynamical systems theory) and motor learning (e.g., practice and feedback schedules) is emerging, further research is warranted. That research must use outcome measures that are functionally meaningful.

As a factor in outcome studies, the placebo effects of biofeedback cannot be underestimated. For example, one study compared actual EMG biofeedback, simulated EMG (therapist muscle activity was being fed to the patient), and no feedback in a group of 24 hemiparetic patients. The authors found that the two feedback conditions resulted in significant increases in muscle function (increased EMG amplitude and ROM) compared with the control group, but no significant difference was seen between the true and sham (placebo) biofeedback (Hurd, Pegram, & Nepomuceno, 1980).

STUDY QUESTIONS

1. Define biofeedback, electromyographic (EMG) biofeedback, and electrogoniometric biofeedback
2. What is the major reason an occupational therapist would use biofeedback?
3. What does the EMG signal represent?
4. What factors are important to consider in selecting electrodes for EMG biofeedback? In placing electrodes for EMG biofeedback?
5. Define artifact. What will cause artifact to appear in the processed signal?
6. What is the function of the third (common) electrode used in EMG biofeedback?
7. Describe procedures used to reeducate movement speed control.
8. Describe an EMG biofeedback procedure used to reeducate a weak muscle.
9. Describe how a treatment session would be organized for a poststroke patient to develop controlled scapular rotation.
10. Describe how a treatment session could be organized to develop recruitment of wrist extensors of a person with a spinal cord injury.

REFERENCES

Agency for Health Care Policy and Research. (1994). *Post-stroke rehabilitation clinical practice guideline.* Washington, DC: Author.

Basmajian, J. V. (1980). Electromyography-dynamic gross anatomy: A review. *American Journal of Anatomy, 159,* 345–360.

Basmajian, J. V., & Blumenstein, R. (1983). Electrode placement in electromyographic biofeedback. In J. V. Basmajian (Ed.), *Biofeedback—Principles and practice for clinicians* (pp. 363–377). Baltimore: Williams & Wilkins.

Basmajian, J. V., & De Luca. C. J. (1985). *Muscles alive: Their functions revealed by electromyography* (5th ed.). Baltimore: Williams & Wilkins.

Bergveld, P. (1980). *Electromedical instrumentation: A guide for medical personnel.* New York: Cambridge University Press.

Brown, D. M., & Nahai, F. (1983). Biofeedback strategies of the occupational therapist in total hand rehabilitation. In J. V. Basmajian (Ed.), *Biofeedback—Principles and practice for clinicians* (2nd ed., pp. 90–106). Baltimore: Williams & Wilkins.

Brown, D. M., DeBacher, G., & Basmajian, J. V. (1979). Feedback goniometers for hand rehabilitation. *American Journal of Occupational Therapy, 33,* 458–463.

Cohen, B. A. (1983). Basic biofeedback electronics for the clinician. In J. V. Basmajian (Ed.), *Biofeedback—Principles and practice for clinicians* (2nd ed., pp. 317–329). Baltimore: Williams & Wilkins.

DeBacher, G. (1983). Biofeedback in spasticity control. In J. V. Basmajian (Ed.), *Biofeedback—Principles and practice for clinicians* (2nd ed., pp. 111–129). Baltimore: Williams & Wilkins.

DeWeerdt, W., & Harrison, M. A. (1986). Electromyographic biofeedback for stroke patients: Some practical considerations. *Physiotherapy, 72*(2), 106–108.

Greenberg, S., & Fowler, R. S. (1980). Kinesthetic biofeedback: A treatment modality for elbow range of motion in hemiplegia. *American Journal of Occupational Therapy, 34*(11), 738–743.

Harris, F. A. (1980). Exteroceptive feedback of position and movement in remediation for disorders of coordination. In L. P. Ince (Ed.), *Behavioral psychology in rehabilitation medicine: Clinical applications* (pp. 87–156). Baltimore: Williams & Wilkins.

Hurd, W. W., Pegram, V., & Nepomuceno, C. (1980). Comparison of actual and simulated EMG biofeedback in the treatment of hemiplegic patients. *American Journal of Physical Medicine,* 59(2), 73–82.

Ince, L. P., & Leon, M. S. (1987). Measurement of success in EMG biofeedback treatment of the upper extremity: Quantitative vs qualitative data and the use of an operant model. *Clinical Biofeedback and Health,* 10(2), 151–156.

Kelly, J. L., Baker, M. P., & Wolf, S. L. (1979). Procedures for EMG biofeedback training in involved upper extremities of hemiplegic patients. *Physical Therapy,* 59(12), 1500–1507.

Middaugh, S., & Miller, C. (1980). Electromyographic feedback: Effect on voluntary muscle contraction in paretic subjects. *Archives of Physical Medicine & Rehabilitation,* 61(1), 24–29.

Miller, N. E. (1978). Biofeedback and visceral learning. *Annual Review of Psychology,* 29, 373–404.

Mulder, T., & Hulstyn, W. (1984). Sensory feedback therapy and theoretical knowledge of motor control and learning. *American Journal of Physical Medicine,* 63(5), 226–244.

Mulder, T., Hulstyn, W., & Van Der Meer, J. (1986). EMG feedback and the restoration of motor control: A controlled group study of 12 hemiparetic patients. *American Journal of Physical Medicine,* 65(4), 173–188.

Newell, K. M., & Walter, C. B. (1981). Kinematic and kinetic parameters as information feedback in motor skill acquisition. *Journal of Human Movement Studies,* 7, 235–254.

Phillips, C. S. (1986). *Movements of the hand.* Liverpool: Liverpool University Press.

Reiner, S., & Rogoff, J. B. (1980). Instrumentation. In E. W. Johnson (Ed.), *Practical electromyography* (pp. 338–393). Baltimore: Williams & Wilkins.

Schenkman, M., & DeCartaya, V. R. (1987). Kinesiology of the shoulder complex. *Journal of Orthopaedic and Sports Physical Therapy,* 8, 438–450.

Schleenbaker, R. E., & Mainous, A. G. (1993). Electromyographic biofeedback for neuromuscular reeducation in the hemiplegic stroke patient: A meta-analysis. *Archives of Physical Medicine & Rehabilitation,* 74(12), 1301–1304.

Schmidt, R. A., & Young, D. E. (1991). Methodology for motor learning: A paradigm for kinematic feedback. *Journal of Motor Behavior,* 23(1), 13–24.

Scholz, J. (1990). Dynamic pattern theory—Some implications for therapeutics. *Physical Therapy,* 70(12), 827–843.

Wells, K. F. (1955). *Kinesiology* (2nd ed). Philadelphia: W. B. Saunders.

Wolf, S. L., Baker, M. P., & Kelly, J. L. (1979). EMG biofeedback in stroke: Effect of patient characteristics. *Archives of Physical Medicine & Rehabilitation,* 60, 96–102.

Wolf, S. L., Baker, M. P., & Kelly, J. L. (1980). EMG biofeedback in stroke: A 1-year follow-up on the effect of patient characteristics. *Archives of Physical Medicine & Rehabilitation,* 61(8), 351–355.

Wolf, S. L., & Binder-Macleod, S. A. (1983). Electromyographic biofeedback applications for the hemiplegic patient: Changes in upper extremity neuromuscular and functional status. *Physical Therapy,* 63(9), 1393–1403.

Yack, H. J. (1984). Techniques for clinical assessment of human movement. *Physical Therapy,* 64(12), 1821–1830.

Young, D. E., & Schmidt, R. A. (1992). Augmented kinematic feedback for motor learning. *Journal of Motor Behavior,* 24(3), 261–273.

33
Physical Agent Modalities

Robert E. Post, Susan L. Lee, and Dorie B. Syen

OBJECTIVES

After studying this chapter, the student will be able to:
1. Understand the physical concepts that underlie the use of physical agent modalities.
2. Understand the physiological changes that occur from applying heat, cold, sound, and electricity to biological tissues.
3. Appreciate the use of physical agent modalities to prepare patients to engage in occupation.
4. Understand which modalities are indicated for particular patient problems and the rationale for their use.
5. Know the contraindications and precautions for each modality.

The American Occupational Therapy Association's (AOTA) position paper on the use of physical agent modalities received a positive vote in its Representative Assembly in March 1991. The paper stated that modalities may be used as an adjunct to, or in preparation for, treatment to improve occupational function. The use of modalities alone is not within the scope of occupational therapy. The use of modalities is currently not an entry-level skill. The position paper further states that the occupational therapist who uses these modalities must have documentation of knowledge of the theoretical background and the technical skills necessary for the proper use of modalities. Theoretical background should be obtained from college-level physics and physiology courses. Technical skills can be acquired from continuing education courses. Furthermore, the occupational therapist must be aware of, and comply with, all state laws and regulations, because these have precedence over AOTA's policies and positions (AOTA, 1991).

This chapter is an introduction to the physical principles, effects, administration, applications, precautions, contraindications, and documentation requirements related to superficial thermal modalities, ultrasound, and electrotherapy.

SUPERFICIAL THERMAL MODALITIES

Superficial Heat

In general, heat is used for chronic or subacute conditions, because it may exacerbate the inflammation and swelling typical of acute musculoskeletal injuries (Feibel & Fast, 1970; Schmidt, 1979). Superficial heat is used as an adjunctive treatment to provide sedation, analgesia, and increased superficial soft tissue extensibility before therapeutic exercises and activities (Fond & Hecox, 1994).

BIOPHYSICS OF HEAT TRANSFER

Heat is transferred within the body and between the body and the outside environment according to a temperature gradient. That is, heat moves from warmer to cooler objects. Two mechanisms that describe heat transfer are conduction and convection. Conduction of heat energy occurs when two objects of different temperatures are in contact, such as the application of a hot pack to the skin. Heat will transfer from the warmer hot pack to the cooler skin. If the heat source is not replenished, it will become cooler as the cool object becomes warmer. Convection of heat energy occurs when the heat source is replenished, such as immersing a limb in a hot whirlpool. New warmer water continuously flows past the skin, maintaining original temperature of the heat source and maintaining the amount of heat to the skin.

Competent cutaneous and subcutaneous vascularity and hemodynamics permit the skin and hypodermis to respond to increased temperatures by flushing the warmer areas with relatively cooler blood. Normal vascular responses limit the depth of heat penetration from superficial heat modalities (Abramson, 1961; Greenberg, 1972). The magnitude of change in tissue

GLOSSARY

Ampere—A unit of electrical current; 1 ampere (amp) is the electrical charge (number of electrons) that are moved by 1 volt through 1 ohm of resistance.

Capacitive current flow—The shift of ions by the application of a negative charge over an excitable membrane such that positive intracellular ions are drawn to the inner surface of the membrane and positive extracellular ions are drawn away from the outer surface of the membrane.

Carrier frequencies—Background medium frequencies of some electrotherapeutic instruments that are modulated to produce either bursts of polyphasic wave activity of uniform amplitude (Russian current) or beats of polyphasic interferential waveforms.

Chronaxie—The minimum duration of a current stimulus, at a given amplitude, that is required to stimulate an excitable membrane to threshold.

Current density—The amount of current flow (am-

perage) at the conducting electrode divided by the area of the electrode, expressed as current per unit area of the electrode.

Ohm—Unit of resistance to an electrical current.

Pulse—Unit of an electrical stimulation current waveform that has one or two phases, and amplitude and duration.

Pulse amplitude—The vertical dimension of the pulse, expressed in volts or amps.

Pulse duration—The horizontal dimension of the pulse, expressed in seconds, milliseconds, or microseconds.

TENS—Acronym for transcutaneous electrical nerve stimulation; all clinical electrical stimulation of nerve is transcutaneous; however, the popular use of the term is related to stimulation for pain modulation.

Tetany—Fusion of individual muscle fiber twitches by the required frequency of electrical stimuli to produce a smooth, sustained muscle contraction.

temperature will also depend on the rate of application of the thermal source and the amount of exposed body area. For example, if heat is applied too quickly, the patient may be burned, because the heat cannot be dissipated quickly enough. Also, larger body areas exposed to heat may cause increases in core temperature and other reflex changes such as increased heart rate (Lehmann & deLateur, 1990).

PHYSIOLOGICAL EFFECTS

Physiological effects of heat transfer in the body will in part depend on the depth of effective tissue temperature changes. Superficial heat applications to the skin ranging from 40 to 45°C increase skin temperature from the normal 34.1 to 45.0°C. If the vascular response is normal, this tissue temperature rise may only extend to 0.5 cm below the skin surface. Changes in tissue temperature deeper than 0.5 cm are significantly less (Michlovitz, 1990).

Vascular Changes

Heat causes an increase of blood flow to the area as a result of the following mechanisms. Release of histamine, prostaglandins, and bradykinin at the site causes relaxation of the smooth muscle of blood vessels and increases capillary permeability. The stimulation of sensory thermoreceptors in the skin produces both direct reflexive vasodilation and vasodilation by spinal reflex, resulting in decreased sympathetic activity and relaxation of vascular muscle tone (Guyton, 1986).

Systemic Effects

Sufficiently warm blood reaching the thermoregulatory centers of the hypothalamus produces such sys-

temic effects as increased metabolism and general perspiration (Guyton, 1986).

Soft Tissue Changes

Adequately heating the skin increases its elasticity and decreases its viscosity, which may facilitate softening of cutaneous scars. However, the scar area should be carefully assessed for neurovascular compromise, because damage to the area may occur if the heat is excessive. The limited depth of therapeutic tissue temperature rise will not have a direct effect on other soft connective tissues such as tendon, ligament, or fascia.

Protective Muscle Guarding and Pain

Cutaneous thermoreceptor stimulation with superficial heat decreases pain by closing the pain gate mediated at the spinal cord (see below for further discussion). The perception of pain relief and relaxation and comfort from heat application may decrease protective muscle guarding, further reducing musculoskeletal pain.

CLINICAL EFFECTS

Superficial heat is applied to produce the physiological effects described above—notably, analgesia, sedation, and relief from muscle guarding—to facilitate patient activities and therapeutic exercise.

SPECIFIC MODALITIES

Hot Packs

Commercial hot packs are canvas-covered silicone gels that are stored in a unit with water heated to

71°C. Six to eight layers of terry cloth are placed between the patient and the hot pack to protect against skin burn. The patient's skin is checked after 5 min; it should feel warm but not be red. If the skin is red, or if the patient complains of burning, remove the hot packs to air out the skin and towel layers; possibly add another layer of toweling. The skin temperature peaks between 8 and 10 min (Lehmann & deLateur, 1990). The total treatment time is 15 to 20 min.

Paraffin

Paraffin is available commercially for both clinic and home use. Paraffin is premixed with mineral oil; in combination, they have a low specific heat. This permits the skin to tolerate higher temperatures (47.0 to 54.4°C) than those applied by moist heat (Michlovitz, 1990). The patient washes and thoroughly dries his hand before dipping it into the paraffin bath 8 to 10 times, while avoiding cracking the paraffin cast by finger movement. The hand is then wrapped in a plastic bag and a towel for 10 to 15 min. The cast is then peeled off; the paraffin may be reused after squeezing it dry of perspiration. Paraffin is especially useful for treating irregular surfaces such as the digits of the hand and foot.

Fluidotherapy

Fluidotherapy uses a convection device that circulates heated dry cellulose particles (Fig. 33.1). The patient places his extremity in the convection chamber, which is sealed at the opening around the limb. The patient may now exercise within the device while receiving the heat treatment. The total treatment time is about 20 min.

Hydrotherapy

Whirlpool is the most commonly used hydrotherapy modality. Whirlpool may be used with a range of water temperatures, from cold to hot. In addition to its thermal effects, the whirlpool offers the advantage of the mechanical effects of buoyancy, resistance, and water agitation. Buoyancy and resistance can facilitate therapeutic exercise within the whirlpool. Agitation can provide the effects of mechanical massage and facilitate debridement and healing of skin wounds. Whirlpool, like fluidotherapy, is a convective thermal modality. Full-body immersions in hot water should be monitored closely because of the possibility of undesired systemic effects. Whirlpool use requires a setting that is adequately ventilated, and the tank must be cleaned and sanitized between patients.

PRECAUTIONS

Because heat may increase edema, the therapist must carefully weigh the expected benefits of the treat-

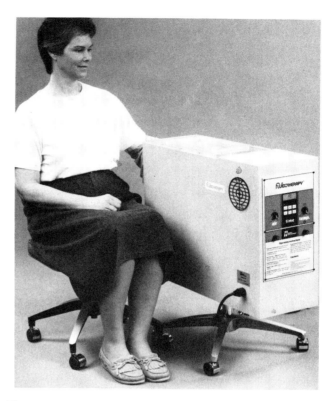

Figure 33.1. Fluidotherapy units contain finely divided particles that are suspended in heated air. Its therapeutic effects include heat, massage, and desensitization.

ment against the possible side effect of increased swelling. Techniques that can be used to ameliorate partially increased edema caused by superficial heat application include elevating the limb receiving the hot pack and active movement while immersed in the whirlpool or fluidotherapy unit. Patients with diminished skin sensation or skin with compromised vascularity, including scars, should be monitored closely for signs of excessive heating. Patients with labile blood pressure, vertigo, and seizure disorders should not be left unattended when receiving whirlpool or fluidotherapy when entire limbs or the full body is treated.

CONTRAINDICATIONS

Therapeutic hot or very warm temperatures should not be used for patients with severe neurovascular compromise of the skin. Patients with open wounds should not use paraffin baths (Lehmann & deLateur, 1990).

Superficial Cold (Cryotherapy)

Cooling occurs when heat is removed from body tissues. The amount of cooling that occurs depends on the temperature difference between the body and cooling agent, exposure time, and thermal conductivity of the area being cooled. Also, cooling agents applied by convection in a manner that maintains the thermal gradient, such as the cold whirlpool, have greater cooling effects. Therapeutic cold is used for the treatment of musculoskeletal pain; muscle guarding; spasticity; and the effects of acute inflammation, including pain and swelling (Griffin & Karselis, 1982; Hecox, 1994a).

PHYSIOLOGICAL EFFECTS

Vascular

Cold application decreases local tissue blood flow by stimulating sympathetic nerves to vasoconstrict. Vasodilation and shunting of blood from deeper soft tissues to the skin occur following the period of vasoconstriction to protect the skin from thermal damage. This accounts for the flushing of the skin within 10 to 15 min of cold application (Guyton, 1986; Hecox, 1994b).

Systemic Changes

If sufficiently cooled blood reaches the thermoregulatory center of the hypothalamus, systemic effects such as general piloerection and shivering occur (Guyton, 1986).

Peripheral Nerves

Cold applied over peripheral nerves decreases conduction velocity and synaptic activity (Brown, 1984). This mechanism may explain relief of pain both by inhibiting the activity of pain-mediating nerves and by damping peripheral nerve activity related to painful spasticity (Bishop, 1977; Clark & Edholm, 1985; Mense, 1978).

Connective Tissue

When cooled, connective tissues and other soft tissues show increased viscosity and decreased elasticity with generally increased mechanical stiffness (Lehmann, Warren, & Scham, 1974).

CLINICAL EFFECTS

Cold applications produce temporary relief from neuromusculoskeletal pain, edema, and muscle guarding and spasticity. As an adjunct to functional activities and therapeutic exercise procedures, cold applications are commonly used for promoting active and passive mobility and for postexercise soreness and swelling.

SPECIFIC MODALITIES

Cold Packs

Commercial cold packs are typically vinyl pouches that contain silica gel and are stored in a freezer. The cold packs are wrapped in a damp towel and applied to the patient for 15 min. The temperature of the cold pack storage is -12.2 to $-9.4°C$; however, the temperature of the cold packs themselves may be much warmer.

Ice Packs

Ice packs are plastic bags filled with crushed ice. The ice packs are also applied within a damp towel. The temperature of the ice pack application is colder than cold packs.

Ice Massage

Ice massage is usually performed over small areas. The therapist uses ice that was formed in a paper cup and frozen with a wooden stick (tongue depressor) for a handle or a commercially available thermal probe. The ice is applied in small, overlapping circles for 5 to 10 min until skin flushing and numbness occur.

Contrast Baths

Contrast baths use alternating baths of hot and cold water. Temperature ranges from 40.6 to 43.3°C for hot water and 15 to 20°C for cold water. The treatment consists of 30 to 60 sec of cold water immersion alternating with 3 min of hot water immersion, repeated for a total treatment time of 30 min. The treatment begins and ends with 3 min of hot water immersion. Contrast baths are used for neuromusculoskeletal conditions in which neurovascular disorders prevail. Here, contrast baths are used for "vascular exercises" because of the anticipated alternation of vasoconstriction and vasodilation associated with alternating the water temperature immersions. Contrast baths have been advocated for the treatment of reflex sympathetic dystrophy of the hands and feet. The clinical effectiveness of contrast baths is not supported in the literature.

Vapocoolant Sprays

Fluori-methane (Gebauer Chemical Co., Cleveland, OH) is the vapocoolant most commonly used for this technique of superficial cold application. The rationale for its use is that spraying the skin with a vapocoolant, using a spray and stretch technique, over "trigger points" associated with myofascial pain syndromes permits the involved muscle and limb to be stretched and moved through a greater functional range of motion (Travell & Simons, 1992). The brief cooling of the skin does not result in the effects of deeper tissue cooling. The mechanism for the observed effects of the treatment may be counterirritation and reflexive muscle relaxation by stimulating cutaneous sensory nerves. The technique of application is to spray the painful area at a 30° angle of incidence, 18 inches away, at a rate of 4 inches/sec, repeating two to three times (Travell & Simons, 1992).

PRECAUTIONS

Individuals with compromised local neurovascular response to cold should be monitored closely. Cold applications could damage skin unable to respond by reflexively flushing the cooler areas with warmer blood.

CONTRAINDICATIONS

Individuals with extreme hypersensitivity or allergy to cold and those with severe Reynaud's disease should not be treated with cold therapy (Fond, 1994). Also, patients with replantations, crush injuries, and healing wounds should not have those areas treated with cold (Lehmann & deLateur, 1990).

ULTRASOUND

Ultrasound therapy is the use of acoustic energy that penetrates the skin and is used in physical rehabilitation for both deep heating and nonthermal deep soft tissue stimulation effects. By use of a hand-held transducer, ultrasound is applied over the skin surface, and as a result of the sound energy penetrating the deeper target soft tissues, the anticipated clinical effects include pain relief, increased soft tissue extensibility, decreased edema, vasodilation of deeper vascular structures, and wound healing (Sweitzer, 1994).

Biophysics of Ultrasound

Ultrasound wave energy, which is produced above the range of audible frequencies (20 to 20,000 Hz), is created by passing an electrical current through a synthetic crystal within the applicator head (Fig. 33.2). The electrical energy is transduced into sound energy by causing the crystal to vibrate at a specific frequency. The two commonly used therapeutic ultrasound frequencies are 1 and 3 MHz.

Ultrasound transmits poorly through air, but transmits well through fluid media and solids such as those found in the body. When ultrasound wave energy transmits within the body tissues, it creates mechanical oscillations of tissue molecules. The concentration of ultrasound energy within the body tissues may sufficiently stimulate those molecules to produce heat within a therapeutic range (Taylor-Mullins, 1990).

Attenuation (lessening of effect) is the result of a combination of absorption, reflection, refraction, and deflection of sound waves as they pass through the body. Intrinsically homogeneous tissues, such as fat, tend to transmit ultrasound with little attenuation (Sweitzer, 1994). Greater attenuation of ultrasound waves occurs at interfaces of nonhomogeneous tissues and materials with different densities, such as between tendon and bone, muscle and fascia, and ligament and bone (Sweitzer, 1994). More absorption of ultrasound energy occurs at those tissue interfaces that will consequently generate a higher tissue temperature rise (Ziskin, McDiarmid, & Michlovitz, 1990). The amount

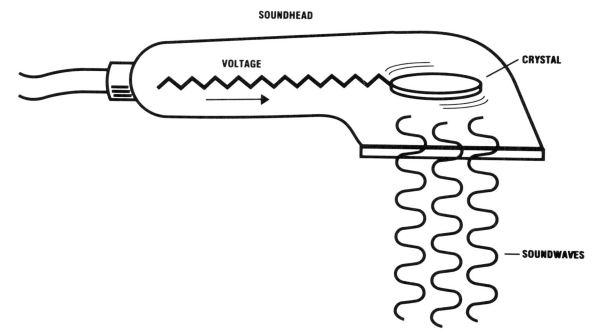

Figure 33.2. A schematic representation of the production of ultrasound.

of tissue temperature rise is affected by the rate that ultrasound energy is applied, thermal conductivity of the tissues, and the response of the local blood flow to dissipate the heat (Sweitzer, 1994).

The depth of penetration of therapeutic ultrasound is generally 1 to 5 cm. Effective depth of penetration, without attenuation, is inversely proportional to the frequency of the generated ultrasound (Griffin & Karselis, 1982). Ultrasound at 1 Mz will penetrate to 5 cm, while 3 MHz delivery will penetrate 1 to 2 cm (Gann, 1991).

The intensity of ultrasound, expressed in Watts, is directly related to the ultrasonic energy created at the ultrasound transducer head. Ultrasound intensity may be shown as a total number Watts at the transducer or as the density of the wattage per unit area of the ultrasound applicator head. This is expressed as Watts per square centimeter. A higher intensity means a greater rate of ultrasonation of body tissues and a faster rate of tissue temperature rise at the tissue interfaces.

Physiological Effects

The physiological effects are categorized as thermal and nonthermal effects.

THERMAL EFFECTS

The thermal effects of ultrasound are the same as those produced by other heat modalities. However, they occur in deeper soft tissue structures.

Connective Tissues and Soft Tissues

Heating of deeper soft tissue structures, such as tendon, ligament, and articular capsule, is possible with ultrasound. The effect is to increase the elasticity of those structures temporarily by heating (Griffin & Karselis, 1982).

Vascular

Heating with ultrasound can increase local blood flow by producing a reflex vasodilation (Lota, 1965).

Peripheral Nerves

Pain relief following ultrasound may be the result of direct stimulation of peripheral nerves or, secondarily, by increasing local tissue metabolism (Szumski, 1960). The effects of ultrasound on nerve conduction velocity is variable and may depend on the intensities used. The possible mechanisms are not fully understood (Sweitzer, 1994).

NONTHERMAL EFFECTS

Observed effects of ultrasound when used in a mode that does not produce heat (pulsed mode, e.g.) have been attributed to mechanisms including cavitation and acoustic streaming (Ziskin et al., 1990). Cavitation refers to the phenomenon of alternating expansion and compression of gas bubbles in the blood or tissue fluids within an ultrasonic field. Acoustic streaming is the movement of tissue fluids along margins of cells from the mechanical pressure of the ultrasound waves.

Arteriolar vasoconstriction and vasodilation are suspected to occur in the presence of nonthermal ultrasound (Hogan, Burke, & Franklin, 1982; Hogan, Franklin, & Fry, 1982). Enhanced connective tissue regeneration secondary to increased fibroblastic activity has also been suggested as an effect of nonthermal ultrasound (Griffin & Karselis, 1982).

Clinical Effects

The expected clinical effects of ultrasound are consistent with the identified physiological effects. The thermal effects of ultrasound are expected to produce increased short-term extensibility of connective tissues in preparation for exercises and activities that include stretching of connective tissue structures to permit improved function (Griffin & Karselis, 1982). Pain relief and reduced inflammation following ultrasound therapy have been reported. Possible mechanisms include the effects of direct ultrasound stimulation of pain-mediating nerves (Williams, McHale, & Bowditch, 1987) and decreased erythema and swelling associated with inflammation caused by vascular responses to nonthermal ultrasound (Middlemast & Chatterjee, 1978). Ultrasound is used for pain modulation and to alleviate inflammation to provide an opportunity for more effective exercise intervention and to permit functional activities. Finally, ultrasound therapy has been shown to enhance indolent wound healing (Stratton, Heckmann, & Francis, 1984) and tendon repair (Enwemeka, 1989).

Treatment Parameters

Ultrasound is applied according to the parameters below. Care should be taken to report these parameters when documenting an ultrasound treatment.

INSTRUMENTATION AND DOSAGE DETERMINATION

Frequency

Choice of frequency is determined by the depth of the tissues to be treated (Docker, 1987). A frequency of 3 MHz is appropriate for superficial, subcutaneous tissues within a depth of 1 to 2 cm. For tissues at a depth of 3 to 5 cm, 1 MHz ultrasound is required.

Duty Cycle

Duty cycle refers to the percentage of time during the treatment that ultrasound energy is actually being introduced into the body. Continuous ultrasound means that the energy is flowing 100% of the treatment time. Pulsed ultrasound is expressed as a percentage of the treatment time that the energy is actually being introduced into the body. For example, a 20% duty cycle indicates that the ultrasound energy is occurring in pulses, evenly spaced, accounting for 20% of the total treatment time (Fig. 33.3). Therefore, over the course of a 5-min pulsed ultrasound treatment, much less ultrasound energy is being introduced than in the continuous mode.

Intensity and Duration

The intensity required to elevate tissue temperature to a therapeutic range of 40 to 45°C ranges from 1.0 to 2.0 W/cm^2 applied continuously for 5 to 10 min (Dyson, 1987; Ziskin et al., 1990). The patient report of mild sensory stimulation or warmth is a suggested guideline for establishing the upper intensity level. Individuals with sensory impairment should be treated more cautiously. Finally, decreasing the intensity over superficial bony prominences is generally practiced. The amount of tissue temperature rise also depends on the effective radiating area of the transducer head relative to the tissue area to be treated (Sweitzer, 1994).

TECHNIQUES OF APPLICATION

A water interface where the ultrasound transducer contacts the skin is required to permit the transmission of the ultrasound waves to the body. This is accomplished with a commercial water-based transmission gel or cream or by immersing the body part to be sonated, with the transducer, in a container of water.

The latter technique requires that the sound head be within 1 cm of the skin, but not in direct contact. For both methods, the transducer is slowly and continuously moved over the target tissues so that temperature hot spots within the tissue do not develop from a buildup of ultrasound energy.

Contraindications and Precautions

Contraindications and precautions for ultrasound therapy that produces a tissue temperature rise are consistent with those for any heat application, including superficial heat (see above). Because ultrasound may elevate the temperature of deep tissues, additional contraindications include ultrasonation over internal organs; areas of infection, tumor, and thrombophlebitis; and the epiphyses of growing bones (Sweitzer, 1994; Ziskin et al., 1990).

ELECTROTHERAPY

Electrotherapy is the use of electrical currents to stimulate excitable membranes of nerve and muscle and other soft tissues to facilitate the return of function in patients with physical impairments and disabilities. Electrotherapy is used by occupational therapists as an adjunctive modality to promote muscle activity and modulate pain to enable the patient to engage in the occupational performance tasks that are important for his lifestyle.

Many electrotherapeutic devices and techniques have been developed and advocated over the past 60 years. The dramatic advances in microcircuitry and other electronic technology over the past 15 years have produced new generations of sophisticated electrotherapeutic instruments. Unfortunately, clinical research has not kept pace with the technology. This has often led to poorly supported claims, by both clinicians and

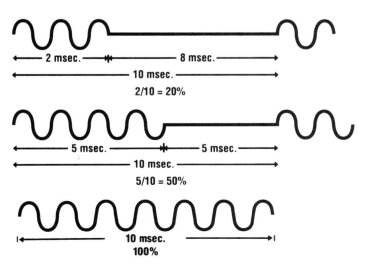

Figure 33.3. The duty cycles determine the on time of the ultrasound.

manufacturers, of the clinical benefits of using the various instruments. Research is slowly evolving, and it is the responsibility of the clinician using electrotherapeutic devices to be familiar with the relevant literature. Finally, the clinician must make every effort to assess and evaluate critically the clinical effects and outcomes of all interventions, including electrotherapy.

Basic Electricity in Electrotherapy

Uniform terminology has been established for electrotherapy to clarify the concepts and standardize the language used by clinicians and manufacturers (Section on Clinical Electrophysiology, 1990). Important terms are defined below.

Current. The flow of electrons through a conductive medium, such as biological tissues and fluids; it is measured in **amperes** (amp).

Voltage. The potential or electromotive force that drives the current; it is measured in volts (V). Current flows from the negative pole of the power source (voltage potential), through the intervening circuit, to the positive pole of the power source.

Resistance. The opposition to current flow; it is measured in **ohms.**

The relationship among these terms is that 1 V of electromotive force is required to drive 1 amp of current through a resistance of 1 ohm. Ohm's law states that voltage (*V*) is proportional to both current (*I*) and resistance (*R*), such that $V = I \times R$.

ELECTROTHERAPEUTIC WAVEFORMS AND CURRENT PARAMETERS

Electrotherapeutic currents can be schematically represented according to the dimensions and features of the waveforms produced by various generators. Current waveforms commonly used today include direct current (DC), monophasic and biphasic pulsed, and medium frequency (interferential and Russian) currents (Fig. 33.4). All currents can be described as having one or more negative or positive phases, which reflect the constant or changing polarity of the current.

Direct Current

Direct current, or Galvanic current, is a continuous flow of current, of one polarity (monopolar or unidirectional), and unchanging in amplitude (Fig. 33.4*A*). Direct current is either negative or positive and is most commonly used for wound healing and iontophoresis (i.e., use of electrical currents for percutaneous drug delivery) (Cummings, 1991). **Low-voltage** (<100 V) generators are used to produce direct currents.

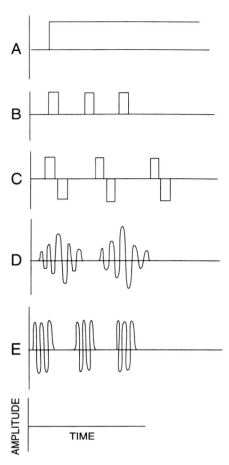

Figure 33.4. Schematic representations of commonly used electrotherapeutic current waveforms. **A,** Direct current. **B,** Monophasic pulsed. **C,** Biphasic pulsed. **D,** Interferential beats. **E,** Russian bursts.

Monophasic Pulsed Current

Monophasic pulsed current is of one polarity (negative or positive) (Fig. 33.4*B*). A monophasic **pulse** of current has a horizontal dimension, or a fixed time duration, called **pulse duration,** averaging 40 to 60 μsec. This dimension is often but inappropriately called "**pulse** width." **Pulse duration** is the amount of time that the current is flowing per **pulse** (Newton, 1991). The vertical dimension of the **pulse** is the **pulse amplitude,** which is the adjustable level of the magnitude of the current per **pulse. Pulse amplitude** may also be displayed in volts. Voltage is proportional to current, because voltage drives current. **High-voltage** generators are capable of producing voltage potentials >100 V. Clinical **high-voltage** generators do not usually exceed 500 V and produce a maximum of 2.5 amps of current.

Biphasic Pulsed Current

Each **pulse** of biphasic current has one negative and one positive phase (Fig 33.4*C*). The phase duration is often adjustable between 25 and 250 μsec. The amplitude is adjustable within a limited range using a **high-voltage** generator.

Interferential Current

The interferential current waveform is produced by combining two medium-frequency alternating currents. Alternating current (AC) describes current flow that is uninterrupted and constantly changing polarity, such as a sinusoidal wave with equal numbers of negative and positive phases. Medium-frequency currents, which range from 3500 to 5000 cycles per second (Hz), are used to create interference currents (Kloth, 1991). Two medium-frequency alternating currents **(carrier frequencies)** of slightly different frequencies are superimposed, which will demonstrate a consistent pattern of constructive and destructive wave interference. The result of this interference is the production of a "beat" or packet of a polyphasic waveform (Fig. 33.4*D*).

Russian Current

Russian current is a medium-frequency (2500 Hz) current, so-named because of its development in the former Soviet Union. Russian current is produced by allowing the 2500 Hz alternating current **(carrier frequency)** to flow for 10 msec, alternating with 10-msec of electrical silence. The result is 50 10-msec periods, or "bursts," of polyphasic current flow per second (Fig. 33.4*E*).

In addition to describing the current waveform by **pulse** or phase duration and amplitude and by the waveform—monophasic, biphasic, or polyphasic (more than two phases, such as medium-frequency waveforms)—the following terms are used to describe the current delivery characteristics.

Rise Time

Rise time is the amount of time for each current **pulse** or phase amplitude to go from zero current flow to peak current amplitude. Most clinical generators have a fixed, nearly instantaneous current rise time to ensure that the rate of stimulus development is adequate for the excitable nerve membrane to reach the threshold for an action potential to occur (Guyton, 1986).

Ramp Time

Ramp time, sometimes called surge time, is the time for successive current stimuli (**pulses**, beats, or bursts) gradually to reach the desired current amplitude. Some instruments permit an adjustable ramp time, others are preset. Ramping a current allows electrically induced muscle contractions gradually to build up tension development proportional to the gradual increase in amplitudes of successive electrical stimuli that are producing the contractions.

Stimulus Frequency

The rate of successive electrical stimuli (**pulses**, beats, or bursts) are adjustable and typically range from 1 to 120 stimuli per second (Hz).

Duty Cycle

In electrotherapeutics, duty cycle is the ratio of the time the current is on to the time the current is off. For example, a treatment protocol in which electrical stimuli are delivered for 10 sec followed by a 50-sec off period illustrates a 1:5 duty cycle.

Electrophysiological Principles

Excitable membranes, notably nerve and muscle, may be electrically stimulated to produce an action potential if the stimulus parameters are adequate. The flow of electrons (electrical current) between the electrodes of the current generating instrument create an ionic current flow in biological tissues when those electrodes are applied to the skin. The electrically induced ionic flow includes an outward **capacitive current flow** at the nerve or muscle membrane (Kukulka, 1992). This capacitive current outflow causes a gradual depolarization from the resting membrane potential. A 15 to 20 mV depolarization is required to cause an action potential (Griffin & Karselis, 1982). In addition, the rate of stimulus application and, therefore, the rate of depolarization must be sufficiently fast to prevent accommodation of the membrane (Guyton, 1986). In the case of nerve membrane, for which critical threshold is reached by the stimulus, a single action potential will be propagated in both directions from the point of stimulation, along the peripheral motor nerve axon or sensory dendrite (Mehreteab, 1994b).

The strength-duration curve explains the electrical stimulus requirements to depolarize selectively a variety of peripheral nerve and muscle membranes (Mehreteab, 1994b) (Fig. 33.5). Analysis of the curve shows that relatively short-duration electrical stimuli (such as the short-duration **pulses** delivered by pulsed monophasic **high-voltage** instruments, pulsed biphasic generators, and the short-duration phases of the polyphasic waveforms produced by interferential and Russian current generators) will selectively stimulate

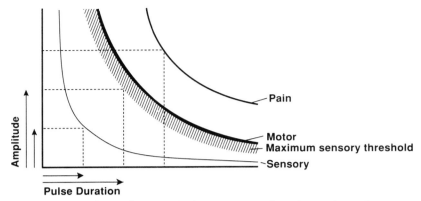

Figure 33.5.   The strength-duration curve of an electrical stimulus.

larger diameter nerves (Alon, 1991). Progressively more intense stimuli, achieved by increasing stimulus durations and amplitudes, are required to depolarize smaller diameter nerves and denervated muscle membrane (Mehreteab, 1994b). Large diameter nerves are associated with nonnoxious cutaneous sensory modalities and motor nerves linked to large motor units. Small diameter cutaneous sensory nerves are associated with pain pathways.

The frequency of stimulus delivery to motor nerves determines the quality and amount of muscle tension development. Normal, volitional motor recruitment is asynchronous. Initially, small motor units are recruited at varying and slowly increasing frequencies, gradually supported by larger motor units according to the size principle of recruitment (Guyton, 1986). In contrast, electrical stimulation of motor nerves results in synchronous motor unit recruitment, whereby all available motor units are simultaneously stimulated by the particular stimulus characteristics contributing to the strength of the contraction. The synchronous nature of electrically stimulated muscle contraction requires that the stimulus frequency (**pulse** rate, beat rate, or burst rate) be sufficiently high to fuse individual muscle twitches into a tetanic contraction consistent with the mechanisms of temporal wave summation (Guyton, 1986). The average rate of stimulus delivery to produce **tetany** is approximately 40 Hz (Griffin & Karselis, 1982).

Techniques of Application

ELECTRODES

Appropriate electrodes attached to the lead wires from the electrical stimulation device are required to provide adequate transition from electronic current flow to ionic current flow when the body is placed within the circuit of the device. Those electrodes must be able to conduct a current efficiently and be of adequate size and configuration to conform to the body area to be treated. Electrode materials commonly used include sponges over metal plates, karaya gum electrodes, silicon rubber, carbon, and self-adherent polymer electrodes. Electrodes may be reusable or pregelled for single use. Patient skin sensitivity may determine which electrode material is best.

ELECTRODE SIZE

For any given magnitude of current output, the size of the electrodes in contact with the skin will determine the **current density** at the electrode-skin interface (Cook & Barr, 1991). Small electrodes increase the **current density,** while large electrodes decrease it. Higher **current density** has the effect of increased current intensity under that electrode. Therefore, uneven electrode contact with the skin may unintentionally intensify the current at those points of electrode contact, possibly resulting in patient discomfort or burns, especially if direct current is used.

ELECTRODE PLACEMENT

Electrodes of both ends of an electrical circuit must be in contact with the patient. Closely spaced electrodes tend to cause more of the current to flow between the electrodes with less effect on subcutaneous tissues. Conversely, electrodes should be spaced far enough apart for the current to affect deeper target nerves or other tissues.

Motor nerve stimulation generally requires either the monopolar or bipolar technique of electrode placement. Monopolar technique is the use of only one pole or side of the circuit (active electrode) of the electrical stimulator to stimulate the target nerve entering the muscle or muscle group. The other pole or side of the circuit (dispersive electrode) is placed away from the target muscle or muscle group. The dispersive electrode is necessary to complete the electrical circuit, not for specific or purposeful stimulation. Therefore, the dispersive electrode is larger than the active electrode to diffuse the current under that electrode, rendering it ineffective. Monopolar techniques are often used when a probe electrode is used to stimulate small muscles.

The bipolar technique requires both electrodes or sides of the circuit to be in contact with the target muscle or muscle group. Both electrodes are of the same size. This technique is more appropriate for stimulating large muscles or muscle groups.

Commonly used electrotherapeutic currents, such as pulsed, interferential, and Russian currents, rarely produce significant skin irritations and are unlikely to produce electrochemical burns, because of the virtual lack of polar or thermal effects (Alon, 1991). Direct and interrupted direct currents with relatively long **pulse durations** may cause severe electrochemical skin burns. Therefore, the skin under the electrodes must be frequently checked.

Physiological Responses

The nature of clinically common electrotherapeutic currents (high-voltage pulsed, biphasic, interferential, and medium-frequency Russian) are such that they will selectively stimulate large diameter peripheral nerves axons and dendrites, owing to the relationship between magnitudes of the **pulses** and/or phases contained in these waveforms and the strength-duration curves. Large diameter cutaneous sensory nerves are initially stimulated, because these nerves are superficial. This results in the characteristic patient report of a "tingling" sensation. Increasing the current amplitude will stimulate deeper, large diameter motor nerves, causing a muscle contraction. Large diameter motor nerves are associated with large motor units and type II muscle fibers (Kukulka, 1992). Therefore, clinical motor nerve stimulation primarily recruits type II muscle fibers, which are phasic, easily fatigued, and volitionally recruited with intense physical activity (English & Wolf, 1982). Long-term electrical stimulation of motor nerve has been observed to cause temporary metabolic, ultrastructural, and membrane changes in type II muscle fibers such that they temporarily take on type IIa muscle fiber characteristics of longer twitch durations and resistance to fatigue (Altman, Hudlicka, & Tyler, 1979).

Electrical stimulation of motor nerve to produce muscle contractions has also been shown to increase local blood flow by increasing muscle vascularity (long-term response) (Myrhage & Hudlicka, 1978) and by immediate, but transient, reflexive vasodilation (Currier, Petrilli, & Threlkeld, 1986).

Neuromuscular electrical stimulation has been shown to increase isometric muscle strength. However, such strength gains do not seem to exceed those obtained through volitional exercise (Currier & Mann, 1983). Also, improvements in other determinants of physical performance, particularly in patient populations, following such strength gains have not been demonstrated.

Several studies have shown that electrical stimulation of soft tissue enhances soft tissue regeneration of open wounds, either by reported bacteriostatic effects of electrical stimulation (Barranco & Berger, 1974) of infected wounds or by accelerating collagen synthesis and reepithelialization (Carley & Wainapel, 1985).

Clinical Effects

The practical applications of electrical stimulation include the treatment of pain, muscle weakness, spasticity related to central nervous system disorders, muscle holding (guarding) related to musculoskeletal injuries, edema, and indolent soft tissue wounds.

ELECTRICAL STIMULATION FOR PAIN MODULATION

The occupational therapist can use electrical sensory stimulation to decrease the patient's pain before, during, or after the performance of therapeutic activities or during routine activities of daily living.

Two major models of pain modulation are used to explain the observed effects of electrical stimulation. First, the gate-control model (Melzack & Wall, 1965) describes a neural mechanism at the segmental levels of the spinal cord that enables nonpainful sensory input from the skin to impede pain impulses from being transmitted to higher centers of pain perception. In this model, local electrical stimulation of large diameter, non–pain-mediating cutaneous sensory afferents closes the gate at the spinal cord level to the further transmission of pain nerve impulses arriving at the spinal cord.

The second model states that the body can be stimulated to release endogenous opiate substances, which are naturally produced by the nervous system (Basbaum & Fields, 1978). Electrical stimulation of sensory nerves has been shown to increase circulating levels of these neuropharmacologic agents (enkephalins and endorphins) and, therefore, decrease reported pain (Hughes et al., 1984).

Electrical Stimulation for Pain Gate Control

Electrical stimulation for pain gate control is also called conventional transcutaneous electrical nerve stimulation (**TENS**) stimulation. The stimulus parameters call for a short **pulse duration** at a frequency of 50 to 100 Hz. Electrodes are often placed at the site of pain, along a dermatome, or at the location of the spinal nerve root (Mannheimer & Lampe, 1984). Current amplitude is increased within limits of sensory perception. Pain suppression should be expected to be nearly immediate. The portability of the stimulation device can permit functional activities while enjoying pain relief.

Electrical Stimulation to Release Endogenous Opiates

The stimulus parameters for electrical stimulation to release endogenous opiates include a long-duration **pulse** and a frequency of 1 to 4 Hz (Weisberg, 1994). The current amplitude is adjusted so that a mild motor response is observed. Electrode placement includes the sites noted for a conventional **TENS** setup (Gersh, 1992). The analgesic effects of this mode of application occur within 20 to 60 min (Mannheimer & Lampe, 1984). Generally, the analgesic effects of the release of endogenous opiates last longer (1 to 2 hr) than the effects of pain gate closure, from which pain may return immediately following cessation of the stimulating current.

ELECTRICAL STIMULATION TO IMPROVE MUSCLE STRENGTH

Impairments of muscle performance may have several causes. Muscle with its nerve supply intact (innervated muscle) may be weak because of disuse atrophy from limb immobilization, motor control deficits with or without spasticity, pain with movement, or denervation (interrupted peripheral nerve supply to the muscle). Electrical stimulation is commonly used to improve muscle performance leading to improved functional capacity.

The use of electrical stimulation to "strengthen" muscle by inducing girth changes and improving the ability of muscle to generate isometric tension has been studied (Currier & Mann, 1983; Selkowitz, 1985). The effects of such muscle changes from electrical stimulation on functional performance and clinical outcomes have not been established. Other rationales and techniques of electrotherapy for improving muscle function have been proposed.

Techniques of muscle facilitation leading to muscle reeducation are used to improve motor performance following disease and injury (Crastam, Larson, & Previc, 1977; LeDoux & Quinones, 1981; Bogataj & Gros, 1989). In this context, neuromuscular electrical stimulation is used to provide sensory, kinesthetic, and proprioceptive stimuli to central-processing mechanisms, inducing muscles to contract to move a joint. The variety of sensory feedback facilitates recovery of

volitional movement. Electrical stimulation used in this way assists and encourages volitional contraction of weak or dysfunctional muscles, whereby the electrically assisted activity is gradually replaced by active exercises, which in turn leads to functional strength gains. The stimulation procedure involves using the appropriate waveform to stimulate motor nerve without stimulating pain fibers (short-duration, monophasic- or biphasic-pulsed currents; Russian or interferential currents).

Painful movement often discourages purposeful activities, and what appears to be muscle weakness may be joint or muscle pain leading to an unwillingness or painful inability to move. Successful electrical stimulation for pain modulation often results in a rapid recovery of muscle function and movement.

Peripheral denervation of muscle leads to profound muscle atrophy and weakness. If reinnervation of muscle occurs, full functional return may be expected. Prolonged muscle denervation often results in fibrotic tissue replacement of the contractile muscle proteins (Spielholz, 1991). Electrical stimulation of denervated muscle requires the use of current waveforms with long-duration **pulses,** i.e., interrupted DC. This is necessary because denervated muscle membranes have a longer **chronaxie** and require a stronger stimulus, according to the strength-duration curve (Fig. 33.5), to achieve threshold (Spielholz, 1991). Electrical stimulation of denervated muscle is not often performed and is controversial because of a lack of documented clinical benefits.

FUNCTIONAL ELECTRICAL STIMULATION

Functional electrical stimulation (FES) is the use of electrical stimulation of innervated muscle to cause the muscle to function as a dynamic brace. FES is often referred to as orthotic substitution. The uses of FES include support of shoulder subluxation associated with strokes, drop foot caused by weakness of pretibial muscles, and scoliosis (Baker, 1991). Also, FES for tetraplegic patients to accomplish grasp-and-release activities has been advocated. Portable neuromuscular stimulators are most appropriate. The treatment protocol includes using tetanizing **pulse** frequencies and on-demand or preset duty cycles that produce appropriately timed muscle contractions. For example, FES for ankle dorsiflexion during gait may be used instead of a molded orthosis. The electrical stimuli are triggered by a foot switch that is activated at the heel-off period of gait. This allows the pretibial muscles to be stimulated to dorsiflex the ankle to permit the limb to swing through. Heel contact with the floor at the beginning of stance phase switches the current off when dorsiflexion is not needed.

TREATMENT OF SPASTICITY

Electrical stimulation is used in the treatment of neurological patients with spasticity and patients with local muscle guarding or holding related to musculoskeletal disorders. The intended benefits of electrical stimulation are to provide a temporary decrease of muscle hyperactivity to permit therapeutic exercises and purposeful activities. Depending on the method of application of electrical stimulation, the reduction of muscle spasticity may last from 10 min to 3 hr. The models that direct this use of electrical stimulation include methods of application that stimulate either the agonist (spastic muscle) or the antagonist of the spastic muscle (Mehreteab, 1994a).

The rationale for stimulating the antagonist is that the opposing spastic muscle is inhibited according to a neurophysiological mechanism similar to reciprocal inhibition, called posttetanic depression (Tan, Apgar, & Marangoz, 1978). Stimulation of the spastic muscles is also performed to cause either sensory habituation of cutaneous reflexes leading to inhibition of muscles underlying the stimulated skin or fatigue of the spastic muscles by a continuous tetanizing current flow (Mehreteab, 1994a).

Electrical stimulation is also used to decrease local muscle guarding and holding accompanying musculoskeletal injuries. Frequently, pain is linked to the muscle guarding, causing a pattern of mutual reinforcement, often referred to as to the "pain-spasm-pain" cycle. Electrical stimulation to relieve musculoskeletal pain can promote improved muscular activity and movement, leading to an interruption of this cycle and decrease the muscle guarding. In addition, the above stated mechanisms and procedures for the relief of neuromuscular spasticity by stimulating the agonist may be applied to muscle guarding.

TREATMENT OF EDEMA

Electrical stimulation is used for the treatment of edema caused by prolonged bed rest, generalized weakness, local musculoskeletal trauma, venous insufficiency, and nonocclusive lymphedema. Two mechanisms are generally advanced to explain the observed effects of electrical stimulation on edema. First, neuromuscular electrical stimulation, which produces mechanical pumping and return of venous and extravascular fluids, is used to cause rhythmic movement of the edematous limb. This protocol requires the use of any appropriate current (monophasic- or biphasic-pulsed or medium-frequency currents) at a tetanizing frequency and the appropriate on-off periods to promote muscle contractions and limb movement with minimal fatigue.

Second, direct current using the negative pole is thought to repel negatively charge blood solids and proteins. This shift in the osmotic gradient allows fluids to be absorbed out of the edematous site (Newton, 1991). This treatment protocol requires that the negative electrode be placed over the edematous area and the positive dispersive electrode be placed away from the site. The recommended maximum DC electrode **current density** is 0.5 milliamps/cm^2 to prevent electrochemical skin burns (Cummings, 1991).

CONTRAINDICATIONS AND PRECAUTIONS

The occupational therapist must be familiar with the patient's current and past medical history before the use of any physical agent, including electrotherapeutic currents, to ascertain that such treatments will be used appropriately and safely. The following contraindications and precautions can be generalized to use of all types of electrotherapy devices.

Demand cardiac pacemakers. Electrical current could block the response of the pacemaker to cardiac failure. Electrotherapy is considered a contraindication for such patients.

Active cancer. Electrical stimulation may increase cell growth in the area of a cancerous lesion (Delitto & Robinson, 1989).

Stimulation of the carotid sinus. Electrical stimulation at the bifurcation of the common carotid artery in the anterior neck may lead to blood pressure changes and cardiac arrhythmias, and is contraindicated (Delitto & Robinson, 1989; Barr, 1991).

Local infections. Electrical stimulation may lead to increased local metabolism and inflammation in certain conditions (Delitto & Robinson, 1989). Not contraindicated when electrical stimulation is used for wound healing.

Decreased cutaneous sensation. Electrochemical burns may occur when using DC or long-duration DC on patients with sensation inadequate to report impending skin injury.

Pregnancy. The safety of electrical stimulation use over the trunk during pregnancy has not been established.

Transcranial electrical stimulation. The safety of this procedure on patients with cerebral vascular disorders or seizure disorders has not been established (Barr, 1991).

Electrical stimulation of the anterior chest wall. This procedure should be avoided because of the possibility of interference with heart function (Delitto & Robinson, 1989; Barr, 1991).

The stability of medical conditions, such as severe high blood pressure, peripheral vascular disease, and cardiac disorders must be ascertained before the use of electrotherapeutic intervention. Also, electrical stimulation of individuals with small body mass, including small children, should be carefully considered, particularly when planning techniques with large spacing between electrodes. Patients with excessive adipose tissue may required greater stimulus amplitudes to reach target muscles. This may precipitate adverse autonomic reactions (Delitto & Robinson, 1989). Finally, patient understanding, cooperation, and compliance is necessary when applying electrical stimulation.

Documentation

Conscientious clinical practice requires that the patient's problems that are to be treated with electrical stimulation be accurately determined, measured, and documented—before and after treatment periods—to know the effectiveness of the intervention. The parameters of the electrical stimulus and the treatment protocols must be documented as well. The following features of the electrical stimulation program should be included in the documentation.

1. Current waveform (DC, pulsed monophasic or biphasic, medium-frequency interferential or Russian);
2. **Pulse duration** and phase duration (if adjustable);
3. Stimulus frequency;
4. Duty cycle;
5. Polarity (if appropriate);
6. Electrode placement (monopolar or bipolar setup);
7. Treatment duration;
8. Elicited physiological response;
9. Patient tolerance, reaction and clinical effect.

STUDY QUESTIONS

1. How does an occupational therapist appropriately incorporate physical agent modalities into a comprehensive treatment program?
2. For what conditions should you use heat versus cold?
3. How is ultrasound produced?
4. What are the thermal and nonthermal effects of ultrasound on the body?
5. Which parameters affect the strength of an electrical stimulus required to depolarize a nerve?
6. Describe two techniques and their rationales for using electrical stimulation for pain modulation.
7. List some common conditions that may be treated with neuromuscular electrical nerve stimulation.
8. What are the contraindications and precautions for electrical stimulation, ultrasound, and superficial thermal modalities?

REFERENCES

Abramson, D. I. (1961). Changes in blood flow, oxygen uptake and tissue temperatures produced by the topical application of wet heat. *Archives of Physical Medicine & Rehabilitation, 42,* 305–311.

Alon, G. (1991). Principles of electrical stimulation. In R. M. Nelson & D. P. Currier (Eds.), *Clinical electrotherapy* (pp. 35–103). Norwalk, CT: Appleton & Lange.

Altman T. J., Hudlicka, O., & Tyler, K. R. (1979). Long-term effects of tetanic stimulation on blood flow, metabolism, and performance of fast skeletal muscle. *Journal of Physiology (London), 295,* 36–44.

American Occupational Therapy Association. (1992). Position paper: Physical agent modalities. *American Journal of Occupational Therapy, 46,* 1090–1091.

Baker, L. L. (1991). Clinical uses of neuromuscular electrical stimulation. In R. M. Nelson & D. P. Currier (Eds.), *Clinical electrotherapy* (pp. 121–170). Norwalk, CT: Appleton & Lange.

Barr, J. O. (1991). Transcutaneous electrical nerve stimulation for pain management. In R. M. Nelson & D. P. Currier (Eds.), *Clinical electrotherapy* (pp. 261–315). Norwalk, CT: Appleton & Lange.

Barranco, S., & Berger, T. (1974). In vitro effect of weak direct current on *Staphylococcus aureus. Clinical Orthopedics, 100,* 250–255.

Basbaum, A. I., & Fields, H. L. (1978). Endogenous pain control mechanisms: Review and hypothesis. *Annals of Neurology, 4,* 451–457.

Bishop, B. (1977). Spasticity: Its physiology and management. IV: Current and projected treatment procedures for spasticity. *Physical Therapy, 57,* 396–401.

Bogataj, U., & Gros, N. (1989). Restoration of gait during two to three weeks of therapy with multi-channel electrical stimulation. *Physical Therapy, 69,* 319–327.

Brown, W. (1984). *The physiological and technical basis of electromyography.* Stoneham, MA: Butterworth.

Carley, P., & Wainapel, S. (1985). Electrotherapy for acceleration of wound healing: Low intensity direct current. *Archives of Physical Medicine & Rehabilitation, 66,* 443–446.

Clark, R., & Edholm, O. (1985). *Man and his thermal environment.* London: Edward Arnold.

Cook, T. M., & Barr, J. O. (1991). Instrumentation. In R. M. Nelson & D. P. Currier (Eds.), *Clinical electrotherapy* (pp. 11–33). Norwalk, CT: Appleton & Lange.

Crastam, B., Larson, E., & Previc, T. (1977). Improvement of gait following functional electrical stimulation. *Scandinavian Journal of Rehabilitation Medicine, 9,* 7–13.

Cummings, J. (1991). Iontophoresis. In R. M. Nelson & D. P. Currier (Eds.), *Clinical electrotherapy* (pp. 317–329). Norwalk, CT: Appleton & Lange.

Currier, D. P., & Mann, R. (1983). Muscular strength development by electrical stimulation in healthy individuals. *Physical Therapy, 63,* 915–921.

Currier, D. P., Petrilli, C. R., & Threlkeld, A. J. (1986). Effect of medium frequency stimulation on local blood circulation to healthy muscle. *Physical Therapy, 66,* 937–942.

Delitto, A., & Robinson, A. J. (1989). Electrical stimulation of muscle: Techniques and appications. In L. Snyder-Mackler & A. J. Robinson (Eds.), *Clinical electrophysiology* (pp. 95–138). Baltimore: Williams & Wilkins.

Docker, M. F. (1987). A review of instrumentation available for therapeutic ultrasound. *Physiotherapy, 73,* 154–155.

Dyson, M. (1987). Mechanisms involved in therapeutic ultrasound. *Physiotherapy, 73,* 116–120.

English, A. W., & Wolf, S. L. (1982). The motor unit—anatomy and physiology. *Physical Therapy, 62,* 1763–1772.

Enwemeka, C. S. (1989). The effects of therapeutic ultrasound on tendon healing. *American Journal of Physical Medicine and Rehabilitation, 6,* 283–287.

Feibel, A., & Fast, A. (1970). Deep heating of joints: A reconsideration. *Archives of Physical Medicine & Rehabilitation, 51*, 481–487.

Fond, D. (1994). Cryotherapy. In B. Hecox, T. A. Mehreteab, & J. Weisberg (Eds.), *Physical agents* (pp. 193–203). Norwalk, CT: Appleton & Lange.

Fond, D., & Hecox, B. (1994). Superficial heat modalities. In B. Hecox, T. A. Mehreteab, & J. Weisberg (Eds.), *Physical agents* (pp. 125–141). Norwalk, CT: Appleton & Lange.

Gann, N. (1991). Ultrasound: Current concepts. *Clinical Management, 11*, 64–69.

Gersh, M. R. (1992). Transcutaneous electrical nerve stimulation (TENS) for management of pain and sensory pathology. In M. R. Gersh (Ed.), *Electrotherapy in rehabilitation* (pp. 149–196). Philadelphia: F. A. Davis.

Greenberg, R. S. (1972). The effects of hot packs and exercise on blood flow. *Physical Therapy, 52*, 273–279.

Griffin, J. E., & Karselis, T. C. (1982). *Physical agents for physical therapists*. Springfield, IL: Charles C. Thomas.

Guyton, A. C. (1986). *Textbook of medical physiology*. Philadelphia: W. B. Saunders.

Hecox, B. (1994a). Clinical effects of thermal modalities. In B. Hecox, T. A. Mehreteab, & J. Weisberg (Eds.), *Physical agents* (pp. 115–124). Norwalk, CT: Appleton & Lange.

Hecox, B. (1994b). Physiological responses to local heat gain or loss. In B. Hecox, T. A. Mehreteab, & J. Weisberg (Eds.), *Physical agents* (pp. 91–114). Norwalk, CT: Appleton & Lange.

Hogan, R. D., Burke, K. M., & Franklin, T. D. (1982). The effect of ultrasound on microvascular hemodynamics in skeletal muscle: Effects during ischemia. *Microvascular Research, 23*, 370–379.

Hogan, R. D., Franklin, T. D., & Fry, F. J. (1982). The effect of ultrasound on microvascular hemodynamics in skeletal muscle: Effect on arterioles. *Ultrasound in Medicine and Biology, 8*, 44–55.

Hughes, G. S., Lichstein, P. R., Whitlock, D., & Harken, C. (1984). Response of plasma beta-endorphins to transutaneous electrical nerve stimulation in healthy subjects. *Physical Therapy, 64*, 1062–1066.

Kloth, L. (1991). Iontophoresis. In R. M. Nelson & D. P. Currier (Eds.), *Clinical electrotherapy* (pp. 221–260). Norwalk, CT: Appleton & Lange.

Kukulka, C. G. (1992). Principles of neuromuscular excitation. In M. R. Gersh (Ed.), *Electrotherapy in rehabilitation* (pp. 3–25). Philadelphia: F. A. Davis.

LeDoux, J., & Quinones, M. A. (1981). An investigation of the use of percutaneous electrical stimulation in muscle reeducation. *Physical Therapy, 61*, 678–682.

Lehmann, J. F., & deLateur, B. J. (1990). Therapeutic heat. In J. F. Lehmann (Ed.), *Therapeutic heat and cold* (pp. 590–632). Baltimore: Williams & Wilkins.

Lehmann, J. F., Warren, C. G., & Scham, S. M. (1974). Therapeutic heat and cold. *Clinical Orthopaedics and Related Research, 99*, 207–245.

Lota, M. (1965). Electronic plethsymographic and tissue temperature studies on effect of ultrasound on blood flow. *Archives of Physical Medicine & Rehabilitation, 44*, 315–322.

Mannheimer, J. C., & Lampe, G. N. (1984). *Transcutaneous electrical nerve stimulation*. Philadelphia: F. A. Davis.

Mehreteab, T. A. (1994a). Clinical uses of electrical stimulation. In B. Hecox, T. A. Mehreteab & J. Weisberg (Eds.), *Physical agents* (pp. 283–293). Norwalk, CT: Appleton & Lange.

Mehreteab, T. A. (1994b). Effects of electrical stimulation on nerve and muscle tissues. In B. Hecox, T. A. Mehreteab, & J.

Weisberg (Eds.), *Physical agents* (pp. 273–281). Norwalk, CT: Appleton & Lange.

Melzack, R., & Wall, P. D. (1965). Pain mechanisms: A new theory. *Science, 150*, 971–976.

Mense, S. (1978). Effects of temperature on the discharge of muscles spindles and tendon organs. *Pflugers Archives, 374*, 159–166.

Michlovitz, S. L. (1990). Biophysical principles of heating and superficial heat agents. In S. L. Michlovitz (Ed.), *Thermal agents in rehabilitation* (pp. 88–108). Philadelphia: F. A. Davis.

Middlemast, S., & Chatterjee, D. C. (1978). Comparison of ultrasound and thermography for soft tissue injuries. *Physiotherapy, 64*, 331–332.

Myrhage, R., & Hudlicka, O. (1978). Capillary growth in chronically stimulated adult skeletal muscle as studied by intravital microscopy and histological methods in rabbits and rats. *Microvascular Research, 16*, 73–76.

Newton, R. M. (1991). High voltage pulsed current: Theoretical bases and clinical applications. In R. M. Nelson & D. P. Currier (Eds.), *Clinical electrotherapy* (pp. 201–220). Norwalk, CT: Appleton & Lange.

Schmidt, K. L. (1979). Heat, cold and inflammation. *Rheumatology, 38*, 391–404.

Section on Clinical Electrophysiology of the American Physical Therapy Association. (1990). *Electrotherapeutic terminology in physical therapy*. Alexandria, VA: American Physical Therapy Association.

Selkowitz, D. M. (1985). Improvement in isometric strength of the quadriceps femoris muscle after training with electrical stimulation. *Physical Therapy, 65*, 186–196.

Spielholz, N. I. (1991). Electrical stimulation of denervated muscle. In R. M. Nelson & D. P. Currier (Eds.), *Clinical electrotherapy* (pp. 121–142). Norwalk, CT: Appleton & Lange.

Stratton, S. A., Heckmann, R., & Francis, R. S. (1984). Therapeutic ultrasound. *Journal of Orthopaedic and Sports Physical Therapy, 5*, 278–281.

Sweitzer, R. (1994). Ultrasound. In B. Hecox, T. A. Mehreteab & J. Weisberg (Eds.), *Physical agents* (pp. 163–192). Norwalk, CT: Appleton & Lange.

Szumski, A. J. (1960). Mechanisms of pain relief as a result of therapeutic applications of ultrasound. *Physical Therapy Review, 40*, 117–122.

Tan, W., Apgar, A., & Marangoz, C. (1978). Decreased post-tetanic potentiation of monosynaptic reflexes by spontaneous tetanization on antagonistic nerves. *Experimental Brain Research, 31*, 499–510.

Taylor-Mullins, P. (1990). Use of therapeutic modalities in upper extremity rehabilitation. In J. M. Hunter, L. H. Schneider, E. J. Mackin, & A. D. Callahan (Eds.), *Rehabilitation of the hand: Surgery and therapy* (pp. 195–220). St. Louis: C. V. Mosby.

Travell, J. G., & Simons, D. G. (1992). *Myofascial pain and dysfunction: The trigger point manual*. Baltimore: Williams & Wilkins.

Weisberg, J. (1994). Transcutaneous electrical nerve stimulation. In B. Hecox, T. A. Mehreteab, & J. Weisberg (Eds.), *Physical agents* (pp. 299–306). Norwalk, CT: Appleton & Lange.

Williams, A. R., McHale, J., & Bowditch, M. (1987). Effects of MHz ultrasound on electrical pain threshold perception in humans. *Ultrasound in Medicine and Biology, 13*, 249–253.

Ziskin, M. C., McDiarmid, T., & Michlovitz, S. L. (1990). Therapeutic ultrasound. In S. L. Michlovitz (Ed.), *Thermal agents in rehabilitation* (pp. 134–169). Philadelphia: F. A. Davis.

The Practice of Occupational Therapy for Selected Diagnostic Categories

*T*hese chapters share the expertise and insights of therapists active in treating patients with these disorders. They pull together the previous information and indicate how it applies to patients with a particular diagnosis. But they also present evaluations and treatments that are specific to persons with a given diagnosis. To help in bridging from theoretical book learning to actual practice, the authors have illustrated their chapters with case studies.

Remember, however, that these chapters are only guidelines to assist in learning the application of occupational therapy to patients with physical dysfunction. No two patients are exactly alike in clinical presentation or in values, goals, and occupational functioning. Application to a particular patient starts with paying attention to the uniqueness of the person and his goals. How the therapist applies her knowledge and skills to this unique person is first learned through supervised clinical experience and then through the continued study that accompanies developing expertise in professional practice.

Therapy for neurological disorders is explained in Chapters 34 through 36 and in Chapter 44. Chapter 36, "Degenerative Diseases," also describes in detail treatment of, and precautions for, HIV/AIDS. Chapters 37 through 43 illustrate therapy for orthopedic and cardiopulmonary disorders.

34
Stroke

Anne M. Woodson

OBJECTIVES

After studying the information in this chapter the reader will be able to:
1. Understand the variety of disorders referred to as stroke or cerebrovascular accident as well as the incidence, risk factors, subtypes, and locations of stroke.
2. Understand courses for neurological and functional recovery from stroke, including the factors influencing recovery and the time frame for recovery.
3. Understand the functional context underlying evaluation and treatment of stroke patients and identify methods to evaluate and treat for deficits in performance of daily living tasks.
4. Identify somatosensory and motor impairments of the stroke patient and identify methods for evaluating these deficits and for designing appropriate treatment to improve both movement components and application of movement to functional task performance.
5. Identify visual-perceptual and cognitive impairments of the stroke patient and identify methods to evaluate and treat for impairments in these areas.

Stroke, or cerebrovascular accident (CVA), does not represent a single disorder but rather a variety of disorders characterized by the sudden onset of neurologic deficits brought about by vascular injury to the brain. The most typical manifestation of CVA is **hemiparesis** or **hemiplegia** (mild weakness or complete paralysis) on the side of the body opposite to the site of the CVA. A wide array of neurological deficits may occur in addition to the motor signs. The mechanism, location, and extent of the cerebrovascular lesion determine the symptoms and prognosis for each patient. Although the onset of stroke may appear suddenly, it is usually the consequence of a long-term complex pathological process involving the cerebral circulation

(Rolak & Rokey, 1990). This chapter focuses on stroke patients, but nonvascular brain trauma or disease, such as gunshot wounds or tumors, may manifest many of the same neurological deficits and may be treated similarly.

INCIDENCE AND RISK FACTORS

Stroke is the third leading cause of death in the United States and is the most common cause of chronic neurologic disability in the adult population (Kelley, 1989). It is estimated that 500,000 persons suffer CVAs in the United States each year and that 66% of these survive, bringing the number of stroke survivors in the U.S. population at any one time to approximately 2 million (Toole, 1990). Stroke is the single most common diagnosis among patients seen by the occupational therapist in clinics for the treatment of physically disabled adults or in home care practice (Trombly, 1989).

The most significant risk factors for stroke include advanced age, hypertension, history of cardiac disease, atherosclerosis, diabetes, and history of previous stroke (Rolak & Rokey, 1990). Although the death rate from stroke has declined in the past decade, incidence of stroke has not appeared to decline overall, probably the result of more sensitive diagnostic procedures (Ostfeld & Wilk, 1990). The projected aging of the U.S. population is expected to have an impact on the incidence of stroke, as 66% of stroke victims are age 65 or older (Ostfeld & Wilk, 1990). The incidence of CVA more than doubles with each successive decade beyond the age of 55 (Kelley, 1989).

Subtypes of Stroke

Strokes are usually classified by the mechanism and location of the vascular damage. The two types of etiologies are ischemia and hemorrhage. Ischemia results from a lack of blood flow, depriving brain tissue of needed oxygen. When this condition results in per-

GLOSSARY

Aphasia—Language disorder caused by brain damage that affects the production and/or comprehension of written or spoken language.

Homonymous hemianopsia—Visual field deficit caused by brain damage in which the patient is unable to perceive half of visual field of each eye.

Hemiparesis—Weakness on one side of body caused by brain damage.

Hemiplegia—Paralysis on one side of body caused by brain damage.

Infarction—Tissue death that occurs when the blood supply has been cut off to an area, such as that caused by occlusion of a cerebral vessel.

Motor planning—Ability to organize voluntary movement sequences used to accomplish a goal.

Postural adaptation—The ability of the body to maintain balance automatically and remain upright during alterations in position and challenges to stability.

Shoulder subluxation—Incomplete downward dislocation of the humerus out of the glenohumeral joint caused by weakness, stretch, or abnormal tone in the scapulohumeral and/or scapular muscles.

Synergistic pattern—Stereotyped pattern seen when movement attempted in one joint results in automatic simultaneous contraction of other muscles at other joints.

Unilateral neglect—Failure to notice, orient, or respond to stimuli in the space opposite to the site of brain damage.

---

manent damage, or tissue death, it is referred to as **infarction** (Caplan & Stein, 1986).

Ischemia is caused by systemic hypoperfusion, thrombosis, or embolism. In systemic hypoperfusion, there is a failure of blood pumping such as would occur with shock, hemorrhage, or cardiac arrest. With this type of stroke, symptoms tend to be more global than with other types (Caplan, 1991). Thrombosis is the stenosis or occlusion of a vessel, usually as a result of atherosclerosis. Thrombotic strokes are the most common type, accounting for an estimated 60% of all cases (Rolak & Rokey, 1990). This occlusion is typically a gradual process, often with warning signs, such as transient ischemic attacks (TIAs), preceding. Embolism refers to dislodged platelets, cholesterol, or other material that travels and blocks a vessel. Emboli probably cause 30% of all strokes and usually occlude distal cortical vessels, resulting in cortical deficits (Rolak & Rokey, 1990).

CVAs caused by hemorrhage account for only 10% of all strokes, but they can be the most catastrophic (Rolak & Rokey, 1990). In hemorrhagic strokes, blood is released outside of the vascular space, cutting off pathways and leading to pressure injuries to brain tissue (Caplan & Stein, 1986). Hemorrhages are referred to as subarachnoid or intracerebral and may be caused by arteriovenous malformation (AVM) or aneurysm. Symptoms usually occur suddenly, and initial mortality is high.

Location of Involvement

Each survivor of a CVA presents with a unique combination of deficits determined by the location and severity of the lesion. Lesions are often localized either as anterior circulation strokes, which present signs and symptoms of hemispheric dysfunction, or as posterior circulation strokes, which display signs and symptoms

of brainstem involvement (Simon, Aminoff, & Greenberg, 1989). The anterior circulation consists of the internal carotid arteries and their branches: the anterior and middle cerebral arteries. The frequency of occlusions of the middle cerebral artery and its branches reflects the fact that this vessel supplies 85% of cerebral hemispheric blood flow (Simon et al., 1989). The posterior circulation consists of the vertebral artery, the basilar artery, and their branches, including the posterior cerebral arteries.

Another distinction related to location of CVA is whether the lesion results from large artery disease or small penetrating artery disease. The syndromes associated with anterior or posterior circulation strokes occur with **infarction** of the large, major cerebral blood vessels. Lacunar strokes are very small **infarctions** that occur only where small arterioles branch off the larger vessels in deeper portions of the brain, such as the basal ganglia, internal capsule, thalamus, and pons. These vessels become subject to damage over a long period and eventually may thrombose, causing small infarcts or lacunae in the specific regions they supply. Lacunar strokes can produce distinctive syndromes (Levine, 1987) and have a good prognosis for almost complete recovery (Rolak & Rokey, 1990).

The exact site of the lesion in the brain can be determined by one of the several computerized diagnostic systems now available such as computerized tomography (CT), positron emission tomography (PET), and magnetic resonance imaging (MRI) (Levine, 1987).

RECOVERY FROM STROKE

Despite a rapidly expanding knowledge base on stroke pathophysiology, no generally accepted specific medical treatment exists for acute brain ischemia and **infarction.** Most current forms of medical treatment are designed to reduce complications of a recent stroke or prevent recurrences (Biller, 1992). Outcome following stroke is influenced by many factors, including cause, location and severity of stroke, age, and preexisting medical disorders (Simon et al., 1989). The degree and time course of recovery from stroke are not easy to predict (Chollet et al., 1991). Gains in function after stroke are often attributed to "spontaneous" recovery in the brain or to interventions that influence neural mechanisms (Bach-y-Rita & Balliet, 1987). It is difficult to distinguish between the two, however, because most patients receive some sort of intervention early poststroke and attempt their own forms of readaptation to their environment (Bach-y-Rita & Balliet, 1987).

A similar model for stroke recovery describes two types of functional recovery. Intrinsic recovery involves return of neural control, such as return of voluntary movement to a paralyzed limb. Adaptive recovery involves using alternative or compensatory strategies for functioning, such as using the unaffected hand for dressing or walking with a cane or walker. The majority of patients gain some degree of both intrinsic and adaptive recovery (Langton Hewer, 1990).

Mechanisms that have been studied and suggested for the return of neurological function after CVA reinforce the concept of plasticity of the central nervous system or the ability of the nervous system to modify structural organization and functioning over time (Chollet et al., 1991). A study of regional cerebral blood flow with PET in recovered hemiplegic patients suggested that ipsilateral (uninvolved) motor pathways may play a role in the recovery of motor function after stroke, supporting clinical observations of possible bilateral cerebral control of the motor function of one side of the body (Chollet et al., 1991). Additional evidence that the ipsilateral, healthy corticospinal system contributes to movement and recovery of movement following brain damage is found in descriptions of decreased strength and subtle motor abnormalities in the uninvolved arm following stroke (Brodal, 1973; Jones, Donaldson, & Parkin, 1989). A case study of a small group of patients who had recovered movement and function after a first stroke and then suffered a second stroke on the opposite side from the first found that the second stroke resulted in bilateral paralysis (Fisher, 1992).

Experimental and clinical studies such as these suggest the complexity of the nervous system, the importance of individual differences in recovery, and the justification of therapeutic interventions to influence recovery (Moore, 1986).

Functional Recovery

Much attention has been and continues to be given to the functional outcomes of stroke patients.

Function, in this case, refers to the components of task performance as well as performance of specific life tasks. The predicted course of return of motor function progresses from proximal to distal movement and from mass, patterned, undifferentiated movement to fine, isolated movement (Brunnstrom, 1970; Twitchell, 1951). This sequence of recovery was supported in a longitudinal study of 20 hemiplegic patients followed from the 1st week of stroke to 1 year after the stroke (Fugl-Meyer et al., 1975). Patients often do not regain full function of the upper extremity. Studies have found only 14 to 16% of stroke survivors with initially severe motor loss regained good arm function (Parker, Wade, & Langton Hewer, 1986; Wade et al., 1983). Most studies, however, looked at recovery of upper extremity function within narrow time limits (up to 6 months poststroke) and usually examined return of movement removed from a functional context. Reliable, simple measures of arm function after stroke are not well developed (Parker et al., 1986), making reports of functional recovery difficult to validate. Hand function seems to be the most difficult motor function to restore even with intensive therapy. This could be related to the hand's rich innervation from the large Betz cells of the cortex, which seem to be adversely affected by any substantial loss (Basmajian, 1989).

Important aspects of functional recovery include the amount of assistance required to carry out daily living tasks and whether a stroke survivor can resume function at home. A large retrospective study found that 6 months poststroke, 47% of 494 stroke survivors were totally independent (based on ratings on the *Barthel Index of ADL* skills), 9% were dependent, and 44% were partially independent. It also was found that only 27% of acute stroke patients could walk independently 1 week poststroke; but 60% could walk independently 3 weeks poststroke, and 85% could walk independently by 6 months poststroke (Wade & Langton Hewer, 1987). In a study of 282 stroke patients in an acute rehabilitation program, 75% were discharged to home and showed substantial gains in functional status based on ratings of 18 activities of the *Functional Independence Measure* (FIM) (Wilson, Houle, & Keith, 1991). The Framingham study, a longitudinal study of 148 long-term stroke survivors, found that 78% of survivors were independent in ambulation 6 months or more after the stroke, 68% were independent in activities of daily living, and 85% were living at home (Gresham et al., 1979).

Few studies exist that look at recovery of home management, vocational, leisure, or community skills. One study found that only 36% of stroke survivors maintained their previous level of sexual activity (Fugl-Meyer & Jääskö, 1980). Another study showed that among stroke patients who had driven a car before their stroke, 58% did not resume driving poststroke (Legh-Smith, Wade, & Langton Hewer, 1986). A study that looked at 56 subjects at least 1 year poststroke gave a picture of typical stroke survivors at home. In general, these individuals were sedentary and felt isolated from friends and unable to pursue previous socialization, leisure, and entertainment activities. They were not involved in the routine care of the home and lacked endurance and confidence in their abilities (Tangeman, Banaitis, & Williams, 1990).

Factors Influencing Recovery

Research in stroke outcomes has sought to identify characteristics and indicators that predict survival rate, neurologic recovery, functional recovery, length of hospitalization, and discharge disposition (Wilson et al., 1991). No single factor has been identified from numerous prospective studies that can accurately predict outcome. The type, size, and site of the brain lesion, of course, influence the extent and course of recovery. The presence and severity of coexisting disease, such as diabetes, heart disease, and peripheral vascular disease, can impede optimal functional recovery. One study of recovery of mobility after stroke found that more than 30% of those patients who had reduced mobility 2 to 7 years poststroke had causes other than stroke, particularly arthritis and dementia, as the primary deterrents to mobility (Collen & Wade, 1991). Coma immediately following stroke and history of previous stroke are associated with less favorable functional outcomes (Wilson et al., 1991).

Much of the literature on stroke has claimed no clear relationship exists between age, sex, or side of stroke and functional outcome (Wilson et al., 1991). Some studies have indicated, however, that advancing age adversely affects recovery after stroke (Andrews et al., 1984; Granger, Hamilton, & Fiedler, 1992). The U.S. Department of Health and Human Services (1990) noted that older persons in general have more limited functional capability in the population at large. It reported that difficulties with activities of daily living (ADLs) and instrumental activities of daily living (IADLs) are infrequent under age 65 but increase thereafter and climb sharply after age 80. Thus many older stroke survivors may have had preexisting functional limitations.

Prognosis for recovery of function in young patients, on the other hand, is considered more favorable. In a retrospective study of 202 stroke patients between the ages of 16 to 45, 54% had no residual disability or had minor impairments and were able to return to their previous level of activity; 30% had moderate sequelae that limited their previous activities; and 14% had severe sequelae that prevented return to previous activities (Bogousslavsky & Pierre, 1992).

Analyses of effect of side of lesion on outcome yield conflicting conclusions. Some studies have indicated that left hemiplegics improve with rehabilitation, but show a lesser degree of improvement in self-care independence, social adjustment, and recovery of motor function 6 months poststroke than do right hemiplegics, presumably because of unilateral spatial neglect (Denes et al., 1982). However, this difference has not been confirmed by all studies (Mills & DiGenio, 1983; Wade, Langton Hewer, & Wood, 1984), indicating that other unidentified variables may be interacting with the affected side to cause different results in separate studies (Trombly, 1989).

The presence of urinary and bowel incontinence, visuospatial deficits, cognitive impairments, and depression have all been found to be associated with decreased levels of functional performance in groups of stroke patients (Barer, 1989; Jongbloed, 1986; Mayo, Korner-Bitensky, & Becker, 1991; Reding & Potes, 1988). Factors that may positively impact outcome include good family support and sufficient financial resources for continued therapy (Evans, Bishop, & Matlock, 1987).

Reding and Potes (1988) discussed the difficulty of systematically predicting stroke outcome because of the wide range of deficits seen in stroke patients. They recommend categorizing patients into three subgroups based on neurological deficits: (1) patients with motor deficits only; (2) patients with motor deficits and somatosensory deficits; and (3) patients with motor deficits, somatosensory deficits, and homonymous visual deficits. They found significant differences in functional outcomes and time after stroke required to achieve these outcomes. The patient group with only motor deficits achieved higher levels of function in a shorter period of time than the other two groups (Reding & Potes, 1988). Predictions about recovery are not sufficiently accurate to be used as a basis for clinical decisions for the management of individual patients (Lincoln et al., 1990).

Time Frame for Recovery

It has traditionally been reported that the major recovery of function following stroke occurs during the first 3 to 6 months poststroke and that little recovery can be expected 6 or more months poststroke (Caplan & Stein, 1986; Langton Hewer, 1990; Licht, 1975). Wade (1992) further indicated that recovery occurs fastest in the first few weeks poststroke and then slows down but continues for at least 6 months. Later recovery of function can be attributed to adaptation or learning rather than to neurologic recovery (Wade, 1992). Research supporting central nervous system plasticity challenges adherence to such a generalized time frame for recovery, citing laboratory studies that document the occurrence of functional recovery 5 years after a stationary brain lesion (Bach-y-Rita, 1981).

One possible explanation for the widespread reporting of time limits on recovery is that postacute therapy intervention for stroke patients is often discontinued within 3 to 6 months poststroke, because of limitations in access, funding, or documented progress (Tangeman et al., 1990). Therapists are inclined to discontinue treatment when a patient has plateaued or no longer shows progress in established functional goals after what is considered an adequate amount of time.

The period immediately after stroke requires significant adjustments by both the patient and his family; these cannot be expected to occur rapidly. Patients report that the stress of the acute stroke phase often prevents them from optimally attending to and benefiting from inpatient rehabilitation. They report that after a period at home or in their postdischarge setting, they gained a greater understanding of how the stroke affected their daily lives. The postacute period is often characterized by a renewed interest in improving skills or in deterioration of skills gained during therapy (Tangeman et al., 1990). There is a tendency, because of the acute onset of stroke, to regard stroke recovery as following a circumscribed, acute course rather than as a chronic, changing condition. As Isaacs (1982) stated, "the stroke patient dramatically typifies the failure of our health care system to identify and respond to continuing needs, as well as a certain lack of medical curiosity in studying the continuing changes in human behavior and physiological function that follow from an assault on brain tissues" (p. 310). It remains a challenge for therapists to attend to the continuing needs of stroke patients over an extended period of time within the confines of current available labor, financial reimbursement, and access guidelines.

ASSESSMENT

The occupational therapist's goal is to increase the stroke patient's independence in occupational performance tasks. The challenges inherent in assessing the stroke patient include the wide variation in individual symptoms, impairments, course of recovery, comorbid conditions, motivation, and expectations. No two stroke patients will present with the same set or degree of impairments, regardless of similarities in site or type of lesion. Generalities about right versus left CVAs and thrombotic versus hemorrhagic strokes are useful only as guides for careful investigation of a patient's strengths and deficits and their impact on functional performance.

The functional context should guide the selection of assessment tools and methods. A vast array of evaluations exists to address the various aspects of stroke disability. If therapists were to routinely administer all tests suitable for strokes to each patient, little time would be left for treatment. Therefore, rather than use an inductive reasoning process, the therapist must use a deductive one by starting with the self-care evaluation (Trombly, 1989). Every stroke patient is evaluated for level of independent functioning in daily living skills. Observation of performance during this evaluation suggests to the therapist probable deficits in components of independent functioning. Those probabilities are then tested directly by administration of selected tests. Evaluation also indicates residual abilities, which will be the key to restoration of function (Trombly, 1989).

Areas to be evaluated include sensation; mechanical and physiological components of movement, such as passive range of motion, soft tissue or joint abnormalities, and muscle tone; and voluntary movement in the upper extremity, including strength, control, endurance, and ability to function. In addition, information concerning factors that affect the ability of the patient to progress or learn must be gathered (Trombly, 1989). These factors include the presence of speech and language disorders and visual-perceptual or cognitive deficits. Emotional status of the patient and level of adaptation to the stroke by the patient and his family will affect outcome and need to be evaluated, as does the patient's degree of motivation to recover (Trombly, 1989).

The assessment and subsequent treatment planning for the stroke patient must take into account the setting for treatment, time elapsed since stroke onset, the expected discharge disposition, and the patient's prestroke level of functioning. Settings in which occupational therapists usually evaluate and treat stroke patients are acute care hospitals, rehabilitation units or facilities, outpatient clinics, skilled nursing facilities, and patients' homes.

If the patient is being seen in an acute care setting, it is important to consider the increasing trend for shorter hospitalization periods. The current Health Care Finance Administration (HCFA) recommended length of hospital stay for the diagnostic related group (DRG) of cerebral vascular disorder is 7.5 days (Kosecoff et al., 1990). Assuming that an occupational therapist is not consulted immediately after the patient is admitted, therapy in this setting may last for only a few days. The therapist must, therefore, set priorities, streamline the evaluation process, and assume a triage role, i.e., determine how best to prepare the patient for the next level of care.

Often the stroke patient is transferred to a rehabilitation setting shortly after the CVA, a national trend referred to as "quicker-and-sicker" admissions (Kosecoff et al., 1990). Inpatient rehabilitation stays are also becoming briefer, with the outcome objective being to assist the patient to return to his preonset living arrangement. It is no longer expected that patients discharged to home will be totally independent in self-care; mobility; or home management, leisure, and vocational tasks. These patients are frequently capable of achieving further gains and could appropriately be followed for continued therapy in an outpatient setting (Davidoff et al., 1991) or home health setting. It is not unusual for patients suffering mild CVAs to be diagnosed in a medical emergency or outpatient clinic and then sent home if their condition is judged stable. These patients receive all rehabilitation intervention as outpatients or through home health services.

Daily Living Skills

The patient's ability to perform the self-care, recreational, and vocational tasks that he hopes to continue are evaluated by observation (Wade & Langton Hewer, 1987). It is important to observe patient performance, because there can be a difference between what a patient is able to do and what he actually does. As mentioned above, evaluation to determine a patient's level of occupational functioning is administered early to predict answers to the following questions: (1) Where will the patient live and what physical adaptations will be necessary? (2) How much and what type of assistance will the patient need from others? (3) What roles will the patient be able to fulfill and how will he spend his time? (Wade, 1992).

Methods for assessing basic activities of daily living are discussed in Chapter 4. Evaluation of other areas of occupational performance is done as warranted by the patient's improvement (Trombly, 1989). It should be remembered that a patient's performance in the structured clinical setting may not indicate his performance in the home setting. For example, patients who can put on and remove clothes during therapy sessions may not be able to locate and retrieve their clothes in a cluttered closet, select clothing appropriate for specific weather conditions, or initiate the dressing routine without prompting (Campbell et al., 1991). Conversely, a patient may be unable to master simple meal preparation in the unfamiliar environment of an occupational therapy clinic kitchen but may readapt easily to this task upon return to home. A home evaluation can help determine what resources and means a patient has to achieve independence in tasks as well as assessing safety and accessibility (see Chapter 5). When appropriate, driving and return to work potential may be evaluated.

The ability to drive rates high on an individual's list of everyday skills (Jones, Giddens, & Croft, 1983). Those patients who want to resume driving should be evaluated by an occupational therapist specializing in driver evaluation. Although the social importance of driving is recognized, it is not known with certainty which deficits necessitate the use of adaptive driving aids or render a stroke survivor unfit to drive (Lings & Jensen, 1991). Standard evaluation procedures do not exist for determining the ability of cerebrally injured patients to return to driving (Galski, Bruno, & Ehle, 1992). In general, **hemiparesis** alone is not the major concern in returning to drive, because vehicles can be adapted to compensate for most motor deficits seen poststroke (Lings & Jensen, 1991). Perceptual, cognitive, and behavioral factors such as reduced awareness, inadequate scanning of the environment, distractability, and attentional deficits seem to be more predictive of poor driving performance (Galski et al., 1992). A suggested model for driving evaluation includes (1) a predriver evaluation, i.e., a battery of neuropsychologic and perceptual tests; (2) a simulator evaluation; and (3) a behind-the-wheel evaluation, both on a protected course and in traffic (Galski et al., 1992).

Communication and coordination with all members of the rehabilitation team and with family members are important to gather as much information as possible regarding ADL performance and to ensure patient success and safety. Occupational therapists planning to work with patients on feeding, for example, need to determine if dysphagia is present, because patients with dysphagia are at risk for aspiration (Chapter 44). Warning signs include decreased levels of alertness, history of aspiration, impaired gag reflex, dysarthria, nasal regurgitation, sensation of obstruction or choking, frequent coughing while eating, and wet-hoarse voice quality (Czyrny, Hamilton, & Gresham, 1990; Daniel & Strickland, 1992).

Somatosensory Deficits

When evaluating for sensory deficits or any other deficits in the stroke patient, it is important to remember that sensation is a component of function and not a focus for treatment, except as it relates to the ability to perform usual daily living tasks. The term *sensorimotor functioning* is often used to indicate the interrelationship of sensation and movement. Somatosensory integration is necessary for organized, purposeful motor behavior; if sensory information is not rapid and accurate, the motor system can react but cannot effectively anticipate or plan (Warren, 1991). Impaired sensation is also closely associated with the presence of less easily recognized parietal lobe syndromes of **unilateral neglect,** spatial and body disorientation, and **motor planning** difficulties, all of which are serious impediments to rehabilitation success (Anderson, 1971).

One of the first steps in testing for sensation may be to determine the patient's effectiveness in communicating and his yes/no reliability. An expressively aphasic patient can nod, gesture, point to written or pictured cues, or select a stimulus object from an array of objects. Yes/no reliability can be estimated by asking several simple true-or-false questions on subjects familiar to the patient, such as spouse's name, home town, or the color of his shirt. If receptive **aphasia** is present, testing with standard procedures may not be possible. Information may be gained, however, from observing a patient's reactions to the testing. The presence of protective sensation (flinching when pricked with a sharp pin) can be documented as grossly intact even if discriminatory perception cannot be determined.

Patients who have had mild CVAs with intact primary sensory awareness may need to be tested for more subtle discriminatory problems using the two-point discrimination test (Callahan, 1990) or the *Moberg Pick-up Test* (Dellon, 1981; Moberg, 1958). Such testing is indicated when motor return is good but hand dexterity remains impaired.

Motor Deficits

Occupational therapy is concerned with assisting the hemiplegic patient to regain movement, not for its own sake, but for the performance of purposeful activities. Movement is complex in that it is an integration of sensorimotor, cardiovascular, cognitive, and psychosocial factors, resulting in a response to the environment (Warren, 1991). Because all of these factors can be affected in varying degrees by a stroke, movement should not be evaluated or treated in isolation. Occupational therapists are most often involved with the evaluation and treatment of motor deficits in the upper extremity of the stroke patient, but effective evaluation and treatment include consideration of trunk and lower extremity movement and **postural adaptation.** Evaluation of the involved upper extremity should look at the mechanical and physiological deterrents to movement, the degree and quality of active or voluntary movement, and the extent of useful function resulting from movement.

POSTURAL ADAPTATION

Postural adaptation refers to the ongoing ability to remain upright against gravity during changes in body position (Warren, 1990). Because so many daily living skills depend on this skill (putting on socks, getting in and out of a bathtub, and participating in sports), the recognition and treatment of deficits in **postural adaptation** is an appropriate component of occupational therapy for stroke patients. Evaluation and treatment that focus on the patient securely supported in bed or in a wheelchair fail to address the majority of usual daily tasks that involve dealing with the force of gravity. In **hemiplegia,** bilateral integra-

tion and automatic postural control are decreased, so that the hemiplegic patient must devote considerably more effort to remaining upright, decreasing his ability to focus on purposeful tasks (Warren, 1991). When engaging in a challenging activity, the hemiplegic patient will often resort to a developmentally lower-level compensatory strategy to help maintain stability (Warren, 1990). Chapter 7 describes methods for evaluating **postural adaptation.**

MECHANICAL AND PHYSIOLOGICAL COMPONENTS

Mechanical factors to consider include passive range of motion and possible movement restrictions in the joints and soft tissues of the extremity. Limitations in passive range of motion may result from an individual's anatomy and lifestyle or from premorbid conditions such as arthritis. Limitations may result more directly from the stroke, with the sudden and prolonged immobilization of joints occurring with paralysis, weakness, or spasticity in muscles. In the shoulder, adhesions, subluxation, tendinitis, and bursitis are common complications of **hemiparesis,** and all can result in limited range of motion (Andersen, 1985; Caillet, 1981). Prolonged stereotyped positioning of joints, such as occurs with spasticity, without counteracting movement results in shortening of muscles, tendons, and ligaments and restriction in movement and eventual contractures. Goniometry measurement of passive range of motion is usually not indicated unless treatment is specifically aimed at increasing passive motion, such as when trying to eliminate an elbow flexion contracture. Comparison of the involved extremity to the uninvolved helps determine whether limitations are preexisting. Edema that may occur secondary to loss of muscle action and reduced circulation can further limit passive joint motion. Any of the above conditions can lead to pain, which can result in further loss of movement as the patient attempts to avoid any movement that causes pain (Warren, 1991).

Abnormal tone is an important component of movement deficits in **hemiplegia.** Typically, patients exhibit individual patterns of both spasticity and hypotonicity in the same extremity, resulting in the imbalances that impair controlled movement. Evaluations for muscle tone are described in Chapter 7.

Evaluation of **shoulder subluxation** can be done by palpation; the patient's arms hang freely while the examiner palpates bilaterally for the separation between the acromion and the head of the humerus. The distance separating the two is evaluated in finger breadths, i.e., the number of fingers that can be inserted in the space (Prevost et al., 1987; Trombly, 1989). The distance separating the acromial angle and the lateral epicondyle of the humerus can also be measured in millimeters (Prevost et al., 1987). Clinical methods of evaluating subluxation correlate highly with objective radiologic testing (Prevost et al., 1987).

Evaluation of pain usually relies on patient self-report as well as observation of facial expressions and behaviors such as withdrawal or protection of a painful joint or extremity. Patients should be asked specifically where the pain occurs, when the pain occurs (with movement, at rest, after certain activities or at certain times of day), and how they would describe the pain (burning, aching, sharp, etc.). The intensity can be graded by asking the patient to rate the severity of the pain from 0 to 10, with 10 being the most painful (Daniel & Strickland, 1992). The *Ritchie Articular Index* can be used to document shoulder pain in stroke patients (Bohannon & LeFort, 1986). The involved shoulder (positioned in 45° of abduction with the elbow held at 90° of flexion and forearm pronated) is rotated laterally toward an end point of 90°, and the patient's responses are graded on a 4-point scale according to their responses: no pain is rated 0; complaint of pain, 1; complaint of pain and wince, 2; and complaint of pain, wince, and withdrawal, 3 (Bohannon & Andrews, 1990).

VOLUNTARY MOVEMENT

Determining the amount and quality of voluntary movement a patient can produce is one of the first steps in assessing the movement potential of a patient (Warren, 1991). The patterns of motion available will be different for each individual. Movement can change dramatically or subtly with time or according to the status of other deficits, requiring careful reassessment throughout treatment. It will be helpful for treatment planning if during the evaluation of motor control the therapist notices such things as the following.

1. *Is the patient able to perform automatic movement* (i.e., movement that is habitual or in response to a familiar object) but not voluntary movement, indicating preservation of subcortical motor control functions but loss of cortical ones? A patient in whom automatic movement is preserved will easily adjust to disturbances of balance (equilibrium reactions), and his body will follow as his head moves (righting reactions).

2. *Do proximal segments (neck, trunk, shoulder, hip) stabilize as needed* to provide firm support for movement of the distal parts? If not, treatment should begin here (Trombly, 1989).

3. *Can voluntary movement be performed unassisted against gravity* or is assistance required in the form of positioning, support, or facilitation? Begin by requesting unassisted movement of individual joints against gravity. Demonstration of the desired movement or passive movement to ensure comprehension is allowed before the patient's attempt (Daniel & Strickland,

1992). If the movement cannot be elicited unassisted, position the extremity in a gravity-eliminated position, provide support, and/or provide various facilitation techniques. Evaluation involves altering conditions as necessary to encourage muscle activation and actively searching for muscle activity (Carr & Shepherd, 1987). If voluntary movement is elicited it should be documented as assisted or unassisted and should be quantified in terms of the amount of active range of motion present (i.e., 25%, 50%, 100%).

4. *Can voluntary movement be performed in an isolated fashion* or only in a **synergistic pattern?** Following stroke, a muscle may be able to contract as a synergist, if not in its prime mover function (Carr & Shepherd, 1987). In motor patterns typical in **hemiplegia,** movement initiated in one joint will result in automatic contraction of other muscles linked in synergy with that movement. This results in limited, stereotyped movement patterns rather than adaptive, selective motions. Typical stereotyped patterns are described as flexor or extensor synergy patterns, based on the motion occurring at the elbow (Brunnstrom, 1970; Caldwell, Wilson, & Braun, 1969). There is considerable variation in synergistic patterning, and many abnormal stereotyped patterns seen may result from compensatory movements, unnecessary movement, muscle tension resulting from exertion or stress, or in response to gravity (e.g., pronation). When isolated muscle action can be controlled, it can be combined in a multitude of synergies that are adaptive to the task being performed rather than stereotyped (Warren, 1991).

5. *The presence, speed, and precision of reciprocal movement should also be noted* (Caldwell et al., 1969). Reciprocal movement is the ability to perform agonist/antagonist motion in individual joints by requesting both movements in succession (Daniel & Strickland, 1992). Abnormal patterns of muscle activation in hemiparetic patients can be seen as difficulty in the ability to control activation as well as deactivation of agonist/antagonist muscle pairs to produce, for example, the rapid alternating movements necessary to brush teeth (Bourbonnais & Vanden Noven, 1989).

Several methods for evaluating poststroke voluntary movement have been described, including Brunnstrom's and Bobath's procedures (Chapter 24). Fugl-Meyer et al. (1975) have standardized and quantified Brunnstrom's method for evaluating motor control in stroke patients (Table 34.1). The evaluation of the upper extremity is divided into 33 details; each detail examined is graded 0 (unable), 1, or 2 (performed faultlessly or within normal limits, as defined for each specific task), resulting in a maximum total score of 66 points (DeWeerdt & Harrison, 1985; Fugl-Meyer et al., 1975). The Fugl-Meyer assessment has validity in

Table 34.1 Brunnstrom Fugl-Meyer Test: Assessment of Motor Function of the Upper Extremity in Hemiplegia

Test 1. Reflex activity (can reflexes be elicited or not?)
   1. flexors
   2. extensors
Test 2. Dynamic flexor and extensor synergies
   3. scapular elevation
   4. scapular retraction
   5. shoulder abduction (to 90°)
   6. shoulder external rotation
   7. elbow flexion
   8. forearm supination
   9. shoulder adduction and internal rotation
  10. elbow extension
  11. forearm pronation
Test 3. Motions that mix the flexor and extensor synergies
  12. hand to lumbar spine
  13. shoulder flexion from 0 to 90° (elbow at 0°)
  14. pronation and supination of forearm with the elbow actively flexed to about 90°
Test 4. Volitional movements with little or no synergy dependence
  15. shoulder abduction from 0 to 90° with elbow extended and forearm supinated
  16. shoulder forward flexion from 90 to 180° with elbow extended and forearm pronated
  17. pronation and supination of the forearm with the elbow straight and the shoulder flexed
Test 5. Normal reflex activity
  18. scored as being hyperactive (0) to not (2)
Test 6. Different functions of the wrist
  19. wrist stability (shoulder, 0°; elbow, 90°)
  20. wrist flexion and extension (shoulder, 0°; elbow, 90°)
  21. wrist stability (shoulder, 30°; elbow, 0°)
  22. wrist flexion and extension (shoulder, 30°; elbow, 0°)
  23. circumduction of the wrist
Test 7. Seven details of function of the hand
  24. mass flexion of the fingers
  25. mass extension of the fingers
  26. grasp with extended metacarpophalangeal joints of digits 2–5 and flexion of the proximal and distal interphalangeal joints (hook grasp)
  27. grasp with pure thumb adduction (lateral prehension of a playing card or paper)
  28. grasp with opposition of the thumb pulp against the pulp of the index finger (palmar pinch of a pencil)
  29. grasp of a cylinder-shaped object
  30. a spherical grasp (tennis ball)
Test 8. Coordination and speed: Finger to nose test is repeated five times in succession as rapidly as possible; the following details are assessed
  31. tremor
  32. dysmetria
  33. speed

that actual recovery of stroke patients parallels the test items (DeWeerdt & Harrison, 1985; Fugl-Meyer et al., 1975), and the test has high intrarater ($r = 0.99$) and interrater ($r = 0.96$ to 0.99) reliability for the upper extremity function test (Duncan, Propst, & Nelson, 1983).

STRENGTH, ENDURANCE, AND COORDINATION

It was traditionally recommended that manual muscle strength be tested only in CVA patients who regain isolated muscle control because of the facilitory effect of added resistance on reflex controlled muscle (Trombly, 1989). However, careful assessment of available voluntary motion involves the determination of muscle strength present to move a joint through range against gravity and with gravity eliminated. Clinically, muscle weakness, ranging from less-than-normal strength to total inability to activate muscles, has been recognized as a limiting factor in the rehabilitation of stroke patients (Carr & Shepherd, 1987; Duncan & Badke, 1987; Trombly & Quintana, 1985). Because clinical studies suggest that strengthening of hemiplegic upper extremity musculature may be an appropriate therapeutic goal (Bohannon, 1987; Bohannon & Smith, 1987; Trombly, 1992), baseline assessment of initial levels of muscle strength, using the motor assessment evaluations described above, is necessary if such treatment is to be provided.

Reduced endurance, seen as the decrease in ability to sustain movement or activity for practical amounts of time, is an important limiting factor in the motor performance of stroke patients and affects the patient's ability to participate fully in his rehabilitation program (Warren, 1991). Decreased endurance can be the result of physical fatigue and/or mental fatigue caused by the exertion required to move weakened limbs (Brodal, 1973) or the result of comorbid cardiac conditions (see Chapter 6).

Muscle coordination, defined as "the harmonious action of muscles, permitting free, smooth and efficient movements under perfect control" (Roper, 1978, p. 74), is a high-level achievement both in normal human development and in recovery from **hemiplegia.** It is, however, a factor affecting the quality of voluntary movement that is frequently evaluated following stroke. Both gross motor coordination of the upper extremity and fine motor coordination or dexterity of the hand should be considered. Assessment of bilateral arm movements, both simultaneous and alternating, gives additional information of higher-level coordinated functioning (see Chapter 7).

FUNCTIONAL ABILITY

Many tests exist to assess the functional ability of the involved upper extremity. Some of these are task-oriented tests, others test active motion by simulating useful activity. One difficulty in measuring function after stroke is that, because premorbid measures that can be used as controls are rarely available, a patient's performance must be judged against the "normal" general population (Wade, 1989). The tendency to use the patient's unaffected arm as a baseline is flawed because of the normal differences in performance ability between dominant and nondominant arms (Bornstein, 1986) and because of performance deficits in the uninvolved arms of hemiplegic subjects compared with neurologically unimpaired subjects (Bell, Jurek, & Wilson, 1976; Jebsen et al., 1971; Spaulding et al., 1988). Because the arm undertakes a wide range of functioning, any single test assesses only a portion of the actual possible functions (Wade, 1989). Therapists must choose tests that seem best suited for the individual patient.

One functional test developed specifically for use with stroke patients is the *Action Research Arm* (ARA) test (Lyle, 1981). The test is divided into four categories—grasp, grip, pinch, and gross movement—and has 19 items overall, which are graded on a 4-point scale. This test is hierarchical in the sense that if the patient passes the hardest item in each category, he will be able to do the other items within that category and these need not be tested (DeWeerdt & Harrison, 1985). This test provides ordinal-level scores and has intrarater ($r = 0.99$) and retest ($r = 0.98$) reliability. It can be completed in a short period of time but requires considerable equipment. The *Brunnstrom–Fugl-Meyer* (BFM) and ARA tests are highly correlated (DeWeerdt & Harrison, 1985).

The *Frenchay Arm Test* was developed as a battery of 25 functional tasks used to study recovery after stroke (DeSouza, Langton Hewer, & Miller, 1980). It has since been abbreviated; one version includes 7 of the original tasks (Wade et al., 1983) and another uses 5 tasks (Heller et al., 1987). The test takes little time to administer and does not require much special equipment. A published study shows the test to have validity and reliability (Heller et al., 1987). It has, however, relatively low sensitivity, with few patients scoring in the middle range (Wade, 1989).

A test developed by occupational therapists specifically to evaluate a patient's motor ability to use his hemiplegic upper extremity for purposeful tasks is the *Functional Test for the Hemiplegic/Paretic Upper Extremity* (Wilson, Baker, & Craddock, 1984a, 1984b). This test consists of 17 tasks, which are divided into 7 functional levels that range from absence of voluntary movement to selective and coordinated movement (Table 34.2). The tasks and levels follow a pattern of increasing difficulty and complexity and reflect Brunnstrom's view of sequential motor recovery in **hemiplegia.** Each task is graded on a pass-or-fail basis, and specific guidelines for grading have been given (Wilson et al., 1984b). The patient is scored at the highest functional level (1 to 7) at which he can successfully complete all tasks. This test was found to

have interrater reliability ($r = 0.976$) and to integrate objective component measures (such as active range of motion and sensation) and functional performance of the hemiplegic arm (Wilson et al., 1984a).

A more recent study found strong correlation between scores on the *Functional Test for the Hemiplegic/Paretic Upper Extremity* and the *Fugl-Meyer Test* (Filiatrault et al., 1991). The *Functional Test for the Hemiplegic/Paretic Upper Extremity* can be administered in approximately 30 min and can be given in a variety of settings. Disadvantages of this test are that it does not provide specific information about why a patient has failed a task (Wilson et al., 1984a), and it has low sensitivity to changes (Filiatrault et al., 1991).

Tests that focus specifically on hemiplegic upper extremity function, such as those listed above, appear to correlate poorly with tests of overall ADL functioning. A comparison of scores on the *Barthel Index* and both the *Fugl-Meyer Test* and the *Functional Test for the Hemiplegic/Paretic Upper Extremity* showed low correlation ($r = 0.60$ and 0.61, respectively) between independence in activities of daily living and upper extremity function (Filiatrault et al., 1991). Filiatrault et al. (1991) concluded that variables such as cognitive or perceptual disorders and the learning of compensatory techniques contribute to the variance associated with ADL independence, but because they account for only approximately 36% of the shared variance, these variables should not be used to predict activities of daily living abilities.

Motor Learning Ability

Motor learning ability refers to a patient's ability to learn and organize movement for adaptation to his environment (Warren, 1991). Proponents of a motor learning model of rehabilitation believe that regaining the ability to perform purposeful motor tasks involves a learning process that includes a recognizable goal, practice, and feedback (Carr & Shepherd, 1987). In this context, factors that affect a patient's ability to learn (or relearn) must be assessed, including **motor planning** ability, visual-perceptual performance, language or cognitive disorders, and emotional adjustment.

MOTOR PLANNING

Motor planning deficits, referred to as apraxia, are deficits of skilled, organized movement sequences used to accomplish a goal that cannot be explained by motor or sensory impairments. These deficits are best identified during performance of daily living tasks. Clinical manifestations of **motor planning** difficulties include the following:

Table 34.2 Functional Test for the Hemiplegic/Paretic Upper Extremity

Patient Name: _____ Patient No.: _____

Level	Task	Date: Grade	Time	Date: Grade	Time	Date: Grade	Time
1	Patient is unable to complete higher-level tasks						
2	A. Associated reaction						
	B. Hand into lap						
3	C. Arm clearance during shirt tuck						
	D. Hold a pouch	(15 sec)		(15 sec)		(15 sec)	
	E. Stabilize a pillow						
4	F. Stabilize a jar						
	G. Stabilize a package						
	H. Wring a rag						
5	I. Hold a pan lid while pouring from pan						
	J. Hook and zip a zipper						
	K. Fold a sheet						
6	L. Blocks and box						
	M. Box on shelf						
	N. Coin in coin gauge						
7	O. Cat's cradle						
	P. Light bulb						
	Q. Remove rubber band from hand						

1. Failure to orient the head or body correctly to a task;
2. Failure to orient the hand properly to objects and/or poor tool use;
3. Difficulty initiating or carrying out a sequence of movements;
4. Failure to make anticipatory movement adjustments;
5. Movements characterized by hesitations and perseveration (Warren, 1991);
6. Movements that can be performed only in context, i.e., in the presence of a familiar object or in a common situation that elicits a gesture such as waving good-bye.

These deficits are most pronounced during learning situations, such as when training in wheelchair propulsion or one-handed buttoning, and in activities with multiple steps, such as making a sandwich.

VISUAL-PERCEPTUAL PERFORMANCE

The visual system is a complex interrelationship of almost all parts of the central and peripheral nervous system; any type or degree of brain damage would, therefore, be expected to have some impact on the functioning of the visual system (Moore, 1992). Chapter 9 describes assessments of visual-perceptual functions.

The most common visual disturbance associated with stroke is **homonymous hemianopsia.** Hemianopsia is a visual field deficit in which the patient is unable to see part of his visual field while looking straight ahead (Trombly, 1989). Left **homonymous hemianopsia** means that the patient has lost the perception of vision in the nasal field of the right eye and the temporal field of the left eye. (Bannister, 1973). Because the role of the occupational therapist is to evaluate for function and dysfunction as a basis for treatment rather than to diagnose the underlying conditions (Abreu & Toglia, 1987), many researchers advocate greater use of visual specialists—ophthalmologists and optometrists—to evaluate visual disorders of patients with brain injury (Bouska, Kauffman, & Marcus, 1990; Cool, 1987; Gianutsos, Ramsey, & Perlin, 1988; Warren, 1993a, 1993b).

Deficits in visual attention in stroke patients are commonly referred to as **unilateral neglect** or hemi-inattention. Unilateral visual neglect (or failure to notice, orient, or respond to stimuli located on one side) is associated with poor functional recovery (Halligan, Mareshall, & Wade, 1989). Visual inattention is much more common in right CVA damage than in left, and incidence is estimated at 33 to 85% in right CVA patients, and 0 to 25% in left CVA patients (Stone et al., 1991). Observation of the patient in the performance of activities of daily living can provide information about the integrity of the visual fields (Warren, 1993b) and the presence of **unilateral neglect.** Patients with significant field deficits or **unilateral neglect** may display behaviors such as failure to notice food on one side of their tray, running into things on one side, or turning their heads to one side to view objects.

COGNITION

Cognitive dysfunction is often felt to be a cause of failure to achieve rehabilitation goals. It is also a source of safety concerns in areas of function such as mobility, self-feeding, and self-medication, which all impact discharge planning (Osmon et al., 1992). Cognitive impairment can be assessed during evaluation and treatment of performance in daily living skills by focusing on the adaptive abilities of planning, judgment, problem solving, and initiation, which are as important in every functional routine as the physical components (Campbell et al., 1991). When evaluating stroke patients, the therapist must choose standardized neuropsychologic tests (as described in Chapter 9) that control for the patient's problems that could impinge on results. For example, in the presence of communication disorders, tests must be able to differentiate between an inability to communicate and cognitive deficits (Trombly, 1989).

SPEECH AND LANGUAGE

The ability to resume or relearn usual activities can be significantly affected by disturbances in the ability to communicate or to comprehend verbal or written information. **Aphasia** refers to an acquired language disorder that results from neurologic impairment that can affect various language modalities, including auditory and reading comprehension, oral and written expression, and gestures (Halper & Mogil, 1986). A simplified clinical classification of **aphasia** recognizes fluent and nonfluent **aphasias,** based on the patient's ability to produce spontaneous speech (Goodglass & Kaplan, 1983), and evaluates the patient's comprehension, or ability to name objects, repeat phrases, and follow written and oral commands (Czyrny et al., 1990). Using this scheme, global **aphasia** refers to a nonfluent **aphasia** in which the patient is unable to name objects, repeat phrases, or follow commands. Other nonfluent **aphasias** include Broca's **aphasia,** or expressive **aphasia,** in which the patient can follow commands but cannot name or repeat and

transcortical motor **aphasia** in which the patient can follow commands and repeat phrases but cannot name objects (Czyrny et al., 1990). Patients with nonfluent **aphasias** may be able to sing familiar songs or speak in other automatic ways, such as praying (Goodglass & Kaplan, 1983) or swearing. Patients with nonfluent **aphasias** may also have agraphia, or the inability to express in writing what they wish to convey.

In the fluent **aphasias,** patients can produce spontaneous speech, but understanding of language is limited. In Wernicke's **aphasia,** or receptive **aphasia,** a patient can speak but cannot name objects, repeat phrases, or follow commands. Other fluent **aphasias** include transcortical sensory **aphasia** in which the patient can repeat phrases but not name objects or follow commands, anomic **aphasia** in which the patient can repeat phrases and follow commands but cannot name objects, and conduction **aphasia** in which the patient can follow commands but cannot repeat phrases and often cannot name objects (Czyrny et al., 1990). Patients with fluent **aphasias** may have alexia, or the inability to understand written language, and, therefore, the inability to read.

Dysarthria is a speech disorder characterized by slurring of speech, drooling, or decreased facial expression caused by paralysis or incoordination of the speech musculature (Trombly, 1989). Oral apraxia is another communication problem following stroke in which the patient has difficulty initiating and sequencing the movements necessary to produce speech. In these disorders, the patient is able to understand and express symbolic language.

The functions and dysfunctions of speech and speech musculature are evaluated by the speech language pathologist. The occupational therapist needs to learn the results of this evaluation and coordinate efforts with the speech language pathologist to evaluate, instruct, or communicate most effectively with the patient (Trombly, 1989).

EMOTIONAL ADJUSTMENT

The majority of patients will have natural emotional reactions to their stroke, including denial, anxiety, anger, and depression (Czyrny et al., 1990). Mood disorders or psychosocial dysfunction is common and does not merely represent expected grief response to loss of function (Stern & Bachman, 1991), as these disorders have been found to be present even in stroke survivors with good physical recovery (Labi, Phillips, & Gresham, 1980). The incidence of depression following stroke is common; one study determined that 26% of patients had symptoms of major depression and 20% had symptoms of minor depression, with prevalence highest between 6 months and 2 years poststroke (Robinson & Price, 1982). Depression in stroke is both a physiological result associated with biochemical changes in the brain and a situational reaction to the personal losses experienced as patients realize, with time, that they will not fully recover. The boundaries between the organic causes and the reactive changes are not clear-cut clinically (Kaufman & Becker, 1991). Evaluation of the patient's and his family's adjustments to the stroke, to rehabilitation, and to the prospect of living with the aftermath of the stroke can be done through interview and observation (Trombly, 1989) and through the sharing of information with other members of the rehabilitation team (see Chapter 10).

TREATMENT

A careful interpretation of the evaluation results helps determine patients' major areas of dysfunction for treatment and intact areas of function available to promote increased independence. Occupational therapy goals for poststroke patients may include the following:

1. Improve independence in daily living tasks;
2. Promote increased somatosensory perception and/or compensatory and safety techniques in response to loss of sensation;
3. Promote optimum biomechanical and physiological components of motion and prevent development of secondary movement restrictions;
4. Increase voluntary movement, control, and functional use of the involved upper extremity;
5. Promote **postural adaptation** and improved **motor planning;**
6. Improve visual-perceptual performance through remedial and/or compensatory techniques;
7. Improve cognitive functioning;
8. Facilitate emotional adjustment to stroke;
9. Motivate participation in the rehabilitation program.

Treatment goals and strategies must be considered in the context of functional outcomes, i.e., performance in daily living tasks. In this age of streamlining and cost-cutting of health care delivery, a major dilemma in planning and administering treatment for stroke patients is how to address multiple complex problems in as little time as possible. Stroke patients often experience many problems, but the length of time allotted for treatment is shrinking. The challenge of designing integrated, effective treatment programs can be simplified with careful selection of activities that simultaneously address several deficit areas (Warren, 1991). A functional approach to treatment includes (1) an emphasis on the effects of patient assets and deficits on the performance of daily living tasks, (2) analysis of components of function (motor, sensory, cognitive, etc.) that are necessary for the performance of each task, and (3) promotion of components that lead to successful performance of tasks and achievement of higher levels of function. This functional approach has the advantages of efficiency, of motivating patients by directly relating treatment to familiar and meaningful activities, and of better securing justification and reimbursement for continuing occupational therapy treatment.

Therapy should begin as soon as possible after the CVA, and treatment can include mobilizing the patient out of bed after his neurologic and medical status are stabilized (Czyrny et al., 1990). The setting for treatment (acute hospital, rehabilitation unit, outpatient clinic, nursing home, or home care) as well as the patient's age, severity of stroke, available support system, and time elapsed since onset of stroke all influence treatment planning. Treatment is facilitated in an atmosphere that reduces stress and enhances learning. Sources of stress for stroke patients can include pain and discomfort, fear of falling, inability to communicate effectively, and distractions and overstimulation in treatment settings. Learning is enhanced when distractions are minimized and interest maintained so that concentration and effort increase. Therapists should promote an individual's best learning style by providing a combination of visual, auditory, and kinesthetic cues without bombarding the patient with too much stimulation. Treatment should be relevant to a patient's age and lifestyle (Warren, 1991).

General Treatment Precautions

In the acute stage, ascertain the patient's medical status and stability daily. Between 10 and 12% of stroke patients have simultaneous myocardial **infarction,** 40% have hypertension, and 60% have been found to have electrocardiographic abnormalities (Schuchmann, 1983). The therapist should determine whether cardiac precautions apply for a particular patient and monitor accordingly, watching for signs of cardiac distress and blood pressure changes including dizziness, dyspnea, chest pain, excessive fatigue, and altered heart rate or rhythm (Trombly, 1989; see Chapter 43). Patient safety during and after treatment is a concern. Both right and left hemiplegic hospitalized patients have been found to have more falling accidents than do other patients, possibly because of stroke patients' ambiguity concerning the range of what can and cannot be done without help (Diller & Weinberg, 1970). Before attempting transfers, be aware of the patient's balance status and assistance needs. To avoid injury or pain, a weak shoulder should never be used for lifting or pulling the patient. Be aware of appropriate precautions in regard to insensitive skin, visual field deficits, or **unilateral neglect.** Avoid feeding activities with the patient who has dysphagia or low levels of alertness (Daniel & Strickland, 1992). Educating family members and other health care workers as well as the patient regarding safety concerns is important.

Daily Living Skills

The occupational therapist's primary goal in stroke rehabilitation is to improve independence in daily living tasks and hence to improve the patient's quality of life. It continues to be controversial as to whether the patient should be taught compensatory one-handed techniques for self-care independence before regaining motor control of the involved upper extremity (Trombly, 1989). It is the opinion of some that if compensatory treatment is encouraged too early, the effectiveness of restorative treatment will be lessened, because the patient will fail to relearn bilateral movements and will instead develop unilateral habits (Bobath, 1978; Carr & Shepherd, 1987). They believe that preferential use of the sound side of the body for weight-bearing and functional tasks makes development of normal motor control less possible (Trombly, 1989). Another view is that ADL training results in success at a faster rate and is, therefore, more economical and more satisfying to the patient, who again feels competent (Sine et al., 1981).

Unfortunately, this issue has become an either-or proposition rather than developing into a coordinated eclectic approach. The majority of stroke patients seem to benefit from both compensatory and remediative treatment strategies. ADL training focusing entirely on one-handed techniques encourages disregard and "learned nonuse" of the involved extremity, which may impede progressive improvements in motor control following stroke (Taub et al., 1993). The patient should be taught to involve the affected arm in ADL tasks, such as putting on a shirt, which involves motor functions (moving the arm away from the body to put on a sleeve, extending at the elbow to push the hand through the sleeve, stabilizing one side of the shirt to button); somatosensory experiences (the texture of the shirt, the position of the affected arm); necessary **postural adaptations** (anterior pelvic tilt, trunk rotation, weight shifting); visual-perceptual skills (locating the shirt in the visual field, distinguishing top from bottom, finding the sleeve opening); and cognitive and emotional components (sequencing, attention span, frustration tolerance, success). In this way, the patient can work on those activities that are most motivating to him, and the therapist can directly address the specific component deficits that make these activities difficult for the patient. All other treatment activities can be justified, to the patient or to a third-party payer, as directly linked to improving ADL skills, e.g. a floor game to work on balance needed to reach over to put socks and shoes on or hand exercises to strengthen the muscles needed to squeeze a tube of toothpaste.

Of concern in recent research is the generalization or transfer of treatment methods and training to daily living skills (Toglia, 1991; Wagenaar et al., 1992; Walker & Lincoln, 1991). Several authors believe that independence in daily living tasks is best achieved by direct, specific training or close simulation rather than relying on the transfer or generalization of treatment effects to tasks not specifically trained (Campbell et al., 1991; Neistadt, 1992; Wagenaar et al., 1992; Walker & Lincoln, 1991).

Several studies discerned a hierarchy of achievement of self-care skills (Wade & Langton Hewer, 1987). The ability to dress independently comes relatively late in recovery (Basmajian, 1989). Results of a study showed that 31% of stroke survivors needed help with dressing and 49% required assistance with bathing (Wade & Langton Hewer, 1987). Another study of 150 stroke patients assessed at 1 month and 2 years after stroke, found that 41 and 36%, respectively, still required assistance to dress (Edmans & Lincoln, 1987). Aspects of dressing that are particularly difficult for CVA patients to master are putting a sock and shoe on the affected foot, lacing shoes, and pulling up trousers or pants (Walker & Lincoln, 1990). A study that investigated the relationship between dressing abilities and cognitive, perceptual, and physical deficits found that, in general, lower extremity dressing correlates more with motor performance and upper extremity dressing correlates more with cognitive or perceptual performance (Walker & Lincoln, 1991).

As the patient progresses, occupational performance tasks other than basic-self care may need to be addressed. Homemaking and home-management skills are practiced with those patients who have sufficient motor, cognitive, and perceptual abilities to enable success and safety in these tasks (Trombly, 1989). Avocational interests, including adapted methods of continuing familiar hobbies, is an important area for treatment. Many stroke survivors are faced with increases in leisure time because of inability to resume vocational roles; however, a reduction in social and leisure activities has been found to be a common sequel to stroke (Jongbloed & Morgan, 1991).

For those patients who expect to resume working, prevocational or vocational evaluation and appropriate work readiness training may be necessary. A study of 79 working-age stroke patients who underwent comprehensive inpatient rehabilitation with an emphasis on prevocational and vocational goals found that 49% were able to return to work—work was defined to include full- and part-time competitive employment, homemaking, and full-time university studies (Black-Schaffer & Osberg, 1990). The study found that a greater percentage of patients with **aphasia** were unable to return to work, and that 58% of those patients who returned to work acknowledged that their jobs required modifications (Black-Schaffer & Osberg, 1990). The factors found to be generally predictive of likelihood to return to work included independence in self-care, younger age, greater education, stable marital status, and high cognitive capacities (Weisbroth, Esibill, & Zuger, 1971).

Somatosensory Deficits

The primary importance of somatosensory input is to provide rapid and accurate feedback necessary to guide motor activity during daily living tasks (Dannenbaum & Dykes, 1988). In a study of 271 hemiplegic patients, 82 (30%) showed sensory defects, and these patients remained in a more dependent category of achievement in rehabilitation (Anderson, 1971). Kinesthesia and proprioception are important in relearning normal movement patterns (Leo & Soderberg, 1981). Tactile sensation enables coordinated, dexterous movement and is important in spontaneous use of the limb. Stereognosis, or texture and shape discrimination, improves manipulative ability and allows hand function independent of vision (Trombly, 1989).

Treatment for sensory dysfunction of stroke patients has not been systematically developed, although therapists attempt remediation as well as compensation for these deficits (Trombly, 1989). Remedial treatment involves the presentation of the stimulus, response by the patient, exact feedback, and practice (Weinberg et al., 1979). Compensatory treatment involves substituting intact senses for those lost or dysfunctional. Therapists must determine the appropriateness of either type of treatment for individual patients. For example, sensory retraining would be a lower priority for patients with minimal voluntary movement or poor cognitive skills. Success in remedial or compensatory techniques may be limited if the patient is hemianoptic and/or has **unilateral neglect.** Based on a pilot program of 6 poststroke patients, Dannenbaum and Dykes (1988) concluded that rehabilitation of severe sensory deficits requires a high degree of patient cooperation in a well-structured program linked to functional tasks. They also noted that such a program is justified in stroke rehabilitation, since research data suggest that function is possible with reduced or missing cutaneous sensation, because some subset of the preexisting afferent inputs is likely to remain and because lack of training can lead to a learned nonuse phenomenon and further deterioration.

Yekutiel and Guttman (1993) conducted a controlled trial in which 20 hemiplegic patients 2 or more years poststroke received systematic sensory training for the hemiplegic hand for 6 weeks. Their sensory reeducation program included exploring with each patient the nature and extent of sensory loss, emphasizing

sensory tasks in which the patient could succeed, selecting sensory tasks of interest to the patient that promoted learning, encouraging constant use of vision and the uninvolved hand to teach tactics of perception, promoting concentration with frequent rests and changes of subject, and avoiding in training any task or object used in the evaluation of sensation. At the end of the training period, the treated group showed significant gains in all sensory tests evaluated before and after training, whereas the control group showed no changes.

Treatment to restore tactile awareness should be structured so that repeated sensory inputs are provided to gain a larger cortical representation for those skin surfaces needed to perform daily tasks (Dannenbaum & Dykes, 1988). The areas of skin surface most used for interaction between the patient and his environment and of the most concern in rehabilitation are the fingertips, toes, and palms. Therapists should provide repetitive stimulation of high enough intensity to be appreciated but should avoid aversive stimuli to prevent withdrawal reactions or increased spasticity (Dannenbaum & Dykes, 1988; Eggers, 1984). One method of providing stimulation is to encourage the patient to use the involved hand as soon as possible in ADLs. Weight bearing on the affected hand on different surface textures such as foam, carpeting, sand, and toweling can be used for patients with limited distal movement (Eggers, 1984). Patients can be assisted in handling objects of different sizes, shapes, and textures. The holding surfaces of commonly used utensils such as cups, forks, and pens can be adapted to provide greater than normal tactile input by enlarging, reshaping, or adding a textural surface such as Velcro (Dannenbaum & Dykes, 1988). Sensory ability is important for function, not just to detect contact against the skin but to monitor the pressure necessary to hold objects of various weights and textures (see Chapter 23).

Redevelopment of Motor Control

Because movement is the physical means by which an individual interacts with his environment, therapy to regain motor control should be goal directed and should build on each patient's movement abilities as well as remediating movement impairments. Various treatment approaches that can be applied to improving the motor performance of stroke patients are described in Chapters 24 and 25. Therapists usually use an eclectic approach and employ a variety of techniques in concert or in sequence rather than in a mutually exclusive fashion. This approach better equips the therapist to address the infinite variety of neurologic symptoms encountered in stroke patients (Harris, 1978). Treatment should address **postural adaptation,** the mechanical and physiological components of movement of the involved upper extremity, the quantity and quality of voluntary movement, and the use of the extremity in functional activities.

POSTURAL ADAPTATION

The effect of postural reflexes on movement and function has been considered an important treatment concern following CVA (Bobath, 1978; Brunnstrom, 1970). Warren (1984), however, found in a comparative study of the asymmetrical tonic neck reflex in adult hemiplegic subjects and normal subjects that the intensity of the reflex, as measured by electromyographic biofeedback, did not differ between the two groups. This suggests that the use of brainstem-level reflexes should be viewed as a normal response to nervous system distress rather than a symptom of pathology (Warren, 1984). In this context, the appearance of primitive reflexes or other dysfunctional **postural adaptations** is a signal that the person is experiencing spatiotemporal stress (Gilfoyle, Grady, & Moore, 1981) caused by gravity (fear of falling, effort to move), by the complexity of the movement asked for, or by the body position required in combination with challenging skilled movements (Trombly, 1989). The patient with paralysis and/or spasticity will be stressed with every postural adjustment and movement and will adapt by using more primitive patterns of adjustment to help stabilize and mobilize his body (Warren, 1990). Treatment to improve postural control for the performance of daily living activities involves reestablishing the prerequisites for mature **postural adaptation,** including the ability

1. To produce full range of movement in the trunk and extremities;
2. To differentiate body parts from one another, such as rotating the shoulders independently of the hips;
3. To stop and hold movement at mid-range to stabilize against gravity;
4. To distribute and redistribute postural tone in body segments automatically to support movement;
5. To move both sides of the body symmetrically (Warren, 1990).

Various techniques can be used to accomplish these goals as long as the therapist has a clear understanding of each patient's particular strengths and weaknesses, i.e., stability and mobility. Application of a developmental treatment approach was endorsed by Warren (1990), because it focuses on weight shift, rotation, midline and proximal stability, and progression from using the upper extremities for support to performing skilled activities. Van Sant (1991) argued against the use of intertask developmental sequences (i.e., motor milestones) for adult patients but supported the use of intratask sequences (e.g., rising from a chair and

reaching to grasp an object). The incorporation of transitional movement patterns (i.e., strategies to change body positions such as from supine to side lying or seated to standing) and the use of strategically placed activities allow patients to practice effective postural adjustment while focusing on task accomplishment (Warren, 1990).

MECHANICAL AND PHYSIOLOGICAL COMPONENTS OF MOVEMENT

Mechanical and physiological complications involving the shoulder are a frequent consequence of stroke (Roy, 1988). The incidence of shoulder pain in hemiplegic patients has been estimated to be as high as 80% (Griffin & Reddin, 1981). Development of a painful shoulder can interfere with stroke rehabilitation, including self-care activities (Andersen, 1985). Despite numerous hypotheses and studies, the mechanisms underlying shoulder pain in **hemiplegia** remain poorly understood (Poulin de Courval et al., 1990). Possible causes include prolonged immobilization of the shoulder, trauma to the joint structures, subluxation of the glenohumeral joint, or a combination of these problems (Andersen, 1985).

Immobilization of the hemiplegic upper extremity, caused by decreased active movement, spasticity, or both, can lead to tightening and eventual shortening of soft tissues, resulting in pain with stretch. Shoulder-hand syndrome, or reflex sympathetic dystrophy, is present in 10 to 15% of hemiplegic patients with painful shoulders and is thought to have a neurovascular origin (Poulin de Courval et al., 1990) such as loss of the muscular physiologic pump of the upper arm (Caillet, 1981). It is characterized by deep, burning pain in the shoulder and hand, trophic changes such as changes in skin color and temperature, limitation of movement, and edema (Swan, 1954).

Trauma to shoulder joint structures can be brought on by impingement or traction. The normal scapulohumeral rhythm may be impaired by increased tone in the shoulder girdle adductors or weakness in scapular protraction. If the humerus moves actively or passively in forward flexion or abduction without adequate upward rotation of the scapula, the humerus can be blocked from full range of motion (ROM) by the acromion, which causes impingement on the supraspinatus and joint capsule; inflammation; and pain of the bursae, biceps tendon, or rotator cuff muscles (Andersen, 1985). In one study, rotator cuff injuries were found to be a frequent clinical finding in the painful hemiplegic shoulder (Najenson, Yacubovich, & Pikielni, 1971). Caillet (1981) also reported that **hemiplegia** can aggravate latent shoulder bursitis and tendinitis; arthritic conditions can also be exacerbated. Any of these painful conditions can lead to further immobility, because the patient refuses to move the shoulder, and may result in adhesive capsulitis or frozen shoulder (Wadsworth, 1986). A study in which arthrographies were performed on painful, paralyzed shoulders found capsular constriction typical of frozen shoulder in 23 of 30 hemiplegic subjects (Rizk et al., 1984).

Trauma to the shoulder caused by traction is usually the result of improper handling, positioning, or passive ROM exercises. This can occur when the hemiplegic arm is pulled on or used as a lever during transfers; when the patient rolls in bed, twisting his affected arm in an awkward position; or when a care provider exercises the affected arm without ensuring proper scapular rotation. **Unilateral neglect** has been suggested as a possible contributing factor to shoulder trauma and pain, but a prospective study was unable to establish a relationship, although pain was found to be significantly more frequent in left hemiplegics (Poulin de Courval et al., 1990). Brachial plexus injury has been reported in stroke patients, although positive identification is difficult because it is often masked by symptoms of **hemiplegia,** such as flaccidity and sensory impairment (Andersen, 1985).

Subluxation of the glenohumeral joint occurs secondary to weakness or spasticity of the scapulohumeral and/or scapular muscles (Trombly, 1989). The structure of the glenohumeral joint itself, designed for mobility rather than stability, contributes to subluxation with impairment of the support musculature. In normal shoulders the glenoid fossa is oriented upward, forward, and lateral so that the head of the humerus remains locked in contact with the fossa surface. The typical orientation of the hemiplegic glenoid fossa is downward, backward, and medial and the humerus is thus susceptible to subluxation from the pull of gravity. Subluxation may or may not be associated with pain.

Treatment of complications of the hemiplegic shoulder centers around prevention and treatment of symptoms and underlying causes to promote function. Securing an accurate history regarding previously existing injuries or conditions is necessary. Any patient with shoulder pain that persists and consistently interferes with function or progress in therapy should be referred to specialists best qualified to diagnose and treat specific shoulder problems.

Therapists must emphasize the risks of pain, contractures, and loss of function inherent in keeping the paretic limb in one position for extended periods. The combination of positioning for comfort and muscle imbalances brought on by spasticity and weakness can lead to the development of a "typical" positioning pattern for the hemiplegic upper extremity: shoulder adduction and internal rotation, elbow flexion, forearm pronation, and wrist and finger flexion. Proper arm positioning in bed as well as seated or standing should be taught from the beginning to the patient, his family, and his care providers. In a supine position, the patient's involved upper extremity should be supported behind the scapula with a small pillow or towel, the shoulder should be slightly flexed and abducted, the elbow extended or slightly flexed, the forearm in a neutral or supinated position, and the wrist in a neutral position with the hand open. When the patient is lying on the unaffected side, the scapula should be protracted with the arm forward and supported with pillows, the elbow extended or slightly flexed, the forearm and wrist in a neutral position, and the hand open. When the patient is lying on the affected side, the shoulder and arm should be forward (so that the patient is not lying on it) and externally rotated with palm up and hand open. While seated, tables, wheelchair lapboards, armrest trays, pillows, and other assistive positioning devices can be used (Andersen, 1985; Daniel & Strickland, 1992). Therapists should emphasize that such positions not only prevent contractures and possible damage to the arm but also are positions of function; the "typical" hemiplegic position of the arm, described earlier, is not useful for many (if any) activities.

Proper handling of the upper extremity during ADLs and exercise is another important aspect of treatment. The best approach is to teach the patient as early as possible to be responsible for the positioning of his arm during transfers, bed mobility, and other activities involving changes of position. Using gait belts or draw sheets to assist the patient in moving his body rather than using the affected arm as a handle will greatly reduce the risk of shoulder injury. Placement of an assistant's hand on the scapula during movement helps provide support and guidance (Andersen, 1985). The patient can also be taught techniques such as clasping both hands together and reaching forward with both arms while attempting transfers or while rolling in bed to ensure arm protection (Andersen, 1985; Bobath, 1978; Eggers, 1984; Gee & Passarella, 1985). Active and passive range of motion can lead to shoulder injury and/or pain unless care is taken that movement is done correctly. The goal of range of motion exercises and activities should be achievement or maintenance of pain-free functional range of motion rather than maximum range. Functional shoulder range of motion is defined as shoulder flexion to 100°, abduction to 90°, lateral rotation to 30°, and medial rotation to 70° (Griffin, 1986). Passive movement to which the patient is not attending has no place in the early care of the stroke patient (Carr & Shepherd, 1987).

The patient needs to concentrate on relearning movement by feeling and thinking about the movement. If performing passive ROM, the therapist should ensure proper scapulohumeral rhythm by relaxing and mobilizing the scapula before elevation of the arm and by manually assisting upward rotation of the scapula (Bobath, 1978). The humerus should be laterally rotated during abduction to prevent impingement of the supraspinatus between the greater tubercle of the humerus and the acromion process. The use of overhead pulleys as a method for self-ranging of the shoulder has been associated with the development of shoulder pain and should be avoided because neither correct scapular nor humeral rotation occurs and the force may be excessive (Kumar et al., 1990; Trombly, 1989). Better methods of teaching self-ROM involve having the patient clasp both hands together while leaning forward to reach for the floor and, with arms supported on a table, pushing both hands forward (Eggers, 1984). The advantage of these activities is that they can easily be given a functional context (such as dusting a table), and the patient is able to monitor his own pain threshold and is, therefore, less apprehensive about movement of the arm (Andersen, 1985). During active ROM of the shoulders, the therapist should encourage and assist with scapular protraction and upward rotation; placement of activities in front of the patient at or below waist level will promote these movements (Andersen, 1985).

The use of slings as a treatment measure for subluxation of the hemiplegic shoulder is controversial (Andersen, 1985). Reasons given for using slings are to reduce the subluxation of the glenohumeral joint, to provide support for the arm, to protect against trauma, and to prevent or reduce pain. Carr and Shepherd (1987) found that x-rays taken of hemiplegic shoulders in slings did not reveal significant reduction of subluxation. Bobath (1978) maintained that flexor spasticity in the upper extremity is reinforced with the use of a sling. If considering a sling, therapists should ask the following questions:

1. Does pain or edema increase when the arm is in a dependent position?
2. Is active movement or function present in the arm that would be prevented with use of a sling?
3. How is the patient's balance during standing, walking, or transfers affected by the use of or lack of a sling?
4. To provide enough support for the arm, would a sling impair circulation or cause excess pressure on the neck?
5. Will the patient or caretaker be able independently to put on and take off a sling correctly? (Andersen, 1985).

Use of other adaptive devices (listed above) for arm support may be preferred while the patient is seated; a sling could be used for some patients with painful or flaccid arms when they are standing or ambulatory.

Hand edema is a frequent complication of **hemi-plegia.** Edema control techniques include elevation of the hand, massage, and use of pressure gloves (Daniel & Strickland, 1992). Patients with minimal voluntary movement should avoid keeping the extremity in a dependent position for long periods of time. Prolonged hand edema can lead to limited passive movement, pain, and soft tissue contractures. Hand edema and pain combined with trophic changes are early signs of shoulder-hand syndrome and should be addressed vigorously to prevent further loss of functional potential (Trombly, 1989). Active, active-assistive, or passive movement should be carried out several times daily. In some instances, splints may be used to provide more functional positioning for hemiplegic hands and to prevent or correct contractures.

THERAPY TO REGAIN VOLUNTARY MOVEMENT AND FUNCTION

Therapy to regain motor control involves treatment of the positive as well as the negative symptoms (Trombly, 1989). The major neuromuscular reeducation approaches differ mainly in what is emphasized as the major neuromotor problem following brain insult (Warren, 1991). Bobath (1978) emphasized spasticity or increased muscle tone as the major deterrent to voluntary motor control in adult **hemiplegia** and her neurodevelopmental treatment (NDT) approach focuses most on inhibitory handling techniques that guide patients toward more normal patterns of movement and posture. Brunnstrom's (1970) Movement Therapy and the proprioceptive neuromuscular facilitation (PNF) approach of Knott and Voss (1968) consider instead motor weakness and decreased control as primary targets for remediation, stressing facilitory techniques to promote functional movement. The dilemma facing therapists in planning treatment is whether to take an inhibitory or facilitory approach (Warren, 1991): whether to normalize tone before eliciting voluntary motor responses (or to try to increase muscle responses first) or whether simultaneously to inhibit spasticity and elicit motor responses (Trombly, 1989). Most therapists combine techniques to address each patient's dominant movement problem without exacerbating other motor problems (Warren, 1991). Motor learning techniques and EMG biofeedback can also be used to promote voluntary movement and function.

Success in restoring voluntary movement in the hemiplegic upper extremity has been limited, perhaps due to limited knowledge about the nature and components of movement deficits after stroke (Basmajian, 1989; Parker et al., 1986; Trombly, 1992). Research that examines and measures components of movement provides new insight into the rationale behind therapy. For example, one study of 20 hemiplegic patients treated with exercise and biofeedback therapy found improved function without significant decreases in spasticity as measured by electromyography (Takebe et al., 1976).

In a literature review on agonist activation, Bourbonnais and Vanden Noven (1989) found that evidence did not support a major role for the spasticity of the antagonist in limiting the production of agonist muscle force. They theorized that the muscle dysfunction seen in hemiplegic patients with spasticity may be more a factor of restraint imposed by the passive mechanical properties of antagonist muscles and surrounding tissues and/or by inappropriate, ungraded cocontractions of antagonists. A quantitative study of the EMG activity of both agonist and antagonist forearm muscles during voluntary isometric contraction in stroke patients and control subjects found both agonist recruitment and antagonist inhibition to be impaired in the paretic forearms (Hammond et al., 1988).

The regaining of voluntary movement involves relearning movement along a continuum from involuntary motion to mass, stereotyped movement to voluntary isolated movement and to voluntary, automatic movement (Trombly, 1989). Treatment also proceeds from a level of assisted and facilitated movement to unassisted motion against gravity to reciprocal patterns and to complex adaptive patterns of movement. Regaining function of the hemiplegic upper extremity involves guiding and extending combinations of muscle action into meaningful tasks (Carr & Shepherd, 1987).

Motor learning research supports the use of activity-based intervention to improve the performance of stroke patients (Sabari, 1991). Patients should repeat desired motor patterns in a manner that maintains their alertness and motivation, i.e., using a variety of modalities and activities. Repeating tasks that are uninteresting or nonfunctional will result in fast, imprecise, and improper motor control (Bach-y-Rita & Balliet, 1987). It is important to promote functional use of the involved upper extremity early and consistently, because a gap usually exists between moving and doing. Typical hemiplegic upper extremity synergy patterning cannot be used for function in the manner that lower extremity patterns can be used for ambulation (Savinelli et al., 1978).

Patients tend to have difficulty translating their limited upper extremity movement into functional use; they will report that their arm is "dead" or "useless," despite sufficient arm movement for simple activities. Movement may return spontaneously, but it appears that function or purposeful use of the arm is enhanced with therapeutic intervention and practice. In a comparative clinical study, Taub et al. (1993) concluded that motor ability in stroke patients can be significantly improved by interventions aimed at overcoming learned nonuse. In this experiment, the unaffected upper extremities of chronic stroke patients were restrained in slings during waking hours for two weeks. This group also received therapy during this time that encouraged intensive practice of functional movements with the impaired arm. A comparison group received procedures designed to encourage use of the impaired arm, but without practice and without restraint of the unimpaired arm. The restraint subjects showed greater improvement on measurements of motor function than the control group and showed carryover of improvement to life tasks and maintenance of gains during a 2-year follow-up period.

Therapists should review the wide range of possible functions of the upper extremity to best select activities patients can succeed in. In normal function, the hand performs mainly as a prehensile tool while the arm places the hand in a wide variety of different and precise positions (Savinelli et al., 1978). Bard, Hirschberg, and Tolleson (1964) proposed a classification of useful function of the upper extremity, including (1) nonmanipulatory activities, (2) prehension activities, and (3) skilled individual finger movements such as typing. Nonmanipulatory activities, in which the movements occur in the arm, forearm, and trunk, can be incorporated into functional activities by stroke patients who have limited movement or no voluntary hand movement.

Relatively little literature exists that describes the results of treatment designed specifically to increase function of the hemiplegic hand. Typical problems preventing function in the hemiplegic hand include

1. Spasticity and muscle tone imbalance;
2. Decreased wrist control or stabilization;
3. Limited finger extension for preparation for grasp and for release;
4. Decreased thumb extension, abduction, and opposition;
5. Lack of individual finger movement;
6. Absent or weak intrinsic muscle power;
7. Loss of sensation.

While various methods to improve hand movement have not been shown conclusively to improve hand function in studies of groups of stroke patients (Trombly & Quintana, 1985; Trombly et al., 1986), the use of specific neurophysiological and biomechanical techniques have been observed to benefit individual patients (Woodson, 1987). Findings in a study using a joint movement tracking test, force tracking test, and EMG monitoring on 16 spastic hemiparetic patients suggest that careful manual stretch of finger flexors of the hemiparetic hand can be used to increase controlled active finger extension movement (Carey, 1990).

The use of splinting for the hemiplegic hand has generated much discussion and investigation, but there exists no consensus regarding the rationales for splinting or not splinting the hemiplegic hand (Neuhaus et al., 1981). Rationales cited for the use of orthotics for the hemiplegic hand include

1. A biomechanical approach, which suggests using orthotics as a means of preventing deformity and achieving proper positioning of the hand (Caldwell et al., 1969);
2. A neurophysiological approach, which looks at using orthoses to promote better balance of muscle tone in the involved extremity (Bobath, 1978; Charait, 1969; Doubilet & Polkow, 1977; McPherson, 1981; McPherson et al., 1982; Snook, 1979);
3. A combination of these (Neuhaus et al., 1981).

Little has been written on the use of orthotics to allow or enhance directly functional movement of the hemiplegic hand. Functional goals for splinting the hemiplegic hand could include the following.

1. To provide prolonged, preferred (facilitory or inhibitory) positioning, e.g., mild stretch on wrist and finger flexors, such as provided by a static hand splint, has been suggested as leading to decreased flexor tone and increased active extension (McPherson, 1981; Snook, 1979)
2. To substitute for or stabilize a weak component to achieve or improve prehension; a dorsal or volar wrist splint can be used to provide stability, improve grasp, and promote increased hand use for those patients who have active finger movement but limited wrist extension.
3. To help train in a correct pattern or movement, because in attempting to accomplish a task, hemiplegics will frequently use incorrect, unnecessary or excessive motor patterns (Carr & Shepherd, 1987); a dorsal extension splint for the thumb interphalangeal joint, e.g., will prevent excessive flexion and help the patient achieve and relearn a more precise and efficient pad-to-pad pinch.

Therapists select appropriate activities for improving hemiparetic arm function after determining each patient's specific movement abilities and disabilities and determining the possible role of the involved arm in ADL tasks. For example, patient A, who tests at level 4 of the *Functional Test for the Hemiplegic/ Paretic Upper Extremity,* can actively flex his shoulder 60°, flex his elbow 100°, has a gross grasp of 3 lb, and a weak lateral pinch of 0.5 lb. He has minimal elbow, wrist, and finger extension and weak shoulder lateral rotation and forearm supination. He has the functional problems of limited range of reach; difficulty maintaining a functional position; difficulty performing reciprocal movements; and poor prehension ability because of lack of wrist stability, minimal finger extension

(reach and release), and limited pinch prehension. Daily living tasks that are difficult because of his upper extremity **hemiparesis** include lower extremity dressing, clothing fasteners, and opening containers.

Patient A has the ability to perform nonmanipulatory activities with his involved arm and is encouraged in these activities to promote use of his involved arm. Examples of these activities include arm placement and weight bearing for balance, weighting of objects on a work surface such as stabilizing a paper while writing with the uninvolved hand, using a shoulder adduction clamp by which an object is held between the adducted upper arm and the trunk, using a forearm hook by which the elbow is kept at 90° of flexion to hold an object such as a bag, using a finger hook by which the fingers are flexed to form a hook to hold a cane or bag, and push and pull activities for which the fixed hand is used to push and pull objects such as when wiping a table with a cloth (Bard et al., 1964).

Prehension activities that patient A can attempt include supportive activities (holding onto a walker or rail), stabilizing activities (holding a jar while opening with uninvolved hand, pinching one side of trousers while closing or opening the zipper), and transportive activities (moving an object from one place to another, such as bringing a cracker to the mouth). To increase his ADL independence, patient A can be guided to begin using his involved hand to hold onto a grab bar for support, to help pull up and push down pants, or to assist the uninvolved hand in reaching for and putting on socks. These treatment activities would incorporate this patient's abilities to use his hemiparetic arm while promoting improvement in deficient areas (increasing range of reach or placement, strengthening elbow extension and lateral pinch, etc.).

STRENGTH, ENDURANCE, AND COORDINATION

Strengthening of weak muscles is traditionally not emphasized in the regaining of motor control in stroke patients because of the observation that increased effort leads to increased spasticity in hemiparetic muscles, which is, therefore, assumed to decrease functional performance (Bobath, 1978). Resisted exercise for spastic or overactive muscles without equivalent strengthening of their antagonists is thought to reinforce the disabling muscular imbalance (Carr & Shepherd, 1987). Studies using objective measures of movement components, however, indicate that therapists should more carefully consider conditions in which paretic muscles can be strengthened to help rather than hurt the patient (Bourbonnais & Vanden Noven, 1989). Trombly and Quintana (1985) found in EMG studies of hemiplegic hands that resisted grasp recruited maximum percentages of output from the flexors but also recruited the antagonistic extensors. More studies are needed to determine the effectiveness of specific clinical strengthening methods in rehabilitating stroke patients.

Because decreased physical and mental endurance can limit participation and performance in therapy, treatment should be carefully graded to compensate for and improve reduced endurance. Length of treatment sessions and need for rest periods should be monitored to meet patients' needs. To avoid fatigue in therapy, the patient may be required to perform only critical elements of a task, and the therapist could assist with setup and completion of the task (Warren, 1991). For example, the patient may be able to put a shirt on but be too tired to complete buttoning. As he improves in skill and endurance, he would be required to perform more steps of the task. Energy requirements increase with activities that demand unsupported sitting, standing, and mobility.

Coordinated movement is the product of successful control of the strength, range, speed, direction, and timing of movement. Because almost all purposeful activity involves coordination, encouraging use of the affected extremities in self-care tasks or leisure activities is an appropriate way to improve coordination. Treatment should progress from unilateral activities, in which the patient can concentrate fully on control of his hemiparetic arm, to bilateral simultaneous activities, in which both arms perform the same movement together (such as lifting and carrying a box and catching and throwing a large ball), to bilateral alternating activities, in which both arms perform different movements at the same time (such as sorting and assembling nuts and bolts). Grading fine motor activities involves progressing from gross to precise manipulation tasks and attempting more difficult patterns of grasp and pinch. Because hand control for hemiplegic patients becomes more difficult as the arm moves away from the body, the placement of activities should be varied. Writing is a highly coordinated task that is frequently a goal for stroke patients who need to at least be able to sign documents. Writing training may be necessary if a patient plans to use his hemiparetic hand or needs to use his noninvolved nondominant hand.

Treatment to Improve Learning Ability

Because occupational therapists are primarily involved in the teaching of skills, they must address the learning process to help patients improve performance in daily living skills (Gentile, 1987). Learning to dress, e.g., involves performing the task effectively and efficiently in a variety of circumstances or contexts (Carr & Shepherd, 1987). In this approach, therapists can best assist hemiplegic patients by imparting problem-solving techniques and by helping them develop their own effective movement strategies to deal with objects and structures in their environment (Sabari, 1991). Some of the areas of focus to improve learning ability include **motor planning**; visual-perceptual and cognitive performance; and emotional adjustment.

MOTOR PLANNING

Motor planning deficits are serious learning disorders and are some of the most difficult aspects of stroke rehabilitation (Duncan & Badke, 1987). Because of the complexity of this impairment, the emphasis of treatment should be on teaching compensatory skills rather than on remediation (Warren, 1991). Suggestions for treatment include breaking down the motor task into basic steps, explaining clearly the components of a task, and having the patient practice the steps (Duncan & Badke, 1987). Begin with one-step tasks and gradually increase the number of steps required. Language can play a facilitory role in planning movement; it assists in the sequencing of actions required for a task, helps focus concentration, and reduces perseveration (Warren, 1991). Therapists can help patients use language to facilitate **motor planning** by having them verbalize what they are going to do in step-by-step fashion and then describe what they have done so that they can identify mistakes (Warren, 1991), e.g. "I have taken the cap off the toothpaste. Now I need to pick up my toothbrush and put toothpaste on it." Therapists should instruct in the style that will best facilitate a patient's individual learning ability (Warren, 1991). With aphasic patients, e.g., minimize the use of words and focus more on visual or kinesthetic cues to help them relearn a task.

Relearning is also facilitated by creating, as closely as possible, the functional context or routine for the motor activity (Warren, 1991). In a clinical setting, therapists frequently require patients to perform familiar tasks in unfamiliar surroundings using unfamiliar objects and unfamiliar motor techniques. For example, learning to get into a bathtub by transferring from a wheelchair to a tub bench in a large, accessible bathroom may be safer and preferable in many cases, but it will not necessarily be easy for a patient to learn. The fact that many stroke patients fail to achieve independence in self-care activities during an inpatient stay but perform better than predicted after they return home may be an indication of the importance of a familiar environment and routine for relearning tasks. The relearning of a specific motor component of an activity is often enhanced by the use of an appropriate object to give the movement a recognizable goal. Placing a cup in a patient's hand may result in better hand-to-mouth movement than when the movement is done without the cup.

VISUAL-PERCEPTUAL AND COGNITIVE DEFICITS

Much has been written about the visual-perceptual and cognitive deficits that follow stroke, and hypotheses have been made concerning the underlying mechanisms. Chapters 26 and 27 cover these areas in detail. Relatively little research has examined the effectiveness of treatment for these problems (Abreu & Toglia, 1987; Herman, 1992; Neistadt, 1990; Warren, 1993b). Results of a study (Weinberg et al., 1977) suggest that visual-perceptual deficits must be confronted and patients educated for treatment to be effective. Sharing results of objective evaluations with the patient and family, giving feedback on the effects of visual or cognitive deficits on functional performance, and teaching patients to recognize and correct errors in performance have been suggested for increasing a patient's awareness of his deficits (Warren, 1993b).

The study by Weinberg et al. (1977) compared the performance of two groups of right CVA patients who had visual neglect. The experimental group received a specific training program designed to increase visual scanning to the left, the control group received standard rehabilitation, including daily occupational therapy. After 1 month, both groups were retested with a battery of reading-related tasks. The group that received training showed much more improvement than the control group. The visual-scanning training program used anchoring (providing a cue such as a line on the left, or impaired side, to indicate starting position), decreased the density of stimuli (facilitating response by increasing the distance between targets), paced the patient's tracking pattern (to slow down the tendency of gaze to pull to the right), and provided feedback on performance (Weinberg et al., 1977). Patients should be reminded to use compensatory motor techniques such as moving their eyes, turning their head and neck, or adjusting posture to better search their environment. Therapists can manipulate environments by placing conspicuous stimuli in neglected space and decreasing distractions from the favored side. If a task cannot be performed at all in the neglected space, it may be attempted in a central space, then gradually moved to the left (Herman, 1992).

To ensure transfer of training skills for improving visual and cognitive functioning, Toglia (1991) recommended a multicontext treatment approach of practicing strategies in multiple environments with varied tasks and movement demands. Therapists can provide a stronger learning event by reinforcing visual-perceptual and cognitive experience with sensorimotor experience, such as combining a visual searching task with touching the targets (Warren, 1993b). Weinberg et al. (1979) found in a comparative study that a training program

in tactile sensory awareness and spatial organization combined with training in scanning and academic skills yielded better results than a traditional treatment program provided to a control group. They concluded that layered treatment produces greater generalization than a single treatment.

A study of the transfer of training effects for visual inattention using single-case studies of five right brain damage stroke patients found a significant positive effect of visual-scanning training on visual-scanning behavior. This effect, however, appeared to be restricted to the task that was specifically trained (e.g., reading); no evidence could be found in this sample for any transfer of training effects to the domain of gross motor skills (e.g., wheelchair navigation) (Wagenaar et al., 1992). To extend training beyond the confined space required for paper-and-pencil tasks, computer activities, or reading activities, therapists should attempt to broaden the visual-scanning field as much as possible. Use of blackboards, pegboards, and large tabletop games require a patient to turn his head or change body positions to accomplish a task, thus reinforcing these compensatory skills for use in extrapersonal space for activities such as locating food items on a shelf and home and community mobility (Warren, 1993b).

EMOTIONAL ADJUSTMENT

Emotional lability is common poststroke (Fordyce, 1971). The patient may cry, laugh, or express anger out of proportion to events in the external environment. He and his family need to be reassured that lability is a symptom of the stroke and that control will improve with time (Carr & Shepherd, 1987). The therapist can instruct the patient in techniques such as deep breathing or redirecting attention to help him modify his behavior (Carr & Shepherd, 1987).

It may be unproductive to expect compliance to treatment instructions when patients and their families are coping poorly with the losses associated with stroke (Evans et al., 1992). The hemiplegic patient and his family need assistance in making a healthy emotional adjustment. Methods include providing support and encouraging those involved to verbalize their ongoing reactions to hospitalization, lifestyle changes, changes in body image, and disease progression (Daniel & Strickland, 1992; see also Chapter 20). Patients and families are often frustrated because they lack important information or have unrealistic expectations regarding stroke. Therapists should reinforce the efforts of the rehabilitation team and assist patients and families in their comprehension of the progression and prognosis of stroke (Daniel & Strickland, 1992).

Methods to reintegrate the patient into his community should be explored (transportation options, architectural barriers, assistance from family or friends, access to senior citizen centers, etc.), because failure to resume premorbid social activities has been significantly correlated with depression in stroke patients (Feibel & Springer, 1982). Investigation and promotion of leisure skills, home management, or volunteer community roles should be considered for stroke survivors who must face loss of employment.

EFFECTIVENESS OF THERAPY

No definitive study has established the effects of specific therapeutic procedures on improving the function of poststroke patients. This may partly be the result of the heterogeneous nature of stroke survivors and the diverse and profound impairments secondary to stroke. Applying rigid, stereotyped therapies to such a varied population cannot help but have dubious results (Basmajian & Gowland, 1987).

Some studies have reported the effects of rehabilitation in general on stroke patients. Logigian et al. (1983) compared traditional (biomechanical and rehabilitative) and facilitation (neurodevelopmental) approaches with therapeutic exercise in occupational and physical therapy programs for stroke patients and found them equally beneficial in terms of gains in functional independence and muscle strength. Dickstein et al. (1986) also compared traditional therapy that included exercise and functional activities (biomechanical and rehabilitative approaches) with PNF and NDT in 131 patients over a 6-week period. Improvement was noted in ADL performance and ambulation nondifferentially across groups. Little to no improvement was seen in wrist or ankle dorsiflexion strength or range of motion across all treatment groups, and extremity muscle tone increased in all three groups. Similarly, Jongbloed, Stacey, and Brighton (1989) found no statistically significant differences between two treatment groups receiving either a functional treatment approach or a sensorimotor integrative treatment approach when assessed at specified intervals for function in self-care and mobility, meal preparation, and sensorimotor integration.

Lord and Hall (1986) compared long-term effectiveness of traditional functional retraining with neuromuscular retraining techniques in poststroke patients. Two groups of patients were matched according to early prognostic indicators; in one group neuromuscular retraining techniques were emphasized and in the other group treatment was restricted to traditional functional retraining. Unlike previous studies, this study evaluated rehabilitation outcome as long-term function within a home or nursing home environment instead of function at the time of discharge from a rehabilitation unit. At least 8 months post-CVA, patients and/or families completed a telephone questionnaire regarding current functional abilities. No statistically significant differences in skill levels were found, with the exception of slightly greater independence in self-feeding in the neuromuscular-retraining group. Rehabilitation hospitalization was noted to be significantly longer in the neuromuscular-retraining group (68.3 versus 28.57 days)

A quantitative review of studies on the effectiveness of rehabilitation therapy for patients who have suffered a CVA indicated that the average patient who received focused rehabilitation services performed at a higher level than approximately 65.5% of patients in comparison or control conditions. Although treatment effects were small, they were significantly practical in that small improvements in independent functioning can make the difference between discharge to home and institutionalization. Improvement in performance appears related to early initiation of rehabilitation treatment (Ottenbacher & Jannell, 1993).

One difficulty in determining treatment effectiveness in the stroke population is the wide range of combinations of functional deficits and the inability to single out specific variables when analyzing the effects of treatment. A suggested method of research to determine treatment effectiveness in the heterogeneous stroke population is the single-case experimental design, in which measurements are taken frequently and treatments alternated as indicated within individual patient programs. In this way, it is argued, a better perspective can be gained on both the relative effectiveness of treatment methods and the different patterns of functional recovery (Wagenaar et al., 1992).

STUDY QUESTIONS

1. What are the subtypes of stroke and their causes?
2. Describe the predicted course of return of motor function in stroke patients.
3. What factors influence recovery of functional performance in stroke survivors?
4. What should occupational therapists evaluate in every stroke patient?
5. How do somatosensory deficits impact movement and occupational performance?
6. What are the mechanical and physiological components of movement that should be evaluated in the stroke patient?
7. What variables should be considered when evaluating for voluntary movement in the hemiplegic patient?
8. What factors can affect a stroke patient's ability to learn and organize movement? Describe how a deficit in each of these factors would impair the performance of functional tasks.
9. Name six occupational therapy goals for poststroke patients and describe how they all can

STUDY QUESTIONS (continued) ——————

be addressed while performing a daily living task such as dressing.
10. What methods can be used to prevent development of a painful hemiplegic shoulder?

REFERENCES

Abreu, B. C., & Toglia, J. (1987). Cognitive rehabilitation: A model for occupational therapy. *The American Journal of Occupational Therapy, 41*, 439–448.

Andersen, L. T. (1985). Shoulder pain in hemiplegia. *American Journal of Occupational Therapy, 9*, 11–19.

Anderson, E. K. (1971). Sensory impairments in hemiplegia. *Archives of Physical Medicine and Rehabilitation, 52*, 293–297.

Andrews, K., Brocklehurst, J. C., Richards, B., & Laycock, P. J. (1984). The influence of age on the clinical presentation and outcome of stroke. *International Rehabilitation Medicine, 6*, 49–53.

Bach-y-Rita, P. (1981). Brain plasticity and rehabilitation in hemiplegia. *Scandinavian Journal of Rehabilitation Medicine, 13*, 73–83.

Bach-y-Rita, P., & Balliet, R. (1987). Recovery from stroke. In P. W. Duncan & M. B. Badke (Eds.), *Stroke rehabilitation: The recovery of motor control* (pp. 79–107). Chicago: Year Book.

Bannister, R. (1973). *Brain's clinical neurology* (4th ed.). New York: Oxford University Press.

Bard, G., Hirschberg, G. G., & Tolleson, G. C. B. (1964). Functional testing of the hemiplegic arm. *Journal of American Physical Therapy Association, 44*(12), 1081–1086.

Barer, D. H. (1989). Continence after stroke: Useful predictor or goal of therapy? *Age Aging, 18*, 183–191.

Basmajian, J. (1989). The winter of our discontent: Breaking intolerable time locks for stroke survivors. *Archives of Physical Medicine and Rehabilitation, 70*, 92–94.

Basmajian, J. V., & Gowland, C. (1987). The many hidden faces of stroke: A call for action [Commentary]. *Archives of Physical Medicine and Rehabilitation, 68*, 319.

Bell, E., Jurek, K., & Wilson, T. (1976). Hand skill measurement: A gauge for treatment. *American Journal of Occupational Therapy, 30*, 80–86.

Biller, J. (1992). Medical management of acute cerebral ischemia. *Neurologic Clinics, 10*, 63–85.

Black-Schaffer, R. M., & Osberg, J. S. (1990). Return to work after stroke: Development of a predictive model. *Archives of Physical Medicine and Rehabilitation, 71*, 285–290.

Bobath, B. (1978). *Adult hemiplegia: Evaluation and treatment* (2nd ed.). London: William Heinemann Medical Books.

Bogousslavsky, J., & Pierre, P. (1992). Ischemic stroke in patients under age 45. *Neurologic Clinics, 10*, 113–124.

Bohannon, R. W. (1987). Relationship between static strength and various other measures in hemiparetic stroke patients. *International Rehabilitation Medicine, 8*, 125–128.

Bohannon, R. W., & Andrews, A. W. (1990). Shoulder subluxation and pain in stroke patients. *American Journal of Occupational Therapy, 44*, 506–509.

Bohannon, R. W., & LeFort, A. (1986). Hemiplegic shoulder pain measured with the Ritchie Articular Index. *International Rehabilitation Medicine, 9*, 379–381.

Bohannon, R. W., & Smith, M. B. (1987). Assessment of strength deficits in eight paretic upper extremity muscle groups of stroke patients with hemiplegia, *Physical Therapy, 67*, 522–525.

Bornstein, R. A. (1986). Normative data on inter manual differences on three tests of motor performance. *Journal of Clinical and Experimental Neuropsychology, 8*, 12–20.

Bourbonnais, D., & Vanden Noven, S. (1989). Weakness in patients with hemiparesis. *American Journal of Occupational Therapy, 43*, 313–319.

Bouska, M. J., Kauffman, N. A., & Marcus, S. E. (1990). Disorders of the visual perceptual system. In D. A. Umphred (Ed.), *Neurological rehabilitation* (pp. 552–585). St. Louis: C. V. Mosby.

Brodal, A. (1973). Self-observations and neuroanatomical considerations after stroke. *Brain, 96*, 675–694.

Brunnstrom, S. (1970). *Movement therapy in hemiplegia*. New York: Harper & Row.

Caillet, R. (1981). *The shoulder in hemiplegia*. Philadelphia: F. A. Davis.

Caldwell, C. B., Wilson, D. J., & Braun, R. M. (1969). Evaluation and treatment of the upper extremity in the hemiplegic stroke patient. *Clinical Orthopedics and Related Research, 63*, 69–93.

Callahan, A. (1990). Sensibility testing: Clinical methods. In J. M. Hunter, L. H. Schneider, E. J. Mackin, & A. D. Callahan (Eds.), *Rehabilitation of the hand: Surgery and therapy* (3rd ed., pp. 594–610). St. Louis: C. V. Mosby.

Campbell, A., Brown, A., Scheldroth, C., Hastings, A., Ford-Booker, P., Lewis-Jack, O., Adams, C., Gadling, A., Ellis, R., Wood, D., Dennis, G., Adeshoye, A., Weir, R., & Coffey, G. (1991). The relationship between neuropsychological measures and self-care skills in patients with cerebrovascular lesions. *Journal of the National Medical Association, 83*, 321–324.

Caplan, L. R. (1991). Diagnosis and treatment of ischemic stroke. *Journal of the American Medical Association, 266*, 2413–2418.

Caplan, L. R., & Stein, R. W. (1986). *Stroke—A clinical approach*. Stoneham, MA: Butterworth.

Carey, J. R. (1990). Manual stretch: Effect on finger movement control and force control in stroke subjects with spastic extrinsic finger flexor muscles. *Archives of Physical Medicine and Rehabilitation, 71*, 888–894.

Carr, J. H., & Shepherd, R. B. (1987). *A motor relearning programme for stroke* (2nd ed.). Rockville, MD: Aspen Systems.

Charait, S. E. (1969). A comparison of volar and dorsal splinting of the hemiplegic hand. *American Journal of Occupational Therapy, 22*, 319–321.

Chollet, M., DiPiero, V., Wise, R. J. S., Brooks, D. J., Dolan, R. J., & Frackowiak, R. S. J. (1991). The functional anatomy of motor recovery after stroke in humans: A study with positron emission tomography. *Annals of Neurology, 29*, 63–71.

Collen, F. J., & Wade, D. T. (1991). Residual mobility problems after stroke. *International Disability Studies, 13*, 12–15.

Cool, S. J. (1987). Occupational therapy and functional optometry: An interaction whose time has come. *Sensory Integration Special Interest Section Newsletter, 10*, 1–5.

Czyrny, J. J., Hamilton, B. B., & Gresham, G. E. (1990). Rehabilitation of the stroke patient. *Advances in Clinical Rehabilitation, 3*, 64–96.

Daniel, M. S., & Strickland, L. R. (1992). *Occupational therapy protocol management in adult physical dysfunction*. Rockville, MD: Aspen Systems.

Dannenbaum, R. M., & Dykes, R. W. (1988). Sensory loss in the hand after sensory stroke: Therapeutic rationale. *Archives of Physical Medicine and Rehabilitation, 69*, 833–39.

Davidoff, G. N., Keren, O., Ring, H., & Solzi, P. (1991). Acute stroke patients: Long-term effects of rehabilitation and maintenance of gains. *Archives of Physical Medicine and Rehabilitation, 72*, 869–873.

Dellon, A. (1981). *Evaluation of sensibility and re-education of sensation in the hand*. Baltimore: Williams & Wilkins.

Denes, G., Semenza, C., Stoppa, E., & Lis, A. (1982). Unilateral spatial neglect and recovery from hemiplegia. *Brain, 105,* 543–552.

DeSouza, L. H., Langton Hewer, R. L., & Miller S. (1980). Assessment of recovery of arm control in hemiplegic stroke patients. I: Arm function tests. *International Rehabilitation Medicine, 2,* 3–9.

DeWeerdt, W. J. G., & Harrison, M. A. (1985). Measuring recovery of arm-hand function in stroke patients: A comparison of the Brunnstrom-Fugl-Meyer Test and the Action Research Arm Test. *Physiotherapy Canada, 37,* 65–70.

Dickstein, R., Hocherman, S., Pillar, T., & Shaham, R. (1986). Stroke rehabilitation: Three exercise therapy approaches. *Physical Therapy, 66,* 1233–1238.

Diller, L., & Weinberg, J. (1970). Evidence for accident-prone behavior in hemiplegic patients. *Archives of Physical Medicine and Rehabilitation, 51,* 358–363.

Doubilet, L., & Polkow, L. S. (1977). Theory and design of a finger abduction splint for the spastic hand. *American Journal of Occupational Therapy, 31,* 320–322.

Duncan, P. W., & Badke, M. B. (1987). Therapeutic strategies for rehabilitation of motor deficits. In P. W. Duncan, & M. B. Badke (Eds.), *Stroke rehabilitation: The recovery of motor control* (pp. 161–197). Chicago: Year Book.

Duncan, P. W., Propst, M., & Nelson, S. G. (1983). Reliability of the Fugl-Meyer assessment of sensorimotor recovery following cerebrovascular accident. *Physical Therapy, 63,* 1606–1610.

Edmans, J. E., & Lincoln, N. B. (1987). The frequency of perceptual deficits after stroke and their relation to functional abilities. *Journal of Clinical Rehabilitation, 1,* 273–281.

Eggers, O. (1984). *Occupational therapy in treatment of adult hemiplegia.* London: William Heinemann Medical Books.

Evans, R. L., Bishop, D. S., & Matlock, A. L. (1987). Pre-stroke family interaction as a predictor of stroke outcome. *Archives of Physical Medicine and Rehabilitation, 68,* 508–512.

Evans, R. L., Hendricks, R. D., Haselkorn, J. K., Bishop, D. S., & Baldwin, D. (1992). The family's role in stroke rehabilitation. *American Journal of Physical Medicine and Rehabilitation, 71,* 135–139.

Feibel, J. H., & Springer, C. J. (1982). Depression and failure to resume social activities after stroke. *Archives of Physical Medicine and Rehabilitation, 63,* 276–278.

Filiatrault, J., Arsenault, A. B., Dutil, E., & Bourbonnais, D. (1991). Motor function and activities of daily living assessments: A study of three tests for persons with hemiplegia. *American Journal of Occupational Therapy, 45,* 806–810.

Fisher, C. M. (1992). Concerning the mechanism of recovery in stroke hemiplegia. *Canadian Journal of Neurological Sciences, 19,* 57–63.

Fordyce, W. (1971). Psychological assessment and management. In F. H. Krusen, F. J. Kottke, & P. M. Ellwood (Eds.), *Handbook of physical medicine and rehabilitation* (2nd ed.). Philadelphia: W. B. Saunders.

Fugl-Meyer, A. R., & Jääskö, L. (1980). Post-stroke hemiplegia and sexual intercourse. *Scandinavian Journal of Rehabilitation Medicine, 7,* 158–166.

Fugl-Meyer, A. R., Jääskö, L., Leyman, I., Olsson, S., & Steglind, S. (1975). The post-stroke hemiplegic patient. I. A method for evaluation of physical performance. *Scandinavian Journal of Rehabilitation Medicine, 7,* 13–31.

Galski, T., Bruno, R. L., & Ehle, H. T. (1992). Driving after cerebral damage: A model with implications for evaluation. *The American Journal of Occupational Therapy, 46,* 324–332.

Gee, Z. L., & Passarella, P. M. (1985). *Nursing care of the stroke patient: A therapeutic approach.* Pittsburgh: AREN Publications.

Gentile, A. M. (1987). Skill acquisition: Action, movement, and neuromotor processes. In J. H. Carr, R. B. Shepherd, J. Gordon,

A. M. Gentile, & J. M. Held (Eds.), *Movement science: Foundations for physical therapy in rehabilitation* (pp. 93–154). Rockville, MD: Aspen Systems.

Gianutsos, R., Ramsey, R., & Perlin, R. (1988). Rehabilitative optometric services for survivors of acquired brain injury. *Archives of Physical Medicine and Rehabilitation, 69,* 573–578.

Gilfoyle, E. M., Grady, A. P., & Moore, J. C. (1981). *Children adapt.* Thorofare, NJ: Slack.

Goodglass, H., & Kaplan, E. (1983). *The assessment of aphasia and related disorders* (2nd ed.). Philadelphia: Lea & Febiger.

Granger, C. V., Hamilton, B. B., & Fiedler, R. C. (1992). Discharge outcome after stroke rehabilitation. *Stroke, 23,* 978–982.

Gresham, G. E., Phillips., T. F., Wolf, P. A., McNamara, P. M., Kannel, W. B., & Dawber, T. R. (1979). Epidemiologic profile of long-term stroke disability: The Framingham study. *Archives of Physical Medicine and Rehabilitation, 60,* 487–491.

Griffin, J., (1986). Hemiplegic shoulder pain. *Physical Therapy, 66,* 1884–1893.

Griffin, J., & Reddin, G. (1981). Shoulder pain in patients with hemiplegia. *Physical Therapy, 61,* 1041–1045.

Halligan, P. W., Marshall, J. C., & Wade D. T. (1989). Visuospatial neglect: Underlying factors and test sensitivity. *Lancet, 2,* 908–911.

Halper, A. S., & Mogil, S. I. (1986). Communication disorders: Diagnosis and treatment. In P. E. Kaplan, & L. J. Derullo (Eds.), *Stroke rehabilitation* (pp. 233–252). Stoneham, MA: Butterworth.

Hammond, M. D., Fitts, S. S., Kraft, G. H., Nutter, P. B., Trotter, M. J., & Robinson, L. M. (1988). Co-contraction in the hemiparetic forearm: Quantitative EMG evaluation. *Archives of Physical Medicine and Rehabilitation, 69,* 348–351.

Harris, F. A. (1978). Facilitation techniques in therapeutic exercise. In J. V. Basmajian (Ed.), *Therapeutic Exercise* (pp. 93–137). Baltimore: Williams & Wilkins.

Heller, A., Wade, D. T., Wood, V. A., Sunderland, A., Langton Hewer, R., & Ward, E. (1987). Arm function after stroke: Measurement and recovery over the first three months. *Journal of Neurology, Neurosurgery and Psychiatry, 50,* 714–719.

Herman, E. W. M. (1992). Spatial neglect: New issues and their implication for occupational therapy practice. *The American Journal of Occupational Therapy, 46,* 207–216.

Isaacs, B. (1982). The continuing needs of stroke patients. In F. C. Rose (Ed.), *Advances in stroke therapy* (pp. 305–312). New York: Raven Press.

Jebsen, R. H., Griffith, E. R., Long, E. W., & Fowler, R. (1971). Function of normal hand in stroke patients. *Archives of Physical Medicine and Rehabilitation, 52,* 170–174.

Jones, R. D., Donaldson, M., & Parkin, P. J. (1989). Impairment and recovery of ipsilateral sensory-motor function following unilateral cerebral infarction. *Brain, 112,* 113–132.

Jones, R., Giddens, H., & Croft, D. (1983). Assessment and training of brain-damaged drivers. *American Journal of Occupational Therapy, 37,* 754–760.

Jongbloed, L. (1986). Prediction of function after stroke: A critical review. *Stroke, 17,* 765–776.

Jongbloed, L., & Morgan, D. (1991). An investigation of involvement in leisure activities after a stroke. *American Journal of Occupational Therapy, 45,* 420–427.

Jongbloed, L., Stacey, S., & Brighton, C. (1989). Stroke rehabilitation: Sensorimotor integrative treatment versus functional treatment. *American Journal of Occupational Therapy, 43,* 391–397.

Kaufman, S. R., & Becker, G. (1991). Content and boundaries of medicine in long-term care: Physicians talk about stroke. *The Gerontologist, 31,* 238–245.

Kelley, R. E. (1989). Cerebrovascular disease. In W. J. Weiner,

& C. G. Goetz (Eds.), *Neurology for the non-neurologist* (2nd ed., pp. 52–66). Philadelphia: J. B. Lippincott.

Knott, M., & Voss, D.E. (1968). *Proprioceptive neuromuscular facilitation: Patterns and techniques* (2nd ed.). New York: Harper & Row.

Kosecoff, J., Kahn, K. L., Rodgers, W. H., Reinisch, E. J., Sherwood, M. J., Rubenstein, C. V., Draper, D., Roth, C. P., Chew, L., & Brook, R. H. (1990). Prospective payment system and impairment at discharge: The quicker and sicker story revisited. *Journal of the American Medical Association, 264,* 1980–1983.

Kumar, R., Metter, E. J., Mehta, A. J., & Chew, T. (1990). Shoulder pain in hemiplegia: The role of exercise. *American Journal of Physical Medicine and Rehabilitation, 69,* 205–208.

Labi, M. L., Phillips, C., & Gresham, G. E. (1980). Psychosocial disability in physically restored long-term stroke survivors. *Archives of Physical Medicine and Rehabilitation, 61,* 561–565.

Langton Hewer, R. (1990). Rehabilitation after stroke. *Quarterly Journal of Medicine, 76,* 659–674.

Legh-Smith, J., Wade D. T., & Langton Hewer, R. (1986). Driving after a stroke. *Journal of the Royal Society of Medicine, 79,* 200–203.

Leo, K. C., & Soderberg, G. L. (1981). Relationship between perception of joint position sense and limb synergies in patient with hemiplegia. *Physical Therapy, 61,* 1433–1437.

Levine, R. L. (1987). Diagnostic, medical and surgical aspects of stroke management. In P. W. Duncan, & M. B. Badke (Eds.), *Stroke rehabilitation: The recovery of motor control* (pp. 1–42). Chicago: Year Book.

Licht, S. (1975). *Stroke and its rehabilitation.* Baltimore: Waverly Press, Inc.

Lincoln, N. B., Jackson, J. M., Edmans, J. A., Walker, M. F., Farrow, V. M., Latham, A., & Coombes, K. (1990). The accuracy of predictions about progress of patients on a stroke unit. *Journal of Neurology, Neurosurgery and Psychiatry, 53,* 972–975.

Lings, S., & Jensen, P. B. (1991). Driving after stroke: A controlled laboratory investigation. *International Disability Studies, 13,* 74–82.

Logigian, M. K., Samuels, M. A., Falconer, J., & Zagar, R. (1983). Clinical exercise trial for stroke patients. *Archives of Physical Medicine and Rehabilitation, 64,* 364–367.

Lord, J. P., & Hall, K. (1986). Neuromuscular re-education versus traditional programs for stroke rehabilitation. *Archives of Physical Medicine and Rehabilitation, 67,* 88–91.

Lyle, R. C. (1981). A performance test for assessment of upper limb function in physical rehabilitation treatment and research. *International Journal of Rehabilitation Research, 4,* 483–492.

Mayo, N. E., Korner-Bitensky, N. A., & Becker. R. (1991). Recovery time of independent function post-stroke. *American Journal of Physical Medicine and Rehabilitation, 70,* 5–12.

McPherson, J. J. (1981). Objective evaluation of a splint designed to reduce hypertonicity. *American Journal of Occupational Therapy, 35,* 189–194.

McPherson, J. J., Kreimeyer, D., Aalderks, M., & Gallagher, T. (1982). A comparison of dorsal and volar resting hand splints in the reduction of hypertonus. *American Journal of Occupational Therapy, 36,* 664–670.

Mills, V. M., & DiGenio, M. (1983). Functional differences in patients with left or right cerebrovascular accidents. *Physical Therapy, 63,* 481–488.

Moberg, E. (1958). Objective methods for determining the functional value of sensibility in the hand. *Journal of Bone and Joint Surgery, 40,* 454–459.

Moore, J. C. (1986). Recovery potentials following CNS lesions: A brief historical perspective in relation to modern research data on neuroplasticity. *American Journal of Occupational Therapy, 40,* 459–463.

Moore, J. C. (1992, November). *Evaluation and treatment of visual dysfunction associated with head trauma.* Paper presented at a workshop sponsored by the Rehabilitation Institute, Kansas City, MO.

Najenson, T., Yacubovich, E., & Pikielni, S. (1971). Rotator cuff injury in shoulder joints of hemiplegic patients. *Scandinavian Journal of Rehabilitation Medicine, 3,* 131–137.

Neistadt, M. E. (1990). A critical analysis of occupational therapy approaches for perceptual deficits in adults with brain injury. *American Journal of Occupational Therapy, 44,* 299–304.

Neistadt, M. E. (1992). Occupational therapy treatment for constructional deficits. *American Journal of Occupational Therapy, 46,* 141–148.

Neuhaus, B. E., Ascher, E. R., Coullon, B. A., Donohue, M. V., Einbond, A., Glover, J. M., Goldberg, S. R., & Takai, V. L. (1981). A survey of rationales for and against hand splinting in hemiplegia. *American Journal of Occupational Therapy, 35,* 83–90.

Osmon, D. C., Smet, I. C., Wingarden, B., & Gandhavadi, B. (1992). Neurobehavioral cognitive status examination: Its use with unilateral stroke patients in a rehabilitation setting. *Archives of Physical Medicine and Rehabilitation, 73,* 414–418.

Ostfeld, A. M., & Wilk, E. (1990). Epidemiology of stroke, 1980-1990: A progress report. *Epidemiologic Reviews, 12,* 253–256.

Ottenbacher, K. J., & Jannell, S. (1993). The results of clinical trials in stroke rehabilitation research. *Archives of Neurology, 50,* 37–44.

Parker, V. M., Wade, D. T., & Langton Hewer, R. (1986). Loss of arm function after stroke: Measurement, frequency & recovery. *International Rehabilitation Medicine, 8,* 69–83.

Poulin de Courval, L., Barsauskas, A., Berenbaum, B., Dehaut, F., Dussault, R., Fontaine, F. S., Labrecque, R., Leclerc, C., & Giroux, F. (1990). Painful shoulder in the hemiplegic and unilateral neglect. *Archives of Physical Medicine and Rehabilitation, 71,* 673–676.

Prevost, R., Arsenault, A. B., Dutil, E., & Drouin, G. (1987). Shoulder subluxation in hemiplegia. A radiologic correlational study. *Archives of Physical Medicine and Rehabilitation, 68,* 782–785.

Reding, M. J., & Potes, E. (1988). Rehabilitation outcome following initial unilateral hemispheric stroke: Life table analysis approach. *Stroke, 19,* 1354–1358.

Rizk, T. E., Christopher, R. P., Pinals, R. S., Salazar, J. E., & Higgins, C. (1984). Arthrographic studies in painful hemiplegic shoulders. *Archives of Physical Medicine and Rehabilitation, 65,* 254–256.

Robinson, R. G., & Price, T. R. (1982). Post-stroke depression disorders: A follow-up study of 103 patients. *Stroke, 13,* 635–641.

Rolak, L. A., & Rokey, R. (1990). *Coronary and cerebral vascular disease: A practical guide to management of patient with atherosclerotic vascular disease of the heart and brain.* Mount Kisco, NY: Futura.

Roper, N. (1978). *New American pocket medical dictionary.* New York: Churchill Livingstone.

Roy, C. W. (1988). Shoulder pain in hemiplegia: A literature review. *Clinical Rehabilitation, 2,* 35–44.

Sabari, J. S. (1991). Motor learning concepts applied to activity-based intervention with adults with hemiplegia. *American Journal of Occupational Therapy, 45,* 523–530.

Savinelli, R., Timm, M., Montgomery, J., & Wilson, D. J. (1978). Therapy evaluation and management of patients with hemiplegia. *Clinical Orthopaedics and Related Research, 131,* 15–29.

Schuchmann, J. A. (1983). Stroke rehabilitation: Minimizing the functional deficits. *Postgraduate Medicine, 74*, 101–111.

Simon, R. P., Aminoff, M. J., & Greenberg, D. A. (1989). *Clinical Neurology*. Norwalk, CT: Appleton and Lange.

Sine, R. D., Holcomb, J. D., Roush, R. E., Liss, S. E., & Wilson, G. B. (1981). *Basic rehabilitation techniques: A self-instructional guide* (2nd ed.). Rockville, MD: Aspen Systems.

Snook, J. H. (1979). Spasticity reduction splint. *American Journal of Occupational Therapy, 33*, 96–101.

Spaulding, S. J., McPherson, J. J., Strachota, E., Kuphal, M, & Ramponi, M. (1988). Jebsen hand function test: Performance of the uninvolved hand in hemiplegia and of right-handed, right and left hemiplegic persons. *Archives of Physical Medicine and Rehabilitation, 69*, 419–422.

Stern, R. A., & Bachman, D. L. (1991). Depressive symptoms following stroke. *American Journal of Psychiatry, 148*, 351–356.

Stone, S. P., Wilson, B., Wroot, A., Halligan, P. W., Lange, L. S., Marshall, J. C., & Greenwood, R. J. (1991). The assessment of visuo-spatial neglect after acute stroke. *Journal of Neurology, Neurosurgery and Psychiatry, 54*, 345–350.

Swan, D. M. (1954). Shoulder-hand syndrome following hemiplegia. *Neurology, 4*, 480–482.

Takebe, K., Kukulka, C. G., Narayan, M. G., & Basmajian, J. V. (1976). Biofeedback treatment of foot drop after stroke compared with standard rehabilitation techniques (part 2): Effects on nerve conduction velocity and spasticity. *Archives of Physical Medicine and Rehabilitation, 57*, 9–11.

Tangeman, P. T., Banaitis, D. A., & Williams, A. K. (1990). Rehabilitation of chronic stroke patients: Changes in functional performance. *Archives of Physical Medicine and Rehabilitation, 71*, 876–880.

Taub, E., Miller, N. E., Novack, T. A., Cook, E. W., Fleming, W. C., Nepomuceno, C. S., Connell, J. S., & Crago, J. E. (1993). Technique to improve chronic motor deficit after stroke. *Archives of Physical Medicine and Rehabilitation, 74*, 347–354.

Toglia, J. P. (1991). Generalization of treatment: A multicontext approach to cognitive perceptual impairment in adults with brain injury. *American Journal of Occupational Therapy, 45*, 505–516.

Toole, J. (1990). *Cerebrovascular disorders* (4th ed.). New York: Raven Press.

Trombly, C. A. (1989). Stroke. In C. A. Trombly (Ed.), *Occupational therapy for physical dysfunction* (3rd ed., pp. 454–471). Baltimore: Williams & Wilkins.

Trombly, C. A. (1992). Deficits of reaching in subjects with left hemiparesis: A pilot study. *American Journal of Occupational Therapy, 46*, 887–897.

Trombly, C. A., & Quintana, L. A. (1985). Differences in response to exercise by post-CVA and normal subjects. *American Journal of Occupational Therapy, 5*, 39–58.

Trombly, C. A., Thayer-Nason, L., Bliss, G., Girard, C. A., Lyrist, L. A., & Brexa-Hooson, A. (1986). The effectiveness of therapy in improving finger extension in stroke patients. *American Journal of Occupational Therapy, 40*, 612–617.

Twitchell, T. E. (1951). The restoration of motor function following hemiplegia in man. *Brain, 74*, 443–480.

U.S. Department of Health and Human Services. (1990). Functional status of noninstitutional elderly: Estimates of A.D.L. & I.A.D.L. difficulties, NMES research findings 4 (DHHS publication no. PHS 90-3462). Washington, DC: U.S. Government Printing Office.

Van Sant, A. F. (1991). Should the normal motor developmental sequence be used as a theoretical model to progress adult patients? In M. J. Lister (Ed.), *Contemporary management of motor control problems: Proceedings of the II Step Conference* (pp. 95–97). Alexandria, VA: Foundation for Physical Therapy.

Wade, D. T. (1989). Measuring arm impairment and disability after stroke. *International Disability Studies, 11*, 89–92.

Wade, D. T. (1992). Stroke: Rehabilitation and long term care. *Lancet, 339*, 791–793.

Wade, D. T., & Langton Hewer, R. (1987). Functional ability after stroke: Measurement, natural history and prognosis. *Journal of Neurology, Neurosurgery and Psychiatry, 50*, 177–182.

Wade, D. T., Langton Hewer, R., & Wood, V. A. (1984). Stroke: Influence of patient's sex and side of weakness on outcome. *Archives of Physical Medicine and Rehabilitation, 65*, 513–516.

Wade, D. T., Langton Hewer, R., Wood, V. A., Skilbeck, C. E., & Ismail, H. M. (1983). The hemiplegic arm after stroke: Measurement & recovery. *Journal of Neurology, Neurosurgery and Psychiatry, 46*, 521–524.

Wadsworth, C. T. (1986). Frozen shoulder. *Physical Therapy, 66*, 1878–1883.

Wagenaar, R. C., VanWieringen, P. C. W., Nelelenbos, J. B., Meijer, O. G., & Kuik, D. J. (1992). The transfer of scanning training effect in visual inattention after stroke: Five single-case studies. *Disability and Rehabilitation, 14*, 51–60.

Walker, M. F., & Lincoln, N. B. (1990). Reacquisition of dressing skills after stroke. *International Disability Studies, 12*, 41–43.

Walker, M. F., & Lincoln, N. B. (1991). Factors influencing dressing performance after stroke. *Journal of Neurology, Neurosurgery and Psychiatry, 54*, 699–701.

Warren, M. (1984). A comparative study on the presence of the asymmetrical tonic neck reflex in adult hemiplegia. *The American Journal of Occupational Therapy, 38*, 386–392.

Warren, M. (1990). A developmental treatment approach for adults with postural dysfunction. *Occupational Therapy Practice, 1*, 53–62.

Warren, M. (1991). Strategies for sensory and neuromotor remediation. In C. Christensen, & C. Baum (Eds.), *Occupational therapy—Overcoming human performance deficits* (pp. 632–662). Thorofare, NJ: Slack.

Warren, M. (1993a). A hierarchical model for evaluation and treatment of visual perceptual dysfunction in adult acquired brain injury, Part 1. *The American Journal of Occupational Therapy, 47*, 42–54.

Warren, M. (1993b). A hierarchical model for evaluation and treatment of visual perceptual dysfunction in adult acquired brain injury, Part 2. *The American Journal of Occupational Therapy, 47*, 55–66.

Weinberg, J., Diller, L., Gordon, W. A., Gerstmann, L. J., Leiberman, A., Lakin, P., Hodges, G., & Ezrachi, O. (1977). Visual scanning training effect on reading-related tasks in acquired right brain damage. *Archives of Physical Medicine and Rehabilitation, 58*, 479–486.

Weinberg, J., Diller, L., Gordon, W. A., Gerstmann, L. J., Leiberman, A., Lakin, P., Hodges, G., & Ezrachi, O. (1979). Training sensory awareness and spatial organization in people with right brain damage. *Archives of Physical Medicine and Rehabilitation, 60*, 491–496.

Weisbroth, S., Esibill, N., & Zuger, R. R. (1971). Factors in the vocational success of hemiplegic patients. *Archives of Physical Medicine and Rehabilitation, 52*, 441–446.

Wilson, D. B., Houle, D. M., & Keith, R. A. (1991). Stroke rehabilitation: A model predicting return home. *Western Journal of Medicine, 154*, 587–590.

Wilson, D. J., Baker, L. L., & Craddock, J. A. (1984a). Functional test for the hemiparetic upper extremity. *The American Journal of Occupational Therapy, 38*, 159–164.

Wilson, D. J., Baker, L. L., & Craddock, J. A. (1984b). *Protocol—Functional Test for the Hemiplegic/Paretic Upper Extremity*. Unpublished manuscript. County Rehabilitation Center, Rancho Los Amigos, Occupational Therapy Department, Downey, CA.

Woodson, A. M. (1987). Proposal for splinting the adult hemiplegic hand to promote function. *Occupational Therapy in Health Care, 4,* 85–96.

Yekutiel, M., & Guttman, E. A. (1993). A controlled trial of the retraining of the sensory function of the hand in stroke patients. *Journal of Neurology, Neurosurgery and Psychiatry, 56,* 241–244.

35

Traumatic Brain Injury

Anna Deane Scott and Patricia Weber Dow

OBJECTIVES

After studying this chapter the student will be able to:
1. Describe a diffuse axonal injury and explain its clinical consequences.
2. Describe the two common focal lesions and differentiate their clinical consequences.
3. Explain the precautions associated with care of the comatose brain-injured patient in the intensive care unit.
4. Describe the process of evaluation of the comatose patient as conducted by the occupational therapist.
5. Explain the rationale for the goals of occupational therapy intervention at each level of return to cognitive awareness.

The rehabilitation of individuals who have sustained a traumatic brain injury requires an understanding of normal brain function and information about the nature of brain injury and the most vulnerable structures. An appreciation of the particular characteristics of the patient in the context of his familial and social environment is important in understanding that head injury is a unique experience for each individual. In addition, it is necessary to be aware of successful intervention strategies for recovery of function to select the most appropriate strategy for each case. As stated in the Preface to this book, prerequisite knowledge of neuroanatomy and neurophysiology is assumed. Information regarding normal function will be presented only as necessary for understanding problems and intervention strategies.

The incidence of traumatic brain injury has steadily increased over the years. The National Institute of Neurological and Communicative Disorders and Stroke (1984) reported more than 400,000 new head-injured people admitted to hospitals each year in the United States. Literature from the National Head Injury Foundation (1993) estimated the number of head injuries to be closer to 2 million per year. This number includes

the 100,000 who die from the initial injury, the large number of pediatric head-injury cases that are generally seen in the emergency room and sent home (Kalsbeek et al., 1980), and the many adults and children who sustain "minor" injuries. Males are twice as likely as females to incur traumatic brain injuries; the highest risk age group is the 15- to 29-year-olds (Gordon, Mann, & Willer, 1993; Rimel, Jane, & Bond, 1990). Although trauma is the cause of brain injury as well as the cause of spinal cord injury, brain injury as a result of trauma is 40 times more likely to occur than spinal cord injury (Kalsbeek et al., 1980). The major causes of traumatic brain injury, in descending order of frequency, are motor vehicle accidents, violence (including gunshot wounds and assaults), falls or being hit by falling debris, and pedestrian accidents (Gordon et al., 1993). Although surveys and studies vary in results, they generally indicate that over half of the traumatic brain injury patients admitted to emergency rooms were intoxicated at the time of injury (Gordon et al., 1993). Patients who were intoxicated when injured had a longer period of hospitalization, an increased duration of agitation, and a lower cognitive status at the time of discharge than those patients who were not intoxicated (Sparadeo & Gill, 1989). Risk-taking behavior is associated with traumatic injury. The majority of patients in one traumatic brain-injury database were unprotected by seat belts or helmets and/or were intoxicated at the time of injury (Gordon et al., 1993). Improved emergency medical treatment has increased the survival rate of persons with severe traumatic brain injuries from 10 to approximately 50% (Lillehei & Hoff, 1985). The increase in survival rates challenges therapists and the medical team to rehabilitate severely injured patients to the fullest possible degree.

MECHANISMS OF INJURY

A traumatic brain injury is usually caused by a dynamic loading or impact to the head from direct

GLOSSARY —————————————————————

Border zone—An area of the brain where arteries meet. It is vulnerable to reduced blood supply.

Diplopia—Double vision.

Dysmetria—A condition seen in cerebellar disorders in which the patient overshoots a target because of an inability to control movement.

Hematoma—A mass of blood confined in an organ or space, caused by a broken blood vessel.

Infarction—A loss of blood supply to tissue, which results in death of the tissue.

Orbital surface—The brain surface located just above the orbits of the eyes.

Transcortical aphasia—A language disorder related to a deficit in the transmission of language between receptive and expressive language areas of the cerebral cortex. Signs of transcortical sensory aphasia are decreased auditory comprehension with good repetition and spontaneous speech production, although it is incomprehensible. Signs of transcortical motor aphasia are good comprehension and repetition, but poor spontaneous speech production.

blows or from sudden movements produced by impacts to other body parts. This loading can result in any combination of compression, expansion, acceleration, deceleration, and rotation of the brain inside the skull (Bakay & Glasauer, 1980).

The type of damage is directly related to the cause and severity of the injury (Katz, 1992). Brain injuries may be diffuse, focal, or both. Motor vehicle accidents and falls involve acceleration and deceleration with rotation of the brain inside the skull. The brainstem is more stable than the cerebrum, which rotates around the brainstem during impact. The rotation places a stretch or shear force on the long axons that transmit information throughout the brain and brainstem (Leech & Shuman, 1982). These injuries are termed diffuse axonal injuries (DAI) and result in coma because of the damage to the axons in the midbrain reticular activating system. Focal lesions involve contusions or lacerations of the brain. Although focal lesions can occur anywhere beneath the impact, they are usually seen at the anterior poles and inferior surfaces of the frontal and temporal lobes and are caused when the brain hits against the skull and scrapes over the irregular bony structures at these locations (Katz, 1992). The occipital and parietal lobes, which have smooth surfaces, are less likely to incur damage. The folds of the dural membranes (especially the falx cerebri and the tentorium) can also cause damage to the brainstem, the medial aspect of the occipital lobe, and the superior surface of the cerebellum (Bakay & Glasauer, 1980).

Cranial nerves can be torn, stretched, or contused. The olfactory nerve (I) is often abraded or torn when the frontal lobes scrape across the **orbital surface** of the skull (Leech & Shuman, 1982). The optic nerve (II) may be damaged directly, or vision can be compromised by injury to the eye, the optic tracts, or the visual cortex (Brandstater et al., 1991). Cranial nerves III, IV, and VI, which control eye movements, are all vulnerable to injury (Brandstater et al., 1991; Leech & Shuman, 1982). The oculomotor nerve (III) is stretched when edema, bleeding, or a tumor expands

the contents of the skull, causing the uncus of the temporal lobe to herniate into the foramen magnum and compress the brainstem (Leech & Shuman, 1982). The abducens (VI) is very long and consequently vulnerable to injury. The facial (VII) and vestibulocochlear (VIII) nerves may be damaged when there are fractures of the temporal bone at the base of the skull (Brandstater et al., 1991; Leech & Shuman, 1982). Cranial nerves V, IX, X, XI, and XII are rarely damaged (Leech & Shuman, 1982).

The skull may fracture from the force of the impact in the area of or at a distance from the actual impact site. The type of fracture depends on the force of the blow and can be linear; stellate; or depressed, which is common and is the result of a forceful blow. The patient with a brain injury from a motor vehicle accident or a fall may have other systemic trauma, such as fractures of the extremities, shoulder girdle, pelvis, or face; cervical fractures with possible spinal cord injury; abdominal trauma; and pneumothorax or other chest cavity trauma.

Secondary effects of the traumatic brain injury can occur immediately or develop within hours or days (Jennett & Teasdale, 1981). Trauma can abolish or disrupt autoregulation of cerebral blood flow, the blood-brain barrier, and vasomotor functions resulting in disordered cerebral energy metabolism, intracranial hypotension, cerebral vasospasm, and increases in intracranial pressure (ICP) and in cerebral edema (Jennett & Teasdale, 1981; Miller, 1985). Other secondary effects of brain trauma include intracranial hemorrhage, ischemic brain damage, uncal herniation resulting in brainstem compression, general systemic reactions to the neural impairment, electrolyte abnormalities, altered respiratory regulation, intracranial infection, and abnormal autonomic nervous system responses (Lillehei & Hoff, 1985; Miller, 1985). Usually by the time the patient is stabilized and occupational therapy ordered, the secondary effects of brain trauma are already present and will influence the patient's ability to respond to therapy.

Hypoxia or anoxia, a reduction or lack of oxygen,

is another cause of brain injury. Anoxic deficits are usually related to cardiovascular or respiratory dysfunction or to cardiac arrest. Brain injury from anoxia produces diffuse loss of cortical neurons with involvement of areas particularly susceptible to lack of oxygen, such as the hippocampus and basal ganglia (Katz, 1992).

CLINICAL SIGNIFICANCE OF INJURY

The consequences of head injury should be differentiated from the outcome following a stroke. A stroke is the result of the blockage of or bleeding from a particular artery that distributes blood to a certain area of the brain and/or brainstem. Brain damage as a consequence of a stroke is limited to the particular cortical area supplied by that artery. Strokes also vary in location and extent of deficit but generally affect one hemisphere with a resultant contralateral hemiplegia that is predictable to some extent. In traumatic brain injury there are many possible areas of damage and consequent impairments. In focal lesions to the lateral side of one hemisphere, the residual problems can be similar to those poststroke and are appropriately evaluated and treated by procedures designed for stroke rehabilitation. In other focal lesions and in diffuse injuries, the residual impairments are very different from those seen in stroke and their distribution cannot be predicted.

The impairments resulting from traumatic brain injury are indeed unpredictable and each individual outcome is unique. The areas of the brain that are most vulnerable to injury were described above, and there is the greatest likelihood that traumatic brain injury will cause damage at those locations. Consequently, therapists need to be aware of the behavioral outcomes associated with diffuse axonal injuries, focal lesions, and anoxia.

Diffuse axonal injuries result in coma, which may quickly reverse if the axonal damage was mild or may continue as a persistent vegetative state if axons were ruptured. Recovery from coma progresses to a period of confusion with impaired attention and anterograde amnesia. When confusion clears, the cognitive impairments are more evident and include diminished mental-processing speed and efficiency as well as difficulty with divided-attention tasks (those that require the patient to respond simultaneously to two different sources of information). There is a reduced capacity for higher-level cognitive functions, including abstract reasoning, planning, and problem solving. Typical behavioral outcomes include impulsivity, irritability, and exaggerated premorbid traits. Sometimes, however, apathy and poor initiative dominate the personality and behavior (Katz, 1992). Diffuse injuries often include

damage to the brainstem and cerebellar pathways, resulting in ataxia, **diplopia,** and dysarthria (Trexler & Zappala, 1988). Once recovery from the diffuse injury progresses, it is easier to identify the result of focal lesions, although impairments related to frontal lobe functions may be a result of both diffuse and focal damage (Katz, 1992).

Focal lesions to the prefrontal and anterior temporal areas interrupt connections to subcortical limbic structures and affect modulation of memory, emotion, and drive (Katz, 1992). Damage to the orbitofrontal areas results in impulsivity that is greater than with diffuse damage, but there are no motor impairments of the extremities or of speech (Trexler & Zappala, 1988). These focal lesions do not affect sensorimotor abilities, praxis, language. or perception (Katz, 1992). Damage to the frontolateral cortex results in hemiparesis as well as impulsivity. Frontolateral lesions result in the most significant attentional impairments. There is decreased accuracy and decreased mental flexibility, which affects the quality of performance (Trexler & Zappala, 1988).

The clinical consequences of anoxic brain damage include dementia and visual agnosia from damage to cortical neurons, persistent amnesia from hippocampal involvement, tone and movement disorders from damage to the basal ganglia, proximal weakness, and **transcortical aphasia** secondary to **infarction** of the vascular **border zone** territory (Horn, 1991; Katz, 1992). Both age and duration of coma have a significant influence on outcome following anoxic brain damage. A study of outcomes for 32 patients with anoxic damage found better outcomes in those who were 25 years or younger and were in coma less than 24 hr. The functional gains achieved in rehabilitation occurred in the first 4 months after the anoxic event (Groswasser, Cohen, & Costeff, 1989). In contrast, after traumatic brain injury, patients 45 years or younger in coma as long as 1 week have the potential for a good recovery and gains in function continue for years after the injury (Katz, 1992).

EARLY CARE AND TREATMENT

Once the severely brain-injured patient is brought to an emergency room, several measures are taken immediately. An adequate airway, if not present, must be established through intubation or tracheostomy. Assisted ventilation may be required. The extent of extracranial injuries, such as fractures, abdominal trauma, and pneumothorax, is assessed. A neurologist or neurosurgeon will evaluate the patient to determine the level of consciousness, severity and extent of the injury, and the presence of intracranial **hematomas.** Computerized tomography (CT) scanning, cerebral angiography, and/or skull x-rays may be used to determine presence of **hematomas** and indications for immediate craniotomy to evacuate a **hematoma** (Miller, Pentland, & Berrol, 1990).

Intensive Care Unit

Following emergency assessment and stabilization, the comatose brain-injured patient is usually taken to the intensive care unit (ICU). The patient will typically then undergo diagnostic procedures; continued monitoring; treatment of systemic and cerebral function; and monitoring of nutrition, fluid, and electrolyte balance in an attempt to minimize the secondary results of the head injury (Jennett & Teasdale, 1981). Diagnostic procedures may include an electroencephalogram, visual-, auditory-, and somatosensory-evoked potentials to analyze cerebral function; measurement of cerebral blood flow; and biochemical analyses (Jennett & Teasdale, 1981; Newlon & Greenberg, 1984). The cardiorespiratory system may be monitored and assisted via frequent vital sign checks, arterial lines, heart monitors, or a ventilator. The intracranial pressure (ICP) can be monitored with a subarachnoid bolt or an intraventricular catheter. Furthermore, a urinary catheter, a nasogastric (n/g) tube for nutrition and medication, and various intravenous (i.v.) lines for medications and management may be used.

The therapist working in ICU should become familiar with this equipment and with the medications used in treatment to control systemic injuries, ICP, spasticity, and seizures. Therapy and patient movement may be limited by the medical paraphernalia, and the patient's response may be affected by the drugs.

Early intervention is crucial to address tone, positioning, stimulation, and the family's concerns. Clinical studies support early, aggressive rehabilitation in the ICU as effective in improving long-term outcome for severely head-injured patients (Cowley et al., 1994; Mackay et al., 1992).

Precautions

The brain-injured patient may be referred for occupational therapy before he is completely medically stable. Because of systemic injuries, secondary effects of the brain injury itself, disturbance of basic body regulatory systems, and the life-support equipment used to treat the patient, precautions may be numerous and must be heeded by the therapist. Typical precautions are described below; other precautions may also be necessary and should be ascertained from the nurse, physician, or patient's chart before initiation of the evaluation.

If less than 1 month has passed since the injury,

the therapist must be alert to drastic systemic changes in the patient in response to stimulation (McGraw & Tindall, 1974; Parsons, Peard, & Page, 1985). A major concern with acute brain trauma is control of intracranial pressure. Sustained increased ICP can be fatal (Jennett & Teasdale, 1981). The patient with an ICP monitor can be readily checked during treatment sessions. The therapist must closely observe patients not on a monitor for pupil changes; decreased neurologic responses; abnormal brainstem reflexes; flaccidity; behavioral changes; vomiting; and changes in pulse rate, blood pressure, and respiration rate. Fluids may be restricted or the patient's head may be positioned in neutral at 30° elevation in an attempt to regulate his ICP (Turner, 1985). Turning the patient's head to one side may obstruct the internal jugular vein and result in a sudden increase of ICP (Boortz-Marx, 1985; Parsons et al., 1985). The neck should be neither flexed nor extended but kept in neutral for maximum venous drainage and decreased ICP. The presence of a family member, gentle touching, quiet talking, and stroking the face have been found to decrease ICP in adults (Mitchell, 1986). Side lying is the most desirable position with the head of the bed elevated. Side lying avoids the increased extensor tone promoted in supine. The prone position is contraindicated with increased ICP, the high Fowler's position of supported sitting at 90° is used as soon as tolerated to help breathing, to provide symmetrical body alignment, and to increase awareness of surroundings (Palmer & Wyness, 1988).

Early posttraumatic epilepsy occurs in 5% of patients with brain injuries, and late-onset epilepsy in 20% of those with prolonged unconsciousness, depressed skull fracture, or intracranial **hematoma** (Jennett & Teasdale, 1981; Schaffer, Kranzler, & Siqueira, 1985). To reduce the chance of a seizure occurring during treatment, tactile stimulation and range of motion are begun slowly to assess the patient's physiological response. His heart rate, blood pressure, and facial color are monitored as well as any autonomic changes such as sudden perspiration or increased restlessness. As the therapist becomes more familiar with the patient's responses, intensity of stimulation is gradually increased. Use seizure precautions by avoiding rapid, repetitive stimuli such as vibration, flickering lights, and an oscillating fan. If a seizure does occur, the therapist should ensure that the airway is open, position the patient on his side to prevent aspiration of stomach contents, and summon medical assistance (Greenberg, Aminoff, & Simon, 1993). The patient's limbs should not be restrained during a seizure.

If the patient has had a craniotomy for evacuation of a **hematoma,** the bone flap may be left off, and the brain may be covered only by scalp to allow the brain to expand. Direct pressure to this site must be avoided.

The patient may have a tear in the dura with subsequent cerebrospinal fluid leak. In this case, the patient initially is treated by head elevation, antibiotics, and precautions against nose blowing (Jennett & Teasdale, 1981; Schaffer et al., 1985).

If the patient has other systemic trauma, such as fractures or chest cavity trauma, appropriate precautions must be taken when stimulating or moving him. Care must also be taken to avoid disturbing i.v. lines, the tracheostomy, the n/g tube, endotracheal or respirator tubes, and traction for extremity fractures. If the patient has an n/g tube, caution must be taken that the patient's head remains above the level of his stomach to avoid regurgitation and aspiration (Miller et al., 1990).

Coma

A brain-injured person may exhibit any of a number of states of altered consciousness, depending on the severity of the injury. Consciousness, unconsciousness, and coma are best viewed on a continuum from complete consciousness to death or complete absence of consciousness. It is important to realize that coma is not a stable state. A person in a coma can fluctuate spontaneously or from stimulation along the continuum toward, and indeed into, varying levels of consciousness. Complete consciousness, the first level, is defined as an awareness, a cognition of self and the surrounding environment; consciousness implies perception, interpretation of this perception, and an appropriate response (Miller & McIntyre, 1984). Such consciousness is a function of an intact cortex. A lesser type of consciousness, arousal, is a state of wakefulness and attention to the environment on primarily a survival, or basic-function, level. Arousal is governed by the ascending reticular activating system (RAS) and may occur despite complete destruction of cerebral hemispheres. The next level on the continuum, clouding of consciousness, is a state of reduced wakefulness, reduced clarity of thought with possible confusion, decreased attention span, and memory lapses. The following stage, stupor, involves unresponsiveness from which the person is aroused only by vigorous stimulation. In the comatose stage, the person cannot be aroused by sensory stimulation, has his eyes closed, and demonstrates an absence of observable interaction with the environment (Plum & Posner, 1972). Coma results from interruption of communication from the RAS to the cerebral hemispheres. It is possible for a person to function in a vegetative state but without consciousness, i.e., the deeper brainstem structures that regulate breathing, reflexes, and heart rate are intact, but the cortex is completely impaired (Bakay & Glasauer, 1980).

COMA SCALES

Various scales have been proposed to facilitate consistent description of coma among the members of the medical team and between research centers, to assess the depth of coma and the inferred severity of the head injury, to monitor and delineate change in the patient's condition, and to predict the patient's eventual outcome as early as possible (Jennett & Teasdale, 1981; Salcman, Schepp, & Ducker, 1981; Stanczak et al., 1984). The most widely used scale is the *Glasgow Coma Scale* (GCS) (Table 35.1), which assesses the following parameters: eye opening in response to a variety of stimuli, best motor response to pressure on the fingernail bed and to supraorbital pressure, and best verbal response. The *Maryland Coma Scale* and the *Comprehensive Level of Consciousness Scale* include such additional areas as eye movements and eye position at rest, brainstem reflexes, posturing and more detailed motor responsiveness, orientation, and intensity of stimulation necessary to elicit motor and verbal responses (Salcman et al., 1981; Stanczak et al., 1984).

Another scale for assessing a patient's level of consciousness or cognitive functioning, developed by Rancho Los Amigos Hospital (Table 35.2), describes levels of a comatose patient's reaction to stimuli or the environment (Malkmus, Booth, & Kodimer, 1980).

MOTOR RESPONSES TO STIMULATION WHILE IN COMA

Patients in the very deepest level of coma will show no observable change in behavior, no movement, no muscle tone changes, and no eye opening in response to auditory, tactile, proprioceptive, or painful stimulation. Such stimulation consists of voices of the

Table 35.1. Glasgow Coma Scale

Eye opening (E)	Spontaneous	4
	To speech	3
	To pain	2
	Nil	1
Best motor response (M)	Obeys	6
	Localizes	5
	Withdraws	4
	Abnormal flexion	3
	Extensor response	2
	Nil	1
Verbal response (V)	Oriented	5
	Confused conversation	4
	Inappropriate words	3
	Incomprehensible sounds	2
	Nil	1
Coma score = (E + M + V) = 3 to 15		

Table 35.2. Rancho Level of Cognitive Functioning Scale

Level I	No response: unresponsive to stimuli
Level II	Generalized response: nonspecific, inconsistent, and nonpurposeful reaction to stimuli
Level III	Localized response: response directly related to type of stimulus but still inconsistent and delayed
Level IV	Confused-agitated: response heightened, severely confused and could be aggressive
Level V	Confused-inappropriate: some response to simple commands, but confusion with more complex commands; high level of distractibility
Level VI	Confused-appropriate: response more goal directed, but cues are necessary
Level VII	Automatic-appropriate: response robot-like, judgment and problem solving lacking
Level VIII	Purposeful-appropriate: response adequate, subtle impairments persist

family, loud noises, touch on the body or face, being moved, and pressure on the fingernail bed or sternum. The motor response will be flaccid. No reflexive movement will be produced either, with the possible exception of purely spinal cord–level reflexes. No pupillary reactions will be present. The damage producing this lack of response is thought to be below the vestibular nuclei in the brainstem, i.e., the pontomedullary area (Davis & Cunningham, 1984).

In the next higher level of coma, the patient responds to internal or external stimulation such as loud noises, painful stimulation, or quick position changes with a generalized motor reflex known as decerebrate rigidity, or extensor posturing. The patient's hips and shoulders extend, adduct, and internally rotate; knees and elbows extend; the forearm hyperpronates; the wrist and fingers flex; the feet plantarflex and invert; the trunk extends; and the head retracts, sometimes exhibiting opisthotonos (Plum & Posner, 1972). This motor pattern is thought to be caused by damage in the upper midbrain and the lower pons (Davis & Cunningham, 1984), sparing the vestibular nuclei; in effect, removing the lower pontine structures from more rostral neural influences (Miller & McIntyre, 1984). Pupillary reactivity and oculovestibular reflexes may or may not be present (Davis & Cunningham, 1984). Spinal-level reflexes and lower brainstem reflexes, such as the asymmetrical tonic neck reflex (ATNR), the tonic labyrinthine reflex (TLR), and the positive supporting reaction, might be seen in their entirety or might simply be influencing the patient's muscle tone (Carr & Shepherd, 1980). The vestibular reflexes are usually operable and assist in the production of increased tone in antigravity (extensor) muscles. The grasp and sucking reflexes may also be elicited at this stage of coma.

The third higher level of coma entails a response to stimulation known as decorticate rigidity, or flexor posturing. This stereotyped pattern of movement consists of adduction, internal rotation, and slight flexion of the shoulder; elbow flexion; forearm pronation; and wrist and finger flexion (Miller & McIntyre, 1984). The patient's lower extremities extend, adduct, and internally rotate as they do in decerebrate rigidity. If flexion of the hip, knee, and ankle is elicited by painful stimulation, this is a spinal reflex known as triple flexion, which indicates damage to the descending motor tracts (Finkelstein & Ropper, 1979). The decorticate response is thought to indicate damage in the internal capsule or cerebral hemispheres, causing an interruption in the corticospinal pathways (Griffith & Mayer, 1990; Plum & Posner, 1972). Midbrain reactions, i.e., neck and body righting reactions, may be elicited at this stage of coma for use in treatment (Carr & Shepherd, 1980).

The fourth level of motor response to stimulation is withdrawal, which includes shoulder abduction and is a more rapid movement than decorticate posturing. For example, the patient withdraws the entire limb when his hand is stimulated. The patient may also show spontaneous, nonpurposeful movement of his limbs. Withdrawal is thought to indicate some function present in the cerebral hemispheres (Griffith & Mayer, 1990).

The fifth-level motor response to stimulation is localization. At this stage, the patient may be said to be "lighter," i.e., he is still comatose, but not as deeply. His responses to stimulation are quicker and becoming more appropriate. The patient may reach over and brush the painful stimulation away, move just the part being stimulated, blink in response to strong light or visual threat, turn toward or away from auditory stimulation, and/or visually track a moving object (Brink, Imbus, & Woo-Sam, 1980). Cortical equilibrium reactions or protective extension reactions may be elicited at this stage. According to Finkelstein and Ropper (1979), limb abduction, or movement away from the body midline (present at this level), is the only movement that is always purposeful and indicates an intact connection from the cortex to that limb.

The sixth and highest level motor response of the patient to stimulation is an appropriate response, i.e., not withdrawing from all touch and stimuli but only from that which is noxious or irritating, and following simple requests or initiating purposeful activity.

The patient can demonstrate any combination of these responses, depending on which areas of the brain are damaged (Jennett & Teasdale, 1981). For example, he may exhibit decerebrate rigidity with his right limbs and localizing response with his left side. He could exhibit bilateral decerebrate posturing. He may initially evidence decorticate posturing on one side and then sink to decerebrate rigidity or flaccidity on that side, which indicates a deterioration in his condition. He may exhibit hemiplegia and have normal muscle tone on the other side.

The terms *decerebrate* and *decorticate* can be easily confused. Some physicians prefer the terms *abnormal extension* and *abnormal flexion* in response to pain (Jennett & Teasdale, 1981) or a description of the limb movement without a label.

PROGNOSIS AND OUTCOME

In recent years, as the number of patients surviving severe traumatic brain injuries has increased, research has focused on finding factors that predict the outcome of such injuries. The reasoning has been that if outcome can be predicted early in coma, expensive medical treatment or rehabilitation could be directed to patients who had the best chance for survival with fewer residual impairments, the effectiveness of medical treatment in decreasing secondary damage could be evaluated, the family could be better prepared to make informed, realistic decisions on immediate and long-term care, and society might be spared the expense of supporting severely impaired survivors (Davis & Cunningham, 1984; Jennett & Teasdale, 1981). There have been many studies that attempted to assess the predictive power of age, clinical observations (such as the GCS, pupillary reactions, and eye movements), data from a CT scan, presence of a surgical lesion, length of posttraumatic amnesia (i.e., the length of time after the accident before the return of continuous memory), presence of brainstem dysfunction, evoked potentials, increased ICP, or a combination of these factors (Braakman et al., 1980; Bricolo, Turazzi, & Feriotti, 1980; Karnaze, Weiner, & Marshall, 1985; Salcman et al., 1981).

No predictive factors have been located that can classify patients within the 1st week or so following head injury into the two categories of death and survival with 100% accuracy. There are falsely pessimistic and falsely optimistic predictions; accuracy ranges from 68 to 98% (Bricolo et al., 1980; Davis & Cunningham, 1984; Lipper et al., 1985). The GCS is useful in predicting outcome. An initial score of 8 or below that is maintained for 6 hr postinjury results in 50% mortality or survival with moderate to severe disability. The length of posttraumatic amnesia (PTA) is another frequently used predictor of outcome. PTA is the time elapsed from injury to recovery of memory for day-to-day events. A PTA of less than 1 hr relates to mild injury, 1 to 24 hr relates to moderate injury, 1 to 7 days relates to severe injury, and greater than 7 days relates to very severe injury (Bond, 1990).

Outcome scales have been developed to allow physicians to correlate "final" recovery levels to early treatment and prognostic indicators. The *Glasgow Outcome Scale* (GOS) is widely used. Its categories are death, vegetative state, severe disability (conscious but dependent), moderate disability (independent but disabled), and good recovery (able to participate in normal social life and could return to work), with 90% accurate assessment of prognosis possible at 6 months postinjury (Jennett & Teasdale, 1981). The GOS does assess some aspects of mental function as well as physical function in assigning outcome categories (Jennett et al., 1981). Some researchers feel more detailed neuropsychologic and/or social factors need to be considered in determining outcome (Hall, Cope, & Rappaport, 1985; Warren & Peck, 1984). When these factors are added, more residual disability is identified than by the GOS and improvements in levels of disability are identified more accurately (Hall et al., 1985). Addition of these factors also allows assessment of continued subtle recovery to be made beyond 6 or 12 months postinjury (Hall et al., 1985; Najenson et al., 1974).

The therapist is not required to predict, but should consider the predictive factors, listed above, when deciding on treatment goals or length of rehabilitation efforts. Cognition, personality, and motivation, all of which may substantially affect quality of survival (Jennett et al., 1981; Newlon & Greenberg, 1984), are also considered in determining treatment goals. Outcome predictions are based on groups of patients, not on individuals who may have family and character strengths that allow them to recover more completely than anticipated.

OCCUPATIONAL THERAPY EVALUATION

When evaluating a newly referred brain-injured patient, carefully note from his medical chart the areas of brain damage, other medical problems, surgical procedures, any precautions that will restrict the evaluation or future therapy, significant past medical history, and current medications. The physician's daily progress notes and the nursing notes are reviewed for the patient's current status and the procedures around which therapeutic evaluation and intervention must be scheduled.

After reviewing the chart, the therapist should talk with the patient's nurse of that day, especially if the patient is in ICU. The nurse will be an invaluable source of information about precautions, patient status and level of responsiveness, the schedule for tests and procedures, and the concerns of the patient's family. The nurse will also be crucial in therapeutic follow-through.

Next, the therapist begins observing any spontaneous patient movement. The patient's eyes may be open or closed. Most traumatic brain injury patients open their eyes spontaneously or to stimulation within the 2nd to 4th week postinjury (Bakay & Glasauer, 1980; Bricolo et al., 1980). Nonpurposeful, roving eye movements or other abnormal movements may be present. Primitive automatic responses of facial grimacing, teeth clenching and grinding, and/or rhythmic chewing may occur spontaneously or in response to stimulation (Bakay & Glasauer, 1980; Plum & Posner, 1972). Spontaneous decerebrate or decorticate posturing or patterned movements are noted. The therapist then proceeds with specific data gathering, as detailed below. During the evaluation and treatment, the therapist describes the procedures to the patient (i.e., what is being done, what movements his body will be taken through, etc.).

The evaluation may need to be done in several brief sessions because of the patient's reduced endurance, other scheduled procedures, or the therapist's decision to gather a representative sample of the patient's responses. The patient can fluctuate between levels of response during the day. He may be at a higher level in the morning and regress with fatigue, or he may evidence brief responses of higher levels scattered throughout predominantly lower-level neurologic responses. The therapist's observations may differ from those of the physicians, nurses, or other allied health team members as each discipline is assessing different aspects of the patient's responsiveness and function. In the process of recovery, not all patients will experience all the stages of recovery described below, as some may show initial responses of a higher neurologic level. Still other patients may stop at one level and plateau there indefinitely. Receptive language skills usually return before nonverbal or performance skills; the patient may be able to hear and understand more than he can demonstrate (Jennett & Teasdale, 1981). The occupational therapy evaluation components will change depending on the patient's stage of coma.

Passive and Active Range of Motion

Joint motions of the upper extremities are assessed. If the patient's tone is severely abnormal, accurate range of motion (ROM) measurements may require two therapists and/or some tone-inhibiting techniques. During passive range of motion (PROM), the therapist also begins to assess the patient's muscle tone, presence of spasticity, reactions to touch and movement, and the nature of any joint limitations discovered (Jennett & Teasdale, 1981). The therapist may discover fractures or dislocations that have not been identified previously. Heterotopic ossification

(HO), the formation of bone in soft tissue and periarticular locations, is a relatively common occurrence in severely brain-injured patients with limb spasticity who are in prolonged coma. Early clinical signs of HO are warmth, swelling, pain, and decreased joint motion. Common joints for HO, in order of frequency of involvement, are the shoulder, elbow, hip, and knee (Spielman, Genarelli, & Rogers, 1983). Range of motion exercises, positioning and splinting are used in the management of HO in addition to medications and forceful joint manipulation under anesthesia. The only precaution regarding PROM in the presence of HO is to avoid exceeding the limit of pain (Citta-Pietrolungo, Alexander, & Steg, 1992).

Sensory Awareness

The therapist assesses the patient's basic sensations by presenting the sensory stimulus and observing any motor response; decrease or change in ongoing posturing or in facial movements; a startle reaction; eye opening; or changes in heart rate, blood pressure, or respirations. The therapist checks the response from both upper extremities, the right and left sides of the face, and the upper trunk and may change the patient's position to see if the response can be altered or magnified. One interesting study described the different posturing patterns elicited from the same comatose patient, depending on the stimulus location and limb position. Initial arm flexion with a painful stimulus produced significantly higher abnormal flexion, whereas initial arm extension produced significantly higher abnormal extension (Barolat-Romana & Larson, 1984). Motor responses may be charted as appropriate, delayed, localized, generalized, abnormal posturing, absent, increased in frequency, or changed in nature secondary to stimulation.

The therapist evaluates the patient's response to pain and other stimuli. Tactile input consists of a variety of textures, touch, and rubbing. Auditory stimuli are loud bells, tapes of familiar voices, hand claps, calling the patient's name, or talking to him. Visual skills such as eye opening, blink to threat, tracking, and focus are assessed using familiar photos, movements, or commands. Visual field neglect and higher-level perceptual skills are difficult to assess before the patient is moving spontaneously or responding specifically to stimulation (Zoltan, 1990).

Olfactory evaluation is done with pleasant and unpleasant odors. Ammonia and vinegar irritate the trigeminal nerve and are avoided. Musk, lemon, almond, fruity, or floral scents can be used (Farber, 1982).

Proprioception and kinesthetic evaluation is grossly done by observing the patient's responses to movement of his head, upper extremities, and trunk.

More discrete testing of these sensations, stereognosis, two-point discrimination, and tactile localization will need to be deferred until the patient is more cognitively alert, approximately at Rancho level V or above. Cranial nerve function must be evaluated continually throughout treatment, as it may influence prognosis and treatment.

Neuromuscular Skills

Assessment of the patient's neuromuscular function includes evaluation of strength, coordination, muscle tone, presence and severity of spasticity, and reflex integration. Traditional muscle strength and coordination tests are usually inappropriate for the head-injured patient with spasticity or abnormal muscle tone or with decreased alertness and ability to cooperate. Instead, observation of spontaneous movements or movements elicited during position changes is necessary to determine muscle strength in the early stages of recovery. Isolated motor control and its quality cannot be assessed until Rancho level IV or V. Then the therapist can begin to observe whether the patient moves in response to command, spontaneously, or only in reaction to a stimulus; whether the movement is in a synergy or is selective; whether the movement is purposeful; whether cerebellar dysfunction is present; and whether there is a disturbance in motor planning. Isolated motor control can be evaluated within a neurodevelopmental framework or, in later stages of recovery, with muscle testing and with tests of hand function and dexterity such as the *Minnesota Rate of Manipulation Test* or the *Purdue Pegboard Test.*

Muscle tone is assessed both passively, using quick stretch, and during position changes through normal transition postures. From handling the patient, the therapist determines whether the patient's head movements are coordinated with his trunk and whether touch and movement increase abnormal tone, posturing, or reflexes.

Types of abnormal posturing were described earlier. Commonly found abnormal reflexes are the ATNR, the symmetrical tonic neck reflex (STNR), the TLR, the positive-supporting reaction, and the extensor thrust (Palmer, 1988). The TLR, STNR, and ATNR influence ROM, strength of spasticity, and the potential for isolated movement. Equilibrium, righting, and protective extension reactions are generally decreased or absent in early stages, as are coordination and control of the head and trunk in static and dynamic positions. Assessment of reflexes and equilibrium reactions is described in Chapter 7.

Oral Motor Evaluation

A prefeeding evaluation is done if the patient shows some response to stimulation (Malkmus et al., 1980). This evaluation includes assessment of tone and motor function of individual facial muscles and tongue movements; jaw mobility; facial, tongue, and mouth sensation; sucking and swallowing; and presence of normal and abnormal oral reflexes. During evaluation and treatment, the patient should be positioned in sitting with neck slightly flexed and with hips and knees in flexion. Pressure to the back of the head is avoided; pillows are placed at shoulder height if head control can be obtained in this way. If the patient cannot be optimally positioned in sitting, this should be noted in the evaluation, and consideration should be given by the therapist to the influence of abnormal limb reflexes or poor head and trunk control on observed oral motor function. Refer to Chapter 44 for assessment and intervention procedures for dysphagia.

Perceptual Evaluation

Perceptual abilities cannot be formally evaluated if the patient is only responding to stimuli in a generalized or localized fashion. However, the therapist can use observation of the patient moving spontaneously to infer possible impairments in this area. The ability to cross the midline, neglect of an extremity, decreased tracking and focus into all visual quadrants, or uncoordinated movement of the body through space would alert the therapist to possible visual-spatial and body integration impairments. Once the patient has begun to respond specifically to external stimuli, his performance during "automatic" physical daily living tasks may indicate possible body schema dysfunction or dyspraxia, his figure/ground and position-in-space awareness and his visual-motor integration may be observed when he reaches for objects on a table or for the bed rail, and his neglect of space or body parts can be observed during spontaneous movement. The patient can also be given gross tabletop activities such as sorting or matching; pegboards; simple imitation of block designs; and shape, color, or form puzzles to evaluate perceptual impairments more exactly.

Specific tests of visual perception generally can be done only when the brain-injured patient is responding at Rancho level VII, i.e., when he is no longer confused. He then has the attention span and short-term memory to understand and follow testing instructions. Testing for perceptual skills is described in Chapter 9.

Cognitive Components

As with perceptual impairments, specific cognitive impairments cannot be evaluated if a patient is exhibiting a generalized, localized, or agitated response to stimulation and the environment. The therapist can observe the presence or absence of certain cognitive skills in patients who are confused. Initiative, length of attention span, concentration, rate of and ability to do information processing, problem solving, sequencing, and appropriateness of response to environmental stimuli can be initially assessed at this time by observing the patient's approach to functional tasks and to simple therapeutic activities.

The patient is usually able to cooperate with standardized tests of cognition after he has recovered some memory function and is no longer confused. However, his responses may continue to be inappropriate when task complexity exceeds his cognitive ability. Neuropsychologic testing is usually done at this time to assess higher-level cognitive impairments fully (Lynch, 1990). The occupational therapist is concerned about aspects of cognitive functioning primarily as they impede the patient's skills in independent living and daily living tasks. Particular aspects of concern include the patient's judgment, ability for new learning, problem solving, abstract thinking, selective attention, and memory (see Chapter 9).

Physical Daily Living Skills

Assessment of physical daily living skills can begin only when the patient is responding more locally to the external environment. When the patient is confused and agitated, he may respond to simple functional tasks such as moving from the bed to the wheelchair or brushing his teeth but be unable to complete enough of the task to offer a true assessment of his physical daily living skills. Once the patient is not agitated, evaluation may be initiated (see Chapter 4). As much as possible, evaluation of these skills is done in the morning to avoid adding to a patient's temporal disorientation. This evaluation is usually the first opportunity for the therapist to begin investigating the patient's perceptual and/or cognitive function. Patient performance in physical daily living skills may be decreased by physical limitations of motor control or tone, low endurance, dyspraxia, poor head control, oral motor dysfunction, perceptual dysfunction, behavioral and cognitive disturbances, or lethargy (Malkmus et al., 1980; McNeny, 1990).

Summary

The evaluation results for a deeply comatose patient consist of the nature, location, frequency, and duration of patient response to various types of stimulation; PROM measurements; assessment of muscle tone and abnormal posturing; and determination of oral motor function and abnormal reflexes. As the patient begins to emerge from a deep coma, the therapist reevaluates those areas and begins to evaluate aspects of daily living skills and elementary perceptual and cognitive skills. As the patient becomes less confused, more formal evaluation of perception, cognition, and independent living skills can be done.

OCCUPATIONAL THERAPY TREATMENT

To determine goals of treatment from the evaluation results, the therapist must consider the interplay of the physical and cognitive impairments identified. Physical impairments will be less limiting to independent functioning in the community than will cognitive impairments, which may reduce the patient's ability for new learning, for problem solving in new unstructured situations, and for learning to compensate for sensory or neuromuscular impairments (Jennett & Teasdale, 1981; Zoltan, 1990). The therapist must also consider the severity of the patient's brain injury and coma as well as preinjury personality, drive, intelligence, and the positive or negative aspects of the patient's family dynamics, which will all influence recovery (Benton, 1979).

The Patient in Deep Coma— Rancho Levels I and II

The goal of occupational therapy with the deeply comatose patient who exhibits flaccidity or posturing is to provide the patient with organized stimulation that attempts to elicit increasingly higher-level and more frequent motor responses. This patient exhibits little spontaneous response to the environment, so the therapist attempts to simplify, structure, and heighten the stimuli to increase the chance of a response being elicited (Malkmus et al., 1980). Each stimulus is thus provided with a desired motor response in mind. The response is verbally requested and/or implied through the therapist's handling. For example, certain oral motor stimulation implies the desired motor response of lip closure, and certain positional changes imply the desired motor response of head righting. As the patient responds more consistently, the therapist attempts to channel those responses into more appropriate patient interaction with the environment. The therapist also begins treating oral motor dysfunction, establishes a positioning program, and provides splints or casts as deemed necessary. Joint occupational and physical therapy sessions are often scheduled to provide optimal treatment, inhibition of abnormal tone, and handling through transitional postures. Frequency of treatment sessions must be carefully coordinated.

Possible long-term goals for the patient in deep coma would be to normalize the patient's abnormal tone, increase the amount of voluntary movement, and increase the level of responsiveness to sensory stimulation. Examples of short-term goals are to increase the patient's level of awareness to tactile sensory stimuli as measured by increased head turning or withdrawal responses, decrease extensor tone through positioning and appropriate sensory stimuli, increase flexor response to stimuli and facilitation, maintain ROM by implementation of optimal positioning and appropriate sensory stimulation during treatment and nursing tasks, and improve his ability to keep his head in midline.

SPECIFIC SENSORY STIMULATION

The use of multisensory stimulation for arousal from coma is a subject of controversy. Conflicting results have been obtained, with some studies promoting sensory stimulation and others promoting caution in its use. Many programs use sensory stimulation for coma patients and report a shorter duration of coma (Mitchell et al., 1990), a greater degree of responsiveness (Hall, MacDonald, & Young, 1992), and improved long-term outcome (Mackay et al., 1992). On the other hand, Wood (1991) stressed the need to provide sensory stimulation under conditions that support selective attention and awareness rather than increased arousal. Sensory stimulation is seen as a means to increase awareness to maintain "cortical tone," which is known as vigilance. Constant stimuli such as a radio or hospital noise become habituated and ignored. Wood (1991) recommended a sensory regulation model in which there is a quiet environment, rest periods, and carefully regulated intensity, frequency, and duration of stimulus presentations to increase vigilance. In a pilot study of the sensory regulation model, the four experimental patients showed greater changes in awareness with that program than the four control patients given the standard unregulated sensory stimulation (Wood et al., 1992).

Tactile, vestibular, olfactory, kinesthetic, proprioceptive, auditory, and visual stimuli are used. Gustatory stimulation may be used if the patient's oral motor status permits. Pleasant and unpleasant, and familiar and unfamiliar stimuli are used; stimuli with emotional significance to the patient may be more likely to elicit a response. Organized stimulation periods are scheduled frequently throughout the day for 15 to 30 min each or until a deterioration in the quality of the patient's responses occurs. These sessions must be spaced to allow for rest and nursing care. Stimulation consists of one or two modalities presented in a consistent and meaningful manner, i.e., the patient is told what the therapist is doing and what is expected of him (Malkmus et al., 1980; Moore, 1980). It is helpful in ICU to draw the curtain around the bed to reduce competing visual and auditory stimuli. Simple, clear verbal feedback is given on every response elicited: "Good, you are pushing your arm forward," or "Your lips are closing, close them more." The patient's response to stimulation may be quite delayed, because

central nervous system (CNS) processing is slowed by the damage sustained, if not prevented altogether. The therapist should wait for a response to the stimulation and, if necessary, repeat the stimulus.

Desired responses at this stage will be that of the patient localizing the stimulus (i.e., turning toward a noise, a change in facial expressions, or increased sucking to olfactory stimuli), making a more normal motor response (pushing painful stimuli away), or evidencing a change in muscle tone. Responses are noted to determine any pattern of more consistent, timely responses. If a particular type of stimulation (especially vestibular or olfactory) causes an increase of posturing or large fluctuations in the patient's status, the precipitating stimulation is reduced in intensity or stopped. The goal is to improve the patient's level of response, not upset his fragile homeostasis.

Tactile stimulation includes rubbing the patient's skin with items of various texture or temperature, applying vibration, and using a firm or moving touch on the patient's limbs with verbal cues to orient the patient to his body (Farber, 1982; Moore, 1980). A daily bath and other physical daily living tasks are excellent sources of varied cutaneous input, especially if verbal orientation to body parts being washed or moved is included. Moving touch at the T^{10} dermatome may be used with a decerebrate patient to facilitate a flexor pattern in the legs. This touch is applied from midline to lateral across the abdomen, with up to five repetitions as necessary (Farber, 1982).

Gentle vestibular stimuli are provided by body position changes (from supine to sitting, sitting to side lying), head and neck movements, rolling, tilting the bed to sitting, side-to-side or anterior-posterior movement of the patient in bed or on a mat, slow spinning, or rocking. Inversion of the head (leaning over while seated, or lying over a large therapy ball) helps reduce hypertonicity. However, this, and other forms of vestibular stimulation are contraindicated in a patient with a tracheostomy, elevated ICP, or seizures. Patient reaction must be closely monitored during and after all vestibular stimulation. Precautions and desired ranges of heart rate, ICP, and blood pressure must be adhered to during stimulation.

Olfactory stimulation can be attempted with noxious or pleasant odors such as sulfur, spices, almond, vanilla, banana, lemon, perfumes, coffee, or other smells familiar to the patient. This stimulation may be more effective when it is done before the patient is fed. The therapist must have an effective concentration of the odor. Saturated cotton balls or a sniff bottle are held close to, but not touching, the patient's nose for 2 to 5 sec (Farber, 1982). This cranial nerve is sometimes injured in head trauma, and thus olfactory stimulation might not elicit a response (Jennett & Teasdale, 1981).

Avoid odors with fumes such as ammonia or artificial vanilla, because they irritate cranial nerve V. This irritation is sensed in the nasal passages and can be wrongly interpreted as having smelled the odor (Varney & Menefee, 1993). In addition, the presence of a tracheostomy or an n/g tube or both will eliminate or reduce the air passing through the nostrils, and thus reduce the effectiveness of olfactory stimuli.

Auditory stimulation consists of tapes of favorite music or familiar voices, bells, loud alerting noises such as clapping hands, direct conversation to the patient, verbal commands, explanations, and feedback. A normal but firm voice is used; a comatose patient does not need to be soothed. During therapy sessions, radios, televisions, and other noises should be eliminated as much as possible so that voice commands for motor responses or the selected auditory stimuli are the most prevalent auditory input to the patient.

Visual stimulation to elicit attention, focus, and visual tracking is provided by brightly colored objects, mobiles over the bed, mirrors, lighting changes during the day and night, using a flashlight in a darkened room, the presence of family members, or by pictures of family, friends, and the patient. Pictures are labeled by the family to assist in orienting the patient to them. Environmental changes from the bed to the therapy room or from indoors to outdoors are important sources of visual stimulation. It is important to get the patient upright and well positioned in a wheelchair to encourage typical visual orientation, provide more normal kinesthetic input to the patient, and facilitate more normal muscle tone (Carr & Shepherd, 1980; Malkmus et al., 1980).

POSITIONING

Early implementation of positioning designed to prevent or reduce contractures, foot drop, or abnormal patterns of muscle tone is essential (Carr & Shepherd, 1980). Some typical abnormal positions seen in patients with severe traumatic brain injuries are abnormally forward head, protracted and forward tipped scapulae with or without elevation, posterior pelvic tilt with unilateral retraction and/or elevation, severe trunk tightness with lack of trunk dissociation from neck and head, hip flexor and adductor tightness, foot plantar flexion, and inversion with lack of dissociation of hindfoot from forefoot.

Patient positioning must be reevaluated frequently. Assistive positioning supports are used intermittently and removed as the patient's neuromuscular status improves. The staff at Elizabethtown Hospital have developed a reusable, adaptable seating system for patients that reduces the expense and time of fabrication and provides immediately available seating for patients (Keener & Sweigart, 1984). For further positioning suggestions, see Charness (1986) and Farber (1982).

The nursing staff and the patient's family must be made aware of the desired bed and wheelchair positioning and of the splint-wearing schedule. For abnormal tone to be reduced and contractures to be reduced or prevented, the positioning must continue throughout the day and night.

Bed

Side lying or semiprone (if permitted) with good body alignment is preferable to supine if the patient is exhibiting abnormal posturing (Carr & Shepherd, 1980; Farber, 1982). The supine position triggers the TLR extensor response. In side lying, the head, resting on a small pillow, should be in neutral and aligned with the trunk; the bottom upper extremity in scapular protraction and humeral external rotation; the top upper extremity in scapular protraction, slight shoulder flexion, and resting on a pillow to avoid horizontal adduction; the bottom elbow flexed, the top elbow extended; wrists in extension; and cones in the hands to decrease spasticity and maintain thumb web spaces. A pillow between the knees will decrease hip internal rotation and adduction. The lower leg also may need pillow support to be aligned with the thigh. The hip and knee are flexed only slightly. Elongation of the lower side of the trunk between the shoulder and pelvis is desirable. A side-lying trunk position may need to be maintained by a pillow or sandbag behind the back and shoulder. Footboards are avoided as they elicit extensor thrust. Splints or special shoes (Farber, 1982) are used that are cut to avoid pressure to the ball of the foot but still maintain ankle flexion to 90° and reduce foot drop in a way that avoids stimulating an extensor thrust.

If the patient must be positioned in supine, a small pillow under the head is used, with small rolled pillows under that pillow to keep the head in midline (if the patient cannot do so). Furthermore, small pillows are placed under the scapulae to protract them, shoulders are positioned in slight abduction and external rotation, elbows are extended, and cones or finger spreaders are used for positioning the fingers (Charness, 1986). If the pelvis is retracted on one side, a small folded towel is placed behind it and that leg is positioned in neutral rotation. Some knee flexion should be encouraged by a small towel roll placed under the distal thigh just above the knee joint.

Wheelchair

Early and correct upright positioning in a wheelchair is helpful in inhibiting abnormal tone, providing normal proprioceptive input, and reducing the likelihood and/or extent of contractures and complications from prolonged bed rest. The pelvis must be positioned correctly before addressing other areas. The pelvis should be in a neutral position or have a slight anterior pelvic tilt and should be symmetrical, without one side retracted or elevated. Weight bearing equally through both buttocks is essential to attainment of more normal tone. Solid seat and back inserts are necessary, as the typical wheelchair seat and back sag and actually facilitate posterior pelvic tilt, unequal weight bearing through both hips, and hip internal rotation and adduction. A small, flat lumbar roll is placed wherever necessary above the pelvis and below the scapula to facilitate anterior pelvic tilt in the patient. If the pelvis is retracted on one side, wedged back pieces may be helpful for positioning. If unequal weight bearing is occurring with habitual elongation of one side of the trunk, an insert under the habitual weight-bearing buttock may be helpful. The back of the chair may be reclined 10 to 15° to position the trunk and head more appropriately. Hip flexion should be 90° and can be achieved by a wedge cushion with the high end at the distal thigh. The seat belt should come from the corners of the seat at a 45° angle and fasten over the lower pelvis/hip area to help maintain the anterior pelvic tilt and equal weight bearing through the buttocks. The patient may need firm pads on the outer aspect of the thighs to reduce excessive abduction or a knee abductor to decrease excessive adduction. If the seat belt cannot keep the patient from scooting forward in the chair, a removable padded bar may need to be placed close to the pelvis and femurs.

The trunk, positioned next, should be symmetrical and in midline with shoulders over pelvis in sagittal, frontal, and horizontal planes. Lateral trunk supports can be used to decrease lateral trunk flexion. Experimentation with the positioning is essential, because patients differ in their trunk control. The therapist must not provide too much trunk support, but only enough to facilitate the patient's normal movement and control. With a solid seat and back, the patient may not require additional trunk support.

A harness, shoulder straps, or a chest strap may be necessary if the patient exhibits forward trunk flexion. These should not fasten directly on top of the shoulders but should extend a little higher up before going through the seat back to fasten. An additional seat belt can also be used, placed horizontally across the anterior superior iliac crests to provide backward pressure (Charness, 1986).

Knees and ankles are flexed to 90°, heels slightly behind the knees in sitting, feet in neutral pronation-supination and inversion-eversion. The footplate should be large enough to support the whole foot. Ankle straps are avoided, because they can encourage increased plantar flexion in some patients; a foot wedge, heel loops, an insert behind the foot, special shoes, toe guards, or a combination may be helpful in decreasing abnormal tone and in achieving weight bearing on the heel.

The ideal upper extremity position is neutral scapular elevation or depression with the scapulae in slight protraction, slight shoulder external rotation, and slight flexion and abduction; elbows are in comfortable flexion; the forearm is in pronation; the wrists are in neutral flexion-extension and neutral ulnar-radial deviation; the fingers are relaxed; and the thumb is radially abducted. Excessive scapular retraction may require contouring of the seat back or reclining the seat unit by about 10°. Positioning of shoulder straps, chest straps, and/or lateral trunk supports may be helpful in obtaining adequate shoulder position.

A lapboard, positioned at the proper height to allow good upper extremity weight bearing, is helpful. The lapboard should not be pushed against the patient's abdomen but placed far enough away so the patient can flex forward slightly at the hips. There should be a cutout so that the lapboard fits around the patient, and the lapboard needs to be large enough to accommodate the whole arm. A V-shaped piece of dense foam can be positioned behind the patient's elbow to decrease elbow flexion and retraction of the arm off the back of the lapboard. A contoured surface for the hands may be added to the lapboard. Hand fixation is avoided, because it usually causes the patient to pull back against the fixation.

Ideally, the head should be in midline, with cervical elongation and the chin tucked in slightly. Care is taken that positioning eliminates chin jutting or neck hyperextension. The position of the patient's shoulders and upper trunk will have an influence on head position. A customized head support may be required (Farber, 1982). Pressure directly to the occipital area of the head elicits increased extensor tone of the head and trunk. Therefore, the pressure to right the head is applied up from the occipital process (to each side of midline) and around the forehead in a back and downward pressure. Such a head support would need to be fastened to a head rest, which is recessed so that the patient's head could not push or rest against it. Lateral head supports may be necessary to position the patient's head adequately.

PASSIVE RANGE OF MOTION

PROM can be difficult when there is increased muscle tone. Inhibitory movements opposite the abnormal tone are done slowly, holding the stretch until muscles relax. Sudden stretch and inappropriate stimulation and handling should be avoided. Scapular mobility should be addressed before upper extremity PROM is done to free the scapula and facilitate normal scapular-humeral movement during the rest of PROM (Palmer & Wyness, 1988). PROM within the limits of pain and positioning are helpful in minimizing contractures from heterotopic ossification (Citta-Pietrolungo et al., 1992). Inhibitory positioning and splinting support the gains made with PROM and help lengthen tight soft tissue structures.

SPLINTING AND CASTING

The goals of splinting and casting are to decrease abnormal tone and increase the patient's functional movement. Splints and casts are, therefore, changed as necessary to meet these goals. The patient's quality of movement is constantly reassessed to determine continued necessity of the splints. Splints can assist in positioning flaccid patients but should be very carefully monitored when used with severely spastic or posturing patients, as abnormal tone can be aggravated and pressure areas created quickly.

Splints to provide maintained pressure and stretch between the thenar and hypothenar eminences or to stretch the fingers in abduction may be helpful in reducing tone. With severe spasticity in elbow, wrist, knee, ankle, or foot, serial casting may be indicated (Malkmus et al., 1980). Serial cylinder casting provides neutral warmth and more even skin pressure and allows for less movement than do splints. Casts are usually left on up to 7 days. Drop-out casts (casts leaving a portion of the limb free to relax out of a tightly contracted position), bivalved casts (casts for maintaining a position that are split in two, with moleskin protecting the edges, so they can be removed during therapy or nursing procedures), and weight-bearing inhibitory casts (casts fabricated to approximate the ideal weight-bearing posture of the foot or hand) can also be used (Carr & Shepherd, 1980; Malkmus et al., 1980). Hill (1994) found casting more effective than traditional treatment of PROM, stretching, and splinting in reducing contractures in a group of 15 head-injured patients. The effect of casting on spasticity was variable. Hill recommended further study.

SPECIFIC THERAPEUTIC PROCEDURES TO IMPROVE NEUROMUSCULAR SKILLS

Specific therapeutic facilitation techniques to stimulate the patient's kinesthetic, vestibular, and proprioceptive senses include neurodevelopmental treatment (NDT) and proprioceptive neuromuscular facilitation (PNF) (see Chapter 24). Such techniques (or modifications thereof) can be combined with quick stretch, tapping over the muscle belly, joint approximation, and the request for an appropriate motor response, thus providing additional tactile and auditory stimulation to the patient (Farber, 1982; Stockmeyer, 1967). Quick ice also can be used to facilitate an individual

muscle response when applied to the muscle belly (Stockmeyer, 1967) or can be used for directionality of motion. ("I am going to put ice on your hand. Pull away from the ice"). Quick ice is perceived as a distinct noxious stimulus when applied to the face, soles of the feet, or palms (Stockmeyer, 1967). Normal precautions with use of ice are observed.

The head, neck, and trunk receive special emphasis in early treatment because of the crucial contribution of these areas to development of visual-spatial awareness and body integration (Moore, 1980). The comatose patient is told in advance of eliciting or changing body position to decrease the possibility of posturing and other stereotypic reactions. If the stimulation causes an increase of posturing, it is stopped temporarily and resumed after the patient has rested.

NDT positions, weight shifting, weight bearing, and transitional movements between positions can be used to increase or decrease muscle tone selectively or to elicit beginning righting reactions. Supine, sidelying, prone, and sitting positions are the most feasible to use with a patient at this level. The prone position may need to be modified for a patient with a tracheostomy. Prone and sitting are best done on a firm surface, such as a mat and may not be possible if the patient cannot be treated in the therapy department. The therapist can, however, incorporate the techniques of weight shifting and weight bearing into treatment in the ICU to change muscle tone and to normalize the patient's proprioceptive input (Charness, 1986; Scherzer & Tscharnuter, 1982).

If using PNF, the therapist first treats the arm that responds to stimulation with the higher-level motor reaction. The patient may be able to respond in only one part of a muscle's range, so the shortened or slightly lengthened positions must each be tried. Verbal instructions to the patient must be as consistent and simple as possible. The patient is instructed to "reach" or "look up" or is simply facilitated into the position and the desired motor response is shaped. Modifications of these techniques may be necessary when working with a patient in the ICU if there are restrictions on his movement.

Because isolated, well-controlled movements in the arms or trunk will not occur in this stage of coma, the therapist must feel the muscle tone changes that signify the beginnings of a voluntary effort. As the therapist handles the comatose patient and becomes more familiar with his pattern of muscle tone, changes occurring in that tone will be more obvious. Movement or pressure in a range where there was no movement before might represent the beginnings of voluntary movement. A sustained push felt near the end of the range is not likely to be the result of quick stretch, which elicits a phasic response earlier in range.

Specific maneuvers to inhibit tone may be necessary with the comatose patient who is posturing. One such inhibition method is axial rotation of the trunk. While the patient is positioned in side lying, the therapist attempts to rotate the thorax on the pelvis, thus breaking up the typical trunk tightness and immobility. This rotation and inhibition of trunk tone will be necessary later for rolling with appropriate patterns of head and neck, for moving from prone to sitting, for upper extremity function, and eventually for equilibrium reactions. Extensor tone can be somewhat lessened by maintenance of hip and knee flexion, avoidance of resistance to the back of the head, and avoidance of the supine position itself. The speed of the therapist's movements and the patient's response to frequent hand position changes should be considered in altering procedures to decrease the patient's tone. Immediately following successful inhibition of tone, the therapist would attempt to facilitate more normal movement in a functional pattern. For example, if trunk extensor tone was reduced while the patient was side lying, the therapist might choose to facilitate upper trunk initiation of rolling to prone, reaching with upper arm, or coming up from side lying to partial sitting.

THERAPY RELATED TO FAMILY NEEDS

The family of these patients usually indicates a need to be involved in the patient's care, to feel they can do something to promote his recovery. Family members can be shown simple PROM exercises to do with the patient. The importance of periods of organized sensory stimulation followed by rest is explained to the family. Auditory and tactile stimulation can be provided by the family, as their voices and touch will be more familiar to the patient at first and may elicit more response than unfamiliar voices (Najenson et al., 1974). Positioning is described and demonstrated to the family, and their participation is encouraged. The family is also a valuable source of information regarding the patient's interests and the activities he enjoys.

The team members also must cope with the family's need for hope and optimism, the reality of the patient's situation, and his probable outcome and residual impairments. Consistency of team members' interactions with the family is essential (see Chapters 10 and 20). Conversations and instructions will have to be repeated frequently, as the family is under considerable stress and flux (Livingston, Brooks, & Bond, 1985; Muir, Rosenthal, & Diehl, 1990).

The Patient at Low Levels of Recovery—Rancho Levels III and IV

Once the patient begins to respond to stimulation with a more localized and adaptive behavioral response, the occupational therapy goal is to refine and direct the patient's response to stimulation. Such localization is seen when the patient pulls at his n/g tube or catheter, focuses on something briefly, or turns his head away when his cheek is stimulated. The therapist attempts to obtain greater consistency in localizing responses and avoiding stereotypic movements, more variety in the patient's responses, and a decreased interval between stimulation and response (Malkmus et al., 1980). The therapist also attempts to increase the patient's ability to follow simple commands; to attend to an activity; and to use common objects such as a spoon, comb, and washcloth. Sometimes the patient will assist with ROM movements or reach for objects.

At this stage of coma, the therapist may be able to identify more precisely motor or sensory impairments by observing the patient's spontaneous repositioning in bed; his periods of restlessness; his neuromuscular response to stimuli of light touch, temperature, pain, sounds, and proprioception; his facial movements in response to family, friends, or stimuli; or his spontaneous response to, or manipulation of, utensils. Specific evaluation and tests are still inappropriate, as the patient is unable to attend consistently to a task or follow commands and has decreased periods of alertness.

The patient is now more responsive to internal and external stimuli, but he still does not initiate activities or remember events and is dependent in most physical daily living skills. He may be moving and repositioning in bed secondary to restlessness, but he continues to require assistance for transfers and other forms of motor activity.

Examples of long-term goals at this stage are to increase and to channel the patient's responsiveness and alertness, increase his ability to move independently, and increase his self-care skills. Short-term goals might be to continue to provide appropriate positioning through splints and casts to maintain PROM; increase the consistency, variety, and quality of response to stimulation; continue normalizing muscle tone through neurorehabilitation techniques; develop more normal movements in head, neck, and trunk during transitional movements; decrease agitation through calming, inhibitory activities or simple repetitive tasks; improve oral motor function through reduction of abnormal oral reflexes; and continue evaluation of cognition and perception.

SENSORY STIMULATION AND POSITIONING

Sensory stimulation, as described above, would continue with the goal of refining the patient's motor responses, e.g., the use of visual stimulation to increase the length of the patient's attentiveness and improve tracking skills. The extent of positioning supports (splints, casts, wheelchair modifications, and bed positioning) would be reduced as much as possible.

PROCEDURES TO IMPROVE NEUROMUSCULAR SKILLS

Treatment of neuromuscular skills continues with NDT, PNF (with resistance applied proximally if necessary to get less associated reactions), and facilitation to specific muscles. At this level, mat activities to elicit head and neck control, rolling, and sitting may be feasible. The patient can be more readily facilitated into positions or transitional movements such as prone, from prone to prone on elbows (for weight bearing through forearms and hands, inhibition of hypertonus, and feedback into the shoulder girdle) (Charness, 1986), prone on elbows with weight shifting side to side and coordinated trunk shortening, from prone on elbows to side lying and back, rolling from prone to supine and back, and sitting with weight shifting in sagittal and frontal planes to facilitate appropriate trunk and upper extremity reactions. The sitting position can be used to elicit upper extremity weight bearing onto a table in front or onto the mat at the patient's side. If the patient has increased hip adductor tone, he may be positioned in sitting over a bolster with weight bearing onto hands in front or on the bolster (Charness, 1986). The patient's feet must be positioned to ensure weight bearing throughout the soles, with hip flexion at 90° or more (Carr & Shepherd, 1980). The above positions are important to attain head and neck, shoulder girdle, and upper trunk control, to free the arms for function, and to develop righting reactions and protective responses. Two therapists may be needed to handle the patient and facilitate appropriate body alignment. If the patient's motor skills are more intact, simple "automatic" games such as throwing or hitting a large ball may be tried. Because of the patient's limited alertness, his praxis cannot be fully assessed at this level.

REDEVELOPMENT OF PHYSICAL DAILY LIVING SKILLS

Rudimentary skills of feeding, face washing, and light grooming are now begun. These basic tasks are overlearned and may draw automatic responses from the patient. Such tasks are normally relegated to subcortical direction (Malkmus et al., 1980; Moore, 1980), which may not have been impaired (Ommaya & Gennarelli, 1976). The attention of the patient is focused on the end result instead of on the process to tap this subcortical direction (Moore, 1980). The therapist may simply hand a wet washcloth to him or put the washcloth in his hand and bring it to his face. The therapist assists as necessary, so that the patient can initiate as much as possible and receive the sensory feedback from the task. These tasks are done at appropriate times of the day to orient the patient. Rest periods are essential, because such patients fatigue rapidly. He is treated in a quiet environment, with minimal and consistent instructions. The variables in the task are reduced, and the tasks are simplified drastically. For example, one dish and one spoon are used in feeding, and the rest of the tray is put out of sight; the patient is not required to bathe himself entirely but merely to wash his face. Once the patient is more consistent and successful at a part of the task, the task can be gradually expanded and made more complex.

PERCEPTION AND COGNITION

Cognitive and perceptual functioning cannot be formally evaluated at this point in the recovery process; such functioning must be inferred from the patient's performance of simple physical daily living skills and his motor responses to the environment. Observation will indicate if the patient notices visitors or objects on both sides or if he exhibits signs of homonymous hemianopia, if he seems to use objects appropriately when handed to him or needs to be shown, if he watches the therapist demonstrating the use of objects, if he visually tracks people and movement, if he is able to sustain attention to a specific task, if he can reach across midline and position himself at midline, and if his spatial and depth perception appears impaired when reaching for objects.

The patient may still have his eyes closed most of the time. If his eyes are open and tracking, he is usually highly distractible and demonstrates a very short attention span and no memory. At this stage, the patient will not show carryover of new learning from treatment session to session. Memory entails attending to the relevant stimuli of an experience, encoding them, storing them appropriately, and then retrieving them. Any or all of these processes can be disrupted by a diffuse, severe traumatic brain injury (Brooks, 1990). The temporal lobes and hippocampus appear to be primarily involved in the encoding of memory, and these areas are frequently damaged (Jennett & Teasdale, 1981; Ommaya & Gennarelli, 1976). The patient with a brain injury will usually not remember day-to-day activities until he is able to produce fairly consistent appropriate responses to external stimulation. Until then, he exists in a fugue-like, confused state.

Treatment of these areas may include simple perceptual activities such as color, form, or shape matching and sorting; simple gross motor catching and throwing games; basic sensory integration activities (within precautions noted above); and simple self-care tasks.

TREATMENT OF THE AGITATED PATIENT

Once the patient begins localizing stimuli, he may become quite agitated and restless as he becomes acutely aware of internal discomfort, pain, internal cognitive confusion and disruption, and external restraints. The patient will usually tear at tubes and restraints, show decreased ability to cooperate with treatment, and may become aggressive. Not all brain trauma patients pass through this phase; those who do may experience this phase for a few days or up to 4 weeks (Malkmus et al., 1980; Reyes, Heller, & Bhattacharyya, 1981). A restless or agitated patient has been found to be more likely to show greater physical improvement than an immobile or sluggishly moving patient (Reyes et al., 1981). Medication to calm the patient should be avoided whenever possible, because the large doses that are necessary also slow the patient's cognitive recovery. However, in some cases, behavior becomes violent and aggressive enough for drug treatment to be considered (Rao, Jellinek, & Woolston, 1985). It is important to remember that the patient is not accountable for the agitation, hostility, or aggressiveness. He is responding to internal cognitive confusion, not specifically to the person who happens to be in the situation with him. At the same time, it is also important to protect yourself from injury.

The goals of occupational therapy during this phase are to decrease the patient's agitation as much as possible by reducing stimuli that agitate the patient and increasing situations or stimuli that calm the patient, to continue to focus his attention on the external environment through engaging his participation in self-care and other automatic tasks, and to attempt to have the patient follow simple commands. Patient cooperation, motivation, and follow-through are minimal. He cannot focus cognitively on his environment and interpret it (Malkmus et al., 1980). Therefore, he cannot learn at this stage. Removal of noxious stimulation, whenever possible, assists in decreasing agitation. Limb restraints are removed during therapy sessions and at other times of constant supervision. An unchanged daily routine can provide structure and predictability and reduce patient confusion.

Inhibitory techniques of repetitive or sustained touch, warmth, rocking, slow rolling, slow vestibular stimulation, and use of the therapist's voice and presence to soothe the patient are helpful (Farber, 1982; Malkmus et al., 1980; Moore, 1980). A change of environment to a quieter place with less stimulation; a drink of juice or a snack (if the patient has normal oral motor activity); tapes of family voices; an explanation to the patient that this is a stage of recovery that will pass; and continual orientation of the patient to where he is, why, and what the therapist is doing with him can also assist in decreasing his agitation. Acknowledgment of the discomfort and gentle redirection of the patient's attention to tasks is useful.

Treatment is done in an individual or structured group setting, using simple and familiar gross motor or daily living tasks, such as face washing, walking, stationary cycling, catching a large ball, throwing bean bags, moving from supine to sitting, and putting on simple clothes such as a T-shirt or pull-on pants. Physical activity, walking or even being wheeled in the wheelchair helps decrease agitation (Baggerly, 1986). The therapist changes the activity frequently at the first sign that the patient is becoming restless or agitated. The patient may also have decreased tolerance to one person working with him; therefore, therapist assignment to the patient at this stage may need to change during a treatment session (Malkmus et al., 1980). Tasks requiring concentration or fine motor precision, such as pegboards and form boards, are avoided during periods of agitation or restlessness (Charness, 1986; Malkmus et al., 1980). The patient will most likely need maximum assistance with self-care tasks because of his short attention span. He also may begin transfers now, depending on his level of muscular involvement.

The patient's orientation may be assessed if he is verbally responsive. However, such assessment should not be pursued if it further agitates the patient. Patients can be aware of their situation early in the recovery process. This awareness may be simply a knowledge that something is wrong even if it cannot be defined or that they should remember something but that they do not. These patients have undergone a total loss of control of their body and actions. Each action is isolated, because the patient cannot remember what came before, yet he struggles to make cognitive sense out of each moment. At this point, the patient needs the therapist to provide consistency and predictability, feedback on reality, calmness, quietness, confidence, acceptance, and consideration of his communications, however nonsensical, inappropriate, or nonverbal. The therapist can gather information on the patient's cognitive status by observing the patient functioning in tasks or by watching his social interactions.

The Patient at Middle Levels of Recovery—Rancho Levels V and VI

As the patient's agitation decreases, he will respond more to the external environment. His responses will be confused and inappropriate at first (Salcman et al., 1981). He is unable to process information at a normal rate or produce an appropriate response to all environmental situations. Later, his response to a given situation may be appropriate but still not completely correct because of poor short-term memory, difficulty in learning new tasks (such as one-handed methods of dressing), persistent confusion, decreased attention span, visual-spatial dysfunction, dyspraxia, and/or inconsistent orientation (Charness, 1986; Malkmus et al., 1980).

Occupational therapy goals in this stage are to increase attention to more specific tasks and salient stimuli; increase the process of sequential organization; increase immediate and short-term memory (i.e., memory of events for up to 1 hr); and increase analysis, association, and categorization (Hill & Carper, 1985; Lundgren & Persechino, 1986). Treatment continues to emphasize improvement of the patient's neuromuscular skills, improvement of his perceptual skills, and his increased ability to do simple physical daily living and homemaking tasks. The therapist continues to structure the patient's environment for him because of the patient's difficulty in structuring the environment himself. Complexity and duration of the tasks are reduced to the patient's level of ability, distractions are kept to a minimum, his immediate environment and schedule are kept as unchanged as possible, and visual memory aids, such as a written daily schedule, are provided (Charness, 1986; Malkmus et al., 1980).

A patient at this level may require almost maximum assistance for independent living skills, exhibit significant neuromuscular impairments, need maximum cuing to orient himself, display severe memory impairment, possibly show confused verbal and mental processes, and have little carryover of new learning. Perceptual impairments may be more apparent and identifiable and preliminary cognitive function can be assessed by observation.

Long-term goals might be to increase the patient's independent functioning in physical daily living and homemaking skills, evaluate equipment needs, increase the patient's cognitive ability to structure his environment, and to store information properly and retrieve it appropriately. Short-term goals might be to improve the patient's voluntary selective movement through continued facilitation of transitional movements and functional positions, increase fine motor control through manipulative activities and exercises for specific muscles, improve motor control of the upper extremities to enable the patient to feed himself with minimal supervision, increase independence in hygiene and dressing through daily training, evaluate perceptual skills more precisely, improve attention and memory through specific cognitive activities and functional tasks, determine the nature of equipment the patient may need after discharge for more independence in daily living skills, and do a home visit to assess architectural barriers and equipment needs.

REDEVELOPMENT OF PHYSICAL DAILY LIVING SKILLS

Self-care training continues as described for Rancho level IV. The task is simplified until the patient is consistently successful in performing it, and then the complexity is gradually increased while the externally provided structure is gradually decreased. Environmental distractions are kept to a minimum. Simple adaptive equipment is provided if necessary. The therapist gathers the items to be used and sequences the task by providing the patient with the appropriate item at the proper time and by giving simplified directions at each step. For example, in dressing, the therapist would first hand the patient his undershorts and then give simple verbal instructions and physical cuing as necessary to have the patient put the shorts over his legs and pull them up. The therapist would not present the patient's T-shirt until the shorts were finished. The clothes chosen initially would be solid colors with minimal fastenings to decrease perceptual confusion. The therapist may also choose to limit the task by having the patient do only one or two steps of the entire task (e.g., put on T-shirt only) if the patient has very low endurance, low frustration tolerance, or limited hip or trunk flexion. The therapist should structure the task and method so that the patient is not reinforcing abnormal movement patterns during his self-care. The position of the patient (i.e., dressing in bed, sitting in the wheelchair, or sitting on the edge of the bed) and the method of dressing would have been selected according to the patient's neuromuscular function.

Gradually, as the patient becomes more successful in dressing, the therapist decreases verbal and physical cuing, gives the patient more than one piece of clothing at once, or increases the speed of the activity (Malkmus et al., 1980). Hygiene training, feeding, and wheelchair transfer training are structured in the same fashion. The therapist would begin with whichever self-care task was most meaningful to the patient and would not add more tasks until reasonable success had been achieved (Charness, 1986).

Because of cognitive impairment, the patient usually continues to require moderate assistance, even if he has only minimal physical impairment. The therapist is prepared to verbalize the task steps repeatedly or to rephrase instructions if the patient appears confused. The anticipated outcome is that the patient will begin to absorb the structure provided to him and internalize it (Malkmus et al., 1980). Generalization of the structure to other tasks is not expected, however, as the patient continues to have comprehensive cognitive impairments and decreased memory at this level.

PROCEDURES TO IMPROVE NEUROMUSCULAR SKILLS

At levels V and VI, therapy to restore motor function can include muscle facilitation and/or strengthening exercises for upper extremity and hand musculature to address isolated dysfunction or overall weakness and activities and/or appropriate NDT or PNF techniques to develop upper extremity stability, mobility, and function. Head control, midline orientation, trunk mobility and rotation, scapular mobility and function, weight bearing, weight shifting, and dissociation of head, neck, and trunk movements are all worked on in therapy until the patient's movement is more normal (Charness, 1986; Scherzer & Tscharnuter, 1982; see also Chapter 24). Following this, activities combining trunk movements and rotation with upper extremity reaching and functional patterns, weight shifting and weight bearing with coordinated upper extremity movements, and righting and equilibrium reactions are worked on.

Once the patient is exhibiting a confused but appropriate response to stimulation in level VI, more detailed sensory and motor evaluations can be done with traditional tests using simplified instructions.

PERCEPTION

Treatment at this level of recovery may consist of matching; sorting; discrimination of differences and similarities in color, size, or shape; very simple three- or four-piece puzzles; tracing; simple figure/ground and visual-motor coordination worksheets; and simple design copying. Sequencing tasks, coding tasks, visual scanning tasks, and more complicated design copying or figure/ground tasks may be done with the patient who is confused but responding appropriately. Formal perceptual testing is usually not possible at this level but can be done in the following stage.

COGNITION AND BEHAVIOR

Formal assessment of the patient's neuropsychologic and behavioral impairments by the team psychologist or neuropsychologist is useful in planning occupational therapy treatment to correspond to and not overtax the patient's current memory status and cognitive abilities. Clinical observations by team members can also assist in informally determining the patient's cognitive status and behavioral problems.

Behavioral sequelae may hamper therapy at this stage. As the patient becomes more alert, his awareness of his situation may increase his irritability, his uncooperativeness, or his mood fluctuations. The patient may be impulsive, easily frustrated, perseverative, and dependent on his family. He will be confused and disoriented at times and will not remember why he is in the hospital. Specific techniques that have been used at this level to reduce confusion and increase more acceptable behavior are behavioral modification programs (Eames, Haffey, & Cope, 1990) and reality-orientation peer groups (Malkmus et al., 1980). The patient may also begin to display secondary emotional and behavioral disturbances in response to the stress of coping with his suddenly altered lifestyle (Hill & Carper, 1985; Malkmus et al., 1980; see also Chapters 10 and 20).

Tests of the duration of posttraumatic amnesia can begin when the patient is responding verbally in a comprehensible fashion. Neuropsychologic tests, however, usually require the patient to be appropriate in his responses, i.e., toward the latter part of level VI or the beginning of level VII (Eson, Yen, & Bourke, 1978). Although results are not definitive, assessment using standardized tests can be done when the patient is confused to provide a preliminary baseline and identify possible deficits (Malkmus et al., 1980). Most tests of posttraumatic amnesia are administered daily and include questions on basic biographical data, orientation in time and space, last memory before and first memory since the accident, and naming of familiar objects with recall requested the following day (Levin, O'Donnell, & Grossman, 1979). Ben-Yishay and Prigatano (1990), at the Institute of Rehabilitation Medicine in New York City, assessed baseline levels of attention, speed of reaction, visual-motor integration, perceptual motor functioning, daily living skills, the patient's understanding of his disability, immediate and short-term memory, academic skills, abstract reasoning, various interpersonal social skills, and the patient's appraisal of his own personality. Results of these tests indicated the patient's ability and willingness to profit from cognitive and interpersonal remediation. These tests are given before intervention is begun and after it has ended. Cognitive impairments have also been measured with such tests as the *Wechsler Adult Intelligence Scale* and the *Wechsler Intelligence Scale for Children*, the *Halstead-Reitan Neuropsychological Test Battery*, the *Revised Benton Visual Retention Test*, and the *Wechsler Memory Scale* (Chadwick et al., 1981; Prigatano et al., 1984). Administration of some of these tests is limited to psychologists.

The patient at level VI usually displays severe immediate (up to 1 min), short-term (up to 1 hr), and long-term (over 1 hr) memory impairment. He is, therefore, unlikely to demonstrate carryover of new learning from day to day or from one setting to another, but he may begin to show carryover of overly familiar tasks of self-care (Malkmus et al., 1980). He appears alert but is highly distractible; he does not initiate functional tasks; he has difficulty solving problems related to simple daily living skills, such as making a phone call; and he displays poor judgment. The patient's language response may include jargon, word finding difficulty, confabulation, or lack of relevance to the conversation.

Ultimately, the goal of cognitive remediation is to prepare the patient for greater independence in living, through maximum improvement in the cognitive skills underlying independent psychosocial, community, and vocational functioning, and successful planning of activities leading toward a goal (Ben-Yishay & Prigatano, 1990). Thus all cognitive remediation, including that done through computer programs, is related to functional skills and practical application (Bracy et al., 1985; Trexler, 1984). In treating cognitive impairment, specific tasks such as simple organizational tasks, map usage, beginning paper-and-pencil tasks such as word recognition or letter cancellation, abstract verbal skills, visual memory tasks, selective attention tasks, and memory drills of letters or numbers may be used (Gianutsos, 1980; Malkmus et al., 1980). The patient may be asked to verbalize all the steps involved in a specific task such as making a sandwich, brushing his teeth, or getting ready to go home on a weekend pass.

Cognitive remediation can be done in individual or in group sessions. The groups must be well structured and guided by the leader as necessary, with good group cohesiveness (Hill & Carper, 1985; Malkmus et al., 1980). The organization and format of one such group in occupational therapy was described by Lundgren and Persechino (1986). Group games suitable for this level would be gross motor games combined with orientation games (i.e., the patient must answer an orientation question in turn), outdoor games such as darts and relays, simple board games, and auditory memory games.

Computers

Recently, computers have been increasingly used to help brain-injured patients attain the goals of cognitive remediation. Computers will not be applicable to every patient. The therapist must carefully assess the patient's abilities and needs and determine the most appropriate tool for optimal cognitive remediation.

The choice of computer programs is governed by the following factors: the skills that the patient needs to improve, the level and consistency of difficulty in the program, the ease of the instructions, the program capacity for keeping data on the patient's performance, the type and amount of feedback provided to the patient, the motivational effect of the program, the consistency of response format, the amount of supervision needed from the therapist (which may be as high as 75% of the computer use time) (Trexler, 1984), and

the control of the variables (speed of task, length of display time, size of stimulus items, nature of prompts).

For treatment at this stage, computer programs would primarily be selected to work on retraining the patient's ability to focus his attention, increase visual scanning, increase his reaction time, improve his visual-motor coordination, improve simple problem-solving skills, and increase frustration tolerance (Bracy et al., 1985). Programs found useful for patients at this stage include those that demand eye-hand coordination and fast reaction time. Also useful are programs that address attention span, visual scanning, other visual motor skills, sequencing, and color discrimination.

The Patient at a High Level of Recovery—Rancho Level VII

When the patient demonstrates fairly consistent appropriate responses to the external environment, the occupational therapy goals are to decrease the external structuring of the patient's environment gradually, increase his purposeful goal-directed behavior, increase his initiation of independent living and daily skills, and increase his responsibility for doing those tasks and for the consequences of his actions (Charness, 1986; Malkmus et al., 1980). The patient is slowly made responsible for coming to therapy sessions on time, gathering the necessary materials and initiating his own exercise program, planning more advanced homemaking and meal preparation activities, dressing and grooming himself appropriately, making his own bed, and keeping a detailed daily log of events. His participation in the decision-making process of his therapy program is increased. He needs to become aware of his physical and cognitive limitations and realistically plan for his future vocational and leisure activities. In addition, therapy concentrates on improving the quality of his neuromuscular skills, cognitive skills, social interactions, and his ability to problem solve in different and new situations.

At this level, the patient continues to exhibit cognitive and behavioral impairments, decreased independence in independent living skills, and inability to function in the community and in unstructured situations.

Long-term goals might be to increase the patient's ability to respond appropriately to and interact with the environment in social, personal, educational, and vocational areas and to enable him to seek employment in a sheltered workshop or another modified job situation.

Examples of short-term goals might be to increase the patient's assumption of responsibility for his own personal needs and decrease external structuring; improve his cognitive skills and perceptual skills and teach compensation skills as necessary through specific spatial and scanning tasks, memory tasks, and organizational tasks; increase his ability to initiate and finish a task; improve his dexterity and his refined balance reactions; improve his praxis; increase his social interaction and its quality through use of groups for social, physical, and community tasks; and plan discharge to coordinate with family and community agencies.

PROCEDURES TO IMPROVE NEUROMUSCULAR CONTROL

Motor problems seen at this stage can include problems of quality of movement as well as continued problems of ataxia, fluctuating tone, or residual spasticity. The patient may exhibit dyspraxia, decreased fine motor control, delayed protective extension or equilibrium reactions, and/or other movement problems. The therapist would continue addressing these problems as necessary with specific facilitation or strengthening techniques, fine motor coordination and dexterity activities, motor sequencing activities, balance activities, and/or timed repetitions to improve the speed of a motor response. Group games or situations can be useful in refining motor responses while providing peer feedback for maladaptive behavior (Charness, 1986; Hill & Carper, 1985; Mercer & Boch, 1983).

PERCEPTION, COGNITION, BEHAVIOR

More formal perceptual and cognitive testing and retraining can be done now, because the patient can follow simple directions (see Chapters 9, 26 and 27). A study of 28 brain-injured patients found that half of the patients lacked controlled eye movements or had eye movements with **dysmetria.** Referral to an ophthalmologist may be needed (Warren, 1993b). With head injury, the visual field loss is often in the superior fields; loss of acuity relates to loss of contrast sensitivity; and the oculomotor system is frequently impaired with poor fixation, deviation of the eyes resulting in **diplopia,** and difficulty in visual scanning. Limitations in complex visual processing will be evident during perceptual evaluation (Warren, 1993a).

Cognitively, the patient's ability to integrate, categorize, sequence, and analyze multiple inputs is assessed (Lynch, 1990). Immediate, short-term and long-term, and verbal memory are also evaluated by a neuropsychologist (Benton, 1979). In this stage of recovery, the patient may demonstrate specific impairments in short- and long-term memory, reasoning, conceptualization, comprehension, abstract thinking, information-processing speed, organization of information, simplification of problems, judgment, and problem solving (Charness, 1986; Dikmen, Reitan, & Temkin, 1983; Gianutsos, 1980). He may display

decreased attention during attempts to store information, decreased use of mental imagery, decreased new learning, inability to locate the salient or relevant details, decreased ability to structure or associate incoming information appropriately, and decreased cognitive flexibility (Scherzer, 1986). These impairments will affect the patient's ability to make coherent decisions, to plan realistically, to structure his behavior or his leisure time, and to make safe decisions in the community (Cervelli, 1990; Malkmus et al., 1980).

Cognitive remediation at this level emphasizes increasing the patient's ability to concentrate on specific tasks, to organize and use information, to remember increasing amounts of information, and to be mentally flexible. The therapist must delineate the patient's cognitive impairment and choose the most appropriate way to remediate the impairment and monitor improvement as well as assess the patient's ability to benefit from such training (Diller & Gordon, 1981). The patient's motivation and his ability to understand the relevance to his personal life are crucial. Cognitive remediation must include systematic use of activities to develop skills, repeated practice by the patient, careful selection and teaching of compensatory cognitive methods and cuing strategies to improve the patient's cognitive skills, and constant, systematic feedback to the patient on his performance. The cognitive remediation program described by Ben-Yishay and Prigatano (1990) is carefully structured and hierarchically arranged in areas of attentional demands (from arousal to cortical content), choice of materials (from simple eye-hand integration to verbal reasoning functions), locus of processing (external buttons and lights to internal processing in the brain), and difficulty level of tasks (easy to hard).

Tasks used by therapists in cognitive remediation at this level may include more complex reading and mathematical tasks or tasks involving increasing analysis of information such as summarizing paragraphs, interpreting proverbs, or ascertaining the meaning of stories or poems. Other examples of tasks are sequential cards depicting an activity such as a picnic, washing a car, and getting ready for school; number and letter sequences; word scrambles; visual memory activities; map reading; simple riddles; jigsaw puzzles; and auditory memory tasks with verbal or written responses requested. Also useful are board games; card games; games and tasks emphasizing problem solving in emergency, social, or community-encountered situations (such as going to a concert, assessing the transportation route, and choosing which friends to call and invite); and planning a trip to two different types of restaurants and discussing the procedures for each in terms of clothing, tipping, and ordering (Anderson & Parente,

1985; Lundgren & Persechino, 1986; Malkmus et al., 1980; Milton, 1985).

Abreu and Toglia (1987) described a cognitive rehabilitation model that emphasized observing how the patient solves a problem or approaches a task, what conditions help his performance, and what conditions lead to difficulty. Cues and strategies could then be selected to improve performance by enhancing the patient's ability to process and organize information. Toglia (1991) is also concerned with the lack of generalization and proposes that transfer of learning be addressed within the process of a multicontext treatment approach. Neistadt (1990) differentiated remedial approaches from adaptive approaches to treatment of perceptual dysfunction. Training in perceptual skills that would generalize across all activities—a remedial approach—is based on the assumption that the brain can recover and reorganize. Training in essential daily life tasks and substituting intact behaviors for impaired ones—an adaptive approach—is based on the assumption that the adult brain has limited potential for repair and reorganization and that generalization is difficult for brain-injured adults. Neistadt (1994) suggested that both the remedial and adaptive approaches will be useful when therapists use clinical judgment based on observation of each patient's level of information processing and ability to transfer learning.

Computer programs carefully matched to the patient's specific deficit areas can be helpful (Bracy et al., 1985). Such programs dealing specifically with retraining perceptual and memory skills are increasingly available (Lynch, 1986). Some advantages of computer use in cognitive retraining are that repetition and drill become challenging because of the program's format, feedback is immediate and consistent, the patient's failures are witnessed only by the computer, data can be tabulated to quantify the patient's improvement, and many programs are available to challenge the patient. Some disadvantages are that computers do not provide social interaction or verbal problem solving, they can lead only to very limited generalization about real-life situations, and the therapist still needs to monitor the patient's work and progress on the various programs.

Behaviorally, the patient may be experiencing continued withdrawal, anger, depression, or denial of his injury. The therapist can help by letting the patient express his feelings, acknowledging the validity of his feelings, showing empathy, supporting the patient within reason, encouraging him to continue to strive for recovery, remaining accessible to the patient, and avoiding judgmental responses to the patient's expressions of anger or depression. Other behavioral changes may include lack of drive or initiation, decreased social restraint, passivity, and decreased frustration tolerance

(Benton, 1979; Jennett & Teasdale, 1981; National Institute of Neurological and Communicative Disorders and Stroke, 1984; Rosenthal & Bond, 1990).

Behavior modification programs may be necessary to address behaviors that are hindering rehabilitation efforts. Family counseling may also be necessary to resolve negative feelings and to cope with the reality of the patient's abilities. A study demonstrated deterioration of relatives' psychiatric and social functioning in the year after the patient's brain injury, in direct correlation to the level of the patient's voiced subjective complaints. These relatives had twice as many psychiatric disturbances as in the normal population (Livingston et al., 1985).

COMMUNITY INTEGRATION

When physical daily living skills and homemaking tasks (such as cleaning, meal preparation, laundry, and solving daily household problems) are being done consistently, the patient must be reintroduced to the community and necessary survival skills. The patient needs to learn how to manage money, write checks, go shopping, use the bank and post office, move in crowds, handle architectural barriers, and go to restaurants; he needs to be able to use public transportation, the telephone, the newspaper, and the phone book; he should know the use and care of his equipment or splints; he needs to use crosswalks and obey traffic lights (American Occupational Therapy Association [AOTA], 1985). Goals of community integration of the patient are to provide increased reality testing and better preparation for an unstructured environment (Malkmus et al., 1980). One suggestion to incorporate memory strategies into the planning of a community outing is to use a form requiring the patient to answer questions such as "Where?" "Why?" "When?" "What time?" "What items are necessary to bring?" and "What method of transportation is to be used?" (Milton, 1985).

The therapist will need to assess carefully the amount of supervision and structuring necessary secondary to the patient's decreased judgment and problem-solving ability. The patient's wheelchair mobility, body control, and/or balance during functional tasks in the kitchen or in the community also must be evaluated carefully. The patient's ability to bend over and get something from a lower cupboard, climb on an escalator, cross the street safely, organize his time adequately, manage his finances, and interact with others in a functional manner must be noted to determine the patient's ability to function independently in the community. The Rehabilitation Institute of Chicago has developed a community skills evaluation, as has Santa Clara Valley Medical Center (AOTA, 1985; Charness, 1986; Occupational Therapy Department, 1985).

The patient also needs to be reintroduced to

avocational interests. Patients may have residual neuro-muscular dysfunction that interferes with resumption of previous leisure activities. His lack of initiative and his cognitive inflexibility may hinder independence in play and leisure skills. The patient can practice anticipating problems he will face in these areas and organizing solutions. Driver training, prevocational skills, and/or vocational skills are taught, if appropriate (Jones, Giddens, & Croft, 1983; Malkmus et al., 1980).

Social skills must also be considered and treated by the whole team, because the postrehabilitation progress of the patient with a traumatic brain injury depends greatly on his family and other social contacts (Oddy & Humphrey, 1980). Social skills retraining following severe head injury develops awareness of appropriate social goals, develops skill in social behaviors, and facilitates successful social interactions. Behavioral learning methods are the most effective for training severely brain-injured individuals to overcome social skill impairments (Giles & Clark-Wilson, 1993).

Driving

The patient's residual physical, cognitive, percep-tual, and visual dysfunction must be thoroughly as-sessed in determining his ability to drive safely. The patient's psychosocial status, including self-control, impulse control, and frustration tolerance, must be carefully considered. A complete history of the patient's medical status, current medications, and previous driv-ing record is also taken. Simulated driving situations on a computer are helpful, if available. Adaptations can be made on a car to compensate for some physical problems, and the patient can be trained to compensate for visual field neglect. However, no compensation can be made for slowed reaction to emergency situations, lack of judgment or problem-solving ability, spatial or directional confusion on the road, impairment in depth perception, or decreased endurance (Jones et al., 1983; McNeny, 1990). Following evaluation, if the patient appears suitable for driving, an on-the-road test, covering all driving situations, is performed in a dual-control car or the patient's own car, with the assistance of an adaptive driving instructor (Jones et al., 1983). The therapist performing a driving evalua-tion should be familiar with the department of motor vehicle regulations applicable in that state or area.

Employment Preparation

A prevocational evaluation is performed, as de-scribed in Chapter 17. If modification of standardized tests is required, the standardized scoring cannot be used, but the results can be described. A variety of job placements, such as an adaptive learning program,

volunteer work, a sheltered workshop, or the patient's former job with modifications, should be considered.

DISCHARGE PLANNING

After hospitalization, the patient could be dis-charged to a number of different settings. The func-tional outcome of the patient, the family's ability to care for the patient, and the wishes of the patient and family are all considered in the team's recommenda-tions. Early in the rehabilitation process, the patient's need for equipment, such as a wheelchair or adaptive equipment, must be assessed. A home evaluation, to determine and discuss necessary modifications and to ascertain what skills need to be taught to the patient to move safely about the home environment, must be made if the patient will return to the family's house. Therapeutic passes give the family a preview of what care will be necessary and also a chance to have the team's help in solving any unanticipated problems that arise with the patient in the home.

As the patient becomes ready to go home, he may still be evidencing decreased responsiveness when fatigued, difficulty operating safely in unfamiliar situa-tions, little flexibility in cognitive processing, concrete and literal interpretation of situations, a shortened attention span, and difficulty in learning new informa-tion or tasks (Anderson & Parente, 1985; Scanlon-Schilpp & Levesque, 1981). The patient may need continued cognitive rehabilitation after discharge, be-cause recovery in this area has been shown to continue for 2 or more years postinjury (Benton, 1979; Dikmen et al., 1983; Najenson et al., 1974). Personality or behavioral changes also may still be present at dis-charge, e.g., disinhibition, low frustration or stress tolerance, reduced insight or judgment, labile affect, irritability, and impulsivity. In the extreme, the patient may experience paranoia, phobias, confusion, or delu-sional ideation (Benton, 1979; Brink et al., 1980). Mental, emotional, and behavioral impairments or changes are more difficult to adjust to than are physical impairments and interfere with successful reintegration into the family, social activity, and community (Benton, 1979; Jennett et al., 1981; Oddy & Humphrey, 1980). The brain-injured patient also must cope with loss of independence and control over his life, embarrassment over residual physical or speech impairment, or de-creased self-esteem.

COMMUNITY PROGRAMS

Following the months of rehabilitation, the head-injured patient who is discharged home to his family may continue outpatient therapy. When more care and physical supervision is required, there are long-term rehabilitation programs available in nursing homes or residential schools. Transitional living programs in a nonmedical setting are designed to increase development of those skills needed for the patient to live independently in progressively more complex living environments, i.e., moving from a small group family house to a supervised group apartment to an independent apartment and independent functioning in the community with help still available from the staff (Centrella, 1985). Day care/day treatment centers are available that emphasize increased independence and preparation for further education or vocational rehabilitation (Cole, Cope, & Cervelli, 1985; Cervelli, 1990). Centers for Independent Living are community-based programs providing or coordinating services to the patient, such as psychosocial evaluation and training, counseling, cognitive retraining, job and education reorientation, and respite care (Epperson-Sebour & Rifkin, 1985).

Self-help groups have been organized to help the patient cope with his psychosocial problems following discharge (Scanlon-Schilpp & Levesque, 1981). The National Head Injury Foundation, formed in 1980, is a valuable resource; there are many state associations and local chapters to assist patients and their families, to disseminate information nationwide on head injuries, and to increase awareness of the needs and advocate improvement in the ongoing treatment of this population. (Their address is 1776 Massachusetts Avenue NW, Suite 100, Washington, DC 20036.)

STUDIES OF THE EFFECTIVENESS OF THERAPY

There is little agreement or evidence concerning when to initiate rehabilitation for comatose brain-injured patients or what rehabilitation measures should be included at various stages of recovery. Most of the available literature on traumatic brain injury has concentrated on proposed medical treatments and assessment of their efficacy and on factors predictive of outcome of severe head injury. More recent publications have described and discussed the mental and behavioral sequelae of these types of injury. The studies that focused on the rehabilitation of the brain injured have primarily reported statistics on the outcome of such patients correlated with the duration of coma and other factors and measured by return to work, social interaction, and degree of autonomy in independent living skills. These publications have contained the authors' opinions on the usefulness and necessity of rehabilitative measures but offer little experimental documentation of different procedures. Unfortunately, articles documenting the effectiveness of specific rehabilitative procedures with the brain-injured patient have been scarce.

Panikoff (1983) documented the sequence of recovery of functional skills (dressing, transfers, gross and fine hand function, wheelchair mobility, basic daily living skills, kitchen skills, and community skills). Recovery sequences of two groups of head-injured patients (one group in coma for 14 days or less, the other in coma for more than 14 days) were compared over a period of 2 years postinjury with significant differences in the groups' performance on six of eight skills at 1 year. The recovery pattern was found to be gross hand function preceding basic daily living skills, followed by social and community skills and fine finger dexterity. No description of the rehabilitation program was offered.

There are a few authors who have described the rehabilitation programs used with their patients and who have presented statistics on the outcome of those patients. Most of these studies had no control groups or other aspects of an experimental design. Najenson et al. (1974) studied the outcome of 169 patients with severe brain injury who underwent a program using postural reflexes, self-care tasks, locomotor tasks, and communicative training. The statistics presented showed that 84% of the patients were independent in daily living skills at discharge. The authors found recovery continuing up to 3 years after injury and stressed the need for continued follow-up of these patients after discharge from a rehabilitation hospital. Gerstenbrand (1972) described a rehabilitation program beginning in the acute stage after trauma that included use of reflexes to influence muscle tone and more active mobilization and socialization techniques later. He briefly stated the results for 170 patients in terms of being back at work and concluded that rehabilitation at full intensity was essential.

Brink et al. (1980) studied 344 children with severe closed head injury, who were comatose more than 24 hr, and who had begun rehabilitation within 3 to 6 weeks postinjury. These authors found that 73% became independent in ambulation and self-care, 10% were partially dependent, and 17% were totally dependent. The nature of the rehabilitation techniques was not specifically described. The study was carried out at Rancho Los Amigos Hospital (Downey, California) and presumably used the Rancho rehabilitation program described in the literature. Jellinek, Torkelson, and Harvey (1982) investigated patients' adjustment to the behavioral and cognitive sequelae of the injury in relation to independence in daily living skills postdischarge. These researchers discovered that patients who were more independent in self-care and mobility experienced less distress and better adjustment than more dependent patients. Cole et al. (1985) described a postdischarge day treatment program and reported 47% of the group attained an improved level of functioning. However, the level to which these patients improved was not specified in terms of community functioning. Mercer and Boch (1983) offered clinical observations but no quantitative measures of improved quality of movement following their sensorimotor integration class with head-injured patients.

Postlesion experience in a mildly stressful, active environment has been found to be more facilitatory to behavioral and motor recovery than a more neutral, passive environment (Herdman, 1983; Walsh & Cummins, 1976). Other authors have emphasized the increased effectiveness of such experience when begun as soon as possible postinjury (Bach-y-Rita, 1981). Cope and Hall (1982) studied two groups of patients with severe brain injuries who were admitted for rehabilitation early (under 35 days postinjury) and later (more than 35 days postinjury) and compared the time required for rehabilitation and the outcome. They concluded that those admitted later required twice as much rehabilitation as those admitted early, despite similar initial injury severity. Outcome at 2 years postinjury was not significantly different between groups.

In a quasi-experimental study, Mackay et al. (1992) found that treatment within a formal trauma rehabilitation program that was started on admission to the acute care facility improved long-term outcome (following patients' subsequent stay in the rehabilitation center) in a group of 17 patients compared with a control group that received a nonformal acute care program. All patients initially had a GCS score of 3 to 8. The formal program included multisensory stimulation, orientation, exercises, and positioning to decrease tone.

Some experimental studies used control groups and documented subtle cognitive impairments caused by a brain injury. However, again, few studies have investigated the efficacy of cognitive retraining with such patients. A few case studies of specific cognitive retraining strategies for patients with head injury are available in the literature. A few studies of larger groups are also available, but they document only changes in patient status not the efficacy of the therapeutic procedures used. Scherzer (1986) studied three groups of patients with severe brain injury who were given physical, cognitive, perceptual, social, and prevocational training and counseling at least 1 year after coma. He determined that the greatest improvement was shown in areas of attention, memory, and complex reasoning, with significant improvements noted also in home life. Prigatano et al. (1984) observed more improvement in a group treated with a neuropsychologic program than in the control group in the areas of performance and memory scores on the *Wechsler Adult Intelligence Scale*. They also documented reduced emotional distress in the treated group.

Even fewer studies have explored the effects of

sensory stimulation or other therapeutic techniques on comatose patients. McGraw and Tindall (1974) found changes in heart rate, respiratory rate, and ICP in 50% of their comatose patient population in response to tactile, auditory, and painful stimulation. No gross movements were noted with these changes, but increased electrical activity was recorded in some patients' cervical muscles. Boortz-Marx (1985) and Parsons et al. (1985) found changes in ICP in response to oral and hygienic nursing procedures with brain-injured patients. Weber (1984) studied three comatose patients and found significant differences in the patients' cortical activity measured after therapy periods and measured after periods of unstructured stimulation and/or activity. The therapy in this study consisted of selected PNF patterns, quick icing, joint approximation, and verbal requests for a motor response.

Documentation of specific treatment techniques has begun, but the studies contain little experimental manipulation of the variables. Baker, Parker, and Sanderson (1983) presented a case study of a head-injured patient who, in addition to other rehabilitation measures, received neuromuscular electrical stimulation to increase ROM and to facilitate voluntary movement. The patient's status improved from wheelchair dependent to independent ambulator for short distances with a quad (four-pronged) cane. Booth, Doyle, and Montgomery (1983) offered descriptive results only of the effects of serial casting on ROM and muscle tone in brain-injured patients.

As is evident, few controlled studies on patients with traumatic brain injury are available. Many factors contribute to such a lack of research, including the philosophical dilemma of withholding therapy from a control group of patients. However, these difficulties need to be surmounted, and research must be conducted on the efficacy of the therapeutic procedures used with head-injured patients, the effect of such procedures on the long-term outcome of the injury, the patient's subsequent quality of life, and the optimum time during the recovery period for therapeutic intervention.

Acknowledgments—We wish to acknowledge the contribution of Ann M. Gillette, whose editing assistance was invaluable in this revision.

STUDY QUESTIONS

1. Why does a patient become unconscious following diffuse axonal injury?
2. Why do some people recover from coma while others remain in a persistent vegetative state?
3. Why is loss of the sense of smell considered a sign of an orbitofrontal focal lesion?
4. Why is contralateral hemiplegia associated with a frontolateral focal lesion?

STUDY QUESTIONS (continued) ━━━━━━━

5. What impairments are associated with an anoxic head injury?

6. Why is increased intracranial pressure dangerous?

7. Why are cognitive problems related to frontal lobe function seen in survivors of both DAI and focal lesions? Who will have the greater difficulties and why?

8. Describe the two sides of the debate concerning use of sensory stimulation in treatment of patients in deep coma.

9. Why are familiar and automatic activities chosen when first retraining self-care activities?

10. In what Rancho level will formal testing of perception and cognition be appropriate and why?

REFERENCES

Abreu, B. C., & Toglia, J. P. (1987). Cognitive rehabilitation: A model for occupational therapy. *American Journal of Occupational Therapy, 41*(7), 439–448.

American Occupational Therapy Association. (1985). *Head injury information packet.* Rockville, MD: Author.

Anderson, J., & Parente, F. (1985). Training family members to work with the head injured patient. *Cognitive Rehabilitation, 3,* 12–15.

Bach-y-Rita, P. (1981). *Brain plasticity as a basis of the development of rehabilitation procedures for hemiplegia.* Martinez, CA: VA Medical Center.

Baggerly, J. (1986). Rehabilitation of the adult with head trauma. *Nursing Clinics of North America, 21*(4), 577–587.

Bakay, L., & Glasauer, F. E..(1980). *Head injuries.* Boston: Little, Brown & Co.

Baker, L. L., Parker, K., & Sanderson, D. (1983). Neuromuscular electrical stimulation for the head-injured patient. *Physical Therapy, 63,* 1967–1974.

Barolat-Romana, G., & Larson, S. J. (1984). Influence of stimulus location and limb position on motor responses in the comatose patient. *Journal of Neurosurgery, 61,* 725–728.

Ben-Yishay, Y., & Prigatano, G. (1990). Cognitive remediation. In M. Rosenthal, E. R. Griffith, M. R. Bond, & J. D. Miller (Eds.), *Rehabilitation of the adult and child with traumatic brain injury* (2nd ed., pp. 393–409). Philadelphia: F. A. Davis.

Benton, A. (1979). Behavioral consequences of closed head injury. In G. L. Odom (Ed.), *Central nervous system trauma research status report* (pp. 220–231). Bethesda, MD: National Institute of Neurological and Communicative Disorders and Stroke.

Bond, M. R. (1990). Standardized methods of assessing and predicting outcome. In M. Rosenthal, E. R. Griffith, M. R. Bond, & J. D. Miller (Eds.), Rehabilitation of the adult and child with traumatic brain injury (2nd ed., pp. 59–76). Philadelphia: F. A. Davis.

Boortz-Marx, R. (1985). Factors affecting intracranial pressure: A descriptive study. *Journal of Neurosurgical Nursing, 17,* 89–94.

Booth, B. J., Doyle, M., & Montgomery, J. (1983). Serial casting for the management of spasticity in the head-injured adult. *Physical Therapy, 63,* 1960–1966.

Braakman, R., Gelpke, G. J., Habbema, J. D. F., Maas, A. I. R., & Minderhoud, J. M. (1980). Systematic selection of prognostic features in patients with severe head injury. *Neurosurgery, 6,* 362–370.

Bracy, O., Lynch, W., Sbordone, R., & Berrol, S. (1985). Cognitive retraining through computers: Fact or fad? *Cognitive Rehabilitation, 3,* 10–23.

Brandstater, M. E., Bontke, C. F., Cobble, N. D., & Horn, L. J. (1991). Rehabilitation in brain disorders. 4. Specific disorders. *Archives of Physical Medicine and Rehabilitation, 72,* S332–S340.

Bricolo, A., Turazzi, S., & Feriotti, G. (1980). Prolonged posttraumatic unconsciousness: Therapeutic assets and liabilities. *Journal of Neurosurgery, 52,* 625–634.

Brink, J. D., Imbus, C., & Woo-Sam, J. (1980). Physical recovery after severe closed head trauma in children and adolescents. *Journal of Pediatrics, 97,* 721–727.

Brooks, D. N. (1990). Cognitive deficits. In M. Rosenthal, E. R. Griffith, M. R. Bond, & J. D. Miller (Eds.), *Rehabilitation of the adult and child with traumatic brain injury* (2nd ed., pp. 163–178). Philadelphia: F. A. Davis.

Carr, J. H., & Shepherd, R. B. (1980). *Physiotherapy in disorders of the brain.* London: William Heinemann Medical Books.

Centrella, J. (1985). *South Valley Ranch: A community re-entry program for head injured adults.* Gilroy, CA: Learning Services Corp.

Cervelli, L. (1990). Re-entry into the community and systems of posthospital care. In M. Rosenthal, E. R. Griffith, M. R. Bond, & J. D. Miller (Eds.), *Rehabilitation of the adult and child with traumatic brain injury* (2nd ed., pp. 463–475). Philadelphia: F. A. Davis.

Chadwick, O., Rutter, M., Brown, G., Shaffer, D., & Traub, M. (1981). A prospective study of children with head injuries. II. Cognitive sequelae. *Psychological Medicine, 11,* 49–61.

Charness, A. L. (1986). *Stroke/head injury: A guide to functional outcomes in physical therapy management* (Rehabilitation Institute of Chicago Series). Rockville, MD: Aspen Systems.

Citta-Pietrolungo, T. J., Alexander, M. A., & Steg, N. L. (1992). Early detection of heterotopic ossification in young patients with traumatic brain injury. *Archives of Physical Medicine and Rehabilitation, 73,* 258–262.

Cole, J. R., Cope, D. N., & Cervelli, L. (1985). Rehabilitation of the severely brain-injured patient: A community-based, low-cost model program. *Archives of Physical Medicine and Rehabilitation, 66,* 38–40.

Cope D. N., & Hall, K. (1982). Head injury rehabilitation: Benefit of early intervention. *Archives of Physical Medicine and Rehabilitation, 63,* 433–437.

Cowley, R. S., Swanson, B., Chapman, P., Kitik, B. A., & Mackay, L. E. (1994). The role of rehabilitation in the intensive care unit. *Journal of Head Trauma Rehabilitation, 9*(1), 32–42.

Davis, R. A., & Cunningham, P. S. (1984). Prognostic factors in severe head injury. *Surgery, Gynecology and Obstetrics, 159,* 597–604.

Dikmen, S., Reitan, R. M., & Temkin, N. R. (1983). Neuropsychological recovery in head injury. *Archives of Neurology, 40,* 333–338.

Diller, L., & Gordon, W. A. (1981). Interventions for cognitive deficits in brain-injured adults. *Journal of Consulting and Clinical Psychology, 49,* 822–834.

Eames, P., Haffey, W. J., & Cope, D. N. (1990). Treatment of behavioral disorders. In M. Rosenthal, E. R. Griffith, M. R. Bond, & J. D. Miller (Eds.), *Rehabilitation of the adult and child with traumatic brain injury* (2nd ed., pp. 410–432). Philadelphia: F. A. Davis.

Epperson-Sebour, M. M., & Rifkin, E. W. (1985). Center for living: Trauma aftercare and outcome. *Maryland Medical Journal, 34,* 1187–1192.

Eson, M. E., Yen, J. K., & Bourke, R. S. (1978). Assessment

of recovery from serious head injury. *Journal of Neurology, Neurosurgery, and Psychiatry, 41,* 1036–1042.

Farber, S. D. (1982). *Neurorehabilitation: A multisensory approach.* Philadelphia: W. B. Saunders.

Finkelstein, S., & Ropper, A. (1979). The diagnosis of coma: Its pitfalls and limitations. *Heart & Lung, 8,* 1059–1064.

Gerstenbrand, F. (1972). The course of restitution of brain injury in the early and late stages and the rehabilitative measures. *Scandinavian Journal of Rehabilitation Medicine, 4,* 85–89.

Gianutsos, R. (1980). What is cognitive rehabilitation? *Journal of Rehabilitation, 46,* 36–40.

Giles, G. M., & Clark-Wilson, J. (1993). *Brain injury rehabilitation: A neurofunctional approach.* San Diego: Singular Publishing Group.

Gordon, W. A., Mann, N., & Willer, B. (1993). Demographic and social characteristics of the traumatic brain injury model system database. *Journal of Head Trauma Rehabilitation, 8*(2), 26–33.

Greenberg, D. A., Aminoff, M. J., & Simon, R. P. (1993). *Clinical neurology* (2nd ed.). East Norwalk, CT: Appleton & Lange.

Griffith, E. R., & Mayer, N. H. (1990). Hypertonicity and movement disorders. In M. Rosenthal, E. R. Griffith, M. R. Bond, & J. D. Miller (Eds.), *Rehabilitation of the adult and child with traumatic brain injury* (2nd ed., pp. 127–147). Philadelphia: F. A. Davis.

Groswasser, Z., Cohen, M., & Costeff, H. (1989). Rehabilitation outcome after anoxic brain damage. *Archives of Physical Medicine and Rehabilitation, 70,* 186–188.

Hall, K., Cope, D. N., & Rappaport, M. (1985). Glasgow outcome scale and disability rating scale: Comparative usefulness in following recovery in traumatic head injury. *Archives of Physical Medicine and Rehabilitation, 66,* 35–37.

Hall, M. E., MacDonald, S., & Young, G. C. (1992). The effectiveness of directed multisensory stimulation versus non-directed stimulation in comatose CHI patients: Pilot study of a single subject design. *Brain Injury, 6*(5), 435–445.

Herdman, S. J. (1983). Effect of experience on recovery following CNS lesions. *Physical Therapy, 63,* 51–55.

Hill, J. (1994). The effects of casting on upper extremity motor disorders after brain injury. *American Journal of Occupational Therapy, 48*(3), 219–224.

Hill, J., & Carper, M. (1985). Greenery: Group therapeutic approaches with the head injured. *Cognitive Rehabilitation, 3,* 18–29.

Horn, L. J. (1991). Rehabilitation in brain disorders: 1) Basic sciences. *Archives of Physical Medicine and Rehabilitation, 72,* S317–S319.

Jellinek, H. M., Torkelson, R. M., & Harvey, R. F. (1982). Functional abilities and distress levels in brain injured patients at long-term follow-up. *Archives of Physical Medicine and Rehabilitation, 63,* 160–162.

Jennett, B., Snoek, J., Bond, M. R., & Brooks, N. (1981). Disability after severe head injury: Observations on the use of the Glasgow Outcome Scale. *Journal of Neurology, Neurosurgery, and Psychiatry, 44,* 285–293.

Jennett, B., & Teasdale, G. (1981). *Management of head injuries.* Philadelphia: F. A. Davis.

Jones, R., Giddens, H., & Croft, D. (1983). Assessment and training of brain-damaged drivers. *American Journal of Occupational Therapy, 37,* 754–760.

Kalsbeek, W. D., McLaurin, R. L., Harris, B. S. H., & Miller, J. D. (1980). The national head and spinal cord injury survey: Major findings. *Journal of Neurosurgery, 53,* S19–S31.

Karnaze, D. S., Weiner, J. M., & Marshall, L. F. (1985). Auditory evoked potentials in coma after closed head injury: A clinical-neurophysiologic coma scale for predicting outcome. *Neurology, 35,* 1122–1126.

Katz, D. I. (1992). Neuropathology and neurobehavioral recovery from closed head injury. *Journal of Head Trauma Rehabilitation, 1*(2), 1–15.

Keener, S. M., & Sweigart, J. E. (1984). Early use of adaptable seating for patients with head trauma. *Physical Therapy, 64,* 206–207.

Leech, R. W., & Shuman, R. M. (1982). *Neuropathology: A summary for students.* New York: Harper & Row.

Levin, H. S., O'Donnell, V. M., & Grossman, R. G. (1979). The Galveston Orientation and Amnesia Test: A practical scale to assess cognition after head injury. *Journal of Nervous and Mental Diseases, 167,* 675–684.

Lillehei, K. O., & Hoff, J. T. (1985). Advances in the management of closed head injury. *Annals of Emergency Medicine, 14,* 789–795.

Lipper, M. H., Kishore, P. R. S., Enas, G. G., da Silva, A. A. D., Choi, S. C., & Becker, D. P. (1985). Computed tomography in the prediction of outcome in head injury. *American Journal of Roentgenology, 144,* 483–486.

Livingston, M. G., Brooks, D. N., & Bond, M. R. (1985). Patient outcome in the year following severe head injury and relatives' psychiatric and social function. *Journal of Neurology, Neurosurgery, and Psychiatry, 48,* 876–881.

Lundgren, C. C., & Persechino, E. L. (1986). Cognitive group: A treatment program for head-injured adults. *American Journal of Occupational Therapy, 40,* 397–401.

Lynch, W. J. (1986). Computer-assisted cognitive retraining. *Journal of Head Trauma Rehabilitation, 1,* 77–78.

Lynch, W. J. (1990). Neuropsychological assessment. In M. Rosenthal, E. R. Griffith, M. R. Bond, & J. D. Miller (Eds.), *Rehabilitation of the adult and child with traumatic brain injury* (2nd ed., pp. 310–326). Philadelphia: F. A. Davis.

Mackay, L. E., Bernstein, B. A., Chapman, P. E., Morgan, A. S., & Milazzo, L. S. (1992). Early intervention in severe head injury: Long-term benefits of a formalized program. *Archives of Physical Medicine and Rehabilitation, 73,* 635–641.

Malkmus, D., Booth, B. J., & Kodimer, C. (1980). *Rehabilitation of the head injured adult: Comprehensive cognitive management.* Downey, CA: Professional Staff Association of Rancho Los Amigos Hospital.

McGraw, C. P., & Tindall, G. T. (1974). Cardio-respiratory alterations in head injury: Patients' response to stimulation. *Surgical Neurology, 2,* 263–266.

McNeny, R. (1990). Deficits in activities of daily living. In M. Rosenthal, E. R. Griffith, M. R. Bond, & J. D. Miller (Eds.), *Rehabilitation of the adult and child with traumatic brain injury* (2nd ed., pp. 193–205). Philadelphia: F. A. Davis.

Mercer, L., & Boch, M. (1983). Residual sensorimotor deficits in the adult head-injured patient. *Physical Therapy, 63,* 1988–1991.

Miller, B. L. & McIntyre, H. B. (1984). Evaluation of the comatose patient. *Primary Care, 11,* 693–706.

Miller, J. D. (1985). Head injury and brain ischaemia—Implications for therapy. *British Journal of Anaesthesiology, 57,* 120–130.

Miller, J. D., Pentland, B., & Berrol, S. (1990). Early evaluation and management. In M. Rosenthal, E. R. Griffith, M. R. Bond, & J. D. Miller (Eds.), *Rehabilitation of the adult and child with traumatic brain injury* (2nd ed., pp. 21–51). Philadelphia: F. A. Davis.

Milton, S. B. (1985). Compensatory memory strategy training: A practical approach for managing persisting memory problems. *Cognitive Rehabilitation, 3,* 8–15.

Mitchell, P. H. (1986). Intracranial hypertension: Influence of nursing care activities. *Nursing Clinics of North America, 21*(4), 563–576.

Mitchell, S., Bradley, V. A., Welch, J. L. & Britton, P. G. (1990). Coma arousal procedure: A therapeutic intervention in the treatment of head injury. *Brain Injury, 4*(3), 273–279.

Moore, J. C. (1980). Neuroanatomical considerations relating to recovery of function following brain lesions. In P. Bach-y-Rita (Ed.), *Recovery of function: Theoretical considerations for brain injury rehabilitation* (pp. 9–90). Baltimore: University Park Press.

Muir, C., Rosenthal, M., & Diehl, L. N. (1990). Methods of family intervention. In M. Rosenthal, E. R. Griffith, M. R. Bond, & J. D. Miller (Eds.), *Rehabilitation of the adult and child with traumatic brain injury* (2nd ed., pp. 433–448). Philadelphia: F. A. Davis.

Najenson, T., Mendelson, L., Schechter, I., David, C., Mintz, N., & Grosswasser, Z. (1974). Rehabilitation after severe head injury. *Scandinavian Journal of Rehabilitation Medicine, 6*, 5–14.

National Head Injury Foundation. (1993). *Every fifteen seconds.* Washington, DC: Author.

National Institute of Neurological Disorders and Stroke. (1984). *Head injury: Hope through research.* Bethesda, MD: National Institutes of Health.

Neistadt, M. E. (1990). Critical analysis of occupational therapy approaches for perceptual deficits in adults with brain injury. *American Journal of Occupational Therapy, 44*(4), 299–595.

Neistadt, M. E. (1994). Perceptual retraining for adults with diffuse brain injury. *American Journal of Occupational Therapy, 48*(3), 225–233.

Newlon, P. G., & Greenberg, R. P. (1984). Evoked potentials in severe head injury. *Journal of Trauma, 24*, 61–66.

Occupational Therapy Department. (1985). *Perceptual motor evaluation for head injured and other neurologically impaired adults.* San Jose, CA: Santa Clara Valley Medical Center.

Oddy, M., & Humphrey, M. (1980). Social recovery during the year following severe head injury. *Journal of Neurology, Neurosurgery, and Psychiatry, 43*, 798–802.

Palmer, M., & Wyness, M.A. (1988). Positioning and handling: Important considerations in the care of the severely head-injured patient. *Journal of Neuroscience Nursing, 20*(1), 42–50.

Panikoff, L. B. (1983). Recovery trends of functional skills in the head-injured adult. *American Journal of Occupational Therapy, 37*, 735–743.

Parsons, L. C., Peard, A. L. S., & Page, M. C. (1985). The effects of hygiene interventions on the cerebrovascular status of severe closed head injured persons. *Research Nursing and Health, 8*, 173–181.

Plum, F., & Posner, J. (1972). *The diagnosis of stupor and coma* (2nd ed.). Philadelphia: F. A. Davis.

Prigatano, G. P., Fordyce, D. J., Zeiner, H. K., Roueche, J. R., Pepping, M., & Wood, B. C. (1984). Neuropsychological rehabilitation after closed head injury in young adults. *Journal of Neurology, Neurosurgery, and Psychiatry, 47*, 505–513.

Rao, N., Jellinek, H. M., & Woolston, D. C. (1985). Agitation in closed head injury: Haloperidol effects on rehabilitation outcome. *Archives of Physical Medicine and Rehabilitation, 66*, 30–34.

Reyes, R. L., Heller, D., & Bhattacharyya, A. K. (1981). Traumatic head injury: Restlessness and agitation as prognosticators of physical and psychologic improvement in patients. *Archives of Physical Medicine and Rehabilitation, 62*, 20–23.

Rimel, R. W., Jane, J. A., & Bond, M. R. (1990). Characteristics of the head injured patient. In M. Rosenthal, E. R. Griffith, M. R. Bond, & J. D. Miller (Eds.), *Rehabilitation of the adult and child with traumatic brain injury* (2nd ed., pp. 8–16). Philadelphia: F. A. Davis.

Rosenthal, M., & Bond, M. R. (1990). Behavioral and psychiatric sequelae. In M. Rosenthal, E. R. Griffith, M. R. Bond, & J. D.

Miller (Eds.), *Rehabilitation of the adult and child with traumatic brain injury* (2nd ed., pp. 179–192). Philadelphia: F. A. Davis.

Salcman, M., Schepp, R. S., & Ducker, T. B. (1981). Calculated recovery rates in severe head trauma. *Neurosurgery, 8*, 301–308.

Scanlon-Schilpp, A. M., & Levesque, J. (1981). Helping the patient cope with the sequelae of trauma through the self-help group approach. *Journal of Trauma, 21*, 135–139.

Schaffer, L., Kranzler, L. I., & Siqueira, E. B. (1985). Aspects of evaluation and treatment of head injury. *Neurology Clinics, 3*, 259–273.

Scherzer, A. L., & Tscharnuter, I. (1982). *Early diagnosis and therapy in cerebral palsy.* New York: Marcel Dekker.

Scherzer, B. P. (1986). Rehabilitation following severe head trauma: results of a three-year program. *Archives of Physical Medicine and Rehabilitation, 67*, 366–374.

Sparadeo, F. R., & Gill, D. (1989). Focus on clinical research: Effects of prior alcohol use on head injury recovery. *Journal of Head Trauma Rehabilitation, 4*(1), 75–82.

Spielman, G., Gennarelli, T. A., & Rogers, C. R. (1983). Disodium etidronate: Its role in preventing heterotopic ossification in severe head injury. *Archives of Physical Medicine and Rehabilitation, 64*, 539–542.

Stanczak, D. E., White, J. G., Gouview, W. D., Moehle, K. A., Daniel, M., Novack, T., & Long, C. J. (1984). Assessment of level of consciousness following severe neurological insult. *Journal of Neurosurgery, 60*, 955–960.

Stockmeyer, S. (1967). An interpretation of the approach of Rood to the treatment of neuromuscular dysfunction. *American Journal of Physical Medicine, 46*, 900–956.

Toglia, J. P. (1991). Generalization of treatment: A multicontext approach to cognitive perceptual impairment in adults with brain injury. *American Journal of Occupational Therapy, 45*(6), 505–516.

Trexler, L. (1984). *Cognitive rehabilitation: Questions and answers.* Framingham, MA: National Head Injury Foundation.

Trexler, L. E. & Zappala, G. (1988). Neuropathological determinants of acquired attention disorders in traumatic brain injury. *Brain & Cognition, 8*, 291–302.

Turner, M. S. (1985). Pediatric head injury. *Indiana Medicine, 78*, 194–197.

Varney, N. R., & Menefee, L. (1993). Psychosocial and executive deficits following closed head injury: Implications for orbital frontal cortex. *Journal of Head Trauma Rehabilitation, 8*(1), 32–44.

Walsh, R. N., & Cummins, R. A. (1976). Neural responses to therapeutic sensory environments. In R. N. Walsh & W. T. Greenough (Eds.), *Environments as therapy for brain dysfunction.* New York: Plenum Press.

Warren, J. B., & Peck, E. A. (1984). Factors which influence neuropsychological recovery from severe head injury. *Journal of Neurosurgical Nursing, 16*, 248–252.

Warren, M. (1993a). A hierarchical model for evaluation and treatment of visual perceptual dysfunction in adult acquired brain injury, Part 1. *American Journal of Occupational Therapy, 47*(1), 42–54.

Warren, M. (1993b). A hierarchical model for evaluation and treatment of visual perceptual dysfunction in adult acquired brain injury, Part 2. *American Journal of Occupational Therapy, 47*(1), 55–66.

Weber, P. L. (1984). Sensorimotor therapy: Its effect on electroencephalograms of acute comatose patients. *Archives of Physical Medicine and Rehabilitation, 65*, 457–462.

Wood, R. L. (1991). Critical analysis of the concept of sensory stimulation for patients in vegetative states. *Brain Injury, 5*(4), 401–409.

Wood, R. L., Winkowski, T. B., Miller, J. L., Tierney, L., & Goldman, L. (1992). Evaluating sensory regulation as a method to improve awareness in patients with altered states of consciousness: A pilot study. *Brain Injury, 6*(5), 411–418.

Zoltan, B. (1990). Occupational therapy evaluation. In M. Rosenthal, E. R. Griffith, M. R. Bond, & J. D. Miller (Eds.), *Rehabilitation of the adult and child with traumatic brain injury* (2nd ed., pp. 284–293). Philadelphia: F. A. Davis.

Degenerative Diseases

Elizabeth M. Newman, Maria Elena Echevarria, and Glenn Digman

OBJECTIVES

After studying this chapter the reader will be able to:
1. State the occupational therapy goals for treatment of persons with degenerative diseases.
2. Provide basic education regarding HIV transmission.
3. Describe the occupational therapy treatment approaches commonly used for six degenerative diseases.
4. Discuss strategies used to promote a meaningful quality of life for persons with degenerative diseases.

Degenerative diseases involve pathology that leads to progressive disability. They provide a unique challenge in all areas of intervention for therapists who work with patients with these diagnoses. The characteristics, evaluation, and treatment of six degenerative diseases—acquired immune deficiency syndrome, amyotrophic lateral sclerosis, muscular dystrophy, multiple sclerosis, Parkinson's disease and postpolio syndrome—are discussed in this chapter. The primary goal of treatment for each is to reduce the effects of disability resulting from symptoms of the disease and to promote a quality of life that the patient finds meaningful.

ACQUIRED IMMUNE DEFICIENCY SYNDROME

Acquired immune deficiency syndrome (AIDS) is a disease in which the immune system's natural defense against opportunistic infections is debilitated. The term AIDS was adopted by the Centers for Disease Control and Prevention (CDC) in 1982, 1 year after a significant number of cases were diagnosed in the United States. The human immunodeficiency virus (HIV) is a retrovirus that destroys CD_4 T-cells (helper Ts), white blood cells responsible for activating the immune system's natural disease-fighting mechanisms. HIV also invades neuronal cells, damaging the central and peripheral nervous systems. The CDC has developed a classification system of the continuum of HIV progression (Table 36.1).

Four primary modes of HIV transmission have been defined.

1. Sexual contact with an infected person in which blood, semen, or vaginal secretions are exchanged.
2. Exposure to blood or blood products, e.g., needle sharing by intravenous drug users, transfusions of blood and blood products between 1977 and mid-1985 (before the development of the HIV antibody tests and screening of the nation's blood supply), and occupational exposure in a health care setting.
3. Infection of patient by health care worker; this is very rare and occurs only when a health care worker fails to follow universal precautions.
4. Transmission from an infected woman to her fetus or newborn via blood or breast milk; about 30% of children born to infected women will develop HIV disease (Hessol & Lifson, 1990).

Precautions

Infection control precautions with HIV patients are critical because of the serious consequences of health care worker infection and the possibility of delivering a serious opportunistic infection to a person with AIDS (PWA). Marcil (1992) reported that the latter is more likely than the former. The CDC (1993) confirmed 33 cases of health care worker occupational exposure and 69 possible occupational transmissions through December 1992. None of these exposures involved occupational, physical, or speech therapists.

Table 36.2 is a comprehensive list of universal precautions concerning HIV. Any therapist providing patient care when the potential of exposure to bodily

GLOSSARY

Akinesia—Impaired ability to initiate voluntary and spontaneous motor responses. It is characterized by the interruption of performance of an ongoing movement (freezing) when attention is distracted.

Bradykinesia—Slowness of body movement. It is a complex phenomenon, consisting of hesitancy in initiating a new movement or stopping an ongoing movement, slowness of execution of movement, and rapid fatigue (Duvoisin, 1991).

Cogwheel rigidity—A series of catches in the resistance during passive movement. As the muscle is passively stretched, the resistance is periodically released during the movement. It is thought to be the combination of rigidity and tremor (Brown, 1980).

Diplopia—Perception of two images when viewing a single object; double vision.

Fasciculations—Involuntary twitching or contraction of muscle fibers that can be seen beneath the skin.

Rigidity—A hypertonicity of agonist and antagonist that offers a constant, uniform resistance to passive movement. The affected muscles seem unable to relax and are in a state of contraction even at rest.

---

fluids exists must follow universal precautions regardless of the patient's suspected HIV status. These universal precautions, as defined by the CDC, protect health care workers and patients from the transmission of a variety of diseases. Likewise, hospital personnel with any type of infectious, or potentially infectious, disease are restricted from working with patients whose immune systems are compromised, including HIV positive (HIV+) individuals (Minerbo, 1992).

An increase in tuberculosis (TB) has been a recent concern in the United States (DiGioia, 1992; Glazer, 1992; Johnson & Chaisson, 1991). People with immune systems compromised by AIDS are particularly vulnerable. TB is transmitted when someone with an active case coughs, thus releasing bacteria into the air. Infection-control measures include wearing a mask and goggles, isolating the patient to his room with negative ventilation (i.e., the pressure in the room is less than that in hallway and adjoining rooms), providing ventilation of air only into the open environment outdoors, using ultraviolet lights in the room to help kill the TB virus in the air (Vareldzis, personal communication, 1993).

Occupational Therapy Intervention

Occupational therapists have much to offer the HIV/AIDS population. However, therapists find that they must deal with two important personal issues before they work with persons who are HIV positive: (1) Fear of the disease, which is best addressed by learning and practicing the universal precautions and realizing it is very unlikely that an occupational therapist will become HIV infected if the precautions are followed, and (2) prejudice toward certain populations affected by the disease. Awareness of prejudice and a commitment to keep its negative effects out of the therapeutic relationship are important first steps.

Evaluation

HIV+ patients will generally present for occupational therapy evaluation and treatment several years postinfection. The patient's status at that time may be changing rapidly. Thus it may be necessary to reevaluate and modify treatment goals frequently. Begin with an evaluation of basic activities of daily living and instrumental activities of daily living, including work roles and leisure activities (see Chapter 4). If those that are important to the patient are deficient, then evaluate the following components of function.

PHYSICAL STATUS

Evaluate muscle strength and tone, endurance, range of motion (Chapter 6), coordination (Chapter 7), sensation (Chapter 8), and feeding and swallowing (Chapter 44) as needed. Perform a vision screen to determine if visual deficits are affecting function. At a minimum, check near and distance acuity plus visual fields. Educate patients that HIV+ people are high risk for cytomegalovirus (CMV) retinitis, which may cause blindness if not detected early (Epps, 1993).

COGNITION

The effects of HIV on cognitive functioning should be considered during all activities of daily living. The effects of decreased memory, dementia, and confusion are of particular concern (see Chapter 9).

PRIMARY CARETAKER ASSESSMENT

Consider stress of the caretaker(s) related to the severity of the disease, prejudice faced by people with AIDS and their significant others, and the fact that the caretaker may be the patient's same-sex partner who fears he, too, is infected.

PSYCHOSOCIAL ASSESSMENT

The serious nature of HIV disease and the likelihood of death require a holistic approach that encourages the patient to take as much control of his life as is important to him. Tigges and Marcil (1992) stress the importance of evaluating and supporting the patient's self-esteem, ability to maintain control over

Table 36.1   Continuum for HIV Progression

Timing	Symptoms	Test Results
	Stage I: Acute Infection	
1 to 12 weeks after initial exposure to HIV	Flu-like, i.e., Fever, pain in joints, lymphadenopathy (Gonzales-Aviles, 1992); Guillain-Barré syndrome (Pizzi, 1990); symptoms last a few days to a few weeks and vary greatly in individuals; 50% of cases develop no symptoms at this stage (Fahrner & Gerberding, 1991)	Two standard tests: Western blot and ELISA test for antibodies to HIV; antibodies develop 3 to 6 months postexposure, therefore, those exposed initially test negative
	Stage II: Asymptomatic Infection	
Extends an average of 8 to 9 years following infection (Hessol & Lifson, 1990; Lui, 1988); lifestyle, i.v. drug use, and increased age negatively affect this period; new treatments are lengthening this period	Most individuals remain symptom free	Measures of CD_4 T-cells show a slow, steady decline; T-cell count usually above 400 for persons at this stage ($N = 1000$); many experts recommend medication that inhibits HIV's effect on T-cells as they approach the 400 level, e.g., AZT
	Stage III: Persistent Generalized Lymphadenopathy	
Varies greatly; begins an average of 8 to 9 years postinfection; may last 1 to 3 years	Painless, chronic enlargement and tenderness of lymph nodes at two or more sites	Continued monitoring of CD_4 T-cell counts, usually between 400 and 200 at this stage; regular medical checkups to rule out presence of opportunistic infections listed in stage IV
	Stage IV: Other Diseases	
Begins 8 to 9 years postinfection on average; average life expectancy 3 to 5 years after first major opportunistic infection; varies greatly	Numerous diseases and opportunistic infections, as the body's immune system is too damaged to fight infections or HIV directly attacking body cells other than the CD_4 T-cell: (A) Constitutional symptoms: Wasting syndrome—fever, night sweats, and diarrhea for > 1 month and weight loss > 10% (Mansell, 1992). Dysphagia caused by oral thrush or other opportunistic infections and hepatitis (Gonzales-Aviles, 1992). Anemia and cytopenia caused by HIV's effect on bone marrow (O'Connell, 1990). (B) Neurological symptoms: May be experienced early after HIV exposure because of HIV directly attacking nerve cells. Central and peripheral nervous system involvement is initial symptom in 10% of cases with 40% of cases eventually experiencing neurological complications (Minerbo, 1992). HIV encephalopathy, encephalitis, dementia, depression, confusion, pyramidal and extrapyramidal symptoms, ataxia, hypertonia, hypotonia, decreased proprioception, decreased sense of touch, peripheral neuropathies, and strokes. (C) Opportunistic infections: *Pneumocystis carini* pneumonia, tuberculosis, oral candiasis (thrush), cytomegalovirus. CMV retinitis produces visual deficits in 10 to 15% of patients. (D) Associated neoplasms: Kaposi's sarcoma (KS), invasive cervical cancer, and tumors of the brain and spinal cord.	A CD_4 T-cell count ≤ 200 or a specified opportunistic infection listed above is the CDC guideline for AIDS classification as of January 1993; many people develop these serious opportunistic infections before their CD_4 T-cell count drops to 200

Table 36.2 Universal Precautions

The National Rehabilitation Hospital (NRH) has adopted a policy in which any person involved with patient care must adhere to universal precautions. Medical history and exam cannot identify all patients infected with human immunodeficiency virus (HIV-AIDS), hepatitis B (HBV), or any other blood-borne pathogens; you must treat **ALL** patients as potentially infectious—you must use these universal precautions when contacting blood/body fluids of **ANY** patient. Blood and body fluids refer to:
blood, tissue, semen, vaginal secretions, cerebrospinal fluid, pleural fluid, amniotic fluid, and other body fluids containing visible blood such as sputum, feces, urine, and vomitus.

Use the following universal precautions.
1. Consider blood and body fluids of all patients as potentially infectious.
2. Wash hands before and after contact with all patients, after removal of gloves, and after contact with any contaminated items.
3. Wear gloves when contact with blood/body fluids, mucus membranes or nonintact skin is likely, when handling items or surfaces soiled with blood/body fluids, and when performing venipuncture or other vascular access procedure.
4. Wear gowns, masks and protective eyewear during procedures that are likely to generate splashes of blood/body fluids.
5. Place used needles and sharp items directly into a puncture-resistent container. DO NOT RECAP NEEDLES.
6. Handle all linen and trash soiled with blood/body fluids as potentially infectious (wear gloves and/or other protective barriers).
7. Bag all laboratory specimens. Wear gloves when handling specimens.
8. To clean up blood/body fluid spills:
   a. Wear gloves.
   b. Use paper towels to soak up the blood/body fluid.
   c. Prepare a fresh solution of 1:10 bleach (1 part bleach to 9 parts water) or use an approved germicide.
   d. Pour the bleach or germicide on the spill and leave on the area for 10 min.
   e. Wear gloves and soak up the bleach or germicide with paper towels and dispose of properly.

his life, sense of competency and achievement, and motivation to maintain quality of life.

Kielhofner's (1985) model of human occupation provides a useful tool for structuring assessment and treatment with this population. The model's holistic incorporation of performance skills (performance subsystem), habits, roles, and routines (habituation subsystem) plus personal goals, values, motivation, interest, and feelings (volitional subsystem) is useful in considering all aspects of the patient's life while promoting maximum control of the treatment process by the patient.

Schindler (1988) discussed the impact of AIDS on psychosocial development. She noted that most PWAs are 20 to 45 years old, the stage of adult development that is typified by the task of intimacy versus self-absorption. At this time, one's energies most commonly focus on "sexual intimacy . . . to love and to work" (Erikson, 1980, pp. 101–102). The key developmental task is to become independent and develop a lasting commitment to another person, cause, institution, and/or work. PWAs face a major challenge to their ability to work and establish sexual intimacy. Occupational therapy assessment should address the areas of intimacy and work and develop strategies for helping the patient continue to experience satisfaction and competence in these areas. Discussion of safe sex practices, positioning, and alternative means for expressing affection provides avenues for helping PWAs continue to enjoy intimacy in relationships.

Treatment

A substantive body of research now exists that supports the position that rehabilitation can decrease the negative effects of HIV. LaPerriere et al. (1992) reported that aerobic exercise training increases cellular immunity in HIV+ patients. Florijn (1992) reported that a program of gymnastics, endurance training, and relaxation delayed the progression of HIV morbidity. Schlenzig et al. (1989) noted that physical exercise can improve both the immunological and psychological function of HIV infected patients. Spence et al. (1990) determined that progressive resistive exercise significantly increased muscle function, mass, and body weight in HIV+ patients. Antoni et al. (1992) reported that both aerobic exercise and stress management training significantly increased immunologic control of Epstein-Barr virus and human herpesvirus type 6 in HIV+ men. All of these authors cautioned that fatigue and overexertion must be avoided. The patient's physician must monitor the activity level and medically clear all strenuous activity.

More research is needed to address the specific benefits of functional/purposeful activity (occupational therapy) on HIV disease. In the meantime, it is reasonable to believe physical activities aimed at restoring meaningful function have a positive impact on quality of life for the HIV+ person.

Many of the interventions appropriate for HIV disease are familiar to occupational therapists and are detailed in other sections of this book. A description of those services that are unique for persons with HIV disease follows.

PHASE I: PREINFECTION

Occupational therapists have contact with many people in high-risk groups. The goals for this stage are to help people who are HIV negative manage their AIDS phobia and remain uninfected through education about AIDS transmission and safe sex practices. The names of organizations from which therapists can acquire basic information about HIV disease are listed in the supplementary resources for this chapter. Research indicates that programs that stress that high-risk sexual activity may lead to HIV infection are not as effective in changing behavior as those that teach concrete skills for condom use and negotiating safer sex encounters with partners (Valdiserri et al., 1988, 1989).

PHASE II: HIV POSITIVE/PRE-AIDS

LaPerriere et al. (1992) reported that the asymptomatic HIV+ individual may experience fear of social rejection, isolation, uncertainty regarding course of the disease as well as depression, anger, and anxiety brought on by a need to change lifestyle. Activities that offer an opportunity to express feelings constructively are indicated. The need for education regarding HIV disease continues with an emphasis on referral for early medical care, on how to maintain intimacy without spreading HIV, on support for informing significant others regarding HIV+ status, and on maintaining or developing vocational and/or leisure skills that contribute to well-being and stress reduction.

PHASE III: EARLY TO MID-STAGE AIDS

Activities of daily living (ADL) intervention is similar to that offered to other individuals experiencing weakness and reduced endurance. The compromised immune system requires special attention to details like dental, skin, nail, hair, vaginal, and rectal care; nutrition, food, and cooking; and kitchen and bathroom cleanliness. PWAs often find companionship in pets. Safe pet precautions must be taken to decrease the risk of disease transmission from pet to pet owner.

Vocational planning and adaptation are frequently primary areas of concern. According to Title I of the Americans with Disabilities Act of 1990, "HIV positive persons and persons perceived to have HIV or AIDS are protected in the work place" (Montoya, 1992. p. 167). Under most circumstances, job applicants cannot be required to take an HIV antibody test and cannot be denied employment or training if they are otherwise qualified. Employees cannot be denied assignments, promotion, benefits, or leave that are available to other employees. PWAs must be able to perform the essential functions of the job, and employers must offer reasonable accommodations that do not cause undue hardship to keep disabled employees on the job.

PHASE IV: END STAGE DISEASE

The primary focus during end stage disease is to prepare patients with limited life expectancy and their caretakers for the return home and the need for supportive care. Creative expression is used to confront and address issues concerning death, saying farewells to

friends and family, and formalizing a will. Therapists may want to consult frequently with the patient's doctor at this stage so therapist and patient can maintain a realistic perspective of life expectancy with a corresponding adjustment of treatment goals. Therapists should also seek consultation as an outlet for their own feelings (see Chapters 10 and 20).

CASE STUDY I

In 1989, John, age 25 was admitted to an acute care hospital experiencing respiratory distress secondary to *Pneumocystis carini* pneumonia (PCP). He had been hospitalized 3 weeks, with a resolution of the PCP. He was referred for inpatient occupational and physical therapy at that time. He exhibited decreased strength and endurance secondary to deconditioning. He also had moderately impaired sensation (light touch, deep pressure, and proprioception) in both lower extremities because of HIV-related peripheral neuropathy. Before hospitalization he had been working as an assistant chef in an Italian restaurant. He was receiving a small monthly disability check and planned to live with his parents after hospital discharge. He did not plan to return to work.

The results of the initial evaluation were as follows.

Dressing upper extremities. Minimum assistance because of decreased sitting balance and decreased upper extremity strength.

Dressing lower extremities. Moderate assistance as a result of decreased sitting balance and decreased lower extremity strength and sensation.

Bathing. Limited to bed because of an inability to transfer; moderate assistance with bed baths as a result of decreased sitting balance, decreased strength overall, and decreased lower extremity sensation.

Hygiene. Independent after setup in bed.

Transfers. Maximum assistance for squat pivot transfers to and from wheelchair to bed and toilet.

Toileting. Minimum assistance in handling clothing and wiping himself because of decreased sitting balance and decreased lower extremity strength.

Bowel and bladder. Continent

Hobbies. Cooking, meditation to music.

Treatment

Occupational and physical therapy together focused on transfer training, functional ambulatory transfers, and standing balance for ADL. Physical therapy provided leadership in selecting treatment techniques and assistive devices to increase lower extremity functioning. Occupational therapy followed up with bedside treatment, incorporating new transfer and mobility skills into bed, wheelchair, toilet, and other transfers performed for grooming, showering, toileting, and dressing. After basic squat pivot transfers from bed to wheelchair were accomplished, dressing and grooming were then performed out of bed, first at the wheelchair level. As standing balance increased, short periods of standing at the sink to brush teeth and comb hair were included. Showering was then mastered by transferring from wheelchair to shower transfer bench and showering independently with a handheld shower. John and the therapist reviewed *Self Care for PWAs* (Davis, 1988), which emphasizes the importance of dental, skin, nail, hair, and rectal care for those with compromised immune systems. Lower extremity exercises performed in physical therapy soon provided enough lower extremity strength to permit complete independence in lower extremity dressing, squatting briefly over the wheelchair, or while sitting on the side of bed to pull pants up over hips.

After the above basic skills were performed independently at the bedside, therapy was scheduled in the kitchen so John could pursue his favorite vocation/hobby: cooking. John expressed concern that his parents would not let him cook at home for fear he would infect them with HIV. John was assured that those who ate his food faced no risk as long as he was careful. The nutrition section of *A Guide to Self Care for HIV Infection* (AIDS Project Los Angeles, 1991) was reviewed, providing John with facts and techniques to avoid catching or spreading illness from unsanitary food handling while preparing nutritious foods. John began with light cooking tasks, e.g., making tea from the wheelchair level but standing to reach high cupboards and other surfaces. The complexity of tasks was increased as John's endurance improved.

Eventually, he agreed to cook a full Italian meal for his occupational therapist, physical therapist, and physical therapy aide. John seemed surprised that the therapists actually ate his food. Despite the fact that John had been educated about the absolute safety of food prepared by PWAs who follow precautions, he did not seem to appreciate fully that he could still please others with his cooking until his therapists enjoyed a meal with him. When John expressed continuing doubts about his parents letting him cook at home, they were invited to a meal prepared by John in the occupational therapy department. The therapists reviewed the safe food guidelines with John's parents and reported on John's progress, including the fact he prepared a complete meal that the therapists all enjoyed the previous week. His parents seemed slightly uncomfortable and surprised to see the therapists eating their son's cooking. However, they joined in, becoming more comfortable, and were able to enjoy the meal.

The social worker learned of John's cooking during a team conference. Arrangements were made for John to do volunteer work after he returned home, cooking part-time at a local agency that provided Meals-on-Wheels to home-bound PWAs. A volunteer driver at the agency agreed to provide John with transportation. Car transfers were practiced in occupational therapy. At discharge, John could transfer between wheelchair and car with minimal assistance. He independently directed loading his lightweight wheelchair into the car.

John was contacted at home 2 months after discharge. He reported that his parents let him cook regularly for family meals. They were still uncomfortable with him cooking for their grandchildren when they visited so he did not do this. He explained that he helped cook three meals per week at the volunteer agency and felt this was plenty of cooking. He continued to be independent in transfers and activities of daily living at home.

Women and HIV

AIDS is currently the fifth most frequent cause of death among American women aged 15 to 45. Women make up the fastest growing group of people with AIDS (Center for Women Policy Studies, 1991). Women of color are disproportionately affected.

Wood and Aull (1990) and Pizzi (1992) have discussed a major issue related to providing occupational therapy services to women with AIDS. These women are frequently single parents with limited resources. Their maternal role is critical and surrounded with fear. They fear for their ability to continue caring for their children as their physical and cognitive status declines. Therapy should strongly address functional aspects of the maternal role and reinforce a sense of empowerment and self-respect. They should be enabled to participate in as much of their children's care as possible and to manage the care that they cannot deliver (see Chapter 16). HIV+ women need to be educated that safe sex practices are important after as well as before infection and should be empowered to be able to stipulate that to future sexual partners. They should be taught self-advocacy skills and problem-solving skills relating to finding and using support systems in the community.

CASE STUDY II

This case is a report by an occupational therapist who facilitated a weekly group for PWAs that addressed mobility and equipment needs. The patients were in a long-term care facility and were nonambulatory. Therefore, wheelchair mobility and positioning needs were addressed primarily. Edema control, splinting, feeding, and adaptive equipment were also addressed. At this stage of patient function, wheelchair and equipment needs changed frequently. The goal was to maintain function for as long as possible with or without adaptive equipment. Patients assisted the group process by identifying deficits that needed to be addressed for new admissions or that arose because of deterioration of longer-term patients. The patients often recognized these needs in each other before the therapist did. They also shared their expertise regarding adaptive equipment and methods that had been employed successfully on the unit.

The occupational therapist found that the best way to get patients to attend the group was by reputation, i.e., the patients spread the word that the group was helpful at increasing mobility and independence and decreasing discomfort. Thus patients voluntarily reported to the central recreation room, where the group was held, if they felt a need for help. Those who could not get out of bed requested services through the nurses. The occupational therapist checked each week with the charge nurse regarding admissions, discharges, or priorities the nurse wished to see addressed since the last group meeting.

One day the nurses advised that many patients were depressed because three of their peers on the unit had died during the previous week. The occupational therapist went to the recreation room where several patients were sitting and talking. The therapist greeted them and asked if anyone needed help with wheelchair seating, mobility, or other equipment. Everyone declined services, appearing withdrawn and depressed. The therapist asked a few questions relating to services and equipment that had been addressed at the last meeting to see if follow-up was needed. No one wanted service, and one patient remarked, "We just don't feel like doing anything today." The therapist asked how she could be of assistance, and one woman said she would like the group to sing. After a short pause, she added that she would like the group to sing "The Way We Were." The patients and the therapist began to sing together. First two women, then a few men began to cry; the therapist could not resist crying herself. At the conclusion of the song, the patients thanked the therapist.

The therapist returned to the occupational therapy clinic with ambivalent feelings. She was quite sad, yet somehow felt that she did the right thing at the right time when someone needed and appreciated support. She discussed her feelings with other therapists who also provided services to AIDS patients. They noted that the hospital made working on the AIDS units a voluntary assignment. After discussion, the therapist remembered why she had volunteered, and decided she did the right thing.

AMYOTROPHIC LATERAL SCLEROSIS

Amyotrophic lateral sclerosis (ALS) is a disease that results in the progressive degeneration of the anterior horn cells, or motor neurons, of the spinal cord and the motor nuclei of the brainstem (Bannister, 1992). It is the most common disorder of the motor neuron diseases, and the terms are frequently interchanged (Williams & Windebank, 1991). ALS is also popularly referred to as Lou Gehrig's disease.

In ALS, voluntary muscle control is affected, and early manifestations indicating upper or lower motor neuron involvement vary, depending on the site of the disease process (Bannister, 1992). Initial signs include generalized muscular weakness, fatigue, and **fasciculations** (Smith, 1992). Damage to upper motor neurons results in generalized weakness, spasticity, and exaggerated reflexes. Lower motor neuron damage results in weakness of the extremities, muscle atrophy, and a loss of reflexes. Speech, swallowing, and breathing are affected by destruction of nerves in the bulbar region (Bannister, 1992). While individuals may initially demonstrate evidence of one characteristic, it is likely that both upper and lower motor neuron symptoms will be experienced during the course of the disease (Smith, 1992). Medications can assist in the management of symptomatic features such as **fasciculations,** abnormal tone, and excessive saliva but do not alter the progression. Respirators may be used to assist those who have difficulty breathing (Muscular Dystrophy Association, 1991).

Mentation, sensation, ocular movements, and bowel and bladder control typically remain unaffected. These areas should be viewed as strengths in the development of a treatment plan, especially for individuals who are in the latter stages of ALS.

The disease appears to affect men more than women at a ratio of 1.2:1 (Bannister, 1992). The etiology is unknown. The average age of onset is 57 years with an average lifespan of 3 years. Because there is no cure for ALS, therapeutic intervention is restorative not curative.

Quality of life should be considered during all stages of treatment. Psychological support for the patient and family is an important part of treatment, and all professionals involved will need to help the patient and family, as well as themselves, deal with the ultimate outcome. The limited life expectancy also creates a need for early and accurate assessment, intervention, and education to promote maximal occupational functioning throughout the course of the disease.

Evaluation

Once the patient has identified his various life roles, occupational therapists should determine the patient's level of current functional ability in all relative performance areas. This includes activities of daily living, work, and leisure. Baseline measurements for the following performance components must be established: range of motion, tone, strength, endurance, postural control, skin integrity, and gross and fine motor coordination. Psychosocial components will also have a strong impact on the course and outcome of intervention. Both the patient and family member or caregiver need to be part of the goal-setting and treatment-planning process from the onset to ensure a quality of life that will have meaning for each patient. Consideration needs to be given to the adjustment to the disability, by both the patient and family members. The patient's level of "gadget tolerance" can also influence what forms of restoration will be used, especially in later stages of the disease process.

Treatment

Once baseline data have been established, patient and family education and training in maintenance care should be completed to limit future complications and to maintain maximum levels of performance throughout the various stages. This includes instruction in range of motion, skin care, energy conservation techniques, work simplification, and ergonomics. In addition, adaptations to overcome functional limitations need to be addressed.

Involvement of the upper extremities is more common initially than of the lower extremities (Williams & Windebank, 1991). Atrophy typically begins in the hands with wasting of the thenar and hypothenar eminences (Bannister, 1992). Because the interossei atrophy, finger extension is usually weaker than normal. Universal cuffs, built-up handles and utensils, and splints (i.e., short opponens, metacarpophalangeal extension) may be considered for decreased hand function. Appropriate application of overhead slings or mobile arm supports can in some instances accommodate for decreased proximal strength. Specific activities may also require additional adaptive equipment. Feeding, for example, may be facilitated with use of a plate guard, adaptive utensil, or extended straw. Automated self-feeders are also an option for individuals at a more dependent stage who want to minimize assistance from others. Velcro closures, zipper pulls, and adapted clothing can facilitate ease of dressing. Use of a wheelchair may progress from manual to power operation. Raised seat heights for all surfaces will ease transfers for both patient and caregiver.

As general mobility decreases, the need to be

aware of skin integrity increases. Electric beds and recline/tilt wheelchair systems that allow the patient the opportunity to change position on a regular basis are vital (see Chapter 30). Pressure-relief surfaces for the bed, such as an alternating air pressure pad and pump, and wheelchair must be made available. There are a variety of pressure-relief cushions on the market (Chapter 23). Soft collars assist in supporting the head when neck musculature is weak. Patients may require the use of tall back seating systems for head support and/or lateral supports for trunk control (Smith, 1992).

When dysphagia becomes an issue, consultation with speech-language pathologists and dieticians is important for changes in food consistency to promote easier swallowing and maintenance of proper nutrition. Positioning as prescribed by the occupational therapist should be used during all meals to avoid complications of choking and aspiration (Chapter 44). Compensation methods found useful for swallowing deficits include a long-stemmed spoon that permits food to be placed far back in the mouth to increase the likelihood of swallowing. Swallowing of saliva may also be a problem that can be addressed through suctioning (Smith, 1992). Ultimately, feeding through a gastric tube may be required to ensure that the nutritional needs are met (Williams & Windebank, 1991).

Alternate forms of communication must be established as verbal communication diminishes because of paralysis of face and respiratory musculature. If motor function is sufficiently intact, writing and/or computer keyboarding can be considered for interactions. Adaptations such as encoding particular keys and using a key guard may need to be made to accommodate for dysfunction. Keyboards may be accessed by alternate input methods, such as a head or mouth stick (Smith, 1992). Various environmental-control systems and computer systems are available, and access to these is possible by individuals who have limited function through the development of nontraditional switches (Chapter 31).

CASE STUDY III

A 56-year-old man had been diagnosed with ALS approximately 2 years before coming to the outpatient occupational therapy clinic for equipment assessment and recommendation. He presented with quadriparesis and verbalizations were limited by decreased respiratory capacity. He was dependent in all aspects of self-care and mobility with the exception of power mobility using a pneumatic, or sip and puff, control. The patient and his wife wanted to ensure that he had a method of accessing emergency assistance independently. They also wanted to explore the possibility of being able to read independently via computer. An evaluation of the patient's abilities were made with consideration given to the progression of the disease process. It was determined that a single switch control would be most appropriate, and that activation of the switch could be accomplished

by tongue or facial gesture or via an eye gaze system. Pneumatics were not being considered given his increasing inconsistency with breath control. Although there was potential to achieve his goal, the patient and his wife ultimately decided against pursuing the system because of cost factors. It was important to work with the patient and family to determine what the options were as well as to provide support and validation when it came time to balance the issues of prognosis and long-term financial investment.

MUSCULAR DYSTROPHY

The term *muscular dystrophy* (MD) is used to describe a group of genetically based diseases that results in progressive weakness and degeneration of skeletal muscles. Nine forms of MD have been identified by the Muscular Dystrophy Association (Table 36.3).

Evaluation

Evaluation should include review of all relevant performance areas. If deficiencies are noted, evaluation continues to include specific component areas. A complete manual muscle test should be done to determine not only the extent of weakness but also the availability of strength in remaining musculature. Determination of range of motion is also important because joint malalignment, produced by contractures, can aggravate the effect of already weakened muscles and lead to premature loss of mobility and function (Johnson, Fowler, & Lieberman, 1992). Other areas to assess include endurance, postural control, and coordination.

Treatment

Contractures, which produce deformity and limit function, are disabling in any neuromuscular disease (Johnson et al., 1992). Daily passive and active range of motion, appropriate positioning during all activities, splinting, and bracing are important in the prevention of contractures.

Assistive devices and adaptation of activities, to compensate for weakness, provide means of continued involvement in daily life roles. For example, a patient with limb-girdle MD manifested in the shoulder girdle was able to continue working given adaptation to his environment, upper extremity stabilization and/or support such as overhead slings and mobile arm supports; and instruction and training in work simplification techniques.

With all forms of MD and during all stages, the occupational therapist addresses the patient's ability to achieve mastery and independence in daily activities through education, training, and support of both the patient and family. The goal of treatment is to maintain function and participation in valued roles without, then with, adapted devices.

Table 36.3 Muscular Dystrophies

Type	Usual Age of Onset	Disease Characteristics
Myotonic	20 to 40 years	Weakness of all muscle groups accompanied by spasm after contraction; affects the peripheral muscles first; also affects the heart, eyes, and endocrine glands; progression is slow and can span a normal lifetime
Duchenne	2 to 6 years	General muscle weakness and wasting affecting pelvis and proximal upper and lower extremities; progresses slowly, yet eventually involves all voluntary muscles; survival is rare beyond the early 20s
Becker	2 to 16 years	Symptoms almost identical to Duchenne; however, this is less severe; progress is slower than Duchenne and survival runs well into middle age
Limb-girdle	Late childhood to middle age	Weakness and wasting, affecting shoulder girdle and pelvis first; disease progresses slowly; respiratory and heart function may also be affected and can result in death caused by cardiopulmonary complications
Facioscapulohumeral	Teens to early adulthood	Facial muscle weakness with weakness and wasting of the proximal upper extremities; can progress to the lower extremities and impair gait; advancement is slow with occasional periods of rapid deterioration; lifespan may be normal
Congenital	At birth	Generalized muscle weakness with possible joint deformities resulting from shortening of muscles; progression, if any, is slow, but lifespan may be shortened
Oculopharyngeal	40 to 70 years	Affects muscles of the eyes and throat, drooping eyelids are usually the first sign; dysphagia can lead to choking and aspiration pneumonia, which can affect longevity; patients may experience extremity weakness during the slow course of the disease
Distal	40 to 60 years	Weakness and wasting of distal muscles of the extremities; coordination may be affected; advancement is slow and rarely leads to incapacity
Emery-Dreifuss	Childhood to early teens	Rare form; joint deformities and cardiac abnormalities are common; disease progresses slowly; lifespan is not affected unless there are cardiac complications

MULTIPLE SCLEROSIS

Multiple sclerosis (MS) is a disease process that occurs in the white matter of the central nervous system when demyelination takes place followed by an overgrowth of glial cells that form sclerotic patches (plaques) on nerve fibers and create focal lesions (Bannister, 1992). It is characterized by episodes of remission and exacerbation that vary from case to case.

Manifestations of MS vary, depending on the location of plaques or areas of demyelination, and can include spasticity, weakness, fatigue, incoordination, sensory deficits, dysarthria, and visual dysfunction (Erickson, Lie, & Wineinger, 1989) as well as changes in cognition and judgment.

While the etiology of MS is unknown, there is evidence of certain associated factors that are characteristic in some cases (Bannister, 1992). Precipitating factors include influenza and upper respiratory tract infections, pregnancy, surgery, tooth extraction, and electric shock (Bannister, 1992). Women are affected by the disease 50% more frequently than are men (Lechtenberg, 1988). Onset usually occurs between 20 and 40 years of age.

While there is still no cure for MS, a pilot study in 1981 found that intensive interdisciplinary inpatient rehabilitation decreased the number of functional limitations experienced by a patient with MS in areas such as self-care, bed mobility, transfers, wheelchair mobility, bladder control, and homemaking (Erickson et al., 1989; Mitchell, 1993). The study of 20 chronically disabled individuals with MS indicated that the annual cost of home health aid per patient decreased from $25,909 before rehabilitation to $8,680 following rehabilitation (Erickson et al., 1989). The combined cost of inpatient rehabilitation plus subsequent home care for 1 year was also less than the original cost of home care. While the study was small compared with the total MS population, it indicates the benefit that intervention and adaptation of functional activity can have in the management of symptoms.

Evaluation

One MS center's description of the role of occupational therapy is to

> facilitate health maintenance in the individual's own environment, to maximize potential for noninstitutional living, and to promote the acceptance of the disease and facilitate compensatory and adaptive strategies. Adapting to the continual changes in function is an important goal of the entire program (Linroth, 1990, p. 54).

To adequately meet patients' needs, occupational therapists must assess performance areas in individuals with MS at onset and following each exacerbation to determine any changes in function (Erickson et al., 1989) and to maximize the effectiveness of remaining function. Evaluation of all occupational performance areas should be completed. Specific component areas to evaluate include sensation, the presence or absence of **diplopia,** range of motion, tone, functional muscle strength, endurance, postural control, skin integrity, activity tolerance, coordination, cognitive function and emotional status. One study indicated that the administration of the *Nine-Hole Peg Test* and the *Box and Block Test* significantly improved the detection of change in upper extremity function for prospectively followed patients with MS (Goodkin, Hertsgaard, & Seminary, 1988).

Reporting accurate assessment results relative to work tasks of the typically young MS patient may alter employers' expectations of the patient and ensure that appropriate adaptations occur in the work setting. These patients may be candidates for formalized cognitive training programs. Early and reliable cognitive evaluation results may increase a patient's qualifications to receive disability benefits (Rao et al., 1991).

Treatment

The occupational therapist can help the patient with MS to identify life goals and values and encourage him to take control to direct his rehabilitation and life realistically toward these goals. Training in activities of daily living using acceptable modifications to compensate for weakness and incoordination to enable independence will help the patient to limit his sense of inability and disablement. Therapeutic group activities that include skill development and tasks related to work, home maintenance, and leisure interests and that focus around problem solving and sharing of experi-

ences and reactions can offer the patient both physical and psychological benefits.

Patients' realistic approaches to intervention may be affected by a sense of euphoria or other personality changes that are symptoms of the disease. They should be guided by an objective, informational approach to goal setting. During an acute exacerbation, the individual with MS should rest. When the deterioration has stabilized and there are no new signs of evolution, it is appropriate to begin therapy (Lechtenberg, 1988).

Therapy intervention includes patient and family instruction in daily stretching through full range of motion to prevent muscle shortening and joint contracture (Erickson et al., 1989). Other modalities such as the use of cold, electrical stimulation, and inhibitory positioning can also be used to manage abnormal muscle tone (Erickson et al., 1989).

Decreased muscle strength resulting from anterior horn cell destruction or motor tract involvement cannot be significantly improved, though weakness and reduced endurance secondary to inactivity or disuse can be treated. Exercise and activity that avoid overexertion and rough physical contact can relieve spasticity and maintain muscular function (Poser, 1991). Patient education concerning management of daily life, with an emphasis on a balance between activity and rest, and increasing the patient's awareness of the relationship between exercise and function can diminish the depressive response to the disease and promote a sense of control over outcome.

Because of the tendency to exacerbate symptoms of MS, fatigue should be avoided (Erickson et al., 1989). High body temperatures can also result in an exacerbation of MS; therefore, treatment should be done in cool, nonhumid places. Instruction in energy conservation, work-simplification techniques, and ergonomics should be provided for both the patient and family and incorporated into all activities (Chapter 16).

One patient who was married and had a 15-year-old son was being seen for follow-up after a recent exacerbation. She was employed full-time as a political speech writer and worked 4 out of the 5 days at home on a computer. Cognition was intact, and she was independent both in self-care using adaptive equipment and in the use of a lightweight wheelchair. The patient sat directly on the sling seat of the wheelchair. During evaluation it was discovered that the patient would become increasingly more fatigued toward the end of the day when working at her computer and present with neck and back discomfort. A review of her positioning when working revealed the need for ergonomic intervention. The patient was assessed and provided with a cushion for the wheelchair that maintained appropriate positioning and alignment. She was also provided with bilateral forearm supports that enabled her to work without the strain of using neck and upper back musculature to support the weight of her arms as she became progressively weaker throughout the course of the day.

Lesions in the cerebellum manifest themselves in incoordination and ataxic gait. Weighted cuffs and utensils are used regularly to compensate for intention tremor during daily activities. In some cases, proximal extremity bracing may decrease ataxia in distal segments during activities (Erickson et al., 1989). For patients who rely on a powered wheelchair for mobility, adjustments can be made in joystick sensitivity, rate of acceleration, and turning speed to offset the effects of tremors. There are no proven treatments that directly ameliorate motor control in patients with cerebellar dysfunction.

Most typical with this disease are paresthesias, a type of pins and needles sensation; hyperpathia, an increased sensitivity to pain; and dysesthesia, which is pain elicited by stimuli such as touch or pressure. Total loss of sensation, or anesthesia, is not as common in patients with MS (Lechtenberg, 1988). However, appropriate education, precaution, and instruction in sensory compensation techniques should be given to avoid complications of pressure sores and thermal injury (Chapter 23). To assist in the maintenance of skin integrity when in a wheelchair, timed pressure reliefs and a pressure-relief cushion should be used. When in bed, a regular turning schedule and appropriate bed surface will also prevent decubitus ulcers.

Dysarthria, disturbances in speech including slurring of words, slowing of speech, and difficulty with clarity or rhythm, typically results from an inability to coordinate movements of the tongue, lips, palate, vocal cords, and other elements that are modulated by the cerebellum (Lechtenberg, 1988). Speech pathologists have the responsibility to treat these impairments (Erickson et al., 1989).

Color vision, visual acuity, **diplopia,** and/or nystagmus may be affected by inflammation or demyelination of the optic nerve (Erickson et al., 1989; Lechtenberg, 1988). Use of an eye patch, which is alternated between eyes several times a week, will functionally alleviate the problem of double vision.

Slowed cognitive processing, loss of short-term memory, and reduced capacity to problem solve are a few of the cognitive problems noted with MS patients (Linroth, 1990). A study by Rao et al. (1991) suggested that patients with MS who present with cognitive impairments experience a greater disturbance in activities of daily living than those who do not.

PARKINSON'S DISEASE

Whereas patients with multiple sclerosis have trouble with voluntary movement, patients with Parkin-

son's disease have trouble with involuntary or automatic movement. Three classic symptoms—resting tremor, **rigidity,** and **bradykinesia**—are characteristic of Parkinson's disease (Bannister, 1992; Duvoisin, 1991).

Parkinson's disease rarely affects people under the age of 40 and the average age of onset is 60, with no preference for sex, race, or climate (Duvoisin, 1991; Quintyn & Cross, 1986). The rate of deterioration varies from 2 years up to 20 years. Patients with tremor as the major symptom have a better prognosis than patients with **rigidity** and slowness of movement. The beginning is usually insidious, and the progression is so gradual that it can rarely be dated precisely. Parkinson's disease is believed to affect about a 0.5 million people in the United States or approximately 1% of the population over age 50, and statistics are comparable with other countries (Duvoisin, 1991). The data suggest that the prevalence of the disease has not changed appreciably over the past century. There are many theories, but the cause of Parkinson's disease is a profound mystery. Its symptoms can be successfully treated but there is still no cure. Parkinson's disease is most often a slowly progressive disease.

The tremor is usually the first symptom the patient notices. It usually starts with one hand or one foot. It is a rhythmic and regular shaking with a frequency of 5 to 6 beats per second (Duvoisin, 1991). Most commonly, the tremor appears with a slight pronation/supination of the forearm and a "pill rolling" back and forth movement of the thumb and the fingers. The intensity of the tremor fluctuates and commonly increases with stress. The tremor disappears during sleep (Brown, 1980; Duvoisin, 1991).

Rigidity is a hypertonicity of agonist and antagonist that offers a constant, uniform resistance to passive movement. The affected muscles seem unable to relax and are in a state of contraction even at rest. Parkinson's **rigidity** is commonly manifested as a series of "catches" in the resistance during passive movement. As the muscle is passively stretched, the resistance is periodically released during the movement. This type of **rigidity** is termed **cogwheel rigidity** and it is thought to be the combination of **rigidity** and tremor (Brown, 1980). **Rigidity** develops, especially in the flexor muscles of the trunk and limbs, and produces the typical stooped posture: head bowed; body bent forward; elbows, knees, and hips flexed; thumbs flexed across the palms; and metacarpophalangeal joints flexed with interphalangeal joints extended (Thomas, 1973).

Bradykinesia is slowness of body movement. It is a complex phenomenon consisting of hesitancy in initiating a new movement or stopping an ongoing movement, slowness of execution of movement, and rapid fatigue (Duvoisin, 1991). The term **bradykinesia**

also encompasses a lack of spontaneity and a diminishing in the performance of the automatic movements of which an individual is usually unaware, such as arm swing, eye blink, swallowing of saliva, expressive gestures, and the small movements of postural adjustments. **Bradykinesia** is the basis of the characteristic festinating gait of small, fast, shuffling steps that propels the body forward, which inclines more and more forward as the disease progresses (Adams & Victor, 1977; Webster, 1968). Because automatic balance and equilibrium adjustments are not made by patients with **bradykinesia** (Quintyn & Cross, 1986) and because the center of gravity becomes more and more anteriorly displaced because of the typical forward flexed posture, persons with **bradykinesia** associated with Parkinson's disease tend to fall when ambulating.

Akinesia is the term given to impaired ability to initiate voluntary and spontaneous motor responses (Angel, Alston, & Higgens, 1970). It is characterized by the interruption of performance of an ongoing movement or "freezing" when attention is distracted (Quintyn & Cross, 1986).

In addition to these classic symptoms, additional common symptoms have been reported. Individuals with Parkinson's disease often speak softly in a rapid, even tone. Speech is characteristically monotone with low volume and shows lack of emotional expression, tremulousness, and blocking, all of which parallel motor problems seen in the rest of the body (Hoehn & Yahr, 1967). Effects of autonomic dysfunction seen in Parkinson's disease are excessive sweating, greasy skin, bladder dysfunction, and flushing of the skin (Duvoisin, 1991). These characteristics are a result of deterioration within the substantia nigra, a crucial part of the motor circuitry of the central nervous system.

The brainstem contains the motor centers that strongly influence muscle tone, postural adjustments, and protective reactions (Brown, 1980; Nolte, 1981). The neural connections of the basal ganglia within the brainstem are complex. Data from the motor cortex are transmitted to the corpus striatum, which is modulated by the substantia nigra and subthalamus (Nolte, 1981; Brown, 1980). Impulses are then relayed to the thalamus and then back to the motor center, along with cerebellar data, resulting in motor output. Dopamine, produced in the cells of the substantia nigra, travels up these fibers to the corpus striatum. Dopamine is a chemical messenger that transmits signals to the nerve cells of the striatum. This circuit is the important regulator of automatic movements such as walking, arm swinging, and postural changes. Parkinson's disease is caused by the depletion of dopamine. Normally, neurons from the substantia nigra connect with the striatum, which has the highest dopamine content in the

brain. When these neurons are destroyed, the dopamine content of the substantia nigra is reduced.

Parkinsonism, as noted, is caused by a deficiency of brain dopamine in the substantia nigra, but that deficiency may be the result of various factors. The nerve cells of the substantia nigra may be injured by a tumor, brain injury, stroke, chemical agent, or virus that infects the brain (encephalitis). A functionally comparable state can be caused by drugs that block the action of dopamine in the striatum. The dopamine is then unable to deliver its chemical message, and the result is the same as when dopamine is depleted. Similarly, if the nerve cells of the striatum that normally receive the dopamine lose their ability to receive it, the effect is the same as when dopamine is absent. Drug-induced Parkinsonism is reversible. The Parkinson-like state gradually disappears when the person stops taking the medication or reduces the dosage (Duvoisin, 1991).

The medical treatment for Parkinson's disease is L-dopa in the form of levodopa. The medication replenishes the missing dopamine but does not affect the basic disease process. The level of levodopa in the blood rises slowly, peaks anywhere from 30 min to 2 hr after taking the medication, and slowly falls over a 4- to 6-hr period (Duvoisin, 1991). Many patients find that in peak times they are less symptomatic, more mobile, and more functional. A strong correlation has been made between the effectiveness of medication and the individual's diet (Duvoisin, 1991). Protein delays the absorption of levodopa and may reduce the amount taken up by circulation. Therefore, following ingestion of protein, the patient with moderate to severe Parkinson's disease is apt to be less functional.

Although patients with Parkinson's disease have difficulty initiating movement, particularly in the absence of an external trigger, from the findings of one study it appears that they are able to select correct motor responses, indicating that they do not have a disorder of the perceptual or decision-making systems (Angel et al., 1970). Some patients do seem able to use prior information to guide ongoing movement, once initiated, and do not have to rely totally on visual feedback to compensate for proprioceptive inattention (Bloxham, Mindel, & Frith, 1984). Studies need to be done to test perceptual spatial abilities separately from motor abilities to determine whether Parkinson's patients actually have perceptual deficits.

Evaluation

The evaluation is based on knowledge of typical symptoms of Parkinson's disease. It should include initial interview to identify roles, interests, and habits; activities of daily living and functional mobility status;

sensory motor evaluation, including muscle tone, righting reactions, and other automatic postural movements; evaluation of speed and accuracy of voluntary movement; range of motion and cognition; visual screening; psychosocial assessment; and evaluation of home accessibility. An ongoing evaluation of the effect of medication on function is done, because therapists who work with these patients daily are in a good position to observe behavior indicative of side effects that might otherwise be missed (Blonsky, 1971; Duvoisin, 1991). Evaluation may require adaptation to the individual, depending on cognitive and attention skills.

Treatment

At this time little has been documented on the effectiveness of occupational therapy treatment interventions with Parkinson's patients. The patient and family member or caregiver need to participate in the goal setting and treatment plan to ensure quality of life that is meaningful for the patient. Occupational therapy goals include the following.

1. *Improve initiation and quality of movement, increase mobility, and prevent deformity.* **Rigidity** and **akinesia** produce a stiff, inanimate patient. Mobility of the neck and trunk are important, because head movements lead body movements in the quick adjustments needed in response to disturbances of equilibrium. Proprioceptive neuromuscular facilitation (PNF) techniques such as rhythmic initiation, reversals, and unilateral diagonal patterns used in conjunction with functional activities are beneficial in improving initiation and quality of movement (see Chapter 24D). After the therapist moves the body part several times passively and rhythmically through the pattern of movement, the patient is asked to assist in the movement. After several more repetitions, the therapist withdraws and allows the patient to move independently. Rapid, rhythmical movements rather than resistive ones are most appropriate for developing mobility responses. PNF techniques starting with the trunk, using scapular, pelvic, and trunk patterns decrease **rigidity** and allow for trunk mobility and rotation. Because resistance produces stability, it should be avoided in treatment of the trunk and proximal parts of the limbs.

Tactile, visual, or auditory cues to evoke movement may be needed to enable the patient to initiate movement. Use of these can help the patient compensate for slow initiation. Strategies based on this idea should be taught to the patient and his family. For example, a forward push or tug on the shoulder helps the patient to initiate standing up. A shout "Stop!" helps the patient who is festinating faster and faster to initiate stopping. Music can be used to establish and maintain the rhythm. Initiation of voluntary movement

reduces tremor. This, too, can be used as a compensatory strategy to help the patient gain control over his symptoms. To stop the resting tremor, the patient can be taught to reach for, or grasp, an object providing distal stability that reduces tremor.

2. *Improve psychosocial status.* The Parkinson's patient is faced with several psychosocial problems: physical isolation imposed by the disability, social isolation imposed by the inactive face and voice, and depression. Feedback from a mirror can be used beneficially to help the patient become aware of his facial expression and to make an effort to appear more animated, which is important to facilitate social interaction and to increase feelings of belonging. Persons with Parkinson's disease can voluntarily smile, nod, etc. However, because they must think about doing it, these behaviors are apt to be lost as a person shifts his attention to carrying on the conversation. Counseling for the family is important so that they understand the patient's problems, as the lack of facial expression and the slowness of movement can be misinterpreted as lack of interest or stubbornness. Not to be overlooked is the beneficial effect of interest and attention that active participation in a well-planned and well-supervised group program provides. Day treatment programs can keep the patient active and interacting with others to alleviate depression as well as improve function and provide caregiver respite.

3. *Improve or maintain independent performance of daily living skills for as long as possible.* The early stage of Parkinson's disease, **rigidity** of the trunk, affects functional mobility during activities of daily living. Later, manipulation and dexterity problems appear and affect the patient's ability to dress, bathe, and feed himself. Adaptive equipment to compensate for these impairments is often beneficial to increase independence and overcome functional limitations. Specifically, a raised toilet seat, tub bench, long-handled reacher, built-up handles, Velcro closures, etc. may be helpful.

As mentioned above, one of the side effects of medication is fluctuations in the patient's ability to move. The occupational therapist educates the patient and family to maximize the times when the patient is more physically able to participate in purposeful activities, which can maximize quality of life for that individual.

POSTPOLIO SYNDROME

Postpolio syndrome is characterized by slowly progressive muscle weakness 20 to 40 years after recovery from the initial, acute onset of poliomyelitis. Polio, an acute inflammation of the anterior horn cell, does not cause sensory losses, upper motor neuron signs, or cognitive/perceptual changes. Survivors were left with weakness and atrophy that ranged from involvement of all muscles innervated by spinal or bulbar lower motor neurons, including respiratory muscles, to weakness of one limb or part of one limb (Laurie, 1984). After the initial febrile stage, some recovery of strength was made, and compensatory methods and devices were employed to maximize function and independence. No further deterioration of function was expected (Halstead & Wiechers, 1985). Within the past years, approximately 20 to 25% of postpolio survivors have been experiencing new losses in function because of muscle weakness, atrophy, muscle pain, **fasciculation,** weakness in respiratory muscles, cold intolerance, and sleep apnea (Halstead & Wiechers, 1985; Sharief, Hentges, & Ciardi, 1991). The postpolio syndrome is not caused by reinfection or activation of a latent virus (Maynard & Roller, 1991).

The cause of postpolio syndrome is unknown (Halstead & Gawne, 1993; Sharief et al., 1991). There are several current theories being researched. One theory is that the increased weakness is the result of the normal aging process affecting muscles, ligaments, and joints (Halstead & Wiechers, 1985; Laurie, 1984). It is known that anterior horn cell populations decline up to 20% between the ages of 60 and 90, but this magnitude of loss does not cause clinical weakness in normal persons (Laurie, 1984; Tomlinson & Irving, 1977). However, following the death of anterior horn cells during the febrile stage in polio patients, many muscle fibers served by those anterior horn cells were reinnervated because of sprouting of the terminal axons of neighboring healthy motor neurons. These motor neurons supplied larger numbers of muscle fibers than they were originally designed for. As a result of overwork, these anterior horn cells may age earlier than other such cells (Dalakas, 1985; Weichers, 1985). Because these cells control a greater than normal percentage of muscle function, these age-related losses are enough to produce weakness that interferes with function (Dalakas, 1985; Weichers, 1985).

Another theory is that exercise causes damage to the motor units (Herbison, Jaweed, & Ditunno, 1985). Overuse weakness also can occur in neurologically normal individuals who exceed their limits in intense exercise (Laurie, 1984). Early symptoms of overuse, before lasting weakness occurs, are short-term postexercise fatigue, short-term postexercise weakness, and/or pain in specific muscles after exercise (Laurie, 1984).

The role and safe amount of exercise for postpolio patients are clinical dilemmas. Common sense indicates that energy conservation is important and overuse of muscles contraindicated.

Evaluation

Postpolio patients may require occupational therapy to continue their accustomed life roles and activities of daily living. The occupational therapist evaluates the individual's life roles, activities of daily living, strength, endurance, and range of motion. The need for job or work place modification, assistive devices, and energy conservation education are also assessed.

Treatment

Treatment goals for postpolio survivors are (1) to alleviate emotional distress, (2) to improve functional independence and to facilitate necessary lifestyle changes, and (3) to maintain strength and improve endurance through modification of daily energy expenditure patterns.

Maynard and Roller (1991) identified three patterns of emotional (i.e., attitudes and behaviors) styles of living of postpolio survivors: passers, minimizers, and identifiers. Passers have mild disability that is easily hidden in casual social interactions. The individual passes as nondisabled. Minimizers use some adaptive equipment or compensation techniques but hide their disability. There is strong denial, and such people do not think of themselves as disabled. Identifiers are those with severe disability, often requiring a wheelchair and respiratory equipment, who have had to identify fully with their disability and make major lifestyle adaptations for successful coping.

Passers are the most distressed with the postpolio syndrome and are most likely to be emotionally overwhelmed (Maynard & Roller, 1991). Depression results from the feelings of loss generated by the deteriorating condition and resultant decreased independence as well as the developmental need to adjust to midlife changes. Putting patients in touch with a peer support group if they are not already active in one is important.

Lifestyle changes are necessary to avoid overuse of muscles and to accommodate to the weakness and fatigue (Young, 1991). Patients need to learn their limits of strength and endurance and avoid going to those limits (Young, 1991). It is imperative that they learn to conserve energy and understand the importance of rest. They should be taught the metabolic cost of participating in activities (Chapter 43) so they can make informed choices concerning the activities of their lives. The occupational therapist may be requested to see these patients to evaluate them for revision of adapted techniques for daily living skills and/or to teach work-simplification and energy-conservation methods (Young, 1991). The only approach validly used with this group of patients is collaborative problem solving and gradually introducing new adaptations.

Unfortunately, such patients must now make many adaptations all at once and thus need support as well as ideas. Also, methods and devices are now available that were not when such patients first experienced symptoms.

Methods for increasing independence compensate for the patient's weakness and low endurance. Adaptations also need to be based on joint and muscle protection principles. Because of muscle imbalances, joints have been stressed, and there is a possibility that some of the pain experienced by these patients is caused by osteoarthritis (Young, 1991). Splinting may be needed to protect joints or to place them in alignment to prevent muscle stretch and to improve the mechanical advantage of weak muscles.

Conditioning, aerobic exercises to maintain or improve cardiovascular endurance are important for polio survivors. Swimming, in which the buoyancy of the water removes stress from the joints and tendons, is an especially good conditioning exercise. A vigorous strengthening exercise program is contraindicated, because weak muscles may be damaged or respond poorly to such a program and because the basic problem of these patients is overuse, not disuse. A mild exercise program for strengthening in which resistance is gradually increased can lead to modest but significant improvement in strength. The increases are guided by the patient's level of fatigue or pain, which are indications of overuse. When either of these occurs after engaging in an activity, the activity or exercise is reduced by half or discontinued and rest time is increased.

Acknowledgments—Details for the second case study of HIV were provided by Judith Dicker Friedman, adjunct faculty, New York University Programs in Occupational Therapy.

STUDY QUESTIONS

1. What are the therapeutic goals of therapy, in general, for patients with degenerative diseases?
2. What are the three classic characteristic symptoms of Parkinson's disease?
3. What are the goals of treatment for patients with AIDS?
4. What treatment techniques have been suggested to improve motor control in patients with Parkinson's disease?
5. What symptoms of multiple sclerosis will interfere with the patient's psychosocial adaptation to life situations?
6. Describe the manifestations of amyotrophic lateral sclerosis and how they are addressed in treatment planning and processes.
7. What does the occupational therapist have to offer patients with postpolio syndrome who are experiencing muscular weakness?
8. What are the precautions health care workers must adhere to when working with HIV+ or other infectious patients?
9. Describe potential psychosocial influences that impact patients who are suffering a chronic progressive disease and their families.

REFERENCES

Adams, R. D., & Victor, M. (1977). *Principles of neurology.* New York: McGraw-Hill.

AIDS Project Los Angeles. (1991). *A guide to self care for HIV infection.* Los Angeles: Author.

Angel, R. W., Alston, W., & Higgens, J. R.(1970). Control of movement in Parkinson's disease. *Brain, 93,* 1–14.

Antoni, M., Esterling, B., Schneiderman, N., LaPerriere, A., Ironson, G., Klimas, N., & Fletcher, M. (1992, July 19–24). *Behavioral interventions modulate IgG antibody titers to EBV-VAC and HHV-6 in HIV positive and HIV negative gay men.* Paper presented at the International Conference on AIDS, Amsterdam.

Bannister, R. (Ed.). (1992). *Brain & Bannister's clinical neurology* (7th ed.). New York: Oxford University Press.

Blonsky, E. R. (1971) The changing picture of Parkinsonism. Part 1. Neurological modifications resulting from administration of L-dopa. *Rehabilitation Literature, 32*(2), 34–37.

Bloxham, C. A., Mindel, T. A., & Frith, C. D. (1984). Initiation and execution of predictable and unpredictable movements in Parkinson's disease. *Brain, 107,* 371–384.

Brown, D. R. (1980). *Neurosciences for allied health therapies.* St. Louis: C. V. Mosby.

Center for Women Policy Studies. (1991). *The guide to resources on women and AIDS* (2nd ed.). Washington, DC: Author.

Centers for Disease Control and Prevention. (1993, February). *HIV/AIDS Surveillance Year End Report.* Atlanta: Author.

Dalakas, M. C., (1985). Neuromuscular symptoms in patients with old poliomyelitis: Clinical, virological and immunological studies. In L. S. Halstead & D. O. Wiechers (Eds.), *Late effects of poliomyelitis* (pp. 11–31). Miami: Symposia Foundation.

Davis, W. (1988, April). Self care for PWAs. *AIDS Patient Care, 2*(2), 13–16.

DiGioia, R. (1992, April 4). An outbreak of tuberculosis. *Washington Blade,* 39.

Duvoisin, R. C. (1991). *Parkinson's disease* (3rd ed.). New York: Raven Press.

Epps, C. H. III (1993, November 21). Personal communication.

Erickson, R., Lie, M., & Wineinger, M. (1989). Rehabilitation in multiple sclerosis. *Mayo Clinic Proceedings, 64,* 818–828.

Erikson, E. H. (1980). *Identity and the life cycle.* New York: W. W. Norton.

Fahrner, R., & Gerberding, J. L. (1991). Risk of HIV infection in health care workers. In P. Volberding & M. A. Jacobson (Eds.), *AIDS clinical review 1991* (pp. 215–225). New York: Marcel Dekker.

Florijn, Y. C. (1992, July 19–24). *Physical activity as a therapeutic measure for HIV − infected.* Paper presented at the International Conference on AIDS, Amsterdam.

Glazer, S. (1992, March 17). New drug-resistant TB cases in the district. *Washington Post Health Magazine,* p. 9.

Gonzales-Aviles, A. (1992). The medical aspects of AIDS. In

W. M. Marcil & K. N. Tigges (Eds.), *The person with AIDS* (pp. 73–86). Thorofare, NJ: Slack.

Goodkin, D., Hertsgaard, D., & Seminary, J. (1988). Upper extremity function in multiple sclerosis: Improving assessment sensitivity with Box-and-Block and Nine-Hole Peg tests. *Archives of Physical Medicine & Rehabilitation, 69,* 850–854.

Halstead, L. S. & Gawne, A. C. (1993, February). *Exercise in the post-polio population* (Medical Grand Rounds). National Rehabilitation Hospital, Washington, D.C.

Halstead, L. S., & Wiechers, D. O. (1985). *Late effects of poliomyelitis.* Miami: Symposia Foundation.

Herbison, G. J., Jaweed, M. M., & Ditunno, J. F. (1985). Clinical management of partially innervated muscle. In L. S. Halstead & D. O. Wiechers (Eds.), *Late effects of poliomyelitis* (pp. 1–16). Miami: Symposia Foundation.

Hessol, N. A., & Lifson, A. R. (1990). Predictors of HIV disease progression. In P. Volberding & M. Jacobson (Eds.), *AIDS clinical review 1990* (pp. 63–79). New York: Marcel Dekker.

Hoehn, M. M., & Yahr, M. D. (1967). Parkinsonism: Onset, progression, and mortality. *Neurology, 17*(5), 427–442.

Johnson, E., Fowler, W., & Lieberman, J. (1992). Contractures in neuromuscular disease. *Archives of Physical Medicine & Rehabilitation, 73,* 807–810.

Johnson, M. P., & Chaisson, R. E. (1991). Tuberculosis and HIV disease. In P. Volberding & M. A. Hacobson (Eds.), *AIDS clinical review 1991* (pp. 109–126). New York: Marcel Dekker.

Kielhofner, G. (1985). *A model of human occupation: Theory and application.* Baltimore: Williams & Wilkins.

LaPerriere, A., Antoni, M., Fletcher, M., & Schneiderman, N. (1992). Exercise and health maintenance in HIV. In M. L. Galantino (Ed.), *Clinical assessment and treatment of HIV* (pp. 65–76). Thorofare, N.J.: Slack.

Laurie, G. (Ed.). (1984). *Handbook on the late effects of poliomyelitis for physicians and survivors.* St. Louis: Gazette International Networking Institute.

Lechtenberg, R. (1988). *Multiple sclerosis fact book.* Philadelphia: F. A. Davis.

Linroth, R. (1990). Multiple sclerosis achievement center: A caring environment for a chronic progressive disease. *Occupational Therapy Practice, 2*(1), 53–59.

Lui, K.-J. (1988). A model-based estimate of the mean incubation period for AIDS in homosexual men. *Science, 240,* 1333–1335.

Mansell, P. W. (1992). An introduction to the medical management of HIV infection. In M. L. Galantino (Ed.), *Clinical assessment and treatment of HIV* (pp. 1–8). Thorofare, N.J.: Slack.

Marcil, W. M. (1992). AIDS facts and implications for occupational therapy. In W. M. Marcil & K. N. Tigges (Eds.), *The person with AIDS* (pp. 135–161). Thorofare, N.J.: Slack.

Maynard, F. M., & Roller, S. (1991). Recognizing typical coping styles of polio survivors can improve re-rehabilitation. *American Journal of Physical Medicine & Rehabilitation, 70,* 2–12.

Minerbo, G. M. (1992) Immunologic aspects in HIV. In M. L. Galantino (Ed.), *Clinical assessment and treatment of HIV* (pp. 17–24). Thorofare, N.J.: Slack.

Mitchell, G. (1993). Update on multiple sclerosis therapy. *Medical Clinics of North America, 77,* 231–249.

Montoya, M. A. (1992). The legal and ethical issues of AIDS. In W. M. Marcil & K. N. Tigges (Eds.), *The person with AIDS* (pp. 163–180). Thorofare, NJ: Slack.

Muscular Dystrophy Association. (1991). *Facts about amyotrophic lateral sclerosis.* Tucson, AZ: Author.

Nolte, J.(1981) *The human brain. An introduction to its functional anatomy.* St. Louis: C. V. Mosby.

O'Connell, P. (1990). AIDS: A medical rehabilitation perspective. In M. Pizzi & J. Johnson (Eds.), *Productive living strategies for people with AIDS* (pp. 19–43). New York: Harrington Park Press.

Pizzi, M. (1990). Occupational therapy: Creating possibilities for adults with human immunodeficiency virus infection, AIDS related complex, and acquired immunodeficiency syndrome. In M. Pizzi & J. Johnson (Eds.), *Productive living strategies for people with AIDS* (pp. 125–137). New York: Harrington Park Press.

Pizzi, M. (1992). Women, HIV infection, and AIDS: Tapestries of life, death, and empowerment. *American Journal of Occupational Therapy, 46*(11), 1021–1027.

Poser, C. (1991). Neurologic disease. *Physician and Sportsmedicine, 19,* 80–92.

Quintyn, M., & Cross, E. (1986). Factors affecting the ability to initiate movement in Parkinson's disease. *Physical & Occupational Therapy in Geriatrics, 4*(4), 51–60.

Rao, S., Leo, G., Ellington, L., Nauertz, T., Bernardin, L., & Unverzagt, F. (1991). Cognitive dysfunction in multiple sclerosis: II. Impact on employment and social functioning. *Neurology, 41,* 692–696.

Schindler, V. J. (1988). Psychosocial occupational therapy intervention with AIDS patients. *American Journal of Occupational Therapy, 42,* 507–512.

Schlenzig, C., Jager, H., Rieder, H., Hammel, G., & Popescu, M. (1989, June 4–9). *Supervised physical exercise leads to psychological and immunological improvement in pre-AIDS patients.* Paper presented at the International Conference on AIDS, Montreal.

Sharief, M. K., Hentges, R., & Ciardi, M. (1991). Intrathecal immune response in patients with the post-polio syndrome. *New England Journal of Medicine, 325*(11), 749–755.

Smith, M. (Ed.). (1992). *Handbook of amyotrophic lateral sclerosis.* New York: Marcel Dekker.

Spence, D. W., Galantino, M. L., Mossberg, K. A., & Zimmerman, S. O. (1990). Progressive resistance exercise: Effect on muscle function and anthropometry of a select AIDS population. *Archives of Physical Medicine & Rehabilitation, 71*(8), 644–648.

Thomas, C. L. (Ed.). (1973). *Taber's cyclopedic medical dictionary* (12th ed.). Philadelphia: F. A. Davis.

Tigges, K. N., & Marcil, W. M. (1992). The occupational therapy process. In W. M. Marcil & K. N. Tigges (Eds.), *The person with AIDS* (pp. 105–134). Thorofare, N.J.: Slack.

Tomlinson, B. E., & Irving, D. (1977). The number of limb motor neurons in the human lumbosacral cord throughout life. *Journal of Neurological Science, 34,* 213–219.

Valdiserri, R. O., Lyter, D., Leviton, L. C., Callahan, C. M., Kingsley, L. A., & Rinaldo, C. R. (1988). Variables influencing condom use in a cohort of gay and bisexual men. *American Journal of Public Health, 78*(7), 801–805.

Valdiserri, R. O., Lyter, D. W., Leviton, L. C., Callahan, C. M., Kingsley, L. A., & Rinaldo, C. R. (1989). AIDS prevention in homosexual and bisexual men: Results of a randomized trial evaluating two risk reduction interventions. *Current Science Limited, 3*(1), 21–26.

Webster, D. D. (1968). Critical analysis of the disability in Parkinson's disease. *Modern Treatment, 5*(2), 257–282.

Weichers, D. O. (1985). Pathophysiology and late changes of the motor unit after poliomyelitis. In L. S. Halstead & D. O. Wiechers (Eds.), *Late effects of poliomyelitis* (pp. 1277–1280). Miami: Symposia Foundation.

Williams, D., & Windebank, A. (1991). Motor neuron disease (amyotrophic lateral sclerosis). *Mayo Clinic Proceedings, 66,* 54–82.

Wood, W., & Aull, M. R. (1990). Women and AIDS: Implications for occupational therapists. In M. Pizzi & J. Johnson (Eds.), *Productive living strategies for people with AIDS* (pp. 151–160). New York: Harrington Park Press.

Young, G. R. (1991). Energy conservation, occupational therapy and the treatment of post-polio sequelae. *Orthopedics, 14*(11), 1233–1239.

SUPPLEMENTARY RESOURCES

Suggested Readings

AIDS Project Los Angeles. (1991). *A guide to self care for HIV infection.* (Available from 6721 Romaine Street, Los Angeles, CA 90038; 213-962-1600)

Muscular Dystrophy Association. (1991). *Facts about muscular dystrophy.* Tucson, AZ: Author.

Muscular Dystrophy Association. (1991). *Muscular Dystrophy Association 1991 Annual Report.* Tuscon, AZ: Author.

Pinsky, L. Douglas, P. H. & Metroka, C. (Eds.). (1992). *The essential HIV treatment fact book.* New York: Pocket Books.

Sacramento AIDS Foundation. (1980). *HIV from A to Z: A self-help manual.* (Available from 920-20th Street, 2nd floor, Sacramento, CA 95814; 916-448-2437)

U.S. Department of Health and Human Services. (1984). *Amyotrophic lateral sclerosis: Hope through research.* Bethesda, MD: National Institutes of Health.

Resources

American Parkinson Disease Association, Inc. (116 John Street, New York, NY 10034)

Center for Women Policy Studies. Published *The Guide to Resources on Women and AIDS* (1991) and other information that advocates for improved services for women with HIV/AIDS. (2000 P Street NW, Suite 508, Washington, DC 20036; 202-872-1770)

Impact AIDS Inc. Published *Infection Precautions for People with HIV/AIDS: Household Guidelines* (1989) and other pamphlets and books regarding HIV and safe sex, drug and needle use, women and teens, HIV antibody testing, AIDS in the workplace, and household and grooming guidelines. (3692 18th Street, San Francisco, CA 94110; 415-861-3397)

Latham Foundation. (Latham Plaza Building, Clement and Schiller Streets, Alameda, CA 94501)

National AIDS Clearinghouse of the Centers for Disease Control and Prevention. Has available a comprehensive library of material regarding all aspects of HIV/AIDS. (800-458-5231)

National AIDS Hotline of the Centers for Disease Control and Prevention. Offers information, education, and referral services for many aspects of HIV/AIDS; has a vast national listing of medical, testing, counseling, legal, and other support services regarding HIV/AIDS. (800-342-2437)

National Parkinson Foundation, Inc. (1501 Ninth Avenue NW, Miami, FL 33136)

National Women's Health Network. Advocacy group for women's health issues; published *AIDS—What every woman needs to know* (1989; available in English and Spanish). (1325 G Street NW, Washington, DC 20005; 202-347-1140)

Parkinson Foundation of Canada. (Suite 232, ManuLife Centre, 55 Bloor Street W, Toronto, Ont., Canada M4W 1A6)

Parkinson's Disease Foundation. (William Black Medical Research Building, 640 West 168th Street, New York, NY 10032)

Pets Are Wonderful Support (PAWS). Published *Safe pet guidelines* (1991) and other information specific to pets and PWAs. (P.O. Box 460489, San Francisco, CA 94146)

Project Inform. Provides information regarding current treatments, including clinical trials and alternative treatment for HIV. (1965 Market Street, Suite 220, San Francisco, CA 94103; 415-558-9051)

United Parkinson Foundation. (220 South State Street, Chicago, IL 60604)

37
Orthopaedic Conditions

Jane Bear-Lehman

OBJECTIVES

After studying this chapter, the reader will be able to:
1. State the appropriate evaluation and intervention goals for the stages of fracture healing.
2. Describe the sequelae that may result from immobilization of the injured region and adjacent structures and identify methods to prevent the occurrence.
3. Identify the functional impact and implications of temporary and permanent orthopaedic conditions.
4. Describe the role of the occupational therapist with the chronic pain patient.
5. Identify the similarities and differences in guidelines for occupational therapy practice for the patient with low back pain and for the patient with upper extremity cumulative trauma.

Orthopaedics refers to the specialized branch of medical science that preserves and restores form and function to the skeletal system, its articulations, and supporting structures (Salter, 1983). Orthopaedic conditions include the injuries; diseases; and deformities of bones, joints, and their related structures (muscles, tendons, ligaments, and nerves). These conditions can be caused by traumatic events such as motor vehicle, recreational, and work-related accidents; they may be cumulative in nature, i.e., they occur and persist over time; or they may result from a congenital anomaly. The four main problems treated by orthopaedic surgeons are loss of independent mobility; musculoskeletal deformity; neurologic problems that result from disease or injury to the musculoskeletal system; and pain that may ensue from fractures, neuromuscular injury, and cumulative trauma disorders (Newell & Turner, 1985). Orthopaedic surgery and rehabilitation place equal emphasis on the prevention and the correction of deformity and disability.

This chapter provides an overview of the occupa-

tional therapy evaluations and treatments used with adult patients who have orthopaedic conditions. Specifically, it includes upper extremity and hip fractures and their sequelae, hip surgery secondary to trauma and disease, and pain with a focus on low back pain and upper extremity cumulative trauma disorders. The aim of occupational therapy in orthopaedic rehabilitation is to help the patient achieve maximal function of body and limb and to restore independence. Evaluation and treatment address both the injured and the adjacent parts as is appropriate for the medical and surgical stages.

FRACTURES

As long as orthopaedic surgeons have been treating fractures, there has been a controversy between the "movers" and the "resters." The surgeons prescribing rest as a fracture treatment keep their patients immobilized in traction or plaster for long periods of time after stabilization of the bone (Apley & Solomon, 1982; Salter, 1983). The goal for surgeons of either philosophy is to mobilize the injured structures as quickly as is compatible with the healing process and to return the patient to work and leisure activities (Salter, 1983).

The first goal of fracture treatment is to achieve a precise and effective stabilization for optimum recovery and resolution of function. Closed fractures that are relatively undisplaced and stable may be managed by protection alone without reduction or immobilization. Fractures that are undisplaced but unstable, do not require reduction but do require positioning and immobilization in a cast or an external splint. Surgical reduction is performed to reduce open fractures and those closed fractures for which the bone fragments cannot be approximated accurately by closed manual reduction alone. The bone fragments are brought into a closer anatomical position during surgical reduction and are stabilized by insertion of an internal fixation device such as an orthopaedic nail, pin, screw, rod,

GLOSSARY

Codman's pendulum exercises—Prescribed for most shoulder fractures in the early recovery stages. The patient bends over at the waist, while standing or sitting, so that the trunk is parallel to the floor. The arm assumes a position away from the body, perpendicular to the floor either with or without a sling. In this gravity-assisted position, the patient moves the arm passively or actively, depending on the surgical protocol, forward into humeral flexion and backward into humeral extension, across and away from the body for shoulder abduction and adduction and then in a circle for circumduction (Heppenstall, 1980). Codman's exercises are contraindicated if the upper extremity is edematous; alternatively, an overhead suspension sling or a skateboard is used.

Collar and cuff sling—A circle of material that is placed around the neck; the forearm is placed in the circle and supported only at the wrist. The length of the sling places the radial side of the wrist just below the nipple line (Apley & Solomon, 1982).

Controlled range of motion—Allows for either active or passive movement within a protected, predetermined, and safe arc. Often the allowed movement begins in the middle of the range and is gradually upgraded toward the full arc as healing occurs. A splint can be used to set the boundaries or block unwanted movement.

Delayed wound closure—To allow for further debridement after surgery, the physician elects to close the wound later when there appears to be no further risk of infection (Skotak & Stockdell, 1987).

Percutaneous pins—Long, slender metal rods used for skeletal traction; they extend through the skin surface from the bone either proximal or distal to the fracture site, e.g., Kirschner wire. They are often used along with plaster to fixate a severely comminuted or unstable intraarticular distal radius fracture (Frykman & Nelson, 1990; Szabo, 1993).

Secondary intention healing—A wound that the physician has left to heal spontaneously because of the presence of host tissue injury, contamination, or a foreign body (Skotak & Stockdell, 1987).

Spica cast—A plaster or metal device that the surgeon uses after surgery to position the shoulder or hip into the prescribed angle of abduction and external rotation. A spica cast made from plaster or thermoplastic material may be applied to hold the thumb into radial abduction.

Trendelenburg gait—Results when a weakened gluteus medius muscle forces the patient to lurch toward the injured side to place the center of gravity over the hip; this is also known as an abduction or gluteus medius lurch (Hoppenfeld, 1976). It is characterized by dropping of the pelvis on the unaffected side at heel strike of the affected foot.

Wall climbing—Also known as finger walking or palm gliding. To develop shoulder flexion, the patient faces the wall, placing the injured shoulder's hand on the wall. Then the patient either finger walks or glides the palm toward the ceiling and then toward the floor. For shoulder and scapular abduction, the patient turns so that he is parallel to the wall and abducts his shoulder to place his fingers or palm on the wall for finger walking or palm gliding. There are commercially available finger climbers (e.g., Smith & Nephew Roylan, Inc., Germantown, Wisconsin) that can be mounted on the wall or used on a tabletop with set increments for the finger walk; some climbers can be adjusted at different angles to allow for varying degrees of movement.

compression plate, or external fixator (Figs. 37.1 and 37.2). Surgical repair also can involve prosthetic devices that are implanted to restore joint motion (Apley & Solomon, 1982).

Fracture healing, when the part is immobilized by a cast, splint, or fracture brace (Figs. 37.3 and 37.4), is accomplished through the biological formation of immature woven bone or external callus. The woven bone then consolidates and remodels so that the fracture is repaired with lamellar bone (Apley & Solomon, 1982; Newman, 1986). When more complete bone immobilization is achieved using internal fixation, external callus does not form and direct healing occurs. This requires more time to heal than when external callus forms (Newman, 1986).

Fracture healing has a general time table that is confirmed by x-rays during the treatment course. Consolidation or complete fracture repair has occurred when the callus is ossified, the fracture site is no longer tender and painful, and there is no movement when the fractured bone is manipulated (Apley & Solomon, 1982). The general estimate of healing time for uncomplicated fractures is as follows (Apley & Solomon, 1986):

Upper extremity spiral fracture: 6 to 8 weeks;
Upper extremity transverse fracture: 12 weeks;
Lower extremity spiral fracture: 12 to 16 weeks;
Lower extremity transverse fracture: 24 to 30 weeks.

Rehabilitation begins as soon as the plaster dries, or within 1 or 2 days after reduction. To restore balance, muscles should be active from the start of fracture stabilization. The amount and kind of activity depend on the place and kind of fracture, the method of fracture reduction selected by the orthopaedic surgeon, and in some instances the age of the patient. Clinical experience in the last decade has shown that early specific use of the injured extremity during healing diminishes

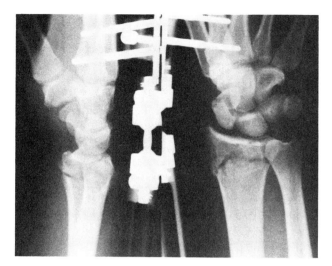

Figure 37.1. Lateral and anterior-posterior x-ray views of an external fixator.

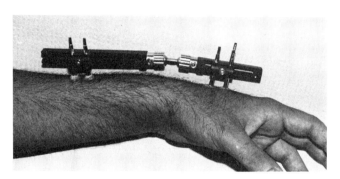

Figure 37.2. An external fixator in place.

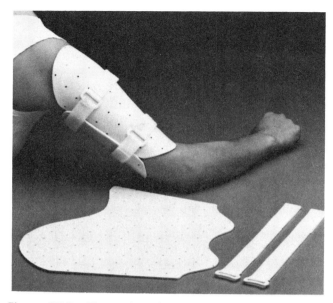

Figure 37.3. Thermoplastic humeral fracture brace to support the length of the humerus during healing.

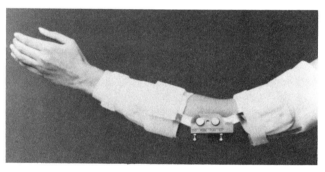

Figure 37.4. Upper extremity fracture brace with an adjustable hinge joint is designed to position the elbow statically in flexion or extension, to block undesirable motion, and to be used for free elbow motion.

or eliminates the need for treatment after immobilization (Salter, 1983). Early movement prevents the unwanted side effects of immobilization: stiff joints, disuse atrophy, and weakness. Figure 37.5 shows the sequence for muscle reeducation after stabilization of upper extremity fractures.

Evaluation

Assessment is a continuous and ongoing process and is carefully coordinated and monitored with the stage of bone healing, the chosen method of reduction and stabilization, and the plan for movement during healing. The surgeon's protocol for treatment of patients may stipulate no movement at the fracture site (as in immobilization) or may require **controlled range of motion,** beginning immediately or within the first 3 to 4 weeks after stabilization (see Fig. 37.5). Physiologic responses can and do occur relatively quickly, necessitating an immediate review and possible alteration of treatment during the acute stage. In early consolidation, when the cast or the fixator is removed and the

controlled movement guidelines are discontinued, the focus of therapy is to restore the loss of motor function of both the injured and the adjacent body parts. The occupational therapy assessment includes the following (see Chapters 4 and 6 for specific procedures).

ACTIVITIES OF DAILY LIVING

Through interview, the quantity and the quality of the patient's performance in activities of daily living (ADL) are ascertained.

Immobilization and Early Mobilization

Identify the areas for which the patient needs to learn an adaptation or obtain assistance during the temporary period of restricted movement.

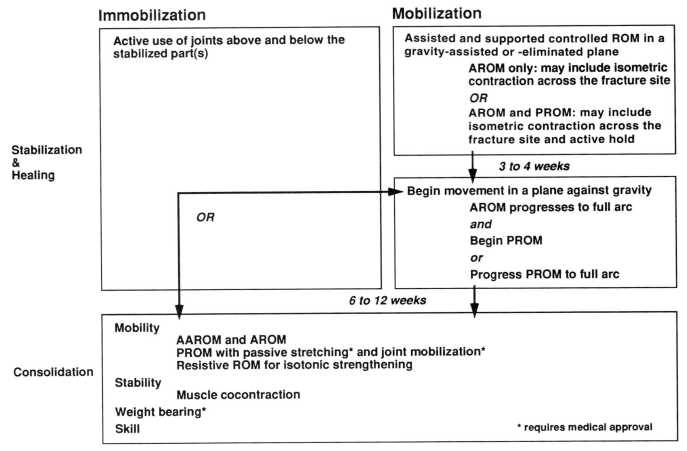

Figure 37.5.   Muscle reeducation sequence to facilitate movement during fracture healing and consolidation.

Early Consolidation

Identify whether the patient is capable of safely reintegrating the injured limb, given the stage of bone healing, into grooming, oral hygiene, bathing, dressing, eating, and communication tasks. Assess the patient's need for assistance and ability to upgrade task performance to correspond with clinical progress.

Work and Leisure

Through interview, identify the components of the patient's instrumental ADL; need to care for others; and home management, educational, vocational, and avocational activities. Guide the patient to resume those tasks that correspond with the achieved clinical status. Teach the use of adaptive equipment and methods as necessary.

Psychosocial Adaptations

Observe how the patient is assuming or resuming societal and family roles and initiating and terminating activities. Be concerned for the patient who magnifies the injury and rehabilitation process and appears to adopt a sick role. Guide your patient to select and to terminate activities that appropriately correspond to the bone healing stage and the rehabilitation goals.

Self-Management

Observe the patient's ability to cope with the injury and actively participate in rehabilitation. Note the patient's self-control in terms of physical limitations and pain reactions. Evaluate the patient's ability to follow written and verbal directions and to adhere to safety precautions. Determine whether your patient is reliant on others for cues to perform activities safely or is self-directed. Consider these observations as you design clinic and home exercises and activities.

ACTIVE RANGE OF MOTION AND PASSIVE RANGE OF MOTION

Immobilization and Early Mobilization

Measurements are conducted on adjacent joints. Active range of motion (AROM) deficits in the adjacent joints that were not present before the fracture need to be remediated. The AROM assessment of injured joints depends on the type of protection and stabilization used and on the orthopaedic surgeon's protocol. If the protocol requires complete rest of the injured bone(s) or joint(s), then range of motion (ROM) measurements are deferred until movement is permissible. If the protocol calls for controlled passive or controlled active movement at the fracture site, then a baseline measure is needed within the prescribed controlled range.

Early Consolidation

Both passive range of motion (PROM) and AROM measurements are conducted. PROM and AROM deficits indicate the need to improve the passive potential and to increase movement. Differences between achieved passive and active scores suggest weakness, pain, or fear of movement. The scores are compared to the surgeon's operative ROM scores, when available, to predict potential limits. Once the joint is stable, the accessory movements at the articular surfaces are assessed to determine the need for joint mobilization and passive stretching.

Edema

Measure the size of the limb above and below the fracture site cirumferentially with a tape measure. If there is access to the fracture site (e.g., when an external fixator is used), record a mid-point circumferential reading. Findings are compared with the uninjured side. When the limb can be immersed in water, volumetric measurements are used. Abnormal findings indicate the immediate need to implement edema reduction and control measures.

Soft tissue damage associated with a fracture results in extracellular edema. Unless this condition is treated quickly, the extracellular fluid will gel and bind down all tissue with adhesions, a condition that retards restoration of movement and function (Apley & Solomon, 1982; Colditz, 1990). The best treatments for this condition are elevation and muscular contraction to pump away the fluid (Hunter & Mackin, 1990; Vasudevan & Melvin, 1979).

Strength

Detailed strength testing with applied resistance is conducted once there is early consolidation. Manual muscle testing, grip and pinch testing can only be assessed if the muscle exertion will not adversely affect the healing bone. Specific manual muscle testing of individual muscles is indicated if neurologic or individual muscle-tendon deficits are suspected. Because of the force required, grip and pinch testing is usually deferred for 2 to 4 weeks following cast removal in forearm fractures.

Sensation

Diminished or abnormal sensory responses occur from edema or neural damage. Test for, and monitor, abnormal touch pressure and vibratory responses. Anticipate an increase in sensitivity over scars and at pin tracks.

Abnormal Signs

Observe the patient for signs of infection: redness, heat, swelling, pain, loss of function, and increased blood flow. Look at the limb's skin color; purple, dusky, or white indicate alterations in circulation as do skin surfaces that are too warm or too cold to the touch. Report abnormal findings to the surgeon.

Complete upper extremity arterial occlusion results in Volkmann's ischemia. Ischemia can be caused by edema or acute elbow flexion that compresses an artery against bone. Signs of ischemia for the forearm fracture include pale, bluish skin color; absence of forearm radial pulse; and decreased hand sensation accompanied by severe pain. Complete occlusion can result in gangrene and loss of a portion of the limb.

Pain

Listen to the patient's complaint of pain. Perception of pain varies from one patient to the next and for the same patient over time. Observe for physical signs that may be causing the pain such as an overly constrictive dressing, splint, or cast or an infection; if present, notify the physician. A well-made, properly fitted cast or fracture brace should provide comfort, never pain (Apley & Solomon, 1982). If the pain interferes with daily activities and exercise, some patients may require the help of prescribed analgesics to diminish or to control the acute pain or they may benefit from some of the pain reduction techniques offered in therapy such as transcutaneous electric nerve stimulation (TENS) or massage. Complaints of pain that are disproportionate to the injury may signal that the patient is coping poorly (see Chapter 10).

Treatment

The patient will experience an increase in localized pain, usually during the initial trials of active or passive movement. As movement is encouraged, the discomfort should subside, but it may not resolve. Persistent pain for 2 hr after a therapy session indicates that the demand in therapy needs to be reduced by half. To determine the patient's perception of pain and response to therapy, the pain analogue scales are used before, during, and after the treatment sessions. On a scale of 1 to 10, with 10 being the most intense pain, the patient identifies the number best associated with the type of pain experienced (Schultz, 1984).

IMMOBILIZATION AND EARLY MOBILIZATION

The occupational therapist emphasizes the benefits of movement of the adjacent parts of the injured extremity, assures the patient that the fracture is safely protected, and teaches the patient how to move the extremity properly to complete self-care, work-related and leisure tasks (Apley & Solomon, 1982). For those patients who have an upper extremity fracture, the therapist may recommend temporary use of the uninjured hand alone to perform ADLs assisted by adaptations such as pump bottles for toothpaste or shampoo, a buttonhook, and a rocker knife. Patients who need to protect a lower extremity fracture may require long-handled devices such as a shoehorn and bath brush and a bath bench for safety.

Early mobilization treatment programs have very specific protocols indicating the timing, type, and quantity of desired movement (see Fig. 37.5). The cautiously controlled movement usually begins in a gravity-assisted or gravity-eliminated plane. The program can include controlled active-assistive range of motion (AAROM) or controlled AROM in mid-range, gradually upgrading to the full ROM arc. Isometric contraction of the muscles that extend across the fracture site is encouraged to facilitate circulation and bone healing. Some protocols require controlled PROM often followed by an active hold, i.e., the therapist passively moves the injured part through the prescribed arc and then asks the patient to isometrically hold the achieved position briefly.

Often the therapist fits the patient with a sling, splint, or fracture brace during healing. A mild compression fracture of the upper end of the humerus may require protection alone, without reduction, as afforded by a sling (Salter, 1983). To add to a patient's comfort while stabilized in an external fixator, the therapist may recommend and then fabricate a supportive static splint. Thermoplastic splinting alone is often used to achieve relative immobilization for fractures of the metacarpals and phalanges. Following the initial treatment of closed reduction of fractures in the shaft of long bones, the surgeon may prescribe a functional fracture brace as shown in Figures 37.3 and 37.4 (Salter, 1983). The lighter weight, thermoplastic fracture brace allows for motion above and below the fracture site and minimizes the effects of prolonged immobilization. The metal hinge controls the amount of movement available (Fig. 37.4). The patient is closely monitored for alignment and controlled movement; the shell is adjusted as limb volume reduces.

Patients whose fractures have been stabilized with an external fixator (Figs. 37.1 and 37.2) or externally exposed pins need to prevent infection and possible osteomyletis by routine pin maintenance. Usually, alcohol or hydrogen peroxide is used to clean the pin; in some protocols the pin is covered with gauze, while in others the area is kept open (Collins, 1993; Skotak & Stockdell, 1987). The surgeon's protocol is followed for wound management procedures for open fractures that are healing with **delayed wound closure** or by **secondary intention healing** (Skotak & Stockdell, 1987).

EARLY CONSOLIDATION

Therapy usually begins with active exercise. It consists of activities to remediate the use of the muscle in the injured region as an agonist, antagonist, and a fixator in static cocontraction (Mennell, 1945). Focus is on redeveloping the function of the injured limb to resume its capacity in mobility, stability, weight bearing, and skill.

Should edema persist even with the efforts of elevation and active muscle contraction, additional methods such as compression gloves or sleeves and retrograde massage are applied. To ameliorate stiffness and pain, the therapist may introduce modalities (e.g., paraffin, fluidotherapy, and heat packs) before or intertwined with exercise or activity (see Chapter 33). If stiffness prevails and the fracture is stable, joint mobilization to facilitate the arthrokinematic accessory movements with passive stretching are performed to increase the passive potential. Splinting or the use of continuous passive movement (CPM) machines are also considerations to increase passive mobility over time (Salter, 1992). Adherent or hypertrophic scar formation after open reduction or soft tissue repair can also limit movement, increase pain, and alter sensation. The therapist teaches the patient deep pressure massage and applies continuous pressure to the scar with agents such as otoform, elastomer, or Silastic gel to facilitate scar remodeling.

SPECIFIC FRACTURES

Shoulder Fracture

The shoulder complex is the most mobile of all joints in the body. It provides a wide range for hand placement, but also provides the important functions of stablization for hand use, lifting and pushing, elevation of the body, and weight bearing (Lehmkuhl & Smith, 1987; Skyhar & Simmons, 1992). The shoulder is considered the most challenging portion of the body to rehabilitate. After traumatic, degenerative, and surgical shoulder lesions, the therapy goals are to relieve pain, restore movement and muscle strength, and maximize function (Skyhar & Simmons, 1992).

It is known that immobilization of the shoulder results in stiffness and pain; therefore, nonoperative and postoperative therapy programs call for a specific regimen of PROM, AAROM, or AROM within a controlled, guarded range. Emphasis is for the patient to resume functional activities, such as eating and performing basic hygiene, using the injured extremity as soon as movement is allowed. Because immobilization quickly results in stiffness, active shoulder motion is begun as soon as the acute pain diminishes in stable shoulder fractures. Unstable shoulder fractures usually require surgical intervention for fixation; most protocols do not start shoulder movement for up to 2 weeks after surgery. Shoulder fractures are closely monitored by x-ray as initial guarded PROM and AAROM begins. There is controversy in regard to PROM. Some physicians and surgeons argue that passive motion is contraindicated, particularly in the elderly (Heppenstall, 1980). Others say that passive movement is not unsafe if the provided range corresponds to the surgeon's prescribed limitations (Skyhar & Simmons, 1992). During the first 6 to 8 weeks, isometric exercises, a stimulant for fracture healing and callus formation, are performed along with **wall climbing** and **Codman's pendulum exercises** (Epps & Cotler, 1985). Stretching and isotonic strengthening do not take place until inflammation has decreased and there is no longer fear of disrupting the fracture (Skyhar & Simmons, 1992).

Shoulder immobilization for 6 to 8 weeks after open reduction and internal fixation in a **spica cast** may be required for serious intraarticular fractures or dislocations. Only movement distal to the shoulder is prescribed. When the cast is removed, shoulder AAROM for flexion, extension, abduction, internal and external rotation, and isometrics begin (Kavanagh, Bradway, & Cofield, 1993). Vigorous stretching and muscle contraction against applied resistive forces are delayed for 2 to 3 months. Isotonic strengthening does not begin until 4 to 6 months after cast removal (Kavanagh et al., 1993).

Prosthetic shoulder replacement, i.e., total replacement of the joint, is a relatively recent procedure. It is accepted that the patient requires PROM and AAROM within the first 2 to 3 days after surgery and that the key to a satisfactory functional result is early passive shoulder forward flexion and external rotation. Some protocols require the use of CPM for forward shoulder flexion for 2- to 3-hr intervals during the first 24 hr (Rockwood, 1990). Codman's exercises are introduced during the first 2 to 3 days after surgery, and the patient is instructed to perform both the Codman's exercises and the passive flexion and external rotation exercises 4 to 6 times per day, beginning with Codman's exercises. Because the subscapularis tendon and rotator cuff are violated during the surgery, some

surgeons introduce external rotation slowly in the first 4 weeks, while others incorporate passive external rotation on the 2nd postoperative day (Rockwood, 1990). The preferred position for passive external rotation exercise is with the humerus adducted. The patient is instructed to use the operated extremity for nonresistive ADLs, namely eating, brushing teeth, and writing (Rockwood, 1990). After suture removal (at 2 weeks), **wall climbing** exercises are added to the program. At 6 weeks, with medical advisement, the program is upgraded to include active resistive exercise and activities to strengthen the rotator cuff muscles and the three parts of the deltoid muscle (Rockwood, 1990). Weight bearing on the injured arm is not allowed for at least 6 months (Arntz, Jackins, & Matsen, 1993; Skyhar & Simmons, 1992).

Fractures of the humeral shaft and humeral neck both respond well to reasonable positioning and early movement. A fracture brace conforming to the length of the humerus may be made in occupational therapy to provide the initial support after a humeral shaft fracture (see Fig. 37.3). The humeral neck fracture requires support in a sling. Codman's exercises are performed to prevent stiffness. For the humeral shaft fracture, there is a risk of radial nerve damage because of the location of the injury relative to the course of the radial nerve (Salter, 1983). Radial nerve injury is characterized by inability to extend the elbow with gravity eliminated or inability to extend the wrist and/ or the digits.

Initial treatment addresses the restoration of shoulder movement in the gravity-assisted or gravity-eliminated plane. Often the weight of the extremity is supported by the therapist, a skateboard, or an overhead suspension sling (see Chapter 22). The therapist provides scapular support while guiding the patient through controlled movement patterns. To enhance scapular-humeral rhythm, proprioceptive neuromuscular faciliation (PNF) may be incorporated into treatment (see Chapter 24D).

Elbow Fracture

Elbow motion gives the individual the capacity to position the hand near or far from the body for manipulation of objects (Hotchkiss & Davlia, 1992; Lehmkuhl & Smith, 1987). These movements are accomplished by two degrees of freedom: flexion and extension at the ulnohumeral joint and pronation and supination at the proximal radioulnar joint.

Supracondylar fractures of the humerus may be treated by immobilization in a removable plaster or thermoplastic splint following open reduction. The elbow is held in 90 to 100° flexion; the arm may be supported in a **collar and cuff sling** (Muckle, 1985).

After the 1st week, the splint is removed daily for gentle, nonresistive, active movement in a gravity-eliminated position. Therapy for elbow fractures emphasizes active, not passive, movement and flexion rather than extension to minimize the risk of ischemia and excessive bone formation (Apley & Solomon, 1982). Many patients achieve close to full movement after 6 to 12 months without specific treatment; some however, may not achieve complete elbow extension even with therapy (Apley & Solomon, 1982; Heppenstall, 1980).

Complex elbow fractures are often treated with open reduction and a well-secured fixation. Active motion begins within 3 to 5 days. Similar to the supracondylar fracture, the elbow fracture is splinted in flexion rather than extension, because if a contracture occurs, the hand can be raised to the face for eating and hygiene (Heppenstall, 1980). In the elderly, elbow fractures are often treated using a **collar and cuff sling** alone and active movement begins early to prevent stiffness and pain. A functional arc of motion for daily activities can be regained; full ROM is not always achieved.

Radial head fractures seldom require immobilization. Undisplaced fractures without loss of joint congruity require protection in a sling for approximately 2 weeks (Salter, 1983). Active pronation and supination exercises are encouraged early. Full supination seems more difficult and painful to achieve than pronation; months of therapy may be required to reach the maximum potential (Hotchkiss & Davila, 1992).

Forearm Fracture

Distal forearm fractures are among the most common of upper extremity injuries. The majority result from a fall on an outstretched hand (protective extension reaction). The fractures of the distal forearm are named for the orthopaedists who first described them: Colles, Smith's, and Barton's fractures (Frykman & Nelson, 1990). These fractures involve the radius and/or the ulna and their articulations. Fixation is often required with **percutaneous pins** and skeletal traction fixators. If there has been extensive injury to the distal radioulnar joint, then the arm is immobilized in a long arm cast, one that extends from the metacarpophalangeal (MP) joints to the mid-humerus, to control for pronation and supination (Cooney & Schutt, 1992). Immobilization for most forearm fractures is 6 to 7 weeks in a short arm cast, one that extends from MP joints to the upper forearm, followed by 2 to 4 weeks in a supportive static splint (Cooney & Schutt, 1992). The short arm cast allows for full proximal and distal interphalangeal flexion and extension but may limit complete MP joint flexion, because it covers the distal

palmar crease. Lateral prehension between the thumb and the index finger is feasible.

Referral for therapy occurs if the patient demonstrates incomplete movement at the joints above and below the cast or if, after cast removal, movement is limited. Therapy begins with active movement. In a stable fracture that has limited movement, passive stretching and joint mobilization is performed. The patient is encouraged to resume functional activities as tolerated. ADL tasks, games, and crafts are frequently used and can be set up to require PNF diagonal and spiral movement patterns. Overhead positioning of a macramé project or use of an inclined board to mount a game incorporates the whole limb into the activity. Strengthening begins 2 weeks after the stabilization is removed. Special emphasis is placed on the development of wrist stability through the use of therapy putty exercises, hand grippers, and tools such as screwdrivers and leather punches that repetitively demand a forceful grasp and wrist stabilization. The ability to bear weight on the consolidated distal forearm begins on softer surfaces by encouraging the patient to lean onto the injured arm as if it were a pillar, and then asking the patient to increase gradually the amount of weight borne by the arm.

For the patient who is stabilized in an external fixator (see Figs. 37.1 and 37.2), depending on the directives of the surgeon, early active motion takes place at the joints immediately above and below the fixator. With approval, active exercise is performed in the whirlpool, providing wound cleansing, increased circulation from the oscillating water, and the opportunity to move in a gravity-eliminated environment. The surgeon may first ask the therapist to loosen the fixator to initiate early wrist flexion and then, in the following weeks, ask her to add wrist extension (Collins, 1993). The arc of movement provided to the patient by the therapist specifically adheres to the surgeon's guidelines; it is judiciously monitored by both therapist and surgeon. After the external fixator is removed, the protocol parallels that of the patient who was stabilized in plaster. Patients require about 9 months to regain maximum wrist motion (Cooney & Schutt, 1992).

Because of inflammation, edema, and extent of damage at the time of injury, there are many complications that can occur with distal forearm fractures. The most serious complication is reflex sympathetic dystrophy (Collins, 1993). The classic symptoms include extreme increase in pain and stiffness; edema; and vasomotor, sudomotor, and trophic changes (Collins, 1993). The sensory status of the skin supplied by the median and ulnar nerves is also monitored because of the risk of damage to these nerves secondary to the distal forearm fracture (Frykman & Nelson, 1990; Wainapel, Davis, & Rogoff, 1981).

The Hip

The hip joint is a large ball-and-socket joint that has three degrees of freedom: flexion and extension, abduction and adduction, and internal and external rotation. Its stability depends on the shape of the articulation between the pelvis (the acetabulum) and the head of the femur. This articulation is interrupted in a fracture or disease. Weak osteoporotic bone in elderly patients can break from a simple fall. The hip joint is a common site for degenerative joint disease and to a lesser extent rheumatoid arthritis. Childhood hip disorders such as congenital dysplasia or Legg-Calvé-Perthes disease may predispose the hip joint to early degeneration in adulthood. Progressive hip pain that interferes with ADL despite medication; rest; reduction in lower extremity loading by the use of a cane, walker, or crutches; and physical therapy indicates the need for hip surgery (Melvin, 1989).

There are a number of surgical procedures for reduction of hip disability and pain. They include osteotomy, arthrodesis or hip fusion, and partial or total hip arthroplasty (THA). To select the procedure, the orthopaedic surgeon considers the patient's physical status, degree of the deformity, and amount of available bone stock as well as the patient's age, occupation, lifestyle, and potential for cooperation in rehabilitation. For younger patients, the physical demand of work and recreational activities are carefully considered. The living arrangements and social support system to which the older patient will return enters into the decision of choice for a procedure. The surgeon may select the least radical procedure to make possible another procedure later, if this should become necessary.

After hip replacement surgery, the occupational and physical therapists teach the patient how to move the operated leg within the ordered weight bearing and movement restrictions. The occupational therapist shows the patient how to perform ADLs safely as well as how to cope with and adapt the environment. The physical therapist directs the patient to regain a normal gait and lower extremity strength and motion, teaches transfer skills, and shows how to use ambulatory devices.

The restrictions for weight bearing and hip movement on the operated leg are directly related to a number of factors, including the severity and location of the fracture, the surgical approach used, the ability of the fixation device or prosthesis to withstand stress, the integrity of the bone, the weight of the patient, and the patient's cognitive status (Goldstein, 1991). The physical therapist teaches the patient to use a walker or crutches for orders that indicate no weight bearing (NWB), touch-down weight bearing (TDWB), or partial weight bearing (PWB) on the operated leg. No body weight can be applied on the operated leg for NWB, 10 to 15% of the body weight can be applied for TDWB, and approximately 30% of the body weight can be used for PWB (Goldstein, 1991). A bathroom scale is used to confirm the amount of weight the patient is applying. A cane is introduced when the medical orders allow for 50% PWB on the operated leg, and the cane or no device is used when full weight bearing (FWB) is allowed (Goldstein, 1991).

Approximately 200,000 hip fractures occur annually in the United States, most in elderly women. Often elderly patients have prior medical complications, including congestive heart failure, coronary artery disease, hypertension, chronic obstructive pulmonary disease, and diabetes, that affect the rehabilitation program (Lowrey & Coutis, 1992).

Hip fractures and other lower extremity fractures are treated with closed reduction and immobilization in plaster or open reduction with internal fixation using pins, nails, screw and plate, or rods (Heppenstall, 1980). Partial joint replacement is the treatment for some fractures of the neck and head of the femur. The femoral head and neck are replaced by a metal prosthesis composed of a metal head and stem, such as an Austin Moore prosthesis. After excision of the femoral head, the stem of the metal prosthesis is inserted distally through the base of the femoral neck, down into the medullary canal of the femur, so that the head articulates with the normal acetabulum. If destructive changes have taken place in both of the components of the hip joint—femur and acetabulum—a THA is necessary.

Occupational Therapy Following Hip Fracture and Surgery

There is great controversy in orthopaedics concerning the rate of progression of weight bearing versus fracture healing versus mobility for patients who have experienced a hip fracture (Goldstein, 1991). Close communication among the members of the rehabilitation team is imperative to provide the patient with the best quality of care and consistency in learning how to function after surgery. Critical to the planned discharge, following a hospital stay of less than 1 week for most, is the therapist's evaluation of the patient's ability to perform basic and instrumental ADL skills safely and independently and his need for adapted equipment and/or assistance of others.

Favorable prognostic indicators for elderly patients to return home after a hip fracture, in addition to general medical condition, include whether they live with someone and whether they have a pattern of social contacts outside the home. In one study, patients who ambulated early and managed dressing, personal hygiene, and toileting during the first 2 postoperative weeks were more likely to return home (Ceder, Thorngren, & Wallden, 1980).

It is best to teach the patient who is restricted to NWB or TDWB to perform ADL tasks while sitting, which conserves energy and increases safety. Grooming can be safely performed in standing once the patient is PWB. For some patients this may be as early as the 1st week, but for others it may be as late as the 3rd or 4th week postsurgery (Goldstein, 1991). For at least 6 weeks, and for some patients even longer, the restrictions are (1) no hip flexion beyond 90°, (2) no hip rotation, (3) no crossing of the operated leg, and (4) no adduction of the operated leg. Because these restrictions preclude the patient from bending over or bringing the foot closer to the hands, adaptations are required to resolve problems in bathing, dressing, functional mobility, and home management (Table 37.1). The patient must be reminded that the operated hip is not to be passively flexed or the leg adducted beyond the midline. Long-handled dressing and grooming devices such as a reacher, dressing stick, shoe horn, and bath brush or sponge are provided, and the therapist teaches the patient to bathe and dress the operated side first, using the devices to avoid bending over or crossing the operated leg. For bathing, if showers are permitted, a nonskid bath mat, grab assist rail, and bath bench are recommended. To get into the bathtub, the patient

1. Stands with his feet parallel to the tub with the operated leg next to the bathtub;
2. Shifts his body weight to the unoperated leg;
3. Uses one hand to hold onto a counter or a grab assist rail for support;
4. Positions the operated leg into hip extension and knee flexion and abducts it to allow the leg to go over the edge of the bathtub;

Table 37.1. Adaptation for ADL after Hip Replacement Surgery

Problem	Adaptation
Bathe feet	Extended-handle bath sponge
Get in and out the bathtub	Nonskid bath mat; bath bench
Don and doff socks	Stocking aide
Don and doff shoes	Extended-handle shoe horn
Don pants	Reacher or dressing stick
Transfer to and from toilet, chair, and bed	Raised toilet seat; increased height of chair and bed
Sit in and rise from a chair	Wedge cushion with thick end of the wedge at the back of the chair
Open and close appliances and cabinets	Relocate frequently used items in the bathroom and kitchen to eliminate the need to bend or to reach; use a reacher

5. Extends the knee on the operated side once the leg is over the tub;
6. Places the foot on a nonskid mat;
7. Transfers his body weight to the operated leg once balance is secure;
8. Lifts the unoperated leg over the edge of the tub and places the foot on the nonskid mat.

Some patients shower standing and require a grab assist bar in the tub area for safety. Others, require the use of a bath bench to conserve energy and to feel secure. The bath bench needs to be high enough so that hip flexion does not go beyond 80 to 90°. To get out of the bathtub, the patient positions himself so that his feet are parallel to the side of the tub and so that he can lead with the operated leg. The same procedure for getting into the tub is used for getting out; it avoids hip adduction, crossing of the operated leg over the unoperated leg, and hip flexion.

To reduce hip flexion during sitting and rising from a seated position, the patient is instructed to use a raised toilet seat, is encouraged to raise bed and chair heights by adding wooden blocks under the furniture legs, and is asked to increase mattress and chair cushion firmness. The mattress is made firmer by inserting a board between the mattress and the box spring; plywood can also be placed under a chair cushion. The patient is encouraged to sit in a reclined position that is enhanced by a wedge cushion or a small rolled pillow or towel set at the junction of the chair's seat and back (McKee, 1975). The patient is instructed not to bend forward, which causes hip flexion, and not to cross his legs while seated.

If the patient sits in a normal-height chair, he is taught to stand up without overflexing the operated hip. In a chair with armrests, the patient scoots to the front edge of the seat, keeping the operated hip extended, and then uses the armrests to push straight up without bending his trunk forward. In a chair without armrests, the patient moves to the side of the chair so that the operated thigh is over the edge and the foot is placed back to the midline of the chair. This puts the operated hip in external rotation; puts the foot closer to the center of gravity, and enables the person to gain momentum to stand up without excessive hip flexion.

The patient needs to stand and walk more than sit. Sitting flexes the hips, whereas standing and walking actively improve hip movement and strength. Once the patient is PWB, he can stand at the kitchen or bathroom counter or home workbench. The patient is advised to have commonly used items relocated to a midrange height to eliminate bending or reaching; such movements cause too much stress on the operated hip.

By 6 weeks, almost all patients will be ambulating with a cane, and some will be unassisted. Most resume their usual methods to perform ADLs. Others, depending on the severity of the fracture and the course of healing, progress slower and have physical restrictions on bending and rotation for a longer time.

Therapy after Hip Surgery Resulting from Disease

The osteotomy is a procedure to change the alignment of the femur to relieve weight bearing on the hip joint. This may be the surgery of choice if it is done in the early stages of the osteoarthritic process and if it is likely that the patient will outlast the known duration of a prosthetic hip replacement (Lowrey & Coutis, 1992). When the osteotomy is done, compression plates are used to stabilize the bone, and the patient can begin early postoperative mobilization with passive movement (Morscher, 1980). The patient, using crutches, is PWB on the operated leg for 6 months, until the bone is healed (Lowrey & Coutis, 1992).

The hip joint arthrodesis fuses the acetabulum with the femoral head at about 25 to 30° flexion and in neutral abduction and rotation. An arthodesis is considered for patients under age 60 who are in good physical condition and who have one painful hip. A candidate for arthodesis is one who is not a candidate for a prosthetic hip implant because of heavy physical demands at work or in recreational pursuits that are beyond the tolerances of an implant.

The patient is mobilized 1 week after the hip fusion and is allowed gradual weight bearing up to FWB in 2 months. Some patients use a cane for a long time after surgery. The patient requires long-handled devices to assist with reaching his feet during bathing and dressing, because of early postoperative flexion restrictions (Seeger & Fisher, 1982). In 6 months, when complete healing is established, the patient may be able to put on a sock and shoe when seated by flexing the knee and reaching behind to pull on a sock or shoe using touch without visual guidance. The arthrodesis does leave the patient with a residual disability, but the hip is strong, stable, and pain free and has adequate endurance for standing at work and participating in active sports such as walking, hiking, sailing, and horseback riding (Liechti, 1978).

A THA surgically replaces the total hip joint that was destroyed from disease or trauma. It is performed using the hip joint implant prostheses developed by Charnley to replace both the acetabular cup and the femoral head with metal or metal-and-plastic implants. The Charnley implant prosthesis has been used for THA in the United States since 1971, and more than 120,000 THAs are performed annually in North America (Lowrey & Coutis, 1992). The Charnley implant was once reserved for older adults, but recent studies have shown favorable results in younger patients (Sarmiento et al., 1990; Unger et al., 1987).

Optimistically, the Charnley implant will last about 25 years (Sarmiento et al., 1990).

During the THA procedure, the greater trochanter is removed with muscle attachments intact and is reflected back for a surgical approach to the hip joint. After the prosthetic placement, the trochanter is wired back into place (Eftekhar, 1978). The postoperative protocol varies, depending on whether the surgeon elected to perform the THA with cement, with no cement, or with a hybrid prosthesis (Salvati, Huo, & Buly, 1991). The cemented femoral procedure usually requires 6 weeks of PWB, and then the patient begins to walk with a cane. The uncemented total hip prostheses, which depends on the ingrowth of porous bone for stability, requires 12 weeks of PWB before a cane is used (Wixson, Stulberg, & Melhoff, 1991). In the hybrid prosthesis, the femoral portion is cemented and the acetabulum is uncemented; a cane can be used after 6 weeks of PWB (Wixson et al., 1991). Success of the THA depends on a special operating room environment to decrease the incidence of infection, exacting surgical technique, and a careful rehabilitation program.

The first 2 months following THA are critical for protection and function of the new hip joint. The postsurgical program is designed to allow for healing of the trochanter and soft tissues and for development of a capsule around the joint for future stability. Until soft tissue is healed and is secure, hip flexion beyond 90°, hip adduction, and hip rotation are avoided. The extremes of these movements during the first 2 months can cause the prosthesis to dislocate. If a dislocation occurs, the hip is surgically realigned, and the patient may be placed in a hip **spica cast** for 3 weeks, delaying rehabilitation (Eftekhar, 1978). To protect the prosthesis, the occupational therapist instructs the patient in adaptive procedures and in methods to modify the environment to allow for safe performance of ADLs and homemaking (see Table 37.1). The techniques used to help the patient following a THA parallel those described earlier for hip fracture surgery, with the additional concern of encouraging hip abduction and carefully adhering to the weight-bearing guidelines based on whether or not cement was used in the procedure.

For at least 3 weeks, and for some patients up to 8 weeks, after surgery, the operated hip is positioned in extension and abduction while supine in bed. A splint or a foam abduction wedge is used while lying down and in sitting to encourage hip abduction. Once the patient achieves 55° hip flexion in physical therapy, the patient can sit reclined on a raised chair using a rolled pillow placed between the seat and the back of the chair and a foam abduction wedge between the legs to encourage hip abduction. The patient learns to transfer from supine to standing without flexing the operated hip beyond 90° by keeping the knees apart (hips abducted) and sliding out of a raised bed to take weight on the unoperated leg; some patients use an overhead trapeze bar during the transfer from supine to standing.

The patient with a cemented or hybrid THA prosthesis usually begins PWB with a walker or crutches immediately after surgery. In some instances these patients can withstand FWB within the first 3 days, however, many orthopaedic surgeons wait 3 weeks before ordering FWB (Goldstein, 1991). The ADL program can be taught in standing and uses the bathing and lower extremity dressing techniques described earlier for fractures (see Table 37.1). The patient with an uncemented THA is usually TDWB for the initial recovery phase and is conservatively progressed to PWB (Goldstein, 1991). This necessitates the learning of ADL tasks from the seated position. Once 50% PWB is ordered, the ADL program is upgraded to allow for standing with a cane. The cane is used until the **Trendelenburg gait** disappears. Older patients walk with a cane for an extended time for reassurance.

Usually after a THA, patients do not receive outpatient therapy following inpatient rehabilitation; many may receive home care occupational and physical therapy for safety assessment, and some also may qualify for home-based rehabilitation. Between the 2nd and 3rd postsurgical month, patients usually resume all routine daily activities with the restrictions about too much hip flexion and no adduction or internal rotation still applicable. For some, this restriction may persist for long period of time. Strenuous sports such as tennis, skiing, or jogging are discouraged. The Charnley prosthesis is designed for walking, not running or other athletic activities. Long term follow-up studies of THA patients showed that most patients have dramatic relief of pain and improved functional performance by 6 months after surgery (Sarmiento et al., 1990).

PAIN

Two common pain problems referred to occupational therapy are low back pain (LBP) from specific and nonspecific causes and arm and hand pain usually following trauma (see Chapter 38) or from stress and strain injuries known as cumulative trauma disorders (CTD). Pain is a personal experience that is real and is expressed by the patient with sensory and emotional adjectives (Kirkaldy-Willis, 1992; Waddell, 1992). Acute pain is proportionate to the physical findings. Chronic pain—pain that lasts for months or years—results in personality changes, causes disassociation from the physical problem, and develops into a different

clinical syndrome (Waddell, 1992). Pain starts out as a physical problem; however, there can be psychological disturbances, depending on how the patient reacts to the pain and the success or the failure of treatment (Raj, 1983; Waddell, 1992). The goal is to alleviate the pain early to prevent emotional changes (Andersson, 1992; Waddell, 1992; Wilkinson, 1992). Pain-alleviating programs are based on the gate control theory of pain (Melzack, 1973; Wall & Cronly-Dillon, 1960). This theory suggests that impulses from large sensory nerve fibers subserving mechanoreceptors stimulate the same transmission cells that pain receptors do and inhibit the perception of pain. The inhibitory effect is believed to be enhanced by concentration on a competing activity. Therefore, to inhibit pain, the occupational therapist shifts the patient's attention from concentration on the movement of the joints and muscles to an enjoyable activity (Kirkaldy-Willis, 1992).

Low Back Pain

Low back pain secondary to work injury has the highest incidence of disability and economic loss in the United States (Kelsey, Mundt, & Golden, 1992; Nordin, 1992; Raj, 1983). The most common cause of LBP is soft tissue strain, resulting from sustained static posture, frequent lifting while twisting, or exposure to vibration (Kelsey et al., 1992; Mooney, 1992; Nordin, 1992; Waddell, 1992). Most episodes of LBP are self-limiting; 90% of patients return to work within 2 months. Approximately 5% of patients, however, have chronic pain and are out of work for more than 6 months (Nordin, 1992). Much medical and therapeutic effort has been directed toward preventing chronicity or reoccurrence once back pain has been experienced (Nordin, 1992). It is believed that by modifying the workplace and changing the behavior of the workers there could be a reduced exposure to etiological factors that cause back pain and injury (Kelsey et al., 1992; Nordin, 1992). To date, primary prevention programs to reduce the incidence of back problems have not been able to solve the problem of reducing the incidence of LBP satisfactorily (Nordin, 1992). These programs are presented to persons at risk for back injury but who have not experienced it.

The primary goal in medically managed back care is to prevent the patient from developing chronic pain. Continued pain, distress, and illness behavior combine to reduce the patient's overall physical activity level, which leads to disuse syndrome or deconditioning (Waddell, 1992). As pain progresses, the objective findings over time may have little to no association with a nociceptive stimulus. Chronic pain and disability become increasingly associated with emotional distress, depression, disease conviction (convince self and others that the disease exists), failure to cope, feelings of catastrophe (total misfortune), and adaptation to chronic invalidity (Waddell, 1992). This situation becomes a self-sustaining condition that is often resistant to traditional medical management alone (Waddell, 1992).

The focus now is to prevent the development of chronic pain syndromes through treatment adapted from the field of sports medicine that calms the pain and relaxes the muscles. Bed rest is replaced with early application of physical therapy modalities, a flexibility program, and actively involving the patient in a graduated, ADL program (Mooney, 1992; Weinstein & Herring, 1993) As physical therapy helps the patient develop dynamic control of the lumbar spine through flexibility training, stretching, and ROM exercises, the occupational therapist directs the patient in performance of activities in a neutral spine position (the midpoint of available range between anterior and posterior pelvic tilt), to maintain ROM and engage the person's attention. The occupational therapist teaches the patient to understand, manage, and protect the low back by using proper body mechanics and alternative techniques to perform activities at home and work (Wilkinson, 1992). As endurance training progresses in physical therapy, the occupational therapist upgrades the quality and the quantity of ADL and work-related task challenges. When return to usual and customary activities is imminent, the treatment addresses safety and prevention of reoccurrence.

The back school concept for educating patients about their back and body mechanics has been part of rehabilitation for many years. The first modern back school began in Sweden in 1969 and was followed by the Canadian Back Education Units in 1974 in Toronto (Andersson, 1992; Mooney, 1992). In the United States, the back school was popularized in the 1970s. The team usually consists of a physician, a physical therapist, an occupational therapist, and in some instances a social worker or psychologist. The basic philosophy is that education in anatomy, spine function, and proper body mechanics for personal daily living and leisure activities will help the LBP patient take responsibility for management of his back. The patient is taught how to live well in spite of back pain and to understand how to prevent reoccurrence or aggravation of symptoms by working and behaving correctly (Andersson, 1992; Mooney, 1992). The programs differ in terms of their target population: chronic LBP patients (the Canadian back school) versus patients with acute pain (the California back school) (Wilkinson, 1992). Descriptive reports support the back school approach as an important adjunct to conservative treatment; however, there are few efficacy studies available to support these claims (Andersson, 1992).

Evaluation

The occupational therapist facilitates the patient's active participation in occupational performance tasks that are safe and correspond with the medical stage. The initial interview incorporates questions about the pain history and pain reaction during activity. This is repeated before, during, and after treatment. Inquiry into ADL performance is conducted to determine the extent of accommodation the person has selected and methods he has chosen for task completion. Observation of actual or simulated performance of ADL tasks may be indicated to understand the patient's functional limitations and decision-making processes. Body mechanics and learning how to perform ADL tasks safely are the primary objectives of occupational therapy. Use of relaxation techniques for stress reduction, biofeedback for motor control, and group educational sessions are often included.

PATIENT EDUCATION FOR BODY MECHANICS

The occupational therapist teaches the principles of body mechanics related to static and dynamic postures as well as transition patterns (e.g., sit to stand and stand to stoop). To facilitate learning, the occupational therapist applies the biomechanical principles to commonly performed tasks and shows the patient how to integrate the principles into everyday tasks. Emphasis is on both cognitive and motor learning to develop the patient's understanding and ability to self-regulate motor activity safely. Therapeutic activities, including games, crafts, and simulated ADL or work tasks, are selected for practice. Using verbal and physical cues initially for feedback, the therapist guides the patient's physical performance during the activities and encourages the patient's development toward self-regulation and correction.

The biomechanical principles involve practices to reduce the load or stresses placed on the spine in various positions and when moving objects. Compression or twisting of the spine is avoided, as are attempts to exert force in positions where the spine is poorly supported. Specifically, the patient is taught to:

1. Incorporate a pelvic tilt in static sitting and standing postures, which unloads the facet joints, aids in pelvic awareness, and decreases muscular tension in the low back;
2. Position the body close to and facing the task, which avoids twisting and bending the trunk and limits excessive loading from upper extremity reaching;
3. Use both legs to turn the body to face the activity, which avoids muscular stress on the spine caused by twisting the body;

4. Maximize lower extremity flexibility and reduce the stress on the lumbar region by using the hip flexors and extensors to lower and raise the body (Nachemson, 1981);
5. Take micro-breaks and walk briefly or stretch every hour, which interrupts sustained periods of static sitting and standing;
6. Balance activity with rest to facilitate endurance, good body mechanics, and safety by incorporating rest periods into the course of the activity or alternating between two work patterns that each challenge different muscle groups.

Activity selection in occupational therapy for the LBP patient is made to allow for both observation and patient practice of body mechanics in the following postures.

Standing

At the bathroom or kitchen sink, the patient places one foot up on the shelf under the sink or on a low stool to achieve a pelvic tilt; this pattern is taught for use in other standing patterns such as cooking or working at a workbench.

Sitting

The body is lowered to sit by flexing the knees and hips, without bending forward at the hips. Guidance and support through the transition are achieved by placing the hands on the chair's armrests. A raised seat reduces pain and stress in acute phases. A slightly reclined sitting posture is preferred. To avoid bending over the work the chair is moved close to the work surface and the work surface may need to be raised or slightly inclined.

Weight Shifting

To avoid excessive reaching, the patient is taught to move the body close to or with the task, e.g., walk with the broom rather than reach with it.

Lifting

For lifting objects from the floor to intermediate heights, the choice of position depends on the size and weight of the object. To pick up a lightweight object such as a newspaper from the floor, the patient faces the newspaper and lowers both knees in a semisquat position (or a ballet position of plié) toward the floor while keeping the back straight and a posterior pelvic tilt. When lifting a large or heavier object or a small child, the patient learns to add more central support by lowering one knee to the floor (half-kneeling) so that the body is positioned close to and facing the object. The goal is to bring and keep the weighted mass as close to the body's center of gravity as possible. A small child is encouraged to climb up into the lap. Once the object or child is grasped securely, the knee on the floor helps push the body up, and then both legs can extend to lift the weight. In the upright position, the patient should achieve balance before carrying the object. If possible, the patient is instructed to lift to an intermediate height such as a chair, briefly rest, and then lift up to carry.

Carrying

The patient is taught to carry balanced, light loads of laundry, groceries, and parcels close to the body. Fanny packs and back packs are often used instead of purses or book bags. However, some find a book bag more comfortable. Infants are best transported in a front or back baby carrier or stroller. Through practice sessions, the therapist helps the patient understand what his achieved and safe load tolerances are over given distances and time. It is important to help the patient translate pounds used in therapy to practical items, e.g., a half gallon of milk weighs 2 lb.

Upper Extremity Cumulative Trauma Disorders

Cumulative trauma disorder, also known as repetitive strain injury (RSI), is a contemporary problem and accounts for 51% of reported occupational illnesses in the United States (Johnson, 1993). It is a class of musculoskeletal disorders in which chronic discomfort, pain, and functional impairment may develop over time as a result of frequent, sustained, and repetitive movements (Browne, Nolan, & Faithful, 1984; Falkenburg & Schultz, 1993; Ferguson, 1984; Guidotti, 1992). It has been suggested that these disorders are associated with the rise in automation and specialization in work. Much faster work rates and the redesign of jobs require a worker to do a single task or a very limited number of tasks tens of thousands of times each day (Bammer & Martin, 1988). Workers whose occupations require repetitive and continuous use of their hands such as in computer keyboarding, repetitive assembly line work, or repetitive crimping, as in the processing industries, are at risk (Bear-Lehman & McCormick, 1985; Pascarelli & Kella, 1993). The dominant hand presents earlier and with more significant symptoms than the subdominant hand unless the design of the workstation is biased to one side (Falck & Aarnio, 1983).

A CTD does not have a single initiating event and the symptoms initially described are usually subjective in nature and are often nonspecific to the musculoskeletal system. The changes initially may manifest as an ache that is present at work but disappears at rest. If the individual avoids repetitive work or the relevant work conditions that aggravate or precipitate the condition are appropriately altered, the CTD will resolve (Stock, 1991). However, if the exposure continues unabated, the symptoms will progress and become more defined to a specific disorder affecting a combination of, or a single component of, the musculoskeletal system. Disorders include neural compression, inflammation of the muscle-tendon unit, and vascular alteration (Stock, 1991). The continuation of exposure to rapid, repetitive, and forceful movements may lead to localized muscle fatigue with ischemia and metabolic change that impairs muscle enzyme function (Stock, 1991). The affected muscles and their tendons are then more susceptible to micro-tears and inflammatory changes, resulting in pain that persists during the work tasks and at rest and jeopardizing the individual's ability to work and perform daily tasks (Stock, 1991). In the severe state, symptoms persist even during rest, sleep is disturbed, and the pain is aggravated by even nonrepetitive movements (Bammer & Martin, 1988; Stock, 1991).

The most common example of a CTD caused by neural compression occurs in the median nerve at the level of the wrist and is known as carpal tunnel syndrome (CTS). An individual who has CTS shows weakness in pinch, clumsiness in hand function, hyperesthesias or paraesthesis in the median nerve distribution in the hand, and may have nocturnal pain. Entrapment of the ulnar nerve at the elbow or within Guyon's canal may also occur secondary to hyperuse of the extensor carpi radialis longus and brevis; similar symptoms are produced but in the ulnar nerve distribution.

de Quervain's tenosynovitis is one of the most common specific muscle-tendon inflammations in CTD. This disorder inflames and effuses the thumb's extensor tendon sheaths. It seems to occur in individuals who use a lot of radial-ulnar hand movement, and it has been described as being associated with excessive spacebar or function key use on the computer keyboard. Two other examples of commonly seen muscle-tendon disorders occur at the elbow: If the long wrist extensors are affected, then it is known as tennis elbow, or lateral epicondylitis, and the tenderness is felt on the lateral side of the elbow at the origin or over the surface of the affected muscle bellies. If the long flexors are affected, then it is known as golfer's elbow, or medial epicondylitis, and the discomfort is along the medial side.

Physical treatment depends on the stage of the CTD (Bammer & Martin, 1988). Work modification, rest breaks, and exercise may quite successfully reverse the symptoms in the earlier stages (Bammer & Martin, 1988; Ferguson, 1984). However, for the many individuals who do not recognize the early symptoms or who do not seek appropriate attention during the early manifestations of symptoms, the therapeutic intervention is more prolonged and the symptoms may not be reversible (Bammer & Martin, 1988; Pascarelli & Quilter, 1994). Treatment addresses rest of the symptomatic region, avoidance of precipitating and aggravating factors, and reconditioning the unaffected proximal musculature, namely the shoulders and upper trunk. Permanent changes in lifestyle and working capacities may ensue for many whose symptoms are progressive and chronic (Bammer & Martin, 1988; Browne et al., 1984; Stone, 1991).

Cumulative trauma disorders cannot be viewed as circumscribed physical phenomena alone. These disorders have a sociological, psychological, and political context that impacts the patient's progress and outcome. Such disorders have unproven etiologies, insidious onsets, few objective signs, and variable symptoms that raise the issue of legitimacy of the conditions and question their work-related status (Reid & Reynolds, 1990). Therefore, the impact of the disorder affects not only the individual and his family but also employers, unions, insurers, and government agencies (Reid & Reynolds, 1990). When the condition is contested, the patient has limited, delayed, or blocked access to medical payments and reimbursement for work time lost usually awarded a person with a compensable injury. Failure to receive this support imposes financial hardship and psychological stress. The individual may appear depressed from the physical effects of the pain and its threat to his persona, career, and daily rhythm of life.

THERAPY

Figure 37.6 shows the series of events that usually take place from the time the patient recognizes and seeks attention for early CTD. Success of the intervention is measured in terms of increasing the person's ability to perform activities with reduced symptoms. The initial treatment effort is to calm the symptoms. Various methods to calm discomfort—rest assisted by splinting and antiinflammatory agents or surgical decompression of the nerve or tenolysis of the tendon to relieve pressure—address the symptoms, not the cause. Once the symptoms are controlled, the cycle, as shown in Figure 37.6, continues unless the precipitating and aggravating factors are removed. These factors are related to the interaction of the physical demands of the job (or hobby) and the design of the workstation and tools.

The occupational therapist assesses the patient's physical and functional abilities beginning with an occupational history since the onset of symptoms. To set the long-term goals for intervention, the therapist needs to know the patient's current status and expected

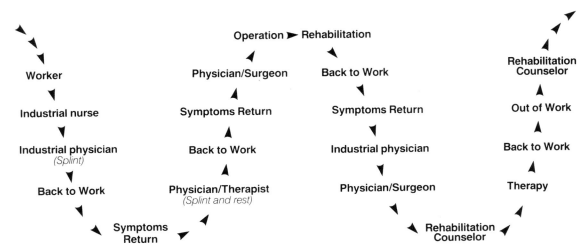

Figure 37.6. The path frequently traveled by patients with a cumulative trauma disorder.

future status relative to work and lifestyle. If return to work is expected, the therapist needs to know what the individual's job demands, work patterns, and environmental conditions are. These conditions can be identified through observation, patient description, review of the *Dictionary of Occupational Titles* (U.S. Department of Labor, 1991), and a job description if a detailed one exists. The upper extremity sensory and motor status is evaluated, and the outcome scores are compared with normative standards. The patient is asked to perform a series of dexterity tests that simulate his job, hobby, and ADL demands. Observations are made relative to patient's preferred patterns of movement, safety, use of rest periods, and response to the tasks in terms of reported pain thresholds and changes in autonomic responses: alteration in breathing and changes in body color or temperature. The assessment of the patient with a CTD follows the general guidelines discussed for upper extremity fractures with special attention to the following.

Activities of Daily Living

Most patients with CTD will experience altered or limited ability to apply pressure, lift, carry, and manipulate components of usual ADL tasks. A detailed inquiry is made to determine the patient's ability to dress, eat, perform personal hygiene, use transportation, maintain the home, write, use the telephone, keyboard on the computer, and do leisure activities. The goal is restoration of safe ADL performance. The program focuses on methods of joint protection and energy conservation to avoid precipitating and aggravating postures and movements (described above). See Chapter 16 for joint protection and energy conservation methods.

The majority of patients with CTD may have

significant functional impairments. The patient often has difficulty with fine motor coordination tasks and needs assistance from the occupational therapist to select adaptive equipment or creatively problem solve innovative solutions to manage such items as fasteners, change purses, dental floss, and pen or pencil. Because of weakness, lifting or carrying is limited to 3 or 5 lb, which severely hinders the patient. A backpack or a waist pack that relies on the support of the larger muscles of the shoulder and trunk to carry groceries, laundry, books, and musical instruments is recommended, as described earlier for the LBP patient.

Lower endurance also affects sustained static patterns, and many patients who have difficulty holding onto the newspaper for more than a few minutes should consider reading the paper on a table. Those who report spontaneously dropping things may need encouragement to use more paper or plastic products in the kitchen, to work over a surface to minimize spillage, or to monitor their hands visually during tasks. Lower tolerance to vibration will limit the amount of time that the person can handle the steering wheel in the car, which may require more frequent balancing of the tires. The vibration from the hair dryer may be irritating to the hands and can be eliminated by mounting the hair dryer on the wall. As the patient experiences improved endurance from therapy, the ADL methods are upgraded with the guidance from the therapist to adhere to the biomechanical principles for joint protection according to his progress.

Work and Leisure

Because of the nature of the CTD disorder, the majority of people affected are in the beginning or first half of their career cycle. Once the symptoms have been reduced and the patient learns how to perform activities with training in biomechanics and joint protection, the issue of return to work is raised. It is critical that the aggravating and precipitating factors that may have caused the symptoms be avoided. Some have advocated programs of work hardening or conditioning for this population (Johnson, 1993), while others firmly believe that such programs are contraindicated (Pascarelli & Quilter, 1994). To toughen up or make stronger the anatomical regions that have been known to be symptomatic in a work-hardening or -conditioning program is probably not possible or safe for the integrity of the muscle-tendon unit. Such an effort will most likely exacerbate an inflammatory response. For successful return to work, the work conditions and methods need to be modified so that the patient is able to work safely and not be put at risk for reinjuring himself. For some, the prospects of job modification and learning new ways to use their hands to reduce the exposure to probable etiolgic factors is possible. Others may benefit from technology, such as a voice-activated computer, to allow them to work without using their hands at the keyboard, obviating exposure to repetitive and continuous hand use. For others, the physical changes may be too severe to allow continuation of their usual and customary work, and unfortunately, there may not be an available reasonable accommodation for their workstation or duties or schedule to enable a safe return with lowered exposure to precipitating factors.

For many patients, the ability to perform physically active sports and to participate in travel with friends and family are hindered. Even sedentary activities like reading and playing cards are difficult to do, as the patient may be unable to hold a book for long. Shuffling and holding cards may not be possible without adaptations. It is vital to identify ways to assist the patient to either continue with important recreational activities or to help the patient select activities that will be both relaxing and meaningful. Swimming, yoga, and ballet are particularly good choices.

Psychosocial Adaptations

For some, the diagnosis of CTD becomes all encompassing and the patient is engulfed solely in the role of patient or claimant. The physical limitations may curtail participation in family and societal roles, although many tasks can still be done with adaptations. The therapist can help the patient develop creative and innovative solutions to maintain roles and to develop new ones.

Self-Management

Pain and the need to cope with the therapeutic process of rehabilitation, because it is not known whether the injury will be covered by worker's compensation and because the employer fails to understand why so much time off is needed, may challenge even the most goal-directed patient. This scenario is quite common, and it is important for the therapist to be aware of the variables beyond the clinical context that may be interfering with the patient's ability to perform. The therapist needs to observe carefully for signs of this stress and help the patient cope, advocate, and/or adapt through patient education. It is of paramount importance that the signs of inadequate coping be identified early and that measures be taken to help the patient so that the rehabilitation process can proceed (see Chapters 10 and 20).

Active and Passive ROM

The therapist must assess the trunk and limb ROM. Alteration in movement occurs in response to pain or lack of movement in one location. It is necessary to measure deficient movement in the spine and the extremities. It is not uncommon to detect decreased neck and shoulder movement among patients with wrist and hand CTD as a result of prolonged postural alterations.

While measuring and then remediating movement, the occupational therapist discourages simultaneous movement or positioning in the same direction across both of the joints in two-joint muscles in the symptomatic region (Lehmkuhl & Smith, 1987). The patient is encouraged to stabilize the wrist in neutral to reduce the tension of the long flexors or extensors as they cross the wrist. Similarly, during wrist flexion or extension action, the digits are held in a relaxed posture. For an activity such as writing, the patient learns to use this pattern by using a 25 to 30° inclined board to write on with an enlarged pen. In addition, the patient is taught that by adjusting the height of an object to be worked on, the wrist is positioned in neutral while the hand is fisted or is pinching.

Edema

Volumetric measures are used to monitor the response to static posture or activity. For sitting, many find increased comfort by resting the forearms and hands on a pillow placed on the lap. Many patients with CTD need to learn how to position their arms and hands when walking (Pascarelli & Quilter, 1994).

Strength

Testing of muscle strength, grip, and pinch are deferred until the patient's symptoms are subacute. Therapy initially focuses on isometric contraction of the muscles in the symptomatic region for those patients with the diagnosis of CTD. If there is also a more specific diagnosis, such a de Quervain's tenosynovitis, then that specific protocol takes precedence. For many CTD patients, it is several weeks before controlled concentric muscle contraction within the patient's tolerance begins in therapy. Extremes of joint range are avoided as are positions that cause simultaneous action at both joints in two-joint muscles (Lehmkuhl & Smith, 1987).

Sensation

In neural entrapment disorders such as CTS, sensory change precedes motor change, and touch-pressure and vibratory sensory studies are more sensitive in detecting the change (Bear-Lehman & Bielawski, 1988; Bell-Krotoski, 1990). Touch-pressure is assessed with the Semmes-Weinstein monofilaments (see Chapter 8). Vibratory perception has been demonstrated to be of clinical value in evaluating early and late signs of nerve entrapment as well as the individual's response and tolerance to vibration (Bear-Lehman & Bielawski, 1988). The vibrometer (Bio-Thesiometer, Bio-Medical Instrument Co., Newbury, Ohio) with a fixed frequency (120 Hz) and variable amplitude is used to detect the vibratory threshold (Dellon, 1983). The threshold level is recorded in volts and is converted to amplitude, measured in microns, using a formula supplied by the manufacturer. Outcome scores are compared with a normative table (Callahan, 1990; Dellon, 1983).

If following rest, splinting, or antiinflammatory agents, the sensory threshold levels continue to be abnormal, then the therapy program addresses sensory reeducation. Altered sensation in the hand will disrupt the patient's feedback, preventing him from regulating force, which may result in use of more force than is required. The patient may be a candidate for biofeedback to discover how to control muscle effort or a sensory protection program to learn how to disperse the force over a larger surface through tool modification.

Pain

The pain profile is administered to document the localized and referred pain pattern and the duration and intensity of the pain. Some patients describe the onset of pain from a specific activity or movement, many will indicate that the pain reaction is often delayed following a precipitating factor. Those with more advanced symptoms may indicate that they are always in pain but that the intensity can rise and that it is not specifically related to an activity or position.

For many patients, therapeutic modalities are an extremely helpful adjunctive treatment (Michlovitz & Wolf, 1990). Local heat through whirlpool, fluidotherapy, paraffin, or heat packs can be used to reduce

pain (Johnson, 1993; see also Chapter 33). Deep heat through acoustic vibration (ultrasound) and electrical stimulation such as galvanic, iontophoresis, and TENS are also beneficial agents. The home program includes the use of those agents that are beneficial to the patient and that can be applied in the home setting, such as cooling with ice packs, local moist heat applications, and TENS.

Positioning

In the acute stages, application of static thermoplastic or soft splints are used to help facilitate the needed rest while allowing movement of adjacent, nonsymptomatic parts. As the patient's condition becomes subacute, the splints are removed, and the patient learns how to safely move the symptomatic region, starting with isometric contractions and moving in midrange. Splints are discouraged during normal activity, because the blockage of a joint or joints will then demand compensation or exaggeration of movement above and below the immobilization. The patient is taught to recruit proximal musculature for power during tasks.

Scar Management

Progression of the inflammatory process and recurrent micro-trauma causes scarring and shortening of the muscle-tendon tissue. Effort is directed toward preventing the inflamed and painful muscle-tendon units from becoming fibrotic. Clinically, this is managed through deep massage and ultrasound to stimulate fibroblast activity on the inflamed tissue (Johnson, 1993). Supportive static splints prevent the inflamed regions from stiffening in a shortened position.

Acknowledgments—The author is indebted to Lillian H. Parent for her mentorship and gift of the opportunity to expand on her work for this chapter. Thanks is expressed to C. J. Schob and to Columbia University for artwork.

STUDY QUESTIONS

1. What are the unwanted side effects of immobilization of any fracture? How can they be prevented?
2. What is a major treatment goal for any patient with an upper extremity fracture?
3. Why is passive motion not used in the treatment of fractures of the elbow?
4. What is the occupational therapist's responsibility if a patient complains of burning pain under a cast? Why?
5. Why should patients with a fractured hip be referred to occupational therapy?
6. What techniques can an occupational therapist

teach a patient with hip pain for whom conservative treatment is recommended?

7. What occupational performance skills can an occupational therapist teach a patient with a hip fracture or total hip arthroplasty?
8. List precautions that must be taught to a patient with a total hip arthroplasty.
9. Describe the body mechanical principles that should be incorporated into the task of lower extremity dressing (sweeping the floor and working at a computer) for the patient with LBP.
10. What is the occupational therapist's role with a patient with an upper extremity cumulative trauma disorder?

REFERENCES

Andersson, G. B. F. (1992). Concept and development of back schools. In M. V. Jayson (Ed.), *The lumbar spine and back pain* (4th ed., pp. 409–415). New York: Churchill Livingstone.

Apley, A. G., & Solomon, L. (1982). *Apley's system of orthopaedics and fractures* (6th ed.). Kent, UK: Butterworth.

Arntz, C. T., Jackins, S., & Matsen, F. A. (1993). Prosthetic replacement of the shoulder for the treatment of defects in the rotator cuff and the surface of the glenohumeral joint. *Journal of Bone and Joint Surgery, 75A*, 485–491.

Bammer G., & Martin, B. (1988). The arguments about RSI: An examination. *Community Health Studies, 12*, 348–358.

Bear-Lehman, J., & Bielawski, T. (1988). The carpal tunnel syndrome: Back to the source. *Rehabilitation Research, 1*, 13–20.

Bear-Lehman, J., & McCormick, E. H. (1985). The expanding role of occupational therapy in the treatment of industrial hand injuries. In F. S. Cromwell (Ed.), *Work-related programs in occupational therapy* (pp. 79–88). New York: Haworth Press.

Bell-Krotoski, J. (1990). Light touch-deep pressure testing using Semmes-Weinstein monofilaments. In J. M. Hunter, L. H. Schneider, E. J. Mackin, & A. D. Callahan (Eds.), *Rehabilitation of the hand* (3rd ed., pp. 585–593). St. Louis: C. V. Mosby.

Browne, C. D., Nolan, B. M., & Faithful, D. K. (1984). Occupational repetition strain injuries. *Medical Journal of Australia, 140*, 329–332.

Callahan, A. D. (1990). Sensibility testing: Clinical methods. In J. M. Hunter, L. H. Schneider, E. J. Mackin, & A. D. Callahan (Eds.), *Rehabilitation of the hand* (3rd ed., pp. 594–610). St. Louis: C. V. Mosby.

Ceder, L., Thorngren, K. G., & Wallden, B. (1980). Prognostic indicators and early home rehabilitation in elderly patients with hip fractures. *Clinical Orthopedics and Related Research, 152*, 173–184.

Colditz, J. C. (1990). Dynamic splinting of the stiff hand. In J. M. Hunter, L. H. Schneider, E. J. Mackin, & A. D. Callahan (Eds.), *Rehabilitation of the hand* (3rd ed., pp. 342–352). St. Louis: C. V. Mosby.

Collins, D. C. (1993). Management and rehabilitation of distal radius fractures. *Orthopedic Clinics of North America, 24*, 365–378.

Cooney, W. P., & Schutt, A. H. (1992). Rehabilitation of the wrist. In V. L. Nickel & M. J. Botte (Eds.), *Orthopedic rehabilitation* (2nd ed., pp. 711–731). New York: Churchill Livingstone.

Dellon, A. L. (1983). The vibrometer. *Plastic and Reconstructive Surgery, 71*, 427–431.

Eftekhar, N. S. (1978). *Principles of total hip arthroplasty.* St. Louis: C. V. Mosby.

Epps, C. H. Jr., & Cotler, J. M. (1985). Complications of treatment of fractures of the humeral shaft. In C. H. Epps Jr. (Ed.), *Complications in orthopaedic surgery* (Vol. 1, 2nd ed., pp. 277–300). Philadelphia: J. B. Lippincott.

Falck, B., & Aarnio, P. (1983). Left-side carpal tunnel syndrome in butchers. *Scandinavian Journal of Work, Environment, & Health, 9*, 291–297.

Falkenburg, S. A., & Schultz, D. J. (1993). Ergonomics for the upper extremity. *Hand Clinics, 9*, 263–271.

Ferguson, D. (1984). The "new" industrial epidemic. *Medical Journal of Australia, 140*, 318–319.

Frykman G. K., & Nelson, E. F. (1990). Fractures and traumatic conditions of the wrist. In J. M. Hunter, L. H. Schneider, E. J. Mackin, & A. D. Callahan (Eds.), *Rehabilitation of the hand* (3rd ed., pp. 267–283). St. Louis: C. V. Mosby.

Goldstein, T. S. (1991). *Geriatric orthopaedics: Rehabilitative management of common problems.* Rockville, MD: Aspen Systems.

Guidotti, T. L. (1992). Occupational repetitive strain injury. *American Family Physician, 45*, 585–592.

Heppenstall, R. B. (Ed.). (1980). *Fracture treatment and healing.* Philadelphia: W. B. Saunders.

Hoppenfeld, S. (1976). *Physical examination of the spine and extremities.* East Norwalk, CT: Appleton-Century-Crofts.

Hotchkiss R. N., & Davila, S. (1992). Rehabilitation of the elbow. In V. L. Nickel & M. J. Botte (Eds.), *Orthopedic rehabilitation* (2nd ed., pp. 733–746). New York: Churchill Livingstone.

Hunter, J. M., & Mackin, E. J. (1990). Management of edema. In J. M. Hunter, L. H. Schneider, E. J. Mackin, & A. D. Callahan (Eds.), *Rehabilitation of the hand* (3rd ed., pp. 187–194). St. Louis: C. V. Mosby.

Johnson, S. L. (1993). Therapy of the occupationally injured hand and upper extremity. *Hand Clinics, 9*, 289–298.

Kavanagh, B. F., Bradway, J. K., & Crogield, R. H. (1993). Open reduction and internal fixation of displaced intra-articular fractures of the glenoid fossa. *Journal of Bone and Joint Surgery, 75A*, 479–484.

Kelsey, J. L., Mundt, D. F., & Golden, A. L. (1992). Epidemiology of low back pain. In M. V. Jayson (Ed.), *The lumbar spine and back pain* (4th ed., pp. 537–549). New York: Churchill Livingstone.

Kirkaldy-Willis, W. H. (1992). *Managing low back pain* (3rd ed.). New York: Churchill Livingstone.

Lehmkuhl, L. D., & Smith, L. K. (1987). *Brunnstrom's clinical kinesiology* (4th ed.). Philadelphia: F. A. Davis.

Liechti, R. (1978). *Hip arthrodesis and associated problems.* Berlin: Springer-Verlag.

Lowrey, C. E., & Coutis, R. D. (1992). Rehabiliation of the hip. In V. L. Nickel & M. J. Botte (Eds.), *Orthopedic rehabilitation* (2nd ed., pp. 779–789). New York: Churchill Livingstone.

McKee, J. I. (1975). Foam wedges aid sitting posture of patients with total hip replacement. *Physical Therapy, 55*, 767.

Melvin, J. L. (1989). *Rheumatic disease in the adult and child: Occupational therapy and rehabilitation* (3rd ed., pp. 519–526). Philadelphia: F. A. Davis.

Melzack, R. (1973). *The puzzle of pain.* New York: Basic Books.

Mennell, J. B. (1945). *Physical treatment by movement, manipulation, and massage.* Philadelphia: Blakiston.

Michlovitz, S., & Wolf, S. (1990). *Thermal agents in rehabilitation.* Philadelphia: F. A. Davis.

Mooney, V. (1992). Rehabilitation of the spine. In V. L. Nickel & M. J. Botte (Eds.), *Orthopaedic rehabilitation* (2nd ed., pp. 765–778). New York: Churchill Livingstone.

Morscher, E. W. (1980). Intertrochanteric osteotomy in osteoarthritis of the hip. In L. H. Riley Jr. (Ed.), *The hip: Proceedings of the Hip Society Eighth Scientific Meeting* (pp. 24–46). St. Louis: C. V. Mosby.

Muckle, D. S. (1985). *An outline of fractures and dislocations.* Bristol, UK: John Wright & Sons.

Nachemson, A. L. (1981, March 22–24). Toward a better understanding of low back injury. In *Proceedings of the Liberty Mutal Back Pain Symposium* (pp. 4–13). Boston: Liberty Mutual Insurance Co.

Newell, R. L. M., & Turner, J. G. (1985). *Orthopaedic disorders in general practice.* Kent, UK: Butterworth.

Newman, F. H. (1986). New developments in fracture management. In R. C. G. Russell (Ed.), *Recent advances in surgery* (pp. 199–214). Edinburgh: Churchill Livingstone.

Nordin, M. (1992). Prevention of back pain in industry. In M. V. Jayson (Ed.), *The lumbar spine and back pain* (4th ed., pp. 551–563). New York: Churchill Livingstone.

Pascarelli, E. F., & Kella, J. J. (1993). Soft-tissue injuries related to use of the computer keyboard. *Journal of Occupational Medicine, 35,* 522–532.

Pascarelli, E. F., & Quilter, D. (1994). *Repetitive strain injury: A computer user's guide.* New York: John Wiley & Sons.

Raj, P. P. (1983). *Practical management of pain.* Chicago: Year Book Medical Publishers.

Reid, J., & Reynolds, L. (1990). Requiem for RSI: The explanation and control of an occupational epidemic. *Medical Anthropology Quarterly, 4,* 162–190.

Rockwood, C. A. Jr. (1990). The technique of total shoulder arthroplasty. In W. B. Greene (Ed.), *Instructional course lectures* (Vol. 39, pp. 437–447). Park Ridge, IL: American Academy of Orthopaedic Surgeons.

Salter, R. B. (1983). *Textbook of disorders and injuries of the musculoskeletal system* (2nd ed.). Baltimore: Williams & Wilkins.

Salter, R. B. (1992). *Continuous passive motion: From its origination to research to clinical applications.* Baltimore: Williams & Wilkins.

Salvati, E. A., Huo, M. H., & Buly, R. L. (1991). Cemented total hip replacement: Long term results and future outlook. In H. S. Tullos (Ed.), *Instructional course lectures* (Vol. 40, pp. 121–134). Park Ridge, IL: American Academy of Orthopaedic Surgeons.

Sarmiento, A., Ebramzadeh, E., Gogan, W. J., & McKellop, H. A. (1990). Total hip athroplasty with cement: A long term radiographic analysis in patients who are older than fifty and younger than fifty years. *Journal of Bone and Joint Surgery, 72A,* 1470–1476.

Schultz, K. S. (1984). The Schultz structured interview for assessing upper extremity pain. *Occupational Therapy in Health Care, 3,* 69–82.

Seeger, M. S., & Fisher, L. A. (1982). Adaptive equipment used inthe rehabilitation of hip arthroplasty patients. *American Journal of Occupational Therapy, 36,* 503–508.

Skotak, C. H., & Stockdell, S. M. (1987). Wound management in hand therapy. In F. S. Cromwell & J. Bear-Lehman (Eds.), *Hand rehabilitation in occupational therapy* (pp. 17–34). New York: Haworth Press.

Skyhar, M. J., & Simmons, T. C. (1992). Rehabilitation of the shoulder. In V. L. Nickel & M. J. Botte (Eds.), *Orthopedic rehabilitation* (2nd ed., pp. 747–763). New York: Churchill Livingstone.

Stock, S. R. (1991). Workplace ergonomic factors and the development of musculoskeletal disorders of the neck and upper limbs: A meta-analysis. *American Journal of Industrial Medicine, 19,* 87–107.

Szabo, R. M. (1993). Extra-articular fractures of the distal radius. *Orthopedic Clinics of North America, 24,* 229–237.

U.S. Department of Labor, Employment and Training Administration. (1991). *Dictionary of occupational titles* (Vols. 1–2, 4th ed. rev.). Washington, DC: U.S. Government Printing Office.

Unger, A. S., Inglis, A. E., Ranawat, C. S., & Johanson, N. A. (1987). Total hip arthroplasty in rheumatoid arthritis: A Long term follow-up study. *Journal of Arthroplasty, 2,* 191–197.

Vasudevan, S. V., & Melvin, J. L. (1979). Upper extremity edema control: Rationale for the techniques. *American Journal of Occupational Therapy, 33,* 520–523.

Waddell, G. (1992). Understanding the patient with a backache. In M. V. Jayson (Ed.). *The lumbar spine and back pain* (4th ed., pp. 469–485). New York: Churchill Livingstone.

Wainapel, S. F., Davis, L., & Rogoff, J. B. (1981). Electrodiagnostic study of carpal tunnel syndrome after Colles' fracture. *American Journal of Physical Medicine, 60,* 126–131.

Wall, P. D., & Cronly-Dillon (1960). Pain, itch and vibration. *American Medical Association Archives of Neurology, 2,* 365–375.

Weinstein, S. M., & Herring, S. A. (1993). Rehabilitation of the patient with low back pain. In J. A. DeLisa (Ed.), *Rehabilitation medicine: Principles and practice* (2nd ed., pp. 996–1017). Philadelphia: J. B. Lippincott.

Wilkinson, H. A. (1992). *The failed back syndrome: Etiology and therapy* (2nd ed.). New York: Springer-Verlag.

Wixson, R. L., Stulberg, D., & Mehlhoff, M. (1991). Total hip replacement with cemented, uncemented, and hybrid prostheses. *Journal of Bone and Joint Surgery, 73A,* 257–269.

38

Impairments of Hand Function

Cynthia A. Philips

OBJECTIVES

After studying this chapter the reader will be able to:
1. Describe the commonly treated hand therapy diagnoses.
2. Understand the principles of hand care.
3. Discuss hand evaluation techniques.
4. Describe the proper postoperative splinting positions for common hand problems.
5. Understand the rationale for appropriate timing of therapeutic exercise and modalities in the treatment of hand problems.

The recent advances in hand surgery, including microvascular surgery, joint implants, and staged tendon repair, require a specialized approach to patient care. The occupational therapist and physician must work closely together in a well-organized therapeutic program. The therapist must have an intimate knowledge of normal hand anatomy and must adhere to the basic principles of wound healing to determine the choice and timing of basic therapeutic modalities. Careful thought must be given to the biomechanical principles of splinting to ensure that the intended purpose of the splint is fulfilled.

Exercises must be done gently and always within the patient's tolerance. Forced passive motion or painful therapy sets up a vicious circle of further injury, leading to increased edema and further scarring and fibrosis. Psychologically the patient becomes fearful and will not exercise. All of this leads to a stiff, useless hand.

Hand therapy should be directed by an experienced therapist who has specialized hand therapy training. A therapist interested in hand therapy should become proficient in general rehabilitation skills and then should seek out specialized hand therapy training and eventually hand therapy certification. This chapter is meant only as a guideline to the treatment of some of the more common hand diagnoses. Treatment procedures will vary, depending on the particular patient's circumstances and the physician's individual approach to management.

EVALUATION

Before treatment can begin, a baseline evaluation is necessary to determine a plan of treatment, monitor the patient's progress, and judge the effectiveness of treatment procedures. An evaluation can be divided into subjective and objective information.

Subjective Information

Subjective information is obtained through speaking with and listening to the patient and by observing and palpating the hand. This type of information is important from a treatment and diagnostic standpoint but cannot be used to make valid statements for research or to assess therapeutic outcome accurately. Subjective information may include the following:

1. History of illness or injury and other pertinent medical information;
2. Posture of the hand: normally, the wrist is in slight dorsiflexion, the digits lie with increasing flexion toward the ulnar side of the hand, the index and middle fingers are slightly supinated, and the fingers lie in the direction of the scaphoid bone. Tendon injuries or certain fractures will disrupt this posture;
3. Condition of the skin, including skin loss, previous injury that has caused scarring, and whether the skin is thin and fragile;
4. Color of the skin;
5. Edema, including whether it is soft and **pitting edema** or hard and **brawny edema;**
6. Sensibility of the hand: the patient describes the way the hand feels, including any pain, numbness, and tingling (if sensibility appears altered, a sen-

GLOSSARY

Arthroplasty—The surgical formation or reconstruction of a joint.

Boutonniere deformity—Flexion of the proximal interphalangeal joint and hyperextension of the distal interphalangeal joint.

Brawny edema—Hard, nonpitting edema.

Claw hand—An intrinsic-minus hand; a deformity seen in a hand with an ulnar nerve injury characterized by hyperextension of the metacarpal joints, especially the fourth and fifth fingers and flexion of the interphalangeal joints.

Closed reduction—Process of manipulating the parts of a fractured bone to align them without surgical intervention.

Coban—A thin elastic bandage made by the 3M Co., which is used for gentle compression.

Cylinder splint—A splint that is fabricated circumferentially around the finger. It is a type of mobilization splint used most often to help decrease proximal interphalangeal flexion contractures.

Dictionary of Occupational Titles—A listing of occupational classifications and definitions (available from the U.S. Government Printing Office).

Dislocation—When the bones making up a joint are no longer in functional contact. Subluxation is when the bones are in malalignment but are not dislocated.

Dorsal blocking splint—A splint fabricated on the dorsum of the hand to prevent full extension at one or more of the finger joints and/or the wrist.

Early controlled mobilization—A technique that uses protective splinting and a specific exercise regime; frequently prescribed to rehabilitate patients with flexor and extensor tendon injuries.

Finger trapping—Taping of finger to adjacent finger or using the adjacent finger to help achieve passive motion.

Mobilization splint—A splint that helps to mobilize a stiff joint.

Neuroma—A mass along the course of a nerve or at the end of a lacerated nerve, which is often painful.

Open reduction—Surgical intervention in which parts of a fractured bone are aligned and some type of bone fixation (i.e., screws, pins, or plates) is used to maintain the alignment during healing.

Percutaneous—Through the skin, i.e., percutaneous pinning to stabilize a fracture.

Pitting edema—Soft swelling that when palpated will leave indentations.

Pull-out wire—Wire used to maintain a tendon avulsion repair intact during healing. The wire holds the tendon to its bony attachment and is pulled out when the attachment is deemed adequately healed.

Staged tendon surgery—A method of tendon reconstruction in which a silastic rod is inserted and sutured distally. This rod is left in place to allow a pseudosheath to form around the rod. The rod is later removed and a tendon graft is used to complete the second stage of the reconstruction.

Sugartong splint—A splint that immobilizes the wrist, forearm, and elbow to prevent forearm rotation. The splint resembles a set of sugar tongs, thus its name.

Swan neck deformity—Hyperextension of the proximal interphalangeal joint and flexion of the distal interphalangeal joint.

Tubigrip—An elastic stockinette.

Tenolysis—The surgical freeing of a tendon from adhesions.

Two-point discrimination—A sensory test in which a person must identify whether he feels one or two points. The distance that the two points can be distinguished is recorded.

Volar plate—A ligamentous structure on the volar surface of the proximal interphalangeal joint which helps to prevent hyperextension of the proximal interphalangeal joint.

---

sory evaluation should be a part of the initial assessment);

7. Pain: determine where the pain is, the frequency of the pain, what aggravates the pain, and what relieves the pain; the patient rates the pain on a scale of 1 to 10, with 1 being slight and 10 being very intense pain;

8. Any deformity;

9. Palpation of the hand to reveal
   a. Any masses or nodules present,
   b. Temperature of the skin,
   c. Texture of the skin (i.e., dry, wet, soft, rough, or scarred);

10. Hand dominance;

11. Patient's family, work, and avocational history (Aulicino & Dupuy, 1990).

Objective Information

Objective measurements lay the foundation for baseline data to determine effectiveness of treatment, to provide a basis for research, and to facilitate more accurate communication among professionals. The clinical assessment committees of the American Society of Hand Therapists (Fess & Moran, 1981) and the American Society for Surgery of the Hand (1983) have provided recommendations for evaluation of range of motion, strength, sensation, volume, dexterity, and coordination.

1. Both active and passive range of motion should be measured using a goniometer. If there is a discrepancy between active and passive range of motion, the problem may be with tendon continuity or tendon glide,

which could be impeded by adhesions or other tendon pathology, rather than the joint or its structures. Goniometer range of motion is recorded following the standards supplied by the American Academy of Orthopedic Surgeons (1965) and as described in Chapter 6.

The American Society for Surgery of the Hand (1983) also recommended recording of total active motion (TAM) and total passive motion (TPM). Total active range of motion is the sum of the angles of the metacarpophalangeal, proximal interphalangeal, and distal interphalangeal joints when the hand is in maximum active flexion, minus any deviation from full extension. Total passive range of motion is the sum of the angles formed by the metacarpophalangeal, proximal interphalangeal, and distal interphalangeal joints when the hand is in full passive flexion, minus any passive extension deficit (Table 38.1). A particular patient's situation (e.g., in the case of severe rheumatoid arthritis) may preclude the usually accepted method of measurement and require an alternative technique. It is important that the therapist documents the changes and consistently uses that technique throughout each reassessment.

Torque-angle range of motion uses a series of increasing forces to make measurements of passive range of motion more objective (Berger-Lee, Bell-Krotoski, & Brandsma, 1990; Berger-Lee et al., 1993; Brand & Hollister, 1993; Flowers & Pheasant, 1988).

2. Grip strength is generally measured using a Jamar dynamometer (see Chapter 6). Lateral, three-jaw (three-point) chuck, and pulp pinch (thumb pad to index finger pad) are measured using a standard pinchmeter (see Chapter 6).

3. Manual muscle testing (see Chapter 6) should be done as a necessary part of a total assessment battery when indicated.

4. Sensory evaluation should be conducted (see Chapter 8).

5. Edema can be evaluated by recording circumferential measurements or volumeter measurements (see Chapter 6). Because reducing edema is a key element in the treatment of the injured hand, it is important to monitor this parameter.

6. Functional capacity evaluation is done using standardized tests (Baxter-Petralia et al., 1990). Standardized evaluations for dexterity and coordination include such tests as the *Jebsen Hand Function Test* (Jebsen et al., 1969), the *Minnesota Rate of Manipulation Test*, the *Purdue Pegboard*, and the *O'Connor Peg Test*. The *O'Connor Peg Test* can be obtained with or without tweezers (Baxter-Petralia et al., 1990). Other tests, such as the *Bennett Hand Tool Test* and the *Crawford Small Parts Dexterity Test*, add the component of working with tools. These tests require a higher level of hand function, including sufficient strength to manipulate and control the tools. See Chapter 7 for a description of some of these tests.

The *Valpar Work Samples* provide a standardized means of determining the patient's ability to do a variety of tasks or to perform various motions necessary to perform his job adequately (Baxter-Petralia et al., 1990; see also Chapter 17).

In most busy clinics, it is not possible to perform a number of objective tests. Therefore, the therapist must choose a battery of tests that is the most appropriate and the most helpful in obtaining the type of data required for planning treatment for a particular patient. Reevaluation should be done on an ongoing basis throughout the patient's treatment program. The frequency of reevaluation depends on the patient's individual circumstances.

TREATMENT

Joint Injuries

Injuries to the joints and their supporting soft tissue structures are among the most common hand injuries. Unfortunately, the full implication of these injuries is not always appreciated. This can often lead to needless disability.

When the therapist is attempting to mobilize joint injuries, there are some aspects of the rehabilitation program that are common to all the injuries discussed here. All exercises must be done gently and within the patient's tolerance. Exercises should not, under any circumstance, increase pain or swelling. In some cases, when swelling of the joint persists, an ice pack or an ice massage may be a useful tool in controlling edema and pain, even after the acute period. **Coban** wrapping is also helpful in reducing and controlling edema. The **Coban** should be wrapped in a diagonal pattern in a distal to proximal direction. The fingernail should be left uncovered to allow observation of any circulatory changes. Proximal interphalangeal joint injuries tend to remain swollen for long periods of time (Nalebuff & Millender, 1985). Therefore, edema control needs to be a part of the general hand therapy program for these and other joint injuries. These injuries often cause a great deal of swelling and pain within the whole hand as well. Therefore, exercises to maintain mobility of

Table 38.1. Example of Recording Total Active Motion and Total Passive Motion

Joint	TAM	TPM
Metacarpophalangeal	0/90	−30/100
Proximal interphalangeal	−30/95	−30/100
Distal interphalangeal	0/50	0/60
Totals	205	200

the rest of the hand and extremity should be done. If the rest of the extremity is not exercised, stiffness and fibrosis may be the result.

The therapist should also pay particular attention to the intrinsic muscles of the hand. Because of the intimate relationship between the injured structures and the intrinsic muscles, exercises to these muscles should be started as soon as it is safe to do so. These exercises can be done in such a way as to prevent undue stress to the injured structures. When exercising the proximal interphalangeal joint, it may be useful to splint the distal joint temporarily as well as to block the metacarpophalangeal joint to prevent it from flexing. This helps to concentrate the flexion and extension power at the proximal interphalangeal joint. Following proximal interphalangeal joint exercises, the distal joint splint is removed and the distal joint is exercised. With proximal interphalangeal joint injuries, it is important that the distal joint also be exercised, because the oblique retinacular ligament may become tight, causing decreased distal joint motion. It should be remembered that although at first glance these injuries may look benign, they are serious. Recovery from these injuries is often prolonged and requires the cooperation and active participation of the patient. The therapist and the physician must educate the patient to maximize his cooperation. Above all, patience and encouragement are necessary throughout the treatment period. The discussion of joint injuries is divided into ligamentous injuries, **volar plate** injuries, and **dislocations.**

LIGAMENTOUS INJURIES

Proximal interphalangeal joint injuries probably occur most frequently. These injuries often occur in athletes. The radial collateral ligament is most commonly injured and frequently involves the **volar plate** (Vicar, 1988). Kiefhaber, Stern, and Grood (1986) tested cadaver joints. They found that with less than a 20° angulation there was a 50-50 chance of a partial versus a complete ligament tear. With stress over 20°, there was complete rupture in all cases and some distal **volar plate** disruption in 92%. An incomplete tear of the ligament implies that the injured joint has enough capsular support remaining to prevent displacement of the joint when adequately stressed (Eaton, 1971).

Of course, the occupational therapist's goal is to maintain joint mobility. However, before the patient can begin motion, a period of rest in the most advantageous position for proper ligamentous healing is required. The joint is immobilized for 10 to 14 days in approximately 15 to 20° of flexion using a dorsal aluminum splint (Belsky, Ruby, & Millender, 1983; Burton, 1980) (Fig. 38.1). The dorsal splint allows the palmar surface to be free and does not block the metacarpophalangeal joint or the distal interphalangeal joint. The

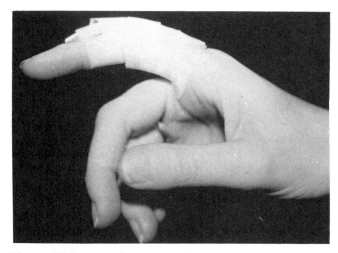

Figure 38.1.   Dorsal aluminum splint to support injured proximal interphalangeal joint in the proper position.

dorsal splint also provides better support and is less likely to be worked loose than a volar splint (Burton, 1980). The therapist should watch that the splint is not causing any pressure over the proximal interphalangeal joint. This is often a vulnerable area for pressure and possible skin breakdown. In some cases, it may be wise to put the whole hand at rest for a few days until the initial pain and swelling have subsided (Belsky et al., 1983). Afterward, only the involved joint is immobilized. The exact length of time for immobilization depends on the amount of pain and swelling and the joint's response to the period of rest (Belsky et al., 1983; Eaton, 1971). If the joint shows instability to stress, immobilization for 3 weeks is required, because this may indicate more extensive damage. Following this period of immobilization, the injured finger may be taped to an adjacent digit to provide support for another 1 to 2 weeks.

Metacarpophalangeal joint ligamentous injuries of the digits occur with much less frequency than the proximal interphalangeal joint ligament injuries. At the metacarpophalangeal joint, it is often the radial collateral ligament that is injured (Belsky et al., 1983; Burton, 1980; Dray, Millender, & Nalebuff, 1979; Eaton, 1971). The mechanism of injury is usually hyperextension of the metacarpophalangeal joint. These injuries often cause large amounts of edema and ecchymosis over the dorsum of the hand and volarly into the palm. The treatment initially is immobilization of the hand from the proximal interphalangeal joint to the mid-forearm. The metacarpophalangeal joints are placed in about 45 to 50° of flexion. Immobilization is continued for approximately 2 to 3 weeks before exercises are started. The exact period depends on the degree of pain and swelling.

Collateral ligament injuries of the metacarpophalangeal joint of the thumb most often occur to the ulnar side and are handled differently from those of the digits. It may be necessary to repair the ligamentous injury of the thumb metacarpophalangeal joint surgically, because soft tissue can become interposed between the bone and the ends of the ligaments (Belsky et al., 1983; Burton, 1980; Eaton, 1971). Without surgical intervention, healing of the ligament would be prevented. The thumb is immobilized for 5 to 6 weeks following repair. The goal is to provide a good stable joint for pinch. Active and active-assisted exercises are started following the immobilization period and are gradually increased as tolerated by the patient. Ligamentous injuries may not be considered stable for up to 10 to 12 weeks. However, the patient may experience some discomfort and weakness for 6 to 12 months following the injury. Therefore, the level of activity allowed is determined on an individual basis. Any exercise program should be designed with this in mind and should progress accordingly.

VOLAR PLATE INJURIES

Injuries to the **volar plate** are caused by hyperextension forces against the extended finger (Belsky et al., 1983; Burton, 1980; Dray et al., 1979; Eaton, 1971). A poorly treated **volar plate** injury can result in a symptomatic **swan neck deformity.** Initially, the finger is splinted with the proximal interphalangeal joint in about 20° of flexion for 2 weeks. When motion is started, a **dorsal blocking splint** is used for an additional 1 to 2 weeks to protect the **volar plate** further (Fig. 38.2). In old **volar plate** injuries that

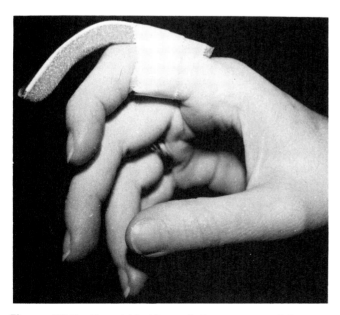

Figure 38.2. Dorsal blocking splinting to prevent full extension while permitting flexion.

have developed symptomatic **swan neck deformities,** surgery may be done. These cases would require immobilization for 3 weeks. A **dorsal blocking splint** is again used for 1 to 2 weeks more.

DISLOCATIONS

Dislocations of the proximal interphalangeal joints often occur during contact sports. The joint can become dislocated in a dorsal, lateral, or volar direction (Belsky et al., 1983; Burton, 1980; Dray et al., 1979; Eaton, 1971). The therapist should remember that when a **dislocation** occurs, there is always associated soft tissue damage. The structures injured depend on the mechanism of the injury. When a dorsal **dislocation** occurs, the major damage is to the **volar plate** (Burton, 1980; Eaton, 1971; Vicar, 1988). There may be an avulsion of a small bone fragment along with the **volar plate.** In these cases, the joint is splinted in 20 to 30° of flexion for about 3 weeks. An active exercise program is then started. A **dorsal blocking splint** may be used for 1 to 2 weeks more. It is important that proper splinting be done, because the sequelae of a poorly treated dorsal **dislocation** may be a **swan neck deformity.**

Another possible complication may be a proximal interphalangeal joint flexion contracture. This may occur if the joint is left in flexion for too long a period of time. Proximal interphalangeal joint flexion deformities are difficult problems. It takes a long time to correct them through either a series of **cylinder splints, mobilization splints,** or a combination of both. Some may ultimately require corrective surgery. For those patients that have surgery, it has been found that continued monitoring may be necessary for at least 6 months postoperatively to prevent recurrence of the deformity. It is also necessary to maintain a program of extension splinting during this time. The patient is progressed from extension splinting except for exercise to intermittent splinting for specified periods of time. A night splint is recommended for an additional few weeks, as it is a natural tendency to sleep with the fingers in a flexed position.

Lateral **dislocations** are caused by torsion, angular, or shearing forces placed on the finger that rupture one of the collateral ligaments and a portion of the insertion of the **volar plate** (Eaton, 1971). The finger is splinted with the proximal interphalangeal joint in approximately 20° of flexion for about 2 weeks. Following this period of immobilization, the finger is protected for another 1 to 2 weeks with taping to the finger adjacent to the side of the ruptured ligament. It may be necessary to use a **dorsal blocking splint** to protect the **volar plate.** Joints that are stable to active motion but show instability to lateral stress need to be immobilized for 3 weeks.

A volar **dislocation** involves either incomplete or complete protrusion of the head of the proximal phalanx through the extensor mechanism (Burton, 1980; Eaton, 1971). This injury is splinted in extension for 4 to 6 weeks to allow the extensor mechanism to heal. A splint used at night and/or between exercises may be continued for another 1 to 2 weeks after the therapy program of active exercises has been started. It is again important that proper splinting be done, because the resulting complication of this injury may be a **boutonniere deformity,** or a proximal interphalangeal joint flexion contracture. Therefore, when exercising the injured joint, extension is emphasized along with gentle flexion exercises. The therapist should carefully observe whether the patient can extend the finger well with each repetition of the exercise. If the patient has difficulty with extension, further splinting is necessary.

When a fracture dislocation occurs, the treatment varies depending on the size of the fragment (Eaton, 1971). Surgery is required to repair the joint and soft tissue damage if the fragment is large, causing the joint to be unstable. Postoperatively, the joint is held in plaster with the proximal interphalangeal joint in about 30 to 35° of flexion for approximately 3 weeks before beginning a therapy program. When exercises are begun, a **dorsal blocking splint** is used for another week. On about the 5th week postoperatively, gentle controlled extension exercises are allowed. If after 8 weeks the patient has not gained full extension, a **mobilization splint** may be used to aid in achieving full extension (Belsky et al., 1983; Burton, 1980; Dray et al., 1979; Eaton, 1971) (Fig. 38.3). If a **closed**

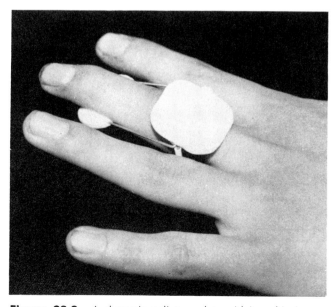

Figure 38.3. A dynamic splint used to aid in achieving or maintaining finger extension.

reduction can be done and joint stability and alignment are satisfactory, the joint is immobilized for 10 days to 2 weeks. A **dorsal blocking splint** is then used for another week before full extension is allowed. **Closed reduction** is the process of manipulating the parts of a fractured bone to align them without surgical intervention.

Dislocations of the metacarpophalangeal joints are rare. When they do occur, it is usually to the index or fifth finger. The **dislocation** is often dorsal and more frequently requires **open reduction,** because soft tissue may become caught in between the joint spaces (Eaton, 1971; Nalebuff, 1975). Following repair, the joint is immobilized for 3 weeks. Active flexion is started but extension is not allowed for 4 weeks. **Dislocation** of the thumb metacarpal results in a major disruption of the soft tissue structures (Belsky et al., 1983; Burton, 1980; Dray et al., 1979; Eaton, 1971). These **dislocations** are generally reduced closed and are held for 3 to 4 weeks before initiating a therapy program. A **dislocation** of the carpometacarpal joint of the thumb usually occurs with such force that the metacarpal shaft is fractured, producing the Bennett's fracture **dislocation.** The fracture may be reduced closed and a Kirschner wire may be placed percutaneously to maintain the reduction. The joint is immobilized for 4 weeks. Gentle exercises are begun at this time and are progressed gradually over the next few weeks.

The mallet deformity also deserves mention. It is a common injury to the distal interphalangeal joint, resulting from elongation, laceration, or rupture of the terminal tendon of the extensor mechanism (Beasley, 1981; Rosenthal, 1990). There may be an interarticular fracture of the distal phalanx in which the tendon avulses a fragment of bone. The distal joint drops into flexion. Generally, the treatment is splinting of the distal joint in extension for 6 to 8 weeks. The patient is instructed in how to change the splint and how to care for the skin to prevent skin breakdown. The patient is taught to be very careful to maintain the joint in extension (Fig. 38.4). If, when the splint is changed, the joint drops into flexion, the splinting must be started all over again.

During the immobilization period, exercises to the proximal interphalangeal joint are done. The result of an untreated mallet deformity may be a **swan neck deformity** brought about by muscle and tendon imbalance. Therefore, following the immobilization period, careful monitoring is required to be sure that extension is maintained. If an extension lag (failure to extend fully) is noted, further splinting is indicated.

Because the profundus tendon attaches to the volar base of the distal phalanx, it can be avulsed from its attachment. This often occurs in sports when a

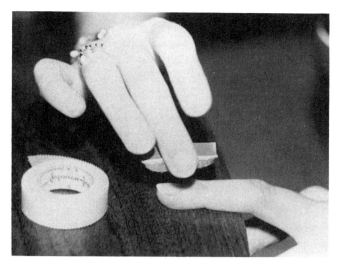

Figure 38.4. Patient changing the aluminum splint, used to maintain extension of the distal interphalangeal joint when a mallet deformity occurs.

player grabs an opponent's jersey. Often the finger is swollen and painful, and there is inability to flex the distal joint actively. The avulsion can occur with or without accompanying bony avulsion. Treatment of this injury is by a surgical repair. Most frequently a **pull-out wire** is used to maintain the repair during healing (Thayer, 1988).

Joint Implant Arthroplasty

When a joint has been irreparably damaged through either trauma or arthritis, it is possible to reconstruct the joint using the various implants now available. The ones most commonly used are the Swanson flexible hinge implants. These implants are made of silicone rubber and act as joint spacers, while the new capsuloligamentous system forms during the healing process (Madden, DeVore, & Arem, 1977; Millender & Nalebuff, 1973; Swanson, 1973; Swanson, Swanson, & Leonard, 1984). Swanson (1973) refers to this as the process of encapsulation. The following is a guideline to the postoperative management of these patients. It should be kept in mind that each patient is unique and treatment may vary. The goal of treatment is to obtain a functional range of motion while maintaining joint stability.

METACARPOPHALANGEAL JOINT INTERPOSITIONAL ARTHROPLASTY

Metacarpophalangeal joint **arthroplasty** is most often done in patients with rheumatoid arthritis. Preoperatively, certain types of deformities are seen. Millender and Nalebuff (1973) described a classification system for these deformities. Postoperatively, the hand

is initially held in a bulky dressing with a plaster splint that supports the metacarpophalangeal joints in extension and some radial deviation to maintain desired joint alignment. If, preoperatively, the patient has limited flexion and minimal or no ulnar deviation, the fingers may be held in some flexion postoperatively (Philips, 1989). On days 1 and 2 following the surgery, the exercises consist of gentle finger pumping (gentle active range of motion) to help reduce edema and provide joint motion. On days 3 to 5, exercises consist of active and active-assisted range of motion to the metacarpophalangeal joints. Metacarpophalangeal joint flexion is stressed by teaching the patient to bring the metacarpophalangeal joints into a shelf-like position and then curl the interphalangeal joints into the palm.

When the patient has good proximal interphalangeal joint motion, he may attempt to substitute this motion for metacarpophalangeal joint flexion. If such substitution is allowed to continue, the patient's final range of motion could be severely compromised. In cases for which this is a problem, the proximal interphalangeal joints can be immobilized during exercise sessions to concentrate flexion and extension at the metacarpophalangeal joint (Philips, 1989; Swanson, 1973; Swanson et al., 1984). The proximal interphalangeal joints may be immobilized either with Alumafoam splints or pieces of splinting material (Fig. 38.5). At about 5 to 7 days after the operation, depending on the amount of pain and swelling, a dynamic splint is fabricated (Madden et al., 1977; Millender & Nalebuff, 1973; Philips, 1989; Swanson, 1973; Swanson et al., 1984). A dorsal splint that provides good wrist support as well as good carpometacarpal support to the mobile fourth and fifth digits is used. An outrigger is positioned to give the metacarpophalangeal joints a gentle, continuous radial pull. Either a high- or a low-profile outrig-

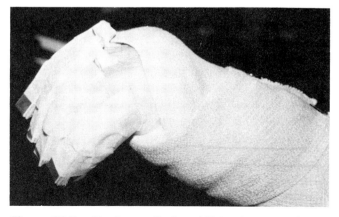

Figure 38.5. Aluminum splint immobilizing the proximal interphalangeal joints to aid in achieving better metacarpophalangeal joint motion following metacarpophalangeal joint arthroplasty.

ger may be used. The elastics must have appropriate tension to provide adequate extension and radial deviation, but they should not be so tight as to restrict flexion. Hyperextension of the metacarpophalangeal joints must be avoided. To be sure that the patient gets full flexion, he may be instructed to remove the cuffs for short periods of time at each exercise session.

Most therapists like to see the patient achieve 45° of flexion at the index finger, 60° at the middle finger, and 70° at the ring and little fingers. If the patient has not gained the desired motion, a volar outrigger may be attached to the splint to provide a flexion pull at the metacarpophalangeal joints. The flexion outrigger is then worn alternately with the extension outrigger. The splint is worn all day for approximately 6 to 8 weeks. The elastics are adjusted, and the splint is modified whenever necessary to maintain proper functioning. At night, the patient wears a resting splint to maintain the position of the hand. This splint is also adjusted as necessary during the postoperative period. The night splint is often worn for another 2 weeks after the dynamic splint has been discontinued. The exact length of time that the patient is involved in the splinting program depends on the condition of the soft tissue at the time of surgery. Patients with rheumatoid arthritis often have poor soft tissue. As a result, exercise programs must be modified and the splinting program increased. The therapist should keep in mind that it is the soft tissue that provides the joint stability.

The exercises are done approximately four times a day for brief periods, approximately 5 min at each session. Several brief sessions of exercise spread out over the entire day are less likely to cause tissue reaction than one long session and the hand is less likely to develop stiffness.

After 2 to 3 weeks, the patient is allowed to begin using the hand for light activities, such as eating, with the splint on the hand. At 6 to 8 weeks, mild resistance may be added to the exercise program for strengthening. Functional use of the hand is also increased at that time. It should be kept in mind that the patient with rheumatoid disease is weakened to begin with. Therefore, the therapist cannot expect the implant to provide normal strength, although strength in many cases is improved. The patient is generally allowed to use the hand for all daily activities at 3 months. This is a gradual, active process and is progressed according to the patient's tolerance. Joint protection principles are taught to the patient during the course of the treatment to allow him to use the newly reconstructed joints safely (see Chapter 40).

There are some considerations when treating patients with metacarpophalangeal joint arthroplasties. In some patients, the fifth finger is more difficult to mobilize than others. The therapist must be sure that the

elastic on the splint for the fifth finger is not too taut. In some cases, it may not be necessary to use an elastic on the fifth finger at all. Of course, this has to be decided on an individual basis.

Another consideration is the proper alignment of the digits. In the normal hand, there is some supination of the digits. Following metacarpophalangeal joint **arthroplasty,** the index finger, especially, may tend to assume a more pronated position (Philips, 1989; Swanson, 1973; Swanson et al., 1984). For this situation, a serpentine-type finger splint may be wrapped around the finger to maintain the digit in some supination (Fig. 38.6). This splint is attached to the outrigger with the elastic and is used in place of the usual finger cuff. Another way to maintain supination is with two finger cuffs that exert tension in opposite directions, creating a force couple (Fig. 38.7).

PROXIMAL INTERPHALANGEAL JOINT ARTHROPLASTY

Much of the postoperative hand therapy management of the patient who has undergone proximal interphalangeal joint **arthroplasty** depends on the soft tissue surgery that is done at the time of the **arthroplasty** (Nalebuff & Millender, personal communication, 1985; Philips, 1989; Swanson, 1973; Swanson et al., 1984). Therefore, the time when motion is begun has to be determined on an individual basis. Proximal interphalangeal joint **arthroplasty** may be done for the following reasons:

1. To reconstruct a stiff, painful proximal interphalangeal joint damaged by trauma, rheumatoid disease, or degenerative joint disease;

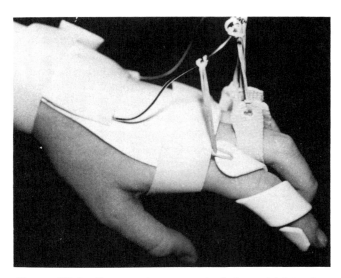

Figure 38.6. Postoperative metacarpophalangeal joint arthroplasty splint with serpentine-type splint attached to help supinate the index finger.

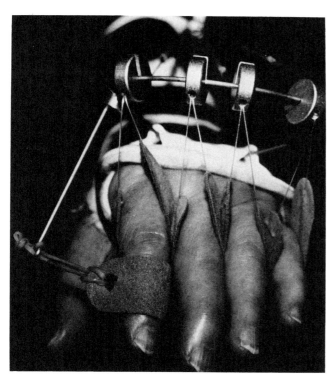

Figure 38.7. Postoperative metacarpophalangeal joint arthroplasty splint, using the force-couple principle for supination of the index finger.

2. To reconstruct a **boutonniere deformity**;
3. To reconstruct a **swan neck** deformity (rarely done).

Stiff Proximal Interphalangeal Joint

When the proximal interphalangeal joint **arthroplasty** is done to relieve pain and stiffness, gentle interphalangeal joint motion may be started as soon as 2 to 3 days postoperatively, depending on the amount of pain and swelling. The patient is held in a plaster splint that supports the proximal interphalangeal joint in extension in between exercise sessions. In cases for which postoperative stiffness appears to be a problem, the proximal interphalangeal joint may be taped down into flexion for at least part of the time in between exercise sessions.

Boutonniere Repair

When an **arthroplasty** is done to repair a **boutonniere deformity,** the extensor mechanism is repaired as part of the procedure. Therefore, the extensor mechanism must be protected in extension, usually with an Alumafoam splint. Gentle active motion is started about 10 to 14 days postoperatively. Between exercise sessions, the finger is placed back in the extension splint. The splint is worn for 4 to 6 weeks, or until the position of the finger has stabilized. It may

be necessary in some cases to delay exercises as long as 4 weeks (Nalebuff & Millender, personal communication, 1985; Swanson, 1973; Swanson et al., 1984).

Swan Neck Repair

Although rarely done, this procedure is undertaken in combination with tendon reconstruction. The finger is held in approximately 20 to 30° of flexion to prevent a recurrent hyperextension deformity. In this situation, a slight proximal interphalangeal joint flexion contracture may be desirable. Range of motion allowing flexion and protected extension may be started about 3 to 5 days postoperatively. The finger is then splinted in between exercise sessions until the position of the joint has stabilized (Swanson, 1973; Swanson et al., 1984).

GENERAL EXERCISE CONSIDERATIONS

Initially, active and active-assisted exercises are done and then increased to gentle passive motion as tolerated by the patient. Care must be taken always to support the metacarpophalangeal joint in extension. This allows all the flexion and extension forces to be placed at the proximal interphalangeal joint. Blocking of the metacarpophalangeal joint into extension may be done by the patient with the other hand or with a piece of splinting material padded with moleskin. Splinting material works well, because it is rigid but also thin enough not to block any proximal interphalangeal joint motion. The hand can be positioned over a book or the edge of a table. When this method is used, the therapist must be sure that the proximal interphalangeal joint motion is not being impeded. Usually at 6 to 8 weeks postoperatively, resistance may be added to the program to improve strength. Therapists often use a foam block for this purpose to provide support to the metacarpophalangeal joints and to prevent ulnar deviation. Functional use of the hand should gradually be increased during this time. At 3 months postoperatively, the patient is usually allowed to use the hand for all activities of daily living.

SILASTIC WRIST IMPLANT ARTHROPLASTY

The postoperative therapy for wrist **arthroplasty** begins the 1st day following surgery when the drain is removed, the dressing is changed, and both volar and dorsal plaster wrist splints are made. At this time, finger range of motion is begun to maintain digital motion. The pumping action of the fingers aids in reducing postoperative edema. The volar and dorsal wrist splints are kept in place for 4 to 6 weeks. During this time, no wrist motion is allowed. If any laxity of the wrist is noted, the wrist will be held longer. Often, a distal ulnar excision is done in conjunction with the wrist **arthroplasty.** An ulnar head implant may or may not be used in these cases. When a distal ulnar excision is done, either a **sugartong splint** or another form of plaster splinting is used to ensure good capsular healing (Goodman et al., 1980).

Generally, wrist exercises are begun at 4 weeks. The goal of the surgery is a stable, pain-free wrist. Motion, therefore, is purposely limited to 25 to 30° of dorsiflexion and 25 to 30° of palmar flexion. Exercises are done carefully with that goal in mind. For the 1st week following initiation of the exercise program, the exercises are gentle, protected active-assisted motion. Exercises are then progressed to active and gentle passive range of motion. Gradually, after approximately 6 to 8 weeks postoperatively, resistance can be added to the exercise program for strengthening. At this point, splinting is discontinued and the patient can begin using his hand unprotected for light activities of daily living. Activities of daily living are increased as strength returns. In special cases, when any laxity of the wrist is noted, a dynamic wrist splint is fabricated to provide controlled, protected motion (Fig. 38.8). This splint is worn during the day, and a resting wrist splint is worn at night. At approximately 12 weeks, the patient may resume normal activities. However, to prevent too much stress to the wrist, it is recommended that the patient wear a wrist cock-up splint indefinitely whenever heavier tasks are performed.

THUMB CARPOMETACARPAL JOINT IMPLANT ARTHROPLASTY

Implant **arthroplasty** of the carpometacarpal joint of the thumb is often done in patients with osteoarthritis. When evaluating these patients for surgery, it is important that the other joints of the thumb be evaluated as well, e.g., an adduction deformity of the

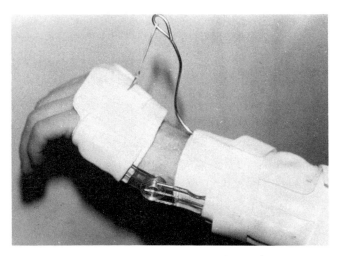

Figure 38.8. Postoperative wrist arthroplasty splint.

metacarpophalangeal joint of the thumb may be an associated problem in patients with carpometacarpal joint arthritis. If the adduction deformity is severe, the adductor pollicis may have to be released to ensure proper balance and seating of the implant. A hyperextension deformity of the metacarpophalangeal joint of the thumb may also contribute to the adduction deformity (Swanson, 1973). If the metacarpophalangeal joint of the thumb is hyperextended, it may be necessary to correct this problem surgically to prevent **dislocation** or subluxation of the implant. Postoperatively, the thumb is held in a plaster splint in palmar abduction for 4 to 6 weeks to ensure good capsular healing.

The goal of treatment is to provide a stable thumb for pinch. Too much motion may lead to joint instability. During this time, range of motion of the fingers is encouraged. When the splint is removed, the patient begins opposition, abduction, and circumduction exercises. Hyperextension of the thumb should be avoided. Dexterity activities are then added to the program and are increased as strength begins to return. Unrestricted use of the thumb is generally allowed at about 12 weeks. Strength takes considerably longer to return. In fact, it may take up to 1 year before the patient feels that he has adequate strength.

Peripheral Nerve Injury

Sensibility of the hand is a complex subject. Obviously, without functioning nerves, the patient would have an essentially useless appendage. Sensibility of the hand encompasses the very essence of human experience. Humans require sensibility of the hand for self-expression; prehension, identification, and evaluation of objects; to protect themselves from harmful stimuli; and to enable them to manipulate the environment. Therefore, every effort must be made to help people with peripheral nerve injuries regain as much useful function as possible.

The type of injury greatly influences treatment as well as later regeneration and the degree of recovery of sensibility and motor control. A sharp laceration, as with glass or a knife will usually have a better prognosis than a crush injury or gunshot wound, also the more proximal the injury, the poorer the prognosis. Pure motor or pure sensory nerves generally have a better outcome than do mixed nerves (Frykman, 1993). Age is also a factor in the final results. Children recover a much higher level of sensibility than do adults, given the same injury.

The radial, ulnar, and median nerves supply sensibility and motor function to the hand. Injury to any one of them can cause significant hand dysfunction. The median nerve supplies sensation to the thumb, index finger, middle finger, and one-half of the ring finger. Loss of this nerve is significant, as the radial side of the hand is used primarily for precision grip and pinch. Loss of sensibility here leaves the hand unable to perform precise activities. Although most of the thenar muscles are also controlled by the median nerve, the motor loss is less significant to function in a median nerve injury than is the loss of sensation. However, the reverse is true with ulnar and radial nerve injuries.

The ulnar nerve innervates the majority of the intrinsic muscles. With an ulnar nerve injury, the therapist would see a typical **claw hand,** because the intrinsic muscles are not able to balance the extrinsic flexors and extensors. In a high ulnar nerve palsy, there would be less clawing, since, at that level, the profundi of the fourth and fifth digits are also not functioning. The functional implications of ulnar nerve loss are significant. The patient would have difficulty grasping larger objects and would lose approximately 75 to 80% of key pinch ability as a result of the loss of the adductor pollicis muscle, which is also innervated by the ulnar nerve (Smith, 1987). When the adductor pollicis is not working, any attempt to pinch an object firmly will often result in flexion of the distal joint of the thumb (Froment's sign) and hyperextension of the metacarpophalangeal joint (Jeanne's sign). Froment's sign results from substitution of the flexor pollicis longus for the adductor pollicis.

The motor loss of a radial nerve injury causes inability to extend the wrist and fingers, making performance of activities of daily living difficult. The superficial branch of the radial nerve, a sensory branch, supplies the lateral part of the thenar eminence and the radial side of the dorsum of the thumb. This area is vulnerable to injury and **neuroma** formation (Tubiana, 1984). This injury is often very painful and difficult to treat. An ill-fitting splint or cast that causes pressure to this area can lead to compression of this nerve and an unhappy patient, because of significant pain.

EVALUATION

The initial evaluation should be done in a quiet, relaxed atmosphere. It should not cause pain and, therefore, should not be done on hypersensitive or painful hands. The patient's active and passive ranges of motion are recorded, and a manual muscle test is administered. Grip and pinch strengths should be recorded for both hands as a comparison.

It is often helpful first to make a drawing of the hand on a piece of paper, noting the location of lacerations and any calluses or other injuries such as burns that would indicate lack of protective sensation. It may be advantageous actually to map out the areas of dysfunction on the patient's hand. Fess (1990) developed a grid for this purpose. The patient then is asked

to describe how the hand feels (Bell, 1978; Callahan, 1990a), including identification of where on the hand the sensibility changes. In this way the therapist obtains information about the degree of sensibility and also may gain insight into the patient's ability to adapt to the altered sensibility. The patient's description and cooperation may also indicate his motivation for sensory reeducation.

Except for electrodiagnostic studies, there are no standardized tests currently available for evaluating sensibility. However, sensory function should be measured and recorded for later comparison. Tests can be classified as threshold tests, functional tests, and objective tests. Threshold tests include vibration and the Semmes-Weinstein monofilaments. Tests for pain, heat, and cold are also included. Functional tests include the *Moberg Pick-Up Test,* **two-point discrimination,** and moving **two-point discrimination** (Callahan, 1990a; Dellon, 1981; see also Chapter 8). Objective tests include nerve conduction studies, the ninhydrin test and the wrinkle test.

Nerve regeneration is generally thought to take place at the rate of approximately 1 inch/month. Therefore, reevaluation following nerve injury should be done approximately every 4 to 6 weeks. Pain is usually an early sign of sensory return (Callahan, 1990a; Dellon, Curtis, & Edgerton, 1972, 1974). The patient's other hand is tested to determine a baseline and to help the patient to become familiar with the testing procedure.

SENSORY REEDUCATION

Dellon (1981) and other authors (Almquist, 1975; Bell-Krotoski, Weinstein, & Weinstein, 1993; Callahan, 1990a, 1990b; Dellon et al., 1974) have shown that the quality of functional sensibility can be improved through a program of sensory reeducation. Sensory reeducation is a program designed for the patient with sensory loss to help him learn to interpret the altered sensory pattern.

Sensory reeducation is begun as soon as possible following the injury. The therapist begins training when light touch has returned to the palm and proximal phalanx (Dellon, 1981; Dellon et al., 1972, 1974; Maynard, 1978; Wynn-Parry, 1981; see also Chapter 23). At this stage, stimulation of the area is done by the patient himself with either a finger of the other hand or an eraser on a pencil. Large objects of various shapes that can be grasped or placed in the palm are next introduced. The patient also is instructed to immerse his hand in substances such as sand or rice. These activities are also done with the normal hand to help the patient in the educational process. As the return of sensibility progresses distally, smaller objects are introduced. These are manipulated with both the normal and injured hands and include such things as nuts and bolts, coins, keys, and other everyday objects. Various textures are added to the program as the patient progresses. Activities of daily living such as buttoning clothing and tying shoes also are encouraged. If the injured hand is the dominant hand, writing skills and manipulation of eating utensils are practiced. As the level of sensibility improves, common objects can be buried in rice or sand. The patient must then try to find these objects and identify them by touch. When possible, tools the patient uses at work are introduced into the treatment program. If the patient's injury is severe and return of protective sensation is not expected, the therapist must instruct the patient in how to care for the hand and to adopt various methods to prevent further injury, such as burns. The patient must continue to use the hand if sensory reeducation is to be effective (Callahan, 1990b).

MOTOR REEDUCATION

After nerve repair, the wrist and fingers are positioned to prevent tension on the repaired area. The exact position depends on the available length of the nerve and is determined by the surgeon at the time of operation. The nerve repair is immobilized from 3 to 5 weeks before motion is allowed (Braun, 1980; Parry, 1980; Smith, 1986). During this period of immobilization, it may be possible to bring the wrist and hand into a more neutral position gradually while they are protected in the splint. The nerve is adversely affected by tension. Rapid stretch will cause the nerve to exceed its elastic limits and may lead to interneural fibrosis (Shultz, 1980). Therefore, it is recommended that the joint not be extended more than 10° per week.

Following immobilization, gentle active exercise should be started along with gentle passive motion to the paralyzed joints to maintain full joint mobility. Exercises for the rest of the extremity also are important to maintain strength of the uninvolved muscles and improve circulation and nutrition in the extremity. Light massage is beneficial for circulation. It also helps to soften scar tissue, increase soft tissue mobility, and maintain the skin in good condition. Any stretching exercises are generally delayed until 8 weeks following the repair (Wynn-Parry, 1981). Splinting is often necessary to prevent deformity that may be caused by muscle imbalance brought about by the nerve injury. The type of splint used depends on the nerve injured and the muscles affected by the loss of nerve function (see Chapter 28). Great caution must be taken to be sure that the correct splint is used. A poorly designed or ill-conceived splint can lead to irreversible deformity.

Atrophy of denervated muscles will take place regardless of good therapy or intermittent electrical stimulation. Currently, the only way to prevent atrophy is to reinnervate the muscles (Taylor Mullins, 1990).

Functional electrical stimulation, however, may be helpful to maintain muscle tone while reinnervation takes place (see Chapter 33).

Tendon Transfers

When irreversible nerve and/or tendon damage occurs, it is possible to restore muscle balance and improve function through tendon transfers. Tendon transfers redistribute the remaining muscle power so that it can be used in the most effective functional combinations. The type of transfers used, of course, depend on the muscles available for transfer. Certain conditions, however, must exist before tendons can be transferred successfully (Beasley, 1975; Omer, 1974; Schneider, 1990; Smith, 1987; Wynn-Parry, 1981). First, joints in the area of the transfer must have adequate passive mobility. In the preoperative stage, it is the responsibility of the therapist to maintain joint mobility through exercise and splinting. Second, soft tissue must be well healed and in good condition. The therapist may help here by using massage and active exercise to uninvolved muscles and joints. This helps improve circulation and nutrition to the extremity and maintain strength of the normal musculature. In some cases, restoration of the soft tissues through various plastic procedures may be necessary before tendon transfers can be done. Third, the proposed transferred muscle must have adequate strength to perform the desired function. Although it is generally agreed that it is easier to train a transferred tendon when synergistic muscles are used, that factor is no longer thought to be a major consideration. The direction of the pull of the transfer is believed to be far more important for the success of the training.

Following the transfer, the hand is immobilized for 3 to 4 weeks. Extensor tendons are generally held at least 4 to 6 weeks, because of the force that is placed on them by the much stronger flexors. A protective splint is then used for an additional 2 to 3 weeks between exercise sessions. The exact period of immobilization depends on the stress to be placed on the transferred tendon. Exercises begin with controlled active motion; any forced manipulation must be avoided. Massage and other edema-control treatments, elevation of the hand, and **Coban** wrap or **Tubigrip** are used. Isotoner gloves are also useful for reducing edema. Active motion of the rest of the extremity also is encouraged.

The therapy program should then progress to gradually increasing resistance for strengthening. When progressing the program, the therapist should watch for any signs of inflammation that would require the intensity of the exercise to be decreased. Proprioceptive neuromuscular facilitation patterns are quite helpful in training certain transferred tendons. Functional activities are introduced into the program at about 4 to 6 weeks after cast removal (Kolumban, 1984; Toth, 1986) (Fig. 38.9). These encourage functional use of the hand and improve strength. In patients who are having difficulty with the retraining process, biofeedback may be a useful adjunct to the treatment program (see Chapter 32). The exact timing for the introduction of various modalities is determined by the surgeon. Generally, the relearning progresses quickly and with little difficulty.

Tendon Repair

Tendon lacerations are among the more common types of hand injuries. Rehabilitation of patients with these injuries offers a special challenge to the therapist. Research on tendon healing and new advances in microsurgical techniques are exciting and make the area of tendon rehabilitation dynamic for both the surgeon and the therapist.

FLEXOR TENDON REPAIRS

Categorizing flexor tendon injuries can best be done by dividing the hand into five zones (Duran & Houser, 1975; Duran et al., 1990; Jaeger & Mackin, 1984; Kleinert, Kutz, & Cohen, 1975; McKay, 1980; Nissenbaum, 1978; Schneider, 1985; Schneider & McEntee, 1986). Zone 1 is the area distal to where the superficialis divides. Zone 2 is the area that begins at the proximal part of the flexor tendon sheath, proximal to the metacarpophalangeal joint and extends to the middle portion of the middle phalanx. This is an especially difficult area in which to restore smooth tendon gliding. Both flexor tendons pass through a tight fibro-osseous canal. This leaves little room for any

scarring. Even a small amount of adhesion formation can disrupt the gliding mechanism and cause decreased range of motion. Zone 3 is the area from the origin of the lumbricals to, but not including, the carpal tunnel. Zone 4 includes the carpal tunnel. Repairs in this area may necessitate placing the wrist in neutral or slight dorsiflexion because of the repair of the transverse carpal ligament. This wrist placement would require the metacarpophalangeal joints to be blocked at about 45 to 60° to ensure that no tension is placed on the repair. In zones 2 and 3, metacarpophalangeal joints are placed in about 35 to 40° of flexion, with the distal interphalangeal joints at 0°. Zone 5 extends from the distal forearm to the wrist, proximal to the transverse carpal ligament.

Another consideration is the position of the hand at the time of injury. If the finger was flexed at the time of the injury, the actual laceration of the tendon will be distal to the skin laceration. If the finger was in extension, the skin laceration will correspond to the tendon laceration.

The therapist also should know how to test individual tendon function. To test for superficialis function, support all the fingers in extension except the one being tested (Fig. 38.10). If the superficialis is intact, the proximal interphalangeal joint should be able to flex. This may not be true, however, for the fifth finger. Baker et al. (1981) concluded that the fifth finger superficialis is functionally deficient in a large portion of the population. To test for profundus function, put the finger in extension and ask the patient to flex the distal joint (Fig. 38.11). If the profundus is intact, he will be able to do so.

Postoperative Management

Early controlled mobilization adds another dimension to the management of tendon repairs in zones

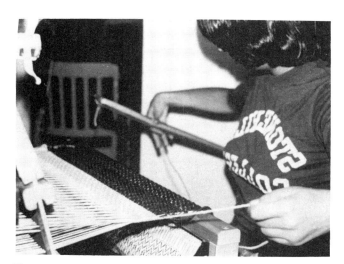

Figure 38.9. Patient performing functional activities to aid in tendon transfer training.

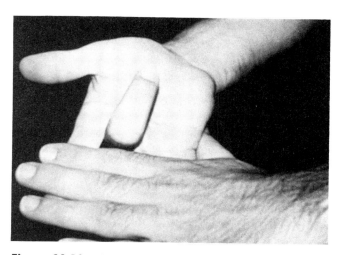

Figure 38.10. Testing for superficialis function.

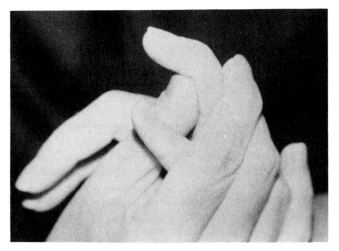

Figure 38.11. Testing for profundus function.

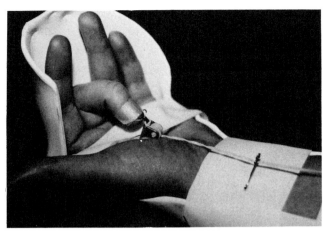

Figure 38.12. Elastic traction used for early flexor tendon mobilization.

2 and 3. The rationale for this method is to influence the favorable remodeling of scar around the tendon. Splints and exercise programs have been developed to accomplish scar remodeling by influencing the biologic processes of collagen synthesis and degradation (Strickland, 1989). Duran and colleagues (Duran et al., 1990; Duran & Houser, 1975) have shown that 3 to 5 mm of extension of the repaired tendon done in a controlled, passive exercise program is generally enough to prevent the formation of firm adhesions in zone 2 repairs. Postoperatively, the wrist is held in about 20 to 40° of flexion and the metacarpophalangeal joints are held in 35 to 40° of flexion, using a **dorsal blocking splint** (Duran et al., 1990; Nissenbaum, 1978; Schneider & McEntee, 1986) (Fig. 38.12). The interphalangeal joints are positioned in 0° of extension to prevent proximal interphalangeal joint flexion contractures. An elastic is attached to the fingernail of the involved finger by means of a suture placed in the nail by the surgeon at the time of the repair or a dress hook cemented to the nail by the therapist. Proximally, the elastic is attached to the wrist with a safety pin that is fastened to the Ace bandage. A safety pin or pulley is often placed distally to allow better profundus gliding. When the finger is flexed, there should not be any tension on the elastic. Often therapists use a modified approach in which they do not use the elastic traction. This helps to decrease the possibility of proximal interphalangeal flexion contracture.

The exercise program begins on days 2 to 5. At this time, the patient is instructed to extend the finger actively within the limits of the splint. He then passively brings the digit into flexion with his other hand. Active finger flexion and passive extension are not permitted (Jaeger & Mackin, 1984; Kleinert et al., 1975; Schneider, 1985; Van Strein, 1990). With the Duran method (Duran et al., 1990; Duran & Houser,

1975), only passive motion within the splint is allowed. Kleinert et al. (1975) suggested that patients be instructed to extend the finger actively within the splint and then allow the elastic to bring the finger into flexion. Using electromyography, It has been shown that during active, unresisted extension the flexors reciprocally relax (Kleinert et al., 1975). At 3 to 4 weeks, the dorsal splint is removed and the traction is attached to a wrist cuff or Ace wrap. At this time, active exercises are started, but the patient is not allowed to use the hand for any strong grasping or any passive extension.

At about 6 weeks, dynamic traction is generally discontinued. Differential tendon gliding exercises are done to provide maximum tendon excursion (Wehbe & Hunter, 1985). Light resistance may be added at 6 to 8 weeks to enhance tendon pull-through if there is moderate to severe adherence of the tendon. If a flexion contracture of the proximal interphalangeal joint appears to be developing, assistive extension and splinting may be started at 8 to 10 weeks. Proximal interphalangeal splinting and modifications within the splint and to the exercises may be started earlier when the contracture is developing (Van Strien, 1990). Throughout treatment, the therapist should be trying to prevent proximal and distal interphalangeal contractures from occurring. Generally, the patient is allowed to resume normal activities at about 12 weeks following repair. It should be noted that because early motion inhibits the formation of firm scar tissue, one complication of early motion is tendon rupture. Therefore, if the patient has good motion early on, the progression of the program should be slowed (Schneider, 1985; Schneider & McEntee, 1986). The fact that the tendon is gliding well indicates that the scarring has been light. Therefore, the tendon juncture is vulnerable to rupture.

STAGED TENDON RECONSTRUCTION

In cases of a severely damaged tendon system, tendon reconstruction may be done in two stages. This technique of **staged tendon surgery** has improved the results of flexor tendon grafting. Hunter (1984; Hunter & Salisbury, 1971; Hunter, Singer, & Mackin, 1990) developed a method of implanting a flexible silicone rod around which a pseudosheath grows. Later, the rod is removed and a tendon graft is placed within the sheath, providing a reconstructed tendon system. A necessary part of the pseudosheath formation is an organized program of passive gliding of the prosthesis. The implant is generally left in place for approximately 3 months before grafting is undertaken. This technique also may be used in some cases for damaged extensor tendons.

Stage One

Mackin and Hunter have published careful guidelines that can be followed in the care of these patients (Hunter, 1984; Hunter & Salisbury, 1971; Hunter & Schneider, 1975; Hunter et al., 1990; Mackin, 1975, 1984; Mackin & Maiorano, 1978). Hunter et al. (1990) developed an active tendon implant to be used as a temporary tendon prostheses. When this surgery is undertaken, the flexor tendons are excised, leaving a stump of the profundus, about 1 cm long, attached to the distal phalanx. A silicone prosthesis is implanted in the finger and sutured to the distal end of the profundus. All potential material for pulley reconstruction is preserved at the time of surgery. Following the surgery, the wrist is placed in about 30 to 35° of flexion with the metacarpophalangeal joints in about 60 to 70° of flexion and the interphalangeal joints in 0° of extension. The hand is maintained in this position in a **dorsal blocking splint** for 3 weeks. During the 1st week, gentle controlled passive flexion of the finger is started. **Finger trapping** also may be done. The therapist must be careful to note any signs of synovitis in the finger. Exercises that are done too vigorously will result in swelling and pain. If these occur, the finger must be rested and infection or failure of the implant must be ruled out. Therefore, the surgeon and the therapist must maintain close communication. At 3 weeks, the protective dorsal splint is removed. If no sign of synovitis is present at 6 weeks, the patient is allowed to return to his normal activities. Generally, 3 months is allowed between stages 1 and 2.

Stage Two

The stage 2 procedure is the introduction of the tendon graft. Following surgery, the patient is protected in a dorsal splint with the hand in the same position as for stage 1. A nail hook and elastic band are attached, and early mobilization is begun. It is recommended that 10 repetitions of passive flexion and active extension be done every hour (Hunter et al., 1990). The elastic must be of the correct tension to allow full interphalangeal extension and also to pull the finger into flexion at rest. The therapist must monitor for the development of flexion contractures of the interphalangeal joints. At about 4 to 6 weeks, the **pull-out wire** is removed and a wrist cuff is used with the elastic traction attached (Hunter et al., 1990; Mackin, 1975, 1984; Mackin & Maiorano, 1978). In some patients, however, it is necessary to protect the hand a bit longer in the dorsal splint in between exercises. This is decided on an individual basis, depending on the patient's circumstances. The cuff is removed at about 6 to 10 weeks, and active flexion exercises are initiated. Active flexion may be started earlier if adhesions are restricting motion. At about 8 to 10 weeks, the patient may be allowed to begin a program of graded activities to improve strength. This would include use of therapy putty and finger-blocking exercises. At 10 weeks, further resistance can be added. Heavy resistance is not allowed until 3 months. Before a staged flexor tendon reconstruction is undertaken, it is important that the therapist see the patient to improve the general condition of the hand by improving passive mobility of the injured finger and active and passive mobility of the uninvolved digits. Every effort must be made to improve the condition of the soft tissue as much as possible before surgery.

EXTENSOR TENDON REPAIRS

Laceration of the extensor tendon is a significant injury and can have a serious effect on hand function. Not only could the patient lose full extension but, because of scarring and a decrease in tendon excursion, he also could lose flexion. The extensor tendons, in contrast to the flexor tendons, do not glide in a synovial sheath, except at the wrist (Jabaley & Heckler, 1980; Rosenthal, 1990). At the wrist, the synovial sheath extends about 1 inch above and 1 inch below the extensor retinaculum. The blood supply to the extensors comes from soft tissue and paratenon rather than from vincula, which is the source of the blood supply for flexor tendons.

Lacerations of the extensor tendons at the level of the distal joint result in a mallet deformity; management of this injury was discussed earlier. Extensor tendon injuries that occur at the level of the proximal interphalangeal joint can result in a **boutonniere deformity,** because the central slip of the extensor digitorum is often lacerated at that level (Jabaley & Heckler, 1980; Lee, 1984; Rosenthal, 1990). The treatment for this injury is immobilization of the proximal interphalangeal joint in full extension for 5 to 6 weeks. Active motion of the metacarpophalangeal joint and the distal interphalangeal joint is allowed during this time. When active motion is started, protective splinting between exercise sessions is usually recommended for another 1 to 2 weeks. When active proximal interphalangeal joint motion is started, extension of the proximal interphalangeal joints must be monitored carefully to be sure that no extensor lag develops. Further splinting would be necessary if a lag does occur.

Extensor tendon injuries to the rest of the hand are immobilized for approximately 4 weeks (Evans & Burkhalter, 1986; Jabaley & Heckler, 1980; Lee, 1984; Rosenthal, 1990). The hand is immobilized in a volar splint that extends from the proximal interphalangeal joints to two-thirds up the forearm. The wrist is held in about 40 to 45° of dorsiflexion with the metacarpophalangeal joints in extension. The proximal interphalangeal joints are free to move. Following this period of immobilization, active and active-assisted exercises are started. At 5 weeks, gentle active flexion is allowed but it must be done carefully. Because the flexors are much stronger than the extensors, vigorous flexion could disrupt the repair. If only the wrist extensors are lacerated, the digits may be left free, and just the wrist immobilized. Immobilization is continued for 3 to 4 weeks.

An exercise found helpful in regaining extension after extensor tendon repair is to tape the proximal interphalangeal joints into flexion (Figs. 38.13 and 38.14). The patient then flexes and extends the metacarpophalangeal joints with the hand in the described position. This helps isolate the long extensors and place the extensor power at the level of the metacarpophalangeal joints. The therapist must remember that the excursion of the extensor tendons can be decreased because of the adherence of the extensor tendons to the surrounding tissues. Therefore, when safe to do so, exercises to enhance tendon gliding should be done.

In some cases, splints to aid in stretching may be necessary. In cases for which an extensor tendon lag persists, a splint is fabricated to support the fingers in extension. In some cases, biofeedback may be useful in treating these injuries. Electrical stimulation is another modality that might be considered to obtain increased tendon gliding.

In carefully selected cases of complex extensor injuries in zones 5, 6, and 7 (from the metacarpophalangeal joints to the wrist), early passive motion has been used successfully. A dynamic splint is fabricated to provide controlled active flexion and passive extension. The splint is fabricated with a built-in stop to allow active flexion within a range of motion that will provide 5 mm of tendon gliding and then passively return the fingers to 0° of extension. The wrist is immobilized at 40 to 45° (Evans, 1986, 1990; Evans & Burkhalter, 1986). Active flexion allows enough metacarpophalangeal joint motion to prevent collateral ligament shortening and enough tendon glide to lengthen adhesions as they are forming, reducing the possible need for **tenolysis** at a later time. Generally, the patient with extensor tendon injuries can expect a good result with careful monitoring.

Extensor Tendon Ruptures with Rheumatoid Arthritis

Extensor tendon rupture is a serious complication of rheumatoid arthritis. It requires a prolonged rehabilitation program of 3 to 4 months or longer to reach the end result. There are thought to be several causes of spontaneous tendon rupture in patients with rheumatoid arthritis (Nalebuff, 1975; Philips, 1989): (1) attrition rupture, when a tendon ruptures secondary to rubbing on a piece of bone, usually the distal ulna; (2) tenosynovitis that infiltrates the tendon; (3) pressure from a hypertrophied synovial membrane beneath the tight dorsal retinaculum; and (4) multiple steroid injections.

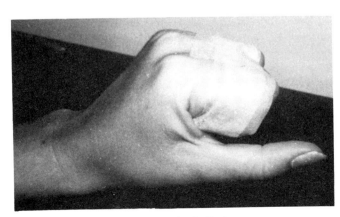

Figure 38.13. Taping exercise in flexion.

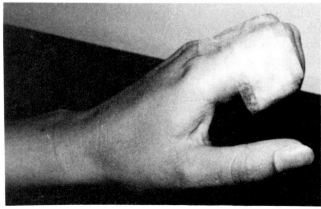

Figure 38.14. Taping exercise in extension.

A single tendon rupture may occur in any digit but is most common in the little finger. This single rupture may cause only a minimal extension lag because of the junctura tendonae that connect the tendons of the fourth and fifth fingers just proximal to the metacarpophalangeal joints (Nalebuff, 1969, 1975). The amount of lag also depends on whether the extensor digiti quinti has ruptured as well (Nalebuff et al., 1988). Patients will often have little disability and may not even see a physician. However, when two tendons rupture, the disability becomes more obvious.

Any acute extensor tendon rupture is treated with urgency, because a single tendon rupture is followed by a second or a third. In patients with rheumatoid arthritis, either tendon transfer (usually the extensor indicis proprius) or adjacent tendon suture is often used to restore tendon function (Nalebuff, 1969). For more complicated ruptures, wrist extensors or the flexor digitorum superficialis tendon may be used. Generally, the poor condition of the soft tissue and the time elapsed between the actual rupture and the surgical repair prevent end-to-end suture. The final results of the repair are, of course, influenced by the number of tendons ruptured and the status of the surrounding joints and soft tissue. Following the transfer, the hand is immobilized for 3 weeks, with the wrist in slight extension and the metacarpophalangeal joints in extension. The proximal interphalangeal joints are free to move. At 3 weeks, the patient is started on gentle, assisted active and passive extension and controlled active flexion. Exercises are increased gradually over the following few weeks, including the previously described taping exercise. The patient wears a protective splint in between exercises for 6 to 8 weeks or longer if a lag develops.

TENOLYSIS

In some patients for whom therapy has failed to restore tendon gliding, it may be necessary to perform a **tenolysis** following a tendon graft or repair. As has been previously mentioned, sometimes the tendon will become bound in scar, preventing it from gliding freely. The **tenolysis** frees the tendon from the scar tissue. Generally, the surgeon waits 3 to 6 months before performing **tenolysis** to see if the patient is able to obtain tendon pull-through without further surgery (Schneider, 1985; Schneider & Hunter, 1975).

Hand therapy after a **tenolysis** begins on the day of the surgery. Range of motion is done briefly several times per day. Care must be taken to teach the patient to exercise gently so as not to increase swelling. The patient is carefully monitored over the next several weeks. During **tenolysis,** there is an interruption of the blood supply to the tendon. This makes the tendon more vulnerable to rupture. Therefore, no resistive

activities are generally allowed before 6 to 8 weeks. The exact time frame is determined by the surgeon and depends on the condition of the tendon at the time of surgery.

Pain Problems

Problems of pain are among the most challenging, and without a doubt, often the most frustrating for all concerned. This is primarily because health care professionals still do not fully understand the mechanisms of pain and how to control it adequately.

REFLEX SYMPATHETIC DYSTROPHY

Reflex sympathetic dystrophy (RSD) appears to be the result of an abnormal response of the autonomic nervous system to trauma. This response triggers a cycle of pain, immobility, swelling, and vasospasm that eventually leads to a stiff, nonfunctioning hand if not treated (Clark, 1978; Erikson, 1978; Lankford, 1990; Morgan, 1980; Omer, 1978). This condition has been called different names: minor causalgia, minor traumatic dystrophy, shoulder-hand syndrome, major traumatic dystrophy, and major causalgia. These, however, all can be classified under the heading of reflex sympathetic dystrophy. This affliction was described in 1864 by Silas Weir Mitchell (Morgan, 1980; Omer, 1978). He reported this condition in Civil War soldiers who sustained gunshot wounds involving injuries to nerves. He termed the resultant pain as causalgia. It is now known that this syndrome does not necessarily result from nerve injury. It can often be the sequela of a minor trauma. It can result from carpal tunnel release, release of Dupuytren's contracture, a crush injury, or fractures. It can be a devastating complication of a Colles fracture.

The predominant symptoms of reflex sympathetic dystrophy are pain and swelling that are out of all proportion to the injury. The patient often describes this pain as burning and stinging. He also may describe it as a constricting or pressure-type pain. This pain often may be exaggerated by motion. As the dystrophy progresses, the hand becomes stiff from lack of motion. There is usually a change in skin color, which often progresses from redness to a wax-like appearance. Often, there is either excessive sweating or dryness of the skin. The hand may at first feel warm, but in later stages, it will feel cool. There will also be progressive atrophy of the skin and muscles. Changes in hair growth and nail growth also may be noted. X-rays of the hand may show demineralization of bone and narrowing of joint spaces. The pain may become so intense that even a breeze across the arm will be unbearable, and it may progress to previously uninvolved areas. It is important to diagnose RSD early to prevent permanent disability. It should be a red flag to the therapist if a patient continues to have pain or develop stiffness that is not consistent with the usual healing process.

These patients often manifest psychological problems and are angry and fearful. Sometimes pushed from doctor to doctor, they may be suspicious and, therefore, not always able to cooperate in their treatment. They expect the medical team to make them better. These patients need to be shown that someone cares about them. They need a lot of emotional support. All treatment must be well coordinated with no inconsistencies among the professionals involved. Because these patients tend to be suggestible, constant, positive reinforcement is beneficial. Various treatment procedures are used in an effort to relieve these unfortunate patients of their pain. Sympathetic blocks are frequently used by the physician to try to break the sympathetic arc. In some cases, it may be necessary to interrupt the sympathetic arc permanently by performing surgical sympathectomy.

The main goals in treating these patients are first to help decrease the pain and second to help increase their range of motion. However, before these goals can be accomplished, a trusting relationship between the therapist and the patient must be established (see Chapter 14).

The program of hand therapy should begin with modalities that will decrease pain. Hot packs or paraffin may be helpful in providing relief and may be used prior to exercises or activities. Some patients may also respond well to ice, either through massage or ice pack. Contrast baths that alternate hot and cold bathing of the extremity also may help to break the pain cycle. Often, a trial of transcutaneous nerve stimulation (TENS) is given. The electrode placement of the TENS unit depends on the area of the pain, the cause of the pain, and the nature of the pain. The electrodes may be placed over the trigger points, the location of the greatest pain, distant or contralateral locations, specific dermatomes or spinal segmental levels, points along the peripheral nerves, or linear pathways (Lampe, 1978; Mannheimer, 1978; Mannheimer & Lampe, 1984; Wolf, 1978; Wolf, Gersh, & Kutner, 1978). In some cases, alternative placement of electrodes may be necessary to produce pain relief. If pain relief is obtained with TENS, the patient may rent or purchase a unit that can be used at home.

Watson and Carlson (1987) developed a stress loading program to help interrupt the process. This program consists of two parts: a scrub portion and a carry portion. The patient scrubs using a brush or a machine called a dystrophile while placing weight on the affected arm. The carry portion requires the patient to carry 1 to 5 pounds of weight throughout the day.

Naturally, once the pain is decreased, a program to improve motion and the general condition of the extremity is much easier to implement. Active exercises and activities are done by the patient as tolerated. Therapy that increases pain is counterproductive and only adds to the patient's anxiety. Splinting to help correct deformities and improve mobility is used as soon as it can be tolerated by the patient. Edema control through elevation, massage, and compression gloves, when necessary, in conjunction with active exercise is also an important part of the treatment. Massage should generally be done by the patient. In combination with massage, the patient is put on a program of systematic desensitization (see Chapter 23).

In cases of painful **neuroma,** the use of percussion and vibration of the **neuroma** along with the desensitization program may be successful in relieving pain in selected patients. In most cases, however, the **neuroma** will need to be surgically removed.

Functional activities are also important in the treatment of pain patients and are introduced as soon as possible. Because these patients often withdraw from social contact, group activities are helpful in getting them back into the mainstream of life (see Chapters 10 and 20). These people often have been out of work for long periods of time. Therefore, vocational counseling and vocational training may be necessary before the patient is able to reenter the work force (see Chapter 17).

CUMULATIVE TRAUMA DISORDERS

Another group of patients seen regularly by the hand therapist are those diagnosed with cumulative trauma disorders (Dobyns, Sim, & Linscheid, 1978; Granjean, 1981; Habes & Putz-Anderson, 1985; Hersherson, 1975; Tubiana, 1983). This encompasses a variety of disorders, including various types of tendinitis, tenosynovitis, tennis elbow, thoracic outlet syndrome, carpal tunnel syndrome, and other pain syndromes and muscle cramps. Repetitive activities done over prolonged periods of time may produce biomechanical stress. These syndromes often may be seen in assembly-line and clerical workers, athletes, and musicians who, over time, are engaged in repetitive activities and are expected to perform at a high level. Treating these people involves a well-organized program and good communication among the patient, the therapist, the physician, and when possible, the patient's supervisor at the workplace (Berryhill, 1990).

Initial treatment involves a thorough evaluation of the patient to obtain baseline data. It is important to get a good work and avocational history from the patient, including motions required and body positions necessary to complete the work or activity. It may also be necessary to verify the patient's job requirements with the patient's supervisor and also through the *Dictionary of Occupational Titles*. In the case of athletes and musicians, it is necessary to discuss with them their practice procedures, the types of equipment they use, and the length of time that they spend practicing or training in their specific area of endeavor.

A medical workup by the patient's physician should be done to rule out any underlying disease process. The therapist should record range of motion, grip, and pinch strength. Circumferential measurements of the upper extremity as well as volumeter measurements should be taken to assess edema. A sensory evaluation also may be needed for some patients (see Chapter 8). The therapist must elicit from the patient information concerning the nature of the pain, the exact site of the pain, when it occurs, what causes it to increase, and what helps to relieve it. It is also important to observe the patient's posture carefully. Poor posture can lead to many problems that may be helped by instruction in postural exercises.

The treatment of these patients can be divided into three phases. The first phase, the acute phase, is geared toward decreasing pain and inflammation. The modalities used include splinting to rest the inflamed area and gentle range of motion of the whole extremity to prevent joint stiffness. Ice and other cold modalities also are used during this period to help reduce inflammation. Ultrasound, phonophoresis, and electrical modalities may be helpful in reducing inflammation and providing an analgesic effect (see Chapter 33). Isometric exercises are also added to help begin strengthening. Massage may be used for edema control and reduction of pain. Phase two is the subacute phase. At this stage the patient is more comfortable. Usually, there is full range of motion. The pain is generally gone, but there may be discomfort at the end range or if the patient attempts to stress the extremity. The use of splints during this phase is gradually decreased and light activities that do not cause pain are added to the patient's program. Massage is continued during this phase to aid in pain reduction and in maintaining tissue mobility.

When the patient is able to perform his activities of daily living without any significant discomfort, he is progressed to the final phase, which is that of conditioning or work hardening. Here, the patient continues to work on flexibility and gradually increasing strength and endurance. One of the modalities that can be used at this stage is the BTE work simulator (Fig. 38.15). This piece of equipment (Baltimore Therapeutic Equipment Co.) has various attachments that simulate a variety of work or life tasks and is computerized to allow collection of accurate records of work performed. The BTE work simulator may be used with other modalities to increase strength and endurance. During this

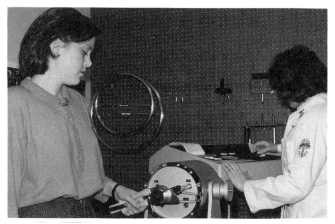

Figure 38.15. Patient being treated on the BTE work simulator.

time, it is important, when necessary and when possible, to suggest tool and/or work site modifications that would help prevent reinjury. These ergonomic modifications might include a different type of handle on a tool or a change in the height of a work table (Johnson, 1990). Ergonomic considerations should be worked out with the patient and his employer. Also, any return-to-work instructions should be well coordinated and communicated to both the patient and his supervisor to prevent misunderstandings. This is particularly true when the patient has been released to do light duty. This could mean different things to different employers and must be specifically outlined to prevent reinjury to the patient. Once the patient has returned to work, it is important to monitor him periodically to make sure that his problem has not recurred and the transition back to work is as smooth as possible.

PSYCHOLOGICAL IMPLICATIONS

It must be kept in mind that people who sustain hand injuries or develop hand problems have to make a number of psychological adjustments to their disability. Their daily lives are interrupted, and their functioning is altered. In many cases, the disability is temporary, and the person eventually will return to his regular routine. However, with more serious problems, the person's life may be permanently changed. He may be unable to perform his usual work or to pursue his various avocational interests. A person may lose self-esteem and become depressed when unable to do regular work. Often, a person who appears to lack motivation is really depressed or may be afraid of returning to the machine on which the injury occurred. The therapist can help the patient set realistic goals and can act as a resource for needed information or referrals to outside agencies. Some patients may require professional psychiatric help to deal with the issues their disability raises. However, the supportive hand therapy environment and the encouragement (not false hope) provided by the therapist can help make the adjustment period much smoother and less traumatic.

Acknowledgments—I would like to thank Lisa DeBlois O'Toole for her assistance in the preparation of this manuscript.

STUDY QUESTIONS

1. List three standardized tests used to document hand function.
2. What are the goals of early treatment of joint injuries?
3. What deformities could develop if proper treatment is not provided for volar or dorsal proximal interphalangeal joint dislocations?
4. What is the goal of dynamic splinting following metacarpophalangeal arthroplasty?
5. Describe the goals of metacarpophalangeal and proximal interphalangeal arthroplasty. How do they differ from the goals of wrist arthroplasty?
6. Following a nerve injury, what are the treatment goals?
7. Why are tendon transfers done?
8. What is the position of hand and wrist splinting immediately following flexor tendon repair? What is the reason for placing the hand and wrist into this position?
9. What is the theory behind early controlled mobilization of flexor tendon repairs in zones 2 and 3?
10. What are the two stages of a two-stage flexor tendon reconstruction?

REFERENCES

Almquist, E. E. (1975). The effect of training on sensory function. In J. Mickon & E. Moberg (Eds.), *Traumatic nerve lesions of the upper extremity* (pp. 53–54). New York: Churchill Livingstone.

American Academy of Orthopedic Surgeons (1965). *Joint motion: Method of measuring and recording.* Chicago: Author.

American Society for Surgery of the Hand (1983). *The hand: examination and diagnosis.* Aurora, CO: Author.

Aulicino, P. L., & Dupuy, T. E. (1990). Clinical examination of the hand. In J. Hunter, L. Schneider, E. Mackin, & A. Callahan (Eds.), *Rehabilitation of the hand* (3rd ed., pp. 31–52). St. Louis: C. V. Mosby.

Baker, D. S., Gaul, J., Williams, V., & Graves, M. (1981). The little finger superficialis: A clinical investigation of its anatomic and functional shortcomings. *Journal of Hand Surgery, 6,* 374–378.

Baxter-Petralia P., Bruening L., Blackmore, S., & McEntee, P., (1990). Physical capacity evaluation. In J. Hunter, L. Schneider, E. Mackin, & A. Callahan (Eds.), *Rehabilitation of the hand* (3rd ed., pp. 93–108). St. Louis: C. V. Mosby.

Beasley, R. W. (1975). Basic considerations for tendon transfer operations in the upper extremity. In American Academy of Orthopedic Surgeons (Ed.), *American Academy of Orthopedic Surgeons Symposium on Tendon Surgery in the Hand* (pp. 163–180). St. Louis: C. V. Mosby.

Beasley, R. W. (1981). *Hand injuries.* Philadelphia: W. B. Saunders.

Bell, J. A. (1978). Sensibility evaluation. In J. Hunter, L. Schneider, E. Mackin, & J. Bell (Eds.), *Rehabilitation of the hand* (pp. 273–291). St. Louis: C. V. Mosby.

Bell-Krotoski, J., Weinstein, S., & Weinstein, C. (1993). Testing sensibility. Including launch-pressure, two-point discrimination, point localization and vibration. *Journal of Hand Therapy, 6*(2), 114–123.

Belsky, M. R., Ruby, L. K., & Millender, L. H. (1983). Injuries of the finger and thumb joints. *Contemporary Orthopedics, 7*(4), 39–48.

Berger-Lee, D., Bell-Krotoski, J., & Brandsma, J. W. (1990). Torque range of motion in the hand clinic. *Journal of Hand Therapy, 3*(1), 7–13.

Berger-Lee, D., Tomancik Voelker, E., Giurintano, D., Novick, A., & Browder, L. (1993). Reliability of torque range of motion: A preliminary study. *Journal of Hand Therapy, 6*(1), 29–34.

Berryhill, B. (1990). Returning the worker with upper extremity injury to industry—A model for physician and therapist. *Journal of Hand Therapy, 3*(2), 56–63.

Brand, P. W., & Hollister, A. (1993). *Clinical mechanics of the hand* (2nd ed.). St. Louis: C. V. Mosby Yearbook.

Braun, R. M. (1980). *Management of peripheral problems.* Philadelphia: W. B. Saunders.

Burton, R. I. (1980). Acute joint injuries. In F. G. Wolfort (Ed.), *Acute hand injuries: A multispecialty approach* (pp. 155–164). Boston: Little, Brown & Co.

Callahan, A. D. (1990a). Sensibility testing: Clinical methods. In J. Hunter, L. Schneider, E. Mackin, & A. Callahan (Eds.), *Rehabilitation of the hand* (3rd ed., pp. 594–610). St. Louis: C. V. Mosby.

Callahan, A. D. (1990b). Methods of compensation and re-education for sensory dysfunction. In J. Hunter, L. Schneider, E. Mackin, & A. Callahan (Eds.), *Rehabilitation of the hand* (3rd ed., pp. 611–621). St. Louis: C. V. Mosby.

Clark, G. L. (1978). Causalgia: A discussion of chronic pain syndromes in the upper limb. In J. Hunter, L. Schneider, E. Mackin, & J. Bell (Eds.), *Rehabilitation of the hand* (pp. 350–355). St. Louis: C. V. Mosby.

Dellon, A. L. (1981). *Evaluation of sensibility and re-education of sensation in the hand.* Baltimore: Williams & Wilkins.

Dellon, A. L., Curtis, R. M., & Edgerton, M. T. (1972). Evaluating recovery of sensation in the hand following nerve injury. *Johns Hopkins Medical Journal, 130,* 235–243.

Dellon, A. L., Curtis, R. M., & Edgerton, M. T. (1974). Re-education of sensation in the hand after nerve injury and repair. *Plastic and Reconstructive Surgery, 53,* 297–305.

Dobyns, J. H., Sim, F. H., & Linscheid, R. L. (1978). Sports stress syndromes of the hand and wrist. *American Journal of Sports Medicine, 6,* 236–254.

Dray, G., Millender, L. H., & Nalebuff, E. A. (1979). Rupture of the radial collateral ligament of a metacarpophalangeal joint to one of the ulnar three fingers. *Journal of Hand Surgery, 4*(4), 346–350.

Duran, R. J., Coleman, C., Nappi, J., & Klerekoper, L. (1990). Management of flexor tendon lacerations in zone 2 using controlled passive motion postoperatively. In J. Hunter, L. Schneider, E. Mackin, & A. Callahan (Eds.), *Rehabilitation of the hand* (3rd ed., pp. 410–413). St. Louis: C. V. Mosby.

Duran, R. J., & Houser, R. G. (1975). Controlled passive motion following flexor tendon repair in zones 2 and 3. In American Academy of Orthopedic Surgeons (Ed.), *American Academy of Orthopedic Surgeons Symposium on Tendon Surgery in the Hand* (pp. 105–114). St. Louis: C. V. Mosby.

Eaton, R. G. (1971). *Joint injuries of the hand.* Springfield, IL: Charles C. Thomas.

Erikson, J. C. (1978). Evaluation and management of autonomic dystrophies of the upper extremity. In J. Hunter, L. Schneider, E. Mackin, & J. Bell (Eds.), *Rehabilitation of the hand* (pp. 356–360). St. Louis: C. V. Mosby.

Evans, R. B. (1986). Therapeutic management of extensor tendon injuries. *Hand Clinics, 2*(1), 157–169.

Evans, R. B. (1990). Therapeutic management of extensor tendon injuries. In J. Hunter, L. Schneider, E. Mackin, & A. Callahan (Eds.), *Rehabilitation of the hand* (3rd ed., pp. 492–511). St. Louis: C. V. Mosby.

Evans, R. B., & Burkhalter, W. E. (1986). A study of the dynamic anatomy of extensor tendons and implications for treatment. *Journal of Hand Surgery, 11A,* 774–779.

Fess, E. E. (1990). Documentation: Essential elements of an upper extremity assessment battery. In J. Hunter, L. Schneider, E. Mackin, & A. Callahan (Eds.), *Rehabilitation of the hand* (3rd ed., pp. 53–81). St. Louis: C. V. Mosby.

Fess, E., & Moran, C. (1981). *Clinical assessment recommendations.* Indianapolis: American Society for Hand Therapists.

Flowers, K. R., & Pheasant, S. D. (1988). The use of torque angle curves in the assessment of digital joint stiffness. *Journal of Hand Therapy, 1,* 69–74.

Frykman, G. K. (1993). The quest for better recovery from peripheral nerve injury—Current status of nerve regeneration research. *Journal of Hand Therapy, 6*(2), 83–88.

Goodman, M. J., Millender, L. H., Nalebuff, E. A., & Philips, C. A. (1980). Arthroplasty of the rheumatoid wrist with silicone rubber: An early evaluation. *Journal of Hand Surgery, 5,* 114–121.

Granjean, E. (1981). *Fitting the task to man: an ergonomic approach.* London: Taylor and Francis.

Habes, D. J., & Putz-Anderson, V. (1985). The NIOSH program for evaluating biomechanical hazards in the workplace. *Journal of Safety Research, 16*(2), 49–60.

Hersherson, A. (1975). Cumulative injury: A national problem. *Journal of Occupational Medicine, 21*(10), 674–676.

Hunter, J. M. (1984). Staged flexor tendon reconstruction. In J. Hunter, L. Schneider, E. Mackin, & A. Callahan (Eds.), *Rehabilitation of the hand* (2nd ed., pp. 288–313). St. Louis: C. V. Mosby.

Hunter, J. M., & Salisbury, R. E. (1971). Flexor tendon reconstruction in severely damaged hands. *Journal of Bone & Joint Surgery, 53A*(5), 829–857.

Hunter, J. M., & Schneider, L. H. (1975). Staged flexor tendon reconstruction: Current status. In American Academy of Orthopedic Surgeons (Ed.), American Academy of Orthopedic Surgeons Symposium on Tendon Surgery in the Hand (pp. 271–274). St. Louis: C. V. Mosby.

Hunter, J., Singer, D., & Mackin, E. (1990). Staged flexor tendon reconstruction using passive and active tendon implants. In J. Hunter, L. Schneider, E. Mackin, & A. Callahan (Eds.), *Rehabilitation of the hand* (3rd ed., pp. 427–457). St. Louis: C. V. Mosby.

Jabaley, M. E., & Heckler, E. D. (1980). Extensor tendon injuries. In F. Wolfort (Ed.), *Acute hand injuries: A multispecialty approach* (pp. 201–210). Boston: Little, Brown & Co.

Jaeger, S. H., & Mackin, E. J. (1984). Primary care of flexor tendon injuries. In J. Hunter, L. Schneider, E. Mackin, & A. Callahan (Eds.), *Rehabilitation of the hand* (2nd ed., pp. 261–272). St. Louis: C. V. Mosby.

Jebsen, R. H., Taylor, N., Trieschmann, R. B., Trotter, M. J., & Howard, L. A. (1969). An objective and standardized test of hand function. *Archives of Physical Medicine & Rehabilitation, 50,* 311–319.

Johnson, S. L. (1990). Ergonomic design of hand-held tools to prevent trauma to the hand and upper extremity. *Journal of Hand Therapy, 3*(2), 86–93.

Kolumban, S. L. (1984). Preoperative and postoperative management of tendon transfers. In J. Hunter, L. Schneider, E. Mackin, & A. Callahan (Eds.), *Rehabilitation of the hand* (2nd ed., pp. 476–481). St. Louis: C. V. Mosby.

Kiefhaber, T. R., Stern, P. J., & Grood, E. S. (1986). Lateral stability of the proximal interphalangeal joint. *Journal of Hand Surgery, 11A,* 661–669.

Kleinert, H. E., Kutz, J. E., & Cohen, M. (1975). Primary repair of zone 2 flexor tendon lacerations. In American Academy of Orthopedic Surgeons (Ed.), *American Academy of Orthopedic Surgeons Symposium on Tendon Surgery in the Hand* (pp. 91–104). St. Louis: C. V. Mosby.

Lampe, G. N. (1978). Introduction to the use of transcutaneous electrical nerve stimulation devices. *Physical Therapy, 58*(12), 1450–1454.

Lankford, L. L. (1990). Reflex sympathetic dystrophy. In J. Hunter, L. Schneider, E. Mackin, & A. Callahan (Eds.), *Rehabilitation of the hand* (3rd ed., pp. 763–786). St. Louis: C. V. Mosby.

Lee, V. H. (1984). Rehabilitation of extensor tendon injuries. In J. Hunter, L. Schneider, E. Mackin, & A. Callahan (Eds.), *Rehabilitation of the hand* (2nd ed., pp. 353–357). St. Louis: C. V. Mosby.

Mackin, E. J. (1975). Physical therapy and staged tendon graft: preoperative and postoperative management. In American Academy of Orthopedic Surgeons (Ed.), *American Academy of Orthopedic Surgeons Symposium on Tendon Surgery in the Hand* (pp. 283–291). St. Louis: C. V. Mosby.

Mackin, E. J. (1984). Therapist management of staged flexor tendon reconstruction. In J. Hunter, L. Schneider, E. Mackin, & A. Callahan (Eds.), *Rehabilitation of the hand* (2nd ed., pp. 314–323). St. Louis: C. V. Mosby.

Madden, J. W., DeVore, G., & Arem, A. J. (1977). A rational post operative management program in metacarpophalangeal joint implant arthroplasty. *Journal of Hand Surgery, 2*(5), 358–366.

Mackin, E. J., & Maiorano, L. (1978). Postoperative therapy following staged flexor tendon reconstruction. In J. Hunter, L. Schneider, E. Mackin, & J. Bell (Eds.), *Rehabilitation of the hand* (pp. 247–261). St. Louis: C. V. Mosby.

Mannheimer, J. S. (1978). Electrode placements for transcutaneous electrical nerve stimulation. *Physical Therapy, 58*(12), 1455–1462.

Mannheimer, J. S., & Lampe, G. N. (1984). *Clinical transcutaneous electrical nerve stimulation.* Philadelphia: F. A. Davis.

Maynard, C. J. (1978). Sensory re-education following peripheral nerve injury. In J. Hunter, L. Schneider, E. Mackin, & J. Bell (Eds.), *Rehabilitation of the hand* (pp. 318–323). St. Louis: C. V. Mosby.

McKay, D. (1980). Flexor tendon injuries. In F. Wolfort (Ed.), *Acute hand injuries: A multidspecialty approach* (pp. 181–191). Boston: Little, Brown & Co.

Millender, L. H., & Nalebuff, E. A. (1973). Metacarpophalangeal joint arthroplasty utilizing the silicone rubber prosthesis. *Orthopedic Clinics of North America, 4*(2), 349–371.

Morgan, J. E. (1980). Sympathetic dystrophy. In F. Wolfort (Ed.), *Acute hand injuries: A multispecialty approach* (pp. 175–179). Boston: Little, Brown & Co.

Nalebuff, E. A. (1969). Surgical treatment of tendon rupture in the rheumatoid hand. *Surgical Clinics of North America, 49*(4), 811–822.

Nalebuff, E. A. (1975). The recognition and treatment of tendon ruptures in the rheumatoid hand. In American Academy of Orthopedic Surgeons (Ed.), *American Academy of Orthopedic Surgeons Symposium on Tendon Surgery in the Hand* (pp. 255–270). St. Louis: C. V. Mosby.

Nissenbaum, M. D. (1978). Early care of flexor tendon injuries: Application of principles of tendon healing and early motion. In

J. Hunter, L. Schneider, E. Mackin, & J. Bell (Eds.), *Rehabilitation of the hand* (pp. 187–196). St. Louis: C. V. Mosby.

Omer, G. E. (1974). Techniques and timing of tendon transfers. *Orthopedic Clinics of North America, 5*(2), 243–252.

Omer, G. E. (1978). Management of pain symptoms in the upper extremity. In J. Hunter, L. Schneider, E. Mackin, & J. Bell (Eds.), *Rehabilitation of the hand* (pp. 341–349). St. Louis: C. V. Mosby.

Parry, E. G. (1980). Nerve injuries. In F. G. Wolfort (Ed.), *Acute hand injuries: A multispecialty approach* (pp. 165–173). Boston: Little, Brown & Co.

Philips, C. A. (1989). Management of the patient with rheumatoid arthritis: The role of the hand therapist. *Hand Clinics, 5*(2), 291–309.

Rosenthal, E. A. (1990). The extensor tendons. In J. Hunter, L. Schneider, E. Mackin, & A. Callahan (Eds.), *Rehabilitation of the hand* (3rd ed., pp. 458–491). St. Louis: C. V. Mosby.

Schneider, L. H. (1985). *Flexor tendon injuries.* Boston: Little, Brown & Co.

Schneider, L. H. (1990). Tendon transfers in the upper extremity. In J. Hunter, L. Schneider, E. Mackin, & A. Callahan (Eds.), *Rehabilitation of the hand* (3rd ed., pp. 669–675). St. Louis: C. V. Mosby.

Schneider, L. H., & Hunter, J. M. (1975). Flexor tenolysis. In American Academy of Orthopedic Surgeons (Ed.), *American Academy of Orthopedic Surgeons Symposium on Tendon Surgery in the Hand* (pp. 157–162). St. Louis: C. V. Mosby.

Schneider, L. H., & McEntee, P. (1986). Flexor tendon injuries: Treatment of acute problems. *Hand Clinics, 2*(1), 119–131.

Smith, J. W. (1986). Peripheral nerve surgery—Retrospective and contemporary techniques. *Clinical Plastic Surgery, 13*(1), 249–254.

Smith, R. J. (1987). *Tendon transfers of the hand and forearm.* Boston: Little, Brown & Co.

Strickland, J. W. (1989). Biologic rationale, clinical application and results in early motion following flexor tendon repair. *Journal of Hand Surgery, 2*(2), 71–83.

Swanson, A. B. (1973). *Flexible implant resection arthroplasty in the hand and extremities.* St. Louis: C. V. Mosby.

Swanson, A. B., Swanson, G., & Leonard, J. (1984). Postoperative rehabilitation in flexible implant arthroplasty of the digits. In J. Hunter, L. Schneider, E. Mackin, & A. Callahan (Eds.), *Rehabilitation of the hand* (2nd ed., pp. 665–680). St. Louis: C. V. Mosby.

Thayer, D. T. (1988). Distal interphalangeal joint injuries. *Hand Clinics, 4*(1), 1–4.

Taylor Mullins, P. A. (1990). Use of therapeutic modalities in upper extremity rehabilitation. In J. Hunter, L. Schneider, E. Mackin, & A. Callahan (Eds.), *Rehabilitation of the hand* (3rd ed., pp. 195–220). St. Louis: C. V. Mosby.

Toth, S. (1986). Therapist's management of tendon transfers. *Hand Clinics, 2*(1), 239–246.

Tubiana, R. (1983). Crampes: Professionnelles du membre superieur. *Annales de Chirurgie de la Main, 2*(2), 134–142.

Tubiana, R. (1984). *Examination of the hand.* Philadelphia: W. B. Saunders.

Van Strien, G. (1990). Post-operative management of flexor tendon injuries. In J. Hunter, L. Schneider, E. Mackin, & A. Callahan (Eds.), *Rehabilitation of the hand* (3rd ed., pp. 390–409). St. Louis: C. V. Mosby.

Vicar, A. (1988). Proximal interphalangeal joint dislocations without fractures. *Hand Clinics, 4*(1), 5–13.

Watson, K., & Carlson, L. (1987). Treatment of reflex sympathetic dystrophy of the hand with an active "stress loading" program. *Journal of Hand Surgery, 12A*, 770–785.

Wehbe, M. A., & Hunter, J. M. (1985). Flexor tendon gliding in the hand. Part I. Differential gliding. *Journal of Hand Surgery, 10A*, 575–579.

Wolf, S. L. (1978). Perspective on central nervous system responsiveness to transcutaneous electrical nerve stimulation. *Physical Therapy, 58*(12), 1443–1447.

Wolf, S. L., Gersh, M. R., & Kutner, M. (1978). Relationship of selected clinical variables to current delivered during transcutaneous electrical nerve stimulation. *Physical Therapy, 58*(12), 1478–1485.

Wynn-Parry, C. B. (1981). *Rehabilitation of the hand* (4th ed.). Kent, UK: Butterworth.

39
Spinal Cord Injury

Laura Devore Hollar

OBJECTIVES ———————————

After studying this chapter, the reader will be able to:
1. Define the basic anatomy, physiology, and terminology of the spinal cord as it pertains to traumatic injuries.
2. Indicate the appropriate tests and procedures used in the occupational therapy assessment.
3. Describe complications and precautions associated with spinal cord injury and the responsibility of the occupational therapist in treatment and prevention.
4. Detail the role of occupational therapy in the three phases of treatment.
5. Provide suggestions for special populations.

An overview of spinal cord injury written several years ago might have described the role of occupational therapy as providing patients with the equipment and skills needed to increase functional independence significantly. As society has changed so has the role of occupational therapy. The occupational therapist now is less of a provider and more of a problem solver. Several years ago it appeared technology would allow all future patients the ability to be independent in most of their self-care skills. With the development of complex **environmental control units,** power-driven hand orthoses, and surgical tendon transfers, the independence available to a tetraplegic patient is remarkable. Today there are few patients taking full advantage of the surgery and technology available (Garber & Gregoria, 1990; McDonald, Boyle, & Schumann, 1989). This has happened for several reasons, including lack of funding, shortened rehabilitation stays, and a change in patient demographics. There are more geriatric patients (Teasell & Allatt, 1989; Yarkony, Roth, Heinemann, & Lovell, 1988), incomplete injuries (Dituinno et al., 1989), and violent crime related injuries (Parsons & Lammertse, 1991). Today's thera-

pist may be faced with developing activities of daily living (ADL) goals for an 80-year-old homeless person or vocational goals for a previous drug dealer. The therapist may also be told by a patient's insurance company that she has only 60 days to rehabilitate a tetraplegic. It is for these reasons that the occupational therapist must act as a resource for her patients. She must educate and encourage patients to be as functionally independent as possible given the constraints of time, resources, and most important, motivation. The therapist must determine priorities in the treatment plan based on patient preference, potential, functional performance, and occupational roles. Today the role of an occupational therapist in spinal cord injury management is to assist the patient in achieving his desired level of functional independence through a variety of skills and equipment.

DEFINITIONS, CLASSIFICATIONS, AND LEVELS OF INJURY

The spinal cord is a cylindrical structure located inside the vertebral column. Motor and sensory information travel between the brain and body via the spinal cord. The spinal cord also plays a major role in most of the body's reflex activity. The cord is composed of spinal tracts (white matter) that surround spinal neuronal cell bodies (gray matter). The gray matter is divided into segments of sensory and motor neurons. Axons that relay sensory information entering and motor information exiting act as conduits between the neurons and the spinal nerve roots. The roots are segmentally located and carry information through the foramina of the vertebral column to skin areas, called dermatomes, and groups of muscles, called myotomes. It is important to note that one nerve root is usually responsible for a very specific skin area yet each muscle may be innervated by more than one nerve root.

When the spinal cord is injured there is a disruption in the motor and sensory pathways at the site of the lesion. Because of the segmental nature of the nerve roots, a thorough evaluation of motor and sensory function can identify the level of lesion. For example, if the spinal cord is completely severed at the level of the sixth cervical nerve root, motor and sensory information below that level will no longer be able to travel to and from the brain. This will result in a paralysis of muscular activity and an absence of sensation below the level of injury. Injury to the cord can be the result of disease, such as amyotrophic lateral sclerosis or multiple sclerosis; congenital deformities; tumors; or trauma. This chapter focuses on trauma-related injuries. The most common causes of traumatic spinal cord injuries are automobile accidents, gunshot and knife wounds, diving accidents, and falls (Parsons & Lammertse, 1991).

Many of the questions asked by patients and therapists new to spinal cord injury are related to terminology. What does incomplete mean? What is the difference between paraplegia and tetraplegia? What is a central cord syndrome? Fortunately, the American Spinal Injury Association (1992) has developed (and regularly revises and updates), standards for neurologic and functional classification of spinal cord injuries. These standards provide internationally accepted terms to define levels and types of injury.

The term tetraplegia has replaced quadriplegia. It is defined as an impairment in motor and/or sensory function in the cervical segments of the spinal cord. It is caused by damage of neural elements within the vertebral canal and cannot be used to describe injuries to peripheral nerves. Tetraplegia results in functional impairment in the arms, trunk, legs, and pelvic organs. The term paraplegia refers to motor and sensory impairment at the thoracic, lumbar, or sacral segments of the cord. Likewise, it only refers to damage to the neural elements inside the vertebral canal. Paraplegia results in sparing of arm function and, depending on the level of lesion, impairment in the trunk, legs, and pelvic organs (American Spinal Injury Association [ASIA], 1992).

There are four levels used to describe a spinal cord–injured person. The neurologic level refers to the lowest segment of the spinal cord with normal sensory and motor function on both sides of the body. Often a patient will have a neurologic level given for each side of the body for example C_{5-6}. The terms sensory level and motor level refer to the most caudal segment of the cord with normal sensory or motor function on both sides of the body. Finally, the term skeletal level refers to the level of greatest vertebral damage (ASIA, 1992).

Two other terms commonly used with spinal cord–injured patients are complete and incomplete injuries. The terms paraparesis and quadriparesis, which used to be used to describe incomplete injuries, are no longer encouraged. The term incomplete injury should be used only when there is partial preservation of sensory and/or motor function below the neurologic level and including the lowest sacral segment. Testing of innervation at the lowest sacral segment is performed by the physician, because it includes anal sensation and sphincter contraction. The term complete injury refers to an absence of sensory and motor function in the lowest sacral segment. A new term that is used for patients with complete injuries who have partial innervation in dermatomes and myotomes below the neurologic level is zone of partial preservation (ASIA, 1992).

There are four clinical syndromes that define a specific type of injury resulting in an unusual impairment of sensorimotor function. A central cord syndrome refers to a lesion that occurs in the cervical region, resulting in greater weakness in the upper limbs than in the lower limbs with sacral sparing. Brown-Sequard syndrome refers to a lesion in which there is ipsilateral proprioceptive and motor loss and contralateral loss of pain and temperature sensation. An anterior cord syndrome refers to a lesion with variable motor and sensory loss and preservation of proprioception. The conus medullaris syndrome is an injury to the sacral cord and lumbar nerve roots. These patients have areflexic bladder, bowel, and lower limbs (ASIA, 1992). All these syndromes can be explained by injury to specific tracts or nerve roots within the spinal cord.

ASSESSMENT

Good evaluation skills are important for an occupational therapist who works with the spinal cord–injured population. The initial occupational therapy evaluation is probably the most important. The evaluation must be thorough and accurate, because the entire medical team often looks to the occupational therapist's muscle and sensory evaluation to identify levels of injury. The initial evaluation is also used to chart progress during the rehabilitation stay and act as justification to the insurance company for a continuation of therapy. The initial evaluation is often the most difficult evaluation to perform, because the newly injured spinal cord patient is usually confused and scared. Therefore, how the occupational therapist approaches the evaluation can affect the results. No matter what psychological state the patient is in, the therapist must present herself as confident, empathetic, and positive. It is best to begin the evaluation with a brief description of occupational therapy and the areas that will be addressed. It is unnecessary to describe equipment or techniques in detail at this time, as this may be overwhelming to the patient. A brief social, vocational, and leisure history are also obtained. Even if this information is already stated in the medical chart, asking a patient about his job, hobbies, or family often opens communication and helps establish a rapport between the therapist and patient. The therapist avoids making any prognostic comments, especially in relation to possible functional gains. It is important to remember that the occupational therapist is only one member of a team of professionals evaluating the patient.

An assessment of a spinal cord–injured patient includes a passive range of motion evaluation, a manual muscle test, and a sensory evaluation (see Chapters 6 and 8). Comments regarding physical conditioning, endurance, and patient and family emotional reactions (see Chapter 10) are also included. The passive range of motion evaluation includes measurements of all upper extremity joints and all digits. The manual muscle test examines muscles of the scapula, shoulder, elbow, wrist, and digits. It may also include grip and pinch strength measurements. It is important to test all muscles regardless of diagnosis because of the possibility of zones of partial preservation or an incomplete injury. There are key muscles that are often used in reference to levels of injury. For example, the biceps is a key muscle for identification of innervation at the C_5 level (ASIA, 1992).

Similarly, the occupational therapist must perform a thorough sensory evaluation of all the dermatomes of the upper body. Sensation is evaluated for light touch, pin prick, joint proprioception, stereognosis, and kinesthesia. As is the case with muscle testing, there are key points for each dermatomal area.

Neurologic, motor, and sensory levels can be determined for the patient when the physician, physical therapist, and occupational therapist confer after completing their evaluations. The identification of these levels and determination of a complete or incomplete injury are key components in determining long- and short-term goals for the patient. The evaluations performed by all members of the team—especially the social worker, psychologist, and nurse—are important in helping the therapist customize goals for each particular patient. Areas that are particularly important to note are patient size and age, family support, employment and educational history, history of drug or alcohol abuse, and previous medical or psychological illness.

Throughout the rehabilitation stay, occupational therapy evaluations will continue to be needed. Reevaluations, which usually consist of a manual muscle test and a sensory test, are performed on a monthly basis for tetraplegics. Specific muscles that are improving are often tested on a weekly or even daily basis. There are other types of evaluations occupational therapists perform in spinal cord injury rehabilitation. These evaluations may assess performance in areas such as vocation (see Chapter 17), ADLs (see Chapter 4), access to home and community (see Chapter 5), leisure time activities (see Chapter 18), and driving. An evaluation is useful to the patient, insurance companies, and other support services such as vocational rehabilitation.

Once the patient has been evaluated, short- and long-term goals are developed. A chart of functional outcomes for each level of spinal cord injury is a useful tool for developing long-term goals (Table 39.1). The chart is used only as a reference and long-term goals are customized for each patient. For example, a patient with a T_{12} paraplegia who is obese may have difficulty handling his body and may not be able to dress independently in his wheelchair. Likewise, an 80-year-old tetraplegic may have difficulty adapting to the technology used for power mobility and control of the environment.

The most important consideration in developing long-term goals is patient involvement. Patients must

Table 39.1. Expected Achievement and Suggested Methods for Spinal Cord–Injured Patients

Last Fully Innervated Level and Key Muscles Added	Movements Patient Can Do	Functional Performance Areas	Technique or Equipment	Long-Term Goal
C_1–C_3 Facial and neck muscles innervated by cranial nerves	Chew Swallow Talk Blow	Self-care	a. Needs ventilator	Directs others for all applicable care, including pressure relief, skin precautions, upper extremity ROM techniques, equipment maintenance, activity and equipment setup procedures, upper extremity positioning in bed and w/c[a]
		Mobility 1. w/c	a. Electronically controlled electric w/c; can use sip and puff or head control b. Appropriate seating system for positioning and safety	Independent with w/c propulsion inside on hard level surfaces Independent with supervision outdoors on hard surfaces Dependent/directs others for assist with architectural barriers
		2. Pressure relief	a. Electronically controlled recline or tilt mechanism	Independent with power recline/tilt w/c
		Communication 1. Word processing	Computer using infrared head pointer, single- or dual-action switches, or mouthstick	Minimal assistance Maximal assistance for mouthstick with only limited use
		2. Telephone	Speaker phone, adapted for automatic dialing	
		Recreation 1. Games	a. Computer games b. Electronic games	Minimal assistance
		2. Art	Mouthstick painting with setup	
		3. Reading	Electronic page turner, or turn pages with mouthstick	Minimal assistance
		4. Other Vocation	Environmental control unit Computer with head pointer, switches, or mouthstick	Minimal assistance
C_4 Diaphragm Trapezius	Respiration Scapular elevation			An externally powered flexor hinge splint and powered mobile arm supports can be used to increase independence
		Self-care 1. Feeding	Long straw with straw holder	Minimal assistance for drinking
		2. Other		Directs others for all applicable care same as C_1–C_3

Table 39.1. Continued

Last Fully Innervated Level and Key Muscles Added	Movements Patient Can Do	Functional Performance Areas	Technique or Equipment	Long-Term Goal
		Mobility		
		1. w/c	Electronically controlled w/c using sip and puff, chin switch, or head control	Independent with w/c propulsion inside and outdoors on hard surfaces Independent with supervision outdoors on uneven terrain Dependent/directs others for assist with architectural barriers
		2. Pressure relief	Electronically controlled w/c with power recline/tilt mechanism	Independent with power recline/tilt w/c
		Communication		
		1. Word processing	a. Computer using infrared head pointer, single- or dual-action switches, or mouthstick b. Mouthstick holder	Modified independent
		2. Telephone	Speaker phone with automatic dialer	Modified independent
		3. Writing	Mouthstick with pencil or pen attached	Modified independent
		4. Note taking in school or business	Adapted tape recorder	
		Recreation		
		1. Art	Mouthstick with brush, or pencil attached	Modified independent
		2. Reading	a. Mouthstick for page turning	Modified independent
			b. Electronic page turner	Minimal assistance
		3. Other	Environmental control unit	Modified independent
C$_5$ Biceps Brachialis Brachioradialis Supinator Infraspinatus Deltoid	Elbow flexion and supination Shoulder external rotation Shoulder abduction to 80–90° Gravity provides shoulder adduction, pronation, and internal rotation			A ratchet splint can be used to increase levels of functional independence
		Self-care		
		1. Feeding	a. Mobile arm support or suspension sling b. Dorsal wrist splint with u-cuff[a] c. Dycem to stabilize plate d. Plate guard or scoop dish e. Stabilized cup or cup holder f. Long straw with straw holder g. Angled spoon or fork	Minimal assistance
		2. Dressing		Moderate assistance with upper extremity Maximal assistance with lower extremity
		3. Grooming	a. Wash mit b. Quad grip hairbrush	Minimal assistance with washing face,

Table 39.1. Continued

Last Fully Innervated Level and Key Muscles Added	Movements Patient Can Do	Functional Performance Areas	Technique or Equipment	Long-Term Goal
			c. Adaptations made to makeup to fit in u-cuff	makeup application, and brushing teeth
				Moderate assistance with brushing hair
		4. Bathing	Quad grip long-handled bath sponge	Moderate assistance with upper extremity
				Maximal assistance with lower extremity
		5. Upper extremity ROM		Maximal assistance
		Mobility		
		1. w/c	Hand-controlled power w/c	Independent on hard surfaces inside and outdoors
				Independent with supervision outdoors on uneven terrain
				Dependent/directs others for assist with architectural barriers
			Manual w/c with projection knobs	Independent on level surfaces for short distances (100 feet or less)
		2. Pressure relief	Power recline or tilt w/c with use of elbow or head switches	Independent with power recline/tilt w/c
				Moderate assistance for side to side in manual w/c
		Communication		
		1. Word processing	Typing stick placed in dorsal wrist splint with u-cuff	Minimal assistance
		2. Writing	Long writing orthosis	Minimal assistance
		3. Telephone	Push button speaker phone using typing stick to press buttons	Minimal assistance
		4. Reading	Turn pages manually using book holder and typing stick in dorsal wrist splint with u-cuff	Minimal assistance
C_6 Pectoralis major Serratus anterior Lattisimus dorsi Pronator teres Radial wrist extensors	Shoulder flexion Reach forward Shoulder internal rotation and extension Shoulder adduction More respiratory reserve (accessory breathing muscles) Pronation Wrist extension (tenodesis grasp)			Wrist driven flexor hinge splint or RIC tenodesis training splint may be used to increase levels of independence and ease
		Self-care		
		1. Feeding	a. May use u-cuff b. Rocker knife or very sharp paring knife for cutting c. Does not need long straw; may use cup with large handle	Modified independent

Table 39.1. Continued

Last Fully Innervated Level and Key Muscles Added	Movements Patient Can Do	Functional Performance Areas	Technique or Equipment	Long-Term Goal
			d. Does not need plate guard	
		2. Grooming	Brushing teeth, shaving, makeup application, hair care can be done using the tenodesis grasp and/or modified equipment	Modified independent
		3. Bathing	a. Shower/tub bench with faucet within reach b. Hand-held shower hose	Minimal assistance
		4. Bowel and bladder care	a. Inserts suppositories with adaptive device b. Adapted handle on dil stick c. Independent transfer to toilet or commode d. Self-catherization e. Apply condom, tubing and storage bag for external drainage system f. Adapted clamp for drainage bag	Male-minimal assistance for intermittent catherization, condom application, leg bag care, and bowel program. Female-maximal assistance for intermittent catheterization
		5. Dressing	a. Dresses lower extremities in bed as described in Chapter 15; uses momentum and substitute movements to turn over, sit up, and pull up clothing b. Uses button hook and zipper pull c. Clothes should be of correct size or larger	Upper extremity: modified independent Lower extremity: pants, minimal assistance; shoes and socks, maximal assistance
		6. Upper extremity ROM		Modified independent
		Mobility		
		1. w/c	Pushes manual w/c with friction material on rims or projection knobs; an electric w/c may be required for long distances	Independent in propelling manual w/c on level surfaces Minimal assistance propelling on uneven surfaces Moderate assistance for architectural barriers Independent driving power w/c
		2. Transfer	Uses a transfer board and partial depression or swivel transfer	Independent
		3. Bed mobility	a. Uses the method described in Chapter 15 b. May require loops attached to the base of the bed	Modified independent for rolling and supine to long sitting Moderate assistance for proning, padding and positioning
		4. Vehicle	Drive using hand controls with adapted steering wheel	Modified independent

Table 39.1. Continued

Last Fully Innervated Level and Key Muscles Added	Movements Patient Can Do	Functional Performance Areas	Technique or Equipment	Long-Term Goal
		5. Pressure relief		Independent side to side
		Communication		
		1. Word processing	Uses u-cuff or tenodesis grasp to hold typing stick	Modified independent
		2. Writing	Uses tenodesis grasp to hold pen or short writing orthosis	Modified independent
		3. Telephone	Uses any telephone with phone holder or uses tenodesis grasp to hold receiver	Modified independent
		Recreation	a. Can turn radio, TV, etc. on and off	
			b. Can play table games with some adaption	
			c. Can participate in some w/c sports	
		Vocation	a. Cannot use hand tools that require strength	
			b. Electronic office machines are well suited to these patients	
			c. Homemaking, can do light cooking and cleaning; needs a w/c-accessible kitchen	Light work, minimal assistance Heavy work, maximal assistance
C_7 Triceps Extrinsic finger extensors Flexor carpi radialis	Elbow extension Active finger extension (tenodesis grasp) Wrist flexion	Self-care 1. Feeding		Modified independent
		2. Dressing	a. Button hook only b. w/c dressing	Modified independent Minimal assistance
		3. Bathing/ grooming	Same as C_6, but easier	Modified independent
		4. Bowel and bladder	Same as C_6, but easier	Male: modified independent Female: modified independent
		Mobility a. w/c	Manual w/c	Independent with propulsion over flat surfaces and inclines Independent/ supervision for rough terrain Doors: modified independent Elevators: independent
		2. Pressure relief		Independent with push ups
		3. Bed mobility		Independent Minimal assistance with padding and positioning
		4. Transfers		Independent
		5. Vehicle	Uses modified car	Modified independent
		Communication	Same as C_6, but easier	Modified independent

Table 39.1.   Continued

Last Fully Innervated Level and Key Muscles Added	Movements Patient Can Do	Functional Performance Areas	Technique or Equipment	Long-Term Goal
		Recreation and vocation	Same as C_6, but easier	
C_8-T_1 Intrinsics, including thumb Ulnar wrist flexors and extensors Extrinsic finger and thumb flexors Extrinsic thumb extensor	Full upper extremity control, including fine coordination and grasp	Self-care, mobility, and communication	Same as C_7, but easier	Same as C_7, except w/c dressing is modified independent and padding and positioning is modified independent
T_6 Top half of intercostals Long muscles of the back	Increased endurance due to larger respiratory reserve Pectoral girdle stabilized for heavy lifting	Self-care Mobility Vocation	No assistive devices a. Uses full braces and a standing aid for physiologic standing only b. Can ambulate with great difficulty, on level surfaces Can work with tools and do fairly heavy lifting from a sedentary position	Independent
T_{12} Full innervation of intercostals Abdominal muscles	Better endurance Better trunk control	Self-care, work, sports, and housekeeping Mobility	Uses w/c for energy conservation Ambulates with difficulty using long leg braces and crutches Can use ride-on snow plow, grass cutter, etc. with hand controls	Independent
L_4 Low back muscles Hip flexors Quadriceps	Hip flexion Knee extension	Mobility Bowel and bladder	Uses canes to prevent deforming effects of gait (recurvatum of knee and lumbar lordosis) that could cause degenerative arthritis; uses short leg braces; w/c may still be a convenience at work and home Bowel and bladder control is not voluntary	Independent in all activities plus ambulation

^{a}w/c, wheelchair; u-cuff, universal cuff.

play an active role in the developing and prioritizing of goals, especially long term (Jordan et al., 1991). The development of short-term goals stems from the therapist's ability to perform an activity analysis. Short-term goals may address functional performance areas and tasks, or they may address underlying problems or the component skills necessary to perform an ADL. For example, for a C_4 tetraplegic to use a mouthstick for word processing on the computer, he must be able to tolerate sitting upright in his wheelchair for significant periods of time. Increasing sitting tolerance at 90° is an appropriate short-term goal for achieving independence in mouthstick computer use. It is important to remember that goals are written to help both the patient and the therapist in directing care. Long-term goals can always be changed and continuous communication with the patient regarding progress toward goals is vital.

TREATMENT

Complications and Precautions

The leading cause of death among tetraplegics and spinal cord–injured patients who are at least 55 years of age is pneumonia (DeVivo et al., 1990a). Although these patients usually contract pneumonia after completing rehabilitation, it is important for the therapist to consider the jeopardized pulmonary status of such patients. In lesions above C_4, damage to the phrenic nerve results in partial or complete paralysis of the diaphragm. These patients require ventilatory support (Hanak & Scott, 1983). Cervical spine injuries can result in paralysis of the accessory breathing muscles such as the intercostals. Most occupational therapists working in spinal cord rehabilitation centers are expected to be familiar with basic **ventilator** operation and must be able to suction secretions and facilitate coughing. Facilitated coughing, also known as assisted coughing, is performed with the patient in a supine position and the therapist's hands placed just below the sternum with one hand on top of the other. The patient is instructed to inhale deeply, and as he exhales pressure is placed by the therapist in an inward and upward direction (Ireland, n.d.). Using proper techniques and following infection control standards are important for respiratory care.

One of the first precautions therapists must consider is spine stabilization. A newly injured patient's spine may not be properly stabilized. Depending on the level and type of vertebral damage, a variety of stabilization procedures are used. Surgical stabilization may involve fusing of the vertebrae, wiring, or insertion of rods or springs. Tetraplegic patients may be placed in a halo device, which is an external fixation device that screws into the skull and maintains a neutral head position (King & Dudas, 1980). Later, they may be placed in hard or soft neck collars for added support and movement restriction. Paraplegic patients may be placed in lumbar jackets, which inhibit trunk flexibility (King & Dudas, 1980). The role of the occupational therapist in spine stabilization is to follow the precautions set by the physician and be sure the spine is stabilized before evaluating the patient or encouraging the patient to participate in any activities.

Postural or orthostatic hypotension is most commonly seen in patients with lesions at the T_6 level and above. The patient may complain of light headedness and dizziness and may faint when moving from a reclined to an upright position. This is caused by a dramatic fall in blood pressure from a disturbance in the vasomotor control system. There is a decrease in the returning blood supply to the heart because of blood pooling in the lower extremities. The therapist must use caution when sitting the patient up and have the patient move slowly and in stages, letting the blood pressure adjust to each increment (Benda, 1983). This can be performed by elevating the head of the bed, using a tilt table, or using a reclining wheelchair. Abdominal binders and elastic stockings are often used to control this problem (Closson et al., 1991).

Immobility and decreased vasomotor tone in the blood vessels may result in pulmonary emboli and thrombophlebitis. The occupational therapist must follow all restrictions set by the physician and inform the nurse or physician of any symptoms. Signs of a pulmonary embolism are a sudden onset of shortness of breath, hyperventilation, apprehension, and cardiac arrhythmias (Benda, 1983). Venous thrombosis can be detected by routine blood flow studies and inspection for swelling and redness in the lower extremities (Benda, 1983).

Heterotophic calcification has been recorded in 15 to 20% of spinal cord injury cases (Zejdlik, 1983). It is a condition in which there is calcification of connective tissue around the joint. Heterotophic ossificans usually appears 1 to 4 months after injury. The symptoms are a warm, swollen extremity and a fever. It is most often seen in the hip and shoulder joints and can result in joint contractures. Although it has not been proven to be effective, daily range of motion is performed in an attempt to prevent or control heterotophic ossificans.

Autonomic dysreflexia is usually seen in patients with lesions at T_6 and above. It is a sympathetic reflex response to adverse stimuli. The most common causes are distended bladder, fecal impaction, pressure sores, ingrown toenails, any infectious process, catherization, or enemas (Benda, 1983). The symptoms include hypertension, headache, sweating, flushing, pupil constriction, nasal congestion, and goose bumps (Benda, 1983). The immediate treatment is to elevate the head and remove the cause (Benda, 1983). Autonomic dysreflexia can result in death if not treated immediately; therefore, the patient and his caregivers must be knowledgeable of the symptoms and treatment.

The spinal cord–injured patient has an inability to regulate body temperature, which can lead to hypothermia or heat stroke (Pierce & Nickel, 1977). Because of decreased sensation, patients may become severely sun burned or frost bitten. Education in the importance of neutral temperatures and the prevention of skin exposure to severe temperatures is an important part of the occupational therapy program (Pierce & Nickel, 1977).

Another leading cause of death among spinal cord–injured patients is septicemia, which usually results from urinary tract infections or pressure sores (DeVivo et al., 1990a). Pressure sores are a common problem for spinal cord–injured people. Most patients do not have the sensory feedback that periodically cues them to shift positions in their wheelchair. The constant pressure caused by maintaining a static position without shifting weight can lead to skin breakdown. All patients must be placed on a weight shifting, pressure-relief schedule. Pressure relief is performed to remove the pressure from the buttock area and allow the capillaries to refill (Trombly, 1989). It is recommended that the patient perform a pressure relief while in his wheelchair for 1 min every 30 min.

Pressure reliefs are performed different ways, depending on the level of injury. Tetraplegics at C_5 and above recline or tilt their wheelchairs. They can be independent in performing pressure relief by the use of a power recline or tilt mechanism, which can be operated by an elbow, head, or pneumatic switch. C_6 tetraplegics may perform pressure relief by bending forward or to each side. Webbing loops can be attached to the wheelchair to help the patient regain his upright position and prevent falling during the shift (Trombly, 1989). Patients at the C_7 level and below have innervation of the triceps and can perform push-ups by extending their arms and raising their buttocks off the seat (Trombly, 1989). While in bed, the patient should also be on a regular turning schedule. Timers with alarms are used with patients who have difficulty remembering to relieve pressure. Padding and positioning are two other important components in decubitus ulcer prevention. While in bed or on a therapy mat, all bony prominences should be padded to prevent skin breakdown. While in the wheelchair, an appropriate seating system and cushion should be used that is customized for each patient (Brown, 1992; Post, 1991; see also Chapters 23 and 30). Daily skin inspection for red areas is usually taught by the rehabilitation nurse using hand mirrors. Occupational therapists are also concerned with skin integrity during treatment and especially during splinting and casting. A small reddened area can quickly become a large sore. During ADL training care is taken to make sure the patient is not rubbing his skin on a surface such as the bed sheet or bumping an area of his body on a piece of equipment such as the wheelchair during a transfer.

Lesions at the T_{12} vertebrae and above usually result in what is termed a spastic paralysis. Upper motor neurons are long neurons that originate in the brain and travel within the spinal cord, where they synapse with lower motor neurons at each segmental level. The brain, via the upper motor neurons, controls the lower motor neurons and prevents them from becoming hyperactive to local stimuli. An injury to the upper motor neurons will result in a lack of this cerebral control over reflex activity (Zejdlik, 1983). In fact, an injury to the spinal cord often results in an increase in transmission within the synaptic stretch reflex (Bishop, 1982). This results in spasticity.

Spasticity develops into clonic or tonic spasms. They are triggered by sensory stimuli such as sudden touch, infection or other irritation (Trombly, 1989). Removing the stimuli may be one way of controlling a spasm, but usually it is not that simple. Management of spasticity is important in maximizing a patient's functional independence. Some patients learn to trigger and use their spasticity to help them in activities such as transferring and dressing. Many patients however are hindered by spasticity. One of the most effective management techniques today is the use of skeletal muscle relaxant medications (Brown, 1992). The intrathecal pump, motor point, and nerve blocks may be used in severe cases (Ditunno et al., 1992). Spasticity can lead to contractures and therefore neutral positioning and regular range of motion are two important treatments the occupational therapist can perform in spasticity management.

Spinal shock is a neurovascular shutdown that occurs immediately after a spinal cord injury. It is characterized by a temporary flaccid paralysis, which is caused by a suppression of all reflex activity. Spinal shock may last for hours, days, weeks, or months. It is important for the occupational therapist to consider the effects of spinal shock when evaluating the patient and during the determination of goals.

Phase I

Also known as the acute phase, the first phase in spinal cord injury rehabilitation is important for education and the prevention of future problems. As described previously, a newly injured patient must be handled with great care, both physically and emotionally.

During the acute phase, patients are usually restricted to their beds. They may be in traction awaiting spine stabilization or recovering from surgery. The occupational therapist begins seeing the patient within 48 hr of admission (Trombly, 1989), which may be in an intensive care unit. The first task is to evaluate the patient within the limits of precautions. As soon as the evaluation has been performed, the patient must be placed on a daily range of motion program. The occupational therapist may need to educate the staff, patient, and family in proper positioning of the upper extremities. While in a supine position, the patient's upper extremities should be placed with the shoulder externally rotated and abducted to 90°. The elbow is flexed and the palms face the ceiling. A pillow may be placed under the forearms to compensate for external rotation restrictions. In side lying, a pillow is placed in a vertical position under the thoracic region of the trunk. The bottom upper extremity is placed in 100° of shoulder flexion. The elbow is flexed or extended with the palm facing the ceiling. The top upper extremity is placed on pillows in a comfortable position in front of the patient.

It is at this time that tetraplegic patients, especially at the C_6 and C_7 level, begin facilitation of a **tenodesis grasp.** During range of motion of the hand, the therapist must keep the wrist extended while the fingers are flexed and the wrist flexed while the fingers are extended (Wilson, 1984). Failure to develop the necessary tightening for a **tenodesis grasp** during the initial stages of rehabilitation can prevent a patient from achieving functional independence (see Table 39.1). Splints may be used to facilitate positioning, but it is important that all joint positioning be done with consideration of future function (Krajnik & Bridle, 1992; see also Chapters 28 and 29).

Another important role of the occupational therapist at this time is to provide the patient with a basic environmental control. Most patients wish to have independent access to the television, telephone, and nurse call system (McDonald, Boyle, & Schumann, 1989). There are many systems available, including pneumatic (sip and puff) and various switches depending on the patients needs (see Chapter 31). By providing this access to patients early in their program, a sense of independence and self-control are immediately facilitated.

Education begins with the first visit by the occupational therapist. The acute phase is the time to educate the patient in the most important basic issues related to his injury. This is a good time to stress the importance of skin management, pressure relief, and daily range of motion (Trombly, 1989). Patients will quickly begin asking questions regarding their prognosis in relation to performance of daily living skills. It is important to encourage patients and describe the level of control that can continue in their life, but use caution in creating a false sense of hope. Education of the family also begins at this time. Questions regarding accessibility at home can help the family begin thinking about home modifications and the discharge plan. Because rehabilitation stays may be as short as 8 weeks, the family must immediately begin planning for discharge. As the patient becomes more medically stable, ADL training and a strengthening program can begin. This is especially useful to patients who are on prolonged bed rest for medical complications such as skin breakdown.

The following is an example of a treatment sequence for a spinal cord–injured patient in the first phase of rehabilitation. The patient is admitted into the intensive care unit of the hospital. He is placed in traction as he awaits surgery to stabilize his spine. The medical personnel evaluate him and orders are received for occupational therapy. The occupational therapist performs the evaluation and begins daily passive range of motion and education. The patient undergoes surgery and orders are resumed for occupational therapy. Nighttime positioning splints are fabricated and an **environmental control unit** is set up, allowing the patient access to the nurse call system and television. Light upper extremity strengthening is begun to increase strength and endurance for phase II. With orders from the physician, the patient is placed in a wheelchair and begins tolerating sitting upright; there is a focus on following the pressure-relief schedule. As the patient becomes medically stable, he is moved out of the intensive care unit. He is able to tolerate being in a wheelchair and can participate in the strengthening activities. He is now ready for phase II.

Phase II

The second phase is also known as the rehabilitation phase. A biomechanical approach is used for strengthening (Trombly, 1989). Strengthening is an important goal in this phase and can be performed by using weights, pulley systems, skateboards, suspension slings, **mobile arm supports,** and modalities such as **EMG biofeedback** and **functional electrical stimulation** (Harnish, 1990; Klose et al., 1990; Trombly, 1989; Wu et al., 1992; Yarkony et al., 1992; see also Chapters 22, 32, and 33).

Regaining independence in activities of daily living is another area of focus during this phase. Instruction followed by trial and error appears to be the most successful method for working on ADLs (Trombly, 1989). Each patient must determine which technique will work for him. Some patients learn by observing others with similar levels of injury, thus many centers use a group approach (Machmer, 1979). Other patients may require step-by-step instruction from the therapist. Time is another important consideration in ADL training. Early morning and mealtimes are the best times to practice bathing, dressing, and feeding (see Chapter 15). It is also important for patients to practice their ADL skills in situations similar to home and work. A patient may be able to dress without difficulty on a firm hospital bed but return home to a soft bed and be dependent. Weekend passes home are beneficial in identifying these problems, and many centers have apartment or work areas set up to simulate the home and work environments.

Bowel and bladder training are two specific ADL areas unique to spinal cord injury. Patients with injuries at C_5 and above will require assistance in both bowel and bladder training. Patients with injuries at C_6 and below can be independent with the use of adaptive equipment (Dailey & Michael, 1977). The rehabilitation nurse usually has the primary role in teaching the patient how to use techniques and adaptive equipment for bowel and bladder emptying. The occupational therapist may need to assist by fabricating and modifying equipment or providing suggestions for positioning. Bladder control is usually regulated through medications and the use of **intermittent catheterization** for emptying (Brown, 1992). Bowel training usually consists of the use of suppositories and/or **digital stimulation.** The therapist's role in all ADL training is to give the patient suggestions for techniques and offer facilitory equipment. She also has the unique ability to perform an activity analysis and can be helpful in problem solving for positioning and techniques with difficult patients. Most important, the occupational therapist can provide emotional support and encouragement through this frustrating time (see Chapter 20).

Education again plays an important role during the rehabilitation phase. Groups are often used to educate patients on a variety of subjects, including accessibility rights, fire safety, environmental temperature management, home modifications, and travel. Educational programs on video are available from some of the major spinal cord injury centers and may be useful. Sexuality is another important area of education. Sexuality may be discussed in a group setting or on an individual basis. Sexual functioning is less affected in female patients who usually resume menstruating within 6 months postinjury (King & Dudas, 1980). Male patients, however, are usually unable to have a psychogenic erection and ejaculate. Male patients with injuries at S_{2-4} have a complete loss of erection. Patients with injuries at all other levels have reflex erections that are uncontrollable (King & Dudas, 1980). Although these may be embarrassing, reflex erections can be useful during **intermittent catheterization** and sexual expression. Advances in technology have provided ways for male patients to sustain an erection during intercourse and improve the chances of fathering children (Brown, 1992; Stien, 1992). It is important that all patients be educated in the equipment and techniques available to them. The four areas that need to be addressed are satisfaction, function, fertility, and desirability (King & Dudas, 1980). The educator must be both knowledgeable and well trained to deal with this sensitive subject (Novak & Mitchell, 1988). Patients must learn that despite this injury they can continue their sexual role (Novak & Mitchell, 1988). Previous patients who have been living successfully with a spinal cord injury are wonderful speakers for all educational groups.

During the rehabilitation phase, the patient is bombarded with treatment. Patients are often participating in physical, occupational, and recreational therapy; attending psychological sessions and support groups; and participating in community outings. The occupational therapist must maximize her designated time. This can be done many ways. As mentioned previously, morning self-care time and mealtimes are good occupational therapy times. During treatment, the occupational therapist can combine several goals. Combining strengthening with practicing an activity of daily living is a useful technique, e.g., instead of having a patient perform repetitive motions with his arms in an overhead arm sling, have him practice page turning at the same time. While the patient is doing daily passive range of motion, the therapist can discuss goals with him, or the motions can be performed during an educational group setting.

Family training also begins in this phase and is composed of both an educational and practical component. The occupational therapist educates the families in range of motion and positioning of the upper extremities, performance of regular pressure relief, and ADLs including transfers and the use of any equipment. It is best to allow family members to practice these techniques and feel comfortable before the patient goes home even for a weekend pass. This is especially true regarding use of complex pieces of equipment and when a spastic extremity is ranged. Families should also be involved in the purchasing of any major equipment, including the wheelchair and bathroom equipment. Home modifications are discussed and determined by what is appropriate for both the patient and his family. A wheelchair prescription must consider not only mobility and positioning but transportation and home accessibility as well as a place of attachment for various pieces of adapted equipment. Good communication with a patient's family is often a key ingredient in the success of rehabilitation.

Patients react to the rehabilitation phase in many different ways. Patients are often angry, frustrated, and depressed. Patients may also be in denial or act apathetic. Fortunately, many patients work through or put aside these feelings and manage to focus on therapy (see Chapters 10 and 20 for suggestions to facilitate this process). For all patients the devastation of a spinal cord injury is still very new and even the most positive patient is likely to have difficult periods. It is important to try to work with each patient on an individual basis within their psychological means (Brown, 1992; Lammertse & Yarkony, 1991). This is a difficult task for many therapists, because the patient's psychological status may affect the physical attainment of functional goals.

An example of a treatment plan in phase II begins with a focus on strengthening. The patient must work on strengthening weak muscles, especially of the scapula and shoulder. This is done by using **functional electrical stimulation, EMG biofeedback,** Swedish aide (overhead pulley system), skateboards, and active or active-assistive range of motion. Daily passive range of motion is continued. Once the patient has developed a strong foundation, light ADL activity training is begun. This may include turning pages, self-feeding with a **mobile arm support** for part of the meal, or bed mobility. As the patient continues to gain strength, the more difficult ADLs are added. During all of phase II the patient is participating in education and support groups. He also is going on community outings and, toward the end of this phase, may go home for a weekend. As the patient is able to perform basic ADLs appropriate for his level of injury and is getting ready for discharge he moves into phase III.

Phase III

The third phase of rehabilitation is also known as the discharge phase. The discharge phase is a time for patients to prepare for return home. It usually includes the last 3 to 4 weeks of inpatient rehabilitation. Independence is the key focus during this time. The emphasis is taken off of strengthening and learning basic skills and placed on perfecting skills already learned. It is important that the therapist begin encouraging the patient to work more independently. This is a good time to let the patient decide what areas he feels need to be practiced before returning home.

Other areas of treatment that often take place in this phase are the driving evaluation and vocational evaluation. It is important that these evaluations not be performed too early in rehabilitation so that the patient can be assessed for his true level of independence. During this phase, the occupational therapist can evaluate the patient for functional independence in a work setting. It is important to keep in mind that the majority of spinal cord–injured patients do not return to work (Alfred, Fuhrer, & Rossi, 1987). Of those who do return, most do not begin until at least 2 years after discharge. Studies have shown that most spinal cord–injured patients are not ready to deal with vocational issues during inpatient rehabilitation or during the first few months after discharge. Priorities are on medical needs and adjustment to family and home. Issues such as transportation, availability of an attendant, and availability of job opportunities make employment more difficult for the disabled. Current government social policies also create financial disincentives (Alfred et al., 1987; Crisp, 1990; Lammertse & Yarkony, 1991). The occupational therapist can provide vocational support during inpatient rehabilitation by discussing future employment options and the use of vocational rehabilitation services. It is often helpful to facilitate communication with a vocational rehabilitation counselor from the patient's home environment who may be useful to the patient as a resource

in the future. Driving evaluations and training are also performed by occupational therapists. Modifications can be made to automobiles and vans to allow patients with injuries at C_5 and below to drive (Brown, 1992). A thorough driving evaluation must consider visual, cognitive, and physical abilities before being initiated. Driving evaluations should be performed by therapists who have had extensive training in this area.

Education is again an important component of this phase. Time management techniques are useful to this population, given the effort required for performance of daily activities. Assertiveness training and how to instruct caregivers and attendants are other important educational programs. Patients should also be educated in the community services and support groups available to them after discharge.

The discharge phase is a difficult time for both the patient and the therapist. Therapists often feel responsible for their patients, especially those with higher, more involved injuries. It is difficult to discharge a patient, if the therapist realizes that the patient may be returning to a dysfunctional environment. Patients may also be anxious about their discharge from this safe, supportive environment. By allowing the patient the opportunity to demonstrate his independence and regain control over his life, both the patient and the therapist are well prepared for the discharge.

As stated above, the focus of phase III is fine-tuning. The treatment sequence for this phase involves continued daily passive range of motion (PROM) as appropriate and ADL training in more advanced skills such as wheelchair dressing. A driving evaluation is performed and vocational issues discussed. The patient is encouraged to work independently, verbally direct all necessary assistance, and practice a typical daily routine as it will be postdischarge. The therapist prepares for the discharge by making sure the patient has the necessary equipment and by setting up outpatient therapy if appropriate.

Postdischarge Treatment

Spinal cord–injured patients may be seen on an outpatient basis for upgrading, which may include vocational training and tendon transfers. Some patients continue to gain strength for up to 2 years after their injury (Ditunno et al., 1992). This increase in strength may allow the patient to become more independent. Patients may be placed in an outpatient program to learn how to use new movement or for intensive ADL training. Orthotic training is another area that may be performed during inpatient rehabilitation and/or on an outpatient basis. Because of poor patient carryover, the use of a hand orthosis, such as the wrist-driven or ratchet brace, has decreased significantly over the past few years (Shepherd & Ruziecka, 1991). In the past, patients were routinely given these expensive, customized braces. Studies have demonstrated that many braces were never used after discharge (Garber & Gregorio, 1990; Krajnik & Bridle, 1992; Shepherd & Ruziecka, 1991). As a result, most centers have a policy stating that to be placed in a training program, a patient must sign a contract committing himself to using the brace daily during performance of all ADL activities.

The philosophy of tendon transfers has changed over the past few years. The majority of model spinal cord injury centers in the United States do not perform tendon transfers. This may be for several reasons, including a lack of physicians skilled in performing this type of surgery. Patient motivation is a major factor even at centers performing this procedure. Tendon transfers are performed after a patient has been discharged from the rehabilitation program. After several months of rehabilitation, many patients do not wish to undergo surgery with its complications and long recovery period of total dependence. It is important that all patients be educated in both the equipment and surgical procedures available to them so that they can make an educated decision as to whether to pursue these options.

Improvements in medicine have led to an increase in an aging spinal cord injury population (Eisenberg & Saltz, 1991; Lammertse & Yarkony, 1991; Sie et al., 1992). While working with newly injured patients it is important for occupational therapist to consider both the short- and long-term consequences of movement patterns and positioning. There are natural physiologic processes that take place as the body ages. The effect of the disability on this aging process can be seen in many areas, e.g., the continued use of a manual wheelchair can contribute to degenerative joint changes or nerve entrapment in the upper extremities (Lammertse & Yarkony, 1991). Other areas in which the spinal cord injury interacts with aging include respiratory status, bowel motility, and coping mechanisms (Lammertse & Yarkony, 1991). Patients who have aged with a spinal cord injury may begin losing function as their body changes (Lammertse & Yarkony, 1991; Menter et al., 1991). Occupational therapy may be needed to assist with adaptive equipment or new techniques to help this population maintain functional independence.

Problem Solving

SPECIAL POPULATIONS

Treatment of a spinal cord injury is in itself a tremendous challenge for any occupational therapist, but adding a head injury to the diagnosis seems over-

whelming. Because of the traumatic nature of both injuries, this dual diagnosis is not uncommon, e.g., as the result of a motor vehicle accident. Cognitive skills important to spinal cord rehabilitation include problem solving, visual perception, and attention. Because these skills are frequently affected by a head injury, the spinal cord therapist must learn how to accommodate. It is often necessary to begin the head- and spinal cord–injured patient's treatment with a focus on maximizing cognitive functions (see Chapters 27 and 35). The spinal cord therapist will need to adjust the treatment techniques and goals to work within the patient's cognitive abilities. This may include a significant downgrading of long-term goals and an increase in repetition for practicing basic skills.

Having a spinal cord injury and being elderly may be considered a dual diagnosis. The physiological process of aging can make rehabilitation from a spinal cord injury even more difficult (Penrod, Hegde, & Ditunno, 1990; Teasell & Allatt, 1991). Most geriatric spinal cord injuries are attributed to falls that result in lesions at the cervical level (DeVivo et al., 1990b; Teasell & Allatt, 1991; Yarkony, Roth, Heinemann, & Lovell, 1988). The central cord syndrome is common among the elderly spinal cord–injured population. Age at the time of spinal cord injury is another factor that affects treatment techniques and goal setting. Some important areas to consider include muscle strength, endurance or physical fitness, joint degeneration, skin integrity, cognition, and emotional status (Teasell & Allatt, 1991). The geriatric population may require downgrading of goals given physical and cognitive limitations (Penrod et al., 1990; Teasell & Allatt, 1991).

The pediatric population also has goals specific to its needs. This population varies tremendously with age. It is important to consider the developmental level of the child in selecting goals. The therapist must also consider what activities will need to be learned as the child continues to develop (Johnson, 1989). Family education is extremely important with this population. Assisting with transition back into the school environment is another important component of pediatric spinal cord rehabilitation.

Improvement in the management of spinal cord injury immediately after the accident has led to a significant increase in incomplete injuries (DeVivo et al., 1990a). It is important for each patient to be evaluated for the possibility of an incomplete injury. Frequent reevaluations are vital in discovering the return of muscle activity that may be strengthened and become functional. It is important to remember that the gain of even one neurologic level can make a dramatic difference in the level of functional independence. Despite their positive prognosis, patients with incomplete injuries often have a greater difficulty coping with their illness and the uncertainty of return. Ambulatory patients, may receive less empathy from fellow patients and staff members. It is important to consider the devastation of any paralysis even if it affects only bowel, bladder, or hand function. Long-term goal setting for incompletely injured patients is difficult, because their muscle and sensory picture may be changing weekly or even daily. Long-term goals can be changed, and so it is best to set them at a lower functional level and upgrade them as the patient improves.

TIME LIMITATIONS

One of the most frustrating aspects of spinal cord injury rehabilitation is the time limitation. The amount of time for rehabilitation is determined by the medical staff and the insurance company. Most spinal cord–injured patients without major medical complications will be in the hospital for 2 to 4 months. The therapist must maximize the time allotted for each of her patients by using patient-directed, prioritized goals. Each patient is educated at the beginning of rehabilitation about the areas he can choose to work on. The patient then indicates which are most important to him. Those are worked on first. This is often difficult for therapists who may see different priorities for the patient. One study asked C_{5-6} patients and occupational therapists to prioritize goals. The patients listed development of work tolerance, muscle strengthening, and bowel and bladder control as the most valued. Occupational therapists listed development of adaptive devices, feeding, socialization, wheelchair mobility, driver education and bowel and bladder control as the priority goals (Taylor, 1974). Goals that are selected and prioritized by the patient not only will assist in motivation during rehabilitation training but also will result in better carryover after discharge. Using the entire rehabilitation team is another important way to maximize rehabilitation time. The physical therapist and nurse are two of the most important team members with whom the occupational therapist should work closely. For example, a component of an ADL activity such as balance and bed mobility skills required for dressing may be practiced during physical therapy. Communication with team members is vital in successful rehabilitation.

FUNDING AND EQUIPMENT

Occupational therapists have a tendency to over-equip their patients. As medical costs have increased, patients and their insurance companies have become more aware of the cost of equipment (Smith, 1988). As a result, occupational therapists must be more resourceful. Two options for reducing the cost of medical equipment are fabricating the equipment from low-cost items and using over-the-counter items. Before providing a patient with a piece of equipment, it is important to make sure the patient wants it and will be willing to use it. A tremendous amount of occupational therapy equipment given to patients is never used (Garber & Gregorio, 1990; McDonald et al., 1989; Shepherd & Ruziecka, 1991). If a patient needs a piece of equipment and funding is a problem, the occupational therapist can help figure a way to fabricate it or substitute. For example, there are **environmental control units** available at consumer electronic stores that are simple to install and to use and cost a fraction of the more complex units. Imaginative, resourceful occupational therapists can turn a simple hair clip into a catheter holder or a pillow into an elbow splint. The key point in the use of equipment for spinal cord injury rehabilitation is to use imagination and creativity in providing patients with equipment they not only need but also want.

Being an advocate for the patient is another important aspect of spinal cord injury rehabilitation. Many patients are not able to afford expensive home or vehicle modifications. It is important to assist patients in identifying available support services in the area and encourage patients to seek funding assistance. Community fund-raisers planned by family members or friends are often successful, especially for funding of a particular item.

CONTRACTURES AND SHOULDER PAIN

Paralysis and spasticity are two contributing factors to joint contractures. There are patterns of spasticity that are frequently seen in patients with different levels of injuries. Spasticity of an agonistic muscle, coupled with paralysis of an antagonistic muscle can lead to a joint contracture. One of the most frequently seen contractures is an elbow flexion contracture in tetraplegics, especially at the C_5 level. The elbow is flexed and supinated. This can be a nonfunctional position for a patient and should be prevented or treated as quickly as possible. Commonly used occupational therapy techniques for correction of contractures include splinting and serial casting. Elbow and pronation splints can be fabricated and are available prefabricated (see Chapter 28). Serial casting is commonly used but is performed with extreme caution for circulatory problems and skin breakdown, because many patients do not have sensation in the extremity being casted.

Chronic upper extremity pain is a common ailment in tetraplegia and paraplegia (Brittell & Mariano, 1991; Sie et al., 1992). It is located most often in the shoulder joint of tetraplegics and paraplegics or related to the carpal tunnel of paraplegics (Sie et al., 1992). Energy conservation and joint protection methods can be useful techniques to prevent pain related to overuse.

Some patients however have severe pain immediately post injury and during their entire rehabilitation (Brittell & Mariano, 1991; Sie et al., 1992). Working with a patient with chronic shoulder pain is extremely frustrating because for many patients, the pain is so severe it interferes with achievement of goals (Brittell & Mariano, 1991). Daily passive range of motion may be painful but is continued to prevent further joint restrictions, which may lead to further pain. Scheduling daily range of motion after a patient has taken pain medication can be helpful. Soft tissue mobilization and joint mobilization are two techniques frequently used by occupational therapists but have not been proven effective.

An important consideration in preventing shoulder pain relates to the therapist's ability to facilitate patterns of strengthening. Having a thorough understanding of the mechanics of the scapula and glenohumeral joints may assist in treating and preventing shoulder pain. A manual muscle test will illustrate which muscles are intact. By determining the pull of the intact muscles in view of the paralysis of other muscles, the therapist can understand how the joint is responding to movement and spasticity. Proximal strengthening and mobilization of the scapula are critical for safe motion at the shoulder. Likewise, functional activities using the elbow must be supported by stability at the shoulder. Common areas neglected by occupational therapists in strengthening include the scapular muscles and the rotators of the shoulder. By preparing the limb proximally for future distal function, substitution patterns and overuse syndromes may be reduced.

RESEARCH IN SPINAL CORD INJURY

General research related to spinal cord injury is plentiful but is focused on a few specific topics (DeJong & Batavia, 1991). Areas that have recently been studied include the effects of aging (Eisenberg & Saltz, 1991; Lammertse & Yarkony, 1991; Mentor et al., 1991; Sie et al., 1992), the effects of age at the time of injury (DeVivo et al., 1990; Penrod et al., 1990; Teasell & Allatt, 1991; Yarkony, Roth, Heinemann, & Lovell, 1988), employment after injury (Alfred et al., 1987; Crisp, 1990), psychosocial effects of spinal cord injury (Jordan et al., 1991), and new advances in surgical and pharmacological treatment (Bracken, 1992; Delisa, 1992; Janssen & Hansebout, 1989). Occupational therapy research related to spinal cord injury treatment has focused on the follow-up use of equipment (Garber & Gregario, 1990; Shepherd & Ruziecka, 1991; Smith, 1988), the effects of using **functional electrical stimulation** (Yarkony et al., 1992), and **EMG biofeedback** for muscle strengthening (Klose et al., 1990), and positioning issues especially related to wheelchairs (Post, 1991). Analysis of the effectiveness of rehabilitation on spinal cord injury has been studied only in a general sense (Yarkony et al., 1987; Yarkony, Roth, Heinemann, Lovell, & Wu, 1988). Spinal cord injury data centers collect functional independence scores for patients from all over the country (DeJong & Batavia, 1991). These studies have indicated an increase over the years in mobility and independence in self-care postrehabilitation (Yarkony et al., 1987; Yarkony, Roth, Heinemann, Lovell, & Wu, 1988). Most of the specific occupational therapy techniques used have not been studied. Although the invention of new equipment and treatment techniques is exciting, the core of spinal cord injury rehabilitation continues to be basic range of motion, strengthening, and ADL instruction. The techniques and equipment that have been used for years continue to be the basis of spinal cord injury rehabilitation. Unfortunately, these techniques have never been studied for their effectiveness. It appears a greater research focus needs to be placed on the effects of funding on outcome, patient motivation, and the functional use of equipment. Given the financial and time restraints being placed on rehabilitation it is vital that occupational therapists begin researching the techniques used routinely in spinal cord injury management to determine their effectiveness and minimal necessary dosage.

Acknowledgments—The author thanks Cheryl Linden and Gayle Shelden for their assistance and support in developing and reviewing this chapter. The author would also like to thank the occupational therapists from the U.S.A. Regional Spinal Cord Injury Centers for all their suggestions.

STUDY QUESTIONS

1. What is the cause of autonomic dysreflexia? Describe the symptoms and treatment.
2. List five important parts of an occupational therapist's initial evaluation for a spinal cord–injured patient.
3. What is spinal shock? How can it effect assessment and treatment?
4. Why must patients perform pressure relief? Describe the techniques used by a C_4 tetraplegic and a T_{12} paraplegic.
5. What is a tenodesis grasp? What must the occupational therapist do to facilitate a tenodesis grasp?
6. Describe the four major areas of treatment focus during the first phase of spinal cord injury rehabilitation.
7. What physical and psychosocial factors need to be considered during the formation of long-term goals?
8. Radical wrist extensors are added at the C_6 level. How does this affect performance of ADLs?

STUDY QUESTIONS *continued*

9. Describe a typical feeding setup for a C_5 tetraplegic patient.
10. List a short-term goal for each of the following areas of a C_4 tetraplegic's program: self-care, weight shifts, wheelchair mobility, communication, and environmental control.

REFERENCES

Alfred, W. G., Fuhrer, M. J., & Rossi, C. D. (1987). Vocational development following severe spinal cord injury: A longitudinal study. *Archives of Physical Medicine & Rehabilitation, 68*, 854–857.

American Spinal Injury Association, (1992). *Standards for neurologic classification of spinal injury patients.* Atlanta, GA: Author.

Benda, S. (1983). *Spinal cord injury nursing education.* Chicago: American Spinal Cord Injury Association.

Bishop, B. (1982). Neural plasticity. Part 4. Lesion-induced reorganization of the CNS. *Physical Therapy, 62*(10), 1442–1451.

Bracken, M. B. (1992). Pharmacological treatment of acute spinal cord injury: Current status and future prospects. *Paraplegia, 30*, 102–107.

Brittell, C. W., & Mariano, A. J. (1991). Chronic pain in spinal cord injury. *Physical Medicine and Rehabilitation: State of the Art Reviews, 5*, 71–82.

Brown, D. J. (1992). Spinal cord injury: The last decade and the next. *Paraplegia, 30*, 77–82.

Closson, J. B., Toerge, J. E., Ragnarsson, K. T. Parson, K. C., & Lammertse, D. P. (1991). Rehabilitation in spinal cord disorders. Comprehensive management of spinal cord injury. *Archives of Physical Medicine & Rehabilitation, 74*(4-S), 298–308.

Crisp, R., (1990). Return to work after spinal cord injury. *Journal of Rehabilitation, 56*(1), 28–35.

Dailey, L., & Michael, R. (1977). Nonsterile self-intermittent catherization for male quadriplegic patients. *American Journal of Occupational Therapy, 31* 2), 86–89.

DeJong, G., & Batavia, A. I. (1991). Toward a health services research capacity in spinal cord injury. *Paraplegia, 29*, 373–389.

Delisa. J. A. (1992). Clinical rehabilitation research advances in spinal cord injury. *Paraplegia, 30*, 73–74.

DeVivo, M. J., Kartus, P. L., Rutt, R. D., Stover, S. L., & Fine, P. R. (1990a). Cause of death for patients with spinal cord injury. *Archives of Physical Medicine & Rehabilitation, 149*, 1761–1766.

DeVivo, M. J., Kartus, P. L., Rutt, R. D., Stover, S. L., & Fine, P. R. (1990b). The influence of age at time of spinal cord injury on rehabilitation outcome. *Archives of Neurology, 47*, 687–691.

Ditunno, J. E., Stover, L. S., Donovan, W. H., Waters, R. L., & Sniezek, J. E. (1989). Research and training benefits of the model system. In D. F. Apple & L. M. Hudson (Eds.), *Spinal cord injury: The model* (pp. 85–105). Atlanta: Georgia Regional Spinal Cord Injury Care System, Shepherd Center for Treatment of Spinal Injuries, Inc.

Ditunno, J. F. Jr., Stover, S. L., Freed, M. M., & Ahn, J. H., (1992). Motor recovery of the upper extremities in traumatic quadriplegia: A multicenter study. *Archives of Physical Medicine & Rehabilitation, 73*, 431–436.

Eisenberg, M. G., & Saltz, C. C. (1991). Quality of life among aging spinal cord injured persons: Long term rehabilitation outcomes. *Paraplegia, 29*(7), 514–520.

Garber, S. L., & Gregorio, T. L. (1990). Upper extremity assistive devices: Assessment of use by spinal-cord injured patients with quadriplegia. *American Journal of Occupational Therapy, 44*(2), 126–131

Hanak, M., & Scott, A. (1983). *Spinal cord injury.* New York: Springer.

Harnish, L. A. (1990). Functional gains in SCI. *Clinical Management, 10*(2), 35–38,40.

Ireland, F. (no date). *Spinal cord injury care manual for nurses.* New York: Eastern Paralyzed Veterans Association.

Janssen, L., & Hansebout, R. R. (1989). Pathogenesis of spinal cord injury and newer treatments. *Spine, 14*(1), 23–32.

Johnson, J. H. (1989). Children with physical and orthopedic disabilities. In P. N. Pratt & A. S. Allen (Eds.), *Occupational therapy for children* (2nd ed., pp. 510–523). St. Louis: C. V. Mosby.

Jordan, S. A., Wellborn, W. R. III, Kovnick, J., & Salzstein, R. (1991). Understanding and treating motivation difficulties in ventilator-dependent SCI patients. *Paraplegia, 29*(7), 431–442.

King, R. B., & Dudas, S. (1980). Rehabilitation of the patient with a spinal cord injury. *Nursing Clinics of North America, 15*(2), 225–243.

Klose, K. J., Schmidt, D. L., Needham, B. M., Brucker, B. S., Green, B. A., & Ayyar, D. R. (1990). Rehabilitation therapy for patients with long term spinal cord injuries. *Archives of Physical Medicine & Rehabilitation, 71*, 659–662.

Krajnik, S. R., & Bridle, M. J. (1992). Hand splinting in quadriplegia: Current practice. *American Journal of Occupational Therapy, 46*(2), 149–156.

Lammertse, D. P., & Yarkony, G. M. (1991). Rehabilitation in spinal cord disorders: 4: Outcomes and issues of aging after spinal cord injury. *Archives of Physical Medicine & Rehabilitation, 72*, S309–311.

Machmer, P. (1979). Group treatment in the physical rehabilitation of the patient with a spinal cord injury. *AOTA Physical Disabilities Special Interest Newsletter, 2*(3), 1–2.

McDonald, D. W., Boyle, M. A., & Schumann, T. L. (1989). Environmental control unit utilization by high-level spinal cord injured patients. *Archives of Physical Medicine & Rehabilitation, 70*, 621–623.

Menter, R. R., Whiteneck, G. G., Charlifue, S. W., Gerhart, K., Solnick, S. J., ART, Brooks, C. A., & Hughes, L. (1991). Impairment, disability, handicap and medical expenses of persons aging with spinal cord injury. *Paraplegia, 29*, 613–619.

Novak, P. P., & Mitchell, M. M. (1988). Professional involvement in sexuality counseling for patients with spinal cord injuries. *American Journal of Occupational Therapy, 42*(2), 105–112.

Parsons, K. C., & Lammertse, D. P. (1991). Rehabilitation in spinal cord disorders: 1. Epidemiology, prevention, and system of care of spinal cord disorders. *Archives of Physical Medicine & Rehabilitation, 72*, 293–297.

Penrod, L. E., Hegde, S. K., & Ditunno, J. F. (1990). Age effect on prognosis for functional recovery in acute, traumatic central cord syndrome. *Archives of Physical Medicine & Rehabilitation, 71*, 963–968.

Pierce, D. S., & Nickel, V. H. (1977). *The total care of spinal cord injury.* Boston: Little, Brown & Co..

Post, K. M. (1991). From the field: Clinical notes on cushion prescription. *American Journal of Occupational Therapy, 45*(6), 559–562.

Shepherd, C. C., & Ruziecka, S. H. (1991). Tenodesis brace

use by persons with spinal cord injuries. *American Journal of Occupational Therapy, 45*(1), 81–83.

Sie, I. H., Waters, R. L., Adkins, R. H., & Gellman, H. (1992). Upper extremity pain in the postrehabilitation spinal cord injured patient. *Archives of Physical Medicine & Rehabilitation, 73,* 44–48.

Smith, R. (1988). Quality assurance in equipment ordering for the spinal cord-injured client. *American Journal of Occupational Therapy, 42*(1), 36–39.

Stien, R. (1992). Sexual dysfunctions in the spinal cord injured. *Paraplegia, 30,* 54–57.

Taylor, D. P. (1974). Treatment goals for quadriplegic patients. *American Journal of Occupational Therapy, 28*(1), 22–29.

Teasell, R., & Allatt, D. (1991). Managing the growing number of spinal cord-injured elderly. *Geriatrics, 46*(6), 78–89.

Trombly, C. A. (Ed.). (1989). *Occupational therapy for physical dysfunction* (3rd ed.). Baltimore: Williams & Wilkins.

Wilson, D. J., McKenzie, M. W., Barber, L. M., & Watson, K. L. (1984). *Spinal cord injury: A treatment guide for occupational therapists* (2nd ed.). Thorofare, NJ: Slack.

Wu, L., Marino, R. J., Herbison, G. J., & Ditunno, J. F. Jr. (1992). Recovery of zero-grade muscles in the zone of partial preservation in motor complete quadriplegia. *Archives of Physical Medicine & Rehabilitation, 73,* 40–43.

Yarkony, G. M., Roth, E. J., Cybulski, G., & Jaeger, R. J. (1992). Neuromuscular stimulation in spinal cord injury: I: Restoration of functional movement of the extremities. *Archives of Physical Medicine & Rehabilitation, 73,* 78–86.

Yarkony, G. M., Roth, E. J., Heinemann, A. W., & Lovell, L. L. (1988). Spinal cord injury rehabilitation outcome: The impact of age. *Journal of Clinical Epidemiology, 41*(2), 173–177.

Yarkony, G. M., Roth, E. J., Heinemann, A. W., Lovell, L., & Wu, Y. (1988). Functional skills after spinal cord injury rehabilitation: Three-year longitudinal follow-up. *Archives of Physical Medicine & Rehabilitation, 69,* 111–114.

Yarkony, G. M., Roth, E. J., Heinemann, A. W., Wu, Y., Katz, R. T., & Lovell, L. (1987). Benefits of rehabilitation for traumatic spinal cord injury. *Archives of Neurology, 44,* 93–96.

Zejdlik, C. M. (1983). *Management of spinal cord injury.* Monterey, CA: Wadsworth Health Sciences Division.

SUPPLEMENTARY RESOURCES

Suggested Readings

American Occupational Therapy Association. The following resource guides (all published in 1992) are helpful: *Spinal Cord Injury; Accessibility & Architectural Modifications; Seating & Wheeled Mobility; Computer;* and *Drivers Education.* (Available from the AOTA, Rockville, MD)

Cunningham, B., & Kelsch, C. (1991). *Patient and family teaching with the spinal-cord injured patient.* Gaithersburg, MD: Aspen Systems.

Park, T. S., Phillips, L. H., & Peacock, W. J. (1989). *Management of spasticity in cerebral palsy and spinal cord injury.* Philadelphia: Hanley & Belfus.

Parsons, K. F., & Fitzpatrick, J. M. (1991). *Practical urology in spinal cord injury.* New York: Springer-Verlag.

Rehabilitation Institute of Chicago. (1986). *Spinal cord injury: A guide to functional outcomes in occupational therapy.* Gaithersburg, MD: Aspen Systems.

Shelden, G. M. (1988). Treatment options for shoulder pain in quadriplegia. *AOTA Physical Disabilities Special Interest Newsletter, 11*(3), 1.

Smith, R. (1989). Mouthstick design for the client with spinal cord injury. *American Journal of Occupational Therapy, 42*(1), 36–39.

Weingarden, S. I., & Martin, C. (1989). Independent dressing after spinal cord injury: A functional time evaluation. *Archives of Physical Medicine & Rehabilitation, 70,* 518–519.

Whiteneck, G., Adler, C., Carter, R. E., Lammertse, D. P., Manley, S., Menter, R., Wagner, K., & Wilmot, C. (1989). *The management of high quadriplegia.* New York: Demos.

Wolf, S. L., & Fisher, W. M. (1987). The use of biofeedback in disorders of motor function. In J. P. Hatch, J. G. Fisher, & J. D. Rugh (Eds.), *Biofeedback studies in clinical efficacy* (pp. 153–177). New York: Plenum.

Videos

Rancho Los Amigos Research and Education Institute. *Starting Over* (Parts 1–3). Downey, CA: Author.

Rehabilitation Institute of Chicago. (1990). *Challenged life: Spinal cord injury.* Chicago: Author.

40
Arthritis

Judy R. Feinberg and Catherine A. Trombly

OBJECTIVES

After studying this chapter, the reader will be able to:
1. Understand the differences in clinical features and etiology between rheumatoid arthritis and osteoarthritis.
2. Know which assessments are used for patients with arthritis.
3. Recognize the typical rheumatoid hand deformities, understand their pathodynamics, and be able to describe **joint protection** techniques.
4. Know the occupational therapy goals and treatments appropriate for a patient with rheumatoid arthritis or osteoarthritis.

This chapter focuses only on the two most common rheumatic diseases: rheumatoid arthritis (RA) and osteoarthritis (OA), also known as degenerative joint disease. The reader should know that there are more than a hundred different rheumatic diseases, most of which may produce inflammation of one or more joints (i.e., arthritis). While occupational therapy treatment of inflammatory arthritis may be similar in many cases, therapists who encounter patients with arthritic conditions other than rheumatoid or osteoarthritis should read the appropriate professional literature before initiating evaluation or treatment programs.

RHEUMATOID ARTHRITIS

Rheumatoid arthritis is a systemic disease characterized by remissions and exacerbations that vary in duration and severity among people (Schumacher, 1988). Joint inflammation is the dominant clinical manifestation of this generalized disease of connective tissue (Salter, 1983), but the disease may also involve the lungs, heart, blood vessels, and eyes (Melvin, 1989). In the United States, the prevalence of rheumatoid arthritis is estimated between 0.3 and 1.5% of the population, depending on the stringency of the criteria used to classify (Schumacher, 1988). Women are affected two to three times more often than men, and onset is usually between the 20th and 40th year of age (Salter, 1983; Schumacher, 1988).

Etiology is unknown. There are at least two theories, which are not mutually exclusive, that are being studied: the infection and the autoimmunity theories. The infection theory hypothesizes that a virus may be the cause. Polyarthritis occurs during many bacterial, spirochetal, and viral infections (Schumacher, 1988). The autoimmune theory holds that there is a disruption of the immune process, resulting in a continuous immunologic response to a persistent antigen, which could be altered γ-globulin in the diseased joint (Salter, 1983). In 70% of the cases, a rheumatoid factor can be demonstrated by a blood test in patients who have had the disease for some time. However, the rheumatoid factor is also positive in 1 to 3% of the normal population. Because RA sometimes clusters in families, there may also be a genetic predisposition to the disease (Melvin, 1989). Psychological stress is not a causative factor but may precipitate the onset of symptoms and aggravate the disease once it is established (Salter, 1983). There is no cure for rheumatoid arthritis at this time.

Because of the chronic nature and often degenerative course of the disease, those treating patients with RA should follow the philosophy applied in the care of patients with any degenerative disease: maintain the patient's physical, psychological, and functional abilities as long as possible through an ongoing, carefully planned treatment program. Integrated team management is essential (Barrows, Berezny, & Reynolds, 1978; Edmonds, 1978; Feinberg & Brandt, 1984; Gross et al., 1982) and has been found to be a statistically important factor in the improvement of patients with rheumatoid disease, although a priori differences

GLOSSARY

Affective tone—The expression of feelings through voice tone and body posture.

Behavioral terms—Words that describe a specific behavior or action of the patient that is observable and measurable.

Bony spurs—Focal bony growth (osteophytes) at the joint margins in response to an inflammatory process.

Contracting—Development of a written or verbal agreement between the patient and therapist delineating certain behaviors or goals and any rewards for accomplishment or consequences of failure.

Crepitus—A grating, crunching, or cracking sound or sensation that occurs during joint or tendon motion.

Energy conservation principles—Guidelines for performing important occupational performance tasks in such a way as to conserve personal energy.

Intrinsic plus hand—Characterized by flexion of the MP joints and extension of the PIP and DIP joints, resulting from shortening of the intrinsic hand muscles.

Joint protection—The process by which stress on joints is reduced during activities for the purpose of reducing pain and inflammation and preserving the integrity of the joint structures.

Morning stiffness—A period of prolonged stiffness after a long period of immobility associated with various arthritides, in particular RA; it is indicative of systemic involvement.

Platform crutches—Crutches that are designed to divert stress from the wrist and finger joints to the forearms during weight-bearing. This is an example of using larger joints instead of smaller ones, a joint protection principle.

Self-instruction—The process by which the patient directs and controls the learning process after appropriate educational materials are introduced.

Trigger finger—An inconsistent limitation of finger flexor or extensor motion caused by either a nodule on a tendon or a narrowing of the tendon sheath.

Visual analogue scale—A line with increments marked and anchored on both ends by statements indicating extreme positions, e.g., a 10-cm line, marked in 1-cm increments, with a statement of "no pain" at the left end and "severe pain" or "worst pain ever experienced" at the right end of the line.

in groups could have accounted for the detected differences (Feinberg & Brandt, 1984). The team at one successful multipurpose arthritic center consists of a rheumatologist, nurse educator, physical therapist, occupational therapist, and social worker (Gross et al., 1982); however, other allied health professionals such as psychologists, dieticians, and vocational rehabilitation counselors may be added to the team as circumstances indicate.

Symptoms of RA are variable but include pain, **morning stiffness,** limited movement of involved joints, malaise, fatigue, wasting of the muscles around the joints, and anemia (Edmonds, 1978). The disease begins with inflammation of the synovial lining of the joints (Edmonds, 1978; Schumacher, 1988). The five characteristic manifestations of inflammation (redness, swelling, heat, pain, and loss of function) become progressively more evident (Salter, 1983). Rheumatoid arthritis usually affects multiple joints, and the distribution tends to be symmetrical. The most commonly involved joints, in order of frequency, are those of the hands, wrists, knees, elbows, feet, shoulders, and hips. The metacarpophalangeal (MP) joints of the thumb, index, and middle fingers; the proximal interphalangeal (PIP) joints of the index, middle, and ring fingers; and the metatarsophalangeal joints of the four small toes are characteristically involved in early stages of the disease.

Once the active disease process burns out, the patient may be left with residual joint deformities and resultant limitations of function (Edmonds, 1978;

Salter, 1983; Schumacher, 1988). The primary objective of treatment is to prevent or minimize joint deformity so that patients can continue to lead comfortable, productive lives.

Occupational therapists help the patient understand his disease pathology and its effects on his life tasks (American Occupational Therapy Association [AOTA], 1986). Through assessment and treatment, the occupational therapist seeks to improve the patient's ability to perform daily activities, prevent loss of function, and facilitate successful adaptation. The therapist helps the patient to develop the problem-solving skills needed to make adaptations throughout life. The occupational therapist also treats the physical and psychosocial impairments that limit, or partially limit, the patient's occupational performance.

Evaluation

In response to a request for services, the occupational therapist reviews the chart, observes and interviews the patient concerning occupational performance, and may use screening tests to determine if referral for occupational therapy is indicated (AOTA, 1986). A patient who risks losing function because of pain, fatigue, loss of strength or endurance, changes in joint range of motion (ROM), or loss of coping skills or whose function may be improved is considered an appropriate candidate for occupational therapy services. Assessment includes determination of areas of occupational dysfunction important to the person through a structured interview such as the *Canadian*

Occupational Performance Measure (COPM) (Law et al., 1991); a review of medical history and status of the patient's disease; tests to document manifestations of the disease, including ROM evaluation, strength testing, and daily living skills evaluations; environmental analyses to determine the impact of the environment on the patient's ability to function; evaluation of the patient's psychosocial status; and identification of the patient's personal goals, interests, and expectations. Sensory evaluation should be done if systemic involvement includes polyneuropathies or nerve compression (Schumacher, 1988).

ACTIVITIES OF DAILY LIVING

Occupational performance is evaluated as described in Chapter 4. It may be useful in assessing the occupational functioning status of people with arthritis to go beyond the regular scoring categories to obtain a more accurate picture of the person's functional status. A person with arthritis may report independence in a given activity yet the activity may be difficult or painful to complete. The therapist should elicit this information so that it can be considered in planning appropriate interventions. Also one should not assume that the newly diagnosed patient without joint deformities will be able to perform all occupational tasks. Pain and stiffness may create considerable impairment. Conversely, the end stage patient with multiple deformities may have adapted to the limitations imposed by the disease over time and be able to perform all necessary tasks with relative ease.

In assessing occupational functioning, the therapist need not ask the patient to demonstrate all tasks. Not only would that be fatiguing but, because of the chronic nature of the disease, verbal reports are usually quite accurate. One study of 45 RA patients found that patients appeared more willing to admit difficulties with self-care in a self-administered questionnaire than in a personal interview (Spiegel, Hirshfield, & Spiegel, 1985), and this can save time in a comprehensive evaluation. The *Assessment of Motor and Process Skills* (AMPS) allows an accurate estimate of ability to do instrumental activities of daily living (IADL) based on performance of three tasks. This instrument also provides information concerning impairments of motor or process (cognitive) skills that may be interfering with ability to do IADL (Fisher, 1993).

STRENGTH

The systemic nature of rheumatoid arthritis, along with atrophy of disuse, produces muscle weakness (Pahle & Raunio, 1969). Use of manual muscle testing involving resistance is controversial. On the one hand, it is necessary to know the patient's strength, especially

the comparative strength of muscles around a joint. On the other hand, resistance causes harm to the diseased tissue, which causes pain. Pain causes the patient to protect the part and results in an unreliable test of strength. Furthermore, some rheumatologists prohibit any resistance beyond that which is necessary for self-care, because of the deforming forces of muscle contraction when joint structures are stretched and weakened (Wozny & Long, 1966). Others feel that knowledge of the level of muscle strength and of the effectiveness of strengthening exercises is important (Vignos, 1980). The muscle test, if done, should be done isometrically, not isotonically. Isotonic movement against resistance tends to increase inflammation and pain in arthritic joints (Vignos, 1980).

ENDURANCE

Endurance is evaluated as outlined in Chapter 6 or by taking note of the patient's limits of endurance during daily activities. The patient must learn to evaluate this for himself, since he must learn to rest before fatigue becomes a factor in the performance of activities.

RANGE OF MOTION

Range of motion (ROM) is typically limited in RA. Initially, joint swelling diminishes joint mobility and stretches ligaments and joint capsules. Subsequently, contractures of muscles and other connective tissues may occur. Measurement of range of motion is limited to active motion in patients in the active stage of the disease. Because range of motion can be affected by the generalized stiffness characteristic of RA, the duration of the patient's **morning stiffness** and the time of day of the evaluation should be noted. Range of motion is measured as described in Chapter 6.

PAIN

Pain is a common symptom of RA that limits ROM, pinch, and grasp, and subsequently, occupational performance. Severity and location of pain should be recorded. The severity of pain can be graded based on its occurrence during activity. It is graded mild if it occurs only with stressful activity such as picking up a heavy object, moderate if it occurs with active motion, and severe if it occurs even at rest (Feinberg & Brandt, 1981). Another effective method of quantifying pain is to ask the patient to indicate the level of pain on a **visual analogue scale** (Huskisson, 1974).

HAND FUNCTION

Assessment of hand function, and the function of the upper extremity insofar as it serves hand function, is of particular importance. Both the prehensile and nonprehensile functions of the hand should be evaluated (Melvin, 1989). Prehensile functions are pinch and grasp; nonprehensile functions are those that use the hand statically, held either flexed (hook grasp) or extended (e.g., tucking in clothing, smoothing sheets, sorting coins on a surface) (Melvin, 1989). In RA, the prehensile functions are potentially deforming. Therefore, if nonprehensile functions can be substituted, the joints may be protected from deformity.

A number of hand function tests exist, but these tests focus only on the prehensile functions. One is the *Jebsen Hand Function Test* (Jebsen et al., 1969; see also Chapter 7). Another hand function test was recently reported; it is currently undergoing development and standardization (Backman, Mackie, & Harris, 1991). The *Arthritis Hand Function Test* consists of 11 items designed to measure pure and applied strength and dexterity. Items include measurement of grip and pinch strength, the *Nine-Hole Peg Test*, and timed functional tasks. The entire battery takes about 20 min to administer. Early validity and reliability testing indicates that this may be a promising instrument for evaluating hand function in people with arthritis.

An electronic standardized test to measure hand movement (active and passive), strength (pinch, grip, and finger extension), and manipulative ability (holding, placing, and twisting) has been devised (Walker, Davidson, & Erkman, 1978). Values obtained for women with arthritis were compared with those for normal subjects. The subjects with arthritis were found to have severely compromised active motion (50% of normal), strength (ranged from 10% of normal for grip to 25% of normal for pinches), and manipulation (50% of normal).

Although the Jamar dynamometer provides an accurate assessment of grip strength and has published norms, the shape and hardness of the instrument can cause pain and inhibit the application of force by persons with inflammatory arthritis. Measurement of grasp and pinch strength should be done using an adapted sphygmomanometer (Melvin, 1989). A recent paper provided a regression equation for converting sphygmomanometer readings to equivalent Jamar scores (Agnew & Maas, 1991). The following formula converts sphygmomanometer readings (in millimeters of mercury) to Jamar scores (in kilograms per centimeter squared): sphygmomanometer score × 0.154 − 0.865 = Jamar score. Conversely, Jamar score × 4.472 + 26.568 = sphygmomanometer score. For example, to convert a patient's sphygmomanometer score of 80 mm: multiply 80 by 0.0154 then subtract 0.865. The score of 80 mm Hg is equal to a score of 11.455 kg/cm^2 on a Jamar dynamometer.

DEFORMITIES OF THE HAND AND WRIST

The location of pain, hot and inflamed joints, swelling, tendon rupture, nodules, **crepitus,** and subluxations or dislocations should be recorded in such a way as to allow comparison from evaluation to evaluation. Some clinics use photography to supplement written descriptions.

Nodules or Synovial Thickening

Nodules or synovial thickening may be found along the extrinsic finger flexors or extensors. Flexor nodules are more common. A flexor nodule can become caught inside one of the flexor tendon sheaths, producing a **trigger finger.** These **trigger fingers** may simply be mildly irritating to the patient or can be quite painful. Clinically, flexor nodules are detected when the patient or therapist notes a snapping or catching of the digit during motion or by a discrepancy between active and passive motion of the digit. To test for the presence of a nodule, observe as the patient actively moves the finger. If the above clinical signs are seen or reported by the patient, palpate for the presence of a nodule along the tendon surface. Flexor nodules are commonly felt around the area of the distal palmar crease.

Tendon Rupture

Rupture of a tendon is uncommon but can occur in patients with significant chronic synovitis. Tendon rupture occurs either from attenuation of the tendons from the disease process itself or from attrition of the tendons over subluxed bones. Finger extensors usually rupture over the distal end of the ulna, whereas the extensor pollicis longus tendon commonly ruptures at Lister's tubercle. Flexor tendon ruptures occur less commonly but can occur at any level from the wrist distally. Tendon ruptures are identified by individual muscle testing when the muscle function is noted to be absent during attempted active motion. Ulnar dislocation of the finger extensor tendons at the MP joints can also result in a lack of ability by the patient to extend the digits actively; however this can be distinguished from tendon rupture, because the intact tendons can be seen in the "valleys" between the MP joints. Because of this position, they lose mechanical advantage to extend the fingers.

Typical Deformities of the Wrist and Hand

Ulnar deviation and volar subluxation of the wrist and MP joints and thumb hyperextension are characteristic of RA. The exact cause of deformity is not yet fully understood, but it appears that hypertrophy of the synovium caused by the inflammation process pushes against the joint structures from within. The ligaments become stretched, and when the swelling of the synovium subsides, the ligaments are left lax. The ligamentous abnormality changes the force moments of the tendons, and their pull becomes deforming (Kay, 1979).

These deformities and the underlying mechanisms thought to produce them are being described in detail not only so that they may be evaluated but also because it is hypothesized that normal use of the hands produces forces that promote the deformities. Although one study that compared deformities of dominant and nondominant hands (based on the assumption that the dominant hand is subject to greater stress during daily activity and, therefore, would have significantly greater deformity) found no significant difference in the frequency or type of deformities between the two hands (Hasselkus, Kshepakaran, & Safrit, 1981). The findings might be explained by noting that whereas the dominant hand is used more often for dexterous tasks involving pinch and grasp, the nondominant hand is used for stabilization and is, therefore, also equally subjected to deforming static pinch and grasp forces. Until studies are done that actually document the amount and type of dominant and nondominant hand usage and demonstrate that there is or is not a causal relationship between hand use and development of deformities, therapists should probably continue to base arthritis treatment on the assumption that there is, indeed, a relationship between hand use and the development of deformities.

Deformities of the Wrist

Volar subluxation of the hand in relation to the ulna is caused by erosion of the intercarpal ligaments and eventually volar displacement of the extensor carpi ulnaris (Swezey, 1971–1972) which, in effect, causes this muscle to act as a flexor force.

Commonly, the wrist radially deviates as the result of a loss of support of the radial and ulnar ligaments, volar displacement of the extensor carpi ulnaris (ECU), and predominant action of the radial muscles— flexor carpi radialis, extensor carpi radialis brevis, and extensor carpi radialis longus (Melvin, 1989; Tubiana, Thomine, & Mackin, 1984). Loss of ligamentous support allows the proximal carpal bones to sublux ulnarly and the distal carpal bones to rotate in a radial direction, which results in the radial deviation (Melvin, 1989; Pahle & Raunio, 1969). The fingers, especially the index finger, then ulnarly deviate in an effort to realign the index finger with the radius. This then completes the zigzag deformity: wrist radial deviation with MP ulnar deviation. However, this sequence of

events has been disputed because of the clinical observation that the ulnar drift at the MP joints seems to occur first, which means that factors other than wrist radial deviation influence finger deviation (Tubiana et al., 1984).

Deformities of the Metacarpophalangeal Joints

Volar subluxation of the fingers appears to develop in the following manner (Kay, 1979). Synovitis of the MP joint stretches the extensor mechanism. The extensor hood is thinner radially, and the hypertrophied synovium tends to herniate on the radial side of the extensor tendons. The hood is pushed distally, which causes the extensor tendons to slip ulnarly off the tops of the joints to the valleys between. This places them below the joint axes; therefore, their force becomes a flexor force (English & Nalebuff, 1971; Kay, 1979). In addition, the large volar forces generated at the mouth of the flexor tunnels (sheaths) during pinch or grasp cause mechanical damage to the metacarpoglenoidal ligaments supporting them, and the tunnel mouths are displaced volarly (Smith et al., 1964). A new equilibrium of forces develops between the pull of the flexors and the supporting structure: the rim of the phalanx and the MP collateral ligaments. If the rim wears down, or the ligaments are stretched, the deformity of volar subluxation results (Smith et al, 1964).

Ulnar deviation deformity develops when the tissues surrounding the joint, especially the radial collateral ligaments, become permanently stretched because of the proliferation of the synovium (Swezey, 1971– 1972). Normally, the ulnar interossei exert a stronger pull than the radial ones do (Kay, 1979; Melvin, 1989; Smith et al., 1964). This, combined with the pull of the flexor tendons on the mouths of the tendon sheaths in an ulnar direction, contributes to the force that causes the dynamic ulnar deviation (Smith et al., 1964). In time, the ulnar intrinsics become shortened, creating a constant pull toward ulnar deviation.

Abnormal laxity of the radial collateral ligament at the MP joint is evaluated by placing each of the patient's MP joints in full passive flexion. Each digit is then pushed in an ulnar direction. In a normal hand the digit should have minimal or no movement laterally. If the radial collateral ligament is stretched the finger can be easily displaced in an ulnar direction.

Deformities of the Interphalangeal Joints

The deformities of the interphalangeal (IP) joints caused by rheumatoid arthritis are swan neck deformity and boutonniere deformity (Swanson, 1972). A swan neck deformity (**intrinsic plus hand**) is a combination of PIP hyperextension and distal interphalangeal (DIP) flexion caused by tight interossei that pull abnormally on the extensor tendons and cause hyperextension of the hypermobile PIP joints (English & Nalebuff, 1971; Swezey, 1971–1972) (Fig. 40.1). This deformity may be flexible or fixed. To test for flexibility, support the MP joint in extension and have the patient flex the PIP joint (English & Nalebuff, 1971). If the patient is able to flex the PIP joint fully, the deformity is flexible and the volar plate that prevents hyperextension is only slightly stretched. If PIP flexion is limited or impossible with the MP joint extended but can be accomplished with the MP joint flexed, a fixed deformity caused by tight intrinsics is present. The intrinsic muscles are on stretch when the MP joints are extended and the interphalangeal joints are flexed. The earliest sign of a swan neck deformity may be a resting posture of MP flexion or a slight cupping of the hand. Early detection of tightness of the intrinsics is important so treatment can be instituted. Tightness of the intrinsics can be detected by noting whether a difference exists in the amount of flexion of the PIP joints when the MP joints are flexed or extended (Melvin, 1989).

A fixed swan neck deformity also may be caused by sticking lateral bands secondary to local inflammation at the PIP joint. In this case, PIP flexion is impossible, regardless of the position of the MP joint (English & Nalebuff, 1971).

A boutonniere deformity is a combination of PIP flexion and DIP hyperextension caused by attenuation of the lateral bands of the extensor digitorum, which slip volarly (English & Nalebuff, 1971; Swezey, 1971–1972) (Fig. 40.2) and then act to flex the PIP joint. The relationship between the flexor digitorum profundus and the extensor digitorum is changed, and the extensor acts unopposed at the DIP joint (Swezey, 1971–1972). To test for shortening of the lateral bands, hold the PIP extended and passively try to flex the DIP. If DIP

flexion is difficult or impossible, there is shortening of the lateral bands (Swezey, 1971–1972).

Deformities of the Thumb

Deformity patterns of the rheumatoid thumb have been described by Nalebuff (1968). The most common thumb deformity involves flexion of the MP joint with hyperextension of the IP joint (type I) (Fig 40.3). This results from stretching of the joint capsule and collateral ligaments at the MP joint. Often there is a compensatory abduction of the carpometacarpal (CMC) joint to achieve approximation of the pads of the thumb and index finger during pinch and grasp activities. A type II deformity involves MP hyperextension, IP joint flexion, and CMC joint subluxation or dislocation into adduction. This deformity is initiated by synovitis of the CMC joint. Type III and IV deformities are less common and begin with synovitis of the MP joint. A type III deformity develops from attenuation of the ulnar collateral ligament and thus presents as MP joint lateral deviation with secondary CMC joint adduction. A type IV deformity looks similar to a type II deformity,

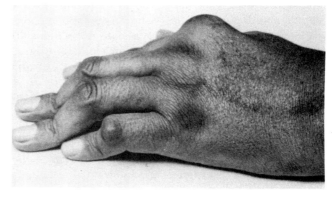

Figure 40.2. Boutonniere deformity (PIP flexion with DIP hyperextension).

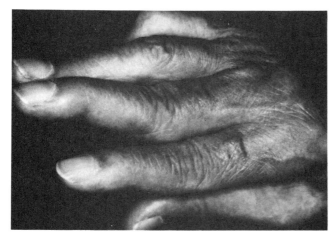

Figure 40.1. Swan neck deformity (PIP hyperextension with DIP flexion).

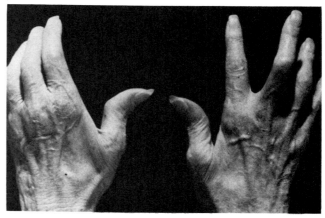

Figure 40.3. Example of a Nalebuff type I thumb deformity.

but there is no CMC involvement. Revision of Nalebuff's classification in 1984 added a type V deformity. This is described as a mutilans deformity or collapse and shortening of the phalanges with total instability (Nalebuff, 1984).

CASE STUDY: RHEUMATOID ARTHRITIS PATIENT

Susan is a 37-year-old female who appears younger than her stated age. She has had symptoms of RA for the past year and was recently evaluated by a rheumatologist who referred her to occupational therapy for assessment and treatment. She has mild swelling of the MP, PIP, and wrist joints bilaterally with no evidence of joint deformity. Her ROM was only slightly limited at the time of testing. She gave a history of being very active. She works full-time as a secretary, is married, has a 10-year-old daughter, and enjoys several recreational sports activities. In an informal discussion with the therapist she minimized her symptoms and felt that she did not need therapy at this time. However, when a detailed assessment of her occupational performance was done, she admitted to having a great deal of pain and difficulty completing many self-care, homemaking, and work activities. Her family and friends have been helping her a great deal, and she has given up participation in all her prior sports activities.

This case represents a typical early RA patient. On physical examination her joints appear as though she should have minimal problems performing her daily activities, and in casual conversation, she avoids talking about her arthritis or the multitude of problems presented by it. However pain, stiffness, and fatigue can significantly limit occupational performance, and in the early stages of her psychological adjustment to her RA, she is likely to deny or be depressed about her functional difficulties. These patients will usually admit to difficulties when the therapist explains the reasons for and completes a detailed functional assessment. The therapist should not assume that no problems exist when physical limitations are not initially obvious. Patient education and treatment such as provision of adaptive equipment may need to be staged out over time, when the patient is better able to accept the therapeutic intervention. It is likely that this patient will receive some benefit from this early intervention. She may or may not be ready to participate in a therapy program, but minimally, she will learn what occupational therapy has to offer her in the future.

Treatment

Treatment addresses the problems identified by evaluation and is guided by the progression of the disease. The disease progresses from the acute phase (characterized by synovial inflammation and proliferation, illness, and pain) to the subacute, noninflammatory phase to the chronic stage in which the disease is burned out but the deformities remain. In all stages, fatigue and exacerbation of pain are avoided. Specific goals depend on the identified problems of the particular patient. These may be any or all of the following:

1. Maintain joint mobility;
2. Prevent joint deformity;
3. Maintain or increase strength;
4. Maintain or increase functional ability;
5. Develop the habit of balancing activity with rest;
6. Develop problem-solving skills to modify daily activities at home and at work to protect joints and conserve energy;
7. Promote psychosocial adjustment to chronic disability.

MAINTAIN JOINT MOBILITY

During the acute stage of the disease, the patient should be instructed in active ROM exercises to be done in three or four short sessions each day. It is essential to put all joints through range of motion at least once daily to maintain mobility (Swezey, 1989). Exercises are best done when pain has been diminished by drugs or moist heat application (see Chapter 33) and when **morning stiffness** has subsided (Glass, 1978).

Stretching at the limit of range is not recommended in the acute phase, because it may add additional stress to structures already on maximal stretch as a result of intraarticular swelling (Melvin, 1989). In the postinflammatory stage, gentle passive ROM may be done to provide gentle, prolonged stretch to prevent the muscles and connective tissues from shortening into fixed deformities (Glass, 1978). Once again, moist heat application before exercise is recommended. Duration of pain provides a guideline for the amount and types of exercises to be done. Pain or discomfort resulting from exercise should not last for more than 1 hr following the exercise session (Melvin, 1989). If pain exceeds 1 hr, the number of repetitions and/or the number of exercise sessions should be reduced by half.

In a trial of 30 patients with RA (McKnight & Schomburg, 1982), an air splint that applied a constant, uniform external pressure (40 mm Hg) to all portions of the hand was applied for 20 min with the wrist in neutral and the fingers in extension and then for 20 min with the fingers flexed into a fist. After a single treatment, mobility increased by 45%, and after five treatments it increased 63%, which was a significant improvement over the control (contralateral) hands. The mechanism involved in producing the effect is not known.

PREVENT JOINT DEFORMITY

Principles of **joint protection** are based on the theory that forces involved in use of the hand contribute to structured joint changes and disease activity that fosters deformity (Cordery, 1965; Hasselkus et al., 1981). The principles of **joint protection** are listed in Table 40.1. The patient has to learn the application of these principles through supervised practice. Avoidance of positions of deformity is a particularly important principle to be aware of when the hands are used

Table 40.1. Principles of Joint Protection

1. Maintain muscle strength and joint range of motion.
2. Avoid positions of deformity as well as external pressures and internal stresses in the direction of deformity.
3. Use the largest, strongest joints available for the job.
4. Use each joint in its most stable anatomical and functional plane.
5. Use correct patterns of movement.
6. Avoid holding one position for any undue length of time.
7. Avoid starting an activity that cannot be stopped immediately if it proves to be beyond capability.
8. Respect pain as a signal to stop the activity.

functionally, because the forces generated during grasp and pinch become increasingly deforming as resistance increases. The hand should be used in nonprehensile functional ways if possible. Joints may need to be supported in a splint to counteract the deforming pull of the muscles (Fig. 28.15). Movements should be done in a direction opposite to the potential deformity. Pressure that pushes the MP joints in an ulnar direction should be particularly avoided. Some examples are as follows:

1. To open jars, stabilize the jar on a wet towel or nonskid pad, place the palm of the right hand on the jar lid, press down, and turn in a radial direction (this may mean using the nondominant hand); another solution is to use a wall-mounted jar opener.
2. Press water from a cloth or sponge rather than wring it.
3. Hold a knife with the blade protruding from the ulnar side of the hand, which pushes the hand toward radial deviation (Fig. 40.4); the knife should be sharp to offer less resistance.
4. Hold stirring spoons so that the bowl of the spoon is on the ulnar side of the hand.
5. Smooth towels, clothes, bed sheets, etc., by using the ulnar border of the hand.
6. When using the hands to assist standing up, apply pressure on the heel of the hand only and avoid putting pressure on the radial side of the index finger.
7. Use adapted tools and utensils in which the handles are angled to eliminate wrist deviation (Tichauer, 1966) and ulnar deviation of the MP joints, e.g., use of a knife with a handle at a 90° angle to the blade prevents ulnar deviation during the cutting process by allowing a dagger grip but still keeping the length of the blade in contact with the food to be cut.

Further testing needs to be done in the laboratory and clinic to establish the effectiveness of these measures to prevent deformities.

The proximal joints are stronger than the distal

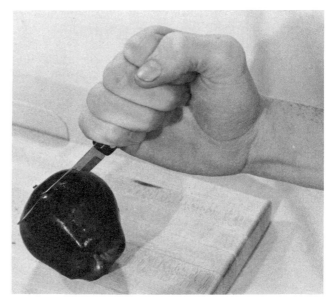

Figure 40.4. Cutting an apple using a dagger grip on the knife to push the fingers in a radial direction during cutting.

ones, and their use protects the weaker joints. Examples demonstrating the principle of using the strongest, largest joints available to do a task are as follows:

1. Slip a purse, shopping bag, or tote bag over the forearm instead of carrying it in the hand.
2. Carry pots, casseroles, and heavy objects by putting one hand and forearm flat underneath and steadying the object with the other (Fig. 40.5); long, insulated oven mitts are, of course, required to transport hot items safely in this manner.
3. Use forearm **platform crutches** instead of standard crutches, which require the body weight to be transported by the hands during ambulation.

Examples of using each joint in its most stable and functional plane are (1) avoid twisting the knees when standing up by first pushing straight up from the chair or bed and then turning and (2) use a splint to hold the fingers in good alignment and to prevent ulnar deviation during hand usage (Fig. 40.6). If constructed from thermoplastic materials, the splint may hinder some activities such as writing but will greatly enhance other activities such as lifting and grasping and relieve the patient from the need to monitor activity constantly from a **joint protection** standpoint (Quest & Cordery, 1971). Detailed, illustrated directions for construction of this type of splint have been published (Quest & Cordery, 1971). A soft version is also sold commercially.

Two major treatment methods to prevent deformity are patient education and splinting.

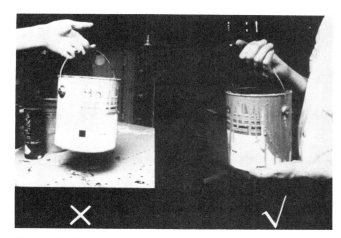

Figure 40.5. Demonstration of how to distribute a load over a larger area and to use largest joint available for a task.

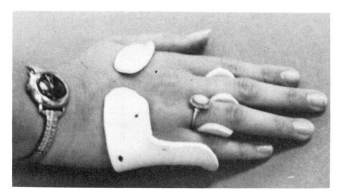

Figure 40.6. Splint to prevent ulnar deviation of the MP joints during hand use.

Patient Education

Patient education is an important treatment method used with RA patients throughout the course of their disease. **Energy-conservation principles,** work simplification techniques, exercise programs, and **joint protection** techniques are taught to the patient who must learn these management techniques and then continue to practice them throughout his lifetime.

Patient education can be effectively completed in a group format in which patients and their families can share ideas and benefit from others' questions and experiences. Educational support groups should be kept small and should include patients at similar stages of the disease so that the relevance of material presented can be maximized for all group members. Groups can also be helpful in facilitating psychological adjustment. Issues of disturbance of self-image, job status, family relationships, and coping mechanisms can be addressed through group therapy (Krawitz & Wolman, 1979; see also Chapter 20). Local Arthritis

Foundation chapters often sponsor support groups or public forums that combine education and social objectives in an effective manner.

Before starting patient education, the therapist should assess the psychological readiness of the patient to learn about disease management (Melvin, 1989). Pain, concerns about the disease process, and the effects of medication may interfere with the learning process.

When instructing the patient, attention should be paid to the instructional process as well as the patient's specific needs and methods of coping with his disability (Melvin, 1989). One process for designing an instructional program has been described (Furst et al., 1987). It suggests that instructional sessions should have specific goals stated in **behavioral terms** and should clearly present the material through discussion, audiovisuals, and demonstration. Opportunities to problem solve relative to the patient's own life tasks and to practice the principles under various conditions also should be included. The information may have to be repeated, because it is not all retained at once. Written information should be provided for future reference (Edmonds, 1978; Melvin, 1989).

Encouraging but not conclusive evidence was presented in support of an instructional program that was based on use of a workbook in conjunction with group or tutorial interactive sessions (Furst, Gerber, & Smith, 1985; Furst et al., 1987). The topics covered were energy-conservation and **joint protection** techniques. The workbook has an introduction that describes the disease, and the remainder of the text is divided into four units: positioning, rest, activity analysis for energy conservation, and **joint protection.** Each unit contains didactic information and illustrations of the techniques, practice assignments to apply learned techniques, and a self-evaluation section. The instructor's guide includes suggestions for teaching the techniques and topics to emphasize in each session. It is designed to be a 6-week program of 1-hr group or individual sessions. Part of the success of the workbook program must be attributed to careful delineation of behavioral objectives, e.g., "patient will demonstrate inclusion of 2 daily 1-hour lying down rest periods" (Furst et al., 1987, p. 105).

A recent study compared the relative effectiveness of three teaching modalities: **self-instruction, self-instruction** with practice, and **self-instruction** with practice and **contracting** (Budesheim et al., 1987). Compliance, as measured by increase in the number of exercises performed and the frequency of the performance of the exercises, significantly improved in all three groups with no significant differences among them. These results suggest that a structured, systematic method of teaching concepts important to self-management for patients with arthritis may be more important than the specific method used.

Splinting

Joint inflammation is often aggravated by joint use. In rheumatoid arthritis and other destructive arthropathies, aggravated joint inflammation results not only in greater pain and disability but also causes progressive joint and tendon damage (Swezey, 1971–1972). Joint rest by means of immobilization can reduce joint inflammation (Partridge & Duthie, 1963). Therefore, it is common for the physician to prescribe the use of resting hand splints as part of the treatment program for the arthritis patient (Fig. 40.7).

The type of splint, position of the splint, and wearing schedule are determined by the reasons for and goals of splinting. Exact position of the wrist and finger joints varies somewhat by practitioners (Davis & Janecki, 1978; Kay, 1979; Melvin, 1989; Pahle & Raunio, 1969; Smith et al., 1964). In general, the wrist should be in 10 to 30° of extension and slight ulnar deviation with the finger joints slightly flexed and aligned straight but not crowded. Splints should be lightweight, durable, comfortable, cosmetically appealing, and easy to apply and remove. If the patient is to be independent in the application and removal of the splint, the Velcro straps should be longer than the circumference of the splint to leave a tab or loop for gripping. This is particularly important if the patient is to wear bilateral orthoses.

In addition to resting a joint to reduce pain and inflammation, splints can provide support, prevent stress, and correct or reduce joint contractures. It is important that both the therapist and the patient be aware of how any given splint affects nonsplinted joints in people with RA, i.e., immobilizing one joint may increase stress to a previously uninvolved or less involved joint (Melvin, 1989). For example, a patient with mild synovitis of the wrist only may be best served with a wrist splint (either rigid or flexible with volar support) to be worn during stressful activities. However this splint, while it alleviates stress on the wrist, may

cause an exacerbation of symptoms at the MP or PIP joints if hand use when the splint is applied is not properly monitored. Dynamic splinting is generally reserved for preoperative or postoperative management and is contraindicated for acutely inflamed joints.

Research on the efficacy of hand splints in arthritis management is scant. While there has been some work that demonstrates that splinting is effective in reducing inflammation (Partridge & Duthie, 1963) and in reducing joint pain (Feinberg & Brandt, 1981), there has been no research as to whether early splinting prevents deformities. However, if it is accepted that joint inflammation causes swelling and swelling in turn stretches the capsular structures, which then allows deformities to occur, then it would seem to follow logically that if joint inflammation is diminished via splint use, then the sequence of events from which deformities occur is affected. Nonetheless, a controlled study to determine if splinting prevents deformity needs to be done.

MAINTAIN OR INCREASE STRENGTH

Exercise for strengthening is avoided during periods of acute systemic illness and when the joints are inflamed (Melvin, 1989; Swezey, 1993). During more quiescent times, isometric exercise is the exercise of choice, because it is least likely to produce pain (Glass, 1978; Melvin, 1989). As few as six isometric contractions per day (held for 6 sec) have been demonstrated to increase muscle strength significantly (Machover & Sapecky, 1966; Rose, Radzyminski, & Beatty, 1957). The goal is to maintain the static holding ability of muscle so that proper positioning can be maintained during functional activities (Swezey, 1993). Strengthening exercises should follow a period of warmup and are done only when pain and stiffness are at a minimum (Swezey, 1993).

Resistive exercise for patients with RA is controversial. Some authorities advocate avoidance of resistance because resistive exercise can neither improve weakened joint structures nor reposition the tendons and because the disease has changed the relationship of the tendons to the axes of movement, causing the forces during resistive isotonic exercise to be deforming (Flatt, 1983). However, Swezey (1993) stated that there is not enough research to support whether resistive exercises are helpful or harmful in cases of myositis. But, to be cautious, he deferred resistive exercises until serum enzymes are at or near normal to avoid exacerbating the myositis. Both Flatt (1983) and Swezey (1993) advocate graduated exercise programs and protection of supporting joint structures during exercise.

It has been recently demonstrated that aerobic exercise by people with arthritis results in an increased

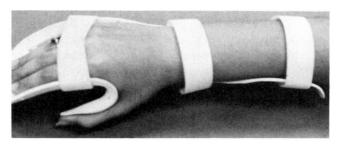

Figure 40.7. Resting hand splints commonly prescribed for night use in the treatment of rheumatoid arthritis.

aerobic and ADL capacity and is enthusiastically accepted by the patients (Harkcom et al., 1985; Minor et al., 1989). Water exercise has also been shown to increase strength and endurance in arthritis patients (Danneskiold-Samsoe et al., 1987). While these reports are positive, it is probably prudent to be selective in recommending such exercise regimens for arthritis patients. For the present, therefore, isometric exercise can be prescribed to tolerance to maintain strength around involved joints, but endurance training should probably be viewed with cautious skepticism (Nicholas, 1993).

In general, activities to maintain and increase strength should be gently resistive and done for short periods of time within the limits of pain and fatigue. **Joint protection** principles should be adhered to when choosing an activity (Melvin, 1989). Activities that require reaching to pick up objects are good choices for the upper extremities, trunk, and neck. It is important that the patient be kept interested in moving actively throughout the day but within limits. Care should be taken that the repetitive exercise or activity is not exacerbating the disease. Finally, the activity or exercise program should be designed so that it can be easily incorporated into a home program.

MAINTAIN OR INCREASE FUNCTIONAL ABILITIES

Principles and methods of self-care and homemaking activities for patients with limited range of motion are described in Chapters 15 and 16. Essentially, the methods involve the use of long handles to extend reach, **joint protection,** and energy conservation. Some other suggestions include the following. A warm morning bath or shower helps the patient overcome **morning stiffness.** Sleeping on flannel sheets in the winter also may help relieve pain and stiffness in the morning. Zippers with large teeth and ring pull tabs and convex buttons on shanks used with vertical buttonholes have been found easiest to manage by women with RA (Dallas & White, 1982). A chair with elevated seat height has been found to decrease significantly the stress on hips and knees when rising (Burdett et al., 1985). Patients with advanced inflammatory polyarthritis may develop such severe deformities and muscle weakness that a powered wheelchair becomes a necessity (Bossingham & Russell, 1980).

It is important that the patient learn how to protect his joints during occupational performance tasks (Edmonds, 1978). Any means of substituting for grasp or reducing the force required during functional activities are sought (Fig. 40.8). Many devices that are not specially made for people with arthritis but make daily tasks easier are routinely available in the marketplace. For example, a jar opener or book holder are easily

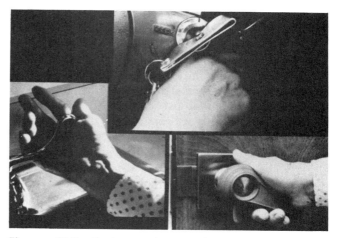

Figure 40.8. Devices to increase leverage and decrease force when turning a faucet, a car ignition, and a door knob.

purchased in the community. It is important that people with arthritis learn to problem solve in their daily activities and to make simple adjustments to maximize their independence and reduce stress on their joints. This education should be a major part of the occupational therapy treatment program.

Sex is a functional task and should be discussed with the patient in relation to **joint protection** and avoidance of pain. Sex presents difficulty to the patient with RA because of pain and joint limitations (Greengross, 1979). The difficulty may not only be related to the mechanics but also may have to do with fear about the effect sex will have on the condition; guilt feelings connected to the idea that the disease is punishment for some previous wrong; role anxieties related to a change in role caused by the disease; or feelings of anger, depression, or a poor self-image. There is also a concern with the inability to obtain or use certain types of contraceptive methods because of physical limitations. There may be worry that the disease is hereditary. Sexual counseling beyond the information concerning **joint protection** should be available to the patient (Greengross, 1979). Regarding the mechanics, it is recommended that the patient take pain medication beforehand, use cushions to support painful limbs, use positions that are found to be most comfortable, and make other methods of sexual satisfaction an important aspect of intimacy (Frederick, 1979; Greengross, 1979; Onder, Lachniet, & Becker, 1973). Sexual intercourse should be avoided during periods of fatigue and during flare-ups of the disease (Krawitz & Wolman, 1979).

Gainful employment can provide the patient with psychosocial and physical benefits as well as financial benefits. In a study of 306 RA patients, almost half had stopped working within 10 years of the diagnosis (Yelin, Henke, & Epstein, 1987). Those who had or were able to switch to a less physically demanding job and those who were able to exercise control over the pace of their job activities were more apt to continue working. These findings suggest that people with RA require flexible working conditions to remain in the labor force. As a result of the implementation of the Americans with Disabilities Act of 1990, it is possible that more people with arthritis will be able to remain in the workforce, because employers are required to make reasonable accommodations in work schedules and job tasks if the person with RA is qualified to do the essential functions of the job (see Chapter 17).

The therapist works with the patient to solve problems related to **joint protection** and energy conservation while working. The day's routine and specific tasks are reviewed, and each is analyzed to ensure that energy is conserved and joints are protected. The occupational therapist may also work with the employer to recommend reasonable accommodations for the patient's needs and requirements to facilitate continued employment.

Home evaluation and home modifications may be necessary to facilitate daily life tasks. Assessment focusing on safety and accessibility of work areas can be completed by a home visit or by providing the patient with a detailed checklist.

Recreational activities to maintain endurance and to overcome the depression associated with chronic disability and pain, yet which are nonstressful to joints, should be promoted. Swimming is one especially good activity for most persons (Swezey, 1993).

BALANCE ACTIVITY WITH REST

The total day of the patient with RA must be examined to develop a plan for activity balanced by rest. At times of greater disease activity, more rest is required. When the disease is quiescent, activity may be increased. Involving the patient in interesting activities in occupational therapy provides the opportunity for the patient to learn to gauge his own endurance and to learn to rest before fatigue occurs. Fatigue may not only cause careless use of joints but also requires a longer rest-recovery period, which means longer immobilization. This balance of rest and activity is carried over to home planning also.

Frequent, short rest periods are more beneficial for these patients than one long one. Similarly, a slow steady rate of work is preferable to rushing. People with arthritis have limited energy and, therefore, need to use **energy-conservation principles:** omit all unnecessary effort, carefully plan tasks, be well organized, eliminate unnecessary steps, and use laborsaving devices. For example, keeping the necessary equipment and supplies concentrated in the area where they are most often used avoids unnecessary steps.

Duplication of cleaning materials in different parts of the house eliminates the need to collect and carry them from place to place. Lightweight, electric appliances and convenient, packaged foods are also labor-saving devices.

Living with Rheumatoid Arthritis

Because RA is a chronic condition, the patient and his family must adjust and incorporate the necessary management program into their lifestyles. It is imperative that the person with arthritis assume the responsibility for the ongoing management of the disease. One major component of effective self-management is patient education. A large part of the role of the occupational therapist in arthritis health care is patient education. The therapist must instruct the patient in principles of **joint protection** and energy conservation, proper use of splints and adaptive equipment, and the need to balance activity and rest.

Compliance is a major problem in the management of chronic diseases. It has been estimated that at least 50% of patients with RA are noncompliant with therapy irrespective of the nature of the intervention (Belcon, Haynes, & Tugwell, 1984). Because patient outcome is affected by both the efficacy of the treatment and the extent of patient compliance, occupational therapists need to use approaches to increase the likelihood of compliance. The more active a patient is in planning and controlling his own regimen, the greater the chance of successful compliance (Hasselkus, 1987). The therapeutic alliance between the therapist and the patient is important in obtaining patient cooperation. In a study designed to examine the effect of the interaction between the patient and the occupational therapist on subsequent splint use, splint use was greater in a group of patients who were treated by a therapist using compliance-enhancing behaviors (Table 40.2) (Feinberg, 1992). These behaviors included the use of principles of patient education, mutual sharing of expected outcomes related to splint use, encouraging the patient to assume responsibility for splint use, and the use of an **affective tone,** which inspired trust and confidence in the therapist's knowledge and skills.

Effectiveness

The effectiveness of occupational therapy provided in the patient's home was the focus of a study completed in Canada (Helewa et al., 1991). A complete arthritis assessment and treatment program was administered during a 6-week period to a group of 53 RA patients and compared with a control group who received no treatment during that time period. Functional scores for the experimental group were significantly higher than those of the control group at follow-up,

Table 40.2. Clinical Suggestions for Enhancing Patient Compliance

I. Apply learning principles to patient education.
1. Patients remember best instructions presented first.
2. Emphasized instructions are recalled better.
3. The fewer the instructions, the greater the proportion remembered.
4. Pace the amount of information to avoid overload.
5. Use simple, understandable language without medical jargon.
6. Individualize teaching methods to the patient.
7. Reinforce essential points by review, discussion, or summary.
8. Ask the patient to repeat essential elements of the message.
9. Provide written instructions for home reference.
10. Devise mechanisms for helping patients to remember advice given.

II. Assess the patient's expectations and experience concerning the following:
1. The clinical encounter.
2. His beliefs and misconceptions about the cause, severity, or symptoms of the illness and susceptibility to complications or exacerbations.
3. Goals of treatment.
4. Perceptions about the costs and risks versus the benefits of treatment.
5. Existing health-related knowledge, skills, and practices.
6. Degree of adaptation to the disease.
7. Sense of self-efficacy or lack of control and hopelessness.
8. Learning limitations.
9. Extent of family involvement and influence.

III. Encourage the patient to assume responsibility for disease management.
1. Use behavioral contracts if necessary.
2. Use other motivational techniques.
3. Encourage the patient that he can be successful with self-management.

IV. Use a facilitating affective tone.
1. Listen to the patient.
2. Be approachable.
3. Appear knowledgeable.
4. Inspire trust and confidence.
5. Be enthusiastic and expect positive results.

indicating the efficacy of occupational therapy when delivered in the home setting.

OSTEOARTHRITIS (DEGENERATIVE JOINT DISEASE)

Degenerative joint disease, or osteoarthritis, is the most common rheumatic disease (Schumaker, 1988). Unlike RA, osteoarthritis is not a systemic disease. It may be limited to one joint or may involve multiple joints. Deformities arise because of changes in the bone, not because of changes in the biomechanics of joint structure and muscle pull. Osteoarthritis is characterized by progressive loss of articular cartilage

and by reactive changes at the margins of the joints and in subchondral bone. Data suggest a role for biochemical, biomechanical, inflammatory, and immunologic factors in the development of pathologic changes characteristic of osteoarthritis. Men and women are equally affected; however, women are more likely to have moderate to severe disease (Swanson & Swanson, 1985). Prevalence of osteoarthritis increases with age, and the disease is almost universal in people 65 years or older.

Osteoarthritis may be classified as primary (idiopathic) or secondary. Genetic factors play a role in primary OA, particularly in the development of OA of the distal interphalangeal joints of the hands (Heberden's nodes). Etiologic factors in secondary OA include congenital or developmental defects, trauma, inflammation, endocrine and metabolic diseases, and prolonged occupational stress. Common sites of OA are the hands, cervical spine, lumbar spine, hips, knees, ankles, and feet (Quinet, 1986).

Symptoms include progressively developing joint pain, stiffness, and enlargement with limitation of motion. Pain on passive motion and **crepitus** are prominent findings. Clinical symptoms do not necessarily correlate with the degree of radiological involvement of the joints. Patients with severe radiographic findings may report little or no pain or discomfort, and conversely, a patient with only minor radiographic changes can be disabled by pain (Melvin, 1989).

Primary OA of the hands is characterized by the development of **bony spurs** at the medial and dorsolateral surfaces of the DIP and PIP joints. These are called Heberden's nodes at the DIP joint and Bouchard's nodes at the PIP joint. These spurs may develop slowly over months or years or the onset may be rapid and associated with pain and inflammation. Involvement of the first carpometacarpal joint leads to tenderness at the base of the first metacarpal and a squared appearance. Occupational therapy treatment for hand involvement includes the following:

1. Splinting to decrease pain;
2. **Joint protection** techniques to prevent pain;
3. Provision of adapted techniques and equipment to maximize independence;
4. Postoperative splinting and mobilization in late stage disease.

Splinting may be used to rest a painful joint or to stabilize it during activity. For example, a CMC splint worn during activity can provide support and reduce stress to the joint (Fig. 40.9). Use of a soft wrap or nylon-spandex stretch gloves may provide pain relief and diminish **morning stiffness** if worn at night. The effectiveness of splints and wraps vary with the individual and the activities that cause the pain. Be-

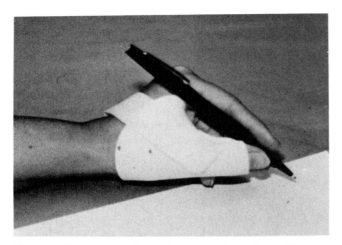

Figure 40.9. CMC splint to decrease pain during activity.

cause the primary goal is to provide symptomatic relief, if relief is not attained with these devices, then they should be discontinued. Moist heat application may be used to decrease discomfort. If heat is not helpful, cold application should be tried.

Range of motion limited by osteophytes will not improve with exercise; however, flexibility exercises done in the morning may help decrease generalized stiffness. Adaptive devices such as built-up handles or jar openers may increase function, and patients should learn adaptive methods to accomplish activities that, if done in the usual manner, aggravate the involved joint, e.g., strong pinching when there is CMC involvement. For severe CMC disease, joint arthroplasty or arthrodesis may be necessary (see Chapter 38).

Occupational therapy may also be used in the management of OA of the hips and knees. Work simplification and **joint protection** techniques are aimed at minimizing stress on the involved weight-bearing joints. Patients may be limited in their ability to ambulate or stand for extended periods of time; therefore, education about work simplification is important. Sitting down and rising up from low surfaces may be particularly difficult or painful, thus provision of elevated toilet seats or adaptations to other chairs may be indicated. Self-care activities such as putting on and removing shoes and socks and bathing the feet may require adaptations for the patient to accomplish these tasks independently.

Occupational therapy is also generally included as part of the postoperative rehabilitation program following total hip or total knee replacement surgery (see Chapter 37). Temporary postoperative limitations either the result of postsurgical precautions or limited joint mobility often necessitate patient education and provision of adaptive equipment such as long-handled bath sponges and shoe horns, sock aids, and reachers to accomplish lower extremity self-care activities. Results of a series of surveys sent to 163 patients at 2, 6, and 10 weeks following hip replacement surgery indicated that at 2 weeks, 73% were using the bathing or toileting aids provided; 50% were using them at 6 weeks; and 37% were still using them at 10 weeks (Haworth, 1983). Another retrospective survey found that most patients reported having used the equipment for 2 to 3 months following hip surgery, and about 33% continued to use adaptive equipment beyond the 3-month precautionary period (Seeger & Fisher, 1982). The patients in this survey reported that the raised toilet seat and reacher were the most useful items. Ideally, patients should not require continued use of these devices beyond the postoperative rehabilitation period. The fact that many patients continued to use adaptive equipment may indicate that these patients had other joint limitations (e.g., the other hip or knee) or that they simply found that these devices made completion of daily tasks easier. Regardless, it would appear that efficacy is validated by the initial and continued use of the adapted devices provided by occupational therapy in the postoperative management of total hip arthroplasty.

CASE STUDY: OSTEOARTHRITIS PATIENT

Sarah is a 72-year-old widow with a diagnosis of primary osteoarthritis involving her CMC and DIP joints bilaterally. She is a retired teacher who enjoys cooking, reading, needle crafts, and gardening. These activities have become increasingly difficult for her. She finds that her pain steadily increases relative to the duration of the activity, yet she does not want to give up any of her current interests. Her primary care physician has referred her to occupational therapy for assessment and treatment.

Following assessment, the occupational therapist fitted her with bilateral CMC joint splints made of a thermoplastic material for use during stressful activities such as gardening. She was instructed in ways to reduce stress to her joints, including limiting the time she participates in any one activity. She was also provided with a book stand for use when she reads so that she will not have to hold a book for extended periods of time. She was made aware of other adaptive devices that she may find helpful in the future.

This is a typical case example of a patient with primary osteoarthritis. Functional problems may be limited to a few activities, and often they can be quickly and easily addressed through education, splinting, and/or provision of adaptive equipment in a single occupational therapy session.

STUDY QUESTIONS

1. What are the five characteristic manifestations of inflammation?
2. What assessments are considered in the evaluation of patients with RA?
3. How is it determined that the intrinsic muscles of the fingers have become abnormally shortened?

4. Describe the underlying process of the ulnar deviation deformity of the MP joints.
5. Discuss the controversy concerning use of resistive exercise with RA patients.
6. What are the occupational therapy goals for patients with RA?
7. What are the positions of deformity that RA patients are educated to avoid?
8. List the principles of joint protection.
9. What is the difference in etiological factors between primary and secondary osteoarthritis?
10. What are the goals of occupational therapy treatment for the patient with osteoarthritis?

REFERENCES

Agnew, P. J., & Maas, F. (1991). Jamar dynamometer and adapted sphygmomanometer for measuring grip strength in patients with rheumatoid arthritis. *Occupational Therapy Journal of Research, 11*, 259–270.

American Occupational Therapy Association. Commission on Practice. (1986). Roles and functions of occupational therapy in the management of patients with rheumatic diseases. *American Journal of Occupational Therapy, 40*, 825–829.

Backman, G. C., Mackie, H., & Harris, J. (1991). Arthritis Hand Function Test: Development of a standardized assessment tool. *Occupational Therapy Journal of Research, 11*, 245–255.

Barrows, D. M., Berezny, L. M., & Reynolds, M. D. (1978). Physical and occupational therapy for arthritic patients: A cooperative effort among hospital departments. *Archives of Physical Medicine & Rehabilitation, 59*(2), 64–67.

Belcon, M. C., Haynes, R. B., & Tugwell, P. (1984). A critical review of compliance studies in rheumatoid arthritis. *Arthritis and Rheumatism, 27*, 1227–1233.

Bossingham, R. G., & Russell, P. (1980). The usefulness of powered wheelchairs in advanced inflammatory polyarthritis. *Rheumatology Rehabilitation, 19*, 131–135.

Budesheim, G. C., Black, S. O., Vogel, K., & Hassenein, R. (1987). A comparison of the relative effects of self-instruction, contracting, and practice on knowledge and compliance to an arthritis treatment regimen (Abstract C). *Arthritis and Rheumatism, 30*, S207.

Burdett, R. G., Habasevich, R., Pisciotta, J., & Simon, S. R. (1985). Biomechanical comparison of rising from two types of chairs. *Physical Therapy, 65*, 1177–1183.

Cordery, J. (1965). Joint protection: A responsibility of the occupational therapist. *American Journal of Occupational Therapy, 19*, 285–294.

Dallas, M. J., & White, L. W. (1982). Clothing fasteners for women with arthritis. *American Journal of Occupational Therapy, 36*, 515–518.

Danneskiold-Samsoe, B., Lynsberg, K., Risum, T., & Telling, M. (1987). The effect of water exercise therapy given to patients with rheumatoid arthritis. *Scandinavian Journal of Rehabilitation Medicine, 19*, 31–35.

Davis, J., & Janecki, C. J. (1978). Rehabilitation of the rheumatoid upper limb. *Orthopaedic Clinics of North America, 9*, 559–568.

Edmonds, J. (1978). The management of rheumatoid arthritis. *Australian Family Physician, 7*, 925–935.

English, C. B., & Nalebuff, E. A. (1971). Understanding the arthritic hand. *American Journal of Occupational Therapy, 25*, 353–358.

Feinberg, J. R. (1992). Effect of the arthritis health professional on compliance with use of resting hand splints by patients with rheumatoid arthritis. *Arthritis Care and Research, 5*, 17–23.

Feinberg, J., & Brandt, K. D. (1981). Use of resting splints by patients with rheumatoid arthritis. *American Journal of Occupational Therapy, 35*, 173–178.

Feinberg, J. R., & Brandt, K. D. (1984). Allied health team management of rheumatoid arthritis patients. *American Journal of Occupational Therapy, 38*, 613–620.

Fisher, A. G. (1993). Assessment of IADL skills: An application of many-faceted Rasch analysis. *American Journal of Occupational Therapy, 47*(4), 319–329.

Flatt, A. E. (1983). *Care of the rheumatoid hand*. St. Louis: C. V. Mosby.

Frederick, B. B. (1979). *Body mechanics instruction manual: A guide for therapists*. Redmond, WA: Express Publications.

Furst, G. P., Gerber, L. H., & Smith, C. B. (1985). *Rehabilitation through learning: Energy conservation and joint protection. A workbook for persons with rheumatoid arthritis* (Publication No. 017-045-00107-4). Washington, DC: U.S. Government Printing Office.

Furst, G. P., Gerber, L. H., Smith, C. C., Fisher, S., & Shulman, B. (1987). A program for improving energy conservation behaviors in adults with rheumatoid arthritis. *American Journal of Occupational Therapy, 41*, 102–111.

Glass, J. (1978). Physical medicine in rheumatology. *Australian and New Zealand Journal of Medicine, 8*(Suppl. 1), 168–171.

Greengross, W. (1979). Sex and arthritis. *Rheumatology Rehabilitation, 18*(Suppl. 1), 68–70.

Gross, M., Brandt, K. D., Feinberg, J., Korba, E., Rankin, M., & Roche, V. (1982). Team care for patients with chronic rheumatic disease. *Journal of Allied Health, 15*(11), 239–247.

Harkcom, T. M., Lampman, R. M., Banwell, B. F., & Castor, C. W. (1985). Therapeutic values of graded aerobic exercise training in rheumatoid arthritis. *Arthritis and Rheumatism, 28*, 32–39.

Hasselkus, B. R. (1987, February 19). Emerging trends in geriatric care. *Occupational Therapy Week*, 5–6.

Hasselkus, B. R., Kshepakaran, K. K., & Safrit, M. J. (1981). Handedness and hand joint changes in rheumatoid arthritis. *American Journal of Occupational Therapy, 35*, 705–710.

Haworth, R. J. (1983). Use of aids during the first three months after total hip replacement. *British Journal of Rheumatology, 22*, 29–35.

Helewa, A., Goldsmith, C. H., Lee, P., Bombardier, C., Hanes, B., Smyth, H. A., & Tugwell, P. (1991). Effects of occupational therapy home service on patients with rheumatoid arthritis. *Lancet, 337*, 1453–1456.

Huskisson, E. C. (1974). Measurement of pain. *Lancet, 2*(7889), 1127–1131.

Jebsen, R. H., Taylor, N., Trieschmann, R. B., Trotter, M. J., & Howard, L. A. (1969). An objective and standardized test of hand function. *Archives of Physical Medicine & Rehabilitation, 50*, 311–319.

Kay, A. G. L. (1979). Management of the rheumatoid hand. *Rheumatology Rehabilitation, 18*(Suppl. 1), 76–81.

Krawitz, M., & Wolman, T. (1979). Group therapy in rheumatoid arthritis. *Pennsylvania Medicine, 82*(12), 35–37.

Law, M., Baptiste, S., McColl, M.A., Opzoomer, A., Polatajko, H., & Pollock, N. (1991). *Canadian Occupational Performance Measure*. Toronto, Ont.: Canadian Association of Occupational Therapists.

Machover, S., & Sapecky, A. J. (1966). Effects of isometric exercise on the quadriceps muscle in patients with rheumatoid arthritis. *Archives of Physical Medicine & Rehabilitation, 47*, 737–741.

McKnight, P. T., & Schomburg, F. L. (1982). Air pressure splint effects on hand symptoms of patients with rheumatoid arthritis. *Archives of Physical Medicine & Rehabilitation, 63,* 560–564.

Melvin, J. L. (1989). *Rheumatic diseases in the adult and child: Occupational therapy and rehabilitation* (3rd ed.). Philadelphia: F. A. Davis.

Minor, M. A., Hewett, J. E., Webel, R. R., Anderson, S. K., & Kay, D. R. (1989). Efficacy of physical conditioning exercise in patients with rheumatoid arthritis and osteoarthritis. *Arthritis and Rheumatism, 32,* 1396–1405.

Nalebuff, E. A. (1968). Diagnosis, classification and management of rheumatoid thumb deformities. *Bulletin of the Hospital for Joint Diseases, 24,* 119–138.

Nalebuff, E. A. (1984). The rheumatoid thumb. *Clinics in Rheumatic Diseases, 10,* 589–608.

Nicholas, J. J. (1993). Rehabilitation of patients with rheumatic diseases. In W. N. Kelley, E. D. Harris, S. Ruddy, & C. B. Sledge (Eds.), *Textbook of rheumatology* (4th ed., pp. 1728–1744). Philadelphia: W. B. Saunders.

Onder, J., Lachniet, D., & Becker, M. C. (1973). Sexual counselling, arthritis, and women. *Arthritis Foundation Allied Health Professions Section Newsletter, 7*(3–4), 1–6.

Pahle, J. A., & Raunio, P. (1969). The influence of wrist position on finger deviation in the rheumatoid hand. *Journal of Bone and Joint Surgery, 5,* 664–676.

Partridge, R., & Duthie, J. (1963). Controlled trial of the effect of complete immobilization of the joints in rheumatoid arthritis. *Annals of Rheumatic Diseases, 22,* 91–99.

Quest, I. M., & Cordery, J. (1971). A functional ulnar deviation cuff for rheumatoid deformity. *American Journal of Occupational Therapy, 25,* 32–37, 40.

Quinet, R. J. (1986). Osteoarthritis: Increasing mobility and reducing disability. *Geriatrics, 41*(2), 36–50.

Rose, D. L., Radzyminski, S. F., & Beatty, R. R. (1957). Effect of brief maximal exercise on the strength of the quadriceps femoris. *Archives of Physical Medicine & Rehabilitation, 38,* 157–164.

Salter, R. B. (1983). *Textbook of disorders and injuries of the musculoskeletal system.* Baltimore: Williams & Wilkins.

Schumacher, H. R. (Ed.). (1988). *Primer on the rheumatic diseases* (9th ed.). Atlanta: The Arthritis Foundation.

Seeger, M. S., & Fisher, L. A. (1982). Adaptive equipment used in the rehabilitation of hip arthroplasty patients. *American Journal of Occupational Therapy, 36,* 503–508.

Smith, E. M., Juvinall, R. C., Bender, L. F., & Pearson, J. R. (1964). Role of the finger flexors in rheumatoid deformities of the metacarpophalangeal joints. *Arthritis and Rheumatism, 7,* 467–480.

Spiegel, J. S., Hirshfield, M. S., & Speigle, T. M. (1985). Evaluating self care activities. Comparison of a self-reported questionnaire with an occupational therapist interview. *British Journal of Rheumatology, 24,* 357–361.

Swanson, A. B. (1972). Flexible implant arthroplasty for arthritic finger joints. *Journal of Bone and Joint Surgery, 54A,* 435–355.

Swanson, A. B., & Swanson, G. DeG. (1985). Osteoarthritis in the hand. *Clinics in Rheumatic Diseases, 11,* 393–420.

Swezey, R. L. (1989). Rehabilitation medicine and arthritis. In D. J. McCarty (Ed.), *Arthritis and allied conditions* (11th ed., pp. 797–825). Philadelphia: Lea & Febiger.

Swezey, R. L. (1971–1972). *Dynamic factors in deformity of the rheumatoid arthritic hand* (Bulletin on the Rheumatic Diseases). Atlanta: The Arthritis Foundation.

Swezey, R. L. (1993). Rehabilitation medicine and arthritis. In D. J. McCarty & W. J. Koopman (Eds.), *Arthritis and allied conditions* (12th ed., pp. 887–917). Philadelphia: Lea & Febiger.

Tichauer, E. R. (1966). Some aspects of stress on forearm and hand in industry. *Journal of Occupational Medicine, 8*(2), 63–71.

Tubiana, R., Thomine, J. M., & Mackin, E. (1984). *Examination of the hand and upper limb.* Philadelphia: W. B. Saunders.

Vignos, P. J. (1980). Physiotherapy in rheumatoid arthritis. *Journal of Rheumatology, 7,* 269–271.

Walker, P. S., Davidson, W., & Erkman, M. J. (1978). An apparatus to assess function of the hand. *Journal of Hand Surgery, 3,* 189–193.

Wozny, W., & Long, C. (1966). Electromyographic kinesiology of the rheumatoid hand. *Archives of Physical Medicine & Rehabilitation, 47,* 702–703.

Yelin, E. H., Henke, C. J., & Epstein, W. (1987). The work dynamics of the person with rheumatoid arthritis. *Arthritis and Rheumatism, 30,* 507–512.

41
Burns

M. Irma Alvarado

OBJECTIVES

After studying this chapter, the reader will be able to:
1. Define first-degree, second-degree, and third-degree burn.
2. Describe the general course of treatment of burn patients.
3. Outline the occupational therapy program for achieving functional outcomes for the burned patient and his family.
4. Describe isolation techniques and the importance of their observance.
5. State the rationale behind positioning the burned patient.
6. State the purpose of constant pressure against healing burn scar and describe the treatment options for various body areas.

The National Fire Data Center, under the auspices of the National Fire Prevention and Control Administration, estimates 2,600,000 reported fires and 30,000,000 unreported fires annually (American Burn Association, 1984). Each year approximately 7,500 people die and 310,000 are seriously injured in fires.

Mortality curves have dramatically improved and the median lethal dose for patients without inhalation injury is burns covering about 75% of **total body surface area** (TBSA) (Salisbury, 1992). Significant advances in the care of burned patients have improved survival rates while decreasing the length of hospitalization for all types of burns (Feller & Jones, 1984). These advances include improved medications to reduce or to prevent burn wound infection, improvement in many life support measures, the use of biological dressings for immediate covering in extensive burns, and vigorous rehabilitation measures to reduce the morbidity of severe burns (Salisbury, Newman, & Dingeldein, 1983). Burn care specialists are no longer satisfied with just survival in the treatment of burns (Dimick, 1984).

Cromes and Helm (1992) reported an increase in attention to the multifaceted rehabilitation needs of patients with burns over a 5-year span when comparing their national survey with a previous study. Burn care programs in the United States are similar, and most of them use occupational therapists in the rehabilitation of the burn patient (Purdue, 1984). The goal is to help patients reach their maximum rehabilitation status (Dimick, 1984).

Comprehensive care of a burn patient requires the special skills and knowledge that come with a multidisciplinary team effort and the coordination of responsibilities of all personnel for optimum care. Because many body systems are involved in a severe burn injury, resulting in physical and psychosocial consequences, the burn care team includes several medical specialists, nurses, physical and occupational therapists, a nutritionist, and a social worker (DiGregorio, 1984), respiratory therapists, and psychologists.

The acute nature of a burned patient's illness can last weeks into months with a therapeutic regimen that may extend beyond 2 years after the initial trauma. Cromes and Helm (1992) determined in a comprehensive survey that the average length of hospitalization was 9 days for patients with burns covering 0 to 10% TBSA, 18 days for patients with burns covering 11 to 20% TBSA, 29 days for patients with burns covering 21 to 40% TBSA, and 42 days for patients with burns covering more than 40% TBSA. The average duration of physician follow-up is 4.7 months for patients with mild burns, 11.5 months for patients with moderate burns, and 24.8 months for patients with severe burns.

Immediate treatment for burns can occur in a doctor's office or in the emergency room of a hospital (Hummel, 1982). However, patients with major burn injuries require hospitalization in a specified burn care facility. The American Burn Association (1993) listed 138 burn care facilities in the United States and 21 in

GLOSSARY

Acute phase—The acute phase covers the period of resuscitation and stabilization of the patient that is influenced by the extent of the total body surface area involved.

Advance directive—Legal document containing the patient's or legal guardian's wishes regarding the patient's medical care.

Blocking, or capener, splint—A splint that blocks motion at one joint while allowing tendon excursion and motion at an adjacent joint to prevent excessive force to the injured tendon during motion (see Chapters 28 and 38).

First-degree, superficial burn—Tissue destruction involving only the epidermis with local pain and erythema, but no blistering present.

Hypertrophic scarring—A red, raised, rigid tangled mass of collagen fibers that develops to bridge a wound to form a scar.

Reverse or protective isolation—Isolation procedures designed to protect the patient from cross-contamination by people or objects.

Rule of Nines—A systematic method for determining percentage of total body surface area burned by assignment of multiples of nine to body parts.

Second-degree, partial-thickness burn—Superficial, partial-thickness burns are red and moist burns with blister formation and intact tactile and pain sensation; usually heal within 14 to 21 days. Deep partial-thickness burns involve the epidermis and portions of the dermis. Because of slow, unstable reepitheliazation, healing is extended over a period of time, and therefore, excision and skin grafting are usually indicated.

Sulfamylon—One of a wide variety of topical antibacterial agents used in the treatment of burn wounds popularized in the mid 1960s. Silver sulfadiazine is now generally the topical agent of choice in most burn units.

Third-degree, full-thickness burn—Tissue destruction involving the epidermis and dermis through the subcutaneous tissue. The wound appears dry and inelasticity necessitates escharotomy or fasciotomy to relieve pressure and prevent edema formation.

Total body surface area—Defines the bodily extent of burn injury for determining severity and medical management.

Canada at which burn care physicians report the presence of beds designated for acute burn care. Some hospitals have burn programs in which there is a method of consistent management for burn patients. This includes designated staff and an available physician with specialized skills in the treatment of burn injury. A burn unit within a hospital refers to beds set aside for the exclusive use of burn patients, who are treated only by trained personnel.

BURN INJURY

A burn wound is a tissue response to heat. Common sources of heat are thermal, chemical, or electrical. The resultant problems and their resolution are a direct result of the heat source and the duration of contact that determines the depth and extent of the trauma to the tissue.

Burn Size Assessment

The extent of a burn injury is estimated by the percentage of **total body surface area** burned. A common method of estimating TBSA burned is the **Rule of Nines.** In adults, the percentage of TBSA is calculated by this formula: head and neck equal 9% (4.5% on each surface); each upper extremity is 9% (4.5% on each surface), for a total of 18%; anterior trunk is 18%; posterior trunk is 18%; each lower extremity is 18% (9% each surface), equaling 36%;

and the genitalia are 1%, for a total of 100%. The extent of burn injury is calculated according to the percentage each body area burned represents.

Although the **Rule of Nines** is practical, it provides only a gross estimate. Exact estimates are obtained by use of the Lund-Browder charts. The Lund-Browder system accounts for body changes that occur during normal growth and development for infants, toddlers, and young children, children ages 10 to 15, and adults over 15 years old. Major burns are those considered to involve more than 25% of TBSA with deep second- and third-degree burns or more than 10% with third-degree burns (Helm, 1983).

Symptoms

The depth of trauma is based on the intensity of heat delivered to the skin or tissue surface. A **first-degree, superficial burn** is an injury that involves only the superficial outer layer of the epidermis and can heal in 2 to 3 days. It is a painful burn. Sunburn is an example of this type of injury (Abston & Rinear, 1986).

A **second-degree, partial-thickness burn** is characterized by redness and blisters. This type of burn injury involves the epidermis and some of the underlying dermis. The epithelial structure of sebaceous and sweat glands and hair follicles, because they are deeply embedded in the dermis, usually survive and are a source of regeneration of new epidermis to reepithelialize the wound. Second-degree, superficial, partial-thickness burns are painful burns that can heal within 10 to 21 days. Second-degree, deep, partial-thickness burns that do not heal in 3 weeks require skin grafting.

Third-degree, full-thickness burns are characterized by a hard, dry surface. The entire skin thickness and deep epithelium have been traumatized. The surfaces are inelastic and anesthetic because the sensory nerve endings may be destroyed. Because there is no ability for spontaneous healing or regeneration of the epithelium, a skin graft must be placed on the area to promote healing (Salisbury et al., 1983).

Flame injuries may cause the most severe burns because of their depth and extent. Scald burns from hot liquid, a common burn injury among the very young, may be superficial or deep in a limited area. Chemical burns may penetrate into tissues until the chemical substance is washed away (Abston & Rinear, 1986).

Burns of electrical etiology constitute a small proportion of patients admitted for treatment, but they have unique characteristics. Although the extent of thermal burns can be identified and is predictable, the extent of electrical burns may not be. They usually have an entry and exit point, and the skin between those points may appear normal. However, the passage of current beneath the skin may have damaged muscles, nerves, and vascular supply between those points. Edema also may compromise vascular supply, which affects muscle and nerve, resulting in peripheral nerve injury.

Many of the procedures applied to the treatment of thermal burns can be applied to the treatment of electrical burns (Abston & Rinear, 1986). Acutely, amputations, peripheral neuropathy, and entrapment syndrome occur more commonly in electrically induced trauma than in thermal burns. Clinicians must be vigilant, because peripheral neuropathy, quadriplegia, paraplegia, and entrapment syndromes may have an insidious onset and become manifest days to months after the original injury. Both patients with electrical burns and those with thermal burns are subjected to two types of trauma: the injury that is caused by the acute injury and complications that occur because of poor positioning, bulky dressings, intramuscular injections, and neurotoxic medications (Rosenberg & Nelson, 1988). The sequelae of electrical burns are progressive muscular fibrosis, contracture, and loss of function. Patients suffering electrical injuries often require intensive and extensive rehabilitation procedures.

Whatever the extent of a burn injury, maximal therapy is administered until further evaluations can be completed. In some facilities, if the patient's condition indicates that survival is not possible, and when the patient and family accept the futility of maximal therapy, then the patient receives comfort care—a protocol that maintains the patient pain free and mentally and physically as comfortable as possible while not prolonging a difficult death (Frank & Wachtel, 1984). **Advance directives** provide a mechanism for patients and their families to exercise their rights in decision making regarding the patient's medical care. These documents delineate the patient's or legal guardian's wishes regarding the patient's medical care and become a part of the patient's medical record.

ACUTE MANAGEMENT AND REHABILITATION

Treatment usually begins in the emergency room, where resuscitation to correct fluid, electrolyte, and protein deficits is instituted to maintain fluid balance without overloading the circulatory system, which can result in excess edema formation (Pruitt, 1981).

Deep burns result in edema that may invade adjacent tissues, leading to ischemic necrosis and contractures. Edema begins to form within 6 hr postinjury in third-degree burns and may result in capillary damage. The elasticity of the skin is lost, and the resultant eschar formation does not stretch, which may result in pressure great enough to cause venous occlusion or ischemia in the affected body part. Pressure in the trunk, extremities or digits is relieved by escharotomy.

The hospitalized patient is cared for by specialists who recognize that medical complications may involve the respiratory tract from inhalation injury, cardiovascular and renal dysfunction, and/or acute gastroduodenal ulceration from stress and the hypermetabolic state characteristic of a severely burned patient. To counteract the hypermetabolism, a high-calorie diet is required until skin coverage is complete and body fluids are no longer being lost (Dingeldein, 1983).

Topical antibacterial creams and ointments, when used as burn wound dressings, help control burn wound sepsis, soften or debride eschar (the coagulated burn slough), and permit active movement when out of splints and positioning devices or before skin grafting. The size and severity of the patient's injury determines the type of dressings that are applied over any topical antibacterial ointment or cream. The smaller or more superficial the wound, the lighter the dressing, thus facilitating independence in self-care and management. Patients' wounds may be dressed with bulky dressings secured with surgical netting or gauze, and these dressings may be covered with elastic wraps. Pads or occlusive dressings that do not stick to the burn wound may be applied over the open wound or over a topical agent.

The patient's wounds may also be treated via the open technique (i.e., without dressings), which requires patients to be in a warm environment to prevent heat loss (shivering) and to lower metabolic needs—a reason burn units may be kept warmer than other hospital areas (Hartford, 1984).

The **acute phase** of burn care generally depends on the extent of **total body surface area** involved but has been significantly shortened over time. Surgeons assess depth of burn injury, manage metabolic complications, use effective antibiotics, topical antimicrobials, and biological and synthetic skin coverings, and use aggressive debridement techniques that include early application of skin grafts.

Heimbach (1987) described the current status of early excisional therapy. Excision can be performed either by removing the burned tissue and subcutaneous fat to the level of attached fascia (fascial excision) or by sequentially removing thin slices of burned tissue until a viable bed remains (sequential excision). The benefits of early excision and grafting of burn wounds are decreased painful wound debridement procedures and decreased incidence of wound infections and associated complications, thus reducing length of hospitalization for the patient and family.

The patient's own skin must be used for autografting, because it is the only skin cover the patient's body will not reject (Smahel, 1977). Cell culture autografts were discovered and developed in Green's laboratories. These unique techniques permit keratinocytes derived from a small, full-thickness (skin) biopsy to be cultured rapidly under laboratory conditions into layered sheets of human epidermis. Clinical application began in 1979 and has continued to date with indications for use in conjunction with meshed split thickness autografts to provide permanent wound coverage of full-thickness burns larger than 30% TBSA (Biosurface Technology, 1989).

Biological dressings used for temporary coverage of open wounds exert both mechanical and physiologic effects by protecting the wound, maintaining microbial control, and hastening wound maturation. Biological dressings may be allografts or homografts (skin from the same species), xenografts (skin from another species), amnion (fetal membrane), or collagen-synthetic bilaminate, a totally synthetic, biologically inert, membrane (Pruitt & Levine, 1984).

Synthetic skin coverings such as Biobrane and Op-site are used to cover the burn wounds, offering a protective barrier against infection and severe fluid loss for extensively burned patients.

Skin grafting with newer, more aggressive techniques to achieve wound cover, along with the increased use of biological dressings or synthetic dressings results in pain relief and physiological and psychological improvement for the patient. The patient's joints are positioned to prevent deformity, and he continues to exercise and perform self-care within the limits of his physical capacity, location of the synthetic or biological skin graft, and its specific management protocol.

A burn injury destroys the protective skin covering, leaving an open wound with the tissue becoming a medium for bacterial growth within 24 hr of the trauma. Until the burn wound is closed through healing or grafting, it is essential to prevent bacterial contamination of the wound (Sheretz, 1983). Burn wound infection can convert a superficial wound into a full-thickness injury. Prevention of infection is a primary goal in burn units and **reverse or protective isolation** is used by all persons coming in contact with the patient to avoid infection.

Each facility may have its own procedures; however, the general guidelines for strict isolation are as follows:

- The patient is placed in a private room;
- All staff wash their hands before patient treatment;
- A barrier gown or apron is donned before entering the patient's room;
- Gloves are donned after hand washing;
- Mask and cap are worn for wound care;
- The door is closed at all times.

After leaving the patient, the gown and mask are removed and placed in an appropriate receptacle and hands are washed again to prevent spread of infection between patients. Disposable equipment is used whenever possible. Other equipment, including splints and occupational therapy media supplies and equipment, must be sterilized according to institutional standards before they are used with another patient (Sheretz, 1983).

Life support measures and treatment techniques that isolate the patient from infection tend to result also in social isolation, itself psychologically stressful (Bernstein, 1976). The occupational therapist provides some social involvement at every visit, the goals of which may be positioning for reduction of edema or fitting and adjusting splints. Treatment rationales are explained to the patient and family to ensure functional outcomes when the wounds have healed or skin cover is achieved. This is evidence to the patient that his recovery is anticipated. The occupational therapist can foster the patient's efforts in his own treatment from the first visit.

The burn wound is cleansed and dressed daily, usually by nursing or rehabilitation services therapy personnel. Shower trolleys with water sprays, ordinary shower or bath routines are used in some centers, whereas in other centers, full body immersion and mechanical debridement is done in a bathing tank. Antibacterial ointment dressings are applied daily after cleansing, and this is an optimum time, while the tissues are soft and moist, for the patient to do active motion (Helm et al., 1983).

In cases of extensive burns, the patient will have some full-thickness wounds in the pregraft stage, whereas other body parts are in the healing stage or in the postgraft stage. Rehabilitation goals are to prevent deformity and maintain range of motion and specific procedures are used for each burned area until total skin coverage is achieved.

Patients with psychological or social problems that predate their burn injuries are more likely to have psychological-behavioral problems in the **acute phases** of care (Kolman, 1984). This circumstance may negatively impact the patient's and family's initial rehabilitation. Early identification of problems that are addressed by the whole team on a consistent basis can facilitate the recovery process (see Chapter 10).

Severely burned patients, aggravated by stress, may exhibit a variety of behaviors and responses because of pain, shock, fear, anxiety, excitation, delirium, and/or hallucinations. The patient may focus on the pain (Malt, 1980). There is no direct correlation between the extent of injury and the psychological adjustment problems of the patient. When prolonged treatment is necessary, the continuing stress may lead to depression or hostility toward the personnel responsible for the patient's care (Kolman, 1984). A burned patient's response to personnel may create hostility and resentment among the staff (see Chapter 20). Daily contact with emotionally distraught, disfigured, and critically ill patients may provoke strong emotions and anxiety in professionals working with them. The occupational therapist has the opportunity to discuss management of negative feelings regarding patient care situations during team meetings in a nonjudgmental manner. Clinical improvement in expression of emotional stress is often observed when most of the patient's burn wounds have healed or have been covered with skin grafts (Bernstein, 1976).

OCCUPATIONAL THERAPY FOR THE BURNED PATIENT AND FAMILY

Rehabilitation begins as soon as the patient is resuscitated and stabilized (**acute phase**) and continues through the remainder of a patient's hospital treatment (subacute phase), discharge, and return for clinic follow-up (convalescent phase). The patient's transition through the acute and subacute phases depends on the extent of burn injury and the occurance of associated vascular, respiratory, or septic complications. From the moment the occupational therapist comes in contact with the burned patient and family, her assessment leads to the establishment of short- and long-term goals for functional restoration. The goals are to prevent contracture and deformity by maintaining range of motion, muscle function, and strength; to promote performance of physical daily living skills; and to educate the patient and family to facilitate recovery. Early initiation of this process facilitates the patient's and family's understanding of what is expected from all to return the patient to maximum function. The long-range goal is to return the patient to pretrauma functional ability. Knowledge of the patient's occupation and its physical requirements, his leisure activities, and age may indicate an approximate extent of function before the injury. These goals are accomplished via a comprehensive program of contracture prevention.

The usual occupational therapy evaluations, such as goniometric measurement of range of motion and manual muscle testing, are not feasible for a patient with extensive burns during the **acute phase.** Any body segments unaffected by the injury may be evaluated and a comparison may be made with burned segments to establish an information base. The patient's medical history contains information about any preexisting conditions, such as developmental anomalies or arthritis, that might indicate less than normal strength and range of motion. If a patient's history and occupation indicate functional ability up to the time of the burn, the therapist might assume that range of motion and strength were within normal limits. A baseline evaluation using goniometric measures is done as soon as the patient is able to move actively or be taken through passive range of motion (see Chapter 6).

Physicians test for sensation in burn patients to discriminate between second- and third-degree burns, because it is known that second-degree burns are very painful, whereas third-degree burns, in which the free nerve endings are destroyed, do not cause pain (Perry, Heidrich, & Ramos, 1981). An occupational therapist would not repeat the sensory test because the findings are not functionally related at the acute stage of treatment.

As the patient's condition permits, active participation in personal daily living self-care such as eating and daily hygiene using adapted methods or equipment is facilitated by the therapist. This includes positioning to accomplish these tasks such as sitting in bed or a chair at bedside. Early active involvement and education of the patient and family are key to a successful rehabilitation program. This intervention helps avoid progressive dependency and passivity and promotes self-esteem, self-reliance, and independence in carrying out the plan of care and home program.

Perioperative Treatment

Before placement of skin grafts, the surgeon and the occupational therapist may confer to plan the positioning devices to be used after the grafting procedure. Splints may be made before surgery or in the operating room (Salisbury, Reeves, & Wright, 1984). The extremity can be placed in the splint and the grafts laid over the open wound without sutures or dressings, or they may be secured with tape (Hartford, 1984). The newly placed graft survives on plasma until it links up with the capillaries in the dermis. During this phase, movement can destroy the capillary linkage, causing the graft to be lost; therefore, any movement before 5 to 7 days may be detrimental (Robson, 1983). A splint immobilizes the part while the graft takes and decreases the chance that the graft will be lost (Salisbury et al., 1984).

The surgeon has the responsibility to decide when the grafted area(s) can be mobilized. The therapist should expect that after the 4th day a determination will be made about exercising the grafted body part. Active or assisted range of motion should continue for those joints not being immobilized for grafting procedures (Hartford, 1984).

Postgraft Treatment

As the patient's wounds heal and the grafts begin to take, the occupational therapist can then do formal assessment measures for range of motion, muscle strength, and prehension (see Chapters 6 and 7). Reinnervation of the grafted area may begin within 2 weeks after the graft is placed, as the nerve fibers enter vacant neurilemma sheaths of the graft. Because sensory return depends on the accessibility of neurilemma sheaths in the donor graft, sensation may be diminished. Touch, pain, temperature, and two-point discrimination return at varying rates (Smahel, 1977). Sensory testing is indicated at this time (see Chapter 8). All joints must be kept mobile, and the patient is taught to avoid heat, friction, and trauma to the grafted areas (Reeves, 1983). At this stage, positioning continues.

POSITIONING

To be effective, all positioning must be enforced from the 1st day of treatment. The primary goal is deformity prevention, which requires maintenance of a consistent positioning program and use of a variety of positioning devices throughout the patient's hospitalization. Prophylactic and consistent positioning and splinting methods prevent deformity if followed until

the patient's burn scars have matured and functional range of motion and joint mobility are maintained. After discharge from hospital, prevention of deformity requires continued positioning and splinting of the burned areas until active scar development has ceased.

The occupational therapist uses the protocol practiced in the burn unit in which she is working. If a patient is able to cooperate with the goals of the positioning program, i.e., to avoid potentially deforming positions, devices may be worn only during rest times or at night to maintain functional gains in range of motion. Positioning methods include the use of splints, specialized beds, and attachments such as air fluidized beds, foam cutouts, traction, and other devices to maintain the burn patient in optimum position. The general rule is to position the body segment opposite to the anticipated deformity (Table 41.1, Fig. 41.1).

Positioning for when the patient is in the prone or supine positions are similar, except that in prone position the forehead should be supported on a contoured piece of foam rubber to maintain an airway and to keep the neck in slight extension (Evans & Parks, 1982). The deforming position for a burn on the face, neck, or chest is neck flexion. The eyelids and mouth as well as the neck and shoulders can be deformed by neck flexion contractures. The antideformity position places the neck in neutral or slight extension by use of a mattress with a cutout area or use of a thermoplastic neck conformer (Fig. 41.2).

The use of the neck conformer, following partial- or full-thickness burns has decreased the incidence and severity of neck contractures in patients with severe burns from an expected 37% to only 9% (Huang, Blackwell, & Lewis, 1978). The thermoplastic neck conformer reported by Willis (1970) was used in the **acute phase** over **Sulfamylon** gauze and in the postgraft phase without padding. Two neck conformers were made: one for the patient in the supine position and the other for the upright position. Since the introduction of that neck conformer, other neck conformers have been developed (Leman, 1986; Sandel & Khaleeli, 1981). Neck conformers can be modified to provide total contact support as well as position for height and range of motion of the neck. These modifications often depend on the patient's medical and social needs and the therapist's resources (Fig. 41.3).

Neck conformers and other full-contact splints are removed for airing and cleansing of the skin and activity; they are always cleaned and dried before reapplication. Neck conformers can also be removed for eating meals for periods not to exceed 1 hr if the patient is uncomfortable or cannot eat with the splint in place.

The deforming position for burns in the shoulder

Table 41.1. Positioning for Function

Body Part Burned	Anticipated Deformity	Position/Positioning Device	Schedule
Head/Face	Eye ectropion	Face mask	All times except meals
	Mouth microstomia	Mouth spreader or incorporate mouth spreader with face mask	All times when out of mask
	Closure of nares	Nasal obturators	All times except bath and meals if breathing is impeded
	Loss of ear cartilage	No pillows or pressure to ear helix	All times while on bed rest
Neck	Flexion	Short mattress	All times while on bed rest

	Lateral scar banding	Neck splint: Foam
		       Wastusi
		       Thermoplastic or clear plastic conformer
			All times except bath and meals

Shoulder	Elevation
	Protraction
	Adduction
	Internal rotation
		Supine: Small roll between scapulae
		    Adduction troughs or small wedges
		    Shoulders abducted 90° and in forward flexion 45°
			Maintain while patient is on bed rest

		Prone: Short mattress length head to 2 inches proximal to malleolus for foot positioning Optional: separate foam piece for head	Maintain while patient is on bed rest
		Axilla pads	All times except exercise and bath
		Foam positioner	Night only for adults or as per patient ROM maintenance
		Airplane splint	
Elbow	Flexion with elbow pronation	Flexion conformer Three-point extension splint (if contracture <90° exists)	All times except bath, exercise, postop; all times until first dressing change and therapist assessment
Hand		Elevate hand on pillows or upper extremity positioning with wedges or arm troughs	All times while on bed rest

	Claw hand—MCP hypertension
	PIP and DIP flexion
	Thumb IP flexion and adduction
	Flattened palmar arch
		Resting hand splint: MCP 75° flexion
		    PIP and DIP 0°
		    Thumb radial or palmar abduction
		    Wrist 30° extension
			All times except bath and exercise

	Palmar burns—PIP and DIP flexion
	Thumb IP flexion and adduction
		Dorsal hand splint: PIP and DIP 0°
		    MCP 0°
		    Thumb radial adduction
		    Wrist 30° Extension
			Postop all times until first dressing change and therapist assessment

Trunk	Scoliosis	Align with shoulders and hip	All times while on bed rest
	Kyphosis	During sitting: upright posture with buttocks well seated in chair and table-top placement to facilitate shoulder positioning	Maintain while sitting
Hip	Flexion Adduction	Hips in neutral position and up to 15° abduction Foam positioner between lower extremities No prolonged sitting with burns across anterior pelvis	All times while on bed rest

Table 41.1.   Continued

Body Part Burned	Anticipated Deformity	Position/Positioning Device	Schedule
Knee	Flexion	Extended with no pillows under knees or heels	All times while on bed rest
		No "frog-leg" positioning (hip abducted and externally rotated with knees flexed)	All times while on bed rest
	Hyperextension	Extension splint: Conforming Three point Knee immobilizer	All times except bath, exercise, and ambulation
		Elevate lower extremities while sitting	Postop: all times until first dressing change or therapist assessment
Ankle	Equinovarus: foot plantar flexion and inversion	Foot board/foam block at end of mattress	All times while on bed rest
		Foot splints that incorporate ankles, i.e., AFO ankle-foot orthosis	All times except bath and exercise Postop all times until first dressing change or therapist assessment
Foot	Equinovarus: foot plantar flexion and inversion	Foot in neutral position: plantar grade on foot board or in splint	All times while on bed rest
	MTP hyperextension	Foot plates/AFO	All times except bath and exercise Can ambulate while in splint

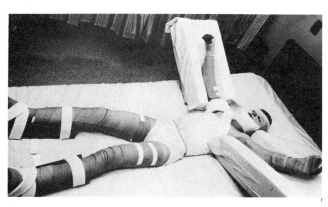

Figure 41.1. Bed positioning for person with burns of all four limbs.

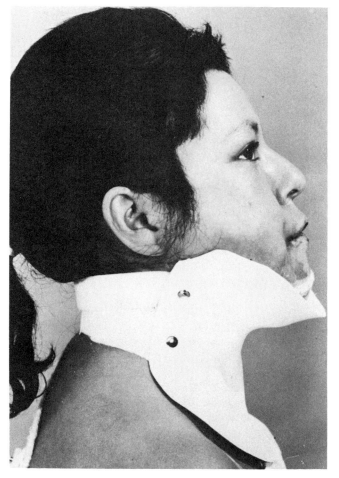

Figure 41.2. Thermoplastic neck conforming splint.

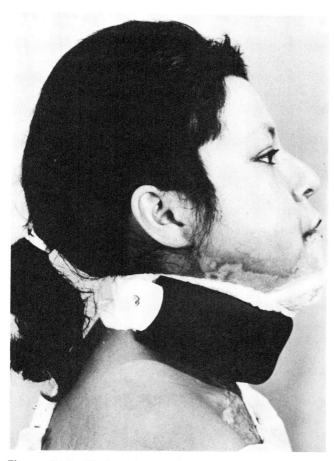

Figure 41.3. Variant of neck splint.

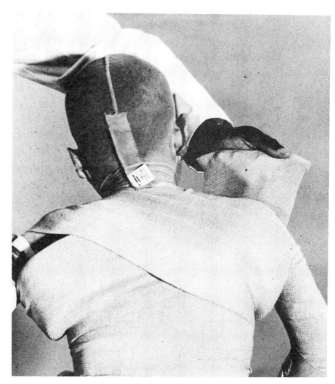

Figure 41.4. Semicircular axilla foam pads held in place by elastic bandage applied in a figure-of-eight pattern.

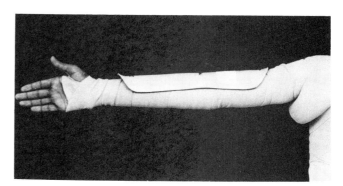

Figure 41.5. Arm conforming splint.

or axillary region is shoulder elevation, protraction, internal rotation, and arm adduction. To counteract this, the arm is positioned in 90 to 110° of abduction and external rotation. Consistent and careful monitoring of the arm position by the patient, family, nursing staff, and therapist is essential to prevent brachial plexus injury caused by excessive traction on the arm. Placement in abduction may be maintained by use of arm troughs (Heeter, 1986), by placing the outstretched, abducted arms into mattress cutouts, on pillows or foam wedges supported on a bedside table, or by use of an airplane splint (Fig. 28.17). In the upright position, semicircular sponges are placed in the axilla and secured with an elastic wrap (Evans & Parks, 1982) (Fig. 41.4).

The deforming position for the elbow is flexion, thus the antideformity position is elbow extension with forearm in supination. The elbow can be maintained in extension using a simple three-point-pressure principle splint or a thermoplastic conformer placed over the flexor surface of the joint (Fig. 41.5). Care is taken not to hyperextend or apply any mechanical force that

stresses the elbow joint into hyperextension; 5 to 10° of elbow flexion are permitted.

People experiencing thermal injuries tend to put their hands to their face protectively, which results in dorsal surface burns. Recommendations for positioning hands with dorsal burns are the antideformity (Salisbury et al., 1984), or safe, positions (Hummel, 1982). The position of deformity for the burned hand is wrist flexion, metacarpophalangeal (MP) hyperextension, and proximal interphalangeal (PIP) flexion with the distal interphalangeal (DIP) joint in slight flexion or hyperextension as in a boutonniere deformity, thumb adduction, and flattened palmar arch. This is an intrinsic minus hand. The deformity can rapidly occur if the burned hand rests unsplinted or is not in an elevated position. The resting hand splint is fabricated to position the burned hand in the antideformity position, which places the wrist in 0 to 45° of extension, the MP joints into 70 to 90° of flexion, and the PIP and DIP joints in full extension, where all lateral ligaments are taut and less likely to shorten. The thumb should be abducted and extended at the carpometacarpal (CMC) joint with the MP and IP joints extended (DiGregorio, 1984; Salisbury et al., 1984). Maintaining full range of motion at the thumb CMC joint is a primary goal. The therapist is vigilant, watching for signs of volar subluxation of the thumb and, should it occur, providing positioning and support to this joint, using opposing mechanical force with splinting.

Burns on the dorsum of the hand may threaten the integrity of the extensor mechanism. Deep second- and third-degree burns can destroy the joints, because of thermal trauma or because of fibrosis of joint capsules and loss of continuity of the extensor tendons. Neither active nor passive motion should place tension on the extensor mechanism, as this tension can cause the extensor mechanism to be damaged. Tension would be placed on the extensor mechanism when the patient actively makes a tight fist or when the therapist moves the fingers passively into total flexion; therefore, these are avoided. Acute flexion of the MP and IP joints simultaneously can result in disruption of the central slip, creating a boutonniere deformity that will require surgical repair. One method recommended for exercising the burned hand is to flex one joint while the other joints remain in extension. Muscle testing positions for MP, PIP, and DIP flexion may be used (see Chapter 6), i.e., MP flexion is done with the PIP and DIP joints in neutral or extension, the PIP joint is flexed slightly with the MP and DIP joints in neutral extension, and the DIP joint is flexed with the MP and PIP joints in neutral extension (Salisbury et al., 1984). A **blocking, or capener, splint** can be used to position the digits during these exercises or during supervised activity.

For burns on the volar surface of the hand, the position of choice is with the wrist in neutral (0 to 30° of extension), the MP joints in neutral (0°), and the fingers extended and abducted. The thumb is extended and abducted to prevent contracture of the flexor tendons (Heeter, 1986; Salisbury et al., 1984).

When circumferential burns involve the dorsal and volar surfaces of the hand, it will be necessary to alternate these two positions equally by using a day splint and a night splint (Salisbury et al., 1984). Careful observation of burn scar contractile forces, use of effective exercise and activities of daily living regimes, and consistent documentation of range of

motion are essential for maximizing functional gains on a daily basis.

For thumb range of motion, the CMC joint is held in neutral while thumb MP flexion is done with the IP joint in neutral. Thumb IP flexion can be done with the CMC and MP joints in neutral. Maintenance of thumb opposition is necessary for functional hand grip and prehension; therefore, full range of motion of extension and radial and palmar abduction must be maintained.

Lateral burns of the trunk may cause a hemithoracic scar, resulting in scoliotic contracture or a convexity of the truncal curve toward the contralateral side. The trunk should be positioned in a straight line so that the shoulders and hips are aligned to prevent development of an incipient contracture toward a scoliosis-like position (Evans & Parks, 1982).

The position of deformity for the hip is flexion and adduction. Therefore, hips are positioned in extension and approximately 15° of symmetrical hip abduction. For patients with severe burns, continual trauma to the anterior hip area such as from needlesticks to obtain blood, arterial line placement, extended positioning in hip flexion such as sitting up in bed require great vigilance to keep the hips and legs in position. Preventing a hip flexion contracture prevents contractures along the entire lower extremity.

A burned knee, like a burned elbow, tends to develop a flexion deformity, especially when the popliteal area (flexor surface) is involved. The antideformity position is knee extension, which can be maintained by a three-point-pressure principle splint (Evans & Parks, 1982) or a posterior leg conforming splint (Fig. 41.6). Hyperextension of the knee is avoided and like the elbow, a slight degree of flexion may make the patient more comfortable and, therefore, more compliant with his program.

The deforming position for the ankle is plantar flexion. The ankle should be maintained in neutral to allow for weight bearing and comfortable walking. A foot board or a posterior splint can be used to support

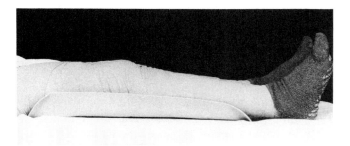

Figure 41.6. Leg conforming splint.

the foot (Reeves, 1983). When the patient is in prone position, if a short mattress is used, the feet are placed over the mattress edge to maintain the ankle joint in the neutral position (Evans & Parks, 1982).

EXERCISE

It is essential, in addition to maintaining proper positioning, for the burned patient to perform active movement from the day of admission to prevent deformity and contracture, the most disabling sequelae of burns. Daily contraction of all muscles and movement of uninvolved joints is essential to maintain joint awareness (Evans, 1966). During periods of strict positioning, before and after grafting, it is important that the patient initiate some voluntary active motion of those body parts that are not being immobilized, either in or out of splints. Active range of motion should be done after cleansing or after analgesics, when the patient is more comfortable. Splints and positioning devices are removed several times daily for the devices to be cleansed so that they do not become reservoirs for bacteria (Salisbury et al., 1984). At these times, active exercise should be supervised by the therapist. The patient is taught to move unsplinted body parts every 2 hr for up to 10 repetitions of movement each time. An activity list can be kept at the bedside to remind the patient and health care personnel to follow the treatment program.

The unconscious patient is exercised using the diagonal patterns of proprioceptive neuromuscular facilitation for gentle, passive motion of limbs (see Chapter 24D) at least once a day. Passive motion should be done slowly and gently and never beyond tissue resistance or pain tolerance. Mild sustained motions, rather than vigorously repeated motions, are used to avoid additional damage to the wound or healing areas (Helm et al., 1983).

Most alterations in the musculoskeletal system occur secondary to the acute injury and are not the direct result of it. It is important to anticipate potential deformities and to use measures to prevent them to ensure that the time of hospitalization and rehabilitation is not extended. Evans (1991) reported that heterotophic bone formation in thermal burns is a rare (1 to 3%) but functionally important complication. In clinical management, painful inflamed joints and resistance to motion are recognized as heralds of heterotophic calcification. During exercise of acutely burned patients stretching the joint's edematous pericapsular structures might precipitate this complication. Evans (1991) pointed out that the overriding goal of therapy is to maintain the range of motion and muscle function; this can be accomplished through controlled and as-

sisted active motion, gentle terminal stretch, and resistance. Once heterotophic calcification or ossification is recognized, stretching the affected joint should be avoided, but restricted passive and active assisted motion should continue (Evans, 1991).

Full-thickness burns over the shoulder, anterior elbow, and hip as well as any flexor surfaces of joints are subject to hypertrophic scar and have resulted in bridging of the joints with heterotophic bone. This has occurred in patients who were unable to participate in an active therapy program or who were resistant to such participation. Heterotophic bone formation is rarely seen when patients are started in programs that emphasize early mobilization. Radiographs of joints that do not yield to usual measures for increasing range of motion should be taken, because if heterotophic bone is present, surgical excision is required to restore range of motion (Evans & Parks, 1982). However, active motion should be encouraged in the available range until surgery can be done (Crawford et al., 1986).

The greatest obstacle to prevention of contracture and maintenance of functional range of motion is the patient's anticipation of pain when moving a burned extremity. If a patient is allowed to be immobile for a few days, he will become fearful of moving and avoid any active or passive motion. One sequence for gaining patient cooperation was described by Evans (1966). The therapist approaches the patient and describes what needs to be done and why, meanwhile surveying the patient to identify joints without burns. Then the patient is coached to do active and active assisted motion with the unburned joints. The patient is then taught to do isometric exercises, or muscle setting, in any unburned parts. Next, the patient is encouraged to do isometric contraction under burned areas. As the patient learns that some muscle contraction can be done without extreme discomfort, he should be able to begin to cooperate with maintaining muscle awareness. Then the patient is asked to perform some active, or active-assisted, motion with a burned body part.

Because partial-thickness burns expose nerve endings (Helm et al., 1983), a patient with a large second-degree burn may experience more pain than a patient with a deeper burn injury (Perry et al., 1981). Areas with superficial second-degree burns may be actively or passively exercised to maintain range of motion.

After the skin grafts are healed, the patient can begin a program of active motion to restore range of motion and function. In the case of hand grafts, the patient begins by moving each of the finger joints carefully. A program of hourly repetitions of these exercises is established. Games and activities are introduced to encourage development of functional strength and dexterity (Salisbury et al., 1984).

The advent of cultured skin grafting provides the therapist with a challenge for providing range of motion to body areas that may be immobilized for varying periods of time because of prolonged healing time and fragile wounds. Jones, as reported by Egan (1992), noted that recovery and rehabilitation with cultured skin require painstaking patience and gentle therapy and concluded that cultured skin cells produce fragile skin. She compared functional outcome in 12 patients with partial-thickness second-degree to full-thickness third-degree hand burns. After immobilization of 6 to 8 days, she found that both groups rated good to excellent finger movement, surface texture, and tissue. However, cultured skin patients who were mobilized 10 to 15 days postgrafting had poorer results, including joint contractures.

Despite the use of static and dynamic splinting, passive range of motion exercises, and pressure devices to counteract the contracting forces of burn scar, a significant number of patients are left with soft tissue contractures and permanent disability. One treatment that appears to be beneficial is use of continuous passive motion (CPM) machines, which move a body part through range and provide low-load stress at end range. CPM is thought to have cumulative positive effects on collagen remodeling, joint motion, and pain reduction (Covey, 1988). Continuous passive motion devices are available in portable, battery-operated units that allow the patient to engage in activity during CPM treatment or mounted units that provide continuous passive motion while the patient is sitting or lying in bed. The use of continuous passive motion devices allows for motion in a variety of ranges, thus freeing the therapist from spending many hours on exercise to maintain range of motion. The challenge to the therapist is to be knowledgeable regarding the patient's status on a day-to-day basis as the opportunities to assess, teach, and rehabilitate are dynamic and ever changing.

Following skin grafting to the lower extremities, the patient is not permitted to ambulate until stable venous drainage has been achieved in the grafted area, or the graft may be lost. After 6 days, the patient ambulates with the lower extremities double-wrapped in elastic bandages. This time period, as previously discussed, varies according to the patient's condition and physician preference. Interdisciplinary consultation is a must. As the patient's ambulatory status improves, he attends the occupational therapy clinic where more advanced personal daily living skills such as cooking and cleaning can be practiced and work evaluation can begin. Specific modalities are introduced for elimination of specific deficits (Reeves, 1983).

BURN SCAR PRESSURE THERAPY

The early result of burn wound healing may be satisfactory, but in a few months a smooth skin graft or healing burn wound can become contracted scar. **Hypertrophic scarring** and the contractures that follow closure of a deep burn wound are a frustrating sequelae of healed burns (Reid et al., 1987). Hypertrophic scars become apparent 6 to 8 weeks after spontaneous healing or after a second- or third-degree burn wound is grafted. Their clinical significance varies with the anatomical site (Abston, 1987). If skin grafts are placed over joint surfaces, the hypertrophic scar tends to involve the flexor surface.

When the deep reticular portion of the dermis is disturbed, **hypertrophic scarring** begins. Increased vascularity in the grafted area leaves a bright red healing wound. Collagen fibers develop to bridge the wound and begin to form an immature or active scar, which is a red, raised, rigid tangled mass that may take years to reach maturity. These deformities can be avoided through a program of pressure therapy, positioning, and exercise until the burn scar reaches maturity.

Continuous gentle pressure influences the arrangement of the collagen fibers so that they align in parallel rows rather then in rope-like whorls, as happens without pressure application to the burn scar. As long as the scar is active, it can be influenced by pressure and positioning. Once the scar becomes mature, surgical correction is indicated if a deformity exists. The optimal outcome is a mature burn scar that approximates the unburned skin color, is flattened, and is pliable.

Scar management is another component of the continuing splinting, positioning, and exercise program. After the autografts take or burn wounds over each body area begin to heal, the area is wrapped in elastic bandages or tubular compression bandages such as Tubigrip (Seton Healthcare Inc., Moorestown, NJ) to control **hypertrophic scarring** and to prevent contracture. This product is available in continuous tubes and in a variety of circumferences to fit all patients. Prefabricated gloves are also available. The tubular compression bandages may be used until custom-fitted garments are received or in lieu of these garments, and according to patient preference and financial resources. Tubigrip allows modifications and can be changed frequently. Other options for early application of pressure on forming scars can be accomplished by using Coban (3M Medical-Surgical Division, St. Paul, MN), a self-adherent wrap.

After the patient's body weight stabilizes, skin grafts are stable, and open wound dressings are minimal, custom-made pressure garments are ordered to replace the elastic bandages or tubular bandages, which are used until the pressure garments are received and fitted to the patient.

The use of pressure therapy in the form of custom-made Lycra garments following burn injury is a well-established procedure, the aim being to minimize the overgrowth of the healed area by limiting the supply of oxygen and nutrients to collagen tissue and hasten the maturing of the scar (Reid et al., 1987).

There remain quesitons concerning the amount of interface pressure indicated for adequate scar treatment. Research by Reid et al. (1986) indicated that 15 to 40 mm Hg is the therapeutic range necessary for influencing scar maturation. However, some authors have reported good clinical results with as little as 4 mm Hg and others have advocated pressures up to 55 mm Hg, (Baur, Parks, & Laison, 1977; Larson et al., 1974; Rose & Deitch, 1983).

It is also generally accepted that early application of pressure garments is necessary, commencing within approximately 2 weeks postgrafting or when spontaneous healing has occurred (Harries & Pegg, 1989). Although pressure garments have been used routinely for most burn patients since the mid-1970s (Linares, Larson, & Baur, 1976), recent studies have indicated that not all burns require the use of pressure garments. Burns that heal in 1 to 2 weeks do not require pressure garments, but the patient can be offered them to alleviate itching and protect healing skin until redness and itching subsides. Burns that require 2 to 3 weeks to heal need to have pressure garments applied. Many manufacturers of custom-fit anti-burn scar garments also produce interim (noncustom) supports for use between healing and the fitting of a custom support. Information specific to each company's measurement techniques is available from the individual manufacturers (Ward, 1991).

A survey of therapists and suppliers was conducted to determine the importance of various factors used in selection of anti-burn scar supports (Ward, 1991). Important factors were time for obtaining a burn scar support after ordering, the willingness of the manufacturer to make nonstandard custom supports and provide special options, the provision of measurement materials and forms by a company, and the cost of the supports. The data from this survey also implied that a majority of burn centers are using multiple companies to supply their pressure supports, a practice that increases the therapist's treatment alternatives (Ward, 1993). Each burn scar management program is unique to the population served, available resources and materials, and the expertise of the occupational therapist.

Pressure garments are available to cover all body areas, and many options are available. Most companies provide instructions in measuring and ordering or pro-

vide trained staff to come to the burn clinic for this purpose. Because the pressure garments are worn continuously, two sets are ordered to permit laundering one set while the other is worn. The garments are removed only for bathing or during exercise if they interfere with exercise movements. Patients are taught the necessary hygiene and cleanliness requirements for use of the garments. Instructions are also given on the use of skin moisturizers and sun screens to lubricate the skin and thus prevent skin breakdown. Any lubricant that does not irritate the patient's skin is acceptable. Those that do not contain perfumes and contain a sun protection factor (SPF) of at least 15 are recommended (Hurwitz, 1988).

A silastic face pad, silicone or foam insert, or clear plastic face mask provides consistent conforming pressure to the facial features, particularly for scars around the nose and mouth. The silastic face pad or insert is worn under the pressure garment. A plastic transparent face mask is another choice to treat facial scars. The process requires making a plaster mold from a negative impression taken from the patient's face. The plastic mask is then fabricated on this plaster mold. Often the negative impression is taken in the operating room while the patient is anesthetized (Derwin-Baruch, 1993).

Splinting may be a necessary adjunct to exercise and pressure to increase the mouth opening and prevent oral microstomia caused by facial scarring. The conforming pressure of splints over burn scars helps to prevent or soften the active hypertrophic scar. Conforming splints can be used over any body part and may be worn either under a pressure garment or applied over the garment and secured with elastic wrap or straps. Any conforming positioning device or splint is worn according to the patient's therapy schedule.

For burn scar management in areas such as the shoulder, neck, and axilla, where it is difficult to fit thermoplastic materials, a flexible silastic insert or silicone gel sheet can be applied. These inserts are worn under pressure dressings, garments, and splints.

To control **hypertrophic scarring** in the axilla, foam crescents (see Fig. 41.4) are secured in the axilla with elastic bandages. These can be applied as soon as open areas are minimal, but can be applied only after a thorough assessment of skin and range of motion have been made and patient and his family fully understand the rationale for use. Caution is advised because of the potential for compression to the brachial plexus by elastic wraps that are applied too tightly. Axilla pads are worn over a pressure garment.

Flexion contracture of the elbow caused by hypertrophic scar is controlled by serially splinting the elbow into extension, using an anterior thermoplastic conformer (see Fig. 41.5). The successful use of a spring-tension device to exert prolonged low-load pressure also has been reported useful to correct elbow flexion contracture (Richard, 1986). These splints serve a dual purpose: to position the extremity and to provide an opposing force to the position of comfort assumed because of unchecked **hypertrophic scarring.**

The occupational therapist's primary responsibility is to be acutely aware of the skin condition and functional status of the patient's hand. Coban adhesive compression dressings, Tubigrip, and interim gloves are used to desensitize the hands and control edema, thus their use usually precedes measurement for custom-ordered gloves. Commercially available pressure garment gloves are ordered when the hand edema has subsided. Gloves are also useful to prevent the skin between the finger web spaces from becoming scarred and adherent, defined as burn scar syndactly. Gloves can be ordered with slant inserts between the fingers or a detachable web spacer gauntlet for added pressure to this area. Elastomer inserts have been used by some therapists to improve finger and thumb web spaces (Malick & Carr, 1980); others use materials graded for providing progressive pressure to unyielding burn scars. Silicone elastomer products come in a variety of forms, including putty, sheets, and Otoform (Smith & Nephew Rolyan, Germantown, WI). Pressure and positioning can also be combined by using materials such as telfa gauze, adhesive elastic, elastic bandages, and pliable rubber tubing in graded sizes stretched through the web spaces. The use of these materials depends on the patient's skin condition and tolerance to the pressure media.

Treatment for the prevention of scarring over the dorsum of the foot, which can lead to hyperextension of the metatarsal joints, is by use of a thermoplastic foot plate. An outline pattern of the patient's foot, marking the anatomic landmarks at the metatarsalphalangeal (MTP) heads and arch is taken. The splint is cut from the pattern, marked, then contoured to the patient's foot to provide flexion of the MTP joints and support to the arch of the foot. This splint is usually worn only at night if the patient can wear high-top tennis shoes that provide adequate support during the day for activity. The pressure exerted from wrapping the metatarsals into flexion when the foot plate is applied onto the sole of the foot for night wear combined with secure lacing of the shoe for day wear, especially if the patient is wearing a pressure garment, ensure adequate pressure for burn scar compression to this area at all times.

Wound healing continues as the patient convalesces. As long as the burn scars are immature, the use of pressure media for scar suppression is necessary until the scar has reached maturity and poses no threat to the patient's functional ability. A 7-year study

(Perkins, Bruce Davey, & Wallis, 1987) of a variety of materials and techniques was undertaken at the burns unit at the Adelaide Children's Hospital in South Australia. The authors determined that contact media reduce both the maturation time of a scar and improve its cosmetic appearance (Perkins et al., 1987). Research has proven that the longer the pressure garments are worn, the fewer number of contractures and ultimate surgical releases of contractures are needed (Huang et al., 1978). An assessment of the length of time the garments and splints were worn showed that the majority (70%) of the patients who wore them for only 6 months required follow-up surgery, whereas only 23% of those who wore splints and garments for 6 to 12 months required surgery. Of the patients who followed the wearing program for more than 12 months only 15% required additional surgery. The savings in fewer inpatient hospitalizations and the trauma of surgery are impressive, but of greater interest is the information that the program is truly preventative and of great benefit for restoration of function following a burn injury. Therefore, following hospital discharge, patients should be monitored on a regular basis for 1 year or more or until the skin grafts mature and there is no evidence of hypertrophic scar activity (Covey, 1988).

Discharge Planning and Functional Outcomes

The occupational therapist devises a home program for the patient's positioning, pressure, exercise, and activity regimen. Education includes the rationale for every aspect of the home program as well as an explanation of the consequences of noncompliance with the program. A therapeutic relationship established with the patient and family when the home program was introduced and implemented according to their learning style, level of receptivity, and comprehension continues as the patient, family, and staff prepare for hospital discharge and follow-up. This relationship is dynamic and essential for a successful outcome for the patient and family.

Jenkins and Stanwick (1991) surveyed pediatric burn units to determine topics covered in discharge teaching, methods used, and obstacles encountered. They found that the topics addressed and the personnel involved in discharge teaching has changed little in 10 years. Subjects addressed in discharge education programs, in rank order of those taught, were active and passive exercise, splints, pressure garments, skin care, follow-up care, positioning techniques, appearance, emergency contact, scarring, and emotional aspects. Obstacles in patient and family education were identified as time constraints, language and sociocultural barriers, lack of receptivity by clientele, lack of educational materials and planning, and inadequate funding. Videotaping was identified as increasingly used for program delivery. This medium is readily available to hospital-based therapists, the home therapist, and the patient's family. Videotaping the patient provides documentation with respect to specific exercises and actual range of motion achieved during the early phase of treatment.

Psychosocial and physical barriers related to the patient's psychological and physical mobility status are also taken into consideration to plan and implement a successful reentry into the home community. The patient's goals and support systems are factors that impact the necessity for the type of retraining, preparation, and community experience that the interdisciplinary team carries out. Finally, a formal review session and follow-up allow the therapist to evaluate the patient's and family's responses and to modify the plan when further intervention is warranted or goals are achieved (Dobner & Mitani, 1988).

Occupational therapy evaluation identifies problems that may limit the patient's function in the community. The occupational therapist can use the following definitions from the Rehabilitation Committee of the American Burn Association in preparing and reporting the patient's discharge evaluation. Burn impairment is a measure of the burn individual's physical and mental difference from accepted standards. Burn disability refers to the impact that the measured impairment has on the individual's activities in the interpersonal, family, school, work, social, and recreational environments and may change as the environments change. Rating a person's impairment using the *Guides to the Evaluation of Permanent Impairment* (Doege & Houston, 1993) published by the American Medical Association requires calculating individual body segment impairments (such as range of motion), taking into account amputation and ankylosis, and combining them sequentially into whole person impairments. Some agencies may not require this type of rating, but once a rater has these objective data, it is easy to convert to other rating methods (Engrav, Dutcher, & Nakamura, 1992). To this end, the occupational therapist maintains a record of range of motion assessments taken at admission, pregrafting, postgrafting, and discharge from hospital.

Furthermore, the occupational therapist can contribute information that assesses the burned person's health status as part of the team effort for facilitating community reentry. The *Sickness Impact Profile* (Bergner, Bobbit, & Carter, 1981) has been used in burn care outcome studies. It assesses three major dimensions: physical functioning (ambulation, mobility, and body care and movement), psychosocial functioning (social interaction, alertness behavior, emotional be-

havior, and communication), and independent categories (sleep and rest, eating, work, home management, and recreation and pastimes). The assessment takes 20 to 30 min to administer and provides for a comprehensive overview of the patient's functioning. The *Burn Specific Health Scale* was modeled, in part, on the *Sickness Impact Profile* at the Baltimore Regional Burn Center. It is considerably shorter in length and is specific to burn injury. This general measure of functioning is an 80-item self-report instrument that measures domains of postinjury functioning such as physical functioning (mobility and self-care, hand function, and role activities), emotional, and social functioning (Pruzinsky et al., 1992).

As a member of the burn team, the informed and attentive occupational therapist can be responsive to the patient's need for benefits. Competition for health care benefits is fierce and proper documentation of disability is necessary. Thoughtful and complete reporting can greatly improve a patient's chances of obtaining fair and appropriate benefits (Salisbury, 1992).

As the occupational therapist practices within a variety of settings, with differing patient populations and resources, treatment programs reflect her creativity at patient care planning to meet functional goals. The following are examples of how therapists can implement programs to meet ever-changing scenarios and provide cost- and energy-efficient activities and treatments while using sound evaluation, reporting, and research practices.

An innovative approach to patient care uses the guided group work principle within a burn care setting as an adjunct to maximizing the patient's return to function. For example, the staff at a burn/trauma center created a formalized patient group based on the concept of communal dining. Their goals were to provide patients with a group setting as a safe arena for socializing, thus overcoming the isolation that frequently occurs in burn treatment. A designated group coordinator arranged the logistics and invited patient participants with input from the entire team who were aware of the program's purpose and suggested patient participants. The daily structured activity of getting to and from the dining room and participating in an activity of daily living with others positively impacted the patient's orientation and mobility status and allowed interaction with fellow burn patients, family members, visitors, and staff (Kasden, Slater, & Goldfarb, 1989).

Fletchall and Hickerson (1991) demonstrated that patients with upper extremity amputations resulting from burns can benefit from early prosthetic fit (within 30 days of amputation), as evidenced by decrease in edema, good stump shape, transference of phantom sensation to the prosthesis, no skin breakdown, and an independent return to preamputation activities. They studied seven patients aged 6 to 55 years. Five patients had other body surface areas burned in addition to the amputated extremity; the average TBSA burned was 17.85%. All patients underwent occupational therapy intervention from the day of admission. Treatment included edema control, educating the patient about future functional abilities to be gained with prosthesis use, establishing goals with definitive time frames, controlling scar formation, and providing a sensory desensitization program. After final prosthetic fitting, time before return to preamputation activities averaged 2 to 5 months and time before return to work averaged 4 months.

Another facet of maximizing the amputee patient's return to his preinjury lifestyle is work hardening. The program begins with a physician's prescription. Evaluation of the patient for the program is ideally initiated when wounds are completely healed, tolerance for pressure garments is 23 hr per day, outpatient therapy goals have been completed, and permanent prosthetics have been provided for the amputee. The basic components of the program are physical reconditioning, job simulation, skin care and prosthetic education, evaluation, and monitoring of work-related behaviors and attitudes. It is a graded 4- to 6-week program, with 5-day-a-week participation. The goal is to increase to an 8-hr period, thus simulating an actual workday (Zeller, Sturm, & Cruse, 1993).

SUMMARY

Occupational therapy for burn patients is primarily aimed at prevention of the deforming sequelae of burn injury, maintenance of daily living skills, and use of adaptive coping skills. Patients and their families use their own as well as learned coping and adaptive mechanisms to help them deal with the physical and emotional trauma of repeated surgeries and uncomfortable procedures. The occupational therapist constantly draws on her knowledge of physiology, anatomy, psychology, splinting, adaptive equipment, and daily living skills to provide the most advanced and effective occupational therapy treatment possible to each patient (Haley, 1993). With current knowledge and practice, patients and their families have a good prognosis for functional recovery.

STUDY QUESTIONS

1. How is the Rule of Nines used in burn injury assessment?
2. Define first-degree, second-degree, and third-degree burns.
3. What is the purpose of surgical escharotomy or fasciotomy in the treatment of burn injury?
4. What is the rationale for using isolation techniques in burn care?
5. What goals do occupational therapists pursue with burn-injured patients and their families?
6. What is heterotophic bone formation and what range of motion methods does the occupational therapist employ when it is recognized?
7. What is the general rule for positioning or splinting the burn patient?
8. Describe the antideformity splinting positioning choice for the burned hand.
9. What is the aim of burn scar pressure therapy and generally when is it begun and discontinued?
10. What subjects do occupational therapists routinely address in the patient's and family's discharge education program?

REFERENCES

Abston, S. (1987). Scar reaction after thermal injury and prevention of scars and contractures. In J. A. Boswick Jr. (Ed.), *The art and science of burn care* (pp. 359–371). Rockville: MD: Aspen Systems.

Abston, S., & Rinear, C. (1986). Burns. In G. S. Parcel (Ed.), *Basic emergency care of the sick and injured* (3rd ed., pp. 138–146). St. Louis: C. V. Mosby.

American Burn Association. Committee on the Organization and Delivery of Burn Care. (1993). *Burn care resources in North America.* (Available from the American Burn Association, 800-548-2876)

American Burn Association. (1984). *Burn care services in North America.* (Available from the American Burn Association, 800-548-2876)

Baur, P. S., Parks, D. H., & Larson, D. L. (1977). The healing of burn wounds. *Clinics in Plastic Surgery, 4,* 389–407.

Bergner, M., Bobbit, R. A., Carter, W. B., & Gilson, B. S. (1981). The Sickness Impact Profile: Development and final revision of a health status measure. *Med Care, 19,* 787–805.

Bernstein, N. R. (1976). *Emotional care of the facially burned and disfigured.* Boston: Little, Brown & Co.

Biosurface Technology. (1989). *Cultured autograph service orientation manual.* (Available from Biosurface Technology, One Kendall Square, Building 200, Cambridge, MA 02139)

Covey, M. H. (1988). Application of CPM devices with burn patients. *Journal of Burn Care and Rehabilitation, 9(5),* 496–497.

Cromes, G. F., & Helm, P. A. (1992). The status of burn rehabilitation services in the United States: Results of a national survey. *Journal of Burn Care and Rehabilitation, 13(6),* 656–662.

Derwin-Baruch, L. (1993). UVA therapists meet the challenge of scar management. *OT Week, 7(15),* 15–17.

DiGregorio, V. R. (1984). (Ed.), *Rehabilitation of the burn patient.* New York: Churchill Livingstone.

Dimick, A. R. (1984). Pathophysiology. In S. V. Fisher & P. H. Helm (Eds.), *Comprehensive rehabilitation of burns* (pp. 16–27). Baltimore: Williams & Wilkins.

Dingeldein, G. P. Jr. (1983). Complications of thermal injury. In R. E. Salisbury, N. M. Newman, & G. P. Dingeldein Jr. (Eds.), *Manual of burn therapeutics* (pp. 95–105). Boston: Little, Brown & Co.

Dobner, D., & Mitani, M. (1988). Community reentry program. *Journal of Burn Care and Rehabilitation, 9*(4), 420–421.

Doege, T. C., & Houston, T. P. (Eds.). (1993). *Guides to the evaluation of permanent impairment* (4th ed.). Chicago: American Medical Association.

Egan, M. (1992, July 23). A functional analysis of thermal injuries to the hand treated with cultured epithelial cells, preserving lives, challenging therapists. Focus: Burn treatment. *OT Week*, 12–15.

Engrav, L. H., Dutcher, K. A., & Nakamura, D. (1992). Burn impairment. *Clinics in Plastic Surgery, Burn Rehabilitation and Reconstruction, 19*(3), 569–598.

Evans, E. B. (1966). Orthopaedic measures in the treatment of severe burns. *Journal of Bone and Joint Surgery, 48A*(4), 643–669.

Evans, E. B. (1991). Heterotopic bone formation in thermal burns, *Clinical Orthopedics, 263*, 94–101.

Evans, E. B., & Parks, D. H. (1982). Burns. In V. L. Nickel (Ed.), *Orthopedic rehabilitation* (pp. 345–359). New York: Churchill Livingstone.

Feller, I., & Jones, C. A. (1984). Introduction—Statement of the problem. In S. V. Fisher & P. A. Helm (Eds.), *Comprehensive rehabilitation of burns* (pp. 1–8). Baltimore: Williams & Wilkins.

Fletchall, S., & Hickerson, W. L. (1991). Early upper-extremity prosthetic fit in patients with burns. *Journal of Burn Care and Rehabilitation, 12*(3), 234–236.

Frank, H. A., & Wachtel, T. L. (1984). Life and death in a burn center. *Journal of Burn Care and Rehabilitation, 5*(4), 339–342.

Haley, R. (1993). Massachusetts OTs find diversity on burn unit. *OT Week, 7*(15), 18–19.

Harries, C. A., & Pegg, S. P. (1989). Measuring pressure under burn pressure garments using the Oxford Pressure Monitor. *Burns, 15*(3), 187–189.

Hartford, C. E. (1984). Surgical management. In S. V. Fisher & P. H. Helm (Eds.), *Comprehensive rehabilitation of burns* (pp. 28–63). Baltimore: Williams & Wilkins.

Heeter, K. H. (1986). Arm hammock for elevation of the thermally injured upper extremity. *Journal of Burn Care and Rehabilitation, 7*(2), 144–152.

Heimbach, D. M. (1987). Early burn wound excision and grafting. In Boswick, J. A. Jr. (Ed.), *The art and science of burn care* (pp. 65–73). Rockville, MD: Aspen Systems.

Helm, P. A., Kevorkian, G., Lushbaugh, M., Pullium, G., Head, M. D., & Cromes, G. F. (1983). Burn injury: rehabilitation management in 1982. *Journal of Burn Care and Rehabilitation, 4*(6), 411–422.

Huang, T. T., Blackwell, S. J., & Lewis, S. R., (1978). Ten years of experience in managing patients with burn contractures of axilla, elbow, wrist and knee joints. *Plastic and Reconstructive Surgery, 61*(1), 70–76.

Hummel, R. P. (1982). Care of the burn wound. In R. P. Hummel (Ed.), *Clinical burn wound therapy: A management and prevention guide* (pp. 85–110). Boston: John Wright.

Hurwitz, S. (1988). The sun and sunscreen protection: Recommendations for children. *Journal of Dermatologic Surgery Oncology, 14*(6), 657–660.

Jenkins, H. M. L., & Stanwick, R. S. (1991). A survey of pediatric discharge educational programs in North American burn units. *Journal of Burn Care and Rehabilitation, 12*(3), 243–248.

Kasden, J. A., Slater, H., & Goldfarb, I. W. (1989). "Diner's Club" An innovation in the rehabilitation of the burn patient. *Journal of Burn Care and Rehabilitation, 10*(3), 276–277.

Kolman, P. B. (1984). Managing psychopathology in burn patients. *Journal of Burn Care and Rehabilitation, 5*(3), 239–243.

Larson, D. L., Abston, S., Willis, B., Linares, H. A., Dobrkovsky, M., Evans, E. B., & Lewis, S. R. (1974). Contracture and scar

formation in the burn patient. *Clinics in Plastic Surgery, 1*, 653–666.

Leman, C. J. (1986). The triple-component neck splint. *Journal of Burn Care and Rehabilitation, 7*(4), 357–360.

Linares, H. A., Larson, D. L., & Baur, P. S. (1976). Influences of mechanical forces on burn scar contracture and hypertrophy. In T. J. Krizek & J. E. Hoopes (Eds.), *Symposium on basic science in plastic surgery* (Vol. 15, pp. 101–127). St. Louis: C. V. Mosby.

Malick, M. H., & Carr, J. A. (1980). Flexible elastomer molds in burn scar control. *American Journal of Occupational Therapy, 34*(9), 603–608.

Malt, U. (1980). Long-term psychosocial follow-up studies of burned adults: Review of literature. *Burns, 6*(3), 190–197.

Perkins, K., Bruce Davey, R., & Wallis, K. (1987). Current materials and techniques used in a burn scar management programme. *Burns, 13*(5), 406–410.

Perry, S., Heidrich, G., & Ramos, E. (1981). Assessment of pain by burn patients. *Journal of Burn Care and Rehabilitation, 2*(6), 322–326.

Pruitt, B. A., & Levine, N. S. (1984). Characteristics and uses of biologic dressings and skin substitutes, *Archives of Surgery, 119*, 12–322.

Pruitt, B. A. (1981). Fluid resuscitation. *Journal of Burn Care and Rehabilitation, 2*(5), 263–294.

Pruzinsky, T., Rice, L. D., Himel, H. N., Morgan, R. F., & Edlich, R. F. (1992). Psychometric assessment of psychologic factors influencing adult burn rehabilitation. *Journal of Burn Care and Rehabilitation, 13*(1), 79–88.

Purdue, G. F. (1984). Reflections on modern burn care. *Journal of Burn Care and Rehabilitation, 5*(1), 58–61.

Reeves, S. U. (1983). Occupational therapy in burn care. In R. E. Salisbury, N. M. Newman, & G. P. Dingeldein Jr. (Eds.), *Manual of burn therapeutics* (pp. 179–195). Boston: Little, Brown & Co.

Reid, W. H., Evans, J. H., Naismith, R. S., Tully, A. E., & Sherwin, S. (1987). Hypertrophic scarring and pressure therapy. *Burns, 13*(Suppl.), S29.

Richard, R. L. (1986). Use of Dynasplint to correct elbow flexion burn contractures: A case report. *Journal of Burn Care and Rehabilitation, 7*(2), 151–152.

Robson, M. C. (1983). Reconstruction and rehabilitation from admission: A surgeon's role at each phase. In N. R. Bernstein & M. C. Robson (Eds.), *Comprehensive approaches to the burned person* (pp. 35–48). New Hyde Park, NY: Medical Examination.

Rose, M. P., & Deitch, E. A. (1983). The effective use of a tubular compression bandage, Tubigrip, for burn scar therapy in the growing child. *Journal of Burn Care Rehabilitation, 4*, 197–201.

Rosenberg, D. B., & Nelson, M. (1988). Rehabilitation concerns in electrical burn patients: A review of the literature. *Journal of Trauma, 28*(6), 808–812.

Salisbury, R. (1992). Burn rehabilitation: Our unanswered challenge. The 1992 presidential address to the American Burn Association. *Journal of Burn Care and rehabilitation, 13*(5), 495–505.

Salisbury, R. E., Newman, N. M., & Dingeldein, G. P. Jr. (1983). *Manual of burn therapeutics: An interdisciplinary approach.* Boston: Little, Brown & Co.

Salisbury, R. E., Reeves, S., & Wright, P. (1984). Acute care and rehabilitation of the burned hand. In J. M. Hunter, L. H. Schneider, E. J. Mackin, & A. D. Callahan (Eds.), *Rehabilitation of the hand* (2nd ed., pp. 585–595). St. Louis: C. V. Mosby.

Sandel, E., & Khaleeli, C. R. (1981). Use of the thermoplastic total contact and the foam Watusi ring neck splint. *AOTA Physical Disabilities Special Interest Newsletter, 4*(2), 3.

Sheretz, R. J. (1983). Isolation practices. In R. E. Salisbury,

N. M. Newman, & G. P. Dingeldein Jr. (Eds.), *Manual of burn therapeutics* (pp. 267–271). Boston: Little, Brown & Co.

Smahel, J. The healing of skin grafts. *Clinics in Plastic Surgery,* 4(3), 409–424.

Ward, R. S. (1991). Pressure therapy for the control of hypertrophic scar formation after burn injury: A history and review. *Journal of Burn Care and Rehabilitation, 12*(3), 257–262.

Ward, R. S. (1993). Reasons for the selection of burn-scar-support suppliers by burn centers in the United States: A survey. *Journal of Burn Care and Rehabilitation, 14*(3), 360–367.

Willis, B. (1970). The use of Orthoplast isoprene splints in the treatment of the acutely burned child. *American Journal of Occupational Therapy, 24*(3), 187–191.

Zeller, J., Sturm, G., & Cruse, C. W. (1993). Patients with burns are successful in work hardening programs, Part 1. *Journal of Burn Care and Rehabilitation, 14*(2), 189–196.

42
Amputation and Prosthetics

Felice Celikyol

OBJECTIVES

After studying this chapter the reader will be able to:
1. Discuss prosthetic components available for upper limb amputations.
2. Describe components appropriate to the level of amputation.
3. State options for formulating appropriate prosthetic prescriptions.
4. Explain the role of occupational therapy for preprosthetic and prosthetic management of upper and lower extremity amputation.
5. Understand the psychosocial implications of amputation and the impact on therapeutic management.

Limb amputation can be categorized as congenital, i.e., present at birth, or acquired, i.e., resulting from trauma, tumors, vascular disease or infection. The child born with a (congenital) limb deficiency has needs that are quite different from those of an adult with an acquired amputation, and these needs change as he develops into an adult. In addition, the needs and expectations of the parents and other family members greatly influence the child. These are some of the issues that impact the pediatric prosthetic therapy program and require separate consideration (see the Suggested Readings for this chapter). Only acquired upper extremity amputation sustained by adults will be addressed in this chapter; a discussion of the role of the occupational therapist in providing therapy for adults with lower limb amputation(s) is also included.

AMPUTATION INCIDENCE, LEVELS, AND CLASSIFICATION

Most upper limb amputations occur as a result of trauma from motor vehicles and machinery accidents, from gunshot wounds, and from electrical burns. The *National Health Interview Survey* of 1983–1985 reported that approximately 4 of every 10,000 people have upper limb amputations in the United States (about 75% are between the ages of 15 and 45); the majority of these are males (LaPlante, 1988). Three times as many people have had lower extremity amputations; 75% these are the result of disease, with peripheral vascular disease and diabetes mellitus being the most common causes in people over 60 years of age.

When amputation is necessary, the surgeon's aim is to preserve as much limb length as possible and still retain healthy skin, soft tissue, blood supply, sensation, muscles, bones, and joints (Banerjee, 1982). A residual limb that is pain free and functional is the final goal.

Amputations are classified by the site of amputation (Department of Prosthetics and Orthotics, 1986). The levels of amputation for the upper extremity are illustrated in Figure 42.1. Often the level of amputation directly affects the actual use of a prosthesis. The higher the level of amputation, the more difficult it is to use a prosthesis, because fewer joints and muscles are available for control. Weight of the prosthesis is a factor, as is the complexity of systems for active control for patients with high amputations. The level of amputation is only one reason for nonacceptance of a prosthesis. Several factors contribute to nonacceptance and many are unique to each person.

REHABILITATION: A TEAM APPROACH

Amputation of an upper limb means losing the ability to hold and manipulate objects, to feel these objects, to communicate through gestures, and be whole in body. This loss can have a profound effect on the person's self-esteem and perception of self (Dise-Lewis, 1989; Racy, 1992). When both upper limbs are amputated, a sense of helplessness may prevail. The complexity of hand function and its meaning to the individual affects his reactions to its loss (Friedmann,

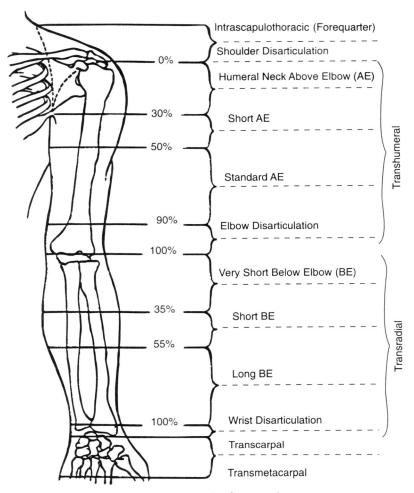

Figure 42.1. Levels of amputation.

1978) and to the expectations he has toward replacement of his arm with a prosthesis. These reactions must be explored and understood by the rehabilitation team.

The primary members of the professional team are the physician, prosthetist, and therapist. The social worker, psychologist, and vocational counselor may be called in as needed. These members should be on an equal footing with the patient who is an active member of the team. The patient is given an opportunity to explain his needs, preferences, and goals. The health care professionals have the responsibility to listen and make realistic recommendations based on the patient's goals. The occupational therapist is critical to the rehabilitation process, because the therapist has the responsibility to provide therapy during the preprosthetic phase and prosthetic period and can also influence the patient's adjustment. Some aspects of the rehabilitation process may be addressed by other team members, e.g., in the acute postoperative management period. This responsibility may vary, depending on the structure of the particular rehabilitation setting, e.g.,

some aspects of postoperative management of the residual limb(s) might be rendered by a physical therapist or a nurse.

PHANTOM LIMB SENSATION

The perception of the presence of the amputated limb is a universally experienced phenomenon and is remarkably real to the patient. This phantom limb sensation is still not clearly understood, but it represents a normal experience and is more common in traumatic amputees. According to Melzack (1989), the "neural system exists within the brain even when the body input is cut off by amputation" (p. 4). These perceptions are stronger with amputations of upper extremities, and the hand and fingers are felt more vividly than the arm.

With time, the distal portions of the phantom limb (hand or foot) may telescope closer to the site of the amputation. This phantom limb sensation often never subsides and is ordinarily accepted by the patient. The patient may view this as an annoyance, as when there is mild burning or tingling sensations, or may think of this as useful, as with learning myoelectric control for externally powered prostheses. Open discussion with the patient regarding this common phenomenon is a must.

PHANTOM LIMB PAIN

Phantom limb pain is even less clear, and its etiology and management remain controversial (Melzack, 1989; Schwell & Bunch, 1992). This pain can be experienced as greatly intensified burning or cramping sensations or shooting pain. Peripheral nerve irritation, abnormal sympathetic function, and psychological factors are thought to be contributory factors and are more common in traumatic amputations.

Often, the pain is experienced as more intense with stress. The therapist is advised to avoid emphasizing the issue of pain when possible. For those with severe pain, analgesics have been used as well as surgery such as nerve blocks and neurectomies. In the rehabilitation setting, limb percussion, ultrasound, and transcutaneous electrical nerve stimulation (TENS) have been used. Some centers have used acupuncture. Psychotherapy, hypnotherapy, and relaxation techniques have also been instituted. However, there is no one approach that has proved to be clearly successful. Fortunately, this is not a common phenomenon.

PREPROSTHETIC THERAPY

Postoperative Care

Postoperative care is required immediately after surgery and addresses wound care, maintenance of skin integrity, joint mobility, reduction of edema, prevention of scarring, and control of pain (Atkins, 1989b; Malone, Fleming, & Robinson, 1984). This usually occurs in an acute care setting and continues in an outpatient setting. Professionals involved in the patient's care are the surgeon, nurse, and physical therapist, with the occupational therapist involved in some institutions. The patient remains in an acute care setting for a relatively short period of time, which can be less than 1 week, barring complications. He then will be admitted to a rehabilitation unit, rehabilitation center, or hand clinic as an outpatient. Inpatient admission may be necessary when multiple amputations or other complications, such as extensive burns, exist.

The preprosthetic therapy program occurs from this postsurgical period until the patient receives the definitive (permanent) prosthesis. This is a preparatory time for emotional healing in addition to the physical healing. An assessment must be conducted before instituting therapy.

Preprosthetic Therapy Program Guidelines

GOAL I

The first goal is to provide the patient with emotional support. Establish an ongoing supportive, trusting relationship with the patient and family to facilitate open discussion. Collaborate with the team regarding patient's needs, and refer the patient for counseling if needed. Introduce the patient to others with similar amputations and like circumstances, if at all possible.

GOAL II

The second goal of preprosthetic therapy is to instruct the patient in limb hygiene and to expedite wound healing. The following interventions can be used.

1. Instruct the patient to wash the limb daily with mild soap and dry it thoroughly;
2. Provide wound cleansing, such as debridement or use of a whirlpool; this may be the responsibility of the physical therapist or nurse;
3. Use creams to massage at the suture line to loosen crust-like formations.

GOAL III

The next goal of therapy is to maximize residual limb shrinkage and to shape the residual limb so that it is tapered at the distal end, which will allow for optimal prosthetic fit. The following interventions can be used to achieve this goal.

1. *Elastic bandage.* The patient is taught to wrap the limb, unless physical or cognitive limitations prevent this. In such a case, a family member or friend must be instructed. Wrap the residual limb in a figure-of-eight diagonal configuration, with more pressure applied at the end of the limb. Never wrap in a circular manner around the limb, because this will cause a tourniquet effect and restrict circulation. The bandage must conform firmly to the limb and must be wrapped from the distal to the proximal direction (Fig. 42.2). The bandage should be worn continuously. If it becomes loose, it should be rewrapped immediately. The bandage must be removed three to four times per day so that the skin can be checked for any redness or pressure; the limb is then rewrapped. The bandage should be replaced with a clean one at least every 2 days. The bandages can be washed using mild soap and should be laid flat to dry. Do not squeeze or machine dry the elastic bandages.

2. *Elastic shrinker.* An elasticized "sock" can be worn in lieu of the bandage if the patient or family members are not reliable in following proper wrapping procedures using the elastic bandage. The shrinker

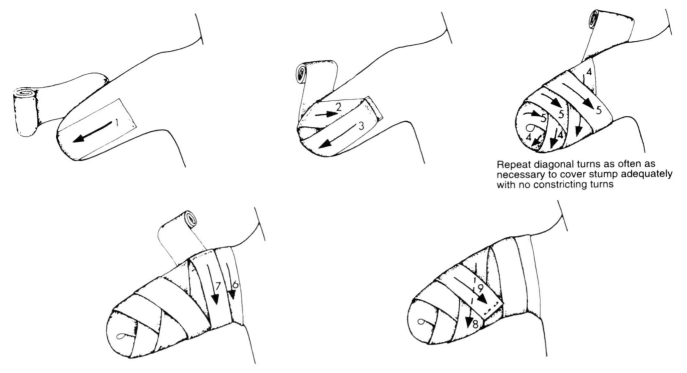

Repeat diagonal turns as often as
necessary to cover stump adequately
with no constricting turns

Figure 42.2. Wrapping techniques for above elbow amputation.

tends to loosen as the limb shrinks. Although this can be less effective than the bandage, the shrinker is better than improper application of the elastic bandage.

3. *Removable rigid dressing.* A socket can be fabricated using plaster bandages or fiberglass casting tape. This may be the method of choice for those unable to wrap the limb (Olivett, 1990); however, it must be replaced or altered as the limb shrinks. A rigid dressing is time-consuming to fabricate.

4. *Immediate postoperative prosthesis.* The immediate postoperative prosthesis (IPOP) is, as the name suggests, applied directly after surgery (Maiorano & Byron, 1990; Malone et al., 1984). This is probably the ideal approach, if the rehabilitation team members are available to ensure success.

5. *Early postoperative prosthesis.* The early postoperative prosthesis (EPOP) is strongly recommended for bilateral amputations (Lehneis & Dickey, 1992) to reduce dependency for self-care activities. This preparatory prosthesis may ensure acceptance and use of the prosthesis. Malone, Flemming, and Robinson (1984) called the first 30 days after amputation the "golden period," because studies support the premise that early fitting tends to ensure acceptance of the prosthesis and its use. They believed that the patient should be fitted with a prosthesis during this period to maximize the chance for prosthetic use.

GOAL IV

The fourth preprosthetic therapy goal should be to desensitize the residual limb and to develop tolerance to touch and pressure in preparation for encasement of the limb in the socket. This goal can be met through the following interventions.

1. Percussion or weight bearing is performed by the patient on the distal end of the amputated limb into various surfaces, graded from very resilient, such as soft foam, to surfaces that offer more resistance and texture, such as layers of felt, rice, and clay (Fig. 42.3); the patient is instructed to push his limb down into the surface in 5-sec intervals and to increase the time as tolerated.
2. Massage is useful as a desensitizing technique but is primarily used to prevent or release adhesions and soften scar tissue.
3. Tapping and rubbing the residual limb and applying a vibrator are also useful approaches.
4. Residual limb wrapping contributes to desensitizing the limb.

GOAL V

The therapist's fifth goal is to provide a physical conditioning regime to increase the range of motion

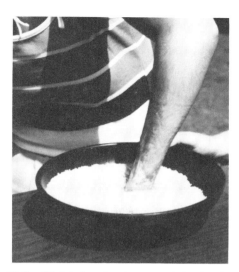

Figure 42.3. Weight bearing into materials of various textures (here, rice) to desensitize limb.

(ROM) of all joints proximal to the amputation and of the contralateral limb, if limitations exist. It is important to at least *maintain* the patient's range of motion. The therapist helps the patient increase the muscle strength of the residual limb and shoulder area as well as the contralateral side, if needed. The therapist should also provide an exercise program to improve or prevent asymmetry of posture. This is of particular importance for patients with high-level amputations, for whom a shift of weight and center of gravity will occur.

As an intervention, the patient can use a customized harness to hold weights or use cuff weights wrapped around the limb. The patient can be instructed in how to use these devices at home. This harness system can also be used with pulley exercise equipment in the clinic or with more sophisticated systems such as the BTE Work Simulator (Olivett, 1990).

GOAL VI

The next goal is to encourage independence in daily living activities. It is important that the patient be as self-sufficient as is reasonable without the prosthesis. There may be times when the patient is without the prosthesis, e.g., if the prosthesis needs to be repaired.

Unilateral Amputation

For those persons with amputation of the dominant limb, change of dominance activities, such as writing, must receive special attention. The patient will automatically use the remaining extremity but instruction in one-handed techniques for a wide variety of activities can be introduced for self-care, home management,

communication, desk activities, and community interaction (see Chapters 15 and 16).

Bilateral Amputation

Establishing some degree of independence is essential for the patient who has undergone bilateral amputation and must be addressed promptly (Lehneis & Dickey, 1992) to allay feelings of dependency and frustration. The therapist can immediately give the patient a cuff that has a pocket in which a utensil or toothbrush can be placed; this is a temporary solution as a substitute for grasp. Early postoperative prosthetic fitting of at least one limb is by far the ideal approach. Adapted devices may be needed (Friedmann, 1989; Heinze, 1988) to assist the patient in performing basic self-care tasks such as eating, toileting, grooming, and some dressing. Use of the feet should be encouraged if at all possible, and/or other modifications of performance can be suggested (such as use of the chin, knees, and teeth) (Edelstein, 1992; Heinze, 1988). The therapist and patient begin to analyze the tasks that must be done and solve problems together. Ordinarily, the longer limb will be chosen as the dominant extremity, but there are instances when the patient will choose to use the shorter limb to be dominant, particularly if there is little difference in length and it had been the dominant limb before the amputation.

GOAL VII

The seventh preprosthetic goal is to discuss the prosthetic choices. If possible, demonstrate the prostheses to help the patient establish realistic expectations. Arrange a meeting with the patient and a former patient or someone with a similar level of amputation and (similar experience, if feasible) so that they can talk candidly about any issues of concern.

GOAL VIII

For patients choosing a myoelectrically controlled prosthesis, the final goal is to conduct muscle site testing. The prosthetist and therapist can collaborate to determine if the patient is a candidate. Evaluate electromyographic (EMG) signal potential to identify optimal location of the control site(s). A special myotester or biofeedback unit can be used. The myotester is used to provide visual and auditory feedback. Train the patient to control the intensity of the muscle contractions and relaxation, and help him isolate the contractions of different muscle groups.

PRESCRIBING THE PROSTHESIS

As a member of the prosthetic team, the occupational therapist also contributes to the prescription of the prosthesis. She had the opportunity to get to know the patient in some depth during the preprosthetic program and thus brings to the team the knowledge of the patient's whole condition (Fleming, 1991). In other words, the occupational therapist knows the extent of the amputation and what it means to the person as well as knowing the patient from a social and cultural perspective. The team considers the following:

1. The patient's preferences for cosmesis and function;
2. The patient's life activities at work, home, and school; for leisure; and in the community;
3. The physical attributes of the residual limb, including length of limb, ROM, strength, and skin integrity;
4. The financial coverage for the prosthesis, such as third-party payment;
5. The patient's motivation and attitude;
6. The patient's cognitive abilities to learn and grasp concepts of prosthetic component controls.

Each prosthetic component must be chosen in regard to these data.

Prosthetic Components

The components of a prosthesis are frequently categorized in the following sequence, from distal to proximal:

1. Terminal devices (TD)
   a. Active prehensors
   b. Passive terminal devices
2. Wrist Units
3. Forearm component or sockets
4. Elbow units or hinges
5. Upper arm component or sockets
6. Shoulder units or hinges

PROSTHETIC CONTROL CHOICES

1. *Body powered (BP):* The elbow and terminal device componentry are activated through body motion, which applies force to pull a cable (Fryer & Michael, 1992).
2. *Externally powered:* The power is usually an electrical motor; the two most common sources of control of the motor are myoelectric and microswitch. The elbow and/or TD can be externally powered.
3. *Passive, cosmetic:* No active motion.
4. *Hybrid systems:* A combination of body powered and electrically powered controls.

TERMINAL DEVICES

A terminal device is the component at the distal end of the arm prosthesis; this device is, in essence, the substitute for the patient's amputated hand. Terminal devices can be hands or hooks and can be subcategorized as active prehensors or passive terminal devices. Terminal devices are considered the most important component of the prosthesis; the other components (for the wrist, elbow, and upper arm) are needed to position the arm in space to enable prehension with the TD.

TD Prehensors—Body Powered Prostheses

Prehensors are active grasping devices and can be a split hook or a mechanical hand. These devices can be classified as operating by a voluntary opening (VO) or voluntary closing (VC) mechanism. For a VO mechanism, the fingers of the device remain closed by a spring (for a mechanical hand) or by rubber bands (for a hook) until tension on the cable causes the terminal device to open. This tension, or pulling, on the cable comes from body movement. The force (amount) of pinch can be increased by the number of rubber bands (approximately 1 lb/band) on the hook and by adjusting the spring mechanism for the hands. For a VC mechanism, the fingers are in an open mode. Tension, or force, on the cable is needed to close the device and must be maintained for sustained grasp on an object.

Voluntary Opening Hooks

The voluntary opening hook is the most frequently used TD, and Hosmer-Dorrance is the primary manufacturer (Fig. 42.4). Hosmer-Dorrance fabricates a variety of hooks in different sizes; there are child and adult sizes and versions for females and males. The hooks are made of aluminum alloy or stainless steel and can have neoprene rubber–lined fingers. Model numbers indicate the size of the device, and letters indicate other attributes. For example, the designation *5XA* can be interpreted this way:

5 is an adult size with canted-shaped fingers;
X means that the device is neoprene lined;
A means that it is made of an aluminum alloy.

The canted shape tends to provide a firmer grasp for cylindrical objects and for picking up flat items from a table. The neoprene lining provides a firmer grip and prevents slippage. Aluminum hooks are lighter in weight (4 oz) than stainless steel (8 oz) and are good for use in light activities. A 7 hook is a stainless steel work hook with a large opening between the fingers to allow the patient to grasp shovel or broom handles. Other contours are made for carrying buckets, holding nails in place for hammering, and holding chisels. Some of these hooks have no neoprene lining, but the inner surfaces of the fingers are serrated for strong grip. The work hook can withstand the rigors of heavy mechanical activity; however, it weighs 10.5 oz.

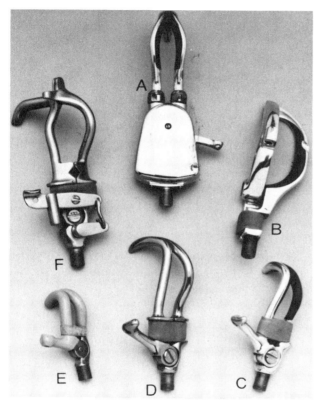

Figure 42.4. Hooks manufactured by the Hosmer-Dorrance Corp. *A*, APRL voluntary closing hook; *B*, contour hook; *C*, child-size 10X aluminum hook; *D*, adult-size 5 stainless steel hook; *E*, child-size 12P hook with plastisol coated fingers; *F*, stainless steel work hook 7 with tool-holding lock.

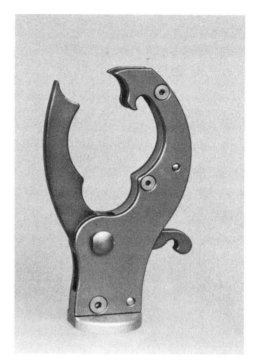

Figure 42.5. The Grip II voluntary closing prehensor manufactured by TRS, Inc.

The adult contour hook allows for a cylindrical grasp and is made of lightweight aluminum. The adult CAPP TD (developed by the UCLA—Child Amputee Prosthetic Project) is another option. The rubber nubbins on its covering provides friction, but it has a weak pinch force. These devices are generally less popular.

Voluntary Closing Hooks

The TRS GRIP voluntary closing terminal device is fast becoming the TD of choice in this category (Fig. 42.5). Strong variable prehension can be achieved, which is controlled by the amount of force the individual is capable of exerting. Tension must be maintained on the cable for sustained prehension. A locking mechanism, which can be manually controlled, is available and can be inserted if requested. These devices are available in aluminum and steel and can be plastic coated. This TD is particularly appealing for people who are active in sports and other recreational activities.

Use of the APRL hook, developed by the Army Prosthetics Research Laboratory, is declining, because it contains more complex inner mechanisms and tends to require more servicing.

Voluntary Opening Mechanical Hands

The Hosmer-Dorrance and the Otto Bock functional hands are the most frequently selected hands. They are available in several sizes and the size is determined by measuring the circumference of the sound hand at the heads of the metacarpals and deducting 0.25 inch. The VO hands operate similarly to the VO hooks except that, in the hand, the thumb and the first two fingers open when the cable is pulled. These fingers oppose in a three-point prehension pattern. With the hook, however, the cable is attached only to the thumb post and thus moves only one finger of the hook; the other finger remains stationary.

Voluntary Closing Mechanical Hands

The APRL VC hand is available only in adult male sizes; the thumb can be manually adjusted and locked in two positions to achieve a 1.5- or 3-inch opening. Otto Bock offers VC hands in several sizes, which weigh less than the APRL hand. The VC hands are not as popular as the VO hands.

Cosmetic Gloves

All prosthetic hands have rubberized coverings (Fryer & Michael, 1992); these gloves are available in a variety of colors and sizes and can be replaced by the prosthetist when damaged. These gloves cover mechanical, passive, and electric hands. Some of the available choices are describe below.

1. A stock glove is one that is ordered by the prosthetist. The skin color choices are made based on a limited selection of small sample swatches. These gloves are the least expensive and are made of polyvinyl chloride (PVC), which is susceptible to staining from contact with newspaper print, clothing dyes, and ink from ballpoint pens. In addition, the glove can deteriorate with temperature extremes and ultraviolet radiation (sunlight).

2. A custom production glove is customized to replicate more closely the patient's remaining hand. A reverse mold of the remaining hand is sent to the manufacturer. There is a wider range of color choices available. Veins and other details are painted onto the glove to render a more realistic covering.

3. A custom sculpted glove, also called an anatomical cover, truly attempts to replicate the individual's remaining hand. It is made of silicone, which can withstand temperature extremes and is not easily damaged (Pillet & Mackin, 1992) (Figs. 42.6 and 42.7). The remaining hand is cast in silicone, which duplicates its contours in great detail. This cast is then reversed to be used as a covering for the prosthetic hand. In addition, a cosmetic restorationist will add to the realistic appearance of the hand by actually painting the glove itself and adding veins and other features on the silicone rubber glove. Of course, this is a very costly procedure.

Passive Cosmetic Hands or Prostheses

Pillet and Mackin (1990) stated that "for some patients the hand not only is a functional tool but also possesses expressive beauty" (p. 1040). Patients will choose a passive cosmetic prosthesis when aesthetics is of prime importance. More often, it is those patients with unilateral amputations, high-level amputations, or partial hand amputations who will make this choice. These prostheses are available to replace a single digit or a total arm, as needed by the amputee with intrascapulothoracic amputation.

The Final Choices: Hooks or Hands?

Fortunately, the patient does not have to narrow his choice to one TD. It is possible to have several hooks and a hand, which can be interchanged. The hook is viewed as more functional for the following reasons:

1. Small items can be grasped with precision;
2. The patient can view the items more easily while using a hook, which is extremely important in providing sensory feedback, because the patient's sense of touch is absent;
3. It weighs less than the hand;
4. It costs less than the hand;
5. It is more reliable and requires less maintenance than the hand;
6. It can fit in close quarters.

Nonetheless, many people prefer the hand, because it is cosmetically more appealing.

With the continued development and refinement of externally powered hands, these TDs are chosen over the mechanical hands, particularly by those with below elbow (BE) amputations as they offer greater pinch force, can be activated with more ease, and do not require a harness. For the individual with bilateral amputations, the body powered hooks continue to be preferred, because function is of greater importance. Occasionally, externally powered hands may be chosen. Some individuals will choose a different TD for each limb, e.g., a body powered hook may be chosen

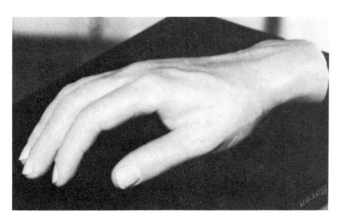

Figure 42.6. An adult male hand prosthesis made to suction fit over the palm.

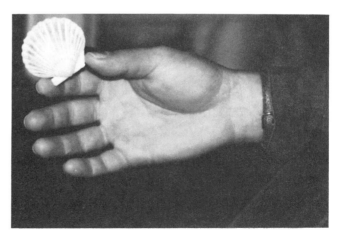

Figure 42.7. Adjustable finger armatures allow the finger positions to be changed and assist in holding objects.

for one side and a myoelectrically powered hand for the contralateral side. How can the ideal TDs be chosen? Listen to the patient and consult with the other team members to get varied perspectives.

WRIST UNITS

The wrist unit provides a means to attach the TD to the forearm. It also provides an important function: The terminal device can be rotated by the individual to positions of supination, pronation, and midposition before engaging in an activity. This is called prepositioning the TD and is an extremely important substitution function for active forearm rotation (supination and pronation), which is reduced or absent.

There are several types of wrist units; the ones described below are the most popular.

1. *Constant friction.* This wrist unit contains a nylon threaded insert that surrounds the stud of the TD to hold it in place. An Allen wrench is used to turn a small set screw that applies pressure against the nylon insert, which causes constant pressure against the stud of the TD. There must be just enough friction to allow the individual to rotate the TD but not so little that the TD inadvertently rotates while it is being activated by the cable pull.

2. *Quick change.* These units provide easy disconnection of different TDs. The TD is pressed down into the wrist to eject the TD or to lock it in position.

3. *Wrist flexion.* There are two versions of this unit: (1) The Hosmer wrist flexion unit can be manually placed in neutral, 30° of flexion, or 50° of flexion. (2) The Sierra wrist flexion unit can be screwed into the wrist unit, is dome shaped, and can be rotated within the wrist to preposition it. It can also be flexed to the same degrees as the Hosmer unit. Wrist flexion units are indispensable for the person with bilateral amputations because of their usefulness in reaching the midline for toileting, dressing, and eating.

4. *Ball and socket.* This unit can be prepositioned universally in positions around the ball, but it cannot be locked in position.

BELOW ELBOW (TRANSRADIAL) COMPONENTS

Forearm Socket Designs

For the forearm socket design, the residual limb is encased in the socket of the prothesis (Fig. 42.8). These sockets are either suspended on the body by a harness system or are self-suspending. The socket design configuration varies according to the residual limb length. For a long limb such as in a wrist disarticulation, the trim line (proximal edge or brim of socket) is cut down toward the distal portion to allow for

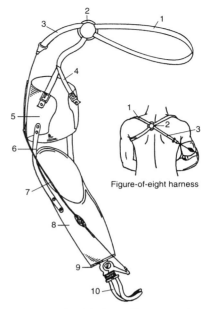

Figure 42.8. A standard below elbow prosthesis. *1,* Axilla loop; *2,* Northwestern University (NU) ring; *3,* control attachment strap; *4,* inverted Y strap; *5,* triceps cuff; *6,* flexible elbow hinge; *7,* cable; *8,* socket; *9,* wrist unit; *10,* TD.

at least 50% active pronation and supination. The prosthetist must be careful not to trim too much, which may compromise the socket stability, particularly for the person who intends to engage in heavy, rigorous activities. For the standard length limb, the socket length will encase two-thirds of the forearm. The supracondylar socket (modified Muenster) is a frequent choice for the short BE limb; the proximal brim grips the humeral lateral and medial epicondyles and the posterior olecranon (Fig. 42.9). In addition, this provides self-suspension for the myoelectrically controlled TD, for which no harnessing is necessary for cable attachment.

Elbow Hinges

Elbow hinges connect the socket to the triceps cuff or pad on the upper arm. These can be flexible (straps of Dacron or leather) or rigid (metal) hinges. Flexible hinges are used for the person with a standard or long residual limb, because they do not restrict forearm rotation. The rigid hinges are used for the short BE limb and offer stability at the elbow joint.

Triceps Cuff

The triceps cuff is used on the upper arm. It is connected to the socket by the elbow hinge. It is part of the harness suspension and serves as a point of attachment for the cable housing of the control attachment strap.

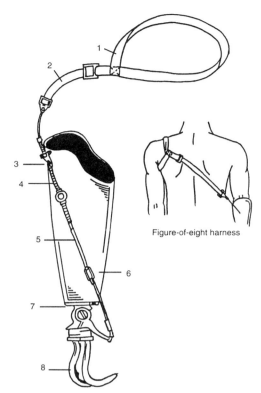

Figure 42.9. A supracondylar prosthesis. *1,* Figure-of-nine harness with axilla loop; *2,* control attachment strap; *3,* lift loop; *4,* housing; *5,* cable; *6,* supracondylar socket; *7,* wrist unit; *8,* TD.

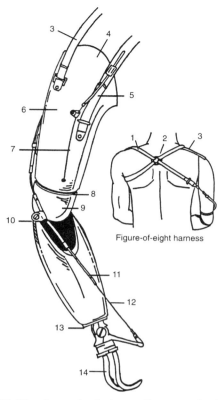

Figure 42.10. A standard above elbow prosthesis. *1,* Axilla loop; *2,* NU ring; *3,* lateral support strap; *4,* control attachment strap; *5,* elastic anterior support strap; *6,* socket; *7,* elbow lock cable; *8,* turntable; *9,* internal lock elbow unit; *10,* lift loop; *11,* housing; *12,* cable; *13,* wrist unit; *14,* TD.

Harness and Control System

The harness serves two purposes: (1) to suspend, or hold the prosthesis firmly on the residual limb and (2) to allow for force (through body motion) to be transmitted to the control cable that operates the terminal device. Three types of harnesses can be used with the BE prosthesis: figure-of-eight, figure-of-nine, and chest strap with a shoulder saddle. The figure-of-eight harness is considered the standard and is most often used (see Fig. 42.8). The axilla loop serves as the anchor point (reaction point) from which the other straps attach. The inverted Y support strap is attached to the anterior support strap of the harness. These attachments are important because they serve to stabilize the socket to the harness and they prevent displacement when the individual is carrying or lifting heavy loads. The chest strap with shoulder saddle is the harnessing system of choice when the patient cannot tolerate the pressure of the axilla loop or when the patient intends to engage in activities that require heavy lifting. With this heavy-duty harness, the pressure is distributed over a larger area via the shoulder saddle.

The figure-of-nine harness is used with the supracondylar socket (see Fig. 42.9). Because the socket configuration allows for self-suspension, only a control attachment strap is needed to attach the axilla loop to the cable control system.

ABOVE ELBOW (TRANSHUMERAL) COMPONENTS

Socket Designs

A great deal of research and development has occurred within the last 10 years in regard to refining socket design (McAuliffe, 1992). The conventional socket edge is generally just near or above the acromion, depending on limb length. On the other hand, the Utah Dynamic Socket, a recent design, is often selected because it provides more rotational stability. A standard above elbow (AE) prosthesis with an internal locking elbow is shown in Figure 42.10.

Elbow Units

There are two available elbow units for the AE prosthesis: (1) for a standard AE or short AE amputation, there is an internal elbow locking unit, which contains an inside locking mechanism, permitting 11 locked positions of flexion; and (2) for a long AE or elbow disarticulation amputation, there is an external elbow locking unit, which has seven locked positions. The external elbow locking unit is used when there is insufficient length to accommodate the internal locking mechanism. Otherwise the upper arm would be much longer than the intact one.

Friction Unit

The friction unit must be passively flexed into position. It is lightweight and is used with passive prosthetic arms. Manual elbow components are also available with a locking mechanism.

External Spring Lift Assist

The external spring lift assist is a clock spring mechanism that is added to the medial side of the elbow. Tightening the mechanism causes increased spring to elbow flexion and assists in initiating this motion.

Shoulder Hinges

The shoulder hinges can be manually positioned into flexion, extension, or abduction-adduction for placement of the arm in space.

SHOULDER DISARTICULATION AND INTRASCAPULOTHORACIC SHOULDER COMPONENTS

The socket designs for shoulder disarticulation and intrascapulothoracic protheses usually consist of a plastic laminated shoulder cap or a frame socket with carbon fiber reinforcements. An endoskeletal passive arm that is lightweight and contains an internal "pylon" shaft, which is covered with resilient foam contoured to the shape of the arm, may also be prescribed for this level of amputation. A chest strap harness suspends the prosthesis. A chin nudge lever attached to the anterior portion of the shoulder cap can be used for locking and unlocking the elbow, or the patient can reach over with the sound hand to lock and unlock a mechanical elbow mechanism.

HARNESS AND CONTROL SYSTEMS

The harness and control systems for an AE amputation are usually of the figure-of-eight or chest strap design. For a shoulder disarticulation (SD) prosthesis, the elbow lock can be activated via a chin nudge lever or a manual elbow lock mechanism.

Externally Powered Prosthetic Components

ELECTRIC TD

Electric powered hands and hooks (commercially available from the prosthetist) can be activated through myoelectric or switch control (Heckathorne, 1992). The electric powered prehensors are heavier (approximately 1 lb) but provide a stronger pinch force (20 to 23 lb) than the body powered types. There are two speed systems: (1) constant speed, whereby muscle contractions cause opening and closing at the same speed and (2) variable speed (proportional control), whereby the speed and pinch force increase in proportion to the intensity of muscle contraction.

ELECTRIC HANDS

The Otto Bock electric hands (Fig. 42.11) are the most popular models and are available in three adult sizes to accommodate males and females. The size is determined by measuring the circumference of the hand at the heads of the metacarpals; the hands are available in 7.5 inches for females and 7.75 and 8 inches for males. The hands can be covered by either a PVC or a Silicone glove. The motor in the hand mechanism drives the thumb and first two fingers as a unit to provide palmar (three-point) prehension. These hands contain a quick disconnect wrist, which allows for easy removal of the hand. The Steeper Hand is another choice (available in two sizes); its features are comparable with the Otto Bock hand.

ELECTRIC HOOKS

The Otto Bock electric Greifer TD is interchangeable with the Otto Bock hand and may be preferred for

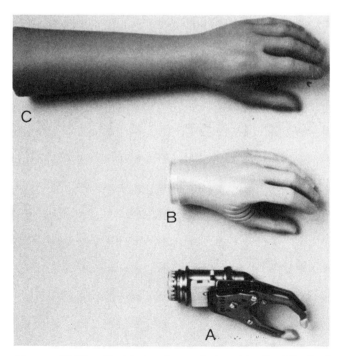

Figure 42.11. Electric hand manufactured by the Otto Bock Co. *A*, Internal mechanism; *B*, hand shell covering; *C*, hand glove.

work that requires high prehension force. It is bulky and encased in a hard plastic shell with no glove covering and is, therefore, less delicate than the hand. It is available in one size. The two fingers move symmetrically in opposition, parallel to one another (Fig. 42.12).

The Hosmer NU-VA Synergetic Prehensor contains motors that drive each of the fingers at different speeds and torque. Therefore, in grasping an object, one finger will close quickly on an object while the other finger applies the force for secure grip. These prostheses are relatively new to the market and may be chosen by an experienced team whose facilities include research and development.

ELECTRIC ELBOWS

There are three electric elbow mechanisms available: the Boston elbow, the NY-Hosmer electric elbow, and the Utah arm. The NY-Hosmer and Boston elbows can be controlled by electromechanical switches or by myoelectric control. Myoelectric control is needed for the Motion Control Utah arm (Fig. 42.13).

The Final Prescription: A Discussion

For an experienced team, there are many options. Table 42.1 gives a quick overview of some of the features that should be considered when prescribing a prosthesis (Datta & Brain, 1992; Edelstein, 1992; Godfrey, 1990; Millstein, Heger, & Hunter, 1986; Roeschlien & Domholdt, 1989; Sears, 1991; Weaver, Lang, & Vogts, 1988).

Motivation is the most important factor in the

acceptance and use of the prosthesis. This is a complex issue, because the patient must choose a prosthesis at the very time when he is most confused and vulnerable. The patient's desire for a prosthesis is strongest after surgery. This may wane as time passes, particularly for the person with a unilateral amputation and as compensatory one-handed techniques are learned. The patient with a bilateral amputation presents a need for function and will probably accept and use the prostheses.

What defines a successful wearer? If the prosthesis is worn and viewed as necessary for any activity, be it for leisure only or purely for cosmesis, it has added to the quality of life and can be viewed as successful. It is not unusual for a patient with a unilateral amputation to use the prosthesis for select activities, which may change as the patient's interests change.

Two sets of prostheses are strongly recommended for the person with high-level bilateral amputations. One pair can be used as a spare should the other set need repairs.

The end goal of a therapeutic program is to ensure the highest level of independence and self-reliance. This does not always assume prosthetic use. The patient may choose no prosthesis but must be exposed to several options before he makes his final choice. However, thorough and early training in the use of the prosthesis can influence prosthetic use as well.

PROSTHETIC TRAINING PROGRAM

The time frames listed below can be used as guidelines for the therapeutic program (Atkins, 1989a). This general guide infers no major complications in

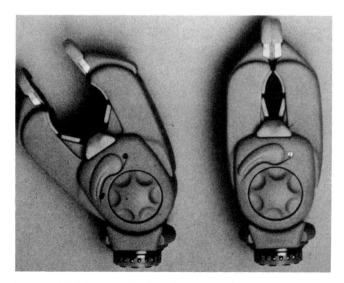

Figure 42.12. Otto Bock's electric Greifer in the open and closed positions.

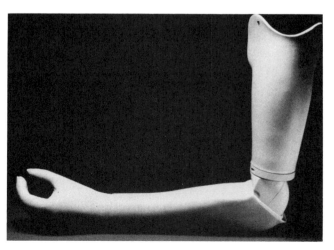

Figure 42.13. Utah arm with myoelectric hand and elbow and Utah dynamic above elbow socket.

Table 42.1. Hooks and Hands Compared

Features	Hooks VO (BP)	VC TRS Grip (BP)	Hands (Myoelectrically Controlled)	Hands VO (BP)
Cosmesis	Considered poor; does not replicate a hand	Poor cosmesis	Cosmetically appealing	Cosmetically appealing
Pinch force	Contingent on number of rubber bands, but more bands also increase the effort required to open	Considered excellent for strong grasp; can achieve >50 lb, contingent on amount of force the individual can exert on the cable	Strong pinch; proportional control allows for variable pinch force up to about 25 lb	Pinch force stronger than VO hook but less than myoelectric hands
Prehension pattern	Precise, fine pinch possible	Fine pinch possible	Cylindrical grasp rather than fine pinch; hand configuration is identical for myoelectric and BP hands	Cylindrical grasp identical to myoelectric hand
Weight	Lighter in weight than hands; aluminum models are even lighter Range: 3.0–8.7 oz	Heavier than VO hooks, but some models are lighter than hands Range: 10–16 oz	Heaviest 16.8 oz	Heavy Range: 10.0–13.8 oz
Durability	Very durable; stainless steel models are even more rugged	Very durable stainless steel TD	Less durable; glove is delicate; control systems may need servicing	Less durable; glove is delicate; spring mechanism may need repairs
Reliability	Little servicing needed	Little servicing needed	Most servicing needed	Needs more servicing than VO and VC TD but less than myoelectric
Feedback	Some proprioceptive feedback experienced from tension on shoulder harness and limb pressure in socket when operating the TD or elbow	Better proprioceptive feedback	Some feedback through intensity of muscle contraction, particularly for proportional control	Feedback similar to VO hook
Ease of use and activation				
Effort to activate	More effort to open	More effort to sustain grasp; can have manual lock	Low effort to activate	Effort to activate
Use in various planes	Difficult at high planes for AE	Similar to VO hook	Very good for BE	Similar to VO hook
Visibility of items being grasped	Very good visibility	Better visibility than hands but less than VO hook	Less visibility than hooks	Less visibility; similar to myoelectric hand
Cost	Low cost	Higher cost than VO but lower than myoelectric	Higher cost for TD and systems	Higher cost than BP hook but lower than myoelectric

regard to the residual limb or prosthesis and no cognitive deficits.

Unilateral BE	6 hr
Unilateral AE/SD	15 hr
Bilateral BE	12 hr
Bilateral AE	20 hr, minimum

Initial Stage of Treatment

The initial stage of treatment can generally be covered in one to two therapy sessions. The therapist should complete the following items during this stage.

1. Evaluate the prosthesis;
2. Introduce the patient to the program goals and sequence, including an overview of the goals for each treatment phase;
3. Review the prosthesis and identify all components, explain the functions of each component, and give the patient an illustration of the prosthesis with all parts labeled;
4. Teach the patient to don and remove the prosthesis;
5. Discuss the wearing schedule with the patient;
6. Teach the patient limb hygiene care;
7. Teach the patient prosthesis care;

8. Begin controls training with the terminal device only.

Evaluation of the Prosthesis

On the first visit after the definitive prosthesis is received, the therapist will complete an evaluation or checkout of the prosthesis. This evaluation can occur with the prosthetist in the amputee clinic, if the prosthesis is delivered in this manner. However, the evaluation must occur before prosthetic training begins. The purpose of the evaluation is to determine (1) compliance with the prescription, (2) comfort of fit of the socket and harness system, (3) satisfactory operation of all components, and (4) appearance (features) of the total prosthesis and its component parts. Refer to Table 42.2 for methods and standards for evaluation (Figs. 42.14-42.16).

First Therapy Session

Generally, patients with unilateral amputations will attend therapy on an outpatient schedule of 2 or 3 days a week; therefore, the first visit is a critical one. The aim from the outset is to minimize negative experiences to ensure prosthetic acceptance and use. The therapist must orient the patient to the overall therapy plan and guide the patient to set realistic goals and expectations. In addition to the prosthetic evaluation, the following must also be covered during the first visit: (1) donning and removing the prosthesis, (2) prosthetic wearing time schedule, (3) hygienic care of the residual limb, and (4) care of the prosthesis. The patient should not leave the clinic without instruction in the first three topics listed.

DONNING AND REMOVING THE PROSTHESIS

Donning and removing the prosthesis can be achieved by one of two methods that simulate putting on a coat or slip-over shirt. To use the coat method, the residual limb is inserted into the socket, which is held in place with the intact hand, the harness and

Table 42.2. Prosthetic Evaluation

Activity	PROSTHESIS		Performance Standards
	Off	On	
Range of motion (BE)			
1. Stump rotation (total range)	_____	_____	Total rotation with prosthesis on should be half that with prosthesis off[a,b]
2. Elbow flexion			
Maximum extension angle (initial flexion)	_____	_____	Active flexion with prosthesis on should be within 10° of range with prosthesis off[b]
Maximum flexion angle	_____	_____	
Range	_____	_____	
Range of motion (AE)			
1. Shoulder flexion	_____	_____	90°
2. Shoulder abduction	_____	_____	90°
3. Shoulder extension	_____	_____	30°
4. Prosthetic elbow: mechanical range		_____	135°
5. Prosthetic elbow: active range		_____	135°
6. Humeral flexion required to flex elbow fully		_____	Should not exceed 45°
Terminal device opening and closing[c]	HOOK	HAND	
1. Mechanical range	_____inches	_____inches	Full opening and closing should
2. Active range (forearm at 90°)	_____inches	_____inches	be obtained in all test posi-
3. Active range (at waist)	_____inches	_____inches	tions for BE, 50% or more for
4. Active range (at mouth)	_____inches	_____inches	movements 3 and 4.
Control System Efficiency[a]			
1. Force applied at TD	_____lb	_____lb	
2. Force applied at harness	_____lb	_____lb	
3. Efficiency = force at terminal device/force at harness	_____%	_____%	Should be 70% or greater.
4. Force required to flex from position of 90°	_____lb	_____lb	Should not exceed 10 lb; should not cause inadvertent TD operation.

Conformance with prescription
_____   1. Is the prosthesis as prescribed? If a recheck, have previous recommendations been accomplished?

Dimensions
_____   2. Is the prosthesis the correct length and do elbow levels coincide? Distal tip of TD should correspond to thumb tip of sound side while patient is standing.

Table 42.2. Continued.

Terminal device and wrist unit

——————— 3. Do the terminal device and wrist mechanism function properly?
——————— 4. If a cosmetic glove is used, is it undamaged, properly color matched, and pulled completely onto the fingers?

Elbow unit

——————— 5. Does cuff fit snugly and not gap? (BE)
——————— 6. Is the forearm set in adequate initial flexion? (AE)
——————— 7. Can the amputee swing his arms while walking and raise his elbow 60° to the side without the elbow locking involuntarily? (AE)
——————— 8. Can the patient use the turntable to position the forearm satisfactorily? (AE)

Harness

——————— 9. Is the axilla loop small enough to keep the cross of the figure-of-eight harness well below the seventh cervical vertebra and slightly to the unamputated side?
——————— 10. Is the axilla loop properly covered and is it comfortable?
——————— 11. Is the control attachment strap below midscapular level and does it remain low enough to give adequate cable travel?
——————— 12. Is the lateral support strap properly positioned? (AE)
——————— 13. If there are additional harness straps, can their use be justified?
——————— 14. Does the front support strap pass through the deltopectoral groove?
——————— 15. Is the elastic front suspensor of adequate length and properly located? (AE)
——————— 16. If a chest strap harness is used, is the saddle of proper size and placement and is the chest strap comfortable?

Cable system

——————— 17. If a hook is to be interchanged with a hand, is the hook-to-cable adapter the proper length?
——————— 18. Is the control cable free from sharp bends?
——————— 19. Is the housing on the control cable long enough to prevent contact of the cable with the patient or with the prosthetic forearm but short enough so it does not interfere with function? (AE)
——————— 20. Does the cable housing cover the cable adequately without restricting forearm flexion?
——————— 21. Is the leather lift loop the proper length and is it positioned to allow adequate terminal device operation after full forearm flexion and heavy enough to withstand buckling during use?
——————— 22. Does the leather lift loop pivot on the screw and grip the cable housing tightly enough to prevent slipping?
——————— 23. Does the elbow lock cable lead directly from the access hole to the deltopectoral groove? (AE)

Socket

——————— 24. Is the socket comfortable, especially when compression force and torque are applied?
——————— 25. Is the residual limb free from abrasions, discolorations, and other signs of irritation immediately after the prosthesis is removed?

Workmanship

——————— 26. Is the general workmanship satisfactory?

Patient's performance and opinion

——————— 27. Can the patient demonstrate effective use of the terminal device, wrist mechanism, and elbow unit?
——————— 28. Does the patient consider the prosthesis satisfactory as to comfort, function, and appearance?

---

[a] This standard applies to medium, well-formed residual limbs but is often exceeded with wrist disarticulation and long below elbow residual limbs. Short or fleshy residual limbs may not be able to attain the 50% standard.
[b] In Muenster sockets, forearm rotation is eliminated and maximum elbow flexion is considerably limited (average 105 to 110°). Furthermore, because of decreased elbow flexion, the measurement of TD opening at the mouth may not apply; however, the TD should open fully at maximum elbow flexion.
[c] Fingers directed medially.

axilla loop are dangling behind the back. The intact arm reaches behind and slips into the axilla loop; a forward shrug of the shoulders positions the prosthesis in place. For the slip-over method, the patient places the prosthesis in front of him, and the noninvolved arm is placed through the axilla loop while the residual limb is placed into the socket. Both limbs are raised to lift the prosthesis and harness over the head and the harness falls into place. Initially, for those patients who are not as limber, have difficulty grasping the concept, or have bilateral amputations, the prosthesis can be placed on a bed or dresser and the patient can lean back and slip into the prosthesis, using a forward shrug to position it in place.

PROSTHETIC WEARING TIME

Developing tolerance to the socket and harness system requires the patient to increase wearing time gradually. The initial wearing time may be 20 to 30 min. The residual limb is examined for redness or irritation each time the prosthesis is removed and should not be put back on until the redness or irritation subsides. If it does not subside after approximately 20 min, this should be reported to the prosthetist for prosthetic adjustment or revision. Otherwise, prosthetic wearing time can be increased in 30-min increments until it can be tolerated a full day. The importance of gradually increasing the wearing time cannot be

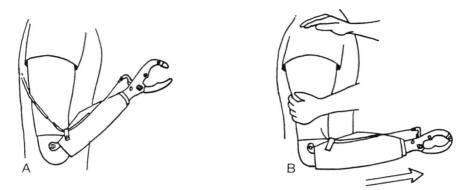

Figure 42.14. Activation of voluntary closing TD. **A.** The VC TD remains open at rest. **B.** The VC TD closes with forward flexion.

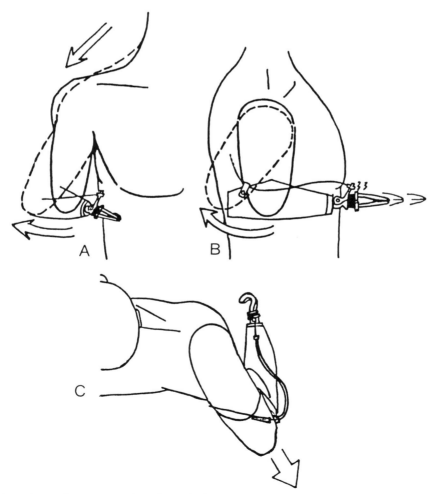

Figure 42.15. Motions (*arrows*) necessary for elbow lock control for an above elbow prosthesis. **A.** Abduction with de- pression. **B.** Extension. **C.** Combined movement pattern of exten- sion, abduction, and depression.

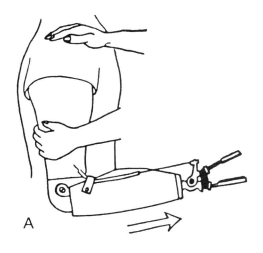

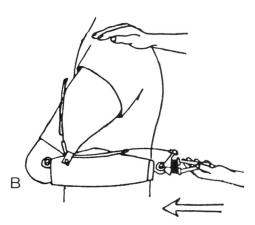

Figure 42.16. A. Teaching activation of voluntary opening TD. When the elbow is locked, the therapist pulls the patient's upper arm forward (*arrow*) to open the TD. **B.** Teaching activation of elbow lock. The therapist pushes the patient's arm back (*arrow*) into extension to lock or unlock the elbow. The arm is brought back to the vertical position between cycles.

overemphasized, particularly for the patient with decreased sensation and scar tissue.

LIMB HYGIENE

Because the residual limb is enclosed in a rigid socket where excessive perspiration can cause skin maceration, it is important to instruct the patient to wash the limb daily with mild soap and lukewarm water and pat dry. It is recommended that the patient wear a T-shirt or equivalent covering so that the harness system of a BP prosthesis is not in direct contact with the skin. This provides padding and also absorbs perspiration. For the same reason, the patient is instructed to wear a sock over the residual limb(s). The patient must examine the skin daily.

CARE OF PROSTHESIS

Mild soap and warm water are recommended to clean the interior of the socket of dirt and perspiration. The socket can also be wiped with rubbing alcohol, which is germicidal, every several weeks. The patient must be cautioned about agents that could stain or damage gloves. The hook is obviously more rugged, but care must be taken when working in areas where there is excessive dirt, grease, or water. The hook and wrist unit must be cleaned. The patient must be especially careful with externally powered components.

Intermediate Stage of Treatment

BODY POWERED PROSTHESIS

The therapy program for the BP prothesis is addressed in two phases: (1) prosthetic controls training and (2) prosthetic functional use training.

Prosthetic Controls Training

Therapy for controls training begins with teaching the operation of each control and component. The patient is expected to practice activation of these. Below elbow prostheses have a single control system that activates, by cable pull, only the TD. Therefore, patients with a BE prosthesis need to learn TD activation and prepositioning of the TD. Above elbow prostheses have a dual-control system for the TD and elbow. Patients with a AE prosthesis must learn elbow activation and use of the turntable and shoulder joints (Table 42.3).

Practice in control drills requires coaching the patient in patterns of reach, grasp, and release for objects that vary in weight, size, texture, and configuration. Ordinarily, the sequence is from hard, larger objects to smaller, fragile ones. The assortment is subject to the therapist's ingenuity. These objects are usually placed on a tabletop for prehension practice and not used within the context of an activity.

To grasp an item, the stationary finger of the TD is placed next to the object and the movable finger closes toward it. The patient can be asked to hold and transport the item to another location. Instruction in determining the most natural and efficient position of the TD and then rotating it before grasping is also given This is called prepositioning the TD.

Eventually, the patient is instructed to perform these motion patterns in different planes, e.g., overhead, at tabletop, and at floor level. Overhead use is the most difficult, particularly for persons with more proximal (AE) amputations and may not be achievable. The person with bilateral amputations must learn to control movement on one side and avoid inadvertently activating the contralateral side. This can easily occur, because the harness system is bilaterally attached.

Prosthetic Functional Use Training

Spontaneous, automatic skillful prosthetic use is a goal for this phase of treatment. Another is completion of activities within a reasonable length of time while using minimal extraneous movement and energy expenditure. Figures 42.17 to 42.20 illustrate bilateral activities. The therapist encourages the patient to use creative problem-solving approaches, which will be useful for future encounters in novel situations. Realistic expectations for prosthetic use for the individual with a unilateral amputation can be for static holding or for stabilization. In addition, the therapist should not expect the patient to complete tasks as quickly with the prosthesis as with the sound, nondominant extremity.

Table 42.3.   Controls Training for Body Powered Prosthetics

Device	Instruction or Intervention

Terminal device
 Body motion to activate TD
  Shoulder glenohumeral flexion on side of TD to be activated
  Scapular abduction (forward roll of shoulder) on side to be activated; bilateral scapular abduction for midline use or with limited strength
	Therapist manually guides the patient through the motion pattern. *Note:* For AE amputation, keep elbow locked in 90° of flexion and teach TD control only (Fig.42.14)

Wrist unit rotation
  Manual prepositioning of TD for supination, pronation or midposition
  For unilateral amputation, the TD is rotated in the wrist unit by using the sound hand
  For bilateral amputation, the TD is rotated by pushing or pulling using the contralateral TD, between the knees, or against a stationary object
	The patient must analyze the task and predetermine how to grasp the object to avoid excessive or awkward body movement such as twisting and bending, e.g., when carrying a tray, the fingers of the hook must be turned with the hook tips toward the person's midline (body) so the hook is in midposition similar to the holding pattern of the sound hand; a jar is held with the fingertips down (pronated) toward floor, while the sound arm opens the top

Elbow unit mechanism *Body motion to activate elbow lock and unlock*	Therapist manually guides the patient through these motion patterns; the patient views himself in mirror for visual feedback (Figs. 42.15 and 42.16)

Table 42.3.   Continued.

Device	Instruction or Intervention

Practice motions
  Scapular depression (push residual limb into socket end)
  Humeral extension/hyperextension
  Humeral abduction
	Begin with the elbow unit in an unlocked position and the elbow in flexion (arm adducted); the forearm is passively pushed back into extension to lock; listen for "click" sounds; this motion may have to be exaggerated during the initial stages

Practice TD activation with elbow locked	Lock elbow; use humeral flexion with scapular abduction to activate TD
Practice elbow flexion and lock at different levels, from full flexion to full extension	Unlock elbow and gravity will pull forearm into extension; use humeral flexion to flex elbow at desired height; when locking the elbow unit, flex the elbow slightly higher than desired, which allows for gravity to pull downward as patient locks elbow
Teach manual control of turntable for internal or external rotation	Unilateral: patient reaches over to rotate upper arm unit; bilateral: patient pulls or pushes against a stationary object in the environment or with opposite prosthesis

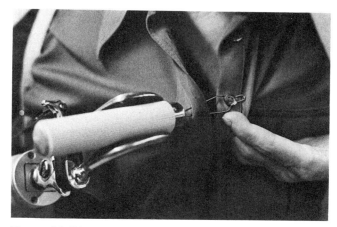

Figure 42.17.   A button hook is a necessary aid for those with bilateral amputations.

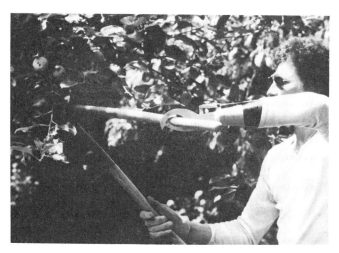

Figure 42.18. Use of the voluntary closing TRS Grip for bilateral activity.

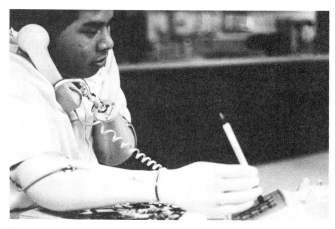

Figure 42.20. Bilateral activity practiced in the occupational therapy clinic. The glove will be put on by the prosthetist after the initial practice phase.

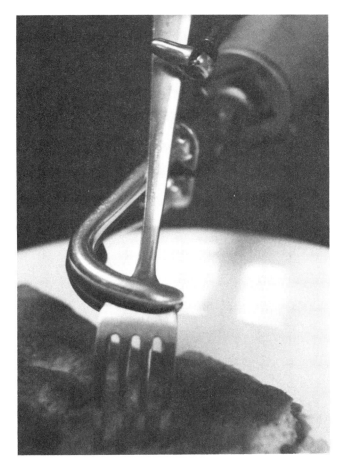

Figure 42.19. Grasping a fork in this manner provides good stability while the sound hand cuts the food.

Table 42.4 suggests how some activities can be accomplished; refer to Atkins (1989a) and Department of Prosthetics and Orthotics (1986) for more comprehensive lists.

Several factors impact the degree of independence for the person with bilateral amputations (Edelstein, 1992; Friedmann, 1989), the major one being the level of amputation. Some adaptations may be necessary for those with high-level bilateral amputations. These may range from a simple button hook or dressing frame (a stand in which coat hooks are inserted to hold clothing) to high-tech solutions such as environmental control units (Lehneis & Dickey, 1992) and computers controlled by breath, voice, or mouthstick. The therapist is advised to encourage foot use when patients show potential and are agile. Persons who have developed this ability at an early age have a high degree of independence. Feet have the advantage of having sensibility, which serves them well in all activities and surpasses prosthetic use.

MYOELECTRICALLY CONTROLLED PROSTHESIS

Myoelectric prostheses are fast becoming standard choices and are frequently prescribed for BE amputations. Figure 42.21 depicts a two-state system whereby two separate muscle groups are used to operate the T.D. The intent is to choose those muscles that physiologically closely correspond to the desired outcome motion and that produce a strong electrical signal when activated. In this case, the wrist flexors and extensors are chosen to produce finger flexion and extension.

For above elbow amputations, the common choices are the biceps and triceps. For higher-level amputations, as in shoulder disarticulation or forequar-

Table 42.4. Functional Activities: Unilateral Upper Limb Deficiency Operation

Task	Prosthesis	Sound Limb
Eating		
1. Cut	Hold fork	Cut with knife
2. Butter bread	Stabilize bread	Spread toward TD
3. Fill glass from faucet	Hold glass	Turn faucet
4. Peel orange	Stabilize orange	Peel
5. Carry tray	Hold side of tray with TD in midposition	Hold opposite side of tray
6. Open milk or juice carton	Stabilize carton	Open top
Dressing		
1. Don and remove prosthesis	Don: amputated limb in socket first	Remove: sound arm out of harness first
2. Don and remove overhead top	Don: prosthesis in sleeve first	Remove: pull sleeve off prosthetic limb first
3. Put clothes on hanger		Place hanger in clothing and hand
4. Buckle belt		Push buckle and prong through
5. Tie bow		Manipulate lace and make loops
6. Button and unbutton sound side cuff	a. Use button hook b. Hold button hole	a. Hold button side cuff with fingertips to palm b. Hold button side cuff with fingertips to palm and maneuver button into hole
7. Use zipper	Hold material	Pull zipper
Desk skills		
1. Write	Stabilize paper	Write
2. Put letter in envelope and seal; open envelope	Hold envelope at end	Seal: insert letter Open: tear at side of envelope
3. Draw line with ruler	Stabilize ruler	Draw line
4. Use paper clip	Hold paper	Apply clip
5. Use phone; take notes	a. Hold receiver with TD b. Hold receiver between chin and shoulder	Write
6. Hold book; turn pages	Stabilize book on table	Turn pages
General skills		
1. Take bill from wallet	Hold wallet	Remove bill
2. Wrap and unwrap package	Stabilize paper and box	Maneuver box, paper, and tie
3. Use key in lock	Grasp knob	Turn key
4. Thread needle	Grasp needle	Thread needle
5. Light match from book of matches	Hold book with cover closed	Remove match and strike

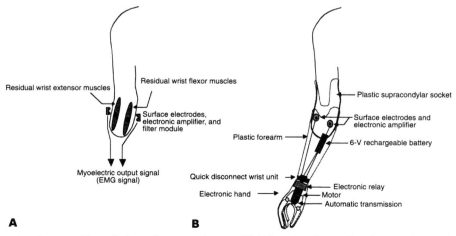

A   **B**

Figure 42.21. Myoelectric control for a below elbow prosthesis. **A,** The muscle contracts and creates an electrical voltage. The electromyographic (EMG) signal is picked up by the surface electrode. The EMG signal is processed by the electronic filters and amplifiers. The signal is transmitted to the relay in the hand.

B, When the electronic relay receives a signal from the residual wrist muscles, the circuit is complete. Electricity from the battery runs the motor to close the hand when the signal is from the wrist flexors. When the signal comes from the residual wrist extensors, the motor will run in the opposite direction to open the hand.

ter amputations, the choices for control may be trapezius, latissimus, infraspinatus, or pectoralis muscles.

Most of the principles and treatment goals previously mentioned for BP prosthesis apply for myoelectrically controlled prosthesis. The therapy program begins with evaluation of the prosthesis, with special emphasis on the control system (Spiegel, 1989):

1. Are the electrodes located over the site offering the best muscle potential control?
2. Is there good contact between the electrodes and the skin? (An imprint should be visible on the skin when the prosthesis is removed, but it should not be deep enough to cause irritation.)
3. Can the patient begin to control the hand in various planes?
4. Can the patient remove and replace the battery from its receptacle with ease?

It is advised that the therapist consult with the prosthetist for guidance with any issues. Donning and removing the prosthesis may require collaboration with the prosthetist to determine the simplest method for the patient. There are times when baby powder or a lubricant can be used to ease donning, but these can inhibit electrode functioning.

Care of the socket requires daily cleansing with a damp cloth and mild soap to remove any residues of powder, lubricants, and perspiration. Other special concerns are care of the batteries, methods for charging the batteries, and operation of the on/off switch. Care of the glove was discussed earlier.

Controls and functional use training goals are similar to those for the BP prosthesis. This assumes that the patient has received muscle site controls training during the preprosthetic period. When a myoelectric tester is used, the goals at this time are to isolate muscle contractions and increase muscle strength (Spiegel, 1989). Figure 42.22 demonstrates functional use for light grasp.

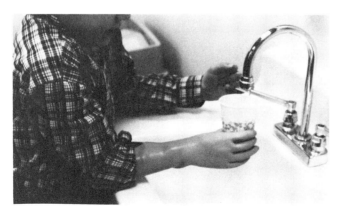

Figure 42.22.   The myoelectric hand can hold delicate objects in bilateral activities.

Final Treatment Stage

In the final stage, prosthetic functional use training is further refined, and daily living skills that are more demanding are introduced at this time. Discharge planning should include exploration of vocational and recreational pursuits and driving and/or the use of public transportation. Visits to the community, home, school, and work are strongly advised. This brings the patient and therapist into the actual environment, away from simulated, static settings.

An adaptation for driving may be a simple knob or driving ring attached to the steering wheel. It is possible to install foot controls for those with very high level bilateral amputations. The therapist can consult companies that do van conversions for the disabled in this case.

Patients may be referred to a self-help group. These organizations vary in their goals, but usually provide a forum whereby people can socially interact and share experiences. Many groups provide ongoing educational programs on new prosthetic developments or on sports and recreational activities. The National Amputee Foundation is one source for information. Sabolich (1992) published personal accounts of patients with amputations, which could serve as sources of encouragement.

SPORTS AND RECREATION

Interest in developing and customizing prostheses for sports and recreational activities has intensified during the past 15 years. Several factors have contributed to this increased interest, one being the attitude of individuals with amputations who are now more rigorously pursuing recreational activities. Two comprehensive references discussing this topic are available: Radocy (1992) and Kegel (1992). Figure 42.23 shows a passive sports device.

Shared and published information inspires ideas for further development. The Americans with Disabilities Act, which requires accessibility changes in the community, helps all people with disabilities expand their participation in all activities. Often, the prosthetist, patient, family, therapist, and physician collaborate to create a customized item, such as the flexible silicone socket that attaches to a violin bow shown in Figure 42.24.

DISCHARGE

At discharge, a follow-up appointment for the clinic is scheduled as determined by the team; this may be 1 month to several months postdischarge. The patient is encouraged to contact the prosthetist for repairs or maintenance as needed and to make an appointment for a clinic visit at any time. As the

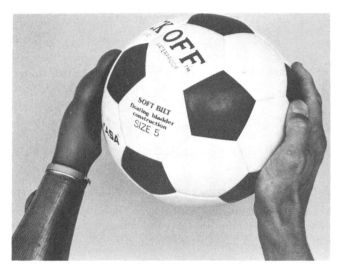

Figure 42.23. TRS's Super Sport Passive Mitt, used for gross grasping patterns.

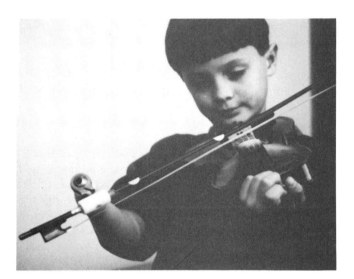

Figure 42.24. The adaptation made to this bow (an attachment to a suction silicone socket) allows for flexibility and stability.

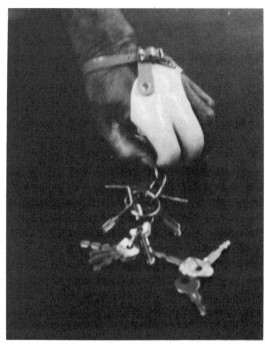

Figure 42.25. Prosthetic finger post provides some function.

patient reestablishes his life and integrates into society, he may decide on a prosthesis with different features. This usually occurs when the decision is made to pursue a change in vocation or participate in additional recreational and sports activities.

PARTIAL HAND AMPUTATIONS

As with any amputation, the surgeon performing a partial hand amputation attempts to preserve length with intact sensibility. At this level, the possibility of retaining residual digits with adequate skin coverage that still have some degree of mobility and sensation is far superior to any prosthesis (Bunnell, 1990). The

principles of preprosthetic therapy (discussed above) apply to this level of amputation as well.

Cosmesis is often of primary concern, and the patient will request a prosthesis that closely replicates his hand. As noted, cosmetic hands (or gloves) are truly artistic endeavors, but they fit over the residual hand and restrict functional use by preventing sensory feedback. For these very reasons, it is not unusual for the glove to be discarded in favor of a partial post or opposition surface (Fig. 42.25). With an opposition post, less skin surface is covered, thereby preserving tactile sensory feedback (Michael, 1992). There are times when the occupational therapist can design and fabricate a temporary functional orthosis or post for trial use in the clinic. This can eventually be translated into a permanent orthosis or prosthesis.

MANAGEMENT OF LOWER LIMB AMPUTATIONS

The preprosthetic and prosthetic therapeutic program for persons with lower limb amputations requires collaboration between the physical and occupational therapists. The physical therapist is responsible for the greater part of the therapy program in relation to skin care, limb wrapping, lower limb strengthening exercises, and ROM in addition to ambulation training (Mensch & Ellis, 1982). Training in some daily living activities may be shared, e.g., limb bandaging, bed mobility, and transfer activities. Often, functional conditioning groups are conducted by an occupational therapist with the following objectives:

1. Instruction in upper extremity strengthening exercises;
2. Instruction in safety precautions related to specific activities;
3. Instruction in energy conservation;
4. Instruction in use of adaptive devices;
5. Review of dietary restriction, when appropriate.

These groups can be conducted with a physical therapist and other team members, e.g., the dietitian could provide information about the diet.

Occupational Therapy Program Guidelines

The occupational therapist should assess physical and cognitive status and obtain information on secondary diagnoses that may impact function. Safety is a major concern with lower extremity amputations, particularly for the geriatric patient. The majority of patients with bilateral lower limb amputations are over age 60, with primary diagnosis of diabetes or vascular disease. Secondary complicating factors that can affect therapy include kidney disease, cardiovascular disease, chronic infection, respiratory disease, and arthritis. In addition, impaired vision and memory deficits strongly influence safe performance in activities of daily living (Andrews, 1987).

The therapist must assess functional activities with an initial focus on areas of personal self-care and mobility. Therapy should be provided to maximize self-reliance in activities of daily living (ADL) in keeping with the patient's lifestyle and goals.

1. ADLs are ordinarily addressed in the following sequence: bed mobility; hygiene and grooming; dressing, including donning and removing the leg prosthesis; and wheelchair propulsion and management. Transfer skills are practiced with and without the prosthesis. Practice sessions include transfers to the bed, toilet, furniture, and car.

2. Homemaking may be an important daily living activity and can include mobility in the kitchen with the wheelchair and/or ambulating with the prosthesis, with or without a device. Home management activities can be taught as appropriate, such as house cleaning and bed making. Home and community visits may also be appropriate and can be done with the patient by the occupational, physical, and/or recreational therapist, who work as a team.

3. The family should be educated in transfer techniques when necessary.

4. Recommendations for home modifications and equipment should be reviewed with the patient and family. Equipment may include such items as a transfer tub bench or seat and toilet safety arm rails. These

rails fit around the toilet and provide a means of arm support so the patient can lower himself down and lift himself up.

5. The therapist makes the referral for driving assessment and training when appropriate. Driving adaptations for a person with a right leg amputation include installation of a left foot accelerator bar and pedal. Hand controls can be installed for persons with bilateral leg amputations.

EMERGING TRENDS IN PROSTHETICS

Significant changes in the area of research and development of upper and lower extremity prostheses have occurred during the past 15 years (Sears, 1992). Materials such as titanium and carbon composites are being used; they are lightweight but strong. Socket designs have been modified to provide better purchase and rotational stability; the Utah Dynamic Socket is an example (see Fig. 42.13). Flexible silicon suction sockets, which provide good purchase on the limb but allow for flexibility, are a breakthrough (see Fig. 42.14). In regard to upper extremity prosthetics, the quest for viable sensory feedback systems continues. Under development are vibrotactile skin systems, electrotactile display mechanisms, nerve stimulation, and extended physiologic systems. However, no practical system is yet commercially available. Terminal device designs continue to receive attention in an attempt to replicate more closely the functions of the hand and to provide hands that weigh less.

Acknowledgments—Very special thanks to Gregory Celikyol for the illustrations and to Susan Souza for word processing. I thank Jack Hodgins for his illustration, and Sudesh S. Jain and Karen Cameron for their helpful comments.

STUDY QUESTIONS

1. Why is the residual limb wrapped with elastic bandaging? How is it done?
2. What are the most common causes of acquired upper and lower limb amputations?
3. Which body movements are required for a patient with an AE amputation to operate a conventional BP terminal device and elbow unit?
4. What are the positive and negative features of a hook? A hand?
5. What are the differences between a VO and a VC terminal device?
6. What is myoelectric control?
7. Why are controls training and use training done?
8. Why might an amputee accept or reject a prosthesis?
9. What are the functional expectations for a person with a unilateral AE limb amputation or a bilateral AE limb amputation?

STUDY QUESTIONS *(continued)*

10. What is the rôle of the occupational therapist in the rehabilitation of the patient with lower extremity amputations?

REFERENCES

Andrews, K. (1987). Lower-limb amputation. In K. Andrews (Ed.), *Rehabilitation of the older adult* (pp. 119–144). London: Edward Arnold.

Atkins, D. J. (1989a). Adult upper-limb prosthetic training. In D. J. Atkins & R. H. Meier III (Eds.), *Comprehensive management of the upper-limb amputee* (pp. 39–59). New York: Springer-Verlag.

Atkins, D. J. (1989b). Post-operative and pre-prosthetic therapy programs. In D. J. Atkins & R. H. Meier III (Eds.), *Comprehensive management of the upper-limb amputee* (pp. 11–15). New York: Springer-Verlag.

Banerjee, S. N. (1982). *Rehabilitation management of amputees.* Baltimore: Williams & Wilkins.

Bunnell, S. (1990). The management of the non-functional hand: Reconstruction versus prosthesis. In J. M. Hunter, L. H. Schneider, E. J. Mackin, & A. D. Callahan (Eds.), *Rehabilitation of the hand* (pp. 997–1017). St. Louis: C. V. Mosby.

Datta, D., & Brain, N. D. (1992). Clinical applications of myoelectrically-controlled prostheses. *Critical Review in Physical Medicine and Rehabilitation, 4,* 215–239.

Department of Prosthetics and Orthotics. (1986). *Upper-limb prosthetics.* New York: New York University Medical Center, Postgraduate Medical School.

Dise-Lewis, J. E. (1989). Psychological adaptation to limb loss. In D. J. Atkins & R. H. Meier III (Eds.), *Comprehensive management of the upper-limb amputee* (pp. 165–172). New York: Springer-Verlag.

Edelstein, J. E. (1992). Special consideration—Rehabilitation without prostheses: Functional skills training. In American Academy of Orthopaedic Surgeons (Ed.), *Atlas of limb prosthetics: Surgical, prosthetic and rehabilitation principles* (pp. 721–728). St. Louis: Mosby Year Book.

Edelstein, J. E., & Berger, N. (1993). Performance comparison among children fitted with myoelectric and body-powered hands. *Archives of Physical Medicine and Rehabilitation, 74,* 376–380.

Fleming, M. H. (1991). The therapist with the three-track mind. *American Journal of Occupational Therapy, 45,* 1007–1014.

Friedmann, L. W. (1978). *The psychological rehabilitation of the amputee.* Springfield, IL: Charles C. Thomas.

Friedmann, L. (1989). Functional skills in multiple limb anomalies. In D. J. Atkins & R. H. Meier III (Eds.), *Comprehensive management of the upper-limb amputee* (pp. 150–164). New York: Springer-Verlag.

Fryer, C. M., & Michael, J. W. (1992). Body-powered components. In American Academy of Orthopaedic Surgeons (Ed.), *Atlas of limb prosthetics: Surgical, prosthetic and rehabilitation principles* (pp. 107–131). St. Louis: Mosby Year Book.

Godfrey, S. (1990). Workers with prostheses. *Journal of Hand Therapy, 3*(2), 101–110.

Heckathorne, C. W. (1992). Components for adult externally powered systems. In American Academy of Orthopaedic Surgeons (Ed.), *Atlas of limb prosthetics: Surgical, prosthetic and rehabilitation principles* (pp. 151–174). St. Louis: Mosby Year Book.

Heinze, A. (Producer). (1988). *Amputation, rehabilitation & pros-*

theses [Videotape]. Washington, DC: Universal Health Associates.

Kegel, B. (1992). Adaptations for sports and recreation. In American Academy of Orthopaedic Surgeons (Ed.), *Atlas of limb prosthetics: Surgical, prosthetic and rehabilitation principles* (pp. 623–654). St. Louis: Mosby Year Book.

LaPlante, M. P. (1988). *Data on disability from the National Health Interview Survey, 1983–1985.* Washington, DC: National Institute on Disability and Rehabilitation Research.

Lehneis, H. R., & Dickey, R. (1992). Fitting and training the bilateral upper-limb amputee. In American Academy of Orthopaedic Surgeons (Ed.), *Atlas of limb prosthetics: Surgical, prosthetic and rehabilitation principles* (pp. 311–323). St. Louis: Mosby Year Book.

Maiorano, L. M., & Byron, P. M. (1990). Fabrication of an early-fit prosthesis. In J. M. Hunter, L. H. Schneider, E. J. Mackin, & A. D. Callahan (Eds.), *Rehabilitation of the hand* (pp. 1048–1056). St. Louis: C. V. Mosby.

Malone, J. M., Fleming, L. L., & Robinson, J. (1984). Immediate, early, and late post-surgical management of upper-limb amputations, *Journal of Rehabilitation, 21,* 33–41.

McAuliffe, J. A. (1992). Elbow disarticulation and transhumeral amputation—Prosthetic principles. In American Academy of Orthopaedic Surgeons (Ed.), *Atlas of limb prosthetics: Surgical, prosthetic and rehabilitation principles* (pp. 255–264). St. Louis: Mosby Year Book.

Melzack, R. (1989). Phantom limbs, the self and the brain. *Journal of Canadian Psychology, 30,* 1–16.

Mensch, G., & Ellis, P. (1982). Physical therapeutic management for lower extremity amputees. In S. N. Banerjee (Ed.), *Rehabilitation management of amputees* (pp. 165–236). Baltimore: Williams & Wilkins.

Michael, J. W. (1992). Prosthetic and orthotic management. In American Academy of Orthopaedic Surgeons (Ed.), *Atlas of limb prosthetics: Surgical, prosthetic and rehabilitation principles* (pp. 217–226). St. Louis: Mosby Year Book.

Millstein, S. G., Heger, H., & Hunter, G. A. (1986). Prosthetic use in adult upper limb amputees: A comparison of the body powered and electrically powered prostheses. *Prosthetics and Orthotics International, 10,* 27–34.

Olivett, B. L. (1990). Adult amputee management and conventional prosthetic training. In J. M. Hunter, L. H. Schneider, E. J. Mackin, & A. D. Callahan (Eds.), *Rehabilitation of the hand* (pp. 1057–1071). St. Louis: C. V. Mosby.

Pillet, J., & Mackin, E. J. (1990). Aesthetic hand prosthesis: Its psychologic and functional potential. In J. M. Hunter, L. H. Schneider, E. J. Mackin, & A. D. Callahan (Eds.), *Rehabilitation of the hand* (pp. 1039–1047). St. Louis: C. V. Mosby.

Pillet, J., & Mackin, E. J. (1992). Aesthetic restoration. In American Academy of Orthopaedic Surgeons (Ed.), *Atlas of limb prosthetics: Surgical, prosthetic and rehabilitation principles* (pp. 227–235). St. Louis: Mosby Year Book.

Racy, J. C. (1992). Psychological adaptation to amputation. In American Academy of Orthopaedic Surgeons (Ed.), *Atlas of limb prosthetics: Surgical, prosthetic and rehabilitation principles* (pp. 707–716). St. Louis: Mosby Year Book.

Radocy, B. (1992). Upper-limb prosthetic adaptations for sports and recreation. In American Academy of Orthopaedic Surgeons (Ed.), *Atlas of limb prosthetics: Surgical, prosthetic and rehabilitation principles* (pp. 325–344). St. Louis: Mosby Year Book.

Roeschlein, R. A., & Domholdt, E. (1989). Factors related to successful upper extremity prosthetic use. *Prosthetics and Orthotics International, 13,* 14–18.

Sabolich, J. (1992). *You're not alone.* Oklahoma City: Sabolich Prosthetic Research Center.

Schwell, M. D., & Bunch, W. H. (1992). Management of pain in the amputee. In American Academy of Orthopaedic Surgeons (Ed.), *Atlas of limb prosthetics: Surgical, prosthetic and rehabilitation principles* (pp. 693–695). St. Louis: Mosby Year Book.

Sears, H. H. (1991). Approaches to prescription of body-powered and myoelectric prostheses. *Physical Medicine and Rehabilitation Clinics of North America, 2*, 361–371.

Sears, H. H. (1992). Trends in upper-extremity prosthetics development. In American Academy of Orthopaedic Surgeons (Ed.), *Atlas of limb prosthetics: Surgical, prosthetic and rehabilitation principles* (pp. 345–356). St. Louis: Mosby Year Book.

Spiegel, S. R. (1989). Adult myoelectric upper-limb prosthetic training, In D. J. Atkins & R. H. Meier III (Eds.), *Comprehensive management of the upper-limb amputee* (pp. 60–71). New York: Springer-Verlag.

Weaver, S. A., Lang, L. R., & Vogts, V. M. (1988). Comparison of myoelectric and conventional prostheses for adolescent amputees. *American Journal of Occupational Therapy, 42*, 89–91.

SUPPLEMENTARY RESOURCES

Suggested Readings

American Amputee Foundation. *National Resource Directory.* (Available from P.O. Box 55218, Hillcrest Station, Little Rock, AR 72225; 501-666-2523)

Amputee Golfer Magazine. (Available from P.O. Box 1228, Amherst, NH 03031)

Canelon, M. F. (1993). Training for a patient with shoulder disarticulation. *American Journal of Occupational Therapy, 47*, 174–178.

Celikyol, F. (1984). Prostheses, equipment, adapted performance: Reflections on these choices for the training of the amputee. *Occupational Therapy in Health Care, 1*(4), 89–115.

Friedmann, L. (1980). Toileting self-care methods for bilateral high-level upper limb amputees. *Prosthetics and Orthotics International, 4*, 29–36.

Garza, P. (1986). Case report: Occupational therapy with a traumatic bilateral shoulder disarticulation amputee. *American Journal of Occupational Therapy, 40*(3), 194–198.

Leavy, J. D. (1980). *It can be done— An upper extremity amputee training handbook.* (Available from P. O. Box 515, Lake Almanor Peninsula, CA 96137)

Sullivan, R., & Celikyol, F. (1974). Post hospital follow-up of three bilateral upper limb amputees. *Orthotics and Prosthetics, 28*(3), 33–40.

Weiss-Lambrou, R., deSart, M., Maureau, R., & Duquette, J. (1985). Toilet independence for severe bilateral upper limb amputee. *American Journal of Occupational Therapy, 39*(6), 397–399.

Wilke, H. H. (1984a). *Using everything you've got!* Chicago: National Easter Seal Society.

Wilke, H. H. (1984b). *Reflections on managing disability.* Chicago: National Easter Seal Society.

Williams, W. (1989). Use of the Boston elbow for high level amputees. In D. J. Atkins & R. H. Meier III (Eds.), *Comprehensive management of the upper-limb amputee* (pp. 211–220). New York: Springer-Verlag.

Washam V. (1973). *The one-hander's book: A basic guide to activities of daily living.* New York: John Day/Intext.

Resources

American Orthotic and Prosthetic Association. (1650 King Street, Suite 500, Alexandria, VA 22314)

Amputee Coalition of America. (6300 River Road, Rosemont, IL 60018-4226)

Amputees in Motion. (P.O. Box 2703, Escondido, CA 92025)

Amputee Sports Association. (11705 Mercy Boulevard., Savannah, GA 31406)

Courses for Therapists and Physicians. (1) Northwestern University, Medical School, Prosthetic and Orthotic Center (Chicago). (2) Institute of Biomedical Engineering, University of New Brunswick: myoelectric control courses (Fredericton, N.B., Canada).

National Handicapped Sports (NHS). Chapters and affiliates are located throughout the United States and Canada. (4405 East-West Highway, Suite 603, Bethesda, MD 20814)

U.S. Amputee Athletic Association. (Route 2, Country Line Road, Fairview, TN 37062)

Sources for Upper Limb Prosthetic Components

Alternative Prosthetic Services. Manufactures silicone components, cosmetic hands and arm anatomical covers. (37 Bridge Street, Brooklyn, NY 11201)

Hosmer-Dorrance Corp. Manufactures body powered components for TD, wrist, elbows, and shoulders as well as prosthetic stock gloves. (561 Division Street, Campbell, CA 95008)

Liberty Mutual Research Center. Manufactures the Boston electronic elbow, electronic control systems, hands, BP components, and gloves. (71 Frankland Road, Hopkinton, MA 01748)

Motion Control. Manufactures the Utah elbow, other elbows, and electronic control systems. (1290 West 2320 South, Suite A, Salt Lake City, UT 84119)

Otto Bock Orthopedic Industry. Manufactures electronic hands and hooks, wrists and elbows, electronic control systems, BP components, and gloves. (3000 Xenium Lane N, Minneapolis, MN 55441)

Ross Prosthetics. Manufactures anatomical hand covers (gloves). (65 Wayne Avenue, White Plains, NY 10606)

Therapeutic Recreation Systems (TRS), Inc. Manufactures VC TD grip/prehensors and sports and recreational components. (1280 28th Street, Suite 3, Boulder, CO 80303-1797)

43
Cardiopulmonary Diseases

Ben Atchison

OBJECTIVES

After studying this chapter, the reader will be able to:
1. Describe common cardiopulmonary conditions that occupational therapists will encounter in rehabilitation.
2. Understand the medical assessments that are specific to this diagnostic population.
3. Interpret the outcome of assessment in terms of occupational performance and establish goals in collaboration with the patient.
4. Describe the therapeutic programming that an occupational therapist would plan for this population.

The function of the cardiopulmonary system has been of interest to health care professionals for centuries. As early as 5 BC, Chinese physicians noted the presence of a patient's pulse (Wilson, 1988) and as early as 384 BC Greek physicians understood that the heart was the center of the vascular system. It was not until the late 19th century that the process of coronary occlusion was accepted, even though Heberden described **angina pectoris** in 1801. A major event in the understanding of cardiopulmonary disease was Herrick's (1912) report of his research that the cause of death in cases of "acute indigestion" was not from gastrointestinal disease but from an occlusion of the coronary arteries. Concurrent with research and advanced knowledge of the coronary disease process was Fick's development of an instrument to measure cardiac output in 1870 followed by Williams's invention of cardiac fluoroscopy in 1896. Finally, in 1903, Einthoven developed the first electrocardiograph (Harvey, 1958). From that point, there have been many advances in medical and surgical treatment of cardiopulmonary diseases. A general overview of treatment for these diseases is presented in this chapter. Students who are interested in specializing in this practice area will need advanced education about specific medical and surgical procedures, including an understanding of pharmacological management.

Rehabilitative regimens for cardiopulmonary diseases has been accepted as beneficial only recently. In 1863, Hilton expressed the widely held opinion that bed rest and inactivity were the best treatments for the cardiac patient (Garrison, 1963). The concept of total bed rest was challenged by studies conducted by the National Aeronautics and Space Administration (NASA), who reported the negative effects associated with cardiopulmonary disease following prolonged bed rest (Vogt, Spencer, & Cardus, 1965). In 1952, Levine and Lown advocated "armchair treatment," which was the first step toward modern cardiac rehabilitation. This was a simple procedure: The patient with an infarction was required to sit in a chair for 1 to 2 hr. Levine and Lown (1952) also described a walking program that the patient was to begin 4 weeks after an infarction.

In 1961, Kornbleau and Michaels designed an exercise program for cardiac patients. The first description of electrocardiographic monitoring of exercise was provided by Cain, Frasher, and Stivelman (1961). In 1968, a major advance in cardiac rehabilitation was made via a detailed report of testing and exercise programs (American College of Sports Medicine, 1986). Wenger's (1987) design of a graduated inpatient program, which the patient followed until discharge from the hospital, provided the framework for modern rehabilitation of patients with cardiopulmonary disorders.

Where is cardiac rehabilitation today? What are some of the common conditions that therapists encounter in treatment of cardiopulmonary diseases? These questions, and others, are addressed in this chapter.

COMMON CARDIOVASCULAR AND PULMONARY CONDITIONS

Cardiopulmonary diseases cover a wide range of diagnoses throughout the life span. The occupational therapist, whether practicing in acute care, outpatient

GLOSSARY

Angina pectoris—Pain around the heart that radiates to the left shoulder and possibly to the left arm. Pain may radiate to the back or to the jaw. It is caused by an inadequate supply of oxygen to the heart muscle.

Atrial fibrillation—Rapid, incomplete, or abnormal contractions of the atria resulting in poor pumping of the blood to the pulmonary artery or the ventricles.

Bradycardia—Abnormally slow heartbeat, defined as heart rate under 60 beats per minute. This may be normal for an elite athlete involved in endurance-type sports.

Cardiac palpitations—Rapid or throbbing pulsations of the heart (premature ventricular contractions) that can be consciously felt by a patient.

Chronic obstructive pulmonary disease—Disease process that causes decreased ability of the lungs to perform ventilatory function. Diagnostic criteria include a history of chronic dyspnea and less than one-half normal predicted maximum breathing capacity.

Congestive heart failure—Condition characterized by weakness, shortness of breath, abdominal discomfort, edema in lower extremities, and reduced blood flow from the left ventricle.

Coronary artery bypass grafting—A surgical procedure that installs an alternate route for the blood to the myocardium to bypass an obstructed vessel. Grafting refers to the transplantation of a vessel, often the saphenous vein, to repair the defect.

Coronary artery disease—A disease process that is the result of an arteriosclerotic process, created by a thickening in the intimal, or inner layer, of the vessel.

Dyspnea—Labored or difficult breathing, often accompanied by chest pain. Wheezing sounds occur because of inelasticity of and secretions in the respiratory tract.

Hypertension—A condition in which blood pressure is higher than that judged to be normal.

Metabolic equivalent level—Measurement of energy expenditure of activities: 1 MET is equal to the amount of energy consumed when an individual is at rest, in a semireclined position and with the extremities supported (basal metabolic rate). This is equal to 3.5 mL of oxygen per minute per kilogram of body weight. Activities are rated in terms of multiples of MET units.

Pursed lip breathing—A method of controlled breathing in which the person purses the lips during exhalation, thereby slowing the exhalation process and improving the carbon dioxide exchange as well as preventing airway collapse.

Syncope—A transient loss of consciousness caused by inadequate blood flow to the brain.

Tachycardia—Abnormally rapid heartbeat, usually defined as over 100 beats per minute.

---

care, home care, or long-term care will encounter individuals with these conditions. It is typical for these conditions to present as secondary diagnoses to other common diagnoses, such as cerebrovascular accident or rheumatoid arthritis. The conditions described in this chapter are those that are often seen in these settings and that are likely to present deficits in occupational performance.

In this section, a general review of common cardiac disorders is provided, followed by a review of those disorders specific to the pulmonary system. It is important to keep in mind that while the diagnostic categories are separated here for purposes of discussion, it is common for both systems to be compromised, hence the term *cardiopulmonary*.

Common Diagnoses

ACUTE MYOCARDIAL INFARCTION

Acute myocardial infarction (MI) is a term used to describe the process of myocardial tissue necrosis. Commonly referred to as a heart attack, it is a condition of sustained myocardial ischemia that is caused by arterial occlusion. Complications include arrhythmia, heart failure, thrombolytic complications, and irreversible damage to the heart structure. Destruction of the cardiac tissue is largely caused by coronary artery occlusion. Coronary artery occlusion is caused by **coronary artery disease** (CAD), which is a progressive destruction of the arterial structure and function. This destruction occurs in a series of changes caused by plaque development or lesions along the inside of the arteries. These lesions are classified, in order of pathologic change, into three types: fatty streak, fibrous plaque, and complicated plaque or lesion (Brannon, Geyer, & Folvy, 1988).

Initial complaints include chest pain, **cardiac palpitations, dyspnea,** and shortness of breath during activity. Recurrent nausea, vomiting, and indigestion also are common. The patient may complain of fatigue and anxiety and occasional vertigo. The patient may have a history of a sedentary lifestyle, emotional stress, tobacco use, and a diet high in fat along with a history of **hypertension** and diabetes. A familial history of cardiac disease is highly probable. Associated conditions often include cardiovascular impairment such as **tachycardia** or **bradycardia** with dependent, presacral or pretibial edema. Respiratory signs include shallow, "crackling," and rapid respirations. Signs of fatigue during activity or at rest can be observed by integumentary changes such as diaphoresis, which results in cold, clammy skin (Guyton, 1986) or pallor.

CONGESTIVE HEART FAILURE

Congestive heart failure (CHF) is a complex syndrome that occurs when the myocardium fails to maintain adequate circulation of the blood for respiration and metabolism (Brannon et al., 1988). Precursors for this condition include myocardial infarction, **hypertension, coronary artery disease, tachycardia** or **bradycardia,** and valvular disease. The primary dysfunction is that of decreased myocardial contractility, which can occur in either the right or left ventricle but typically involves both ventricles. Patients who have left ventricular failure will have associated pulmonary congestion. Right ventricular failure causes congestion in visceral and peripheral tissues. This systemic congestion leads to edema, hepatomegaly, and elevated venous pressure (Brannon et al, 1988).

The patient with CHF demonstrates other cardiovascular deficits such as jugular vein distension; peripheral and dependent edema, i.e., swelling of the lower extremities; elevated blood pressure; cardiopulmonary infection; and/or **angina pectoris.** Respiratory findings include pulmonary edema marked by rapid, shallow respirations; dry, hacking cough; and crackling or wheezing during breathing. The renal and urinary system is often compromised as demonstrated by fluid retention and edema. Dark, amber urine is a common sign. In general, the patient complains of restlessness, lethargy, fatigue, and insomnia; all of which compromise the expenditure of physical energy (Dolan, 1990).

HYPERTENSION

Hypertension (HTN), which refers to an elevation in blood pressure, is defined in the adult as pressure that is consistently greater than 140/90 mm Hg. Blood pressure is a measure of the contraction phase of the heart's output (systolic pressure) and the relaxation phase at which time the chambers are filling with blood (diastolic pressure). The elevation of pressure refers specifically to elevation of pressure in the arteries. Blood pressure is lower at rest and higher with changes in posture, physical activity, and emotional stress.

The most common type of **hypertension** (90% of cases) is referred to as primary or essential **hypertension** (Falvo, 1991). The onset is insidious and is usually determined during a regular physical examination. The pathogenesis is not certain, but several factors are believed to be involved. These include controllable factors such as increased sodium, fat, and calorie consumption; alcohol and tobacco use; emotional stress; and high caffeine intake. Noncontrollable factors, such as family history, race (black), and gender (male) also are associated with primary **hypertension.** Secondary **hypertension,** also referred to as malignant

hypertension, accounts for the remaining 10% of cases and has an abrupt onset, more severe symptoms, and has other associated complications (Falvo, 1991).

The symptoms of essential **hypertension** are often not immediately apparent; hence it is sometimes referred to as "the silent killer." Patients may experience progressively noticeable symptoms that are initially ignored such as light-headedness, dizziness, numbness and tingling in the arms and legs, and occasional nausea. The patient may be experiencing nocturia, urinary frequency, occipital headaches, and fatigue. In more severe cases, intermittent chest pain is noted (Kochar & Woods, 1985).

ANGINA PECTORIS

Angina pectoris refers to the chest pain that occurs when the coronary artery blood supply fails to supply the myocardium with oxygen. The most common cause of angina is arteriosclerosis, although unusual physical activity, stress, eating a heavy meal, tobacco use, and straining while urinating or defecating may also precipitate symptoms (Campbell, 1984).

It is important to note the different types of angina. Stable angina is most typical. It is usually the result of a specific physical or emotional stressor and is effectively treated with nitroglycerin. The duration of chest pain is 3 to 5 min. Unstable angina is unrelated to stress; lasts longer than 20 min; and progressively increases in frequency, intensity, and duration. It is often referred to as preinfarction angina, indicating impending myocardial infarction. Intractable angina is the most severe type, is not amenable to treatment, and incapacitates the patient (Ulrich, 1986).

Patients with angina usually describe the chest pain as crushing, sharp, vise-like, or burning. **Dyspnea** is an associated respiratory symptom along with integumentary changes, leading to diaphoresis and cool, clammy skin (Ulrich, 1986).

CORONARY ARTERY BYPASS GRAFTING

Coronary artery bypass grafting (CABG) is a surgical procedure used to relieve angina caused by arterial circulation blockages, which lead to myocardial ischemia. This procedure involves the grafting of a vein (usually the saphenous vein) to reroute circulation to the myocardium. This increases the myocardial blood supply, which allows the patient to again engage in activity. Although the surgery increases blood flow to the heart muscle, the disease process that caused the blockages is still present. Often, more than one artery is restricted and several grafts may be needed, which are referred to as CABG×2, CABG×3, etc. (Underhill, 1986).

Surgical procedures are usually done after conventional therapies—the use of nitrates such as nitroglycerin and calcium channel blockers—have failed. Angioplasty, also referred to as percutaneous transluminal coronary angioplasty (PTCA), is done to enlarge a narrowed artery and is often used if the success of drug therapy is limited (Jader & Lekander, 1987). For this procedure, a small balloon-tipped catheter is inserted into a vessel and inflated at the site of the occlusion, causing a compression of plaque against the vessel wall, thus freeing the obstruction.

Associated findings may include pulmonary edema, tachypnea, **tachycardia,** and crackling during respiration. Complaints of acute fatigue during activity, **syncope,** vertigo, and nausea are common. Postprandial discomfort (discomfort following a meal) and epigastric discomfort and burning sensations are possible complaints (Dolan, 1990).

CHRONIC OBSTRUCTIVE PULMONARY DISEASE

Chronic obstructive pulmonary disease (COPD) is a progressive, irreversible destruction of the airways that causes **dyspnea** and leads to chronic inflammation and destruction of lung alveoli. Several conditions may be referred to as COPD such as recurring, acute emphysema; asthma; and bronchitis. Airflow obstruction is caused by excessive mucus secretion and/or constriction of the airways, which leads to loss of lung elasticity (Andrews, 1987).

Patients with COPD present with shortness of breath, varying from an unusual increase of respiration after physical exertion to one-word **dyspnea,** in which the patient must catch his breath after each word when he speaks. **Dyspnea** can usually be classified according to how conscious one is of the person's breathing. For example, 0 **dyspnea** would refer to a normal, subconscious awareness of breathing, whereas 4 + refers to one-word **dyspnea.** Other common symptoms include decreased appetite, headaches, insomnia, fatigue, and nausea (Ayres, 1984).

Associated cardiovascular conditions include **atrial fibrillation,** jugular vein distension, and **tachycardia.** Neurologic signs may include tremors, which are an adverse effect of medication; integumentary changes, leading to mottled or discolored skin; and cyanosis (Berkow & Fletcher, 1987).

Common Diagnostic Procedures

Although the occupational therapist does not conduct the diagnostic procedures described here, it is critical that the therapist understands the purpose of each procedure to gain a complete sense of the patient's medical condition as it affects daily treatment.

SERUM ENZYME LEVELS

Analysis of serum enzyme levels is a laboratory procedure that offers conclusive evidence about both the onset of myocardial infarction and other heart diseases and the recovery status. Creatine phosphokinase (CPK) and lactic dehydrogenase (LDH) are two enzymes that are significant for their sensitivity to myocardial ischemia. Elevated levels of these enzymes may indicate a new infarction or complications of a previous infarction (Wolf, 1984).

CHEST ROENTGENOGRAPHY (X-RAY)

The chest x-ray is a noninvasive radiographic procedure that is done to evaluate evidence of lung congestion, hypertrophy of the chambers of the heart, and other structural abnormalities in the chest cavity (Berkow & Fletcher, 1987).

ELECTROCARDIOGRAPHY

Electrocardiography (ECG) records on a graph the electrical conductivity that occurs within the myocardium. An ECG identifies cardiac arrhythmias that allows assessment of the amount and location of myocardial damage and determination of the adequacy of the oxygen supply to the myocardium. In this noninvasive procedure, electrodes (leads) are placed externally on the skin to detect the electrical impulses from the heart, which are transferred to the electrocardiograph (Berkow & Fletcher, 1987).

The advanced occupational therapist who works specifically in an inpatient cardiac rehabilitation program should be trained to read and interpret the 12 dysrhythmias associated with exercise and those that are contraindication to exercise (American Heart Association, 1980).

HOLTER MONITOR

The Holter monitor is a portable FM tape recorder that records ECG signals while the patient completes regular activities during a 24-hr period. Three electrodes are attached externally to the chest, and the recorder is worn on the shoulder or waist. The patient keeps an activity diary for the 24-hr period. At the end of the test, the tape is processed. Sections with dysrhythmias are converted to a paper record, labeled with the activity specified in the diary, and presented for the physician's review. The ability to read ECG changes over a continuous 24-hr period is obviously helpful in determining the heart's functioning in a variety of activities (Corbett, 1982).

CARDIAC STRESS TEST

The cardiac stress test records cardiac activity during graded physical exertion to determine the functional extent of cardiac disease and to advise the patient about the type and amount of physical activity that he is safely able to engage in. The procedure begins with the patient walking on a motor-driven treadmill or pedaling slowly on a stationary bicycle. The intensity (speed and/or resistance or slope) is progressively increased. During the activity, the ECG, blood pressure, and heart rate are monitored to determine the patient's response to exercise (Corbett, 1982).

Occupational therapists in advanced specialty practice may perform this procedure after they have completed extensive training, such as that provided by the American College of Sports Medicine (ACSM). However, regardless of whether the therapist is trained in graded exercise testing, it is important that the therapist who is involved in the treatment of patients with cardiopulmonary diseases have a thorough understanding of what this test measures and the information it provides in regard to the patient's functional abilities.

ECHOCARDIOGRAPHY

The echocardiogram is an ultrasonic diagnostic tool used to record the size, motion, and structure of the heart and its vessels. Ultrasound allows sound waves to be converted to electrical signals, which are then recorded as visual images. These images are displayed on a television screen or oscilloscope. Echocardiograms provide information about valvular defects or other structural abnormalities of the heart such as cardiomegaly (Corbett, 1982).

CARDIAC CATHETERIZATION

Cardiac catheterization is a procedure by which the physician can visualize the coronary circulation. In this procedure, a catheter is passed through a vein in one of the extremities and slipped into the heart. The physician is able to watch the catheter's movements into the heart by way of a fluoroscope. Once in place, the internal pressure of the heart is measured and then dye is forced into the catheter to allow visualization of the heart's action.

Cardiac catheterization is helpful in determining the degree of **coronary artery disease,** congenital heart disease, valvular disease, and myocardial damage. It is also helpful in determining the need for surgery as well as to assess the effectiveness of CABG in postsurgical patients (Dolan, 1990).

PULMONARY FUNCTION TESTS

Pulmonary function tests are used to determine the cause of **dyspnea,** the magnitude of lung disease, and the effectiveness of treatment. The tests measure the amount of air that a patient can inspire and expire as well as his efficiency in moving air into and out of the lungs. The patient is asked to breathe into a device, called a spirometer, that measures breathing function and records it on a spirogram. Two common types of pulmonary function tests include vital capacity (VC) and forced expiratory volume (FEV). Vital capacity measures the maximum volume of air that can be inhaled and exhaled. FEV tests indicate the total amount of air that the individual can forcibly exhale in 1, 2, or 3 sec (Carroll, 1986); the measures are expressed as FEV_1, FEV_2, and FEV_3. These measures provide discrete data about the patient's endurance potential for functional activities, which is useful to the occupational therapist.

ENDURANCE AND ACTIVITY TESTING IN OCCUPATIONAL THERAPY

Individual's who have survived cardiac arrest or complications from cardiac surgery will commonly experience a decline in activity tolerance and endurance. The patient fatigues more quickly, is apprehensive about engaging in activity, and often has a poor appetite, leading to a general decline in physical activity. It is important that the occupational therapist learn how to measure heart rate, blood pressure, and respiratory rate, because all three are reliable indicators of activity tolerance (see Chapter 6).

The heart rate, or pulse, is the alternate expansion and recoiling of an artery, which can be palpated at several sites. The most common sites of palpation are at the radial and carotid arteries. Two factors are responsible for the existence of a pulse. First is the intermittent injections of blood from the heart into the arteries. Second is the elasticity of the artery wall, which makes it possible for the artery to expand with each injection of blood and then recoil. It is important to remember that the pulse is a wave that starts with the contraction of the ventricles. The farther away from the heart the therapist palpates, the longer the interval is. For example, the radial artery pulse does not coincide exactly with ventricular contraction, but the carotid pulse is closer.

In determining the patient's maximal safe response of the heart to varied activity, a rate that is usually used at discharge from cardiac rehabilitation is 75% of maximum heart rate (Nixon et al., 1976). Maximum heart rate is computed by subtracting the patient's age, in years, from 220. A "handicap" of 40 is further subtracted if the subject's true maximum heart rate has not ever been determined by a symptom-limited graded exercise test. It is 75% of that figure that is used as a guideline for the safe maximum heart rate that the patient should have as a result of engaging in exercise or activity. It is important to assess resting heart rate and then the postactivity rate to determine the amount of increase and the amount of time it takes for the patient to recover to the resting level. A prolonged rate of 120 beats per minute (bpm) and above is indicative of cardiac overload (Dolan, 1990).

Blood pressure is measured before, during, and after activity to determine if the heart is responding as it should to activity demands.

A sphygmomanometer is used to measure blood pressure. This instrument includes a cuff that is wrapped around the upper arm of the patient over the brachial artery. Air is pumped into the cuff by means of an attached tube and pump. This pumping exerts pressure against the outside of the artery. Simultaneously, a stethoscope is placed over the brachial artery. Air is added to the cuff until the air pressure exceeds the blood pressure within the artery. By slowly releasing the air in the cuff, the air pressure is decreased until the pulse is heard. At this point, the air pressure in the cuff is approximately equal to the blood pressure within the artery; the value is read off an attached meter. This first sound is the systolic pressure. The systolic pressure indicates the amount of force with which the blood is pushing against the artery walls when the ventricles are contracting. As the cuff pressure continues to drop, a series of increasingly louder sounds can be heard until the sounds become muffled and finally disappear. The lowest point at which the sounds can be heard is equal to the diastolic pressure. The diastolic pressure indicates the force of blood when the ventricles are relaxed and the atria are filling. The diastolic pressure is often the more critical variable, because this number indicates the amount of pressure or strain that the blood vessel walls are constantly subjected to.

Blood pressure is reported as a ratio, e.g., 120/80. The upper number indicates the systolic pressure and the lower number, the diastolic pressure (Andreoli et al., 1983).

Complaint of fatigue is a common problem that reflects increased myocardial oxygen demand (Dolan, 1990). The occupational therapist needs to monitor the patient for signs of fatigue such as cold, clammy skin; dizziness; and shortness of breath.

Metabolic equivalent (MET) **level** assessment is a commonly used measure to indicate endurance and activity tolerance. Used by occupational therapists and others involved in cardiopulmonary rehabilitation, it consists of a table of specific activities and codeterminants of energy expenditures. Energy is measured by the amount of oxygen consumed to maintain metabolic processes (respiration, circulation, peristalsis, temperature, glandular function, etc.) and to carry out activities. It is expressed as a MET level (Thomas, 1973). The amount of energy used when a patient is at rest in a semireclined position is 1 MET, which is equal to 3.5 mL of oxygen per minute per kilogram of body weight. Table 43.1 provides the MET levels for various activities.

COGNITIVE ASSESSMENT

There are reports of cognitive sequelae following survival of cardiopulmonary arrest. Cognitive outcomes studied by Suave (1992) included orientation, attention and concentration, memory, and reasoning. In this study of sudden cardiac death survivors, 62.5% had at least one cognitive deficit, and 73% of these had problems in three or more areas on initial evaluation that tended to persist over time. The occupational therapy evaluation should include an assessment of cognitive function to gain an overall indication of the patient's ability to retain information that is taught in the process of rehabilitation and apply it to everyday activities (see Chapter 9). The patient's ability to understand, e.g., the concept of risks that are associated with the disease, will be a critical factor in the success of rehabilitation.

PSYCHOSOCIAL ASSESSMENT

The literature is replete with reports and discussions of the effects of cardiopulmonary disease on psychological and social well-being. As early as 1951, White recognized the critical complications of mental health following a myocardial infarction. Factors such as depression, low morale, and psychological distress are significant predictors of mortality among post-MI patients (Gentry, Foster, & Haney, 1972). It is important to recognize that those who demonstrate poor adaptation to the initial onset of the disease may have overall adjustment problems during the course of the disease (see Chapters 10 and 20).

Anxiety and stress in patients with cardiopulmonary disease need to be monitored and reduced as much as possible. Anxiety leads to decreased levels of rest, which decreases energy expenditure, thus reducing stamina and increasing symptoms. Uncontrolled anxiety or stress leads to physiologic changes, such as increased catecholamine production, which increases the heart rate and causes vasoconstriction. This consequently creates additional burden on cardiac function. Chemicals released when stress occurs causes the release of fats and sugars into the blood via the liver. This creates increased platelet stickiness and subsequently can speed up the progression of arterial destruction (Campbell, 1984).

It should be recognized that the degree and ways in which stress creates the onset of cardiopulmonary disease is not fully known. It is likely that inappropriate coping methods such as alcohol and tobacco used to reduce stress have led to the actual pathological changes (Gray, Rheinhardt, & Ward, 1969). Learning

Table 43.1. Approximate Metabolic Cost of Activities[a]

Energy Level	Occupational	Recreational
1.5–2 MET[b] 4–7 mL O_2/min/kg 2–2.5 kcal/min[d]	Desk work Auto driving[c] Typing Electric calculating machine operation	Standing Walking (strolling 1.6 km or 1 mile/hr) Flying,[c] motorcycling[c] Playing cards[c] Sewing, knitting
2–3 MET 7–11 mL O_2/min/kg 2.5–4 kcal/min[d]	Auto repair Radio, TV repair Janitorial work Typing, manual Bartending	Level walking (3.25 km or 2 miles/hr) Level bicycling (8 km or 5 miles/hr) Riding lawn mower Billiards, bowling Skeet,[c] shuffleboard Woodworking (light) Powerboat driving[c] Golf (power cart) Canoeing (4 km or 2.5 miles/hr) Horseback riding (walk) Playing piano and many musical instruments
3–4 MET 11–14 mL O_2/min/kg 4–5 kcal/min[d]	Brick laying, plastering Wheelbarrow (220-lb or 100-kg load) Machine assembly Trailer-truck in traffic Welding (moderate load) Cleaning windows	Walking (5 km or 3 miles/hr) Cycling (10 km or 6 miles/hr) Horseshoe pitching Volleyball (6-person noncompetitive) Golf (pulling bag cart) Archery Sailing (handling small boat) Fly fishing (standing in waders) Horseback (sitting to trot) Badminton (social doubles) Pushing light power mower Energetic musician
4–5 MET 14–18 mL O_2/min/kg 5–6 kcal/min[d]	Painting, masonry Paperhanging Light carpentry	Walking (5.5 km or 3.5 miles/hr) Cycling (13 km or 8 miles/hr) Table tennis Golf (carrying clubs) Dancing (foxtrot) Badminton (singles) Tennis (doubles) Raking leaves Hoeing Many calisthenics
5–6 MET 18–21 mL O_2/min/kg 6–7 kcal/min[d]	Digging garden Shoveling light earth	Walking (6.5 km or 4 miles/hr) Cycling (16 km or 10 miles/hr) Canoeing (6.5 km or 4 miles/hr) Horseback (posting to trot) Stream fishing (walking in light current in waders) Ice or roller skating (15 km or 9 miles/hr)
6–7 MET 21–25 mL O_2/min/kg 7–8 kcal/min[d]	Shoveling 10 min (22 lb or 10 kg)	Walking (8 km or 5 miles/hr) Cycling (17.5 km or 11 miles/hr) Badminton (competitive) Tennis (singles) Splitting wood Snow shoveling Manual lawn mowing Folk (square) dancing Light downhill skiing Ski touring (4 km or 2.5 miles/hr), loose snow Water skiing
7–8 MET 25–28 mL O_2/min/kg 8–10 kcal/min[d]	Digging ditches Carrying 175 lb or 80 kg Sawing hardwood	Jogging (8 km or 5 miles/hr) Cycling (19 km or 12 miles/hr) Horseback (gallop) Vigorous downhill skiing

Table 43.1. Continued.

Energy Level	Occupational	Recreational
(7–8 MET, continued)		Basketball Mountain climbing Ice hockey Canoeing (8 km or 5 miles/hr) Touch football Paddleball
8–9 MET 28–32 mL O$_2$/min/kg 10–11 kcal/min[d]	Shoveling 10 min (31 lb or 14 kg)	Running (9 km or 5.5 miles/hr) Cycling (21 km or 13 miles/hr) Ski touring (6.5 km or 4 miles/hr), loose snow Squash (social) Handball (social) Fencing Basketball (vigorous)

10+ MET
32+ mL O$_2$/min/kg
11+ kcal/min[d]
	Shoveling 10 min (35 lb or 16 kg)	Running
		  6 mph = 10 MET
		  7 mph = 11.5 MET
		  8 mph = 13.5 MET
		  9 mph = 15 MET
		  10 mph = 17 MET
		Ski touring (8+ km or 5+ miles/hr), loose snow
		Handball (competitive)
		Squash (competitive)

[a]Includes resting metabolic needs.
[b]1 MET is the energy expenditure at rest, equivalent to approximately 3.5 mL O$_2$/kg body weight/min.
[c]A major increase in metabolic requirements may occur because of excitement, anxiety, or impatience, which are common responses during some activities. The patient's emotional reactivity must be assessed when prescribing or sanctioning certain activities.
[d]Based on a 70-kg person.

how to cope appropriately with inevitable stress is discussed later in this chapter (see also Chapter 20).

The reaction of family members and others in the patient's environment can have a major influence on the patient's recovery. It is common for family members to demonstrate anxiety and an overprotective attitude toward the patient while hoping, at the same time, to provide support and consolation. It is important for the occupational therapist to recognize these as natural reactions and work toward creating opportunities for family and patients to discuss their fears and anxieties about the patient's condition, role changes, and behavioral changes (see Chapters 10 and 20).

After the diagnosis of a cardiac condition, a special concern may be the resumption of sexual activity. In most instances, sexual activity can be resumed, pending physician recommendations. As a guideline, physicians recommend return to sexual activity if a person can walk up and down two flights of stairs without symptoms (Stern, Pascale, & Ackerman, 1977). The patient and spouse should recognize that methods of sexual expression other than intercourse can be used until the patient's dysfunction is resolved. However, persistent sexual dysfunction can occur, which may be related to certain medications such as diuretics, antihypertensives, and sedatives or as a result of persistent anxiety or fear. In any case, the patient and his spouse should receive expert consultation by the physician and a professional trained in sexuality counseling.

OCCUPATIONAL THERAPY INTERVENTION FOR CARDIOPULMONARY DISEASE

Occupational therapy involvement in the treatment of cardiopulmonary disease has historically been hospital based, i.e., acute care. However, because of earlier discharge from hospital care related to the payment system, many more cardiopulmonary patients are followed in home care programs and in outpatient cardiac rehabilitation programs. Participants in cardiac rehabilitation programs include patients who have **coronary artery disease,** patients who have had a myocardial infarction, patients with **coronary artery disease** but who have not had an MI, and patients who have undergone cardiac surgery (before or after an MI) (Wilson, 1988). Cardiac rehabilitation programs consist of four progressive phases.

Phase I: Inpatient Care

The inpatient phase, lasts approximately 5 to 14 days and begins early while the patient is still in the coronary care unit. During this phase, functional assessment of the patient includes tolerance of basic self-care tasks. If the patient is pain free, exhibits no arrhythmia, and has a resting pulse of 100 or less, an activity program is initiated (Mead, 1977). This program begins with light diversional activity and exercise to increase cardiac capacity and reduce anxiety. Activities requiring a maximum of 1.5 METs are allowed (see Table 43.2). The patient is placed in a fully supported sitting position with the proximal extremities supported so that activities or exercise is restricted to the distal parts of the extremities and use phasic movements on a gravity-eliminated plane (Kottke, 1971).

The evening resting pulse rate is a guideline to rehabilitation progress. If it exceeds the morning resting rate by more than 20%, then the program may be progressing too rapidly (Mead, 1977). Over time, the frequency of the activity can be increased as the patient's pulse decreases because of a training effect (see Chapters 6 and 22). At the end of phase I, the patient will have progressed to a 4.0-MET functional capacity.

The overall goals of this phase are to educate the patient about heart disease and recovery, to build patient confidence with activities (Killen, 1986), to provide emotional support to the patient and his family, and to teach the patient the value of continuing the program as an outpatient and developing the psychological readiness to do so.

Phase II: Outpatient/Home Health Care

Phase II may take place in a formal outpatient program or in the home. It may begin as early as 3 to 4 weeks post-MI for patients with stable angina (Erb, Fletcher, & Sheffield, 1979; Mead, 1977) or as late as 8 weeks for others (Cohen, 1975). The goals for this phase include continued physical conditioning through supervised exercise, behavioral counseling and lifestyle modification relative to risk factors, vocational counseling and evaluation, and continued psychological support (Erb et al., 1979; Killen, 1986). Those patients who begin the outpatient program closer to the time of onset continue the supervised step-by-step progression gauged by pulse rate (not to exceed 100/min) and fatigue (disappears 10 to 20 min after activity) (Mead, 1977).

Because the availability of formal cardiac rehabilitation programs is geographically uneven, many patients with recent cardiac events are discharged home immediately after the acute phase, without opportunity for involvement in traditional follow-up cardiac rehabilitation programs. A solid team approach must be instituted. The knowledge the home care nurse has about the specific signs and symptoms, precautions, and medication regimens cannot be underestimated.

It is important for the therapist to feel comfortable to ask questions in order to learn, but it is equally important for her to have the prerequisite knowledge to know what should be asked. For example, if the nurse is concerned with fluid output, why does that concern exist? What does fluid retention have to do with occupational performance? Many questions like these need to be posed and much data must be gathered to know a patient's performance potential.

The home is the most natural environment for the patient, and the occupational therapist has the opportunity to see the Gestalt, or the big picture, of the patient's life. It is similar to looking through a wide angle lens at the patient's environment, home, and family and at the interactions taking place among them as well as at the objects that indicate something about that patient. These are often overlooked in an institutional setting, in which the specific pathology is emphasized. Once the overall picture is clear, the zooming in to the specific factors that impede occupational functioning is easier.

Phase III: Supervised Community Program

After 4 to 6 months, the patient may safely participate in a community program that emphasizes that exercise is only one part of a healthy lifestyle and that a commitment to a change in lifestyle is necessary to maintain cardiac health. The program during phase III consists of not only progressive, monitored exercise but also individualized education, including nutritional counseling, smoking termination, relaxation skills, stress reduction, and determination of vocational readiness.

Supervised physical activity and exercise programs are beneficial to recovery of cardiopulmonary patients for these reasons: They demonstrate to the patient that certain levels of physical activity can be done safely, depression is decreased, the heart and other muscles are conditioned to handle stress and strain (Levy, 1980), and weight is reduced. A graded exercise program is also financially beneficial both to the individual and to society. One study of 123 post-MI patients concluded that a cardiac rehabilitation program of early mobilization and graded exercise and activities significantly reduced the length of hospitalization and improved the level of functional capacity at discharge of the experimental group compared with the controls (Grant & Cohen, 1973).

Phase IV: Maintenance

Phase IV is considered an indefinite phase in that the patient continues to maintain exercise and activity programs that are necessary to his lifestyle and occupation. It is hoped that the patient will develop habits

Table 43.2. Suggested Interdisciplinary Stages for Patients with Cardiopulmonary History and/or Precautions .

Stage/MET Level	ADL and Mobility	Exercise	Recreation
Stage I (1.0–1.4 MET)	*Sitting:* Self-feeding, wash hands and face, bed mobility[c] Transfers Progressively increase sitting tolerance	*Supine:* (A)[a] or (AA)[b] exercise to all extremities (10–15 times per extremity) *Sitting:* (A) or (AA) exercise to *only* neck and lower extremities Include deep breathing exercise	Reading, radio, table games (noncompetitive), light handwork
Stage II (1.4–2.0 MET)	*Sitting:* Self-bathing, shaving, grooming, and dressing in hospital Unlimited sitting *Ambulation:* At slow pace, in room as tolerated	*Sitting:* (A) exercise to all extremities, progressively increasing the number of repetitions[c] NO ISOMETRICS	*Sitting:* Crafts, e.g., painting, knitting, sewing, mosaics, embroidery NO ISOMETRICS
Stage III (2.0–3.0 MET)	*Sitting:* Showering in warm water, homemaking tasks with brief standing periods to transfer light items, ironing	*Sitting:* Wheelchair mobility, limited distances *Standing:* (A) exercise to all extremities and trunk, progressively increasing the number of repetitions[c] *May include* (1) balance exercises and (2) light mat activities without resistance *Ambulation:* Begin progressive ambulation program at 0% grade and comfortable pace	*Sitting:* Card playing, crafts, piano, machine sewing, typing[c]
Stage IV (3.0–3.5 MET)	*Standing:* Total washing, dressing, shaving, grooming, showering in warm water; kitchen/homemaking activities while practicing energy conservation (e.g., light vacuuming, dusting and sweeping, washing light clothes) *Ambulation:* unlimited distance walking at 0% grade, in and/or outside[c]	*Standing:* Continue all previous exercise, progressively increasing 1. Number of repetitions 2. Speed of repetitions *May include* additional exercises to increase workload up to 3.5 MET, balance and mat activities with mild resistance *Ambulation:* Unlimited on level surfaces in and/or outside[c] progressively increasing speed and/or duration for periods up to 15–20 min or until target heart rate is reached[c] *Stairs:* May begin slow stair climbing to patient's tolerance up to two flights *Treadmill:* 1 mph at 1% grade, progressing to 1.5 mph at 2% grade[c] *Cycling:* Up to 5.0 mph without resistance	Candlepin bowling Canoeing—slow rhythm, pace Golf putting *Light* gardening (weeding and planting) Driving[c]
Stage V (3.5–4.0 MET)	*Standing:* Washing dishes, washing clothes, ironing, hanging light clothes, and making beds	*Standing:* Continue exercises as in stage IV, progressively increasing (1) number of repetitions and (2) speed of repetitions *May add* additional exercises to increase workload up to 4.0 MET *Ambulation:* As in stage IV, increasing speed up to 2.5 mph on level surfaces[c]	Swimming (slowly) Light carpentry Golfing (using power cart) Light home repairs

Table 43.2. Continued.

Stage/MET level	ADL and Mobility	Exercise	Recreation
(Stage V, continued)		*Stairs:* As in stage IV and progressively increasing, if increasing to patient's tolerance *Treadmill:* 1.5 mph at 2% grade, progressing to 1.5 mph at 4% grade up to 2.5 mph at 0% grade[c] *Cycling:* Up to 8 mph without resistance[c] May use up to 7–10 lb[c] of weight for upper and lower extremity exercise in sitting	
Stage VI (4.0–5.0 MET)	*Standing:* Showering in hot water, hanging and/or wringing clothes, mopping, stripping and making beds, raking	*Standing:* As in stage V *Ambulation:* As in stage V, increasing speed to 3.5 mph on level surfaces[c] *Stairs:* As in stage V *Treadmill:* 1.5 mph at 4–6% grade, progressing to 3.5 mph at 0% grade[c] *Cycling:* Up to 10 mph without resistance May use up to 10–15 lb of weight in upper and lower extremity exercises in sitting	Swimming (no advanced strokes) Slow dancing Ice or roller skating (slowly) Volleyball Badminton Table tennis (noncompetitive) Light calisthenics

[a] A, active.
[b] AA, active assistive.
[c] Please refer to physician's guidelines.

that are conducive to continued cardiac health maintenance and that he will independently maintain them. Support groups, such as the Broken Hearts, provide an avenue for sharing information and supporting members in maintaining a healthy cardiac lifestyle.

Continued Development of Cardiac Rehabilitation Programs

In 1975, the ACSM initiated a certification program for the various professionals involved in cardiac rehabilitation programs. Their *Guidelines for Graded Exercise Testing and Prescription* (ACSM, 1986) has become a much used protocol for program personnel. In 1985, a preventive and rehabilitative manual was developed to meet the increased need for qualified staff to use in the later phases of cardiac rehabilitation (ACSM, 1986).

The American Heart Association (AHA) supports the development of cardiac rehabilitation programs and services through workshops, seminars, and published material (Wilson, 1988). Their most widely used publication is *The Exercise Standards Book* (AHA, 1979), which includes standards for exercise testing, cardio-

vascular exercise programs, and supervised maintenance programs.

Parmely (1986) defined the American College of Cardiology's recommended services and strategies for cardiac rehabilitation programs. The report includes information about national associations. One such group is the American Association of Cardiovascular and Pulmonary Rehabilitation (AACVPR), which has a wide membership of specialists in clinical cardiac and pulmonary rehabilitation. The *Journal of Cardiopulmonary Rehabilitation* is the official journal of the AACVPR.

SABRES: An Alternative Approach to Cardiac Rehabilitation

One striking feature of most cardiac rehabilitation programs is that they focus on physical reconditioning. Most program protocols focus on exercise programming, with less consideration given to the individual's ability to control the factors that led to the disease in the first place. The importance of psychological assessment is now widely recognized and, in some cases, mandatory for cardiac rehabilitation (Blumenthal & Emery, 1988).

King and Nixon (1988) described a unique approach to cardiac rehabilitation. Their focus was on the individual's lack of adaptation to the physical, psychological, and social stimuli in the external environment that likely led to the disease. Education focused on the importance of homeostatic well-being and emphasized the awareness of the importance of sleep, relaxation methods, proper breathing, and a balance of rest and effort. They suggest the acronym SABRES as an easy method of remembering these factors, which are discussed below.

S STANDS FOR SLEEP

The patient needs to realize that the quality and quantity of sleep are important to the ability to handle effort and emotion during daytime activities. Adequate sleep eases daytime activities and allows the general arousal level to be set at a lower level and in turn assists in performance of daily activities (King & Nixon, 1988). Physiologically, sleep decreases the secretion of cortisol and catecholamine and enables left ventricular healing (Oswald, 1987).

A INDICATES AROUSAL

Each patient learns to become aware of arousal levels and to regulate them (King & Nixon, 1988). This is achieved through a variety of modalities, including body massage, hypnosis, dance therapy, and biofeedback techniques. Some of these interventions have been considered unconventional by Western medical standards, but they are gaining acceptance through research conducted in the field of immunology (Cousins, 1979). Communication skills are also important for arousal management. The ability of a patient to articulate feelings of anxiety, anger, and despair prevent the retention of those feelings, which often contributes to cardiopulmonary stress.

B STANDS FOR BREATHING

Correct breathing is an important aspect of arousal management. By learning to control breathing patterns, a patient can control the autonomic influences that cause coronary artery constriction and thus is able to reduce the heart rate and blood pressure responses to effort. Patients will often hold their breath when performing isometric activity, such as lifting objects. One way to avoid this is to teach **pursed lip breathing** in which the patient purses his lips and makes a hissing sound on exhalation. The patient can also be taught to talk or sing during exertion.

R AND E STAND FOR REST AND EFFORT

Each individual needs to achieve a balance between rest and effort. Nixon and King (1988) provided specific ideas to achieve this balance:

1. Be honest about functional capabilities, to recover healthy respect for fatigue, to know when to go forward, and to acquire the discipline to change course or back off effort when overloaded. [The patient] should learn to keep a reserve of energy in hand for dealing with contingencies and emergencies.
2. Examine exhausting and time-wasting habits and learn to conserve energy. Daily activities should be paced and spaced in such a way as to avoid unnecessary time pressure displacement activity, and the compulsive drive to do several things at once.
3. Avoid angina and become familiar with the effects of different levels and varieties of effort by self-checking the various effects of emotional tension and isometric and isotonic effort, for example:
   a. By using a sphygmomanometer to learn how blood pressure responds to different sorts of effort, both in untired conditions and in various levels of fatigue.
   b. To count heart rate in order to learn about tolerance of effort and to ensure that it is kept within healthy levels.
4. Increase general mobility and body awareness through graded walking programs, promoting stamina rather than speed. Exercise should not be taken after a large meal.
5. When appropriate, fitness training may be taken up as a pleasurable activity to enable patients to return to sport and recreation. Warming up is essential. A healthy training level is usually at 60–70% of the maximum heart rate. Sports that put sudden severe demands upon the left ventricle should be discouraged as well as those that depend upon isometric effort and exposure to cold. "Train, don't strain" is the watchword (p. 382).

OCCUPATIONAL THERAPY INTERVENTION FOR CHRONIC OBSTRUCTIVE PULMONARY DISEASE

The occupational therapist works with individuals with chronic lung disease in various settings, as is the case with cardiac rehabilitation. Intervention may be directly provided in the clinic or in the home. The occupational therapist may also be a part of the pulmonary rehabilitation team that provides a series of classes designed to assist the individual with COPD and family members to better adapt to the debilitating effects of the condition.

In the initial assessment, the occupational therapist determines the functional capacity of the patient to perform occupational activities including work, leisure, and self-care tasks. A particular concern is how the patient approaches activity and how well a balance is achieved in performing activity. It is important to know activity tolerance and methods employed to handle stress of various activities. Persons with COPD often experience energy deficiency early in their day, because they lack the ability to organize and properly pace themselves through activities. The lack of energy available to perform activity leads to general disuse atrophy. It is not uncommon for the patient with COPD to have experienced weight loss as well as a result of general malaise, which leads to a poor appetite. This, in addition to depression and anxiety, is often a major reason for the lack of endurance and strength.

Evaluation of motor performance includes functional mobility, strength, and endurance. The use of an arm ergometer provides the occupational therapist and the patient with an objective measure of upper extremity endurance. This device is used for exercise programming as well. A positive correlation between improved upper extremity endurance and increased abilities in activities of daily living (ADL) has been reported in the literature (Walsh, 1986).

Evaluation of the patient's level of motivation, affect, and personal goals for coping with the disease is critical. Commonly, patients with COPD are caught in a vicious circle of decreased energy: Anxiety about the loss of function and fear of the disease worsening lead to further loss of energy. This leads to depression over their loss of function, which further exacerbates the energy-deficient state.

In a pilot study, Phillips (1986) described a rating scale used to measure changes in performance of ADL following participation in an outpatient pulmonary rehabilitation program. Patients were asked to rate their perceived performance in self-care, household tasks, and outdoor activities. Following this subjective rating, patients were shown energy-conservation procedures and relaxation techniques, taught to do task analysis, and instructed in how to coordinate breathing patterns with the demands of activities. In this study, a postassessment was completed to determine if the intervention resulted in perceived changes of ability as well as physiological changes as measured by FEV testing. Although this study used a small sample, it provided preliminary evidence of positive changes in the patients' function.

Walsh (1986) described an occupational therapy program for persons with COPD. Her treatment protocol included exercise, stress management, and practice in demonstrated techniques of work simplification and motion economy, proper body mechanics, and proper breathing techniques during self-care and household management activities. In addition to individual treatment sessions, patients were provided with an opportunity to share their experiences of coping with various challenges and ways in which they coped.

CASE REPORTS

Two case reports are given in this section. The first illustrates the effects of cardiopulmonary disease on occupational performance for a patient who had undergone CABG and the second discusses the effects of COPD on occupational performance.

CASE I: JT: CORONARY ARTERY BYPASS GRAFT

JT (52 years old) experienced unusual discomfort in his chest for about 1 month. He initially attributed this discomfort to ongoing episodes of gastric upset, commonly referred to as heart burn. However, the over-the-counter antacid tablets he frequently consumed had not provided any relief. His concern led him to seek medical advice.

Following examination by his physician, it was clear that JT's condition was serious. JT had been experiencing the warning signs of angina, which is a hallmark of atherosclerosis. As his doctor explained, JT's cardiac health was compromised by a buildup of plaque in the coronary arteries. He was at risk for a myocardial infarction, because the vessel blockage was life threatening. Traditional therapy, including the use of nitrates to relieve angina and angioplasty to reduce coronary occlusion, would not be effective at this point. **Coronary artery bypass grafting** was recommended.

The findings of JT's physician are those that are commonly associated with patients who are candidates for CABG. In addition to chest discomfort, JT's angina was accompanied by **dyspnea** and acute fatigue during exertion. He had experienced recent episodes of **syncope** and vertigo. His heart burn episodes were characteristic of epigastric discomfort and burning. JT had experienced increased postprandial discomfort as well as discomfort in his back, shoulders, and elbows lasting more than 5 min. A family history of **hypertension** and diabetes had put him at a primary risk for coronary disease.

Laboratory results indicated elevated triglyceride and cholesterol (blood lipids) levels. His physician immediately ordered cardiac catheterization to determine the number and location of bypasses needed. This included an angiogram and left ventriculogram. The angiogram indicated severe blockage to the left main coronary artery. Because this artery branches into the left anterior descending artery and the circumflex coronary artery, both of which nourish the majority of heart muscle, JT had a life-threatening condition. The left ventriculogram provided information about the function of the main cardiac pump, which, on x-ray review, indicated faulty pumping motion.

The surgical procedure was performed by a team made up of a cardiac surgeon, two assistant surgeons, an anesthesiologist, a perfusionist (who operates a heart-lung machine), and several cardiac nurses. The procedure began with an incision to the sternal area to allow access to JT's heart. The internal mammary artery was used as a graft. This artery and the saphenous vein are commonly used, because both are "excess" blood vessels. Grafting was performed under a microscope using sutures as fine as hair. JT's surgeon sutured the graft to the aorta and to the left coronary artery.

Following surgery, JT was transferred to the intensive care unit (ICU) where he was continuously monitored by the cardiac care team. During this time, his immediate family was able to visit him briefly. Initially, they were frightened by the multiple surgical lines coming from all areas of his body. These included intravenous tubing, tubing directly into an artery, a urinary catheter, a nasogastric tube, and tubing to his nose for oxygen. JT also had ECG leads attached, which allowed the cardiac care team to assess his progress closely. Once the family members understood that these procedures are common and temporary, they better understood their value and felt relieved that JT was being watched carefully.

After JT was moved to the recovery unit, a respiratory therapist assisted him with deep breathing exercises to prevent postoperative lung complications such as a collapsed lung, infection, or pneumonia.

After 2 days, JT's initial recovery was going well enough that he was moved to an intermediate coronary care unit. He was ready to begin cardiac rehabilitation. This included physical therapy, which initiated a monitored, graded ambulation program. JT learned how to monitor his own heart rate and to limit upper arm movement to allow safe, sternal healing. Respiratory therapy services continued with inhalation exercises. JT was taught to use a spirometer, which helped to expand and exercise his lungs. Coughing and deep breathing exercises would be discontinued once JT returned to normal respiratory patterns. A nutritionist consulted with JT regarding the necessity to plan low-fat and low-cholesterol meals. He was given specific lists of foods to avoid as well as low-fat cooking tips. A low-sodium diet was recommended as well.

The occupational therapist initiated a program to increase progressively functional performance using self-care activities. The therapists also provided reinforcement of the need to assess heart rate before and after each activity to avoid performing activities that would overfatigue. Initial instruction in work simplification and energy conservation (see Chapter 16) was provided so that JT could begin to incorporate energy-saving steps while performing routine self-care tasks, such as sitting at the sink to perform hygiene activities.

After a total of 5 days, JT was ready to go home. It was decided by his physician that he could benefit from home health care. A follow-up outpatient program, which would provide updated stress assessments and consultation, was considered for a later date. On the date of JT's discharge and return to home, he was scheduled for an initial assessment by a home health care nursing service. The nurse's findings, compiled from physician orders, hospital information, and her own diagnostic assessment, indicated the following areas of concern (Dolan, 1990).

Nursing Assessment

1. Decreased cardiac output related to cardiac dysrhythmia and secondary to surgery.
2. Potential for altered bowel elimination; constipation was related to analgesic use, decreased physical activity, and dietary changes.
3. Anxiety related to surgical recovery, financial concerns, and imminent lifestyle changes.
4. Potential sexual dysfunction related to fear of pain or death during intercourse.
5. Potential for permanent loss of interest in leisure pursuits as a result of fear of pain and concern about wound healing.
6. Potential for ineffective family coping related to disruption of patient's role during recuperation.

A referral to occupational therapy was initiated to address occupational performance functioning. The nurse noted that JT could experience incisional discomfort or redness of the scar and sharp pain during respiration while performing activities. Shortness of breath, productive cough, pedal or pretibial edema, and increased fatigue would also be critical signs to watch for and would need to be reported to the physician. Syncopal episodes, resulting from activities that increase myocardial oxygen demand, would also require physician contact if they persisted.

Occupational Therapy Assessment

MEDICAL/SURGICAL HISTORY

It is critical that the occupational therapist consider the multiple factors associated with recovery from CABG. The findings presented by JT's nurse have both primary and secondary implications for his return to a functional status in occupational perfor-

mance. An understanding of the patient's medications and possible side effects is needed to determine if a patient's response to activity is affected by a certain drug. Knowing the sequelae of recovery from CABG will ensure that needed precautions are taken during treatment planning and implementation.

LIVING SITUATION

On arrival at JT's home, the occupational therapist assessed the physical layout of the house. Observations indicated that it was a two-story house that provided an overall cluttered, yet comfortable, environment. The bedrooms and two full bathrooms were situated on the second floor. The carpeting was a thick shag type, with wooden floors and throw rugs in the kitchen and family room. Much of the furniture in the family room was overstuffed and low to the floor. All these factors were potential concerns in looking at functional mobility.

JT lived with his 48-year-old wife and two teenage daughters (aged 14 and 17). His wife was employed as an office manager for a busy dental practice. His daughters both had active schedules outside of school. JT was on medical leave from his position as chief accountant of a tax preparation firm. He expressed a great deal of concern about whether he would lose his job. He wanted to know how long his medical leave would need to continue. JT's wife was equally concerned about his recovery. She had many questions about how limited his activities should be, what should he do, and what should he not do. In essence, they needed to get an idea of what the future held. Both were concerned about resumption of sexual activity. When would it be safe? Would it ever be safe?

OCCUPATIONAL PERFORMANCE AREAS

The discussion below follows the occupational therapist through her assessment of JT's current functioning in occupational performance areas, including activities of daily living, work and leisure activities.

Activities of Daily Living

JT is independent, but tires easily while grooming, showering, performing oral hygiene, dressing, and eating. He experiences mild postprandial discomfort following meals. He needs standby assistance for stepping into and out of the bathtub in which he currently takes stand-up showers (no physical assistance is required, therapist provides verbal cuing for safety). His medication routine is supervised by his nurse and is in compliance at this time. He has difficulty cleaning himself after toileting because he feels mild discomfort on his sternal incision when he reaches behind himself.

In terms of functional mobility, JT is able to ambulate at a slow pace for approximately 300 feet outside, after which his resting heart rate has increased from 100 to 125 bpm. His blood pressure increases from 126/88 to 130/96.

Sexual expression is not fully addressed during this initial evaluation. It will be explored further when JT feels he is ready to do so.

Work Activities

The therapist evaluates JT's home management responsibilities and his job. JT has not historically performed home management tasks such as clothing care, cleaning, meal preparation, cleanup, and shopping. These activities have traditionally been assigned to his wife. He would like to help her now that he is at home on temporary medical disability. His ability to maintain the home, yard, and other household management tasks is limited at this time, because he is functioning at a 3.6-MET level. These activities require 5+ METs. However, the therapist expects that JT will gradually begin participating in these tasks. JT feels he is able to resume money management responsibilities.

JT recognizes that accounting is his primary vocational skill and, at his age, the best opportunity for him in terms of continued employment. Although he is considered a very competent employee, he is anxious about the potential for returning to work and hopes that his absence will not last too long. JT's disability income is adequate but only extends for a period of 6 months.

Leisure Activities

JT indicates that his primary interests are golfing, playing bridge, reading, and listening to classical music. He enjoys family activities but notes that there have been fewer of these since his daughters entered teenhood and seem to be involved in many other activities. He indicated that although he enjoys these activities, his actual participation is minimal because of long workdays and weekend work.

Assessment of Occupational Performance Components

Based on reports and observations made during the assessment of occupational performance areas, the therapist notes that JT's only motor impairment is endurance for activities. He is functioning at a 3.6-MET level and wants to be able to function at a 6-MET level. Activity tolerance is affected by decreased endurance level and orthostatic hypotension. He is concerned that overactivity may cause further cardiac problems.

JT is alert and well oriented to his environment. He is aware of his disease process, the subsequent surgery, and the prognosis of his recovery. He asks intelligent questions and expresses interest in working with all the team members to develop an appropriate treatment plan. He understands instructions about the home activity program, energy-conservation principles, and other issues related to his overall treatment program.

JT's major life roles include husband, parent, and worker. He has interest in performing each one well and is anxious about his ability to resume these roles effectively. He demonstrates a moderate depression.

JT is highly sociable. He easily interacts with others during interviews and readily engages in discussion about selected topics. He seems to listen well to advice, asks questions for clarification, and summarizes what he has been told.

JT is able to identify those areas of his life that have caused him stress and those that he anticipates will be coping challenges. He is not sure how well he will respond to the demands and needs of his family and employer. He feels very dependent on his family at this time for support and encouragement.

Discussion of JT's Occupational Therapy Program

JT's current functional performance is limited across all categories of occupational performance because of reduced endurance. This limitation is likely to be of a temporary nature, although lifestyle changes and readjustment of priorities in his life will need to be permanent. Based on information from the nurse and the occupational therapy assessment, the following program goals, in JT's terms, have been established:
1. Return to work;
2. Assume home responsibilities;
3. Resume sexual activity;
4. Prevent further heart disease.

To accomplish the first three goals, JT will need to increase his endurance. Therefore, the therapist sets the following goals for JT:
1. Promote a training effect;
2. Grade MET level of activities from 3.6 to 6.0;
3. Teach JT to monitor his responses to exercise and activity;
4. Teach energy-conservation principles and techniques.

For JT to achieve his goal of prevention of further heart disease, the therapist sets the following goals:
1. Learn and practice appropriate lifestyle changes;
2. Develop methods of coping with demands of work and family.

In collaboration with the patient's physician, a progressive activity/exercise program begins to give JT new confidence in the ability of the heart to increase its function. Assessing baseline heart rate and then measuring again postactivity provides the needed information to determine which activities are appropriate and which are not, because heart rate is directly related to the physiological capacity of the cardiopulmonary system. The therapist will teach JT stress-management techniques and breathing exercises to help him reduce anxiety. Anxiety will decrease when JT observes a training effect.

Exercise results in a training effect in which more blood is pumped during each heartbeat (increased stroke volume) and the number of heartbeats are decreased for the same amount of exercise, which indicates improved functional capacity. A patient starts an exercise program at a level of energy expenditure that is safe but puts demand on cardiac output. When the training effect from this activity level is experienced, the frequency, duration, or intensity of the activity is increased. The training effect will occur at successive levels of cardiac output up to a maximal level for a given individual.

The occupational therapist gives JT a chart that lists typical activities during waking hours. He is taught to report any dysrhythmias that occur during any task immediately to the physician. Dysrhythmias can damage the heart by reducing myocardial oxygenation (Dolan, 1990). The therapist tells JT to report any chest pain, as this indicates coronary spasm and decreased myocardial oxygenation. JT must report any shortness of breath, edema, or fatigue, because these are signs of dysfunctional cardiac muscle, which may lead to pulmonary edema and reduced blood oxygenation. JT learns to omit any activities that create frequent **syncope.**

Anxiety results from the ambivalence associated with surgical success. Patients often are fearful that recovery is an illusion. The occupational therapist reinforces the nurse's effort to inform JT about all aspects of his progress toward recovery. Knowledge about wound healing and blood pressure regulation helps alleviate his fear. The therapist encourages JT to express fears concerning his condition.

The occupational therapist does not act as a sex counselor unless credentialed as such. It is important, however, that the therapist provide an opportunity for JT to express his concerns about sexual matters in a private, quiet setting. The therapist expresses a genuine sense of concern, in a nonjudgmental way. She reassures JT that sexual anxiety is common after CABG. The therapist helps JT understand that sex, like any exercise, requires a certain level of exertion (6 METs), which alleviates his fear. A progressive activity and exercise program to increase MET levels is developed as an important part of addressing JT's need for resumption of sexual activity. JT is made aware that certain medications can have adverse physiologic and psychologic effects on sexual behavior, which also helps alleviate his anxiety.

JT and his family need to realize that JT's dependency is temporary and that it is likely he will resume his presurgical activities. The therapist encourages JT and his family to discuss their fears so she can assess their level of coping skills. Knowing the family's positive and negative coping behaviors allows the therapist to suggest alternative actions for negative responses (see Chapter 20). The therapist knows that collaborating with the family in coping is more successful than telling them what to do in response to JT's dependency needs.

CASE II: RP: CHRONIC OBSTRUCTIVE PULMONARY DISEASE

RP is a 68-year-old woman who has a long history of emphysema with a recent exacerbation of her condition. She lives alone in a very cluttered, one-story frame house. Her two adult children live in the area, yet only her son maintains contact with her. He phones her on a daily basis and visits a few times a week to help her.

Medical/Surgical History

RP was discharged from the hospital to be followed by the home care team. She had repeated episodes of emphysema that resulted in chronic inflammation and alveoli destruction, which resulted in an abnormal exchange of oxygen and carbon dioxide.

Nursing Assessment

The nursing assessment indicated that RP experienced 3+ **dyspnea** along with generalized fatigue, loss of appetite, and insomnia. She had a productive cough that produced thick sputum. Her cardiovascular function was compromised as noted by findings of **tachycardia, atrial fibrillation,** and jugular vein distension. The adverse side effects of medication resulted in a resting tremor. RP was depressed, sometimes lethargic, and was quite apprehensive about her condition. The potential for injury existed because she had difficulty recognizing signs and symptoms of acute illness. After conferring with the nurse, the occupational therapist learned that the patient's chest x-ray indicated structural lung damage and her white blood count was elevated, both common findings associated with COPD.

Occupational Therapy Assessment

Because the occupational therapist has studied both the medical and surgical history and the nursing assessment, she can anticipate the occupational performance deficits and potential for exacerbation of these problems. The discussion below follows the occupational therapist in her assessment of RP's functional status in occupational performance areas and components of function.

ACTIVITIES OF DAILY LIVING

The therapist observes that RP is able to complete all activities of daily living independently yet does so with great effort. She tires easily as observed by her slow, deliberate movements marked by shortness of breath as she proceeds through grooming, dressing, and showering. RP has difficulty with functional ambulation, and the therapist notes she has 3+ **dyspnea** while walking throughout her home. RP is unable to climb more than one step without pausing for rest.

WORK ACTIVITIES

RP is unable to perform all home management activities. She relies on her son to do her shopping and household maintenance. She is inconsistent in meal preparation and cleanup, because she is often too tired to prepare all her meals during the day. Her nutritional intake thus is of concern. She is not aware of the potential danger inherent in her cluttered environment and is at risk for falls and injury. The therapist notes that RP needs assistance with money management, because she is anxious about her ability to pay her expenses.

LEISURE ACTIVITIES

RP expresses interest in reading, theater, and socializing with two very good friends. However, she has not kept up with her regular contacts because of her illness. She continues to read a little but generally watches TV. RP sleeps intermittently during the day. She feels any other activity would cause too much fatigue so she avoids anything else.

ASSESSMENT OF OCCUPATIONAL PERFORMANCE COMPONENTS

Sensory integration functioning is intact. In terms of neuromuscular function, RP is experiencing significant decrease in upper extremity proximal range of motion. Upper extremity muscle strength as well as endurance and overall activity tolerance are

significantly affected by her disease process. Because of compensatory trunk flexion patterns, typical of persons with COPD, RP tends to ambulate with a stooped posture.

Basic cognitive orientation is not affected. RP's attention span is limited to approximately 20 min of conversation at which time the therapist recognizes that she has difficulty focusing her attention. Her long-term memory is intact with moderate short-term memory impairment. The therapist must repeat instructions to RP and must break down the information into short segments.

RP expresses concern that she has lost important roles. Once active in the church and her family, she feels that her life is very limited. RP thinks it is important to do things and maintain an active life, but she feels too uncomfortable physically to do anything.

The therapist notes that RP interacts in an appropriate manner, answering questions to the best of her ability and understanding that the information provided is for the development of a treatment program. RP has a significant level of difficulty with coping. She realizes that the disease is creating a great deal of physical and psychological stress for her, which creates even greater anxiety. RP feels she has lost control of her coping mechanisms.

Planning RP's Occupational Therapy Program

Based on all the available data, the occupational therapist develops the following goals with RP:

1. Be able to care for self:
   a. Develop methods to conserve energy;
   b. Employ work simplification principles and techniques in daily routine;
   c. In collaboration with respiratory therapy, teach RP to use controlled breathing techniques such as **pursed lip breathing.**
2. Be able to care for home:
   a. Help RP to define particular home responsibilities that she will need to do such as meal preparation, light household cleaning, and making her bed;
   b. Teach energy-conservation and work-simplification methods (see Chapter 16);
   c. Practice controlled breathing techniques during functional tasks;
   d. Enlist the support of RP's son to help with the needed rearrangement of her furniture and clearing household clutter to ensure safe access through each room.
3. Improve sleeping patterns:
   a. Instruct in and evaluate RP's use of a balanced schedule for work and rest;
   b. Teach relaxation techniques;
   c. Reduce anxiety.
      (1) Teach effective coping strategies to decrease stress and anxiety;
      (2) Involve RP in a pulmonary support group;
      (3) Develop a program of meaningful activity within RP's capabilities.
4. Identify and pursue satisfying social roles.

STUDY QUESTIONS ⎯⎯⎯⎯⎯⎯⎯⎯⎯⎯

1. Describe common complaints of someone who is a candidate for a myocardial infarction.
2. List functional deficits that would likely accompany congestive heart failure.
3. Define and describe hypertension.
4. Why does angina occur? What is the difference between stable and unstable angina?

5. When is coronary artery bypass grafting recommended? What does the procedure consist of?
6. Describe the common diagnostic procedures used to assess cardiopulmonary health status.
7. Develop a matrix that includes the occupational performance areas and components. Describe how cardiopulmonary disease impacts these.

Performance Components	Occupational Performance Areas		
	Work	Leisure	ADL
Sensorimotor			
Cognitive			
Psychosocial			

8. What is a training effect? How is it achieved?
9. In the first case study, JT is involved in a progressive activity program. He will eventually move to a 6.0-MET level of performance. Outline appropriate activities that he will be able to do at MET levels 3.5 and 4.5.
10. Develop an energy-conservation and work-simplification program for RP (the second case study) that includes all ADLs for which she is responsible. Your plan should include specific suggestions for each ADL that are supported by the energy-conservation or work-simplification principle being employed by that suggestion.

REFERENCES

American College of Sports Medicine. (1986). *Guidelines for graded exercise testing and prescription* (3rd ed.). Philadelphia: Lea & Febiger.

American Heart Association. (1979). *The exercise standards book.* Dallas: Author.

American Heart Association. (1980). Cardiopulmonary resuscitation: Advanced life support. *Journal of the American Medical Association, 24*(8), 760–781.

Andreoli, K. G., Fowkes, V. K., Zipes, D. R., & Wallace, D. G. (Eds). (1983). *Comprehensive cardiac care: A text for nurses, physicians, and other health practitioners.* St. Louis: C. V. Mosby.

Andrews, J. L. (1987). Pulmonary disease: Improving the prognosis. *Modern Medicine, 55,* 88–103.

Ayres, S. M. (1984). Chronic bronchitis: A clinical guide. *Hospital Medicine, 20*(5), 213–241.

Berkow, R., & Fletcher, A. J. (Eds.). (1987). *The Merck manual of diagnosis and therapy.* Philadelphia: F. A. Davis.

Blumenthal, J., & Emery, C. (1988). Rehabilitation of patients following myocardial infarction. *Journal of Consulting and Clinical Psychology, 56*(3), 374–381.

Brannon, F. J., Geyer, M. J., & Folvy, M. W. (1988). *Cardiac rehabilitation.* Philadelphia: F. A. Davis.

Cain, H. D., Frasher, W. G., & Stivelman, R. (1961). Graded activity program for safe return to self care following myocardial infarction. *Journal of the American Medical Association, 17*(1) 111–115.

Campbell, C. (1984). *Nursing diagnosis and intervention in nursing practice* (2nd ed.). New York: John Wiley & Sons.

Carroll, P. F. (1986). What you can learn from pulmonary function tests. *RN, 49*(7), 24–27.

Cohen, B. S. (1975). A program for rehabilitation after acute myocardial infarction. *Southern Medical Journal, 68*(2), 145–148.

Corbett, J. V. (1982). *Diagnostic procedures in nursing practice.* Norwalk, CT: Appleton-Century-Crofts.

Cousins, N. (1979). *Anatomy of an illness as perceived by the patient.* New York: W. W. Norton.

Dolan, M. B. (1990). *Community and home health care plans.* Springhouse, PA: Springhouse.

Erb, B. D., Fletcher, G. F., & Sheffield, T. L. (1979). AHA committee report: Standards for cardiovascular exercise treatment programs. *Circulation, 59,* 1084–1090.

Falvo, D. R. (1991). *Medical and psychosocial aspects of chronic illness and disability.* Gaithersberg, MD: Aspen Systems.

Fox, S. M., Naughton, J. P., & Gorman, P. A. (1972). Physical activity and cardiovascular health III. The exercise prescription. Frequency and type of activity. *Modern Concepts in Cardiovascular Disease, 41,* 6–14.

Garrison, F. H. (1963). *An introduction to the history of medicine* (4th ed.). Philadelphia: W. B. Saunders.

Gentry, W. D., Foster, S., & Haney, T. (1972). Denial as a determinant of anxiety and perceived health status in the coronary care unit. *Psychosomatic Medicine, 34,* 39–44.

Grant, A., & Cohen, B. S. (1973). Acute myocardial infarction: Effect of a rehabilitation program on length of hospitalization and functional status at discharge. *Archives of Physical Medicine & Rehabilitation, 54*(5), 201–206.

Gray, R. M., Rheinhardt, A. M., & Ward, J. R. (1969). Psychosocial factors involved in the rehabilitation of persons with cardiovascular disease. *Rehabilitation Literature, 30,* 354–362.

Guyton, A. (1986). *A textbook of medical physiology* (7th ed.). Philadelphia: W. B. Saunders.

Harvey, W. (1958). *De circulatione sanguinis.* Oxford, UK: Blackwell Scientific Publications.

Herrick, J. B. (1912). Clinical features of sudden obstruction of the coronary arteries. *Journal of the American Medical Association, 59,* 2015–2018.

Jader, G. C., & Lekander, B. J. (1987). Open heart surgery: Caring for bypass and transplant patients. *RN, 50*(4), 40–43.

Killen, K. (1986). What is cardiac rehabilitation and how does occupational therapy fit in? *Occupational Therapy News, 40*(10), 15.

King, J. C., & Nixon, P. G. (1988). A system of cardiac rehabilitation: Psychophysiological basis and practice. *British Journal of Occupational Therapy, 51*(11), 378–384.

Kochar, M., & Woods, K. (1985). *Hypertension control for nurses and other health professionals* (2nd ed.). Philadelphia: Springer.

Kornbleau, I. H., & Michaels, E. (1961). Outline of an exercise program for patients with myocardial infarction. *Pennsylvania Medicine, 60,* 1575–1578.

Kottke, F. J. (1971). Common cardiovascular problems in rehabilitation. In F. H. Krusen, F. J. Kottke, & P. M. Ellwood (Eds.), *Handbook of physical medicine and rehabilitation* (pp. 875–913). Philadelphia: W. B. Saunders.

Levine, S. A., & Lown, B. (1952). Armchair treatment of acute coronary thrombosis. *Journal of the American Medical Association, 148,* 1365–1369.

Levy, R. L. (1980). *Medicine for the layman: Heart attacks* (Publication No. 80-1803). Bethesda, MD: National Institutes of Health.

Mead, W. F. (1977). Exercise rehabilitation after myocardial infarction. *American Family Physician, 15*(4), 121–123.

Nixon, P. G., Carruthers, M. E., Taylor, D. J, Bethel, H. J., & Grabau, T. R. (1976). British pilot study of exercise therapy:

Patients with cardiovascular disease. *British Journal of Sports Medicine, 10*(4), 54–61.

Oswald, I. (1987). The benefit of sleep. *Holistic Medicine, 2*, 137–139.

Parmley, W. W. (1986). Position report on cardiac rehabilitation: Recommendations of the American College of Cardiology. *Journal of the American College of Cardiology, 7*, 451–453.

Phillips, M. A. (1986). A subjective ADL rating scale for the pulmonary rehabilitation patient. *Occupational Therapy in Health Care, 3*(1), 79–88.

Stern, M. J., Pascale, L., & Ackerman, A. (1977). Life adjustment, postmyocardial infarction: Determining predictive variables. *Archives of Internal Medicine, 137*, 1680–1685.

Suave, M. J. (1992). Incidence and severity of cognitive deficits in cardiac arrest survivors. *Journal of Critical Care, 21*(3), 293–298.

Thomas, C. L. (Ed.). (1973). *Taber's cyclopedic medical dictionary* (12th ed.). Philadelphia: F. A. Davis.

Ulrich, S. (1986). *Nursing care planning guides: A nursing diagnosis approach.* Philadelphia: W. B. Saunders.

Underhill, S. L. (1986) Coronary heart disease: Myocardial ischemia and infarction. In M. L. Patrick, (Ed.), *Medical surgical nursing: Pathophysiological nursing* (pp. 698–799). Philadelphia: J. B. Lippincott.

Vogt, F. B., Spencer, W., & Cardus, D. (1965). The effects of bedrest on various parameters of physiological functions (NASA Contractor Reports). Washington, DC: National Aeronautics and Space Administration.

Walsh, R. L. (1986). Occupational therapy as part of a pulmonary rehabilitation program. *Occupational Therapy in Health Care, 3*(1), 65–78.

Wenger, N. K. (1987). Future directions in cardiovascular rehabilitation. *Journal of Cardiopulmonary Rehabilitation, 7*, 169–174.

White, P. D. (1951). *Heart disease.* New York: Macmillan.

Wilson, P. (1988). Cardiac rehabilitation: Then and now. *Physician and Sports Medicine, 16*(9), 75–80.

Wolf, K. S. (1984). Management of the cardiovascular surgery patient. In L. S. Brunner & S. D. Suddarth (Eds.), *Textbook of medical surgical nursing* (5th ed., pp. 462–516). Philadelphia: J. B. Lippincott.

Katherine A. Konosky

Dysphagia, or difficulty eating, is a symptom of an underlying disease process (Donner, 1986). Dysphagia affects between 6 and 10 million people per year. The consequences of dysphagia are numerous, including serious medical complications and social isolation. This chapter serves as an introduction for occupational therapists to the evaluation and treatment of patients with dysphagia.

NORMAL SWALLOWING

The ability to feed oneself is one of the primary aspects of self-care (Silverman & Elfant, 1979). To maintain health, human beings require sufficient hydration and nutrition to achieve homeostasis. As a result, two of the basic human drives are controlled by hunger and thirst (Clarke, 1989). Both of these drives necessitate the swallowing of food or fluid to be sated. Swallowing occurs as an orderly physiologic process that transports saliva or ingested material from the mouth to the stomach while protecting the respiratory tract (Dodds, 1988; Kennedy & Kent, 1988). The average human being swallows 1000 times a day, or once during every wakeful minute for saliva management and 50 to 100 times per meal (Dodds, 1988).

Phases of Deglutition

The term *deglutition* is used to describe the semi-automatic action of respiratory and gastrointestinal tract muscles to propel food from the oral cavity to the stomach (Kennedy & Kent, 1988). The process of deglutition is typically broken down into four phases (Groher, 1984; Logemann, 1983) (Fig. 44.1). Each phase is important and is interdependent on the other phases (Palmer et al., 1992). The phases typically identified are preparatory, oral, pharyngeal, and esophageal. A fifth phase should be included that precedes the other phases: the anticipatory phase (Ylvisaker, 1985).

The anticipatory phase is volitional and includes multisensory processing of the food in regard to food appeal and acceptance, hand to mouth patterning, memory for the food item or similar food item, and mouth opening in response to the eating utensil. This phase is believed to be important in developing a preliminary plan about what will need to happen once the food reaches the mouth, this in turn results in the preactivation of specific motor pathways and saliva production (Clarke, 1989). To develop such a plan, the human being gains visual, olfactory, and tactile and proprioceptive information about the food to be eaten by visually inspecting, smelling, and stirring as well as using other strategies to determine if the food is "swallow safe" (Kinny et al., 1989). Bite size and rate of intake for self-feeders is determined during this phase.

The second stage is the preparatory phase. During this phase, food is taken into the mouth and formed into a ball, or bolus. How the bolus is formed depends on the type of food being eaten. Solid food items like peanuts require rotary chewing to mash them before the bolus is formed. Puréed food items such as applesauce and pudding require little oral manipulation to

GLOSSARY

Aspiration—Occurs when material (saliva or food) from the pharynx enters the larynx and falls below the level of the true vocal cords. The amount of aspiration, the substance aspirated, and the general physical condition of the patient determine the effect of the aspiration.

Bite reflex—A primitive reflex in which the patient bites in response to any stimulus and is unable to release volitionally.

Nonoral feeding source—A way of providing nutrition, hydration, and medication without swallowing. A variety of nonoral sources exist, including nasogastric tubes, percutaneous endoscopic gastrostomies, gastrostomies, jejunostomies, and parentral sources.

Rooting reflex—A primitive reflex. When tactile stimulation is given to the facial area, the head turns and the mouth opens. Excessive rooting is suggestive of hypersensitivity or lack of inhibition.

Swallow response—Protects the airway while allowing food to enter the esophagus. Previously, the term *reflex* was used; however, because the behavior is not stereotypic, the term *response* is now used.

Tracheostomy—A surgically created opening in the trachea.

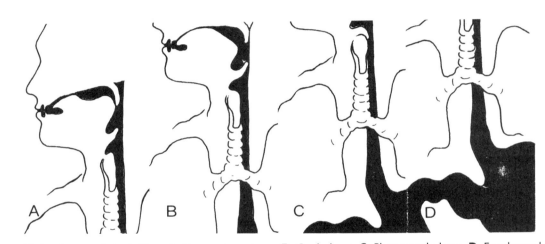

Figure 44.1. Stages of deglutition. **A.** Preparatory phase. **B.** Oral phase. **C.** Pharyngeal phase. **D.** Esophageal phase.

form the bolus. The amount of time required to complete this stage is variable and depends on the individual's emotional state, eating habits, and dentition and food consistency and amount. After it is formed, the bolus is held in the anterior part of the mouth until the oral stage begins.

The oral, or third phase, occurs when the bolus is moved by the tongue from the front of the mouth to the back of the mouth. Typical oral transit time is 1 sec (Logemann, 1983, 1986a). During this stage, oral pressures change and the tongue squeezes the bolus against the soft palate until it reaches the area around the anterior faucial arches.

Normally, when a bolus reaches the area of the anterior faucial arches initiation of the **swallow response** occurs, which is the beginning of the pharyngeal phase (Bass, 1988; Dodds, 1988; Pommerenke, 1928). During the pharyngeal phase, the soft palate elevates to close off the nasopharynx, the larynx elevates and retracts, the epiglottis inverts, the true and false vocal cords adduct, the pharyngeal constrictors contract, and the upper esophageal sphincter relaxes.

Breathing stops during the swallow and the airway is protected from ingested food or saliva by the epiglottis and true and false vocal cords. The pharyngeal stage is involuntary (Dodds, 1988). Normal pharyngeal transit time is 1 sec (Logemann, 1986b).

Once the bolus passes the upper esophageal sphincter, it enters the esophagus and the esophageal phase begins. During the esophageal phase, the upper esophageal sphincter returns to its tonic state, peristaltic contraction of the esophagus assists gravity in propelling the bolus toward the stomach. The time required to complete this phase in normal healthy adults is 8 to 20 sec.

Anatomy and Physiology

To swallow efficiently, the head, neck, and gastrointestinal anatomy and neurophysiology must be intact. If function is even partially altered, a change in swallowing efficiency will occur. An example of this occurs when a dental patient receives novocaine to numb the oral tissue around a cavity. Drooling out of the numbed side occurs, the tongue or cheek may be bitten during mastication, and the preparatory phase duration increases significantly. It is, therefore, important for the therapist treating people with dysphagia to have a working knowledge of normal and abnormal head and neck anatomy and neurophysiology.

The neuroregulation of deglutition is a complex process. Sensory and motor cranial nerves as well as the cortex, midbrain, cerebellum, and brainstem are involved. The swallowing centers of the brainstem process information from the other areas to generate the swallow. Thus the swallowing centers control most of the 26 pairs of muscles that are used when swallowing. The esophageal stage is regulated by the central nervous system, the enteric nervous system, and stretch receptors within the esophagus (Hendrix, 1993b).

DYSPHAGIA

There are many disease processes that may result in dysphagia, including diseases that affect the central nervous system, the peripheral nervous system, the motor end plate, muscles, and the anatomic structures (Buchholz, 1987; Castell & Donner, 1987; Kushner, 1989). Dysphagia may lead to dehydration, malnutrition (Musson et al., 1990), and/or pulmonary complications secondary to **aspiration,** including **aspiration** pneumonia, abscess, airway obstruction, fibrosis, and adult respiratory distress syndrome (Terry & Fuller, 1989). Because the consequences of dysphagia can be life threatening (Donner, 1986; Terry & Fuller, 1989), it is important for health care providers to be aware of key signs and symptoms. These signs and symptoms include coughing or choking during or after mealtime, increased time to complete meals, refusal to eat, difficulty managing secretions, self-modification of diet, weight loss, frequent respiratory tract infections, changed vocal quality during or after eating, vomiting, and complaints of food sticking in the throat (Groher, 1984; Logemann, 1983). A partial review of the literature that discusses the common disease processes and dysphagia characteristics is presented in Table 44.1. If any of the above symptoms are present or if the patient's disease process has a high incidence of dysphagia associated with it, further evaluation of the swallowing function is indicated.

Management

Dysphagia is a complex problem that requires management by a multidisciplinary, experienced team (Musson et al., 1990; Young & Durant-Jones, 1990). The primary team consists of the patient, the patient's family, the primary physician, the clinical nutritionist, the nursing staff, the speech pathologist, and the occupational therapist (Jones & Altschuler, 1987). In addi-

Table 44.1. Dysphagia Characteristics of Various Diagnoses

Disease Process/Diagnosis	Dysphagia Characteristics
Bulimia nervosa	Increased preparatory and oral time
	Decreased pharyngeal constrictor activation (Roberts et al., 1989)
Cancer, head and neck	Swallowing problems vary with type of medical intervention
	Radiation therapy for oral cancer results in dry mouth
	Following laryngectomy, decreased laryngeal closure noted when swallowing (Logemann, 1991)
	Total laryngectomy may result in pharyngeal spasm or stricture (Dziadziola et al., 1992)
	Increased time required to form and propel bolus
	Irradiation may result in edema, inflammation, and fibrosis of tissue (Groher, 1991)
Cerebral vascular accident	
Right hemisphere	Delayed initiation of the swallow response
	Aspiration before initiation of the swallow
	Pharyngeal residue
	No spontaneous compensation for dysfunction (Robbins & Levine, 1988)
Left hemisphere	Oral stage dysfunction
	Difficulty coordinating lips and tongue
	Apraxia
	Spontaneous compensation (Robbins & Levine, 1988)
Lacunes	Diffuse oropharyngeal dysfunction (Buchholz, 1990)
Huntington's disease	Mandibular rigidity
	Slow lingual chorea
	Respiratory chorea
	Laryngeal chorea
	Pharyngeal residue
	Aspiration (Kagel & Leopold, 1992)
Parkinson's disease	Reduced sensory processing with anterior spillage
	Decreased frequency of swallow
	Reduced lingual control with tremor
	Laryngeal and pharyngeal discoordination (Lieberman et al., 1980)
Rheumatoid arthritis, cervical subluxation	Coughing, regurgitation, and hoarseness (Davidson et al., 1977)
Spinal cord injury	
Cervical spondylosis	C_{3-4} osteophyte limits airway protection
	C_{6-7} osteophyte may result in upper esophageal sphincter dysfunction (Crowther & Ardran, 1985)

Table 44.1. Continued

Disease Process/Diagnosis	Dysphagia Characteristics
(Cervical spondylosis, continued)	Spasms reported while swallowing, regurgitation, and choking; voice change (Stuart, 1989) Postoperative dysphagia should not extend beyond 48 hr Regional complications after surgery may be caused by denervation or mechanical obstruction (Welsh, Welsh, & Chinnici, 1987)
Cervical fusion	Edema may result in transient dysphagia Nerve damage that occurs secondary to retractor use may cause long-lasting dysphagia (Welsh et al., 1987)
Tracheostomy	69% aspirate Pulmonary problems common Reduced laryngeal excursion noted (Cameron, Reynolds, & Zuidema, 1973)
Traumatic brain injury (TBI)	Dysphagia occurs in approximately 27% of people with TBI (Winstein, 1983) Dysphagia symptoms by order of occurrence: delayed initiation of the swallow, reduced tongue control, decreased pharyngeal constriction, and laryngeal dysfunction Multiple problems occur more frequently than singular problems Decreased cognition increases the potential for aspiration (Lazarus & Logemann, 1987)

tion, medical specialists in the following areas may be consultants to the team: gastroenterology, pulmonology, laryngology, radiology, dentistry, physical therapy, and therapists specializing in the videofluoroscopic evaluation of deglutition. Together decisions are made regarding evaluation and treatment of the individual with dysphagia. The occupational therapist has an important role within the dysphagia team. Her specialized assessment and treatment skills in the following areas are critical for comprehensive management of the patient with dysphagia: activities of daily living, including feeding and medication intake; adaptive equipment prescription and use; cognition; sensory function, including vision, olfaction, and gustation; motor control of posture, face, and limbs; and psychosocial factors.

All health care workers who are involved in the care of patients with dysphagia should adhere to universal precautions related to bodily fluids (see Chapter 36). In addition, because patients with dysphagia are at greater risk for choking (Ekberg & Feinberg, 1992), training in emergency medical procedures of foreign

body airway obstruction is critical before treating this patient population.

Evaluation

The evaluation process can be broken down into four components: history, prefeeding evaluation, feeding evaluation, and videofluoroscopic evaluation.

HISTORY

A comprehensive history is crucial for accurate assessment and treatment (Buchholz, 1987; Castell & Donner, 1987; Hendrix, 1993a; Kramer, 1988; Logemann, 1986a). The history should be obtained by the dysphagia therapist from the patient, care providers, and the patient's medical record. For the patient's medical history, the evaluating therapist should obtain information about the patient's general health, medications, and nutritional status.

In regard to the patient's general health, frequency of respiratory tract infections, complaints of heartburn or other gastrointestinal complaints, facial fractures, laryngeal trauma, and weight loss should be covered in detail, because these symptoms suggest a potentially life-threatening form of dysphagia or may directly affect oral intake.

Information about any medication the patient is on, the form of the medication (caplet, capsule, tablet, liquid suspension, crushed, or whole), and any difficulty with intake is important to include in the evaluation of the patient's medical history. Some medications enhance swallowing performance, especially the dopaminergic agents, while others, including certain psychotropics (Bazemore, Tonkonogy, & Ananth, 1991) and muscle relaxants, may negatively affect the swallowing function. In addition, certain drugs are known to alter taste, depress appetite, and induce vomiting, all of which may alter oral intake.

When obtaining the patient's nutritional history it is important to include food allergies, food preferences, current method of nutritional intake (Table 44.2), type of diet, level of assistance needed, foods that are difficult to swallow, foods that are easy to swallow, time required to complete a meal, and subjective information about the feeding process. The information obtained during the history component of the evaluation will assist the therapist in tailoring the assessment components to the patient's needs.

PREFEEDING

The prefeeding evaluation consists of observation as well as physical examination. During the prefeeding evaluation, assessment of cognitive status, motor control, respiratory status, oral structural function, oral reflexes, sensation, laryngeal function, and pharyngeal

Table 44.2. Method of Nutritional Intake

Total oral	All nutrition, hydration, and medication are taken orally; patients can be self-fed or fed by care provider
Partial oral	A nonoral feeding source is used to ensure adequate nutrition and hydration and safe medication intake; patients can be self-fed or are fed by a care provider.
Therapeutic feedings	Oral intake is limited and done by therapeutic staff only; primary nutrition, hydration, and medication intake is via a nonoral source
Nonoral	All nutrition, hydration, and medication are given via a nonoral source

function occurs without the presentation of food items (Selly et al., 1990; Sonies et al., 1987; Tuchman, 1989).

The cognitive abilities noted by the therapist during the prefeeding evaluation should include level of arousal, self-discipline (impulse control), judgment, orientation, memory, sequencing, and the ability to follow commands. Emotional state and behavioral management may also influence feeding ability. Combined, these factors may affect resumption of oral feeding and/ or progression of treatment (Logemann, 1990).

Postural control can be observed as the patient is sitting in the clinic. The therapist should note any skeletal deformities, abnormal patterns of muscle tone such as those related to tonic neck reflexes, weakness, and difficulty with postural control. The patient's postural set will influence self-feeding and swallowing abilities. In most cases, the optimal position for eating is sitting upright, trunk in midline, with 90° or more of hip flexion, knee flexion to 90°, with feet flat on a support surface.

Respiratory status information should include breathing pattern, respiration rate, oxygen requirements, if the patient has or had a **tracheostomy,** suctioning requirements, and whether or not the patient uses a respirator. Apnea, bradycardia, choking, coughing, chronic noisy breathing, and recurrent wheezing all suggest possible **aspiration** (Tuchman, 1989).

Sensory evaluation of the olfactory, gustatory, and tactile senses is an important component to the prefeeding assessment. Olfactory and gustatory functions should be screened (Farber, 1982). If alterations are noted, they should be formally tested (Cain et al., 1988; Doty, Shaman, & Dann, 1983). Extraoral and intraoral sensation should be tested for temperature and touch. In addition, the therapist should note any bite marks on the inner surface of the cheek when doing the oral structural evaluation; these may indicate

decreased sensory processing. In the cognitively impaired or nonverbal patient, oral tactile perception can be observed throughout the course of evaluation. Typically, withdrawal from tactile stimulation is suggestive of hypersensitivity, whereas nonresponse suggests hyposensitivity.

The therapist begins the oral structural evaluation by observing whether the face is symmetric at rest. The degree of facial asymmetry may be recorded by photograph or by amount of paralysis (Jongkees, 1973). After observing the patient's face at rest, the patient is asked to imitate various facial movements and the degree of paralysis or strength is recorded (strength testing is deferred if recent facial fracture is reported). Grading facial muscle function may be done as suggested by Kendall and McCreary (1983).

Jaw control is then evaluated. The therapist should gently palpate the temporomandibular joint and ask the patient to open and close his mouth slowly. The therapist should note any popping, asymmetry in opening, or other symptoms of temporomandibular joint dysfunction. The patient's ability to open and close; the patient's ability to perform lateral, graded, and rotary movements; and the patient's jaw strength are quantified.

Labial function is then assessed. The patient is asked to purse (pucker), retract (show teeth while making an *E* sound), and round the lips and to maintain lip closure while simulating chewing. If asymmetry is noted or weakness suspected, formal muscle testing is indicated (Kendall & McCreary, 1983). Coordination of control is assessed by asking the patient to alternate rapidly between rounding and retracting his lips four times as fast as he can. The therapist observes the patient's performance for timing and symmetry of response.

Lingual control is evaluated next. Initially, the therapist should note the appearance of the tongue. People with dysphagia may present with discoloration, coating, enlargement, surgical revisions, tremors, fasiculations, or atrophy of their tongues. The therapist then asks the patient to protrude, retract, elevate, and lateralize his tongue while the therapist records range, deviations (with hemiparesis the tongue will deviate to the weaker side), and speed of movement. Diadochokinetic rate is assessed by asking the patient to rapidly lateralize his tongue and then protract and retract his tongue while the therapist notes any breakdown in patterning and speed of performance.

While observing lingual control, dental condition can be noted. The therapist should look for missing teeth; abnormal wearing patterns on the tooth surfaces, suggesting bruxism, malocclusions, poorly fitting dentures, and missing teeth; and abnormal gum condition (Garcia, Perlmuter, & Chauncey, 1989).

The next structure evaluated is the soft palate or velum. To assess the patient's velar function, the therapist begins by noting the soft palate at rest. Using a tongue depressor, the therapist slightly depresses the tongue to view the palate. Patients may present with hypotonia, tremor, a high palatal vault, or other abnormalities. After viewing the velum at rest, with the tongue depressor in place, the therapist asks the patient to say "ah" for 3 sec while observing for elevation and retraction of the soft palate. Symmetry, amount of excursion, and the ability to maintain the "ah" are recorded. Decreased ability to either perform or maintain elevation suggests weakness.

Laryngeal screening relies on the therapist's subjective ability to assess laryngeal function as a protective mechanism during feeding. The therapist assesses the patient's vocal quality and his ability to cough and clear his throat. The therapist also palpates laryngeal excursion during swallowing as part of the screen. Vocal quality should be assessed throughout the entire evaluation process. The therapist should comment on clarity, wetness, hoarseness, breathiness, and volume of speech as well as changes in vocal quality with fatigue. In addition, the therapist should ask the patient to maintain phonation over a 5-sec interval. If not noted during the history, the patient or a family member should be asked if a change in vocal quality has occurred since onset of disease process or dysphagia. Changes in vocal quality suggest an alteration in vocal cord function, which may result in decreased airway protection when swallowing. Volitional coughing and throat clearing are then assessed, with the therapist commenting on ability and strength of response. Spontaneous coughing or throat clearing should be documented throughout the evaluation including frequency, strength, and whether or not the cough or throat clear was productive in bringing material to the oral cavity. Throat clearing and coughing are protective responses to irritants within the pharynx or larynx.

The therapist then assesses the patient's ability to swallow. The **swallow response** can be screened only during the prefeeding and feeding evaluations, as the structures involved cannot be directly observed. The therapist should sit or stand next to the patient and gently place her fingers as shown in Figure 44.2. The patient is asked to swallow. The therapist counts the time (saying "one, one thousand; two, one thousand; three, one thousand; . . .") from initial posterior tongue movement until laryngeal elevation occurs. If the time exceeds 1 sec the therapist may suspect delayed initiation of the **swallow response.** Delayed initiation of the **swallow response** can only be suspected, because visualization is not possible.

The therapist should continue to palpate for the return of the larynx to its resting position. Following

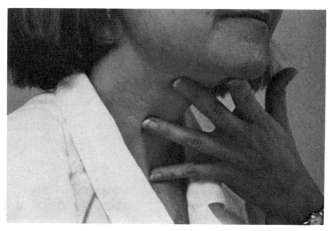

Figure 44.2. Therapist hand position for palpating the swallow response and laryngeal excursion. The first finger is on the chin, the second finger is at the base of the tongue, the third finger is over the thyroid cartilage, and the fourth finger is at the base of the throat (sternal notch).

the swallow, the patient is asked to vocalize, and the therapist records any change in vocalization. A change in vocal quality after the swallow suggests that the material (saliva during the prefeeding evaluation or food during the feeding evaluation) swallowed has entered the laryngeal vestibule and is resting on the vocal cords. If wetness occurs, the therapist should request a second swallow. The patient's ability to retrigger a swallow is noted, and the therapist assesses whether or not vocal quality changed after the second swallow. If vocal quality improves after the second swallow, the material in the larynx has either been swallowed or aspirated.

The last component of the prefeeding evaluation is the assessment of oral reflexes. Normal reflexes examined at this time include the gag and palatal reflexes. It should be noted that the gag reflex is variable among the normal population and an exact relationship between the presence or absence of the gag and swallow function has not been demonstrated. The gag reflex is a protective response that prevents **aspiration** of regurgitated material. The gag reflex is elicited by applying pressure to the tongue, posterior pharyngeal wall, or palate and observing for elevation of the palate, rolling of the tongue, and tearing of the eyes (Logemann, 1983). The therapist should document where the gag reflex was elicited and whether the response was symmetrical or not. Palatal reflexes are more difficult to elicit. The therapist takes a sterile swab and strokes the palate; typically elevation without overt gagging should occur. In addition to the normal reflexes, the therapist should look for the presence of abnormal reflexes, such as the **bite reflex** and the **rooting reflex.**

After finishing the prefeeding assessment, the therapist should summarize areas of impairment, because this information is used to help plan further evaluation and treatment. For instance, if the patient presents with right hemifacial weakness, decreased lingual control with limited movement of the right side of the tongue, and a hypotonic soft palate, the therapist may want to begin the feeding assessment with purées placed on the left side of the mouth.

FEEDING

After completing the prefeeding assessment, the therapist must decide whether a feeding evaluation can be safely done or if a videofluoroscopic evaluation is indicated. In general, people who are currently receiving all nutrition, hydration, and medication orally should undergo a feeding evaluation. Those receiving all nutrition, hydration, and medication via a **nonoral feeding source** should have a videofluoroscopic evaluation of deglutition before taking food by mouth. Patients who are on modified diets, are partial oral feeders, or have had previous videofluoroscopic studies should be evaluated on an individual basis. Decision making at this point is guided by institutional policies and procedures.

During the feeding assessment, the therapist evaluates the patient's performance during the various stages, carefully noting postural control, respiratory function, and alterations in cognition or behavior as they relate to the feeding process. When evaluating a patient's swallowing capabilities, it is important to include various consistencies, a variety of methods of intake, and different bolus sizes (Adnervill, Ekberg, & Groher, 1989; Robbins et al., 1987).

Optimally, patients should be allowed to choose food items of various consistencies. Consistencies used during the feeding evaluation are selected based on information obtained from the history and prefeeding evaluation. If decreased oral control or delayed initiation of the **swallow response** is suspected, the therapist may choose purées and thickened liquids to start with. These consistencies require little bolus formation while providing sensory information to the tongue about taste and texture, and their viscosity prevents premature loss into the pharynx. If upper esophageal sphincter dysfunction or decreased pharyngeal constrictor activity is suspected, thin liquids and thinned purées may be selected because of their fluid state. Consistencies of food items presented during the feeding evaluation may include water, thin flavored liquid (grape juice), slightly thickened liquids (tomato juice), thick liquids (liquids thickened with fruit purée, yogurt, or commercially available thickening agents), purées (strained baby food applesauce), purées with texture (commercial "adult" applesauce), ground foods

(homemade chunky applesauce), soft foods (sautéed apple slices with peel removed), and solid foods (fresh apple).

The range of bolus sizes used depends on the patient's performance with various textures and small bolus size (1/4 to 1/2 teaspoon). If the patient does not exhibit any signs of dysfunction with small boluses, the bolus size can be increased until symptoms occur or a normal bolus size is swallowed without difficulty. Whether the patient self-feeds or not at this time depends on cognitive and motor abilities.

As a food item is presented, the consistency and size of bolus should be recorded along with the patient's response. To assess the anticipatory phase, the therapist observes the patient's hand-to-mouth patterning if self-feeding, awareness of the feeding process, and anticipatory mouth opening in response to the food. Preparatory phase function is determined by the patient's ability to remove food from the utensil, prevent anterior spillage of material, thoroughly masticate food, and swallow the bolus without leaving residue in the cheeks or on the tongue.

Actual bolus formation cannot be seen. The therapist should observe and palpate for posterior tongue movement, which signifies oral phase function, and laryngeal elevation, which signifies initiation of the **swallow response** that begins the pharyngeal phase. Approximate timing should be recorded; however, it may not reflect actual performance, as bolus location and various internal structures cannot be seen.

Throughout the feeding evaluation, the therapist should note any spontaneous coughing, throat clearing, or changes in vocal quality, all of which suggest that material is entering the airway. Common problems noted during the evaluation process and their underlying causes are listed in Table 44.3. Clinical observations of feeding are not definitive in detecting **aspiration** (Linden & Siebens, 1983; Splaingard et al., 1988), differentiating between various pharyngeal stage dysfunctions, and screening for esophageal stage dysfunction.

VIDEOFLUOROSCOPY

Videofluoroscopic evaluation of deglutition should be done by professionals with postgraduate training in this area (American Occupational Therapy Association, 1989). Videofluoroscopic evaluation of deglutition is a highly specialized testing procedure that uses radiographic equipment to view swallowing function dynamically (Linden, 1989; Logemann, 1986a; Rushmer & Hendron, 1951). The ability to visualize the preparatory, oral, pharyngeal, and esophageal stages of the swallow allows for accurate identification of the nature and extent of swallowing dysfunction, including whether or not **aspiration** is occurring and the patient's

Table 44.3. Common Feeding Problems of Patients with Dysphagia

Stage	Problem	Sign or Symptom
Anticipatory	Impulsivity Poor attending	Rapid rate of intake; large bolus size; distracted during meal
Preparatory	Facial weakness	Facial asymmetry; decreased labial seal; inability to remove food from utensil; anterior spillage (food falls out of mouth)
Oral	Decreased lingual control	Decreased tongue strength; poor tongue coordination (slow diadochokinetic rate); pocketing of food (food held between cheek and teeth); multiple anterior-posterior tongue movements (pumping) before swallow; coating on tongue after swallowing
Pharyngeal	Delayed initiation of swallow	Coughing time is greater than 1 sec from palpation of posterior tongue movement until elevation of the larynx is felt; videofluoroscopic evaluation shows delay

response to **aspiration.** In addition, compensatory strategies can be observed and effectiveness of the strategies determined. Manometry (the measurement of pressure changes) is occasionally done simultaneously with fluoroscopy to determine pressure changes, anatomic events, and bolus transit (McConnel & Logemann, 1990).

New technologies continue to be incorporated into the therapeutic milieu. Fiberoptic endoscopic viewing of the pharynx and larynx is starting to be used by therapists to detect **aspiration** and pharyngeal residue after the swallow. One advantage of this method is that the patient is not exposed to radiation. Fiberoptic endoscopic viewing can be used as a screening tool or as a follow-up measure to quantify change (Langemore, Schatz, & Olsen, 1988).

CLINICAL IMPRESSIONS AND RECOMMENDATIONS

Once the feeding evaluation is complete, the therapist must summarize the information obtained, identify problems, and make recommendations to the treatment team. When summarizing this information it is important for the occupational therapist to highlight key information from the history, prefeeding, and feeding components of the evaluation. For example, "Given

the patient's recent 40-lb weight loss, decreased cognitive functioning, and multiple-stage swallowing impairment, the following recommendations are being made . . ." The recommendations section of the therapist's report should include the following information: feeding status, diet and liquid levels, medication form and method of intake, body position during and following feeding, feeding strategies, compensatory strategies, therapeutic exercises, recommended consultations, need for videofluoroscopic evaluation and reevaluation, and long-term therapeutic goals.

The team reviews the recommendations, and decisions are made regarding the course of care (Jones & Altschuler, 1987). Multiple issues can be involved, including risk of complications if a **nonoral feeding source** is recommended (Groher, 1990b); patient and family refusal to accept or comply with recommendations; the time required to feed the patient safely, which may be excessive or burdensome to care providers; whether or not nutritional adequacy can be achieved on the proposed diet; and whether the recommendations take into account the patient's disease process, especially if the disease is progressive. Once consensus is reached, education of the patient and family, communication with other health care providers, and actual treatment can begin.

Patient and Family Education

Throughout the evaluation and treatment process, the patient and his family should receive information and have input as decisions are made. The more information the patient and family have about the patient's dysphagia, the more likely they will be to follow the guidelines established by the rehabilitation team. In addition, the family, armed with accurate information, will be able to support and encourage the patient appropriately.

Treatment

Typically, dysphagia interventions used by allied health care providers are broken down into four areas: diet modification, equipment, compensatory strategies to maximize safety, and remediation and direct treatment. Diet modifications are made in an attempt to allow for safe oral intake and adequate nutrition and hydration. Many dysphagia diets exist (Granger & Craig, 1990; Martin, 1991; Mary Free Bed Hospital and Rehabilitation Center, 1992) with multiple food and liquid levels; therefore, the therapist treating a patient with dysphagia should work closely with a clinical nutritionist to identify the appropriate diet level for a patient or to upgrade a patient's diet.

Progression from nonoral to oral feeding follows

a typical pattern (Logemann, 1983; Mary Free Bed Hospital and Rehabilitation Center, 1992). Initially, the patient receives all nutrition, hydration, and medication via a **nonoral feeding source.** As the patient recovers swallowing abilities or learns compensatory strategies, as indicated by increased ability to manage secretions or change in videofluoroscopic findings, he will receive therapeutic feedings by allied health personnel. When the amount of intake increases and safe feeding behaviors are noted, the patient is permitted to eat under the supervision of other health care providers or trained family members and is identified as a partial oral feeder. Calorie counts are usually initiated at this time by the clinical nutritionist (Kamel, 1990).

As intake improves and calories are consistently sufficient, the **nonoral feeding source** may be used only for hydration and/or medication intake. Eventually, if the patient continues to improve, he will become able to drink enough fluid and take medication so that the **nonoral feeding source** can be removed. It is important that throughout this process the patient be weighed at regular intervals and be monitored for signs of dehydration or malnutrition. Upgrading of the patient's diet, in terms of consistency, should occur as skills develop, with the goal of returning to a normal diet. Meal preparation practice and community outings can reinforce diet modifications, enhance patient education, and motivate the patient.

Equipment used to assist the patient in safe feeding should be issued judiciously, and procedures for its use and cleaning should be clearly communicated to the patient, the patient's family, and the nursing staff.

Treatment techniques used for patients with dysphagia are like any other intervention to improve motor control or maximize safety, as they require careful training, practice, and monitoring. Therapeutic interventions, either compensations or remediation, for problems during each phase of the swallow are listed in Table 44.4. Specific treatment techniques have been outlined in the literature (Brown, Nordloh, & Donowitz, 1992; Bryant, 1991; Davis, 1989; Devorken & Nadol, 1991; Farber, 1982; Kahrilas, Logemann, & Gibbons, 1992; Langley, 1989; Layne, 1990; Logemann, 1983, 1986b; Thomas-Stonell & Greenberg, 1988; Tippett, Palmer, & Linden, 1987; Voss, Ionta, & Myers, 1985).

In addition to specific treatment, oral hygiene and prefeeding and feeding activities can be used to provide stimulation to the oral cavity and reinforce normal patterning. Therapeutic intervention focusing on postural and limb control and cognitive, behavioral, and perceptual remediation, if needed, will enhance dysphagia interventions. Progression of treatment should be made based on individual performance with appropriate grading to ensure safety.

Table 44.4. Compensatory or Remediational Therapeutic Interventions

Problem	Treatment
Impulsivity	*Compensatory:* Supervise feeding; require placement of utensil on table after each bite; present one food item at a time
Poor judgment	*Compensatory:* Use small-bowled utensils to decrease bolus size; for liquids, use of covered cup with small opening or pinch straw to limit amount
Poor attending	*Compensatory:* Feed in a quiet, distraction-free environment
Facial weakness	*Compensatory:* Diet consisting of purées, ground foods with sauce, and thickened liquids for easy control; place food toward back of mouth; place food on stronger side of mouth; tilt head toward stronger side; therapist places finger around lips to assist with closure *Remediational:* Tactile stimulation of face by tapping or quick stretch; facial exercises using a mirror for feedback; electromyographic biofeedback; sucking or blowing activities with increasing resistance
Poor lingual control	*Compensatory:* Diet consisting of food that requires little oral manipulation; place food toward the back of the mouth; tilt head toward the stronger side; forward and backward head movement to assist with bolus propulsion; oral inspection after mealtime to check for residue *Remediational:* Tongue range of motion exercises; resistive tongue exercises; gauze or gum in gauze exercises (gauze, or gum wrapped in gauze, is placed in the patient's mouth with a tail of the gauze sticking out. The therapist asks the patient to move the gauze right to left or forward and back and observes oral manipulation by watching the tail); encourage precise articulation
Swallow delay	*Compensatory:* Diet excludes thin liquids; chin tucked toward chest to maximize airway protection; head rotation to the weaker side *Remediational:* Thermal stimulation (A sterile #00 laryngeal mirror is dipped in iced water for 10 sec, then the therapist strokes the faucial arch 5 to 10 times, and a swallow is requested; the therapist should alternate between the right and left sides; treatment should stop after 5 min or if fatigue occurs as evidenced by increased time before initiation or coughing and choking

CASE STUDY: ASSESSMENT, TREATMENT, AND PROGRESSION

Ms. S was a 36-year-old woman who developed a pontine angioma, which was surgically removed. Following surgery, severe right hemifacial paralysis with sensory loss, trismus (tightening of jaw muscles that limits opening), poor secretion management, frequent episodes of choking and coughing, aphonia with right vocal cord paralysis, decreased ocular control, dizziness, and generalized motor weakness were noted. **Aspiration** pneumonia developed during her acute hospitalization, which resulted in **tracheostomy** and gastrostomy placement. Initial videofluoroscopic evaluation of deglutition showed preparatory phase dysfunction and severe pharyngeal phase dysfunction. The pharyngeal phase impairments included delayed initiation of the **swallow response,** decreased epiglottic inversion, decreased vocal cord adduction, decreased pharyngeal constrictor activity, and limited duration of upper esophageal opening. Combined, these problems resulted in **aspiration** before and after the swallow, residue throughout the pharynx, and only small amounts of food entering the esophagus. Coughing was noted in response to **aspiration,** but it was not effective in clearing material from the trachea.

Treatment initiated to improve secretion management incorporated the compensatory techniques of head turning to the right to occlude the weak side of the pharynx, and the Mendelssohn maneuver (a compensatory technique that increases the duration of upper esophageal opening by maintaining laryngeal elevation after the initial swallow). After 2 to 3 weeks a repeat videofluoroscopic swallowing study was done to assess the effectiveness of the strategies and to determine if oral feedings could be initiated. Results showed sufficient clearing of pharyngeal residue with small boluses of thin liquid but poor clearing with purées.

Therapeutic feedings using water were begun. At this time, Ms. S was discharged from inpatient rehabilitation. She was safely able to continue the therapeutic feedings at home. A repeat videofluoroscopic swallowing study was done after 2 months to see if her swallowing abilities had improved and whether her diet could be modified. Results showed safe intake of liquid and thinned purée consistencies, using the recommended compensatory techniques. Regular puréed or semisolid food items continued to show residue in the pyriform sinuses, despite the use of liquid washes and multiple swallows.

At this time, Ms. S began partial oral feedings with liquids and thinned purées using the compensatory techniques. She progressed to full oral feedings at this diet level, with subsequent removal of her gastrostomy tube. Occasionally, she would attempt to eat soft food items; however, she found that she had difficulty swallowing them and that she would cough them up hours later. A final study was done 1 year after onset with results similar to that of the 2-month study, i.e., if compensatory techniques were not used or if food was solid or semisolid, residual material could be seen throughout the pharynx, which increased her potential for **aspiration.**

Effectiveness of Therapeutic Intervention

Efficacy studies regarding dysphagia treatment by allied health care providers are limited, but overall they support therapeutic intervention. Kasprisin, Clumeck, and Nino-Murcia (1989) indicated that treatment versus nontreatment was effective in decreasing the occurrence of **aspiration** pneumonia in patients with dysphagia. Groher (1987) suggested that diet modification reduced **aspiration** in patients with pseudobulbar dysphagia by increasing sensory processing and heightening awareness. Lazara, Lazarus, and Logemann (1987) found thermal stimulation to be effective in reducing the amount of time required to trigger the **swallow response** in dysphagic patients with delayed initiation of the **swallow response.** Martens, Cameron, and Simonsen (1990) identified increased weight in neurologically impaired patients who were treated for dysphagia by a multidisciplinary team compared with those patients who were not treated for dysphagia. Drooling was found to be reduced with treatment by McCracken (1978).

As the body of knowledge regarding dysphagia evaluation and treatment expands, it will be important for therapists treating dysphagia to review the literature critically. When reviewing dysphagia research, it is important to note how homogeneous the subjects were, because age, cognitive function, and disease process are known to alter swallowing function. The therapist should also examine the methods used for determining dysphagia severity, type of treatment, and length of treatment, as these factors allow the therapist to decide whether the information is applicable to her particular patient. Technologic advances in the near future will further enhance the assessment and treatment of patients with dysphagia by permitting better quantification of impairment and treatment effectiveness.

STUDY QUESTIONS

1. What are the five stages of swallowing and what key events occur during each stage?
2. What is aspiration and why is it harmful?
3. What are the key signs and symptoms that may indicate someone has dysphagia?
4. When evaluating someone with dysphagia the patient history should include which key components?
5. When performing a prefeeding and feeding evaluation what can the therapist not tell about swallowing function?
6. When should a videofluoroscopic swallowing study be requested and what information can be obtained from this procedure?
7. After completion of the swallowing evaluation what information should be included in the recommendations?
8. What treatment activities could be done with someone who has mild right hemifacial weakness? (Hint: be sure to include hygiene activities.)
9. How is progress measured in dysphagia treatment?

REFERENCES

Adnervill, I., Ekberg, O., & Groher, M. (1989). Determining normal bolus size for thin liquids. *Dysphagia, 4,* 1–3.

American Occupational Therapy Association. Commission on Practice. (1989). Occupational therapy in eating dysfunction (Position Paper). *American Journal of Occupational Therapy, 43,* 805.

Bass, N. H. (1988). Neurogenic dysphagia: Diagnostic assessment and rehabilitation of feeding disorders in the neurologically impaired. *Advances in Clinical Rehabilitation, 2,* 186–230.

Bazemore, P. H., Tonkonogy, J., & Ananth, R. (1991). Dysphagia in psychiatric patients: Clinical and videofluoroscopic study. *Dysphagia, 6,* 2–5.

Brown, G. E., Nordloh, S., & Donowitz, A. J. (1992). Systematic desensitization of oral hypersensitivity in a patient with a closed head injury. *Dysphagia, 7,* 138–141.

Bryant, M. (1991). Biofeedback in the treatment of a selected dysphagic patient. *Dysphagia, 6,* 140–144.

Buchholz, D. (1987). Neurologic evaluation of dysphagia. *Dysphagia, 1,* 187–192.

Buchholz, D. (1990, March). *Causes of unexplained neurogenic dysphagia.* Paper presented at the Third Symposium on Dysphagia, Johns Hopkins Medical Institute, Baltimore.

Cain, W. S., Gent, J. F., Goodspeed, R. B., & Leonard, G. (1988). Evaluation of olfactory dysfunction in the Connecticut Chemosensory Clinical Research Center. *Laryngoscope, 98,* 83–88.

Cameron, J. L., Reynolds, J., & Zuidema, G. (1973). Aspiration in patients with tracheostomies. *Surgery, Gynecology, and Otology, 136,* 68–70.

Castell, D. O., & Donner, M. W. (1987). Evaluation of dysphagia: A careful history is crucial. *Dysphagia, 2,* 65–71.

Clarke, K. A. (1989). *Neurophysiology: Applications in behavioral and biomedical sciences.* New York: John Wiley & Sons.

Crowther, J. A., & Ardran, G. M. (1985). Dysphagia due to cervical spondylosis. *Journal of Laryngology and Otology, 99,* 1167–1169.

Davidson, R. C., Horn, J. R., Herndon, J. H., & Grin, O. D. (1977). Brain-stem compression in rheumatoid arthritis. *Journal of the American Medical Association, 338,* 2633–2634.

Davis, J. W. (1989). Prosthodontic management of swallowing disorders. *Dysphagia, 3,* 199–205.

Devorken, J. P., & Nadol, J. C. (1991). Non-surgical treatment of drooling in a patient with closed head injury and severe dysarthria. *Dysphagia, 6,* 40–49.

Dodds, W. J. (1988, March). *Physiology of swallowing.* Paper presented at the Second Symposium on Dysphagia, Johns Hopkins Medical Institute, Baltimore.

Donner, M. J. (1986). Editorial. *Dysphagia 1,* 1–2.

Doty, R. L., Shaman, P., & Dann, M. (1983). Development of the University of Pennsylvania Smell Identification Test: A standardized microencapsulated test of olfactory function. *Neurology, 32,* 489–502.

Dziadziola, J., Hamlet, S., Michou, G., & Jones, L. (1992). Multiple swallows and piecemeal deglutition: Observations from normal adults and patients with head neck cancer. *Dysphagia, 7,* 8–11.

Ekberg, O., & Feinberg, M. (1992). Clinical and demographic data in 75 patients with near fatal choking episodes. *Dysphagia, 7,* 205–208.

Farber, S. (1982). *Neurorehabilitation: A multisensory approach.* Philadelphia: W. B. Saunders.

Garcia, R., Perlmuter, L. C., & Chauncey, H. H. (1989). Effects of dentition status and personality on masticatory performance and food acceptance. *Dysphagia, 4,* 121–126.

Granger, D., & Craig, R. M. (1990). Swallowing disorders and nutritional support. *Dysphagia, 4,* 213–219.

Groher, M. (1984). *Dysphagia: Diagnosis and management.* Stoneham, MA: Butterworth.

Groher, M. (1987). Bolus management and aspiration pneumonia in patients with pseudobulbar dysphagia. *Dysphagia, 1,* 215–216.

Groher, M. (1990a). Managing dysphagia in a chronic care setting: An introduction. *Dysphagia, 5,* 59–60.

Groher, M. (1990b). Ethical dilemmas in providing nutrition. *Dysphagia, 5,* 102–109.

Groher, M. E. (1991). Management: General principles and guidelines. *Dysphagia, 6,* 67–70.

Hendrix, T. R. (1993a). Art and science of history taking in the patient with difficulty swallowing. *Dysphagia, 8,* 69–73.

Hendrix, T. R. (1993b). Coordination of peristalsis in pharynx and esophagus. *Dysphagia, 8,* 74–78.

Jones, P. L., & Altschuler, S. L. (1987). Dysphagia teams: A specific approach to a non-specific problem. *Dysphagia, 1,* 200–205.

Jongkees, L. B. W. (1973). Practical application of clinical tests for facial paralysis. *Archives of Otolaryngology, 97,* 220–223.

Kagel, M. C., & Leopold, N. A. (1992). Dysphagia in Huntington's disease. *Dysphagia, 7,* 106–114.

Kahrilas, P. J., Logemann, J. A., & Gibbons, P. (1992). Food intake by maneuver: An extreme compensation for impaired swallowing. *Dysphagia, 7,* 155–159.

Kamel, P. (1990). Nutritional assessment and requirements. *Dysphagia, 4,* 189–195.

Kasprisin, A. T., Clumeck, H., & Nino-Murcia, M. (1989). The efficacy of rehabilitative management of dysphagia. *Dysphagia, 4,* 48–52.

Kendall, F. P., & McCreary, E. K. (1983). *Muscle testing and function* (3rd ed.). Baltimore: Williams & Wilkins.

Kennedy, J. G., & Kent, R. D., (1988). Physiological substrates of normal deglutition. *Dysphagia 3,* 24–37.

Kinny, D. J., Koheil, R. M., Greenberg, J., Reid, D., Milner, M., Mornan, R., & Judd, P. L. (1989). Development of a multidisciplinary feeding program for children who are dependent feeders. *Dysphagia, 4,* 16–28.

Kushner, H. S. (1989). Causes of neurogenic dysphagia. *Dysphagia, 3,* 184–188.

Langemore, S. E., Schatz, K., & Olsen, N. (1988). Fiberoptic endoscopic evaluation of swallowing safety: A new procedure. *Dysphagia, 2,* 216–219.

Langley, J. (1989). *Working with swallowing disorders.* Oxon, UK: Winslow Press.

Layne, K. (1990). Feeding strategies for the dysphagic patient: A nursing perspective. *Dysphagia, 5,* 84–88.

Lazara, G. L., Lazarus, C., & Logemann, J. A. (1987). Impact of thermal stimulation on the triggering of the swallow reflex. *Dysphagia, 1,* 73–77.

Lazarus, C., & Logemann, J. A. (1987). Swallowing disorders in closed head trauma patients. *Archives of Physical Medicine & Rehabilitation, 68,* 79–84.

Lieberman, A. N., Horowitz, L., Redmond, P., Pachter, L., & Lieberman, M. (1980). Dysphagia in Parkinson's disease. *American Journal of Gastroenterology, 74,* 157–160.

Linden, P. (1989). Videofluoroscopy in the rehabilitation of swallowing dysfunction. *Dysphagia, 3,* 189–191.

Linden, P., & Siebens, A. (1983). Dysphagia: Predicting laryngeal penetration. *Archives of Physical Medicine & Rehabilitation, 64,* 281–284.

Logemann, J. (1983). *Evaluation and treatment of swallowing disorders.* San Diego: College Hill Press.

Logemann, J. A. (1986a). *A Manual for fluoroscopic examination of swallowing*. San Diego: College Hill Press.

Logemann, J. A. (1986b). Treatment for aspiration related to dysphagia. *Dysphagia, 1*, 34–38.

Logemann, J. A. (1990). Factors affecting ability to resume oral nutrition in the oropharyngeal dysphagic individual. *Dysphagia, 4*, 202–208.

Logemann, J. A. (1991, November). *Swallowing disorder after oral cancer treatment*. Paper presented at the American Speech and Hearing Association Seminar, Houston.

Martens, L., Cameron, T., & Simonsen, M. (1990). Effects of a multidisciplinary management program on neurologically impaired patients with dysphagia. *Dysphagia, 5*, 147–151.

Martin, A. W. (1991). Dietary management of swallowing disorders. *Dysphagia, 6*, 129–134.

Mary Free Bed Hospital and Rehabilitation Center. (1992). *Dysphagia policies and procedures*. Grand Rapids, MI: Author.

McConnel, F. M. S., & Logemann, J. A. (1990). The evaluation of swallowing. *Current Concepts in Otolaryngology*, 1–12.

McCracken, A. (1978). Drool control and tongue thrust therapy for the mentally retarded. *American Journal of Occupational Therapy, 32*, 79–85.

Musson, N. D., Kincaid, J., Ryan, P., Glussman, B., Varone, L., Gamarra, N., Wilson, R., Reffe, W., & Silverman, M. (1990). Nature, nurture, nutrition: Interdisciplinary programs to address the prevention of malnutrition and dehydration. *Dysphagia, 5*, 96–101.

Palmer, J. B., Rudin, N. J., Lara, G., & Crompton A. W. (1992). Coordination of mastication and swallowing. *Dysphagia, 7*, 187–200.

Pommerenke, W. T. (1928). A study of the sensory areas eliciting the swallow reflex. *American Journal of Physiology, 84*, 36–41.

Robbins, J., & Levine, R. L. (1988). Swallowing after unilateral stroke of the cerebral cortex: Preliminary experience. *Dysphagia, 3*, 11–17.

Robbins, J., Sufit, R., Rosenbek, J., Levine, R., & Hyland, J. (1987). A modification of the modified barium swallow. *Dysphagia, 2*, 83–86.

Roberts, M. W., Tylenda, C. A., Sonies, B. C., & Elin, R. J. (1989). Dysphagia in bulimia nervosa. *Dysphagia, 4*, 106–111.

Rushmer, R. F., & Hendron, J. A. (1951). The act of deglutition: A cinefluoroscopic study. *Journal of Applied Physiology, 3*, 622–630.

Selly, W. G., Flack, F. C., Ellis, R. E., Phil, M., & Brooks, W. A. (1990). The Exeter dysphagia assessment technique. *Dysphagia, 4*, 227–235.

Silverman, E. H., & Elfant, I. L. (1979). Dysphagia: An evaluation and treatment program for the adult. *American Journal of Occupational Therapy, 33*, 382–392.

Sonies, B. C., Weiffenbach, J., Atchinson, J. C., Brahim, J., Machynski, A., & Fox, P. C. (1987). Clinical examination of motor and sensory function of the adult oral cavity. *Dysphagia 1*, 178–186.

Splaingard, M. L., Hutchins, B., Sulton, L., & Chaudhuri, G. (1988). Aspiration in rehabilitation patients: Videofluoroscopy vs. bedside clinical assessment. *Archives of Physical Medicine & Rehabilitation, 69*, 637–639.

Stuart, D. (1989). Dysphagia due to cervical osteophytes. *International Orthopedics, 13*, 95–99.

Terry, P. B., & Fuller, S. D. (1989). Pulmonary consequences of aspiration. *Dysphagia, 3*, 179–183.

Thomas-Stonell, N., & Greenberg, J. (1988). Three treatment approaches and clinical factors in the reduction of drooling. *Dysphagia, 3*, 73–78.

Tippett, D. C., Palmer, J., & Linden, P. (1987). Management of dysphagia in a patient with closed head injury. *Dysphagia, 1*, 221–226.

Tuchman, D. N. (1989). Cough, choke, sputter: The evaluation of the child with dysfunctional swallowing. *Dysphagia, 3*, 111–116.

Voss, D. E., Ionta, M. K., & Myers, B. J. (1985). *Proprioceptive neuromuscular facilitation: Patterns and techniques*. New York: Harper & Row.

Welsh, L. W., Welsh, J. J., & Chinnici, J. C. (1987). Dysphagia due to cervical spine surgery. *Annals of Otology, Rhinology, & Otolaryngology, 96*, 112–115.

Winstein, C. J. (1983). Neurogenic dysphagia: Frequency, progression, and outcomes in adults following head injury. *Physical Therapy 63*, 1992–1996.

Ylvisaker, M. (1985). *Head injury rehabilitation: children and adolescents*. New York: Harper & Row.

Young, E. C., & Durant-Jones, L. (1990). Developing a dysphagia program in an acute care hospital: A needs assessment. *Dysphagia 5*, 159–165.

Figure and Table Credits

FIGURES

Figure 4.1. Adapted from Law, M., Cooper, B., Letts, L., Rigby, P., Stewart, D., & Strong, S. (1992). *The environment: A critical review of person-environment relations and environmental assessment* (Res. Rept. #92-4). (Available from the Neurodevelopmental Clinical Research Unit, School of Occupational Therapy and Physiotherapy, McMaster University, 1200 Main Street W, Hamilton, Ont. L8N 3Z5 Canada).

Figure 4.2. Reprinted by permission from Law, M., Baptiste, S., Carswell, A., McColl, M., Polatajko, H., & Pollock, N. (1991). *The Canadian Occupational Performance Measure*. Toronto, Ont., Canada: CAOT Publications.

Figure 4.3. Reprinted by permission from *The Klein-Bell ADL Scale*. (1982). Developed and marketed by the Health Sciences Center for Educational Resources of the University of Washington, Seattle.

Figure 4.4. Reprinted by permission from Morgan, V. J. (1992). *The Safety and Functional ADL Evaluation*. Poster presented at the annual conference of the American Occupational Therapy Association, Houston, TX.

Figure 5.1. From Steinfeld, E., Schroeder, S., Duncan, J., Faste, R., Chollet, D., Bishop, M., Wirth, P., & Cardell, P. (1979). *Access to the built environment: A review of the literature* (HUD #660). Washington, DC: U.S. Government Printing Office.

Figure 5.2. From Steinfeld, E., Schroeder, S., Duncan, J., Faste, R., Chollet, D., Bishop, M., Wirth, P., & Cardell, P. (1979). *Access to the built environment: A review of the literature* (HUD #660). Washington, DC: U.S. Government Printing Office.

Figure 7.2. Reprinted by permission from Mathiowetz, V. & Bass Haugen, J. (1994). Motor behavior research: Implications for therapeutic approaches to CNS dysfunction. *American Journal of Occupational Therapy, 48*(8), 733–745.

Figure 7.3. Reprinted by permission from Mathiowetz, V. & Bass Haugen, J. (1994). Motor behavior research: Implications for therapeutic approaches to CNS dysfunction. *American Journal of Occupational Therapy, 48*(8), 733–745.

Figure 7.4. Adapted from Trombly, C. A. (1989). Motor control therapy. In C. Trombly (Ed.), *Occupational therapy for physical dysfunction* (3rd ed., pp. 72–95). Baltimore: Williams & Wilkins.

Figure 7.5. Reprinted by permission from From Twitchell, T. (1965). *The Child with Central Nervous System Deficit*. Washington, DC: U.S. Government Printing Office.

Figure 7.8. Reprinted by permission from Mathiowetz, V. & Bass Haugen, J. (1994). Motor behavior research: Implications for therapeutic approaches to CNS dysfunction. *American Journal of Occupational Therapy, 48*(8), 733–745.

Figure 8.1. Reprinted by permission from Tomancik, L. (1987). *Directions for using Semmes-Weinstein monofilaments*. San Jose, CA: North Coast Medical.

Figure 8.2. Reprinted by permission from Barr, M. L., & Kiernan, J. A. (1983). *The human nervous system: An anatomical viewpoint* (4th ed.). Philadelphia: Harper & Row.

Figure 8.6. Reprinted by permission from Callahan, A. D. (1990). Sensibility testing: Clinical methods. In J. Hunter, L. Schneider, E. Mackin, & A. Callahan (Eds.), *Rehabilitation of the hand* (3rd ed., pp. 594–610). St. Louis, MO: Mosby.

Figure 9.5. Reprinted by permission from Benton, A. L., Hamsher, K., Varney, N. K., & Spreen, O. (1983). *Contributions to neuropsychological assessment—A clinical manual*. New York: Oxford University Press.

Figure 9.6. Reprinted by permission from Goodglass, H., & Kaplan, E. (1972). *The assessment of aphasia and related disorders*. Philadelphia: Lea & Febiger.

Figure 11.3. Reprinted from Eggers, O. (1983). *Occupational therapy in the treatment of adult hemiplegia*. London: William Heinemann Medical Books.

Figure 15.16. Reprinted by permission of the Higland View Cuyahoga County Hospital, Cleveland, OH.

Figure 16.1. Courtesy of Fred Sammons, Inc., Burr Ridge, IL.

Figure 16.2. Courtesy of Fred Sammons, Inc., Burr Ridge, IL.

Figure 16.3. Courtesy of North Coast Medical, Inc., San Jose, CA.

Figure 16.4. Courtesy of North Coast Medical, Inc., San Jose, CA.

Figure 16.5. Courtesy of North Coast Medical, Inc., San Jose, CA.

Figure 16.6. Courtesy of Fred Sammons, Inc., Burr Ridge, IL.

Figure 16.7. Courtesy of Fred Sammons, Inc., Burr Ridge, IL.

Figure 16.8. Courtesy of North Coast Medical, Inc., San Jose, CA.

Figure 16.9. Designed by Lee Heintzman and Gordon Heintzman. Reprinted by permission from Dunn, V. M. (1978). Tips on raising children from a wheelchair. *Accent on Living, 22*(4), 78–83.

Figure 17.1. Reprinted by permission from U.S. Department of Labor. (1982). *A guide to job analysis*. Menomonie: University of Wisconsin Materials Development Center.

Figure 17.2. Courtesy of Work Evaluation Systems Technology (WEST), Long Beach, CA.

Figure 17.3. Reprinted by permission from the Department of Occupational Therapy at the Work Enhancement Rehabilitation Center, Burlington, VT.

Figure 17.4. Courtesy of Work Evaluation Systems Technology (WEST), Long Beach, CA.

Figure 17.5. Courtesy of Valpar International Corp., Tucson, AZ.

Figure 23.1. Reprinted by permission from Dellon, A. (1988). *Evaluation of sensibility and re-education of sensation in the hand*. Baltimore: John D. Lucas.

Figure 24A.1. Reprinted by permission from Willard, H. S., & Spackman, C. S. (1963). *Occupational Therapy* (3rd ed.). Philadelphia: J. B. Lippincott.

Figure 28.4. Reprinted by permission from Bobath, B. (1990). *Adult hemiplegia:*

Evaluation and treatment (3rd ed.). London: William Heinemann Medical Books.

Figure 28.5. Reprinted by permission from General Medical Manufacturing, Norcross, GA.

Figure 28.7. Reprinted by permission from Fred Sammons, Inc., Brookfield, IL.

Figure 28.8. Reprinted by permission from Hill, J., & Presperin, J. (1986). Deformity control. In S. Intagliata (Ed.), *Spinal cord injury: A guide to functional outcomes in occupational therapy* (pp. 49–85). Gaithersburg, MD: Aspen Systems. Copyright © 1986 Aspen Publishers, Inc.

Figure 28.9. Reprinted by permission from Hill, J., & Presperin, J. (1986). Deformity control. In S. Intagliata (Ed.), *Spinal cord injury: A guide to functional outcomes in occupational therapy* (pp. 49–85). Gaithersburg, MD: Aspen Systems. Copyright © 1986 Aspen Publishers, Inc.

Figure 28.10. Reprinted by permission from Hill, J., & Presperin, J. (1986). Deformity control. In S. Intagliata (Ed.), *Spinal cord injury: A guide to functional outcomes in occupational therapy* (pp. 49–85). Gaithersburg, MD: Aspen Systems. Copyright © 1986 Aspen Publishers, Inc.

Figure 28.12. Reprinted by permission from Long, C., & Schutt, A. (1986). Upper limb orthotics. In J. B. Redford (Ed.), *Orthotics etcetera* (3rd ed., pp. 198–277). Baltimore: Williams & Wilkins.

Figure 28.15. Reprinted by permission from LMB Hand Rehab Products, Inc., San Luis Obispo, CA.

Figure 28.17. Reprinted by permission from Long, C., & Schutt, A. (1986). Upper limb orthotics. In J. B. Redford (Ed.), *Orthotics etcetera* (3rd ed., pp. 198–277). Baltimore: Williams & Wilkins.

Figure 28.18. Reprinted by permission from Green, D. P., & McCoy, H. (1979). Turnbuckle orthotic correction of elbow-flexion contractures after acute injuries. *Journal of Bone and Joint Surgery, 61A*(7), 1092–1095.

Figure 28.19. Reprinted by permission from Smith & Nephew Rolyan, Inc., Germantown, WI.

Figure 28.21. Reprinted by permission from LMB Hand Rehab Products, Inc., San Luis Obispo, CA.

Figure 28.25. Reprinted by permission from LMB Hand Rehab Products, Inc., San Luis Obispo, CA.

Figure 28.26. Reprinted by permission from LMB Hand Rehab Products, Inc., San Luis Obispo, CA.

Figure 28.30. Reprinted by permission from Southpaw, Inc., Dayton, OH.

Figure 28.31. Reprinted by permission from Hill, J., & Presperin, J. (1986). Deformity control. In S. Intagliata (Ed.), *Spinal cord injury: A guide to functional outcomes in occupational therapy* (pp. 49–85). Gai-

thersburg, MD: Aspen Systems. Copyright © 1986 Aspen Publishers, Inc.

Figure 28.34. Reprinted by permission from LMB Hand Rehab Products, Inc., San Luis Obispo, CA.

Figure 28.36. Reprinted by permission from Long, C. (1966). Upper limb bracing. In S. Licht & H. Kamenetz (Eds.), *Orthotics etcetera* (pp. 152–248). Baltimore: Waverly Press.

Figure 28.37. Reprinted by permission from Hill, J., & Presperin, J. (1986). Deformity control. In S. Intagliata (Ed.), *Spinal cord injury: A guide to functional outcomes in occupational therapy* (pp. 49–85). Gaithersburg, MD: Aspen Systems. Copyright © 1986 Aspen Publishers, Inc.

Figure 28.40. Reprinted by permission from Long, C., & Schutt, A. (1986). Upper limb orthotics. In J. B. Redford (Ed.), *Orthotics etcetera* (3rd ed., pp. 198–277). Baltimore: Williams & Wilkins.

Figure 28.44. Reprinted by permission from Long, C., & Schutt, A. (1986). Upper limb orthotics. In J. B. Redford (Ed.), *Orthotics etcetera* (3rd ed., pp. 198–277). Baltimore: Williams & Wilkins.

Figure 28.56. Reprinted by permission from Drew, W. E., & Stern, P. H. (1979). Modular adjustment mechanism for the balanced forearm orthosis. *Archives of Physical Medicine & Rehabilitation, 60*(2), 81.

Figure 30.1. Reprinted by permission from McFarland, S. (1991). Prescription considerations and a comparison of conventional and lightweight chairs. *Journal of Rehabilitation Research and Development: Clinical Supplement, 2*, 11.

Figure 31.1. Reprinted by permission from Smith, R. O. (1991). Techological approaches to performance enhancement. In C. Christiansen & C. Baum (Eds.), *Occupational therapy: Overcoming human performance deficits* (pp. 746–786). Thorofare, NJ: Slack.

Figure 31.4. Courtesy of TASH, Inc., Ajax, Ont., Canada.

Figure 31.5. Courtesy of Don Johnston Developmental Equipment, Inc., Wauconda, IL.

Figure 31.10. Courtesy of TeleSensory, Inc., Mountain View, CA.

Figure 31.15. Redrawn by Jeanne Eichler by permission from Dianne Ostdiek (developer), Madonna Hospital, Lincoln, NE.

Figure 31.1. Elgon was designed and built by Gary de Bacher, assistant professor of rehabilitation medicine at Emory University and rehabilitation engineer at the Center for Rehabilitation Medicine, Atlanta, Georgia.

Figure 33.1. Courtesy of Henley International, Houston, TX.

Figure 37.3. Courtesy of Smith & Nephew Roylan, Inc., Germantown, Wisconsin.

Figure 37.4. Courtesy of Smith & Nephew Roylan, Inc., Germantown, Wisconsin.

Figure 37.6. Reprinted by permission from Bear-Lehman, J., & Bielawski, T. (1988). The carpal tunnel syndrome: Back to the source. *Rehabilitation Research, 1*, 13–20.

Figure 40.1. Reprinted by permission of the Arthritis Foundation. From the AHPA Arthritis Teaching Slide Collection, 2nd ed. © 1988.

Figure 40.2. Reprinted by permission of the Arthritis Foundation. From the AHPA Arthritis Teaching Slide Collection, 2nd ed. © 1988.

Figure 40.3. Reprinted by permission of the Arthritis Foundation. From the AHPA Arthritis Teaching Slide Collection, 2nd ed. © 1988.

Figure 40.5. Reprinted by permission of the Arthritis Foundation. From the AHPA Arthritis Teaching Slide Collection, 2nd ed. © 1988.

Figure 40.8. Reprinted by permission of the Arthritis Foundation. From the AHPA Arthritis Teaching Slide Collection, 2nd ed. © 1988.

Figure 42.1. Adapted from Department of Prosthetics and Orthotics. (1986). *Upper-limb prosthetics.* New York: New York University Medical Center, Postgraduate Medical School.

Figure 42.4. Courtesy of Hosmer-Dorrance Corp., Campbell, CA.

Figure 42.5. Courtesy of TRS, Inc., Brooklyn, NY.

Figure 42.6. Courtesy of Alternative Prosthetic Services, Brooklyn, NY.

Figure 42.7. Courtesy of Alternative Prosthetic Services, Brooklyn, NY.

Figure 42.11. Courtesy of Otto Bock Orthopedic Industry, Minneapolis, MN.

Figure 42.12. Courtesy of Otto Bock Orthopedic Industry, Minneapolis, MN.

Figure 42.13. Courtesy of Motion Control, Salt Lake City, UT.

Figure 42.18. Courtesy of TRS, Inc., Brooklyn, NY.

Figure 42.21. Courtesy of Jack Hodgins, Kessler Institute for Rehabiliation, Inc., West Orange, NJ.

Figure 42.23. Courtesy of TRS, Inc., Brooklyn, NY.

Figure 42.24. Courtesy of Jack Hodgins, Kessler Institute for Rehabiliation, Inc., West Orange, NJ.

Figure 44.1. Reprinted by permission from Mary Free Bed Hospital and Rehabilitation Center. (1992). *Dysphagia policies and procedures.* Grand Rapids, MI: Author.

TABLES

Table 2.1. Adapted from American Occupational Therapy Association. (1993). The philosophical base of occupational therapy. *American Journal of Occupational Therapy, 47*(12), 1119.

Table 3.2. Reprinted by permission from Trombly, C. A., & Quintana, L. A. (1989). Activities of daily living. In C. A. Trombly (Ed.), *Occupational therapy for physical dysfunction* (3rd ed., pp. 386–410). Baltimore: Williams & Wilkins.

Table 3.3. Adapted from U.S. Department of Health and Human Services, Health Care Financing Administration. (1989, May). *Medicare outpatient physical therapy and comprehensive outpatient rehabilitation facility manual. 503 Medical review of part B, outpatient occupational therapy (OT) services* (HCFA Publication 9). Washington, DC: U.S. Government Printing Office.

Table 3.4. Adapted from Steich, T. (1992). Legal issues in documentation: Fraud, abuse, and confidentiality. In J. D. Acquaviva (Ed.), *Effective documentation for occupational therapy* (pp. 211–217). Rockville, MD: American Occupational Therapy Association.

Table 5.2. Reprinted by permission from Coulton, C. J. (1979). Developing an instrument to measure person-environment fit. *Journal of Social Service Research, 3,* 159–173.

Table 5.3. Reprinted by permission from Kelly, C., & Snell, K. (1989). *The source book: Architectural guidelines for barrier-free design.* Toronto, Ont., Canada: Barrier-Free Design Centre.

Table 5.4. Reprinted by permission from Canada Mortgage and Housing Corporation. (1989). *Maintaining seniors' independence: A guide to home adaptations.* Ottawa, Ont.: Author.

Table 5.5. Reprinted by permission from Goltsman, S. M., Gilbert, T. A., & Wohlford, S. D. (1992). *The accessibility checklist: An evaluating system for buildings and outdoor settings.* Berkeley, CA: M.I.G. Communications.

Table 6.4. Adapted from Mathiowetz, V., Kashman, N., Volland, G., Weber, K., Dowe, M., & Rogers, S. (1985). Grip and pinch strength: Normative data for adults. *Archives of Physical Medicine and Rehabilitation, 66*(2), 69–74.

Table 6.5. Adapted from Mathiowetz, V., Kashman, N., Volland, G., Weber, K., Dowe, M., & Rogers, S. (1985). Grip and pinch strength: Normative data for adults. *Archives of Physical Medicine and Rehabilitation, 66*(2), 69–74.

Table 7.1. Reprinted from Bohannon, R. & Smith, M. B. (1987). Interrater reliability of a modified Ashworth scale of muscle spasticity. *Physical Therapy, 67,* 207, with permission of the American Physical Therapy Association.

Table 7.2. Adapted from Fiorentino, M. R. (1973). *Reflex testing methods for evaluating CNS development,* (2nd ed.). Springfield, IL: Charles C. Thomas; Hoskins, T., & Squires, J. (1973). Development

assessment: A test for gross motor and reflex development. *Physical Therapy, 53,* 117–126; O'Sullivan, S. B. (1988). Motor control assessment. In S. B. O'Sullivan & T. J. Schmitz (Eds.), *Physical rehabilitation: Assessment and treatment* (2nd ed., pp. 135–158). Philadelphia: F. A. Davis; and Trombly, C. A., & Scott, A. D. (1989). Evaluation of motor control. In C. Trombly (Ed.), *Occupational therapy for physical dysfunction* (3rd ed., pp. 55–71). Baltimore: Williams & Wilkins.

Table 7.3. Reprinted from Mathiowetz, V., Volland, G., Kashman, N., & Weber, K. (1985). Adult norms for the Box and Block Test of manual dexterity. *American Journal of Occupational Therapy, 39,* 389–390.

Table 9.3. Reprinted by permission from Benton, A. L., Hamsher, K. deS., Varney, N. K., & Spreen, O. (1983). *Contributions to neuropsychological assessment—A clinical manual.* New York: Oxford University Press.

Table 9.5. Adapted from Haaland, K. (1993, March). *Typology and assessment of individuals with limb apraxia.* Paper presented at the AOTA Neuroscience Institute conference: Treating Adults with Apraxia, Baltimore; and Haaland, K. (1992, November). *Assessment of limb apraxia.* Paper presented at Educational Resources Conference: Apraxia in children and adults, Boston.

Table 9.6. Reprinted by permission from Goodglass, H., & Kaplan, E. (1972). *The assessment of aphasia and related disorders.* Philadelphia: Lea & Febiger.

Table 9.7. Reprinted by permission from Goodglass, H., & Kaplan, E. (1972). *The assessment of aphasia and related disorders.* Philadelphia: Lea & Febiger.

Table 9.8. Adapted from Sohlberg, M. M., & Mateer, C. A. (1989). *Introduction to cognitive rehabilitation.* New York: Gilford Press.

Table 9.9. Reprinted by permission from Benton, A. L., Hamsher, K. deS., Varney, N. K., & Spreen, O. (1983). *Contributions to neuropsychological assessment—A clinical manual.* New York: Oxford University Press.

Table 9.11. Reprinted by permission from Strub, R. L., & Black, F. W. (1977). *The mental status examination in neurology.* Philadelphia: F. A. Davis.

Table 13.1. Adapted from Gentile, A. M. (1987). Skill acquisition: Action, movement, and neuromotor processes. In J. H. Carr, R. B. Shepherd, J. Gordon, A. M. Gentile, & J. M. Held (Eds.), *Movement science: Foundations for physical therapy in rehabilitation* (pp. 93–154). Rockville, MD: Aspen Systems.

Table 17.2. Adapted from President's Committee on Employment of People with Disabilities. (1993). *ADA Brochure.* (Avail-

able from 1331 F Street NW, Washington, DC 20004).

Table 17.3. Reprinted by permission from Putz-Anderson, V., & Waters, T. (1991, April). *Revisions in NIOSH guide to manual lifting.* Paper presented at the conference National Strategy for Occupational Musculoskeletal Injury Prevention—Implementation Issues and Research Needs, Ann Arbor, MI.

Table 19.1. Adapted from Law, M. (1991). The environment: A focus for occupational therapy. *Canadian Journal of Occupational Therapy, 58,* 171–179.

Appendix to Chapter 19: Reprinted by permission from American National Standard (ANSI A117.1-1986), copyright 1986 by the American National Standards Institute.

Table 21.1. Reprinted by permission from Bonder, B. R. (1994). The psychosocial meaning of activity. In B. R. Bonder & M. Wagner (Eds.), *Functional performance in older adults* (pp. 28–40). Philadelphia: F. A. Davis.

Table 23.1. Modified from Dellon, A. (1988). *Evaluation of sensibility and reeducation of sensation in the hand.* Baltimore: John D. Lucas.

Table 23.2. Data from Barber, L. (1990). Desensitization of the traumatized hand. In J. Hunter, L. Schneider, E. Mackin, & A. Callahan (Eds.), *Rehabilitation of the hand* (3rd ed., pp. 721–730). St. Louis: C. V. Mosby.

Table 24D.1. Courtesy of D. E. Voss, Northwestern Medical School. Figures redrawn by Julie A. Livingston.

Table 24D.2. Courtesy of D. E. Voss, Northwestern Medical School.

Table 25A.1. Reprinted by permission from Carr, J. H., & Shepherd, R. B. (1987). *A motor relearning programme for stroke* (2nd ed.). Rockville, MD: Aspen Systems. Copyright © Butterworth-Heinemann, Ltd.

Table 26.2. Reprinted by permission from Toglia, J. (1991). Generalization of treatment: A multicontext approach to cognitive perceptual impairment in adults with brain injury. *American Journal of Occupational Therapy, 45,* 505–516.

Table 26.3. Adapted from Warren, M. (1993b). A hierarchical model for evaluation and treatment of visual perceptual dysfunction in adult acquired brain injury, Part 2. *American Journal of Occupational Therapy, 47,* 55–66.

Table 26.5. Reprinted by permission from Jarvis, P. E., & Hamlin, D. H. (1991). The use of verbal maps to help people with right cerebral hemisphere lesions compensate for perceptual spatial deficits. *Journal of Rehabilitation, 57*(3), 51–53.

Table 27.1. Data from Ben-Yishay, Y., & Diller, L. (1993). Cognitive remediation in traumatic brain injury: Update and issues.

Archives of Physical Medicine & Rehabilitation, 74, 204–213; Neistadt, M. E. (1988). Occupational therapy for adults with perceptual deficits. *American Journal of Occupational Therapy, 42,* 434–440; Neistadt, M. E. (1990). A critical analysis of occupational therapy approaches for perceptual deficits in adults with brain injury. *American Journal of Occupational Therapy, 44,* 299–304; Toglia, J. P. (1991). Generalization of treatment: A multicontext approach to cognitive perceptual impairment in adults with brain injury. *American Journal of Occupational Therapy, 45,* 505–516; Toglia, J. (1993, March 19, 20). *OT intervention for individuals with constructional apraxia,* paper presented at the AOTA Neurosciences Institute, Baltimore.

Table 27.2. Data from Toglia, J. P. (1991). Generalization of treatment: A multicontext approach to cognitive perceptual impairment in adults with brain injury. *American Journal of Occupational Therapy, 45,* 505–516; Toglia, J. (1993, March 19, 20). *OT intervention for individuals with constructional apraxia,* paper presented at the AOTA Neurosciences Institute, Baltimore.

Table 27.3. Reprinted by permission from Toglia, J. P. (1991). Generalization of treatment: A multicontext approach to cognitive perceptual impairment in adults with brain injury. *American Journal of Occupational Therapy, 45,* 505–516.

Table 27.4. Adapted from Crosson, B., Barco, P. P., Velozo, C. A., Bolesta, M. M., Cooper, P. V., Werts, D., & Brobeck, T. C. (1989). Awareness and compensation in postacute head injury rehabilitation. *Journal of Head Trauma Rehabilitation, 4*(3), 46–54.

Table 27.5. Adapted from Sohlberg, M. M., & Mateer, C. A. (1989). *Introduction to cognitive rehabilitation.* New York: Gilford Press.

Table 27.6. Adapted from Sohlberg, M. M., & Mateer, C. A. (1989). *Introduction to cognitive rehabilitation.* New York: Gilford Press; and Wilson, B. (1992, October). *Approaches to memory therapy.* Paper presented at the conference for Evaluation and Treatment of Disorders of Memory, Attention and Visual Neglect, Philadelphia, PA.

Table 27.7. Data from Glasgow, R. E., Zeiss, R. A., Barrera, M., & Lewisohn, P. M. (1977). Case studies on remediating memory deficits in brain-damaged individuals. *Journal of Clinical Psychology, 33,* 1049–1054; Malec, J., & Questad, K. (1983). Rehabilitation of memory after craniocerebral trauma: Case report. *Archives of Physical Medicine & Rehabilitation, 64,* 436–438; Milton, S. B. (1985). Compensatory memory strategy training: A practical approach for managing persistent memory problems. *Cognitive Rehabilitation, 3*(6), 8–15; Wilson, B. (1982). Success and failure in memory training following a cerebral vascular accident. *Cortex, 18,* 581–594.

Table 28.1. Devised by the staff at Rancho Los Amigos Hospital, Downey, CA.

Table 34.1. Adapted from DeWeerdt, W. J. G., & Harrison, M.-A. (1985). Measuring recovery of arm-hand function in stroke patients: A comparison of the Brunnstrom-Fugl-Meyer Test and the Action Research Arm Test. *Physiotherapy Canada, 37,* 65–70.

Table 34.2. Adapted from Wilson, D. J., Baker, L. L., & Craddock, J. A. (1984). *Protocol—functional test for the hemiplegic/paretic upper extremity.* Unpublished manuscript. County Rehabilitation Center, Rancho Los Amigos, Occupational Therapy Department. Downey, CA.

Table 35.1. Reprinted by permission from Jennett, B., & Teasdale, G. (1981). *Management of head injuries.* Philadelphia: F. A. Davis.

Table 35.2. Adapted from Malkmus, D., Booth, B. J., & Kodimer, C. (1980). *Rehabilitation of the head injured adult: Comprehensive cognitive management.* Downey, CA: Professional Staff Association of Rancho Los Amigos Hospital.

Table 36.2. Reprinted by permission from the National Rehabilitation Hospital, Washington, DC.

Table 36.3. Adapted from Muscular Dystrophy Association. (1991). *Facts about muscular dystrophy.* Tucson, AZ: Author and Muscular Dystrophy Association. (1991). *Muscular Dystrophy Association 1991 Annual Report.* Tuscon, AZ: Author.

Table 39.1. Adapted from Trombly, C. A. (Ed.). (1989). *Occupational therapy for physical dysfunction* (3rd ed.). Baltimore: Williams & Wilkins.

Table 40.1. From Cordery, J. (1965). Joint protection: A responsibility of the occupational therapist. *American Journal of Occupational Therapy, 19,* 285–294.

Table 40.2. From Feinberg, J. R. (1992). Effect of the arthritis health professional on compliance with use of resting hand splints by patients with rheumatoid arthritis. *Arthritis Care and Research, 5,* 17–23.

Table 42.2. Adapted from Department of Prosthetics and Orthotics. (1986). *Upper-limb prosthetics.* New York: New York University Medical Center, Postgraduate Medical School.

Table 43.1. Reproduced with permission. Fox, S. M., Naughton, J. P., & Gorman, P. A. (1972). Physical activity and cardiovascular health III. The exercise prescription. Frequency and type of activity. *Modern Concepts in Cardiovascular Disease, 41,* 6–14. Copyright © 1972 American Heart Association.

Table 43.2. Reprinted by permission from Spaulding Rehabilitation Hospital, Boston.

Table 44.3. Adapted from Logemann, J. A. (1986). Treatment for aspiration related to dysphagia. *Dysphagia, 1,* 34–38; and Mary Free Bed Hospital and Rehabilitation Center. (1992). *Dysphagia policies and procedures.* Grand Rapids, MI: Author.

Index

Page numbers followed by "f" denote figures; those followed by "t" denote tables.

909